Contents

Contributors

Karen Bawel-Brinkly, RN, MS, MSN, PhD
Associate Professor
San Jose State University, School of Nursing
San Jose, California

Carol Bostrom, RN, MSN, APRN, BC
Clinical Assistant Professor
Indiana University, School of Nursing
Indianapolis

Judith A. Halstead, RN, DNS
Executive Associate Dean and Professor
Indiana University, School of Nursing
Indianapolis

Margie Hull, MED, MSN, APRN-BC, CDE-RN
Visiting Lecturer
Indiana University, School of Nursing
Indianapolis

Colleen M. O'Leary-Kelley, PhD, RN
Associate Professor
San Jose State University, School of Nursing
San Jose, California

Virginia Richardson, RN, DNS, CPNP
Associate Professor
Coordinator of Pediatric Nurse Practitioner Program
Indiana University, School of Nursing
Indianapolis

Pat Twedt, RN, MS
Associate Professor of Nursing
Dakota Wesleyan University
Mitchell, SD

Gayle Roux, PhD, RN, NP-C
Associate Professor and Associate Dean for Faculty
Loyola University
Chicago

Lee W. Schwecke, RN, MSN, EDD
Associate Professor
Indiana University, School of Nursing
Indianapolis

Evelyn Stephenson, MSN, RNC
Clinical Assistant Professor
Indiana University, School of Nursing
Indianapolis

Sharon Vinten, MSN, RNC, WN
Clinical Associate Professor
Indiana University, School of
Indianapolis

Mary Ann Wehmer, RN, MSN, CNOR
Nursing Instructor
University of Southern Indiana
Evansville

Sandra Wood, MSN, APRN, BC
Clinical Assistant Professor
Indiana University, School of Nursing
Indianapolis

Reviewers

Wanda M. Baker, RN, MN, FNP
Academic Program Chair
Greenville Technical College
Greenville, South Carolina

Linda D. Barnes, MN, RN, BC
Professor of Nursing
Shoreline Community College
Shoreline, Washington

Carol Ann Blakeman, RN/ARNP, MSN
Professor of Nursing
Central Florida Community College
Ocala, Florida

Kathryne Bornell, CAN
Nursing Student
Purdue University
West Lafayette, Indiana

Mary Ann Breen, RN, MED, MS
Associate Professor, Director AS and Professional Track
Nursing Programs
Rivier College
Nashua, New Hampshire

Jessie Casida, PhD(c), RN, CCRN, APN-C
Assistant Professor
Seton Hall University, College of Nursing
South Orange, New Jersey

Sally L. Gaines, MSN, RN
Nursing Instructor
West Texas A&M University
Canyon, Texas

Janice J. Hoffman, RN, PhD
Instructor
Johns Hopkins University
Baltimore, Maryland

Sharon C. Hunsucker, RN, MSN, ARNP
Assistant Professor of Nursing
Morehead State University
Morehead, Kentucky

Kathy Jorgensen, MA, MSN
Associate Professor
University of South Dakota
Vermillion, South Dakota

Judith A. Kaplan, RN, PhD, LCCE
Associate Professor
Nassau Community College
Garden City, New York

Eileen Kaslatas, MSN, RN
Professor, Nursing Faculty
Macomb Community College
Clinton Township, Michigan

Cindy Kohtz, EdD, RN, CNE
Associate Professor
Methodist College of Nursing
Peoria, Illinois

Linda Ann Kucher, MSN, RN, CMSRN
Associate Professor
Gordon College
Barnesville, Georgia

Patricia Lange-Otsuka, EdD, MSN, APRN, BC
Associate Dean of Nursing, Associate Professor of
Nursing
Hawaii Pacific University
Kaneohe, Hawaii

Cecilia Jane Maier, MS, RN, CCRN
Assistant Professor
Mount Carmel College of Nursing
Columbus, Ohio

Marie Messier, MSN, Med
Associate Professor
Germanna Community College
Locust Grove, Virginia

Louise M. Niemer, PhD, ARNP
BSN Program Director
Northern Kentucky University
Highland Heights, Kentucky

Barbara Patterson, RN, PhD
Associate Professor
Widener University
Chester, Pennsylvania

Janet A. Reilly, RN, BSN, MA
Nurse Educator
Kellogg Community College
Battle Creek, Michigan

Donna Russo, RN, MSN, CCRN
Nursing Instructor
Frankford Hospital School of Nursing
Philadelphia, Pennsylvania

Diane Saleska, MSN, RN
Clinical Assistant Professor, Coordinator Clinical
Skills/Simulations Center
University of Missouri, St. Louis
St. Louis, Missouri

Cheryl Swallow, MSN, RN
Professor of Nursing, Program Coordinator
St. Louis Community College, Forest Park
St. Louis, Missouri

Jo A. Voss, PhD, RN, CNS
Assistant Professor
South Dakota State University
Rapid City, South Dakota

Preface

Overview of this NCLEX-RN® Review Package

This exam review book, the accompanying CD-ROM, and the online resources have been developed to help you prepare for the National Council Licensing Examination for Registered Nurses (NCLEX-RN®). Students will also find this book helpful for review when preparing for course exams, final exams, NCLEX-RN assessment exams, or other standardized or competency exams.

Study resources

This review package includes multiple resources that you can use in any combination to meet your own study and test preparation plans:

- ☐ More than 5,800 "NCLEX-RN style" test questions
  - The book contains more than 4,500 questions with rationales and can be used for traditional study
  - The CD-ROM includes more than 1,300 questions with rationales that provides you with ample opportunity to experience test-taking using computer-administered questions and allows you to customize tests for specific review and practice

- ☐ Questions written for all clinical areas of nursing (childbearing family and their neonate; nursing care of infants, children, and adolescents; nursing care of adults with medical and surgical health problems; and nursing care of clients with psychiatric disorders and mental health problems)

- ☐ Questions organized by health problems to facilitate review for course-specific exams

- ☐ Questions coded by client needs to assure practice in *all* areas of the NCLEX-RN test plan

- ☐ Questions emphasizing integrative processes on the NCLEX-RN test plan

- ☐ Questions with teaching feedback and rationales for both correct and incorrect answers

- ☐ Questions using all NCLEX-RN style questions (multiple choice, multiple response, hot-spot, fill-in-the blank, drag-and-drop/ordered response, and chart/exhibit)

- ☐ Questions written at higher levels of the cognitive domain (application, analysis, synthesis, and evaluation)

- ☐ Questions emphasizing clinical decision making and management of care

- ☐ Questions to provide practice for calculating drug dosages, intravenous drip rates, intake and output, and other questions requiring calculation and reporting of a numerical response to the question

- ☐ Questions emphasizing current nursing practice in the areas of client safety, home care, health promotion, care of the older adult, cancer nursing, end-of-life care, perioperative care, community health nursing, emergency and disaster nursing

- ☐ Six comprehensive tests of 190 questions each designed to resemble the testing format of the NCLEX-RN

- ☐ A description of the current NCLEX-RN test plan

- ☐ A study plan and checklist to guide systematic preparation for the licensing examination

- ☐ Information about developing study skills, taking tests, and managing test anxiety

- ☐ Tips for studying from students who have successfully passed the NCLEX-RN exam

- ☐ Addresses, telephone numbers, and websites for the National Council of State Boards of Nursing, Inc., and each state board of nursing

- ☐ Online resources for students, including tips for test-taking and downloadable NCLEX questions for your portable audio player.

Organization of the book

The review book is organized in three sections. The first section of the book provides information about the licensing exam and how to prepare for and take examinations using "NCLEX-RN style" questions. In the second section of the book, there are four major units—nursing care of the childbearing family and their neonate; nursing care of infants, children, and adolescents; nursing care of adults with medical and surgical health problems; and nursing care of clients with psychiatric disorders and mental health problems. Within each unit, tests are grouped according to health problems and include questions that are matched to the NCLEX-RN test plan. The third section of the book contains six comprehensive exams written to simulate the NCLEX-RN by placing test items in random order of content area. Each test presents a variety of situations commonly encountered in nursing practice, and includes test questions from all components of the NCLEX-RN test plan and all six types of questions used on the licensing exam. Except in the comprehensive tests in Part 3, alternate-format questions (and their answers and rationales) appear in blue to help the reader immediately distinguish them from traditional questions.

The CD-ROM

Additionally, this review package includes a CD-ROM with more than 1,300 questions. The CD-ROM can be used in several ways. For example, you may take a test in the four content areas, arrange a test to present questions in random order, or select questions for particular review and practice. The program also enables you to print out test results to gauge your progress. The CD-ROM simulates the actual NCLEX-RN exam by formatting questions on a computer screen and requiring you to use the keyboard and mouse to enter answers to the questions. It also features a pull-down calculator for use in answering questions that require you to calculate drug doses and drip rates for intravenous infusions.

Using This Review Package for Preparing for Nursing Exams

We suggest that you begin your review by using the practice exams in the book to identify areas of strength and areas in which you need further study. Each exam contains specific questions written in the style of the NCLEX-RN. Answers include rationales for both correct and incorrect answer options to reinforce learning. You may wish to score the results of each practice test and identify areas in which you need further review. To evaluate your results after completing each exam, divide the number of your correct responses by the total number of questions in the test and multiply by 100. For example, if you answered 72 of 90 items correctly, you would divide 72 by 90 and multiply by 100, for a result of 80%. If you answered more than 75% of the items in an area correctly, you are most likely prepared

to answer questions in that area on the NCLEX-RN. If you answered fewer than 75% of the questions correctly, you need to determine why. Did you answer incorrectly because of lack of content knowledge or because you did not read carefully? Use this information to guide your study.

After reviewing the specific content areas in the practice exams, take the comprehensive exams. These exams more realistically reflect the NCLEX-RN because each test presents a variety of situations commonly encountered in nursing practice and across all clinical disciplines. Underlying knowledge, skills, and abilities related to the basic sciences, fundamentals of nursing, pharmacology and other therapeutic measures, communicable diseases, legal and ethical considerations, and nutrition are included in items as needed to plan nursing care for individual clients or groups of clients.

Next, use the CD-ROM to simulate taking computerized adaptive tests. Note how the questions are presented on the computer screen, and practice answering questions without using a pencil. Use the diagnostic features of the CD-ROM to identify areas for further study and develop your own customized test for focused review.

And don't forget to check the online resources available at *http://thepoint.lww.com/*. The study tips will provide you with a foundation to begin your exam preparation. The 250 downloadable NCLEX questions can be put on your MP3 player, allowing you to practice anytime and anywhere.

Acknowledgements

This ninth edition has been developed with the expertise of nationally recognized test item writers. Thanks to Karen Bawel-Brinkley, Carol Bostrom, Judith Halstead, Margie Hull, Colleen O'Leary, Virginia Richardson, Gayle Roux, Lee Schwecke, Pat Twedt, Mary Ann Wehmer, and Sandy Wood for developing questions to prepare students for test-taking success. Thanks also to the Lippincott Williams & Wilkins editorial team, Margaret Zuccarini, Jaime Buss, Brenna Mayer, and Elaine Kasmer for support and design of a user-friendly book.

Diane M. Billings, EdD, RN, FAAN
Chancellor's Professor Emeritus
Formerly Associate Dean, Teaching Learning and Information Resources
Indiana University School of Nursing

Introduction to the NCLEX-RN® Licensing Examination and Preparation for Test-Taking

1

The NCLEX-RN® Licensing Examination

Overview

The National Council Licensure Examination for Registered Nurses (NCLEX-RN®) is administered to graduates of nursing schools to test the knowledge, abilities, and skills necessary for entry-level safe and effective nursing practice. The examination is developed by the National Council of State Boards of Nursing, Inc. (NCSBN), an organization with representation from all state boards of nursing.[1] The same examination is used in all 50 states, the District of Columbia, and United States possessions. Students who have graduated from baccalaureate, diploma, and associate-degree programs in nursing must pass this examination to meet licensing requirements in the United States.

The Test Plan

The NCSBN prepares the test plan used to develop the licensing examination. The test plan is based on an analysis of current nursing practice and the skills, abilities, and processes nurses use to provide nursing care.

Practice Analysis: The Foundation of the Test Plan

The NCLEX-RN test plan is based on the results of a practice analysis conducted every 3 years of the entry-level performance of newly licensed registered nurses and on expert judgment provided by members of the National Council's Examination Committee as well as a Job Analysis Panel of Experts.[1, 2, 4] The job analysis asks newly graduated nurses to rank the nursing activities that they perform on a regular basis. The questions used on the test plan, therefore, include those activities that nurses commonly perform. For example, the 2005 RN practice analysis revealed that nursing practice commonly involved assessing and evaluating client's physical status, treatments, outcomes of interventions, and lab results; administering medication and assessing incompatibilities, side effects, and outcomes; applying principles of infection control; ensuring proper identification of the client; and managing care, including supervision, communication, staff educa-

tion, and discharge planning.[4] Less commonly performed activities included microdermabrasion, leading group therapy sessions, and implementing phototherapy.[4] This information is helpful in anticipating the content emphasis for the questions that will appear on the NCLEX-RN exam.

Test item writers

Nurse clinicians and nurse educators nominated by the Council of State Boards of Nursing to serve as item writers write the test questions on the NCLEX-RN exam. Because the item writers come from a variety of geographical areas and practice settings, the test items reflect nursing practice in all parts of the country.

Test plan details

Test plans, or test blueprints, are developed to indicate the components and the relative weights of the components that will be tested on an exam. Because exams test both content (knowledge) and process (critical thinking, synthesis of information, clinical decision-making), test plans usually have two or three dimensions. The test plan for the NCLEX-RN addresses two components of nursing care: (1) client needs categories and (2) integrated process, such as the nursing process, caring, communication and documentation, and teaching/learning (see Table 1.1). Representative items test knowledge of these components as they relate to specific health care situations in all of the four major areas of client needs. The questions developed for the test plan are written to test nursing knowledge and the ability to apply nursing knowledge to client situations.

Client Needs

The health needs of clients are grouped under four broad categories: (1) safe, effective care environment; (2) health promotion and maintenance; (3) psychosocial integrity; and (4) physiologic integrity. Two of these categories include subcategories of related and specified needs (see Table 1.2). The percentage of test items in each subcategory on the NCLEX-RN examination is shown in Figure 1.1.

Integrated Processes

The NCLEX-RN test plan also is organized according to four integrated processes. These include the nursing process, caring, communication and documentation, and teaching/learning. (See Table 1.1 and Figure 1.1)

The Nursing Process

The NCLEX-RN test plan includes questions from all steps of the nursing process. The five phases of the nursing process are: (1) assessment, (2) analysis, (3) planning, (4) implementation, and (5) evaluation.

Assessment. Assessment involves establishing a database. The nurse gathers objective and subjective information about the client, and then verifies the data and communicates information gained from the assessment.

Analysis. Analysis involves identifying actual or potential health care needs or problems based on assessment data. The nurse interprets the data, collects additional data as indicated, and identifies and communicates the client's nursing diagnoses. The nurse also determines the congruency between the client's needs and the ability of the health care team members to meet those needs.

Planning. Planning involves setting outcomes and goals for meeting the client's needs and designing strategies to attain them. The nurse determines the goals of care, develops and modifies the plan, collaborates with other health team members for delivery of the client's care, and formulates expected outcomes of nursing interventions.

Implementation. Implementation involves initiating and completing actions necessary to accomplish the defined goals. The nurse organizes and manages the client's care; performs or assists the client in performing activities of daily living; counsels and teaches the client, significant others, and health care team members; and provides care to attain the established client goals. The nurse also provides care to optimize the achievement of the client's health care goals; supervises, coordinates, and evaluates delivery of the client's care as provided by nursing staff; and records and exchanges information.

Evaluation. Evaluation determines goal achievement. The nurse compares actual with expected outcomes of therapy, evaluates compliance with prescribed or proscribed therapy, and records and describes the client's response to therapy or care. The nurse also modifies the plan, as indicated, and reorders priorities.

The five phases of the nursing process are equally important. Therefore, each is represented by an equal number of items on the NCLEX-RN and all are integrated throughout the exam. In this book, you will have opportunities to respond to questions involving all five steps of the nursing process.

TABLE 1.1
Test Plan Structure

The framework of Client Needs was selected for the NCLEX-RN examination because it provides a universal structure for defining nursing actions and competencies across all settings for all clients.

Client Needs

Four major categories of Client Needs organize the content of the NCLEX-RN® Test Plan. Two of the four categories are further divided into a total of six subcategories that define the content contained within the two Client Needs categories. These categories and subcategories are:

A. Safe, Effective Care Environment
1. Management of Care
2. Safety and Infection Control

B. Health Promotion and Maintenance

C. Psychosocial Integrity

D. Physiologic Integrity
3. Basic Care and Comfort
4. Pharmacologic and Parenteral Therapies
5. Reduction of Risk Potential
6. Physiologic Adaptation

Integrated Concepts and Processes

The following concepts and processes fundamental to the practice of nursing are integrated throughout the four major categories of Client Needs:

- **Nursing Process**
- **Caring**
- **Communication and Documentation**
- **Teaching/Learning**

Used by permission of the National Council of State Boards of Nursing, Inc., Chicago, IL.

Caring

The caring process refers to interaction between the nurse, client, and family in a way that conveys mutual respect and trust. The nurse offers encouragement and hope to clients and their families while providing nursing care. Questions about the caring process are threaded throughout the licensing exam to test the candidate's attitudes and values for caring for and about clients. In this book, you will have the opportunity to respond to questions that test your ability to apply the caring process in a variety of situations.

(Text continues on page 6.)

TABLE 1.2
Categories and Subcategories of Client Needs

A. Safe, Effective Care Environment

1. *Management of Care*—providing integrated, cost-effective care to clients by coordinating, supervising, and/or collaborating with members of the multidisciplinary health care team. Related content includes but is not limited to:

- Advance Directives
- Advocacy
- Case Management
- Client Rights
- Collaboration with Multidisciplinary Team
- Concepts of Management
- Confidentiality
- Consultation
- Continuity of Care
- Delegation
- Establishing Priorities

- Ethical Practice
- Incident/Irregular Occurrence/Variance Reports
- Informed Consent
- Legal Rights and Responsibilities
- Organ Donation
- Performance Improvement (Quality Assurance)
- Referrals
- Resource Management
- Staff Education
- Supervision

2. *Safety and Infection Control*—protecting clients and health care personnel from environmental hazards. Related content includes but is not limited to:

- Accident Prevention
- Disaster Planning
- Emergency Response Plan
- Error Prevention
- Handling Hazardous and Infectious Materials
- Home Safety
- Injury Prevention

- Medical and Surgical Asepsis
- Reporting of Incident/Event/Irregular Occurrence/Variance
- Safe Use of equipment
- Security Plan
- Standard/Transmission-Based/Other Precautions
- Use of Restraints/Safety Devices

B. Health Promotion and Maintenance

The nurse provides and directs nursing care of the client and family/significant others that incorporates expected growth and development principles, prevention and early detection of health problems, and strategies to achieve optimal health. Related content includes but is not limited to:

- Aging Process
- Ante/Intra/Postpartum and Newborn Care
- Developmental Stages and Transitions
- Disease Prevention
- Expected Body Image Changes
- Family Planning
- Family Systems
- Growth and Development
- Health and Wellness

- Health Promotion Programs
- Health Screening
- High Risk Behaviors
- Human Sexuality
- Immunizations
- Lifestyle Choices
- Principles of Teaching and Learning
- Self-care
- Techniques of Physical Assessment

C. Psychosocial Integrity

The nurse provides and directs nursing care that promotes and supports the emotional, mental, and social well-being of the client and family/significant others experiencing stressful events, as well as clients with acute and chronic mental illness. Related content includes but is not limited to:

- Abuse/Neglect
- Behavioral Interventions
- Chemical Dependency
- Coping Mechanisms
- Crisis Intervention
- Cultural Diversity
- End of Life
- Family Dynamics
- Grief and Loss
- Mental Health Concepts

- Psychopathology
- Religious and Spiritual Influences on Health
- Sensory/Perceptual Alterations
- Situational Role Changes
- Stress Management
- Support Systems
- Therapeutic Communication
- Therapeutic Environment
- Unexpected Body Image Changes

D. Physiologic Integrity

The nurse promotes physical health and well-being by providing care and comfort, reducing client risk potential, and managing the client's health alterations.

3. *Basic Care and Comfort*—providing comfort and assistance in the performance of activities of daily living. Related content includes but is not limited to:

- Alternative and Complementary Therapies
- Assistive Devices
- Elimination
- Mobility/Immobility
- Nonpharmacologic Comfort Interventions
- Nutrition and Oral Hydration
- Palliative/Comfort Care
- Personal Hygiene
- Rest and Sleep

4. *Pharmacologic and Parenteral Therapies*—managing and providing care related to the administration of medications and parenteral therapies. Related content includes but is not limited to:

- Adverse Effects/Contraindications and Side Effects
- Blood and Blood Products
- Central Venous Access Devices
- Dosage Calculations
- Expected Outcomes/Effects
- Intravenous Therapy
- Medication Administration
- Parenteral Fluids
- Pharmacologic Agents/Actions
- Pharmacologic Interactions
- Pharmacologic Pain Management
- Total Parenteral Nutrition

5. *Reduction of Risk Potential*—reducing the likelihood that clients will develop complications or health problems related to existing conditions, treatments, or procedures. Related content includes but is not limited to:

- Diagnostic Tests
- Laboratory Values
- Monitoring Conscious Sedation
- Potential for Alterations in Body Systems
- Potential for Complications of Diagnostic Tests/Treatments/Procedures
- Potential for Complications from Surgical Procedures and Health Alterations
- System Specific Assessments
- Therapeutic Procedures
- Vital Signs

6. *Physiologic Adaptation*—managing and providing care for clients with acute, chronic, or life-threatening physical health conditions. Related content includes but is not limited to:

- Alterations in Body Systems
- Fluid and Electrolyte Imbalances
- Hemodynamics
- Illness Management
- Infectious Diseases
- Medical Emergencies
- Pathophysiology
- Radiation Therapy
- Unexpected Response to Therapies

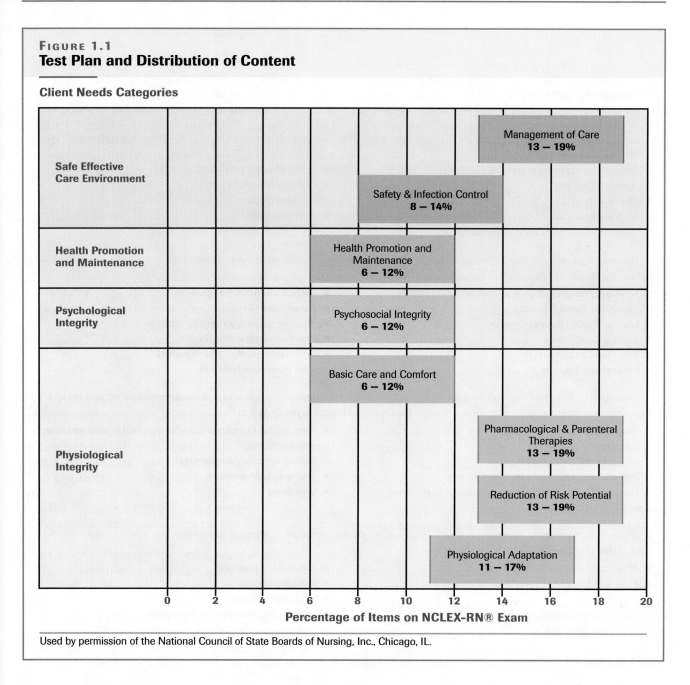

FIGURE 1.1
Test Plan and Distribution of Content

Client Needs Categories

Used by permission of the National Council of State Boards of Nursing, Inc., Chicago, IL.

Communication and Documentation

Another element of the licensing exam test plan evaluates the nurse's ability to communicate with clients, families, and health team members. The test also includes questions about documenting nursing care according to standards of nursing practice. In this book, you will be presented with questions that ask you to determine the most effective way to communicate with clients, families, and other health professionals. You will also have the opportunity to respond to questions that require you to select the appropriate information to document or chart.

Teaching/Learning

An important aspect of nursing care is to teach clients and their families about managing their own health status. Nurses also teach other members of the health care team. Questions in this book are designed to assist you in answering questions about the teaching and learning process for a variety of clients and health care team members.

The Test Questions

Each test item on the NCLEX-RN exam is written to test aspects of nursing care indicated on the test plan. Test questions are written at different levels of the cognitive domain that will test your ability to apply, analyze, and evaluate. There are also a variety of test item formats used on the NCLEX-RN.

Cognitive levels

The test items are written to test a variety of levels of the cognitive domain. The cognitive level of questions refers to the type of mental activity required to answer the question as defined in a taxonomy of the cognitive domain.[3] (See Table 1.3.) The lowest level of the taxonomy is the *knowledge* (or *remember*) level and involves the ability to remember or recall facts about principles, concepts, theories, terms, or procedures. Questions at this level ask you to define, identify, or select responses. The next level of the cognitive domain, *comprehension* (or *understand*) requires understanding data; questions at this level ask you to interpret, explain, or understand examples of the content. The *application* level involves using information in new situations. At this level, you are expected to solve problems, develop or modify nursing care plans, manipulate data, and demonstrate appropriate use of information. *Analysis* requires recognizing and differentiating relationships between parts. Questions at this level ask you to analyze, select, differentiate, or interpret data from a variety of sources, and to think critically and set priorities. The next level of the cognitive domain is *evaluation*. Here you must check data, critique information, or judge the outcome of nursing care. The final level of the cognitive domain is *creation*. At this level, you must be able to generate new approaches to nursing care or develop a unique nursing care plan based on data provided. Test questions can be written to test at all levels of the cognitive domain, but questions that are written for the NCLEX-RN are generally written at application levels and above because nursing requires the ability to analyze data, think critically, and make clinical decisions for client care. This book presents questions at the application level and higher.

Types of test questions

The NCLEX-RN examination uses six types, or formats, of test questions.[1] These include multiple-choice, multiple-response, fill-in-the-blank, hot-spot, chart/exhibit questions, and drag-and-drop/ordered-response. Multiple-choice questions are the most common type of question used on the NCLEX-RN exam, but each exam may include one or more of each of the other types of questions (referred to as *alternate-format questions*). Although each type of question tests your understanding of nursing content, each requires you to respond in a different way. All question types are scored as either correct or incorrect; no partial credit is awarded for any question type.

All six types of questions are used in this review book and CD-ROM to give you opportunity to learn how to answer each type of question. You can also find examples of these types of questions on the NCSBN web site (*www.ncsbn.org*), in the candidate tutorial that precedes each licensing exam at the PearsonVue web site (*www.pearsonvue.com/nclex*), and in the candidates' bulletin that you will receive prior to taking the licensing exam.

Multiple-choice questions

Multiple-choice questions include a situation or scenario, a question, and four answers, only one of which is correct. The situation is a client-based scenario that gives information about the client or care management. The question that follows is based on the information given in the situation. As you answer the question, relate the answer to the background information. Pay particular attention to information about the client's age, family status, health status, ethnicity, or point in the care plan (e.g., early admission versus preparation for discharge).

The question (stem) poses the problem to solve. The question may be written as a direct question, such as "What should the nurse do first?" or as an incomplete sentence, such as "The nurse should…"

The answers (options) are possible responses to the stem. Each stem has one correct option and three incorrect options. The options may be written as complete sentences or may complete the sentence stem stated in the question. (See Figure 1.2.)

TABLE 1.3
Levels of the Cognitive Domain

Knowledge/Remember: Recognizing, recalling
Comprehension/Understand: Interpreting, exemplifying, classifying, summarizing, inferring, comparing, explaining
Application: Executing, implementing
Analysis: Differentiating, organizing, attributing
Evaluation: Checking, critiquing
Creation: Generating, planning, producing

FIGURE 1.2
Sample Single Response Multiple-Choice Question

112. Which of the following actions should the nurse plan to do first when caring for a client who is experiencing spiritual distress?
- ☐ 1. Make a referral to a member of the clergy.
- ☐ 2. Explain the major beliefs of different religions.
- ☐ 3. Suggest reading material.
- ☐ 4. Help the client explore his or her own values and beliefs.

Multiple-response questions

Multiple-response questions are similar to multiple-choice questions, except that they include more than four answers and may have more than one correct response. These questions will ask you to identify all of the answers that are correct ("Select all that apply"). As is true of all test questions on the NCLEX-RN exam, the multiple-response questions will be scored as being either correct or incorrect; no partial credit is given for selecting some of the correct responses. (See Figure 1.3.)

FIGURE 1.3
Sample Multiple-Response Multiple-Choice Question

141. The family of a hospitalized client demonstrates understanding of the teaching about advanced directives when they make which of the following statements? Select all that apply.

☐ **1.** "Advanced directives documents give instructions about future medical care and treatment."

☐ **2.** "If people are not capable of communicating their wishes, health care providers and family together can agree on measures or actions that will be taken."

☐ **3.** "Ethics experts agree that the family is the sole deciding factor when the client is competent."

☐ **4.** "Medical power-of-attorney primarily gives financial access to the designee."

☐ **5.** "Medical power-of-attorney or durable power-of-attorney for health care is a document that lists who can make health care decisions should a person be unable to make an informed decision for himself or herself."

☐ **6.** "Advanced directives documents give details about the client's past medical history."

Hot-spot questions

Hot-spot questions involve identifying the location of a specific item, such as an appropriate injection site, assessment area, or correct part of a waveform. The question will be phrased "Identify the location" or "Select the area." In the book, you should place an X on the illustration provided to identify the proper area. On the actual NCLEX-RN, and on the CD-ROM in the back of this book, you will use the mouse to move your cursor over the area you want to select and then left-click the area. A red "X" will appear over the area you have selected. If you make an error, you can move the cursor to the part of the figure that is the answer you wish to enter. (See Figure 1.4.)

FIGURE 1.4
Sample Hot-Spot Question

58. The nurse performed Leopold's maneuvers on a pregnant client and determined that the fetal position is LOA. Indicate the area where the nurse should place the Doppler to most easily hear fetal heart sounds.

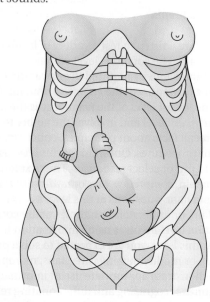

Fill-in-the-blank questions

Fill-in-the-blank questions involve calculations, such as determining a drug dose, calculating an I.V. drip rate, or adding intake-output records. These questions can be answered with a number; if you do not enter a number, you will receive an error message that will prompt you to "enter a numeric answer." When an answer includes a measurement amount such as milliliters (ml), grams (g), or inches, the measurement unit will be stated in the stem of the question and supplied in the answer box. You should not include the unit of measure as part of your answer. The question will indicate if you are to round your answer and, if so, to how many decimal places. (See Figure 1.5.)

FIGURE 1.5
Sample Fill-in-the-Blank Question

55. The physician orders an intravenous infusion of 5% dextrose in 0.25 normal saline to be infused at 2 ml/kg/hour in an infant who weighs 9 lb. How many milliliters per hour of the solution should the nurse infuse?

_____ ml/hr

A drop-down calculator is available within the computer administered NCLEX-RN examination that you can use to calculate your answers. The division sign used is similar to the one used on the Microsoft Calculator (/); be sure to familiarize yourself with the mathematical function keys. To practice calculations required for fill-in-the-blank questions, pull down the calculator on your computer. The CD-ROM accompanying this book has a built-in calculator that approximates the one you will find on the actual test. To avoid calculation errors, be sure that you do not enter numbers rapidly when you are using the calculator.

Chart/exhibit questions

Chart/exhibit questions present data from a chart. The data will be presented from one or more chart "tabs" such as: prescriptions, history and physical, laboratory results, miscellaneous reports, imaging results, flow sheets, intake and output, medication administration record, progress notes, and vital signs. (See Figure 1.6.) You will be asked to use the data to make a nursing decision. For example, you will click on up to three tabs to locate data and then you will interpret the data, validate if the data are correct or sufficient, and then be asked to respond to a question based on the data. When these types of questions are administered by the computer (as in the NCLEX-RN exam), you may be asked to determine which "tab" to use to locate the information that is required to answer the question. In this book and on the accompanying CD-ROM, chart/exhibit questions show data on one particular "tab" and then ask you to use the data to respond to the question.

Drag-and-drop/ordered-response questions

Drag-and-drop/ordered-response questions require you to place information in a specified order. (See Figure 1.7.) For example, the question might ask you to put steps of a procedure in order, provide information about several clients and ask you to determine their priorities for nursing care, or ask you the order in which to teach a client about a procedure or self-care. On the licensing exam, you will drag each response from the left-hand column and drop it into the correct order on the right-hand column. You can move the items around until you have them in the correct order and then click "submit" to enter your answer. The CD-ROM that accompanies this book functions in much the same way, except that you will click on "Next" to proceed to the next question. In the book, you will simply rewrite the answer options in their correct order in the blank spaces provided in the answer column.

Taking the Exam

Computer Adaptive Testing

The NCLEX-RN is administered using computer adaptive testing (CAT) procedures. CAT uses the memory and speed of the computer to administer a test individualized for each candidate. When the examination begins, the computer randomly selects a question of medium difficulty. The next question is based on the candidate's response to the previous question. If the question is answered correctly, an item of similar or greater difficulty is generated; if it is answered incorrectly, a less-difficult item is selected. Thus, the test is adapted for each candidate. Once competence has been determined, the exam is completed at a passing level.

FIGURE 1.6
Sample Chart/Exhibit Question

16. A 13-year-old has been admitted with a diagnosis of rheumatic fever and is on bed rest. He complains of a sore throat. His joints are painful and swollen. He has a red rash on his trunk and is experiencing aimless movements of his extremities. Use the chart below to determine what the nurse should do first.

VITAL SIGNS		
Time	8:00 am	12:00 noon
Temperature	100.4 (X)	98.6 (X)
Respirations	22 (X)	25 (X)
Apical heart rate	110 (X)	150 (X)
Blood pressure	110 (X)	120 (X)

☐ 1. Report the heart rate to the physician.
☐ 2. Apply lotion to the rash.
☐ 3. Splint the joints to relieve the pain.
☐ 4. Request an order for medication to treat the elevated temperature.

FIGURE 1.7
FIGURE 1.7
Sample Drag-and-Drop/Ordered-Response Question

111. A nurse is assigned to the obstetrical triage area. When beginning the assignment, the nurse is given a report about four clients waiting to be seen. Place the clients in the order in which the nurse should see them.

1. A primigravid client at 10 weeks' gestation complaining of not feeling well with nausea and vomiting, urinary frequency, and fatigue.

2. A multiparous client at 32 weeks' gestation asking for assistance with finding a new physician.

3. A single mother at 4 months postpartum fearful of shaking her baby when he cries.

4. An antenatal client at 16 weeks' gestation who has occasional sharp pain on her left side radiating from her symphysis to her fundus.

CAT has several advantages. For example, an exam can be given in less time because candidates potentially have to answer fewer questions. CAT exams also can be administered frequently, allowing a graduate of a nursing program to take the exam following graduation, receive the results quickly, and enter the work force as a registered nurse in less time than is possible with paper-and-pencil exams. Study results also show that, because CAT is self-paced, candidates undergo less stress.

Each NCLEX-RN test is generated from a large pool of questions (a test item bank) based on the NCLEX-RN test plan. The test item bank includes all types of questions, but an individual candidate may or may not receive each type of question, depending on the questions generated from the item bank for each candidate. The exams for all candidates are derived from the same large pool of test items. They contain comparable questions for each component of the test plan. Although the questions are not exactly the same, they test the same knowledge, skills, and abilities from the test plan. All candidates must meet the requirements of the test plan and achieve the same passing score. Each candidate, therefore, has the same opportunity to demonstrate competence. Although one candidate may answer fewer questions, all candidates have the opportunity to answer a sufficient number of questions to demonstrate competence until the stability of passing or failing is established or the time limit expires.

All candidates must answer at least 75 test questions; the maximum number of questions is 265. Each exam also includes 15 "pretest" questions that are being tested for use on subsequent exams. Candidates cannot differentiate "pretest" items from operational items on the exam.

Six hours are available to each candidate for completing the test. This time includes an opportunity to review the online candidate tutorial about the test and to take rest breaks. Although some candidates may finish in a shorter time, others will use the entire 6 hours. The amount of time used during testing is not an indication of passing or failing the examination, but rather, reflects the time required to establish competence for each candidate.

Scheduling the Examination

The first step you must take to schedule your NCLEX-RN exam is to apply to the state board of nursing in the state in which you plan to take the examination. You will then receive an Authorization to Test (ATT). Registration for the exam can be done by mail or online, and confirmation of registration should occur within several days, or immediately if done online. At this point, you can schedule an appointment to take the exam. Check for current information at the NCSBN web site (*www.ncsbn.org*) and the web site of your state board of nursing (see the appendix State and Territorial Boards of Nursing).

Exam Locations

The Council of State Boards of Nursing contracts with vendors in each state to serve as exam sites. Your school of nursing can inform you of the nearest location. You can also contact your state board of nursing for information. (See the appendix State and Territorial Boards of Nursing for the address.) You can also find updated information from the NCSBN at its web site (*www.ncsbn.org*).

Computer Use and Screen Design

Test questions are presented on the computer screen (monitor); you select your answer and use the keyboard or a mouse to enter your answer. The CD-ROM included with this book simulates the NCLEX-RN and provides you with an opportunity to practice taking computer-generated examinations. At every testing site, written directions are provided at each computer exam station. There are also tutorials and practice questions on the computer that you can complete to be sure you understand how to use the computer before you begin the exam.

Exam Security

Each testing site maintains a high level of security for the exam and for the candidate. The exam is administered on a secured file server and uses password security and host site authentication. All exam sites use proctors and video/audio monitoring. Candidates are required to undergo identification verification, which may include showing a photo ID, fingerprint testing, or providing a digital signature. Check with your state board of nursing and the NCSBN for details about exam security in the jurisdiction in which you are taking the exam.

Special Accommodations

Special accommodations for ADA candidates can be made with authorization from the individual state board of nursing and the NCSBN. If approved, the accommodations will be noted on the ATT and implemented at the testing center. Check with your state board of nursing for additional information.

Results Reporting

Computerized testing allows timely reporting of examination results. The results of the examination are first reviewed at the testing site and then forwarded to the state board of nursing within 8 hours. Results are reported to the candidate within 2 weeks. Some jurisdictions have "quick results" services; for a fee, the candidate can obtain "unofficial" results by internet or a 900 number telephone call.

The exam can be retaken within 45 days. Check with your state board of nursing for details. (See the appendix for a listing of state boards of nursing.)

When to Take the NCLEX-RN

Recent research indicates that candidates should take the exam within 6 months of graduating.[5] You should, therefore, plan your own schedule to be prepared to take the NCLEX-RN exam as soon after graduation as is possible. Suggestions for developing a study plan are discussed in Chapter 2 of this book.

Additional Information

For further information about the NCLEX-RN, the test plan, test questions, or exam format, visit the NCSBN web site at *www.ncsbn.org* or write to the NCSBN. For information about the dates, requirements, and specifics of writing the examination in your state, contact your state board of nursing. The addresses and telephone numbers of the NCSBN and each state board of nursing are provided in the appendix. Information can also be obtained from the vendor who has contracted to provide the testing center for the NCLEX-RN exam. The current vendor is Pearson-Vue, and information can be found at their web site (*www.pearsonvue.com/nclex*).

References

1. National Council of State Boards of Nursing, Inc. *www.ncsbn.org*
2. Aucoin, J., and Treas, L. (2005). Assumptions and realities of NCLEX-RN. *Nursing Education Perspectives,* 26(5), 268–271.
3. Anderson, L.W., & Krathwohl, D. (Eds.). (2001). *A Taxonomy for Learning, Teaching, and Assessing: A Revision of Bloom's Taxonomy of Educational Objectives.* New York: Longman.
4. Wendt, A., & O'Neill, T. (2006). *Report of Findings from the 2005 RN Practice Analysis: Linking the NCLEX-RN to Examination and Practice.* Chicago, IL: National Council of State Boards of Nursing.

2 Preparing for and Taking the NCLEX-RN® and Other Nursing Exams

Studying for the NCLEX-RN or other similar exams requires careful planning and preparation. You can make the best use of your time by developing a systematic approach to study that includes these five steps to test for success:

- assessing your study needs
- developing a study plan
- refining your test-taking strategies
- rehearsing test anxiety management skills
- evaluating progress on a regular basis.

Use these five steps as you take your first test in nursing school. Refine your test-taking strategies as you evaluate your progress at each step of the way, so that when you are ready to take the licensing exam you will be an experienced and successful test-taker. Use the Personal Study Plan in Table 2.1 to help develop your own study plan.

Assessing Study Needs

The first step toward test success is to determine your strengths and limitations. Even students who have been successful throughout their academic life and nurses who are excellent caregivers have areas in which they need improvement. Be honest with yourself as you assess your own study needs. These steps can help you in your assessment:

■ Review your success in nursing school. Review your record of achievement in courses in the nursing curriculum. Success on the NCLEX-RN tends to correlate with grades (grade point average) achieved in nursing school. Subjects in which you received high grades, that you found easy to learn, or in which you have had additional clinical practice or work experience are likely to be areas of strength. On the other hand, subjects you found difficult to learn (or in which you did not achieve high grades) should be areas for concentrated review. Also consider content areas that you have not studied for a while. Recent course work will be the most familiar and, therefore, may require the least amount of study. All students, even students who have achieved success in nursing courses, benefit from identifying areas requiring study and spending time practicing test-taking skills. You also can use the practice exams in this book to identify areas needing further study. Begin with the subjects you find most difficult or in which you have the least confidence.

■ Assess your test-taking skills. Using effective test-taking skills contributes to exam success. What have you done in the past to make you confident about taking a test? How do you feel when you are in the exam situation? What has worked in the past to help you be successful? Review these strategies to build on past successes and work on problem areas. Consider additional strategies suggested in the section "Refining Your Test-Taking Strategies," page 15. You can practice these skills by simulating the testing situation using the practice tests and comprehensive exams in this review book.

■ Assess your ability to take tests that require application, analysis, and evaluation. Test questions used on the licensing exam are written at higher levels of the cognitive domain. Many candidates' experience with taking tests has come from taking "teacher-made" tests—tests developed by the faculty at your school of nursing. These tests are commonly written to test students' knowledge and understanding of course content and may not include questions that require application, analysis, or evaluation of course material. Additionally, several of the types of alternate-format questions have recently been added to the exam, and nursing faculty may not yet be designing their own test questions using these formats. Finally, some students are able to "second-guess" the teacher and use this ability to their advantage when taking teacher-made classroom tests. However, it is not as easy to anticipate test questions on standardized and licensing exams, and you will need to develop skills that will help you think critically when presented with an unfamiliar situation. As you prepare to take the licensing exam, spend time on questions where you need to "figure out" the best approach to answering the question. You can use the questions in this book and CD-ROM to be sure you understand the difference between questions that require only recall and understanding and those that require you to apply information to provide client care, make clinical judgments, and initiate nursing actions.

■ Assess your English language skills. Persons for whom English is a second language or who do not have well-developed reading and comprehension skills may require additional practice in reading and answering NCLEX-RN style test questions. If you are one of these persons, plan additional time to practice reading and answering questions, to time yourself when answering questions, and to

TABLE 2.1
Personal Study Plan

Assess Study Needs

1. Review your success in nursing school.

☐ I did best in these courses:

_____
_____

☐ I needed to study harder in these courses:

_____
_____

☐ I took these courses near the beginning of the curriculum:

_____
_____

☐ I scored best on these practice exams in this book:

_____
_____

☐ I am not satisfied with my scores on these practice exams in this book:

_____
_____

☐ I need further study in these content areas:

_____
_____

☐ I need further study in these areas of the nursing process:

_____
_____

☐ I need further study in these areas of client needs:

_____
_____

2. Review your test-taking skills.

☐ I can identify the components of a test question.
☐ I read questions carefully before answering.
☐ I can make reasonable guesses if I am not certain of the correct answer.

3. Review your test-anxiety management skills.

☐ I can do relaxation and deep-breathing exercises.
☐ I can visualize success.
☐ I can give myself positive feedback.
☐ I can concentrate for extended periods of time.

4. Review your computer skills.

☐ I am able to use a computer to read and answer test questions.
☐ I have used the CD-ROM accompanying this book.

Develop a Study Plan

☐ I will study in this location:

_____
_____

☐ I will study at these times and dates:

_____
_____

☐ I have assembled all of the materials I need to study:

_____
_____

☐ I will study with a study group:

_____
_____

Evaluate Progress

☐ I have completed the practice tests in this book.
☐ I have completed the comprehensive tests in this book.
☐ I need to improve my scores in these areas:

_____
_____

☐ I am prepared to take the NCLEX-RN examination.

Strategies for Taking Tests

■ Read the question carefully.
■ Anticipate the correct answer.
■ Read for key words.
■ Base answers on nursing knowledge.
■ Identify the components of the test item.

Strategies for Managing Test Anxiety

■ Mental rehearsal
■ Relaxation
■ Deep breathing
■ Positive self-talk
■ Distraction
■ Concentration

---

validate that you understand the question correctly. If necessary, seek assistance.

■ Assess your ability to take timed tests. Are you always the last one to finish a test? Do you request additional time to complete a test? If so, you will want to practice taking timed tests and doing your best, while completing as many questions as possible. The licensing exam is designed to be completed in 6 hours; only questions completed within that time frame will be scored. As you use the practice questions and tests in this book and CD-ROM, time yourself and, if needed, determine ways that you can increase your speed without sacrificing accuracy.

■ Assess your skills for taking computer-administered exams. Although previous computer experience is not necessary to take the NCLEX-RN, you should familiarize yourself with the differences between taking a paper-and-pencil exam and taking exams administered by the computer. If you have not used a computer before, find a learning resource center at your college, university, library, or hospital where you can become familiar with basic computer keyboard skills. The CD-ROM in the back of this book, which simulates the computerized NCLEX, offers you the opportunity to practice taking computer-administered test questions. Use it to practice reading questions from the computer screen and become acquainted with answering questions in a computerized format. If you are accustomed to underlining key words or making notes in the margins of paper-and-pencil tests, adapt these strategies to reading and answering the questions on the computer screen. Also be sure that you can use a drop down calculator to answer questions requiring the use of math skills.

Developing a Study Plan

Once you have identified areas of strength and areas needing further study, develop a specific plan and begin to study regularly. Students who study a small amount of content over a longer period of time tend to have higher success rates than students who wait until the last few weeks before the exam and then "cram." Consider these suggestions:

■ Identify a place for study. The area should be quiet and have room for your books and papers. This area might be in your home, at your nursing school, at your workplace, or in a library. Be sure your friends and family understand the importance of not interrupting you when you are studying.

■ Establish regular study times. Make appointments with yourself to ensure a commitment to study. Frequent, short study periods (1 or 2 hours) are preferable to sporadic, extended study periods. Plan to finish your studying 1 week before the NCLEX-RN; last-minute cramming tends to increase anxiety.

■ Obtain all necessary resources. As you begin to study, it is helpful to have easy access to textbooks, notes, and study guides.

■ Make the best use of your time. Make review cards that you can carry with you to study during free moments throughout the day. Some students record review notes and listen to the tapes or Podcasts while driving or exercising.

■ Reduce or eliminate stressful situations. Students who are juggling multiple responsibilities (such as working, managing a family, taking courses, planning a wedding, or caring for elderly parents) may find it difficult to find time to study or to concentrate when studying. Managing a variety of stressful situations puts students at risk for failing exams. If possible, reduce the number of stressful situations you are involved in during the time you are preparing to take the NCLEX-RN exam.

■ Develop effective study skills. Study skills enable you to acquire, organize, remember, and use the information you need to take the NCLEX-RN. These skills include outlining, summarizing, applying, synthesizing, reviewing, and practicing test-taking strategies. Use these study skills each time you prepare for an exam.

■ Use study skills with which you are familiar and that have worked well for you in the past. Recall effective study behaviors that you used in nursing school, such as reviewing highlighted text, outlines, or content maps.

■ Study to learn, not to memorize. The NCLEX-RN tests application and analysis of knowledge. When reviewing content, continually ask yourself, "How is this information used in client care?" "What clinical decision-making will be required of this information?" and "What is the role of the nurse in using this information?" Being able to apply information, rather than just being able to list or recognize information, is one of the most important study skills to master.

■ Identify your learning and study style preferences. Each student has a preferred way of learning. For example, some students prefer learning material by listening; they are considered *auditory* learners. If this describes your preference, you will benefit from reviewing taped notes or class lectures. Some students learn best in a visual mode. They learn by reading, reviewing slide presentations, or looking at illustrations. For these *visual* learners, reading and looking at images is helpful. *Kinesthetic* learners, those who like to touch and manipulate to learn, benefit from working with models and manikins to reinforce their learning. While you likely have one learning style and study preference, using a variety of styles will enhance the study experience.

■ Some students prefer to study alone, whereas others benefit from study groups; know which approach works best for you and develop your study plan accordingly. If you participate in a study group, limit the group. The group should develop norms for working together that focus on understanding and applying nursing content, rather than memorizing facts. Every member must come prepared to contribute.

■ Anticipate questions. As you study, formulate questions around the content. Practice giving a rationale for your answer to these questions. If you work in a study group, have each member contribute questions that the entire group answers.

■ Study common, not unique, nursing care situations. The NCLEX-RN tests minimum competence for nursing practice; therefore, focus on common health problems and client needs. Review the *RN Practice Analysis*, published by the National Council of State Boards of Nursing, and the current licensing exam test plan to determine common nursing care activities.[1, 2]

■ Simulate test-taking. The comprehensive tests in Part Three of this book and the CD-ROM are designed to simulate the random order in which questions appear in the NCLEX-RN. Use these resources to focus on areas of common concern in nursing care rather than on the traditional content delineation of adult, pediatric, psychiatric, and childbearing clients. Make additional copies of answer sheets, and retake the exams on which you had low scores.

Refining Your Test-Taking Strategies

Knowing how to take a test is as important as knowing the content being tested. Strategies for taking tests can be learned and used to improve test scores. Here are some suggestions for building a repertoire of effective test-taking strategies:

■ Understand the type of test question and the components of the test item. (See "Types of test questions" on pages 7 to 9 for more information on question types found on the NCLEX-RN exam.)

■ Understand which integrated process (step of the nursing process, caring, communication, documentation, teaching/learning) is being tested. For example, as you read the question, determine whether the question is asking you to set priorities (planning) or judge outcomes (evaluation).

■ Understand client needs. As you read the question, consider the question in the context of client needs. Be sure to understand if the question is asking you to determine what to do "first" or to select the nursing action that is "best."

■ Understand the age of the client noted in the test question. If relevant to answering the question, the age of the client will be specified; consider what information about that age-group will be important to answering the question. If the age of the client is not specified, assume that the client is an adult and base your answers on principles of adult growth and development.

■ Read the question carefully. This is one of the most important aspects of effective test taking. Do not rush. Ask yourself, "What is this question asking?" and "What is the expected response?" If necessary, rephrase the question in your own words. Do not read meaning into a question that is not intended, and do not make a question more difficult than it is. If you do not understand the question, try to figure it out. If, for example, the question is asking about the fluid balance needs of a client with pheochromocytoma and you do not remember what pheochromocytoma is, then try to answer the question based on your knowledge of principles of fluid balance. The exam questions reflect national nursing practice standards and are not written to test knowledge of procedures or practices at specific health care agencies. Thus, it is important to answer the question from the framework of best nursing practice, not unique practices.

■ Determine if the question is asking you to set priorities or place steps of a procedure in a particular order. Read the stem of the question carefully and be clear about the priority (first, last) or order (first, last) in which you are to answer the question.

■ Look for key words that provide clues to the correct answer. For instance, words such as "except," "not," and "but" can change the meaning of a question; words such as "first," "next," and "most" ask you to establish a priority or use an order or sequence of steps. When the question asks you to select all that apply, be sure you are considering each option as having the possibility of being correct.

■ Be certain you understand the meaning of all words in the question. If you see a word you do not know, try to figure out its meaning from a familiar base of the word or from the context of the question.

■ Attempt to answer the question before you see the answers, then look for the answer(s) that is/are similar to the one(s) you generated.

■ Base answers on nursing knowledge. Remember that the NCLEX-RN is used to test for safe practice and that you have learned the information needed to answer the question.

■ If you do not know an answer, make a reasonable guess. Hunches and intuition are often correct. Do not waste time and energy; give yourself permission to not know every question, and move on to the next one. In CAT, you must answer each question before the next item is administered, and because the level of difficulty will be adjusted as you answer each question, it is likely that you will know the answer to one of the next questions.

Strategies for Managing Test Anxiety

All test takers experience some anxiety. A certain amount of anxiety is motivating, but be prepared to control unwanted anxiety. Anxiety can be managed by both physical and mental activities. Practice anxiety management strategies while you are taking the comprehensive examinations in this book, and use them with *each* exam you take in school or elsewhere. Practicing managing test anxiety when taking "low stakes" tests, such as classroom tests, will make managing test anxiety much easier when you are taking the "high stakes" tests such as course or program final exams and, of course, the licensing exam. Commonly used anxiety management strategies include:

■ *Mental rehearsal*—Mental rehearsal involves reviewing the events and environment during the examination. Anticipate how you will feel, what the setting will be like, how you will take the exam, what the computer screen will look like, and how you will talk to yourself during the exam. Visualize your success. Rehearse what you will do if you have test anxiety.

■ *Relaxation exercises*—Relaxation exercises involve tensing and relaxing various muscle groups to relieve the physical effects of anxiety. Practice systematically contracting and relaxing muscle groups from your toes to your neck to release energy for concentration. You can do these exercises during the exam to promote relaxation. Smile! Smiling relaxes tense facial muscles and reminds you to maintain a positive attitude.

■ *Deep breathing*—Taking deep breaths by inhaling slowly while counting to 5 and then exhaling slowly while counting to 10 increases oxygen flow to the lungs and brain. Deep breathing also decreases tension and helps manage anxiety by focusing your thoughts on the breathing and away from worries.

■ *Positive self-talk*—Talking to yourself in a positive way serves to correct negative thoughts (e.g., "I can't pass this test" and "I don't know the answers to any of these questions") and reinforces a positive self-concept. Replace negative thoughts with positive ones, for example, tell yourself, "I can do this," "I studied well and am prepared," or "I can figure this out."

■ *Distraction*—Thinking about something else can clear your mind of negative or unwanted thoughts. Think of something fun, something you enjoy. Plan now what you will think about to distract yourself during the exam.

■ *Concentration*—During the exam, be prepared to concentrate. Have tunnel vision. Do not worry if others finish the test before you. Remember that everyone has his or her own speed for taking tests and that each test is individualized. Do not rush; you will have plenty of time. Focus; do not let noises from the keyboard next to you divert your attention. Do not become overwhelmed by the testing environment. Use positive self-talk as you begin the exam. Some students become bored during the exam and then become careless as they answer questions toward the end of the exam. Practice taking tests of at least 265 questions and discover how long you can focus your attention on the test questions. Practice taking breaks if you begin to lose your concentration.

Evaluating Your Progress

The last step of your study plan is to check your progress. Note if your scores on the practice and comprehensive tests improve. Do not spend time on content you have mastered, on areas in which you obtained high scores on the practice exam, or on areas with which you feel confident. Use the results of your evaluation to set priorities for study on areas needing additional review. As noted above, evaluate your study skills, your test taking abilities, and the use of test-anxiety management strategies as you take *each* test throughout your academic program. Doing so now will prepare you to test for success.

Tips from Students Who Have Passed the NCLEX-RN

Students who have successfully passed the NCLEX-RN offer these tips for preparing for and taking this exam:

■ Study regularly several months before taking the exam. Be sure you are well prepared. Accept responsibility for your study plan—being prepared is up to you!

■ Practice taking randomly generated test questions. Most students are accustomed to taking teacher-made exams that cover several topics in the same content area. When taking the NCLEX-RN examination, however, each question will come from a different topic or content area, and you will need to be prepared to shift your focus to a different practice area for each question.

■ Use practice questions until you can score at least 75% on the exam. Use practice exams with at least 2,000 questions so you test yourself with a wide range of content and types of questions.

■ Use a timer to determine how many questions you can answer in a specified amount of time. Use the timer to be sure you are keeping a steady pace, but not rushing through the test.

■ Schedule to take the exam when YOU are ready but as soon after graduation as is feasible.[3] Candidates who take the exam before they are prepared are not as successful. You are in control of when you take the exam!

■ Make sure you know the date, time, and place the exam will be given; how to get to the exam site; how long it takes to drive there; and where you can park. It may be helpful to visit the exam site and see the room where the exam will be given.

■ Visualize yourself in the room taking the test. Use mental rehearsal to practice anxiety-managing strategies.

■ Organize the information you will need to bring to the testing center the night before the exam. You will need to present your Authorization to Test. You will also need to provide required identification.

■ Make sure you are physically prepared. Get enough rest before the examination; fatigue can impair concentration. If you work, it may be advisable not to work the day before the exam; if you work on a shift that is different from the time of the exam, adjust your work schedule several days ahead of time.

■ Avoid planning time-consuming activities (e.g., weddings, vacation trips) immediately before the exam.

■ Do not use any drugs you usually do not use (including caffeine and nicotine), and do not use alcohol for 2 days before the exam.

■ Eat regular meals before the exam. Remember that high-carbohydrate foods provide energy, but excessive sugar and caffeine can cause hyperactivity.

■ Dress comfortably, in layers that can be added or removed according to your comfort level.

The authors of this review book and CD-ROM offer you our best wishes for success on all of the exams you will be taking throughout your academic career. We are confident that your review and preparation have given you a good foundation for a positive testing experience!

References

1. Wendt, A., & O'Neill, T. (2006). *Report of Findings from the 2005 RN Practice Analysis: Linking the NCLEX-RN to Examination and Practice.* Chicago, IL: National Council of State Boards of Nursing.
2. National Council of State Boards of Nursing. *www.ncsbn.org*
3. National Council of State Boards of Nursing. (2002). *The NCLEX Delay Pass Rate Study.* Retrieved January 5, 2007, from www.ncsbn.org/pdfs/recentNCLEX Research_web_testing017B02.pdf

Practice Tests

1

The Nursing Care of the Childbearing Family

The Preconception Client

1. An antenatal G 2, T 1, P 0, Ab 0, L 1 client is discussing her postpartum plans for birth control with her health care provider. In analyzing the available choices, which of the following factors has the greatest impact on her birth control options?
- [ ] **1.** Satisfaction with prior methods.
- [ ] **2.** Preference of sexual partner.
- [ ] **3.** Breast- or bottle-feeding plan.
- [ ] **4.** History of clotting disease.

2. After the nurse instructs a 20-year-old nulligravid client on how to perform a breast self-examination, which of the following client statements indicates that the teaching has been successful?
- [ ] **1.** "I should perform breast self-examination on the day my menstrual flow begins."
- [ ] **2.** "It's important that I perform breast self-examination on the same day each month."
- [ ] **3.** "If I notice that one of my breasts is much smaller than the other, I shouldn't worry."
- [ ] **4.** "If there is discharge from my nipples, I should call my health care provider."

3. Assessment of a 16-year-old nulligravid client who visits the clinic and asks for information on contraceptives reveals a menstrual cycle of 28 days. The nurse formulates a nursing diagnosis of *Deficient knowledge* related to ovulation and fertility management. Which of the following would be important to include in the teaching plan for the client?
- [ ] **1.** The ovum survives for 96 hours after ovulation, making conception possible during this time.
- [ ] **2.** The basal body temperature falls at least 0.2° F after ovulation has occurred.
- [ ] **3.** Ovulation usually occurs on day 14, plus or minus 2 days, before the onset of the next menstrual cycle.
- [ ] **4.** Most women can tell they have ovulated because of severe pain and thick, scant cervical mucus.

4. Which of the following instructions about activities during menstruation would the nurse include when counseling an adolescent who has just begun to menstruate?
- [ ] **1.** Take a mild analgesic if needed for menstrual pain.
- [ ] **2.** Avoid cold foods if menstrual pain persists.
- [ ] **3.** Stop exercise while menstruating.
- [ ] **4.** Avoid sexual intercourse while menstruating.

5. After conducting a class for female adolescents about human reproduction, which of the following statements indicates that the school nurse's teaching has been effective?

☐ **1.** "Under ideal conditions, sperm can reach the ovum in 15 to 30 minutes, resulting in pregnancy."

☐ **2.** "I won't become pregnant if I abstain from intercourse during the last 14 days of my menstrual cycle."

☐ **3.** "Sperm from a healthy male usually remain viable in the female reproductive tract for 96 hours."

☐ **4.** "After an ovum is fertilized by a sperm, the ovum then contains 21 pairs of chromosomes."

6. A 20-year-old nulligravid client expresses a desire to learn more about the symptothermal method of family planning. Which of the following would the nurse include in the teaching plan?

☐ **1.** This method has a 50% failure rate during the first year of use.

☐ **2.** Couples must abstain from coitus for 5 days after the menses.

☐ **3.** Cervical mucus is carefully monitored for changes.

☐ **4.** The male partner uses condoms for significant effectiveness.

7. Before advising a 24-year-old client desiring oral contraceptives for family planning, the nurse would assess the client for signs and symptoms of which of the following?

☐ **1.** Anemia.

☐ **2.** Hypertension.

☐ **3.** Dysmenorrhea.

☐ **4.** Acne vulgaris.

8. After instructing a 20-year-old nulligravid client about adverse effects of oral contraceptives, the nurse determines that further instruction is needed when the client states which of the following as an adverse effect?

☐ **1.** Weight gain.

☐ **2.** Nausea.

☐ **3.** Headache.

☐ **4.** Ovarian cancer.

9. While discussing reproductive health with a group of female adolescents, one of the adolescents asks the nurse, "Where is the ovum fertilized?" The nurse responds by stating that fertilization normally occurs at which of the following sites?

☐ **1.** Uterus.

☐ **2.** Vagina.

☐ **3.** Fallopian tube.

☐ **4.** Cervix.

10. A 22-year-old nulligravid client tells the nurse that she and her husband have been considering using condoms for family planning. Which of the following instructions would the nurse include about the use of condoms as a method for family planning?

☐ **1.** Using a spermicide with the condom offers added protection against pregnancy.

☐ **2.** Natural skin condoms protect against sexually transmitted diseases.

☐ **3.** The typical failure rate for couples using condoms is about 25%.

☐ **4.** Condom users commonly report penile gland sensitivity.

11. Which of the following would the nurse include in the teaching plan for a 32-year-old female client requesting information about using a diaphragm for family planning?

☐ **1.** Douching with an acidic solution after intercourse is recommended.

☐ **2.** Diaphragms should not be used if the client develops acute cervicitis.

☐ **3.** The diaphragm should be washed in a weak solution of bleach and water.

☐ **4.** The diaphragm should be left in place for 2 hours after intercourse.

12. After being examined and fitted for a diaphragm, a 24-year-old client receives instructions about its use. Which of the following client statements indicates a need for further teaching?

☐ **1.** "I can continue to use the diaphragm for about 2 to 3 years if I keep it protected in the case."

☐ **2.** "If I get pregnant, I will have to be refitted for another diaphragm after the delivery."

☐ **3.** "Before inserting the diaphragm I should coat the rim with contraceptive jelly."

☐ **4.** "If I gain or lose 20 lb, I can still use the same diaphragm."

13. A 22-year-old client tells the nurse that she and her husband are trying to conceive a baby. When teaching the client about reducing the incidence of neural tube defects in newborns, the nurse would emphasize the need for intake of which of the following nutrients?

☐ **1.** Iron.

☐ **2.** Folic acid.

☐ **3.** Calcium.

☐ **4.** Magnesium.

14. When describing a vasectomy to a couple inquiring about this procedure, the nurse would explain that which of the following is clamped or excised?

☐ **1.** Ejaculatory duct.

☐ **2.** Seminiferous tubules.

☐ **3.** Seminal vesicles.

☐ **4.** Vas deferens.

15. A 39-year-old multigravid client asks the nurse for information about female sterilization with a tubal ligation. Which of the following client statements indicates effective teaching?
- ☐ **1.** "My fallopian tubes will be tied off through a small abdominal incision."
- ☐ **2.** "Reversal of a tubal ligation is easily done, with a pregnancy success rate of 80%."
- ☐ **3.** "After this procedure, I must abstain from intercourse for at least 3 weeks."
- ☐ **4.** "Both of my ovaries will be removed during the tubal ligation procedure."

16. When discussing sexual arousal and orgasm with a 25-year-old nulliparous client, which of the following would the nurse include as the primary anatomic female structure involved?
- ☐ **1.** Vaginal wall.
- ☐ **2.** Clitoris.
- ☐ **3.** Mons pubis.
- ☐ **4.** Vulvovaginal glands.

17. A 23-year-old nulliparous client visiting the clinic for a routine examination tells the nurse that she desires to use the basal body temperature method for family planning. The nurse should instruct the client to do which of the following?
- ☐ **1.** Check the cervical mucus to see if it is thick and sparse.
- ☐ **2.** Take her temperature at the same time every morning before getting out of bed.
- ☐ **3.** Document ovulation when her temperature decreases at least 1° F.
- ☐ **4.** Avoid coitus for 10 days after a slight rise in temperature.

18. A couple visiting the infertility clinic for the first time asks the nurse, "What causes infertility in a woman?" Which of the following would the nurse include in the response as one of the most common factors?
- ☐ **1.** Absence of an ovary.
- ☐ **2.** Overproduction of prolactin.
- ☐ **3.** Anovulation.
- ☐ **4.** Immunologic factors.

19. A couple visiting the infertility clinic for the first time states that they have been trying to conceive for the past 2 years without success. After a history and physical examination of both partners, the nurse determines that an appropriate outcome for the couple would be to accomplish which of the following by the end of this visit?
- ☐ **1.** Choose an appropriate infertility treatment method.
- ☐ **2.** Acknowledge that only 50% of infertile couples achieve a pregnancy.
- ☐ **3.** Discuss alternative methods of having a family, such as adoption.
- ☐ **4.** Describe each of the potential causes and possible treatment modalities.

20. A client is scheduled to have in vitro fertilization (IVF) as an infertility treatment. Which of the following client statements about IVF indicates that the client understands this procedure?
- ☐ **1.** "IVF requires supplemental estrogen to enhance the implantation process."
- ☐ **2.** "The pregnancy rate with IVF is higher than that with gamete intrafallopian transfer."
- ☐ **3.** "IVF involves bypassing the blocked or absent fallopian tubes."
- ☐ **4.** "Both ova and sperm are instilled into the open end of a fallopian tube."

21. A 20-year-old primigravid client tells the nurse that her mother had a friend who died from hemorrhage about 10 years ago during a vaginal delivery. Which of the following responses would be most helpful?
- ☐ **1.** "Today's modern technology has resulted in a low maternal mortality rate."
- ☐ **2.** "Don't concern yourself with things that happened in the past."
- ☐ **3.** "In the United States, mothers seldom die in childbirth."
- ☐ **4.** "What is it that concerns you about pregnancy, labor, and delivery?"

22. A 19-year-old nulligravid client visiting the clinic for a routine examination asks the nurse about cervical mucus changes that occur during the menstrual cycle. Which of the following statements would the nurse expect to include in the client's teaching plan?
- ☐ **1.** About midway through the menstrual cycle, cervical mucus is thick and sticky.
- ☐ **2.** During ovulation, the cervix remains dry without any mucus production.
- ☐ **3.** As ovulation approaches, cervical mucus is abundant and clear.
- ☐ **4.** Cervical mucus disappears immediately after ovulation, resuming with menses.

23. When instructing a client about the proper use of condoms for pregnancy prevention, which of the following instructions would be included to ensure maximum effectiveness?
- ☐ **1.** Place the condom over the erect penis before coitus.
- ☐ **2.** Withdraw the condom after coitus when the penis is flaccid.
- ☐ **3.** Ensure that the condom is pulled tightly over the penis before coitus.
- ☐ **4.** Obtain a prescription for a condom with nonoxynol 9.

24. A multigravid client will be using medroxyprogesterone acetate (Depo-Provera) as a family planning method. After the nurse instructs the client about this method, which of the following client statements indicates effective teaching?
- ☐ **1.** "This method of family planning requires monthly injections."
- ☐ **2.** "I should have my first injection during my menstrual cycle."
- ☐ **3.** "One possible adverse effect is absence of a menstrual period."
- ☐ **4.** "This drug will be given by subcutaneous injections."

25. Which of the following instructions should the nurse expect to include in the teaching plan for a 30-year-old multiparous client who will be using an intrauterine device (IUD) for family planning?
- ☐ **1.** Amenorrhea is a common adverse effect of IUDs.
- ☐ **2.** The client needs to use additional protection for conception.
- ☐ **3.** IUDs are more costly than other forms of contraception.
- ☐ **4.** Severe cramping may occur when the IUD is inserted.

26. After counseling a 35-year-old client about breast self-examination and mammography, the nurse determines that the client has understood the instructions when the client states which of the following?
- ☐ **1.** "I should have a mammogram every year once I'm 40."
- ☐ **2.** "I should schedule a mammography examination during my menstrual period."
- ☐ **3.** "Mammography screening is inexpensive."
- ☐ **4.** "Mammography is an extremely painful procedure."

27. After instructing a 40-year-old woman about osteoporosis after menopause, the nurse determines that the client needs further instruction when the client states which of the following?
- ☐ **1.** "One cup of yogurt is the equivalent of one glass of milk."
- ☐ **2.** "Women who do not eat dairy products should consider calcium supplements."
- ☐ **3.** "African American women are at the greatest risk for osteoporosis."
- ☐ **4.** "Estrogen therapy at menopause can reduce the risk of osteoporosis."

28. When developing a teaching plan about sexually transmitted diseases for an 18-year-old female client, which of the following treatments would the nurse need to keep in mind?
- ☐ **1.** Acyclovir (Zovirax) can be used to cure herpes genitalis.
- ☐ **2.** *Chlamydia trachomatis* infections are usually treated with penicillin.
- ☐ **3.** Ceftriaxone sodium (Rocephin) may be used to treat *Neisseria gonorrhoeae* infections.
- ☐ **4.** Metronidazole (Flagyl) is used to treat condylomata acuminata.

29. The physician prescribes raloxifene hydrochloride (Evista) for a 60-year-old woman. The nurse should instruct the client that this drug is useful in preventing which of the following?
- ☐ **1.** Hot flashes.
- ☐ **2.** Osteoporosis.
- ☐ **3.** Hyperglycemia.
- ☐ **4.** Migraine headaches.

30. A couple is visiting the clinic because they have been unable to conceive a baby after 3 years of frequent coitus. After discussing the various causes of male infertility, the nurse determines that the male partner needs further instruction when he states which of the following as a cause?
- ☐ **1.** Seminal fluid with an alkaline pH.
- ☐ **2.** Frequent exposure to heat sources.
- ☐ **3.** Abnormal hormonal stimulation.
- ☐ **4.** Immunologic factors.

31. A 24-year-old woman is being assessed for a malformation of the uterus. The figure below indicates which of the following uterine malformations?
- ☐ **1.** Septate uterus.
- ☐ **2.** Bicornate uterus.
- ☐ **3.** Double uterus.
- ☐ **4.** Uterus didelphys.

The Pregnant Client Receiving Prenatal Care

32. The nurse is reviewing results for clients who are having antenatal testing. The assessment data from which client warrants prompt notification of the provider and a further plan of care?
- [ ] **1.** Primigravida who reports fetal movement 6 times in 2 hours.
- [ ] **2.** Multigravida who had a positive oxytocin challenge test.
- [ ] **3.** Primigravida whose infant has a biophysical profile of 9.
- [ ] **4.** Multigravida whose infant has a reactive nonstress test.

33. A primagravid client at 16 weeks' gestation has had an amniocentesis and has received teaching concerning signs and symptoms to report. Which statement indicates that the client needs further teaching?
- [ ] **1.** "I need to call if I start to leak fluid from my vagina."
- [ ] **2.** "If I start bleeding, I will need to call back."
- [ ] **3.** "If my baby does not move, I need to call my health care provider."
- [ ] **4.** "If I start running a fever, I should let the office know."

34. During a visit to the prenatal clinic, a pregnant client at 32 weeks' gestation complains of heartburn. The nurse knows the client needs further instruction when she says she must do what?
- [ ] **1.** Avoid highly seasoned foods.
- [ ] **2.** Avoid laying down right after eating.
- [ ] **3.** Eat small, frequent meals.
- [ ] **4.** Consume liquids only between meals.

35. The nurse is teaching a new prenatal client about her iron deficiency anemia during pregnancy. Which statement indicates that the client needs further instruction about her anemia?
- [ ] **1.** "I will need to take iron supplements now."
- [ ] **2.** "I may have anemia because my family is of Asian descent."
- [ ] **3.** "I am considered anemic if my hemoglobin is below 11 g/dl."
- [ ] **4.** "The workload on my heart is increased when there is not enough oxygen in my system."

36. Following a positive pregnancy test, a client begins discussing the changes that will occur in the next several months with the nurse. Identify the psychosocial aspect of pregnancy the nurse will incorporate into the plan of care as she educates this client about the changes that occur in the first trimester:
- [ ] **1.** Differentiating the self from the fetus.
- [ ] **2.** Enjoying the role of nurturer.
- [ ] **3.** Preparing for the reality of parenthood.
- [ ] **4.** Experiencing ambivalence about pregnancy.

37. An antenatal primagravid client has just been informed that she is carrying twins. The plan of care includes educating the client concerning factors that put her at risk for problems during the pregnancy. The nurse realizes the client needs further instruction when she indicates carrying twins puts her at risk for which of the following?
- [ ] **1.** Preterm labor.
- [ ] **2.** Twin-to-twin transfusion.
- [ ] **3.** Anemia.
- [ ] **4.** Group B *Streptococcus.*

38. A 30-year-old multigravid client has missed three periods and now visits the prenatal clinic because she assumes she is pregnant. She is experiencing enlargement of her abdomen, a positive pregnancy test, and changes in the pigmentation on her face and abdomen. These assessment findings reflect this woman is experiencing a cluster of which signs of pregnancy?
- [ ] **1.** Positive.
- [ ] **2.** Probable.
- [ ] **3.** Presumptive.
- [ ] **4.** Diagnostic.

39. An antenatal client receives education concerning medications that are safe to use during pregnancy. The nurse evaluates the client's understanding of the instructions and determines that she needs further information when she states which of the following?
- [ ] **1.** "If I am constipated, Milk of Magnesia is okay but mineral oil is not."
- [ ] **2.** "If I have heartburn, it is safe to use Tums, Rolaids, Mylanta, and Maalox."
- [ ] **3.** "I can take Tylenol if I have a headache."
- [ ] **4.** "If I need to have a bowel movement, Ex-Lax is preferred."

40. When preparing a 20-year-old client who reports missing one menstrual period and suspects that she is pregnant for a radioimmunoassay pregnancy test, which of the following would the nurse need to keep in mind about this test?
- [ ] **1.** It has a high degree of accuracy within 1 week after ovulation.
- [ ] **2.** It is identical in nature to an over-the-counter home pregnancy test.
- [ ] **3.** A positive result is considered a presumptive sign of pregnancy.
- [ ] **4.** A urine sample is needed to obtain quicker results.

41. After instructing a female client about the radioimmunoassay pregnancy test, the nurse determines that the client understands the instructions when the client states that which of the following hormones is evaluated by this test?
- [ ] **1.** Prolactin.
- [ ] **2.** Follicle-stimulating hormone.
- [ ] **3.** Luteinizing hormone.
- [ ] **4.** Human chorionic gonadotropin (hCG).

42. Using Nägele's rule for a client whose last normal menstrual period began on May 10, the nurse determines that the client's estimated date of delivery would be which of the following?
☐ **1.** January 13.
☐ **2.** January 17.
☐ **3.** February 13.
☐ **4.** February 17.

43. After instructing a primigravid client about the functions of the placenta, the nurse determines that the client needs additional teaching when she says that which of the following hormones is produced by the placenta?
☐ **1.** Estrogen.
☐ **2.** Progesterone.
☐ **3.** Human chorionic gonadotropin (hCG).
☐ **4.** Testosterone.

44. A client, about 8 weeks pregnant, asks the nurse when she will be able to hear the fetal heartbeat. The nurse should respond by telling the client that the fetal heartbeat can be heard with a Doppler ultrasound device when the gestation is as early as which of the following?
☐ **1.** 4 weeks.
☐ **2.** 8 weeks.
☐ **3.** 15 weeks.
☐ **4.** 18 weeks.

45. A primiparous client at 10 weeks' gestation questions the nurse about the need for an ultrasound. She states "I don't have health insurance and I can't afford it. I feel fine, so why should I have the test?" The nurse should incorporate which statements as the underlying reason for performing the ultrasound now? Select all that apply.
☐ **1.** "We must view the gross anatomy of the fetus."
☐ **2.** "We need to determine gestational age."
☐ **3.** "We want to view the heart beating to determine that the fetus is viable."
☐ **4.** "We must determine fetal position."
☐ **5.** "We must determine that there is a sufficient nutrient supply for the fetus."

46. A 20-year-old married client with a positive pregnancy test states, "Is it really true? I can't believe I'm going to have a baby!" Which of the following responses by the nurse would be most appropriate at this time?
☐ **1.** "Would you like some booklets on the pregnancy experience?"
☐ **2.** "Yes it is true. How does that make you feel?"
☐ **3.** "You should be delighted that you are pregnant."
☐ **4.** "Weren't you and your husband trying to have a baby?"

47. A newly diagnosed pregnant client tells the nurse, "If I'm going to have all of these discomforts, I'm not sure I want to be pregnant!" The nurse interprets the client's statement as an indication of which of the following?
☐ **1.** Fear of pregnancy outcome.
☐ **2.** Rejection of the pregnancy.
☐ **3.** Normal ambivalence.
☐ **4.** Inability to care for the newborn.

48. When caring for a newly diagnosed primigravid client at 10 weeks' gestation who is experiencing breast tenderness, amenorrhea, nausea and vomiting, and urinary frequency, which of the following would the nurse identify as a priority nursing diagnosis?
☐ **1.** *Readiness for enhanced family coping* related to pregnancy confirmation.
☐ **2.** *Ineffective sexuality patterns* related to fear of spontaneous abortion.
☐ **3.** *Compromised family coping* related to the discomforts of pregnancy.
☐ **4.** *Imbalanced nutrition: Less than body requirements* related to increased demands of pregnancy.

49. A client, approximately 11 weeks pregnant, and her husband are seen in the antepartal clinic. The client's husband tells the nurse that he has been experiencing nausea and vomiting and fatigue along with his wife. The nurse interprets these findings as suggesting that the client's husband is experiencing which of the following?
☐ **1.** Ptyalism.
☐ **2.** Mittelschmerz.
☐ **3.** Couvade syndrome.
☐ **4.** Pica.

50. A primigravid client asks the nurse if she can continue to have a glass of wine with dinner during her pregnancy. Which of the following would be the nurse's best response?
☐ **1.** "The effects of alcohol on a fetus during pregnancy are unknown."
☐ **2.** "You should limit your consumption to beer and wine."
☐ **3.** "You should abstain from drinking alcoholic beverages."
☐ **4.** "You may have 1 drink or 2 ounces of alcohol per day."

51. Examination of a primigravid client complaining of increased vaginal secretions since becoming pregnant reveals clear, highly acidic vaginal secretions. The client denies any perineal itching or burning. The nurse interprets these findings as a response related to which of the following?
☐ **1.** A decrease in vaginal glycogen stores.
☐ **2.** Development of a sexually transmitted disease.
☐ **3.** Prevention of expulsion of the cervical mucus plug.
☐ **4.** Control of the growth of pathologic bacteria.

52. When measuring the fundal height of a primigravid client at 20 weeks' gestation, the nurse would anticipate locating the fundal height at which of the following points?
☐ **1.** Halfway between the client's symphysis pubis and umbilicus.
☐ **2.** At about the level of the client's umbilicus.
☐ **3.** Between the client's umbilicus and xiphoid process.
☐ **4.** Near the client's xiphoid process and compressing the diaphragm.

53. A primigravid client visiting the antepartal clinic at 8 weeks' gestation tells the nurse that she wants an amniocentesis because there is a history of hemophilia A in her family. The nurse instructs the client that newer techniques now allow amniocentesis to be performed as early as which of the following?
☐ **1.** 8 weeks' gestation.
☐ **2.** 10 weeks' gestation.
☐ **3.** 12 weeks' gestation.
☐ **4.** 14 weeks' gestation.

54. A 40-year-old gravida 4 client at 10 weeks' gestation and her husband are coming into the clinic to discuss tests that are available during the first or early second trimester to diagnose an abnormality of the fetus. Which of the following tests are appropriate? Select all that apply.
☐ **1.** Electrocardiogram.
☐ **2.** Chorionic villus sampling (CVS).
☐ **3.** Amniocentesis.
☐ **4.** Triple screen.
☐ **5.** External fetal monitoring (EFM).

55. After instructing a primigravid client about desired weight gain during pregnancy, the nurse determines that the teaching has been successful when the client states which of the following?
☐ **1.** "A total weight gain of approximately 20 lb (9 kg) is recommended."
☐ **2.** "A weight gain of 6.6 lb (3 kg) in the second and third trimesters is considered normal."
☐ **3.** "A weight gain of about 12 lb (5.5 kg) every trimester is recommended."
☐ **4.** "Although it varies, a gain of 25 to 35 lb (11.4 to 14.5 kg) is about average."

56. When developing a teaching plan for a client who is 8 weeks pregnant, which of the following foods would the nurse suggest to meet the client's need for increased folic acid?
☐ **1.** Spinach.
☐ **2.** Bananas.
☐ **3.** Seafood.
☐ **4.** Yogurt.

57. The nurse instructs a primigravid client about the importance of sufficient vitamin A in her diet. The nurse knows that the instructions have been effective when the client indicates that she should include which of the following in her diet?
☐ **1.** Buttermilk and cheese.
☐ **2.** Strawberries and cantaloupe.
☐ **3.** Egg yolks and squash.
☐ **4.** Oranges and tomatoes.

58. The nurse is discussing dietary concerns with pregnant teens. Which of the following choices are convenient for teens yet nutritious for both the mother and fetus? Select all that apply.
☐ **1.** Milkshake or yogurt with fresh fruit or granola bar.
☐ **2.** Chicken nuggets with tater tots.
☐ **3.** Cheese pizza with spinach and mushroom topping.
☐ **4.** Peanut butter with crackers and a juice drink.
☐ **5.** Buttery light popcorn with diet cola.
☐ **6.** Cheeseburger with tomato, lettuce, pickle, ketchup, and baked potato.

59. When developing a meal-planning guide about foods rich in riboflavin for a primigravid client, the nurse would expect to instruct the client to include at least two daily servings of which of the following foods?
☐ **1.** Fresh fruit.
☐ **2.** Prunes.
☐ **3.** Potatoes.
☐ **4.** Enriched cereals.

60. The nurse instructs a primigravid client to increase her intake of foods high in magnesium because of its role with which of the following?
☐ **1.** Prevention of demineralization of the mother's bones.
☐ **2.** Synthesis of proteins, nucleic acids, and fats.
☐ **3.** Amino acid metabolism.
☐ **4.** Synthesis of neural pathways in the fetus.

61. When caring for a primigravid client at 9 weeks' gestation who immigrated to the United States from Vietnam 1 year ago, the nurse would assess the client's diet for a deficiency of which of the following?
☐ **1.** Calcium.
☐ **2.** Vitamin E.
☐ **3.** Vitamin C.
☐ **4.** Iodine.

62. Which of the following statements by a primigravid client scheduled for chorionic villi sampling indicates effective teaching about the procedure?
☐ **1.** "A fiberoptic fetoscope will be inserted through a small incision into my uterus."
☐ **2.** "I can't have anything to eat or drink after midnight on the day of the procedure."
☐ **3.** "The procedure involves the insertion of a thin catheter into my uterus."
☐ **4.** "I need to drink 32 to 40 ounces of fluid 1 to 2 hours before the procedure."

63. A 34-year-old multiparous client at 16 weeks' gestation who received regular prenatal care for all of her previous pregnancies tells the nurse that she has already felt the baby move. The nurse interprets this as which of the following?
- ☐ **1.** The possibility that the client is carrying twins.
- ☐ **2.** Unusual because most multiparous clients do not experience quickening until 30 weeks' gestation.
- ☐ **3.** Evidence that the client's estimated date of delivery is probably off by a few weeks.
- ☐ **4.** Normal because multiparous clients can experience quickening between 14 and 20 weeks' gestation.

64. Which diagnostic test would be the most important to have for a primigravid client in the second trimester of her pregnancy?
- ☐ **1.** Culdocentesis to detect abnormalities.
- ☐ **2.** Chorionic villus sampling.
- ☐ **3.** Ultrasound testing.
- ☐ **4.** α-fetoprotein (AFP) testing.

65. When performing Leopold's maneuvers, which of the following would the nurse ask the client to do to ensure optimal comfort and accuracy?
- ☐ **1.** Breathe deeply for 1 minute.
- ☐ **2.** Empty her bladder.
- ☐ **3.** Drink a full glass of water.
- ☐ **4.** Lie on her left side.

66. The nurse performed Leopold's maneuvers and determined that the fetal position is LOA. Identify the area where the nurse would place the Doppler to most easily hear fetal heart sounds.

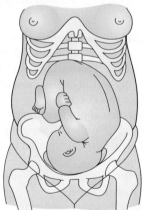

67. The nurse is assessing fetal position for a 32-year-old client in her eighth month of pregnancy. As shown below, the fetal position can be described as which of the following?
- ☐ **1.** Left occipital transverse.
- ☐ **2.** Left occipital anterior.
- ☐ **3.** Right occipital transverse.
- ☐ **4.** Right occipital anterior.

68. Which of the following statements by the nurse would be *most* appropriate when responding to a primigravid client who asks, "What should I do about this brown discoloration across my nose and cheeks?"
- ☐ **1.** "This usually disappears after delivery."
- ☐ **2.** "It is a sign of skin melanoma."
- ☐ **3.** "The discoloration is due to dilated capillaries."
- ☐ **4.** "It will fade if you use a prescribed cream."

69. A 36-year-old primigravid client at 22 weeks' gestation without any complications to date is being seen in the clinic for a routine visit. The nurse expects to assess the client's fundal height for which of the following reasons?
- ☐ **1.** Determining the level of uterine activity.
- ☐ **2.** Identifying the need for increased weight gain.
- ☐ **3.** Assessing the location of the placenta.
- ☐ **4.** Estimating the fetal gestational age.

70. After reviewing the physician's explanation of amniocentesis with a multigravid client, which of the following, if reported by the client as a primary risk of the procedure, would indicate successful teaching?
- ☐ **1.** Premature rupture of the membranes.
- ☐ **2.** Possible premature labor.
- ☐ **3.** Fetal limb malformations.
- ☐ **4.** Fetal organ malformations.

71. A primigravid client at 28 weeks' gestation tells the nurse that she and her husband wish to drive to visit relatives who live several hundred miles away. Which of the following recommendations by the nurse would be best?
- ☐ **1.** "Try to avoid traveling anywhere in the car during your third trimester."
- ☐ **2.** "Limit the time you spend in the car to a maximum of 4 to 5 hours."
- ☐ **3.** "Taking the trip is okay if you stop every 1 to 2 hours and walk."
- ☐ **4.** "Avoid wearing your seat belt in the car to prevent injury to the fetus."

72. The nurse is teaching a woman who is 18 weeks pregnant about seat belt safety. Identify the area that indicates that the client understands where the lap portion of the seat belt should be placed.

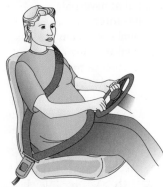

73. Which of the following recommendations would be *most* helpful to suggest to a primigravid client at 37 weeks' gestation who is complaining of leg cramps?
☐ **1.** Change positions frequently throughout the day.
☐ **2.** Alternately flex and extend the legs.
☐ **3.** Straighten the knee and flex the toes toward the chin.
☐ **4.** Lie prone in bed with the legs elevated.

74. Which of the following recommendations would be the *most* appropriate preventive measure to suggest to a primigravid client at 30 weeks' gestation who is experiencing occasional heartburn?
☐ **1.** Eat smaller and more frequent meals during the day.
☐ **2.** Take a pinch of baking soda with water before meals.
☐ **3.** Decrease fluid intake to four glasses daily.
☐ **4.** Drink several cups of regular tea throughout the day.

75. A nurse is eating lunch at a restaurant when she sees a pregnant woman showing signs of airway obstruction. When the nurse asks the woman if she needs help, the woman nods her head yes. Indicate the area where the nurse's fist should be placed to effectively administer thrusts to clear the foreign body from the airway.

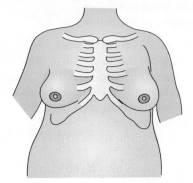

76. When performing Leopold's maneuvers on a primigravid client at 22 weeks' gestation, the nurse performs the first maneuver to do which of the following?
☐ **1.** Locate the fetal back and spine.
☐ **2.** Determine what is in the fundus.
☐ **3.** Determine whether the fetal head is at the pelvic inlet.
☐ **4.** Identify the degree of fetal descent and flexion.

77. A primigravid adolescent client at approximately 15 weeks' gestation who is visiting the prenatal clinic with her mother is to undergo alphafetoprotein (AFP) screening. When developing the teaching plan for this client, the nurse should include which of the following pieces of information?
☐ **1.** Ultrasonography usually accompanies AFP testing.
☐ **2.** Results are usually very accurate until 20 weeks' gestation.
☐ **3.** A clean-catch midstream urine specimen is needed.
☐ **4.** Increased levels of AFP are associated with neural tube defects.

78. Which of the following statements best identifies the rationale for why the nurse reinforces the need for continued prenatal care throughout the pregnancy with an adolescent primigravid client?
☐ **1.** Pregnant adolescents are at high risk for pregnancy-induced hypertension.
☐ **2.** Gestational diabetes during pregnancy commonly develops in adolescents.
☐ **3.** Adolescents need additional instruction related to common discomforts.
☐ **4.** The father of the baby is rarely involved in the pregnancy.

79. An adolescent primigravid client at 20 weeks' gestation weighs 120 lb, having gained only 5 lb since becoming pregnant. She states, "I haven't had any appetite." Which of the following would be the most appropriate nursing diagnosis for this client?
☐ **1.** *Knowledge deficit* about fetal development as evidenced by lack of sufficient weight gain.
☐ **2.** *Noncompliance with diet* related to fear of body image changes.
☐ **3.** *Altered nutrition: Less than body requirements* related to lack of appetite.
☐ **4.** *Chronic low self-esteem* related to poor appetite and decreased weight gain.

80. Which of the following would be included in the teaching plan about pregnancy-related breast changes for a primigravid client?
☐ **1.** Growth of the milk ducts is greatest during the first 8 weeks of gestation.
☐ **2.** Enlargement of the breasts indicates adequate levels of progesterone.
☐ **3.** Colostrum is usually secreted by about the 16th week of gestation.
☐ **4.** Darkening of the areola occurs during the last month of pregnancy.

81. A primigravid client at 32 weeks' gestation is enrolled in a breast-feeding class. Which of the following statements indicate that the client understands the breast-feeding education? Select all that apply.

☐ 1. "My milk supply will be adequate since I have increased a whole bra size during pregnancy."

☐ 2. "I can hold my baby several different ways during feedings."

☐ 3. "If my infant latches on properly, I won't develop mastitis."

☐ 4. "If I breast-feed, my uterus will return to prepregnancy size more quickly."

☐ 5. "Breast milk can be expressed and stored at room temperature since it is natural."

☐ 6. "I need to feed my baby when I see feeding cues and not wait until she is crying."

82. When the nurse is planning a class for primigravid clients about the common discomforts of pregnancy, which of the following physiologic changes of pregnancy would the nurse need to keep in mind?

☐ 1. The temperature decreases slightly early in pregnancy.

☐ 2. Cardiac output increases by 25% to 50% during pregnancy.

☐ 3. The circulating fibrinogen level decreases as much as 50% during pregnancy.

☐ 4. The anterior pituitary gland secretes oxytocin late in pregnancy.

83. When teaching a primigravid client at 24 weeks' gestation about the diagnostic tests to determine fetal well-being, which of the following would the nurse include?

☐ 1. A fetal biophysical profile involves assessments of breathing movements, body movements, tone, amniotic fluid volume, and fetal heart rate reactivity.

☐ 2. A reactive nonstress test is an ominous sign and requires further evaluation with fetal echocardiography.

☐ 3. Contraction stress testing, performed on most pregnant women, can be initiated as early as 16 weeks' gestation.

☐ 4. Percutaneous umbilical blood sampling uses a needle inserted through the vagina to obtain a sample.

84. When teaching a primigravid client how to do Kegel exercises, the nurse explains that the primary purpose of these exercises is to accomplish which of the following?

☐ 1. Prevent vulvar edema.

☐ 2. Alleviate lower back discomfort.

☐ 3. Strengthen the perineal muscles.

☐ 4. Strengthen the abdominal muscles.

85. During a routine clinic visit, a 25-year-old multigravid client who initiated prenatal care at 10 weeks' gestation and is now in her third trimester states, "I've been having strange dreams about the baby. Last week I dreamed he was covered with hair." Which of the following would be the nurse's best response?

☐ 1. "Dreams like the ones that you describe are very unusual. Please tell me more about them."

☐ 2. "Commonly when a mother has these dreams, she is trying to cope with becoming a parent."

☐ 3. "Dreams about the baby late in pregnancy usually mean that labor is about to begin soon."

☐ 4. "It's not uncommon to have dreams about the baby, particularly in the third trimester."

86. A primigravid client at 36 weeks' gestation tells the nurse that she has been experiencing insomnia for the past 2 weeks. Which of the following suggestions would be *most* helpful?

☐ 1. Practice relaxation techniques before bedtime.

☐ 2. Drink a cup of hot chocolate before bedtime.

☐ 3. Drink a small glass of wine with dinner.

☐ 4. Exercise for 30 minutes just before bedtime.

87. Which of the following client statements indicates a need for additional teaching about self-care during pregnancy?

☐ 1. "I should use nonskid pads when I take a shower or bath."

☐ 2. "I should avoid using soap on my nipples to prevent drying."

☐ 3. "I should sit in a hot tub for 20 minutes to relax after working."

☐ 4. "I should avoid douching even if my vaginal secretions increase."

88. To obtain the obstetric conjugate measurement, the nurse practitioner would do which of the following?

☐ 1. Add 1.5 cm to the transverse diameter.

☐ 2. First measure the angle of the pubic arch.

☐ 3. Subtract 1.5 to 2 cm from the diagonal conjugate.

☐ 4. Measure the diameter of the pelvic inlet.

The Pregnant Client in Childbirth Preparation Classes

89. A client asks the nurse why taking folic acid is so important before and during pregnancy. Which of the following would be the nurse's best response?

☐ 1. "Folic acid is important in preventing neural tube defects in newborns and preventing anemia in mothers."

☐ 2. "Eating foods with moderate amounts of folic acid helps regulate blood glucose levels."

☐ 3. "Folic acid consumption helps with the absorption of iron during pregnancy."

☐ 4. "Folic acid is needed to promote blood clotting and collagen formation in the newborn."

90. A client entering the third trimester of her pregnancy is in the office for a routine check-up and teaching, as needed. The nurse should provide anticipatory guidance and discuss which of the following developmental tasks most common to the third trimester? Select all that apply.
- ☐ 1. Differentiating the fetus from the self.
- ☐ 2. Ambivalence concerning pregnancy.
- ☐ 3. Experimenting with mothering roles.
- ☐ 4. Realignment of roles and tasks.
- ☐ 5. Trying various caregiver roles.
- ☐ 6. Concern about labor and delivery.

91. A new antenatal G 6, P 4, Ab 1 client attends her first prenatal visit with her husband. The nurse is evaluating this couple's psychological response to their pregnancy. If they are not adjusting well to the pregnancy, the nurse may see which of the following?
- ☐ 1. The couple are concerned with financial changes this pregnancy causes.
- ☐ 2. The couple expresses ambivalence about the current pregnancy.
- ☐ 3. The father of the baby states that the pregnancy has changed the mother's focus.
- ☐ 4. The father of the baby is irritated that the mother is not like she was before pregnancy.

92. When preparing a prenatal class about endocrine changes that normally occur during pregnancy, which of the following subjects would be included?
- ☐ 1. Human placental lactogen maintains the corpus luteum.
- ☐ 2. Progesterone is responsible for hyperpigmentation and vascular skin changes.
- ☐ 3. Estrogen relaxes smooth muscle in the respiratory tract.
- ☐ 4. The thyroid enlarges with an increase in basal metabolic rate.

93. When developing a series of parent classes on fetal development, which of the following would the nurse include as being developed by the end of the third month (9 to 12 weeks)?
- ☐ 1. External genitalia.
- ☐ 2. Myelinization of nerves.
- ☐ 3. Brown fat stores.
- ☐ 4. Air ducts and alveoli.

94. A primigravid client attending parenthood classes tells the nurse that there is a history of twins in her family. What should the nurse tell the client?
- ☐ 1. Monozygotic twins result from fertilization of two ova by different sperm.
- ☐ 2. Monozygotic twins occur by chance regardless of race or heredity.
- ☐ 3. Dizygotic twins are usually of the same sex.
- ☐ 4. Dizygotic twins occur more often in primigravid than in multigravid clients.

95. During a 2-hour childbirth preparation class focusing on the labor and delivery process for primigravid clients, the nurse is describing the maneuvers that the fetus goes through during the labor process when the head is the presenting part. In which order do these maneuvers occur?

| 1. Engagement |
| 2. Flexion |
| 3. Descent |
| 4. Internal rotation |
| |
| |
| |
| |

96. A primigravid client in a Preparation for Parenting class asks how much blood is lost during an uncomplicated delivery. Which of the following would be the nurse's best response?
- ☐ 1. "The maximum blood loss considered within normal limits is 500 ml."
- ☐ 2. "The minimum blood loss considered within normal limits is 1,000 ml."
- ☐ 3. "Blood loss during a delivery is rarely estimated unless there is a hemorrhage."
- ☐ 4. "It would be very unusual if you lost more than 100 ml of blood during the delivery."

97. Which of the following statements by a primigravid client about the amniotic fluid and sac indicates the need for *further* teaching?
- ☐ 1. "The amniotic fluid helps to dilate the cervix once labor begins."
- ☐ 2. "Fetal nutrients are provided by the amniotic fluid."
- ☐ 3. "Amniotic fluid provides a cushion against impact of the maternal abdomen."
- ☐ 4. "The fetus is kept at a stable temperature by the amniotic fluid and sac."

98. During a childbirth preparation class, a primigravid client at 36 weeks' gestation tells the nurse, "My lower back has really been bothering me lately." Which of the following exercises suggested by the nurse would be most helpful?
- ☐ 1. Pelvic rocking.
- ☐ 2. Deep breathing.
- ☐ 3. Tailor sitting.
- ☐ 4. Squatting.

99. A client is experiencing pain during the first stage of labor. What should the nurse instruct the client to do to manage her pain? Select all that apply.
☐ **1.** Walk in the hospital room.
☐ **2.** Use slow chest breathing.
☐ **3.** Request pain medication on a regular basis.
☐ **4.** Lightly massage her abdomen.
☐ **5.** Sip ice water.

100. During a Preparation for Parenting class, one of the participants asks the nurse, "How will I know if I am really in labor?" Which of the following statements about true labor contractions would be the nurse's best response?
☐ **1.** "Walking around helps to decrease true contractions."
☐ **2.** "True labor contractions may disappear with ambulation, rest, or sleep."
☐ **3.** "The duration and frequency of true labor contractions remain the same."
☐ **4.** "True labor contractions are felt first in the lower back, then the abdomen."

101. After instructing participants in a childbirth education class about methods for coping with discomforts in the first stage of labor, the nurse determines that one of the pregnant clients needs further instruction when she says that she has been practicing which of the following?
☐ **1.** Biofeedback.
☐ **2.** Effleurage.
☐ **3.** Guided imagery.
☐ **4.** Pelvic tilt exercises.

102. After a Preparation for Parenting class session, a pregnant client tells the nurse that she has had some yellow-gray frothy vaginal discharge and local itching. The nurse's best action is to advise the client to do which of the following?
☐ **1.** Use an over-the-counter cream for yeast infections.
☐ **2.** Schedule an appointment at the clinic for an examination.
☐ **3.** Administer a vinegar douche under low pressure.
☐ **4.** Prepare for preterm labor and delivery.

103. During childbirth preparation classes for a group of adolescent primigravid clients, one of the clients asks, "How does the baby breathe inside of me?" The nurse responds by explaining fetal circulation, stating that circulation of oxygenated blood from the placenta begins with which of the following?
☐ **1.** Umbilical artery.
☐ **2.** Foramen ovale.
☐ **3.** Ductus arteriosus.
☐ **4.** Umbilical vein.

104. Which of the following instructions would the nurse expect to include in the teaching plan for a group of primigravid clients attending a parenting class about the placenta and the umbilical cord?
☐ **1.** The highest oxygen content is found in the umbilical artery.
☐ **2.** About 10% of umbilical cords have only two vessels.
☐ **3.** The cord normally inserts in the center of the placenta.
☐ **4.** A nuchal cord usually occurs when the cord is abnormally short.

105. The topic of physiologic changes that occur during pregnancy is to be included in a parenting class for primigravid clients who are in their first half of pregnancy. Which of the following would be important for the nurse to include in the teaching plan?
☐ **1.** Decreased plasma volume.
☐ **2.** Increased risk for urinary tract infections.
☐ **3.** Increased peripheral vascular resistance.
☐ **4.** Increased hemoglobin levels.

106. While preparing a childbirth education class for a group of nursing students, the nurse expects to emphasize the need for continued prenatal care and postpartum well-baby care for all clients. Which of the following should be included in the teaching plan?
☐ **1.** The maternal mortality rate has been steadily increasing in the United States during the past 20 years.
☐ **2.** The infant mortality rate is defined as the number of infant deaths before the age of 12 months per 1,000 live births.
☐ **3.** The perinatal mortality rate is the number of deaths among infants younger than 12 months of age per 1,000 live births.
☐ **4.** The neonatal mortality rate is the number of infant deaths before the age of 12 months per 1,000 live births.

The Pregnant Client with Risk Factors

107. A multigravid client at 32 weeks' gestation has experienced hemolytic disease of the newborn in a previous pregnancy. The nurse would prepare the client for frequent antibody titer evaluations obtained from which of the following?
☐ **1.** Placental blood.
☐ **2.** Amniotic fluid.
☐ **3.** Fetal blood.
☐ **4.** Maternal blood.

108. A client with a past medical history of ventricular septal defect repaired in infancy is seen at the prenatal clinic. She is complaining of dyspnea with exertion and being very tired. Her vital signs are 98, 80, 20, BP 116/72. She has + 2 pedal edema and clear breath sounds. As the nurse plans this client's care, which of the following is her cardiac classification according to the New York Heart Association Cardiac Disease classification?

☐ **1.** Class I.
☐ **2.** Class II.
☐ **3.** Class III.
☐ **4.** Class IV.

109. A primigravid client has completed her first prenatal visit and blood work. Her laboratory test for the hepatitis B surface antigen (HBsAg) is positive. What should the nurse anticipate the plan of care for this newborn to include? Select all that apply.

☐ **1.** Hepatitis B immune globulin at birth.
☐ **2.** Series of three hepatitis B vaccinations per recommended schedule.
☐ **3.** Hepatitis B screening when born.
☐ **4.** Isolation of infant during hospitalization.
☐ **5.** Universal precautions for mother and infant.
☐ **6.** Contraindication for breast-feeding because the mother is HBsAg positive.

110. A new antenatal client is being seen for the first time. She has had asthma since she was a child and it is under control when the client takes her medication correctly and consistently. Which of the following client statements concerning asthma during pregnancy indicates the need for further instruction?

☐ **1.** "I need to continue taking my asthma medication as prescribed."
☐ **2.** "It is my goal to prevent or limit asthma attacks."
☐ **3.** "During an asthma attack, oxygen needs continue to be high for mother and fetus."
☐ **4.** "Bronchodilators should be used only when necessary because of the risk they present to the fetus."

111. A nurse is assigned to the obstetrical triage area. When beginning the assignment, the nurse is given a report about four clients waiting to be seen. Place the clients in the order in which the nurse should see them.

1. A primigravid client at 10 weeks' gestation complaining of not feeling well with nausea and vomiting, urinary frequency, and fatigue.

2. A multiparous client at 32 weeks' gestation asking for assistance with finding a new physician.

3. A single mother at 4 months postpartum fearful of shaking her baby when he cries.

4. An antenatal client at 16 weeks' gestation who has occasional sharp pain on her left side radiating from her symphysis to her fundus.

112. An antenatal client at 22 weeks' gestation is seen in the clinic complaining of right upper quadrant pain radiating to her back. She rates the pain as 9 on a scale of 1 to 10 and says that it has occurred 2 times in the last week for about 4 hours at a time. She does not associate the pain with food. Which of the following nursing measures is the highest priority for this client?

☐ **1.** Educate the client concerning changes occurring in the gallbladder as a result of pregnancy.
☐ **2.** Refer the client to her health care provider for evaluation and treatment of the pain.
☐ **3.** Discuss nutritional strategies to decrease the possibility of heartburn.
☐ **4.** Support the client's use of acetaminophen (Tylenol) to relieve pain.

113. A client in the triage area who is at 19 weeks' gestation states that she has not felt her baby move in the past week and no fetal heart tones are found. While evaluating this client, the nurse identifies her as being at the highest risk for developing which problem?

☐ **1.** Abruptio placentae.
☐ **2.** Placenta previa.
☐ **3.** Disseminated intravascular coagulation.
☐ **4.** Threatened abortion.

114. A 40-year-old client at 8 weeks' gestation has a 3-year-old child with Down syndrome. The nurse is discussing amniocentesis and chorionic villus sampling as genetic screening methods for the expected baby. The nurse is confident that her teaching has been understood when the client states which of the following?

☐ **1.** "Each test identifies a different part of the infant's genetic makeup."

☐ **2.** "Chorionic villus sampling can be performed earlier in pregnancy."

☐ **3.** "The test results take the same length of time to be completed."

☐ **4.** "Amniocentesis is a more dangerous procedure for the fetus."

115. After conducting a presentation to a group of adolescent parents on the topic of adolescent pregnancy, the nurse determines that one of the parents needs further instruction when the parent says that adolescents are at greater risk for which of the following?

☐ **1.** Denial of the pregnancy.

☐ **2.** Low-birth-weight infant.

☐ **3.** Cephalopelvic disproportion.

☐ **4.** Congenital anomalies.

116. A dilatation and curettage (D&C) is scheduled for a primigravid client admitted to the hospital at 10 weeks' gestation with abdominal cramping, bright red vaginal spotting, and passage of some of the products of conception. The nurse anticipates that the client will most likely express which of the following feelings?

☐ **1.** Ambivalence.

☐ **2.** Anxiety.

☐ **3.** Fear.

☐ **4.** Guilt.

117. When providing care to the client who has undergone a dilatation and curettage (D&C) after a spontaneous abortion, the nurse administers hydroxyzine (Vistaril) as ordered, primarily for which of the following reasons?

☐ **1.** To counteract nausea.

☐ **2.** To reduce pain.

☐ **3.** To decrease uterine cramping.

☐ **4.** To promote uterine contractility.

118. On entering the room of a client who has undergone a dilatation and curettage (D&C) for a spontaneous abortion, the nurse finds the client crying. Which of the following comments by the nurse would be most appropriate?

☐ **1.** "Are you having a great deal of uterine pain?"

☐ **2.** "Commonly spontaneous abortion means a defective embryo."

☐ **3.** "I'm truly sorry you lost your baby."

☐ **4.** "You should try to get pregnant again as soon as possible."

119. Rho(D) immune globulin (RhoGAM) is ordered for a client before she is discharged after a spontaneous abortion. The nurse understands that the rationale for administration is to prevent which of the following?

☐ **1.** Development of a future Rh-positive fetus.

☐ **2.** An antibody response to Rh-negative blood.

☐ **3.** A future pregnancy resulting in abortion.

☐ **4.** Development of Rh-positive antibodies.

120. A multigravid client who stands for long periods while working in a factory visits the prenatal clinic at 35 weeks' gestation, stating, "The varicose veins in my legs have really been bothering me lately." Which of the following instructions would be helpful?

☐ **1.** Perform slow contraction and relaxation of the feet and ankles twice daily.

☐ **2.** Take frequent rest periods with the legs elevated above the hips.

☐ **3.** Avoid support hose that reach above the leg varicosities.

☐ **4.** Take a leave of absence from your job to avoid prolonged standing.

121. A multigravid client at 36 weeks' gestation has been diagnosed with condylomata acuminata. Which of the following would the nurse include when teaching the client about the disorder and current therapies?

☐ **1.** Cryotherapy may be used to remove the warts.

☐ **2.** Podophyllin solution may be used to decrease the size of the warts.

☐ **3.** A 25% trichloroacetic acid solution can eradicate the disorder.

☐ **4.** Condylomata acuminata has been associated with ovarian cancer.

122. A primigravid client at 8 weeks' gestation tells the nurse that since having had sexual relations with a new partner 2 weeks ago, she has noticed flu-like symptoms, enlarged lymph nodes, and clusters of vesicles on her vagina. The nurse refers the client to a physician because the nurse suspects which of the following sexually transmitted diseases?

☐ **1.** Gonorrhea.

☐ **2.** *Chlamydia trachomatis* infection.

☐ **3.** Syphilis.

☐ **4.** Herpes genitalis.

123. While caring for a 24-year-old primigravid client scheduled for emergency surgery because of a probable ectopic pregnancy, the nurse would expect to do which of the following?

☐ **1.** Witness an informed consent for surgery.

☐ **2.** Assess the client for massive external bleeding.

☐ **3.** Explain that the fallopian tube can be salvaged.

☐ **4.** Monitor the client for uterine contractions.

124. A 30-year-old G 4, P 3 client at 30 weeks' gestation is admitted to the hospital for evaluation. The client has experienced two neonatal deaths because of hemolytic disease of the newborn. An amniocentesis is to be performed to evaluate bilirubin density. The nurse would obtain a specimen container that is which of the following?

☐ **1.** Dark.
☐ **2.** Clear.
☐ **3.** Green.
☐ **4.** Amber.

Correct Answers and Rationales

The letter in parentheses after each rationale identifies the client need addressed in the item, including management of care (M), safety and infection control (S), health promotion and maintenance (H), psychosocial adaptation (P), basic care and comfort (C), pharmacological and parenteral therapies (D), reduction of risk potential (R), and physiological adaptation (A).

The Preconception Client

1. 3. Birth control plans are influenced primarily by whether the mother is breast- or bottle-feeding her infant. The maternal milk supply must be well established prior to the initiation of most hormonal birth control methods. Low dose oral contraceptives would be the exception. Use of estrogen/progesterone based pills and progesterone only pills are commonly initiated from 4 to 6 weeks postpartum because the milk supply is well established by this time. Prior experiences with birth control methods have an impact on the method chosen as does the preferences of the client's partner; however, they are not the most influential factors. A history of blood clots or thrombophlebitis is the second most important factor as several methods will be eliminated because of their potential to place the client at risk for clotting disorders. (D)

2. 4. The nurse determines that the client has understood the instructions when the client says that she will notify her physician if she notices discharge or bleeding because this may be symptomatic of underlying disease. Ideally, breast self-examination should be performed about 1 week after the onset of menses because hormonal influences on breast tissue are at a low ebb at this time. The client should perform breast self-examination on the same day each month only if she has stopped menstruating (as with menopause). The client's breasts should mirror each other. If one breast is significantly larger than the other, or if there is "pitting" of breast tissue, a tumor may be present. (R)

3. 3. For a client with a menstrual cycle of 28 days, ovulation usually occurs on day 14, plus or minus 2 days, before the onset of the next menstrual cycle. Stated another way, the menstrual period begins about 2 weeks after ovulation has occurred. Ovulation does not usually occur during the menses component of the cycle when the uterine lining is being shed. In most women, the ovum survives for about 12 to 24 hours after ovulation, during which time conception is possible. The basal body temperature rises 0.5° to 1.0° F when ovulation occurs. Although some women experience some pelvic discomfort during ovulation (mittelschmerz), severe or unusual pain is rare. After ovulation, the cervical mucus is thin and copious. (H)

4. 1. The nurse should instruct the client to take a mild analgesic, such as ibuprofen, if menstrual pain or "cramps" are present. The client should also eat foods rich in iron and should continue moderate exercise during menstruation, which increases abdominal tone. Avoiding cold foods will not decrease dysmenorrhea. Sexual intercourse is not prohibited during menstruation, but the male partner should wear a condom to prevent exposure to blood. (H)

5. 1. Under ideal conditions, sperm can reach the ovum in 15 to 30 minutes. This is an important point to make with adolescents who may be sexually active. Many people believe that the time interval is much longer and that they can wait until after intercourse to take steps to prevent conception. Without protection, pregnancy and sexually transmitted diseases can occur. When using the abstinence or calendar method, the couple should abstain from intercourse on the days of the menstrual cycle when the woman is most likely to conceive. Using a 28-day cycle as an example, a couple should abstain from coitus 3 to 4 days before ovulation (days 10 through 14) and 3 to 4 days after ovulation (days 15 through 18). Sperm from a healthy male can remain viable for 24 to 72 hours in the female reproductive tract. If the female client ovulates after coitus, there is a possibility that fertilization can occur. Before fertilization, the ovum and sperm each contain 23 chromosomes. After fertilization, the conceptus contains 46 chromosomes unless there is a chromosomal abnormality. (H)

6. 3. The symptothermal method is a natural method of fertility management that depends on knowing when ovulation has occurred. Because regular menstrual cycles can vary by 1 to 2 days in either direction, the symptothermal method requires daily basal body temperature assessments plus close monitoring of cervical mucus changes. The method relies on abstinence during the period of ovulation, which occurs approximately 14 days before the beginning of the next cycle. Abstinence from coitus for 5 days after menses is unnecessary because it is unlikely that ovulation will occur during this time period (days 1 through 10). Typically, the failure rate for this method is between 10% and 20%. Although a condom may increase the effectiveness of this method, most clients who choose natural methods are not interested in chemical or barrier types of family planning. (H)

7. **2.** Before advising a client about oral contraceptives, the nurse needs to assess the client for signs and symptoms of hypertension. Clients who have hypertension, thrombophlebitis, obesity, or a family history of cerebral or cardiovascular accident are poor candidates for oral contraceptives. In addition, women who smoke, are older than 40 years of age, or have a history of pulmonary disease should be advised to use a different method. Iron-deficiency anemia, dysmenorrhea, and acne are not contraindications for the use of oral contraceptives. Iron-deficiency anemia is a common disorder in young women. Oral contraceptives decrease the amount of menstrual flow and thus decrease the amount of iron lost through menses, thereby providing a beneficial effect when used by clients with anemia. Low-dose oral contraceptives to prevent ovulation may be effective in decreasing the severity of dysmenorrhea (painful menstruation). Dysmenorrhea is thought to be caused by the release of prostaglandins in response to tissue destruction during the ischemic phase of the menstrual cycle. Use of oral contraceptives commonly improves facial acne. (R)

8. **4.** The nurse determines that the client needs further instruction when the client says that one of the adverse effects of oral contraceptive use is ovarian cancer. Some studies suggest that ovarian and endometrial cancer are reduced in women using oral contraceptives. Other adverse effects of oral contraceptives include weight gain, nausea, headache, breakthrough bleeding, and monilial infections. The most serious adverse effect is thrombophlebitis. (D)

9. **3.** Fertilization normally occurs in the outer third of the fallopian tube. Although there have been reports of fertilization outside the fallopian tube, this is not a normal occurrence. (H)

10. **1.** The typical failure rate of a condom is approximately 12% to 14%. Adding a spermicide can decrease this potential failure rate because it offers additional protection against pregnancy. Natural skin condoms do not offer the same protection against sexually transmitted diseases caused by viruses as latex condoms do. Unlike latex condoms, natural skin (membrane) condoms do not prevent the passage of viruses. Most condom users report decreased penile gland sensitivity. However, some users do report an increased sensitivity or allergic reaction (such as a rash) to latex, necessitating the use of another method of family planning or a switch to a natural skin condom. (H)

11. **2.** The teaching plan should include a caution that a diaphragm should not be used if the client develops acute cervicitis, possibly aggravated by contact with the rubber of the diaphragm. Some studies have also associated diaphragm use with increased incidence of urinary tract infections. Douching after use of a diaphragm and intercourse is not recommended because pregnancy could occur. The diaphragm should be inspected and washed with mild soap and water after each use. A diaphragm should be left in place for at least 6 hours but no longer than 24 hours after intercourse. More spermicidal jelly or cream should be used if intercourse is repeated during this period. (R)

12. **4.** The client would need additional instructions when she says that she can still use the same diaphragm if she gains or loses 20 lb. Gaining or losing more than 15 lb can change the pelvic and vaginal contours to such a degree that the diaphragm will no longer protect the client against pregnancy. The diaphragm can be used for 2 to 3 years if it is cared for and well protected in its case. The client should be refitted for another diaphragm after pregnancy and delivery of a newborn because weight changes and physiologic changes of pregnancy can alter the pelvic and vaginal contours, thus affecting the effectiveness of the diaphragm. The client should use a spermicidal jelly or cream before inserting the diaphragm. (R)

13. **2.** Folic acid (folate) can reduce the incidence of neural tube defects in newborns. Adequate intake of folic acid is especially important just before conception and during the first 6 weeks after conception. Folic acid supplements may be prescribed, especially after conception occurs. Foods that are rich in folic acid include fruits and green leafy vegetables. Iron, calcium, and magnesium are not associated with reducing the risk for neural tube defects. Iron is necessary to maintain iron stores during pregnancy and postpartum. Calcium is important for bone density of the mother and bone formation in the developing fetus. Magnesium aids in the synthesis of proteins and fats in the mother. It also is important in promoting cell growth in the fetus. Magnesium can be found in dark green leafy vegetables. (R)

14. **4.** In vasectomy, a common procedure for male sterilization, the vas deferens (ductus deferens) is cut and tied. Coagulation may also be used to create an obstruction in the vas deferens and block the passage of sperm. (H)

15. **1.** Tubal ligation, a female sterilization procedure, involves ligation (tying off) or cauterization of the fallopian tubes through a small abdominal incision (laparotomy). Reversal of a tubal ligation is not easily done, and the pregnancy success rate after reversal is about 30%. After a tubal ligation, the client may engage in intercourse 2 to 3 days after the procedure. The ovaries are not generally removed during a tubal ligation. An oophorectomy involves removal of one or both ovaries. (H)

16. **2.** Although the vaginal wall and cervix may be sensitive structures, the primary anatomic female structure involved in sexual arousal is the clitoris. Composed of erectile tissue with a plentiful arterial blood supply, the clitoris is especially sensitive to foreplay, temperature, and movements of the shaft of the penis against its surface. The mons pubis—the round, fleshy prominence over the symphysis pubis—forms the anterior border of the external reproductive organs. Covered with varying amounts of pubic hair, the mons pubis is not associated with sexual arousal. The vulvovaginal glands include the Skene and

Bartholin glands with ducts that lie within the vestibule. These glands provide lubrication for the urethra and vaginal introitus. They are not the primary anatomic organ associated with sexual arousal because they do not contain the highly sensitive erectile tissues of the clitoris. (H)

17. **2.** The basal body temperature method requires that the client take her temperature each morning before getting out of bed, preferably at the same time each day before eating or any other activity. Just before the day of ovulation, the temperature falls by 0.5° F. At the time of ovulation, the temperature rises 0.4° to 0.8° F because of increased progesterone secretion in response to the luteinizing hormone. The temperature remains higher for the rest of the menstrual cycle. The client should keep a diary of about 6 months of menstrual cycles to calculate "safe" days. There is no mucus for the first 3 or 4 days after menses, and then thick, sticky mucus begins to appear. As estrogen increases, the mucus changes to clear, slippery, and stretchy. This condition, termed spinnbarkeit, is present during ovulation. After ovulation, the mucus decreases in amount and becomes thick and sticky again until menses. Because the ovum typically survives about 24 hours and sperm can survive up to 72 hours, couples must avoid coitus when the cervical mucus is copious and for about 3 to 4 days before and after ovulation to avoid a pregnancy. (H)

18. **3.** The most common factor in female infertility is ovarian dysfunction, particularly anovulation. Other common factors include blocked fallopian tubes and cervical factors, such as infection and inflammation. The causes of infertility can be determined in about 80% to 90% of couples investigated, but in about 10% to 20% of the cases no cause can be found. Less common causes include endometriosis, vaginitis, polycystic ovaries, overproduction of prolactin, immunologic factors, inadequate secretion of progesterone, and stenosis of the cervical os (possibly preventing sperm transport). Immunologic factors do play a role in female infertility; however, they are less common than anovulation. Absence of an ovary is an extremely rare cause of infertility. (H)

19. **4.** By the end of the first visit, the couple should be able to identify potential causes and treatment modalities for infertility. If their evaluation shows that a treatment or procedure may help them to conceive, the couple must then decide how to proceed, considering all of the various treatments before selecting one. Treatments can be difficult, painful, or risky. The first visit is not the appropriate time to decide on a treatment plan because the couple needs time to adjust to the diagnosis of infertility, a crisis for most couples. Although the couple may be in a hurry for definitive therapy, a thorough assessment of both partners is necessary before a treatment plan can be initiated. The success rate for achieving a pregnancy depends on both the cause and the effectiveness of the treatment, and in some cases it may be only as high as 30%. The couple may desire information about alternatives to treatment, but insufficient data are available to suggest that a specific treatment modality may not be successful. Suggesting that the couple consider adoption at this time may inappropriately imply that the couple has no other choice. If a specific therapy may result in a pregnancy, the couple should have time to consider their options. After a thorough evaluation, adoption may be considered by the couple as an alternative to the costly, time-consuming, and sometimes painful treatments for infertility. (H)

20. **3.** The client's understanding of the procedure is demonstrated by the statement describing IVF as a technique that involves bypassing the blocked or absent fallopian tubes. The physician removes the ova by laparoscope- or ultrasound-guided transvaginal retrieval and mixes them with prepared sperm from the woman's partner or a donor. Two days later, up to four embryos are returned to the uterus to increase the likelihood of a successful pregnancy. Supplemental progesterone, not estrogen, is given to enhance the implantation process. Gamete intrafallopian transfer (GIFT) and tubal embryo transfer have a higher pregnancy rate than IVF. However, these procedures cannot be used for clients who have blocked or absent fallopian tubes because the fertilized ova are placed into the fallopian tubes, subsequently entering the uterus naturally for implantation. In IVF, fertilization of the ova by the sperm occurs outside the client's body. In GIFT, both ova and sperm are implanted into the fallopian tubes and allowed to fertilize within the woman's body. (R)

21. **4.** The client is verbalizing concerns about death during childbirth, thus providing the nurse with an opportunity to gather additional data. Asking the client about these concerns would be most helpful to determine the client's knowledge base and to provide the nurse with the opportunity to answer any questions and clarify any misconceptions. Although the maternal mortality rate is low in the United States, maternal deaths do occur, even with modern technology. Leading causes of maternal mortality in the United States include embolism, pregnancy-induced hypertension, hemorrhage, ectopic pregnancy, and infection. Telling the client not to concern herself about what has happened in the past is not useful. It only serves to discount the client's concerns and block further therapeutic communication. Also, postponing or ignoring the client's need for a discussion about complications of pregnancy may further increase the client's anxiety. (H)

22. **3.** As ovulation approaches, cervical mucus is abundant and clear, resembling raw egg white. Ovulation generally occurs 14 days (plus or minus 2 days) before the beginning of menses. During the luteal phase of the cycle, which occurs after ovulation, the cervical mucus is thick and sticky, making it difficult for sperm to pass. Changes in the cervical mucus are related to the influences of estrogen and progesterone. Cervical mucus is always present. (H)

23. **1.** To ensure maximum effectiveness, the condom should always be placed over the erect penis before coitus. Some couples find condom use objectionable because foreplay may have to be interrupted to apply the condom.

The penis, covered by the condom, should be withdrawn before the penis becomes flaccid. Otherwise sperm may escape from the condom, providing an opportunity for possible fertilization. Rather than having the condom pulled tightly over the penis before coitus, space should be left at the tip of the penis to allow the condom to hold the sperm. The client does not need a prescription for a condom with nonoxynol 9 because these are sold over the counter. (R)

24. 3. With medroxyprogesterone acetate, irregular menstrual cycles and amenorrhea are common adverse effects. Other adverse effects include weight gain, breakthrough bleeding, headaches, and depression. This method requires deep intramuscular injections every 3 months. The first injection should occur within 5 days after menses. (R)

25. 4. Severe cramping and pain may occur as the device is passed through the internal cervical os. The insertion of the device is generally done when the client is having her menses, because it is unlikely that she is pregnant at that time. Common adverse effects of IUDs are heavy menstrual bleeding and subsequent anemia, not amenorrhea. Uterine infection or ectopic pregnancy may occur. The IUD has an effectiveness rate of 98%. Therefore, additional protection is not necessary to prevent pregnancy. IUDs generally are less costly than other forms of contraception because they do not require additional expense. Only one insertion is necessary, in comparison to daily doses of oral contraceptives or the need for spermicides in conjunction with diaphragm use. (R)

26. 1. The American Cancer Society recommends an annual mammography screening examination for all women after the age of 40. Some high-risk women may begin annual screening at an earlier age. Some women have never had a mammogram because of fear or misconceptions. Mammography should be scheduled after the client's menses to reduce complaints of breast tenderness. Mammography screening is considered expensive, especially by low-income women. Although some discomfort is common because the breast is placed between two plates during the screening process, the procedure should not be considered extremely painful. (H)

27. 3. Small-boned, fair-skinned women of northern European descent are at the greatest risk for osteoporosis, not African American women. One cup of yogurt or 1.5 oz of hard cheese is the equivalent of one glass of milk. Women who do not eat dairy products, such as women who are lactose intolerant, should consider using calcium supplements. Inadequate lifetime intake of calcium is a major risk factor for osteoporosis. Estrogen therapy, or some of the newer medications that are not estrogen based, can greatly reduce the incidence of osteoporosis. (R)

28. 3. Ceftriaxone sodium (Rocephin) may be used to treat *Neisseria gonorrhoeae* infections and is commonly combined with doxycycline hyclate (Vibramycin). Both the client and her partner should be treated if gonorrhea is present. Acyclovir (Zovirax) can be used to treat herpes genitalis; however, the drug does not cure the disease. *Chlamydia trachomatis* infections are usually treated with antibiotics such as doxycycline or azithromycin (Zithromax). Metronidazole (Flagyl) is used to treat trichomoniasis vaginalis, not condylomata acuminata (genital warts). (D)

29. 2. Raloxifene hydrochloride (Evista), an estrogen receptor modulator, increases bone mineral density without stimulating the endometrium. The drug is useful in preventing osteoporosis in postmenopausal women. This drug is contraindicated for women who smoke cigarettes or who have a history of venous thrombosis. Raloxifene does not prevent hot flashes, hyperglycemia, or migraine headaches. One of its adverse effects is increased headaches. (R)

30. 1. The client needs further instruction when he says that one cause of male infertility is decreased sperm count due to seminal fluid that has an alkaline pH. A slightly alkaline pH is necessary to protect the sperm from the acidic secretions of the vagina and is a normal finding. An alkaline pH is not associated with decreased sperm count. However, seminal fluid that is abnormal in amount, consistency, or chemical composition suggests obstruction, inflammation, or infection, which can decrease sperm production. The typical number of sperm produced during ejaculation is 400 million. Frequent exposure to heat sources, such as saunas and hot tubs, can decrease sperm production, as can abnormal hormonal stimulation. Immunologic factors produced by the man against his own sperm (autoantibodies) or by the woman can cause the sperm to clump or be unable to penetrate the ovum, thus contributing to infertility. (H)

31. 2. A bicornate uterus has a "Y" shape and appears to be a double uterus but in fact has only one cervix. A septate uterus contains a septum that extends from the fundus to the cervix, thus dividing the uterus into two separate compartments. A double uterus has two uteri, each of which has a cervix. A uterus didelphys occurs when both uteri of a double uterus are fully formed. (A)

The Pregnant Client Receiving Prenatal Care

32. 2. Late decelerations during an oxytocin challenge test indicate that the infant is not receiving enough oxygen during contractions and is exhibiting signs of uteroplacental insufficiency. This client would need further medical intervention. Fetal movement 6 times in 2 hours is adequate in a healthy fetus and a biophysical profile of 9 indicates that the risk of fetal asphyxia is rare. A reactive nonstress test informs the health care provider that the fetus has 2 fetal heart rate accelerations of 15 beats per minute above baseline and lasting for 15 seconds within a 20-minute period, which is a reassuring result and an indication of fetal well-being. (M)

33. **3.** At 16 weeks' gestation, a primipara will not feel the baby moving. Quickening occurs between 18 and 20 weeks' gestation for a primipara and between 16 and 18 weeks' gestation for a multipara. Leaking fluid from the vagina should not occur until labor begins and may indicate a rupture of the membranes. Bleeding and a fever are complications that warrant further evaluation and should be reported at any time during the pregnancy. (H)

34. **4.** Consuming most liquids between meals rather than at the same time as eating is an excellent strategy to deter nausea and vomiting in pregnancy but does not relieve heartburn. During the third trimester, progesterone causes relaxation of the sphincter and the pressure of the fetus against the stomach increases the potential of heartburn. Avoiding highly seasoned foods, remaining in an upright position after eating, and eating small, frequent meals are strategies to prevent heartburn. (A)

35. **2.** Iron deficiency anemia is caused by insufficient iron stores in the body, poor iron content in the diet of the pregnant woman, or both. Other thalassemias and sickle cell anemia, rather than iron deficiency anemia, can be associated with ethnicity but occur primarily in clients of African American or Mediterranean origin. Because red blood cells increase by about 50% during pregnancy, many clients will need to take supplemental iron to avoid iron deficiency anemia. A pregnant client is considered anemic when the hemoglobin is below 11 mg/dl. In most types of anemia, the heart must pump more often and harder to deliver oxygen to cells. (R)

36. **4.** Many women in their first trimester feel ambivalent about being pregnant because of the significant life changes that occur for most women who have a child. Ambivalence can be expressed as a list of positive and negative consequences of having a child, consideration of financial and social implications, and possible career changes. During the second trimester, the infant becomes a separate individual to the mother. The mother will begin to enjoy the role of nurturer postpartum. During the third trimester, the mother begins to prepare for parenthood and all of the tasks that parenthood includes. (H)

37. **4.** Group B *Streptococcus* is a risk factor for all pregnant women and is not limited to those carrying twins. The multiple gestation client is at risk for preterm labor because uterine distention, a major factor initiating preterm labor, is more likely with a twin gestation. The normal uterus is only able to distend to a certain point and when that point is reached, labor may be initiated. Twin-to-twin transfusion drains blood from one twin to the second and is a problem that may occur with multiple gestation. The donor twin may become growth restricted and can have oligohydramnios while the recipient twin may become polycythemic with polyhydramnios and develop heart failure. Anemia is a common problem with multiple gestation clients. The mother is commonly unable to consume enough protein, calcium, and iron to supply her needs and those of the fetuses. A maternal hemoglobin level below 11 g/dl is considered anemic. (A)

38. **2.** The plan of care should reflect that this woman is experiencing probable signs of pregnancy. She may be pregnant but the signs and symptoms may have another etiology. An enlarging abdomen and a positive pregnancy test may also be caused by tumors, hydatidiform mole, or other disease processes as well as pregnancy. Changes in the pigmentation of the face may also be caused by oral contraceptive use. Positive signs of pregnancy are considered diagnostic and include evident fetal heartbeat, fetal movement felt by a trained examiner, and visualization of the fetus with ultrasound confirmation. Presumptive signs are subjective and can have another etiology. These signs and symptoms include lack of menses, nausea, vomiting, fatigue, urinary frequency, and breast changes. The word "diagnostic" is not used to describe the condition of pregnancy. (A)

39. **4.** Ex-Lax is considered too abrasive to use during pregnancy. In most instances, a Fleet enema will be given before Ex-Lax. Medications for constipation that are considered safe during pregnancy include compounds that produce bulk, such as Metamucil and Citrucel. Colace, Dulcolax, and Milk of Magnesia can also be used. Mineral oil prevents the absorption of vitamins and minerals within the GI tract. The strategies for heartburn are considered safe and Tylenol may be used as an over-the-counter analgesic. (D)

40. **1.** The radioimmunoassay pregnancy test, which uses an antiserum with specificity for the b-subunit of human chorionic gonadotrophin (hCG) in blood plasma, is highly accurate within 1 week after ovulation. The test is performed in a laboratory. Over-the-counter or home pregnancy tests are performed on urine and use the hemagglutination inhibition method. Radioimmunoassay tests usually use blood serum. A positive pregnancy test is considered a probable sign of pregnancy. Certain conditions other than pregnancy, such as choriocarcinoma, can cause increased hCG levels. (R)

41. **4.** The hormone analyzed in most pregnancy tests is hCG. In the pregnant woman, trace amounts of hCG appear in the serum as early as 24 to 48 hours after implantation owing to the trophoblast production of this hormone. Prolactin, follicle-stimulating hormone, and luteinizing hormone are not used to detect pregnancy. Prolactin is the hormone secreted by the pituitary gland to prepare the breasts for lactation. Follicle-stimulating hormone is involved in follicle maturation during the menstrual cycle. Luteinizing hormone is responsible for stimulating ovulation. (R)

42. **4.** When using Nägele's rule to determine the estimated date of delivery, the nurse would count back 3 calendar months from the first day of the last menstrual period and add 7 days. This means the client's estimated date of delivery is February 17. (H)

43. **4.** The placenta does not produce testosterone. Human placental lactogen, hCG, estrogen, and progesterone are hormones produced by the placenta during pregnancy. The hormone hCG stimulates the synthesis of estrogen and progesterone early in the pregnancy until the placenta can assume this role. Estrogen results in uterine and breast enlargement. Progesterone aids in maintaining the endometrium, inhibiting uterine contractility, and developing the breasts for lactation. The placenta also produces some nutrients for the embryo and exchanges oxygen, nutrients, and waste products through the chorionic villi. (H)

44. **2.** With a Doppler ultrasound device, the fetal heartbeat can be heard as early as 8 weeks' gestation. With a fetoscope, the fetal heartbeat can be heard between 17 and 20 weeks' gestation. (H)

45. **1, 2.** Although ultrasounds are not considered part of routine care, the ultrasound is able to confirm the pregnancy, identify the major anatomic features of the fetus and possible abnormalities, and determine the gestational age by measuring crown-to-rump length of the embryo during the first trimester. At this time, the ultrasound cannot confirm the fetus is viable. The ultrasound will provide information about fetal position; however, this information would be more important later in the pregnancy, not during the first trimester. The ultrasound would provide no information about nutrient supply for the fetus. (H)

46. **2.** This client is expressing a feeling of surprise about having a baby. Therefore, the nurse's best response would be to confirm the pregnancy, which is something that the client already suspects, and then ascertain how the client is feeling now that the suspicion is confirmed. Studies have shown that a common reaction to pregnancy is summarized as ambivalence or "someday, but not now." Such feelings are normal and are experienced by many women early in pregnancy. Offering a pamphlet on pregnancy does not respond to the client's feelings. Telling the client that she should be delighted ignores, rather than addresses, the client's feelings. Also, doing so imposes the nurse's opinion on the client. Ambivalence is a common reaction to pregnancy. Telling the client that she should be delighted may lead to feelings of guilt. Asking the client if she and her husband were trying to have a baby is a "yes–no" question and is not helpful. In addition, it ignores the client's underlying feelings. (P)

47. **3.** Women normally experience ambivalence when pregnancy is confirmed, even if the pregnancy was planned. Although the client's culture may play a role in openly accepting the pregnancy, most new mothers who have been ambivalent initially accept the reality by the end of the first trimester. Ambivalence also may be expressed throughout the pregnancy; this is believed to be related to the amount of physical discomfort. The nurse should become concerned and perhaps contact a social worker if the client expresses ambivalence in the third trimester. The client's statement reflects ambivalence, not fear. There is no evidence to suggest or imply that the client is rejecting the fetus. The client's statement reflects ambivalence about the pregnancy, not her ability to care for the newborn. (P)

48. **4.** The priority nursing diagnosis at this time relates to nutrition, and the necessary health teaching involves a definite need for appropriate nutrition to meet the needs of the growing fetus. Pregnancy places additional demands on the body, and adequate nutrition is important for fetal well-being throughout pregnancy. *Readiness for enhanced family coping* related to pregnancy confirmation is not a priority diagnosis at this time. The developing fetus is the priority; the fetus requires adequate nutrition throughout the pregnancy. Insufficient information is provided in the scenario to support a nursing diagnosis of *Ineffective sexuality patterns* or *Compromised family coping*. (R)

49. **3.** Couvade syndrome refers to the situation in which the expectant father experiences some of the discomforts of pregnancy along with the pregnant woman as a means of identifying with the pregnancy. Ptyalism is the term for excessive salivation. Mittelschmerz is the lower abdominal discomfort felt by some women during ovulation. Pica refers to an oral craving for substances such as clay or starch that some pregnant clients experience. (P)

50. **3.** Maternal alcohol use may result in fetal alcohol syndrome, marked by mild to moderate mental retardation, physical growth retardation, central nervous system disorders, and feeding difficulties. Because there is no definitive answer as to how much alcohol can be safely consumed by a pregnant woman, it is recommended that pregnant clients be taught to abstain from drinking alcohol during pregnancy. Smoking and other medications also may affect the fetus. (R)

51. **4.** An increase in clear, highly acidic vaginal secretions is a normal finding during pregnancy that aids in controlling the growth of pathologic bacteria. Vaginal secretions increase because of the influence of estrogen secretion and increased vaginal and cervical vascularity. The highly acidic nature of the vaginal secretions is caused by the action of *Lactobacillus acidophilus*, which increases the lactic acid content of the secretions. The increased acidity helps to make the vagina resistant to bacterial growth. During pregnancy, estrogen secretion fosters a glycogen-rich environment. Unfortunately, this glycogen-rich, acidic environment fosters the development of yeast (*Candida albicans*) infections, manifested by itching, burning, and a cheese-like vaginal discharge. If the client had a sexually transmitted disease, most likely she would complain of additional symptoms, such as lesions in the genital area or changes in color, consistency, or odor of the vaginal secretions. An increase in vaginal secretions does not help prevent expulsion of the mucus plug. The mucus plug is held in place by the cervix until the cervix becomes ripe. (H)

52. **2.** Measurement of the client's fundal height is a gross estimate of fetal gestational age. At 20 weeks' gestation, the fundal height should be at about the level of the client's umbilicus. The fundus typically is over the symphysis pubis at 12 weeks. A fundal height measurement between these two areas would suggest a fetus with a gestational age between 12 and 20 weeks. The fundal height increases approximately 1 cm/week after 20 weeks' gestation. The fundus typically reaches the xiphoid process at approximately 36 weeks' gestation. A fundal height between the umbilicus and the xiphoid process would suggest a fetus with a gestational age between 20 and 36 weeks. The fundus then commonly returns to about 4 cm below the xiphoid owing to lightening at 40 weeks. Additionally, pressure on the diaphragm occurs late in pregnancy. Therefore, a fundal height measurement near the xiphoid process with diaphragmatic compression suggests a fetus near the gestational age of 36 weeks or older. (H)

53. **3.** Previously it was believed that amniocentesis should not be performed until 14 to 16 weeks' gestation because of risk to the fetus and also to allow for a generous amount of amniotic fluid to form. However, with the newer techniques of amniocentesis analysis, only 1 ml of fluid is required and the test can be performed as early as 12 weeks' gestation, which is especially useful for identifying genetic disorders. Gestation of 8 or 10 weeks will not provide the volume of amniotic fluid needed for testing. (H)

54. **2, 3, 4.** CVS, amniocentesis and triple screen are tests specifically designed to detect fetal abnormalities. Electrocardiogram is never reliable. EFM detects uterine contraction frequency and intensity as well as fetal heart rate. (R)

55. **4.** The National Academy of Sciences Institute of Medicine recommends that women gain between 25 and 35 lb during pregnancy. These guidelines were developed to decrease the risk of intrauterine growth retardation. It is believed that the pattern of weight gain is as important as the total amount of weight gained. Underweight women and women carrying twins should have a greater weight gain. Typically, women should gain 3.5 lb during the first trimester and then 1 lb/week during the remainder of the pregnancy (24 weeks) for a total of about 27 to 28 lb. A weight gain of only 6.6 lb in the second and third trimesters is not considered normal because the client should be gaining about 1 lb/week, or 12 lb during the second and third trimesters. Gaining 12 lb during each trimester would total 36 lb, which is slightly more than the recommended weight gain. In addition, nausea and vomiting during the first trimester can contribute to a lack of appetite and smaller weight gain during this trimester. (H)

56. **1.** Green, leafy vegetables, such as asparagus, spinach, brussel sprouts, and broccoli, are rich sources of folic acid. The pregnant woman needs to eat foods high in folic acid to prevent folic acid deficits, which may result in neural tube defects in the newborn. A well-balanced diet must include whole grains, dairy products, and fresh fruits;

however, bananas are rich in potassium, seafood is rich in iodine, and yogurt is rich in calcium, not folic acid. (R)

57. **3.** Egg yolks and squash and other yellow vegetables are rich sources of vitamin A. Pregnant women should avoid megadoses of vitamin A because fetal malformations may occur. Buttermilk and cheese are good sources of calcium. Strawberries, cantaloupe, citrus fruits (such as oranges), and tomatoes are good sources of vitamin C, not vitamin A. (C)

58. **1, 3, 4.** Dairy products, fresh fruit, vegetables, and foods high in protein (like cheese and peanut butter) are excellent choices. Fried foods, such as chicken nuggets and tater tots, and foods such as cheeseburgers and buttered popcorn are high in fat; carbonated drinks such as diet colas, and foods such as pickles and ketchup contain large amounts of sodium. These foods can lead to an increase in ankle edema and promote weight gain from empty calories. (H)

59. **4.** Riboflavin forms coenzymes needed to release energy. Enriched grain products (e.g., cereals, breads), deep green leafy vegetables, milk, veal, beef, and cheddar cheese are rich sources of riboflavin. Fresh fruit is rich in vitamin C and fiber. Prunes are rich in iron, fiber, and vitamin C. Potatoes are a source of vitamin C and carbohydrates. (C)

60. **2.** Magnesium aids in the synthesis of protein, nucleic acids, proteins, and fats. It is important for cell growth and neuromuscular function. Magnesium also activates the enzymes for metabolism of protein and energy. Calcium prevents demineralization of the mother's bones. Vitamin B6 is important for amino acid metabolism. Folic acid assists in the development of neural pathways in the fetus. (C)

61. **1.** The diet for Vietnamese Americans typically consists of small portions of meat and ample amounts of rice. Fresh milk may not have been readily available in Vietnam, and many Asian clients are lactose intolerant. Therefore, the nurse would need to assess the client's diet for deficiencies of calcium and possibly iron. Traditionally, Southeast Asian diets have an abundance of dark green leafy vegetables, such as mustard greens and bok choy, which contain adequate amounts of vitamin E and vitamin C. Seafood, which contains iodine, is usually adequate in the diets of Southeast Asian women. (R)

62. **3.** Chorionic villi sampling, which can be performed between 8 and 10 weeks' gestation, involves the insertion of a thin catheter into the vagina and uterus to obtain a sample of the chorionic cells. It is a useful diagnostic test to determine trisomy 13, translocations, fragile X syndrome, and trisomy 18. Fetoscopy is performed with a small fiberoptic fetoscope inserted through a small incision into the client's uterus to inspect the fetus for gross abnormalities. There are no food or fluid restrictions necessary before chorionic villi sampling. Ideally, the client should empty the bladder before this procedure. A full bladder would be needed if the client were scheduled to have an ultrasound examination. (R)

63. **4.** Although most multiparous women experience quickening at about 17½ weeks' gestation, some women may perceive it between 14 and 20 weeks' gestation because they have been pregnant before and know what to expect. Detecting movement early does not suggest a twin pregnancy. If the multiparous client does not experience quickening by 20 weeks' gestation, further investigation is warranted, because the fetus may have died, the client has a hydatidiform mole, or the pregnancy dating is incorrect. There is no evidence that the client's expected date of delivery is erroneous. (H)

64. **4.** AFP testing is usually performed between the 15th and 18th weeks of gestation. Abnormally high levels found in maternal serum may be indicative of neural tube defects such as anencephaly and spina bifida. Low levels may indicate trisomy 21 (Down syndrome). Culdocentesis is used to confirm a tubal pregnancy. Chorionic villus sampling is done as early as 10 weeks' gestation to detect anomalies. Ultrasound testing may be done in the first trimester to determine fetal viability and in the third trimester to determine pelvic adequacy and fetal or placental position. (R)

65. **2.** Leopold's maneuvers involve abdominal palpation. The client should empty her bladder before the nurse palpates the abdomen. Doing so increases the client's comfort and makes palpation more accurate. Although breathing deeply may help to relax the client, it has no effect on the accuracy of the results of Leopold's maneuvers. The client does not need to drink a full glass of water before the examination. The client should be lying in a supine position with the head slightly elevated for greater comfort and with the knees drawn up slightly. (H)

66. Because the fetus is determined to be in an LOA, a vertex position, the convex portion of the fetus lying closest to the uterine wall would be located in the lower left quadrant of the abdomen. Placing the Doppler ultrasound over that area would produce the loudest fetal heart sounds. (M)

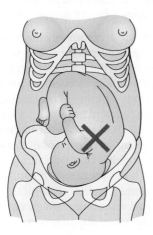

67. **1.** In left occipital transverse lie, the occiput faces the woman's left hip. In left occipital anterior lie, the occiput faces the left anterior segment of the woman's pelvis. In right occipital transverse lie, the occiput faces the woman's right hip. In right occipital anterior lie, the occiput faces the right anterior segment of the woman's pelvis. (A)

68. **1.** Discoloration on the face that commonly appears during pregnancy, called *chloasma* (mask of pregnancy), usually fades postpartum and is of no clinical significance. The client who is bothered by her appearance may be able to decrease its prominence with ordinary makeup. Chloasma is not a sign of skin melanoma. It is not caused by dilated capillaries. Rather, it results from increased secretion of melanocyte-stimulating hormones caused by estrogen and progesterone secretion. No treatment is necessary for this condition. (H)

69. **4.** Assessment of fundal height is a gross estimate of gestational age. By 20 weeks' gestation, the height of the fundus should be at the level of the umbilicus, after which it should increase 1 cm for each week of gestation until approximately 36 weeks' gestation. Fundal height that is significantly different from that implied by the estimated gestational age warrants further evaluation (e.g., ultrasound examination), because it possibly indicates multiple pregnancy or fetal growth retardation. Fundal height estimation will not determine uterine activity or a need for increased weight gain. Ultrasound examination, not fundal height estimation, will locate the placenta. (H)

70. **2.** One of the primary risks of amniocentesis is stimulation of the uterus and subsequent preterm labor. Other risks include hemorrhage from penetration of the placenta, infection of the amniotic fluid, and puncture of the fetus. There is little risk for rupture of the membranes, fetal limb malformations, or fetal organ malformations, if a practitioner skilled in using ultrasound performs the procedure. Fetal limb malformations have been associated with percutaneous umbilical blood sampling. (R)

71. **3.** The client traveling by automobile should be advised to take intermittent breaks of 10 to 15 minutes, including walking, every 1 to 2 hours to stimulate the circulation, which becomes sluggish during long periods of sitting. Automobile travel is not contraindicated during pregnancy unless the client develops complications. There is no set maximum number of hours allowed. The pregnant client should always wear a seat belt when traveling by automobile. The client should be aware of the nearest health care facility in the city to which she is traveling. (R)

72. Seat belt safety is important for pregnant women because proper use reduces maternal mortality in car accidents. Both lap and shoulder belts are to be used. The lap portion of the belt is placed snugly but comfortably to fit under the abdominal bulge. Wearing the lap belt over the abdomen could increase the risk of uterine rupture and fetal complications due to belt tightening as the woman is propelled forward during an automobile accident. The shoulder belt is placed snugly across the shoulder, chest, and upper abdomen. (S)

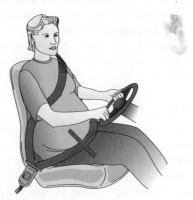

73. **3.** Leg cramps are thought to result from excessive amounts of phosphorus absorbed from milk products. Straightening the knee and flexing the toes toward the chin is an effective measure to relieve leg cramps. Also, decreasing milk intake and supplementing with calcium lactate may help to reduce the cramping. Keeping the legs warm and elevating them are good preventive measures. Changing positions frequently aids venous return but is not helpful in relieving leg cramps. Alternately flexing and extending the legs will not help to relieve the leg cramp. Lying prone in the bed is a difficult position for a client at 37 weeks' gestation to achieve and maintain because of the increase in abdominal size and therefore is not considered helpful. (C)

74. **1.** Eating smaller and more frequent meals may help prevent heartburn because acid production is decreased and stomach displacement is reduced. Heartburn can occur at any time during pregnancy. Contributing factors include stress, tension, worry, fatigue, caffeine, and smoking. Certain spicy foods (e.g., tacos) may trigger heartburn in the pregnant client. The client should be advised to avoid sodium bicarbonate antacids (e.g., Alka-Seltzer), baking soda, Bicitra or sodium citrate, and fatty foods, which are high in sodium and can contribute to fluid retention. Increasing, not decreasing, fluid intake may help to relieve heartburn by diluting gastric juices. Caffeinated products such as coffee or tea can stimulate acid formation in the stomach, further contributing to heartburn. (C)

75. The fist is placed against the middle of the woman's sternum, with backward thrusts until the foreign body is expelled. The pressure from the backward thrusts causes compression of the ribs, further adding to the chest and lung pressure, thereby forcing the foreign body to move upward. (S)

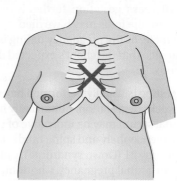

76. **2.** In the first maneuver, which is done with the nurse facing the client's head, both hands are used to palpate and determine which fetal body part (e.g., the head or buttocks) is in the fundus. This first maneuver helps to determine the presenting part of the fetus. In the second maneuver, also done with the nurse facing the client's head, the palms of both hands are used to palpate the sides of the uterus and determine the location of the fetal back and spine. In the third maneuver, one hand gently grasps the lower portion of the abdomen just above the symphysis pubis to determine whether the fetal head is at the pelvic inlet. The fourth maneuver, done with the nurse facing the client's feet, determines the degree of fetal descent and flexion into the pelvis. (H)

77. **4.** Increased AFP levels are associated with neural tube defects, such as spina bifida, anencephaly, and encephalocele. Ultrasonography is used to confirm a neural tube defect only when AFP levels are increased. Because AFP levels are usually highest at 15 to 18 weeks' gestation, this is the optimum time for testing. Performing the test after this time leads to inaccurate results. The client's blood, not urine, is used for the sample. (R)

78. **1.** Prenatal care is commonly the most critical factor influencing pregnancy outcome. This is especially true for adolescents, because the most significant medical complication in pregnant adolescents is pregnancy-induced hypertension. Continued prenatal care helps to allow for early detection and prompt intervention should the complication arise. Other risks for adolescents include low-birth-weight infant, preterm labor, iron-deficiency anemia, and cephalopelvic disproportion. Gestational diabetes can occur with any pregnancy regardless of the age of the mother. Generally, all first-time mothers need instruction related to discomforts. Adolescent mothers have better nutrition when they attend group classes and are subject to peer pressure. No evidence demonstrates that most adolescents lack support systems. Fathers may abandon mothers at any time during the pregnancy; other fathers, regardless of age, are supportive throughout the pregnancy. (H)

79. 3. The most appropriate nursing diagnosis for this client is *Altered nutrition: Less than body requirements* related to lack of appetite. The evidence of gaining only 5 lb since the beginning of pregnancy supports this diagnosis. Additional supportive evidence is the client's statement that she has no appetite. The nurse needs to gather additional data to determine the reason for the client's poor appetite, such as a physiologic or psychological problem. More information is needed to support a nursing diagnosis of *Knowledge deficit, Noncompliance,* or *Chronic low self-esteem.* These nursing diagnoses may be appropriate after the reason for the client's poor appetite is determined. (R)

80. 3. Colostrum is usually secreted by about the 16th week of gestation in preparation for breast-feeding. Growth of the milk ducts is greatest in the last trimester, not in the first 8 weeks of gestation. Enlargement of the breasts is usually caused by estrogen, not progesterone. Darkening of the areola can occur as early as the sixth week of gestation. (H)

81. 2, 4, 6. Understanding of breast-feeding education is demonstrated by statements involving knowledge of the several positions available for comfortable breast-feeding, oxytocin release from the pituitary leading to a let-down reflex and uterine contractions for involution, and feeding cues helpful in successful breast-feeding (because waiting until the infant is hungry and crying is stressful). Breast size does not ensure successful breast-feeding. Mastitis is an infectious process and is not influenced by latching on. Breast milk needs to be stored in the refrigerator or freezer to decrease the risk of bacterial growth. (C)

82. 2. During pregnancy, the circulatory system undergoes tremendous changes. Cardiac output increases by 25% to 50%, and circulatory blood volume increases by about 30%. The client may experience transient hypotension and dizziness with sudden position changes. Early in pregnancy there is a slight increase in the temperature, and clients may attribute this to a sinus infection or a cold. The client may feel warm, but this sensation is transient. The level of circulating fibrinogen increases as much as 50% during pregnancy, probably because of increased estrogen. Any calf tenderness should be reported, because it may indicate a clot. Late in pregnancy, the posterior pituitary gland secretes oxytocin. The client may experience painful Braxton Hicks contractions or early labor symptoms. (H)

83. 1. The fetal biophysical profile includes fetal breathing movements, fetal body movements, tone, amniotic fluid volume, and fetal heart rate reactivity. A reactive nonstress test is a sign of fetal well-being and does not require further evaluation. A nonreactive nonstress test requires further evaluation. A contraction stress test or oxytocin challenge test should be performed only on women who are at risk for fetal distress during labor. The contrac-

tion stress test is rarely performed before 28 weeks' gestation because of the possibility of initiating labor. Percutaneous umbilical cord sampling requires the insertion of a needle through the abdomen to obtain a fetal blood sample. (R)

84. 3. The purpose of Kegel exercises is to strengthen the perineal muscles in preparation for the labor process. These movements strengthen the pubococcygeal muscle, which surrounds the urinary meatus and vagina. No evidence is available to support the idea that these exercises prevent vulvar edema, alleviate lower back discomfort, or strengthen the abdominal muscles. (C)

85. 4. During the third trimester, it is not uncommon for clients to have dreams or fantasies about the baby. Sometimes the dreams are about infants who are malformed or, in this example, covered with hair. There is no evidence to suggest that the client is trying to cope with becoming a parent. Having dreams about the baby does not mean that labor will begin soon. (P)

86. 1. Insomnia in the later part of pregnancy is not uncommon because the client has difficulty getting into a position of comfort. This is further compounded by frequent nocturia. The best suggestion would be to advise the client to practice relaxation techniques before bedtime. The client should avoid caffeine products such as chocolate and coffee before going to bed because caffeine is a stimulant. Alcohol consumption, regardless of the type or amount, should be avoided. Exercise is advised during the day, but it should be avoided before bedtime because exercise can stimulate the client and decrease the client's ability to fall asleep. (C)

87. 3. The client needs further instruction when she says it is permissible to sit in a hot tub for 20 minutes to relax after working. Hot tubs and saunas should be avoided, particularly in the first trimester, because their use can lead to maternal hyperthermia, which is associated with fetal anomalies such as central nervous system defects. The client should use nonskid pads in the shower or bath to avoid slipping because the client's center of gravity has shifted and she may fall. The client should avoid using soap on the nipples to prevent removal of the natural protective oils. Douching is not recommended for pregnant women because it can destroy the normal flora and increase the client's risk of infection. (H)

88. 3. The obstetric conjugate can be estimated by subtracting 1.5 to 2 cm from the diagonal conjugate, which can be measured during a pelvic examination. Transverse diameters of the pelvic inlet are not measured and the pubic arch has no relevance to the obstetrical conjugate. (H)

The Pregnant Client in Childbirth Preparation Classes

89. 1. Folic acid supplementation is recommended to prevent neural tube defects and anemia in pregnancy. Deficiencies increase the risk of hemorrhage during delivery as well as infection. The recommended dose prior to pregnancy is 400 mcg/day; while breast-feeding and during pregnancy, the recommended dosage is 500 to 600 mcg/day. Blood glucose levels are not regulated by the intake of folic acid. Vitamin C potentiates the absorption of iron and is also associated with blood clotting or collagen formation. (H)

90. 3, 5, 6. During the third trimester of pregnancy, experimenting with maternal and caregiver roles and concern about safety and passage through labor and delivery are major foci. Other psychological tasks include preparation of the nursery, being tired of the pregnancy, and being introspective. A woman will begin to see herself as someone different from the fetus in the second trimester. Additionally, the mother may fantasize about the infant during the second trimester and be concerned about her changing body image. She may experience ambivalence about pregnancy in the first trimester. (P)

91. 4. Pregnancy creates changes in the mother and father. Being considerate, accepting changes, and being supportive of the current situation are considered acceptable responses by the father, rather than feeling irritation about these changes. Expressing concern with the financial changes pregnancy and an expanded family include is normal. The first trimester involves the client and family feeling ambivalent about pregnancy and moving toward acceptance of the changes associated with pregnancy. Maternal acceptance of the pregnancy and a subsequent change in her focus are normal occurrences. (H)

92. 4. Thyroid enlargement and increased basal body metabolism are common occurrences during pregnancy. Human placental lactogen enhances milk production. Estrogen is responsible for hyperpigmentation and vascular skin changes. Progesterone relaxes smooth muscle in the respiratory tract. (H)

93. 1. Although sex is not easily discerned at 9 to 12 weeks, external genitalia are developed at this period of fetal development. Myelinization of the nerves begins at about 20 weeks' gestation. Brown fat stores develop at approximately 21 to 24 weeks. Air ducts and alveoli develop later in the gestational period, at approximately 25 to 28 weeks. (H)

94. 2. Monozygotic twinning is independent of race, age, parity, or heredity. Monozygotic twins result from the fertilization of one ovum by two different sperm. Dizygotic twinning occurs with the fertilization of more than one ovum during conception. Dizygotic twins may be of the same sex or different sexes. Dizygotic twinning is correlated with increased parity, becoming pregnant within 1 month after stopping oral contraception, and infertility treatments. A primigravid client is less likely to conceive dizygotic twins. (H)

95.

| 1. Engagement |
| 3. Descent |
| 2. Flexion |
| 4. Internal rotation |

Engagement refers to the fetus' entering the true pelvis and occurs before descent in primiparas and concurrently in multiparous women. If the head is the presenting part, the normal maneuvers during labor and delivery are (in order): descent, flexion, internal rotation, extension, external rotation, and expulsion. These maneuvers are called the *cardinal movements*. They occur as the fetal head passes through the maternal pelvis during the normal labor process. (H)

96. 1. In a normal delivery and for the first 24 hours postpartum, a total blood loss not exceeding 500 ml is considered normal. Blood loss during delivery is almost always estimated because it provides a valuable indicator for possible hemorrhage. A blood loss of 1,000 ml is considered hemorrhage. (H)

97. 2. Although the amniotic fluid promotes normal prenatal development by allowing symmetric development, it does not provide the fetus with nutrients. Rather, nutrients are provided by the placenta. The amniotic fluid does help dilate the cervix once labor begins by pressure and gravity forces. The amniotic fluid helps to protect the fetus from injury by cushioning against impact of the maternal abdomen and allows room and buoyancy for fetal movement. The amniotic fluid and sac keep the fetus at a stable temperature by maintaining a neutral thermal environment. (H)

98. 1. Pelvic rocking helps to relieve backache during pregnancy and early labor by making the spine more flexible. Deep breathing exercises assist with relaxation and pain relief during labor. Tailor sitting and squatting help stretch the perineal muscles in preparation for labor. (H)

99. 1, 2, 4. Pain during the first stage of labor is primarily caused by hypoxia of the uterine and cervical muscle cells during contraction, stretching of the lower uterine segment, dilatation of the cervix and perineum, and pressure on adjacent structures. Ambulating will assist in increasing circulation of blood to the area and relaxing the muscles. Slow chest breathing is appropriate during the first stage of labor to promote increased oxygenation as well as relaxation. The woman or her coach can lightly massage the abdomen (effleurage) while using slow chest breathing. Chest breathing and massaging increase oxygenation and relaxation of uterine muscles. Pain medication is not used during the first stage of labor because most medications will slow labor; anesthesia may be considered during the second stage of labor. Sipping ice water, while helpful for maintaining hydration, will not be useful as a pain management strategy. (H)

100. **4.** With true labor, the contractions are felt first in the lower back and then the abdomen. They gradually increase in frequency and duration and do not disappear with ambulation, rest, or sleep. In true labor, the cervix dilates and effaces. Walking tends to increase true contractions. False labor contractions disappear with ambulation, rest, or sleep. False labor contractions commonly remain the same in duration and frequency. Clients who are experiencing false labor may have pain, even though the contractions are not very effective. (H)

101. **4.** Pelvic tilt exercises are useful to alleviate backache during pregnancy and labor but are not useful for the pain from contractions. Biofeedback (a conscious effort to control the response to pain), effleurage (light uterine massage), and guided imagery (focusing on a pleasant scene) are appropriate pain relief techniques to practice before labor begins. Various breathing exercises also can help to alleviate the discomfort from contraction pain. (H)

102. **2.** Increased vaginal discharge is normal during pregnancy, but yellow-gray frothy discharge with local itching is associated with infection (e.g., *Trichomonas vaginalis*). The client's symptoms must be further assessed by a health professional because the client needs treatment for this condition. *T. vaginalis* infection is commonly treated with metronidazole (Flagyl). However, this drug is not used in the first trimester. In the first trimester, the typical treatment is topical clotrimazole. Although a yeast infection is associated with vaginal itching, the vaginal discharge is cheese-like. Furthermore, because the client may have a serious vaginal infection, over-the-counter medications are not advised until the client has been evaluated. Douching is not recommended during pregnancy because it would predispose the client to an ascending infection. The client is not exhibiting signs and symptoms of preterm labor, such as contractions or leaking fluid. And although the client's complaints are suggestive of a *T. vaginalis* infection, which can lead to preterm labor and premature rupture of the membranes, further evaluation is needed to confirm the cause of the infection. (H)

103. **4.** The umbilical cord normally consists of two arteries and one vein. Oxygen and other nutrients are carried to the fetal circulation by the umbilical vein. The umbilical arteries carry oxygen-poor blood back to the placenta. The foramen ovale is a shunt that allows blood returning from the lungs to mix. The ductus arteriosus allows oxygenated blood via the umbilical vein to be carried to the inferior vena cava. (H)

104. **3.** The umbilical cord normally inserts in the center of the placenta. A velamentous cord does not insert centrally into the placenta, and cord vessels branch out, which can lead to fetal hemorrhage. The highest oxygen content is found in the umbilical vein. Oxygenated blood flows through the umbilical vein to the fetus. Blood leaving the fetus to return to the placenta flows through the two umbilical arteries. About 1% of umbilical cords have only one artery. A nuchal cord occurs when the cord is wrapped around the fetus' neck, commonly because the cord is longer than normal. (H)

105. **2.** During pregnancy, urinary tract infections are more common because of urinary stasis. Clients need instructions about increasing fluid volume intake. Plasma volume increases during pregnancy. The increase in plasma volume is more pronounced and occurs earlier than the increase in red blood cell mass, possibly resulting in physiologic anemia. Peripheral vascular resistance decreases during pregnancy, providing a relatively stable blood pressure. Hemoglobin levels decrease during pregnancy even though there is an increase in blood volume. (H)

106. **2.** Infant mortality rate is defined as the number of deaths of infants younger than 12 months of age per 1,000 live births. Maternal mortality in the United States has been steadily decreasing; however, African American infants have a higher mortality rate than Caucasian infants. The perinatal mortality rate includes all stillborn infants with a gestational age of 28 weeks or more plus all neonatal deaths before 7 days of age per 1,000 of this population. The neonatal mortality rate is the number of deaths of infants younger than 28 days of age per 1,000 live births. (H)

The Pregnant Client with Risk Factors

107. **4.** For the Rh-negative client who may be pregnant with an Rh-positive fetus, an indirect Coombs test measures antibodies in the maternal blood. Titers should be performed monthly during the first and second trimesters and biweekly during the third trimester and the week before the due date. (H)

108. **2.** According to the New York Heart Association Cardiac Disease classification, this client would fit under Class II because she is symptomatic with increased activity (dyspnea with exertion). The New York Heart Association Cardiac Disease Classification identifies Class II clients as having cardiac disease and a slight limitation in physical activity. When physical activity occurs, the client may experience angina, difficulty breathing, palpations, and fatigue. All of the client's other symptoms are within normal limits. (M)

109. **1, 2, 5.** The test result indicates that the mother has an active hepatitis infection and is a carrier. Hepatitis B immune globulin at birth provides the infant with passive immunity against hepatitis B and serves as a prophylactic treatment. Additionally, the infant will be started on the vaccine series of three injections. The infant should not be screened or isolated because the infant is already hepatitis B positive. As with all clients, universal precautions should be used and are sufficient to prevent transmission of the virus. Women who are positive for hepatitis B surface antigen are able to breast-feed. (M)

110. **4.** Asthma medications and bronchodilators should be continued during pregnancy as prescribed before the pregnancy began. The medications do not cause harm to the mother or fetus. Regular use of asthma medication will usually prevent asthma attacks. Prevention and limitation of an asthma attack is the goal of care for a client who is or is not pregnant and is the appropriate care strategy. During an asthma attack, oxygen needs continue as with any pregnant client but the airways are edematous, decreasing perfusion. Asthma exacerbations during pregnancy may occur as a result of infrequent use of medication rather than as a result of the pregnancy. (D)

111.

> **3.** A single mother at 4 months postpartum fearful of shaking her baby when he cries.

> **4.** An antenatal client at 16 weeks' gestation who has occasional sharp pain on her left side radiating from her symphysis to her fundus.

> **1.** A primigravid client at 10 weeks' gestation complaining of not feeling well with nausea and vomiting, urinary frequency, and fatigue.

> **2.** A multiparous client at 32 weeks' gestation asking for assistance with finding a new physician.

The first client to be seen should be the postpartum mother who is fearful of shaking her infant. Postpartum depression is a disorder that may occur during the first year postpartum but peaks at 4 weeks postpartum, prior to menses, or upon weaning. As a single mother, this client may not have support, a large factor putting women at risk. Other factors accentuating risk include prior depressive or bipolar illness and self-dissatisfaction. Second, the nurse should see the 16-week antenatal client, who is likely experiencing round ligament syndrome. At this point in the pregnancy, the uterus is stretching into the abdomen causing this type of pain. The pain is on the wrong side to be attributed to appendicitis or gallbladder disease. Nursing interventions to ease the pain include a heating pad or bringing the legs toward the abdomen. The nurse should next see the primigravid client complaining of not feeling well because she is exhibiting signs and symptoms of discomfort experienced by most women in the first trimester. The multiparous client at 32 weeks' gestation is the lowest priority as she is physically well, while the other clients have physical and psychological problems. In most emergency department situations, she may not be seen by medical or nursing staff but would be given the names of health care providers in the reception area. (M)

112. **2.** The nurse seeing this client should refer her to a health care provider for further evaluation of the pain. This referral would allow a more definitive diagnosis and medical interventions that may include surgery. Referral would occur because of her high pain rating as well as the other symptoms, which suggest gallbladder disease. During pregnancy, the gallbladder is under the influence of progesterone, which is a smooth muscle relaxant. Because bile does not move through the system as quickly during pregnancy, bile stasis and gallstone formation can occur. Although education should be a continuous strategy, with pain at this level, a brief explanation is most appropriate. Major emphasis should be placed on determining the cause and treating the pain. It is not appropriate for the nurse to diagnose pain at this level as heartburn. Discussing nutritional strategies to prevent heartburn are appropriate during pregnancy, but not in this situation. Tylenol is an acceptable medication to take during pregnancy but should not be used on a regular basis as it can mask other problems. (M)

113. **3.** A fetus that has died and is retained in utero places the mother at risk for disseminated intravascular coagulation (DIC) because the clotting factors within the maternal system are consumed when the nonviable fetus is retained. The longer the fetus is retained in utero, the greater the risk of DIC. This client has no risk factors, history, or signs and symptoms that put her at risk for either abruptio placentae or placenta previa, such as sharp pain and "woody," firm consistency of the abdomen (abruption) or painless bright red vaginal bleeding (previa). There is no evidence that she is threatening to abort as she has no complaints of cramping or vaginal bleeding. (M)

114. **2.** Chorionic villus sampling (CVS) can be performed from approximately 8 to 12 weeks' gestation, while amniocentesis cannot be performed until between 11 weeks' gestation and the end of the pregnancy. Eleven weeks' gestation is the earliest possible time within the pregnancy to obtain a sufficient amount of amniotic fluid to sample. Because CVS take a piece of membrane surrounding the infant, this procedure can be completed earlier in the pregnancy. Amniocentesis and chorionic villus sampling identify the genetic makeup of the fetus in its entirety, rather than a portion of it. Laboratory analysis of chorionic villus sampling takes less time to complete. Both procedures place the fetus at risk and postprocedure teaching asks the client to report the same complicating events (bleeding, cramping, fever, and fluid leakage from the vagina). (M)

115. **4.** Additional teaching is needed when the parent says that adolescents are at greater risk for congenital anomalies. Although adolescents are at greater risk for denial of the pregnancy, lack of prenatal care, low-birth-weight infant, cephalopelvic disproportion, anemia, and nutritional deficits and have a higher maternal mortality rate, studies reveal that congenital anomalies are not more common in adolescent pregnancies. (H)

116. **4.** With a spontaneous abortion, many clients and their partners feel an acute sense of loss. Their grieving commonly includes feelings of guilt, which may be expressed as wondering whether the woman could have done something to prevent the loss. Anger, sadness, and disappointment are also common emotions after a pregnancy loss. Ambivalence, anxiety, and fear are not common emotions after a spontaneous abortion. (P)

117. **1.** Hydroxyzine (Vistaril) has a tranquilizing effect and also decreases nausea and vomiting. It does not decrease fluid retention, reduce pain, decrease uterine cramping, or promote uterine contractility. One of the adverse effects of the medication is sleepiness. Ibuprofen may decrease pain from uterine cramping. Oxytocin may be used to increase uterine contractility. (D)

118. **3.** The death of a fetus at any time during pregnancy is a tragedy for most parents. After a spontaneous abortion, the client and family members can be expected to suffer from grief for several months or longer. When offering support, a simple statement such as "I'm truly sorry you lost your baby" is most appropriate. Therapeutic communication techniques help the client and family understand the meaning of the loss, move less stressfully through the grief process, and share feelings. Asking the client whether she is experiencing a great deal of uterine pain is inappropriate because this is a "yes-no" question and doesn't allow the client to express her feelings. Saying that the embryo was defective is inappropriate because this may lead the client to think that she contributed to the fetus's demise. This is not the appropriate time to discuss embryonic or fetal malformations. However, the nurse should explain to the client that this situation was not her fault. Telling the client that she should get pregnant again as soon as possible is not therapeutic and discounts the feelings of the expectant mother who had already begun to bond with the fetus. (P)

119. **4.** Rh sensitization can be prevented by Rho(D) immune globulin, which clears the maternal circulation of Rh-positive cells before sensitization can occur, thereby blocking maternal antibody production to Rh-positive cells. Administration of this drug will not prevent future Rh-positive fetuses, nor will it prevent future abortions. An antibody response will not occur to Rh-negative cells. Rh-negative mothers do not develop sensitivities if the fetus is also Rh negative. (D)

120. **2.** The client with leg varicosities should take frequent rest periods with the legs elevated above the hips to promote venous circulation. The client should avoid constrictive clothing, but support hose that reach above the varicosities may help alleviate the pain. Contracting and relaxing the feet and ankles twice daily is not helpful because it does not promote circulation. Taking a leave of absence from work may not be possible because of economic reasons. The client should try to rest with her legs elevated or walk around for a few minutes every 2 hours while on the job. (R)

121. **1.** Cryotherapy, electrocautery, or laser therapy may be used to remove the genital warts. Podophyllin solution should not be used to decrease their size while the client is pregnant, because fetal malformations may result. A 25% trichloroacetic acid solution can decrease the size of the warts, but because this disease is caused by a virus, the disorder may recur. Condylomata acuminata has been associated with cervical cancer, and the client should have semiannual or annual Pap smears to detect cervical dysplasia. (D)

122. **4.** The client is reporting symptoms typically associated with herpes genitalis. Some women have no symptoms of gonorrhea. Others may experience vaginal itching and a thick, purulent vaginal discharge. *C. trachomatis* infection in women is commonly asymptomatic, but symptoms may include a yellowish discharge and painful urination. The first symptom of syphilis is a painless chancre. (A)

123. **1.** The client may need surgery to remove a ruptured fallopian tube where the pregnancy has occurred, and the nurse is usually responsible for witnessing the signature on the informed consent. Usually, if bleeding is occurring, it is internal. Typically there is only scant vaginal bleeding with no discoloration. The nurse cannot determine whether the fallopian tube can be salvaged; this can be accomplished only during surgery. If the tube has ruptured, it must be removed. If the tube has not ruptured, a linear salpingostomy may be done to salvage the tube for future pregnancies. With an ectopic pregnancy, although the client is experiencing abdominal pain, she is not having uterine contractions. (A)

124. **1.** The optical density of the amniotic fluid is evaluated for bilirubin level with a spectrophotometer. The higher the optical density, the more bilirubin is present in the fluid, indicating that fetal red blood cells are being destroyed. From these findings, the severity of the disease can be estimated. Because light destroys bilirubin, specimens should be kept in a dark container until the analysis is complete. A clear, green, or amber container would allow light to enter, thus destroying bilirubin. (R)

Complications of Pregnancy

The Pregnant Client with Preeclampsia or Eclampsia

1. Several pregnant clients are waiting to be seen in the triage area of the obstetrical unit. Which client is the highest priority?
- ☐ **1.** A client at 13 weeks' gestation experiencing nausea and vomiting three times a day with + 1 ketones in her urine.
- ☐ **2.** A client at 37 weeks' gestation who is an insulin-dependent diabetic and experiencing 3 to 4 fetal movements per day.
- ☐ **3.** A client at 32 weeks' gestation who has preeclampsia and + 3 proteinuria who is returning for evaluation of epigastric pain.
- ☐ **4.** A primigravida at 17 weeks' gestation complaining of not feeling fetal movement at this point in her pregnancy.

2. A laboring client with preeclampsia is prescribed magnesium sulfate 2 g/hr I.V. piggyback. The pharmacy sends the I.V. to the unit labeled *magnesium sulfate 20 g/ 500 ml normal saline*. To deliver the correct dose, the nurse should set the pump to deliver how many milliliters per hour?

_____ ml

3. A 32-year-old multigravida returns to the clinic for a routine prenatal visit at 36 weeks' gestation. She has had a prior pregnancy with pregnancy-induced hypertension. The assessments during this visit include BP 140/90, P 80, and + 2 edema of the ankles and feet. Based on the client's past history and current assessment, what further information should the nurse obtain to determine if this client is becoming preeclamptic?
- ☐ **1.** Headaches.
- ☐ **2.** Blood glucose level.
- ☐ **3.** Proteinuria.
- ☐ **4.** Edema in lower extremities.

4. The nurse is instructing a preeclamptic client about monitoring the movements of her fetus to determine fetal well-being. Which statement by the client indicates that she needs further instruction about when to call the health care provider concerning fetal movement?
- ☐ **1.** "If the fetus is becoming less active than before."
- ☐ **2.** "If it takes longer each day for the fetus to move 10 times."
- ☐ **3.** "If the fetus stops moving for 12 hours."
- ☐ **4.** "If the fetus moves more often than 3 times an hour."

5. A 29-year-old multigravid client at 37 weeks' gestation is being treated for severe preeclampsia. She has magnesium sulfate infusing at 3 grams per hour. The nurse would base her nursing care on which priority nursing diagnosis?
☐ **1.** *Risk for central nervous system injury* related to hypertension, edema of cerebrum.
☐ **2.** *Anxiety* related to fetal and maternal risk.
☐ **3.** *Risk for hepatic injury* related to liver dysfunction.
☐ **4.** *Risk for fetal injury* related to decreased uteroplacental perfusion.

6. At 32 weeks' gestation, a 15-year-old primigravid client who is 5 feet, 2 inches tall has gained a total of 20 lb, with a 1-lb gain in the last 2 weeks. Urinalysis reveals negative glucose and a trace of protein. The nurse determines that which of the following factors increases this client's risk for preeclampsia?
☐ **1.** Total weight gain.
☐ **2.** Short stature.
☐ **3.** Adolescent age group.
☐ **4.** Proteinuria.

7. A primigravid client's baseline blood pressure at her initial visit at 12 weeks' gestation was 110/70 mm Hg. During an assessment at 38 weeks' gestation, which of the following data would indicate mild preeclampsia?
☐ **1.** Blood pressure of 160/110 mm Hg on two separate occasions.
☐ **2.** Proteinuria, more than 5 g in 24 hours.
☐ **3.** Serum creatinine concentration of 1.4 ml/dl.
☐ **4.** Weight gain of 2 lb in the last week.

8. A 19-year-old primigravid client at 38 weeks' gestation is diagnosed with mild preeclampsia and mild peripheral edema, requiring bed rest at home for the past 2 weeks. Which nursing diagnosis would the nurse identify as the priority for this client?
☐ **1.** *Noncompliance* related to poor nutrition and lack of exercise during pregnancy.
☐ **2.** *Delayed growth and development* related to required bed rest and subsequent immobility.
☐ **3.** *Deficient fluid volume* related to fluid shift from intravascular to extravascular space.
☐ **4.** *Situational low self-esteem* related to prolonged bed rest and pregnancy complications.

9. During a home visit to a 16-year-old client at 34 weeks' gestation diagnosed with mild preeclampsia, assessment reveals that the client has gained 2 lb in the past week and her current blood pressure is 130/86 mm Hg. Which of the following assessment findings would provide further evidence to support the client's diagnosis?
☐ **1.** Pounding headache after reading.
☐ **2.** History of urinary tract infection.
☐ **3.** Frequent voiding in large amounts.
☐ **4.** Mild edema in hands and face.

10. When developing the teaching plan for a primigravid client at 30 weeks' gestation diagnosed with mild preeclampsia who is being treated at home, which of the following would the nurse identify as the most appropriate client-centered goal?
☐ **1.** Return visit to the prenatal clinic in approximately 4 weeks.
☐ **2.** Decreased edema after 1 week of a low-protein, low-fiber diet.
☐ **3.** Bed rest on the left side during the day, with bathroom privileges.
☐ **4.** Immediate reporting of adverse reactions to magnesium sulfate therapy.

11. After instructing a primigravid client at 38 weeks' gestation about how preeclampsia can affect the client and the growing fetus, the nurse realizes that the client needs additional instruction when she says that preeclampsia can lead to which of the following?
☐ **1.** Hydrocephalic infant.
☐ **2.** Abruptio placentae.
☐ **3.** Intrauterine growth retardation.
☐ **4.** Poor placental perfusion.

12. After instructing a multigravid client diagnosed with mild preeclampsia how to keep a record of fetal movement patterns at home, the nurse determines that the teaching has been effective when the client says that she will count the number of times the baby moves during which of the following time spans?
☐ **1.** 30-minute period three times a day.
☐ **2.** 45-minute period after lunch each day.
☐ **3.** 1-hour period each day.
☐ **4.** 12-hour period each week.

13. When teaching a multigravid client diagnosed with mild preeclampsia about nutritional needs, which of the following types of diet should the nurse discuss?
☐ **1.** High-residue diet.
☐ **2.** Low-sodium diet.
☐ **3.** Regular diet.
☐ **4.** High-protein diet.

14. In response to a question from a 40-year-old multigravid client diagnosed with mild preeclampsia about the causes of this problem, the nurse teaches the client about the various theories surrounding the conditions associated with preeclampsia. Which of the following, if stated by the client as an associated condition, would indicate the need for additional teaching?
☐ **1.** Multifetal pregnancy.
☐ **2.** Diabetes mellitus.
☐ **3.** Age older than 35 years.
☐ **4.** Iron deficiency.

15. A 17-year-old client at 33 weeks' gestation diagnosed with mild preeclampsia is prescribed bed rest at home. The nurse instructs the client to contact the health care provider immediately if she experiences which of the following?
- [ ] **1.** Blurred vision.
- [ ] **2.** Ankle edema.
- [ ] **3.** Increased energy levels.
- [ ] **4.** Mild backache.

16. One week after her prenatal visit, a primigravid client at 38 weeks' gestation diagnosed with mild preeclampsia calls the clinic nurse complaining of a continuous headache for the past 2 days accompanied by nausea. The client does not want to take aspirin. Which of the following responses by the nurse would be most appropriate?
- [ ] **1.** "Take two acetaminophen tablets. They aren't as likely to upset your stomach."
- [ ] **2.** "I think the doctor should see you today. Can you come to the clinic this morning?"
- [ ] **3.** "You need to lie down and rest. Have you tried placing a cool compress over your head?"
- [ ] **4.** "I'll ask the doctor to call in a prescription for aspirin with codeine. What's your pharmacy's number?"

17. When reviewing the prenatal records of a 16-year-old primigravid client at 37 weeks' gestation diagnosed with severe preeclampsia, the nurse would interpret which of the following as most indicative of the client's diagnosis?
- [ ] **1.** Blood pressure of 138/94 mm Hg.
- [ ] **2.** Severe blurring of vision.
- [ ] **3.** Less than 2 g of protein in a 24-hour sample.
- [ ] **4.** Weight gain of 0.5 lb in 1 week.

18. When preparing the room for admission of a multigravid client at 36 weeks' gestation diagnosed with severe preeclampsia, which of the following would the nurse obtain?
- [ ] **1.** Oxytocin infusion solution.
- [ ] **2.** Disposable tongue blades.
- [ ] **3.** Portable ultrasound machine.
- [ ] **4.** Padding for the side rails.

19. The physician orders intravenous magnesium sulfate for a primigravid client at 38 weeks' gestation diagnosed with severe preeclampsia. Which of the following medications would the nurse have readily available at the client's bedside?
- [ ] **1.** Diazepam (Valium).
- [ ] **2.** Hydralazine (Apresoline).
- [ ] **3.** Calcium gluconate.
- [ ] **4.** Phenytoin (Dilantin).

20. For the client who is receiving intravenous magnesium sulfate for severe preeclampsia, which of the following assessment findings would alert the nurse to suspect hypermagnesemia?
- [ ] **1.** Decreased deep tendon reflexes.
- [ ] **2.** Cool skin temperature.
- [ ] **3.** Rapid pulse rate.
- [ ] **4.** Tingling in the toes.

21. A 28-year-old multigravid client at 37 weeks' gestation arrives at the emergency department via ambulance with a blood pressure of 160/104 mm Hg and +3 reflexes without clonus. The client, who is diagnosed with severe preeclampsia, asks the nurse, "What is the cure for my high blood pressure?" Which of the following would the nurse identify as the primary cure?
- [ ] **1.** Administration of glucocorticoids (Betamethasone).
- [ ] **2.** Vaginal or cesarean delivery of the fetus.
- [ ] **3.** Sedation with phenytoin (Dilantin).
- [ ] **4.** Reduction of fluid retention with thiazide diuretics.

22. Which of the following would the nurse identify as the priority to achieve when developing the plan of care for a primigravid client at 38 weeks' gestation who is hospitalized with severe preeclampsia and receiving intravenous magnesium sulfate?
- [ ] **1.** Decreased generalized edema within 8 hours.
- [ ] **2.** Decreased urinary output during the first 24 hours.
- [ ] **3.** Sedation and decreased reflex excitability within 48 hours.
- [ ] **4.** Absence of any seizure activity during the first 48 hours.

23. When administering intravenous magnesium sulfate as ordered for a client at 34 weeks' gestation with severe preeclampsia, the nurse would explain to the client and her family that this drug acts as which of the following?
- [ ] **1.** Peripheral vasodilator.
- [ ] **2.** Antihypertensive.
- [ ] **3.** Central nervous system depressant.
- [ ] **4.** Sedative-hypnotic.

24. Soon after admission of a primigravid client at 38 weeks' gestation with severe preeclampsia, the physician orders a continuous intravenous infusion of 5% dextrose in Ringer's solution and 4 g of magnesium sulfate. While the medication is being administered, which of the following assessment findings should the nurse report immediately?
- [ ] **1.** Respiratory rate of 12 breaths/minute.
- [ ] **2.** Patellar reflex of +2.
- [ ] **3.** Blood pressure of 160/88 mm Hg.
- [ ] **4.** Urinary output exceeding intake.

25. Which of the following would be the most appropriate nursing diagnosis for a primigravid client at 38 weeks' gestation who was just admitted for eclampsia after experiencing a seizure in her home?
- ☐ **1.** *Risk for injury* related to possibility of further convulsions.
- ☐ **2.** *Deficient knowledge* related to symptoms of preeclampsia.
- ☐ **3.** *Hypertensive crisis* related to severe preeclampsia.
- ☐ **4.** *Situational low self-esteem* related to hospitalization and sedation.

26. As the nurse enters the room of a newly admitted primigravid client diagnosed with severe preeclampsia, the client begins to experience a seizure. Which of the following should the nurse do first?
- ☐ **1.** Insert an airway to improve oxygenation.
- ☐ **2.** Note the time when the seizure begins and ends.
- ☐ **3.** Call for immediate assistance.
- ☐ **4.** Turn the client to her left side.

27. After administering hydralazine (Apresoline) 5 mg intravenously as ordered for a primigravid client with severe preeclampsia at 39 weeks' gestation, the nurse would be alert for which of the following?
- ☐ **1.** Tachycardia.
- ☐ **2.** Bradypnea.
- ☐ **3.** Polyuria.
- ☐ **4.** Dysphagia.

28. A primigravid client with severe preeclampsia exhibits hyperactive, very brisk patellar reflexes with two beats of ankle clonus present. The nurse documents the patellar reflexes as which of the following?
- ☐ **1.** 1+.
- ☐ **2.** 2+.
- ☐ **3.** 3+.
- ☐ **4.** 4+.

29. A 16-year-old unmarried primigravid client at 37 weeks' gestation with severe preeclampsia is in early active labor. Her mother is at the bedside. The client's blood pressure is 164/110 mm Hg. Which of the following would alert the nurse that the client may be about to experience a seizure?
- ☐ **1.** Decreased contraction intensity.
- ☐ **2.** Decreased temperature.
- ☐ **3.** Epigastric pain.
- ☐ **4.** Hyporeflexia.

30. Fifteen minutes after a client experiences an eclamptic seizure, the nurse assesses the client for which of the following?
- ☐ **1.** Polyuria.
- ☐ **2.** Facial flushing.
- ☐ **3.** Hypotension.
- ☐ **4.** Uterine contractions.

31. If a client at 36 weeks' gestation with eclampsia begins to exhibit signs of labor after an eclamptic seizure, for which of the following would the nurse assess?
- ☐ **1.** Abruptio placentae.
- ☐ **2.** Transverse lie.
- ☐ **3.** Placenta accreta.
- ☐ **4.** Uterine atony.

32. For a multigravid client at 39 weeks' gestation with suspected HELLP syndrome, the nurse would immediately notify the physician for which of the following laboratory test results?
- ☐ **1.** Hyperfibrinogenemia.
- ☐ **2.** Decreased liver enzymes.
- ☐ **3.** Thrombocytopenia.
- ☐ **4.** Hypernatremia.

The Pregnant Client with a Chronic Hypertensive Disorder

33. An obese 36-year-old multigravid client at 12 weeks' gestation has a history of chronic hypertension. She was treated with methyldopa (Aldomet) before becoming pregnant. When counseling the client about diet during pregnancy, the nurse realizes that the client needs additional instruction when she states which of the following?
- ☐ **1.** "I need to reduce my caloric intake to 1,200 calories a day."
- ☐ **2.** "A regular diet is recommended during pregnancy."
- ☐ **3.** "I should eat more frequent meals if I get heartburn."
- ☐ **4.** "I need to consume more fluids and fiber each day."

34. After instructing a multigravid client at 10 weeks' gestation diagnosed with chronic hypertension about the need for frequent prenatal visits, the nurse determines that the instructions have been successful when the client states which of the following?
- ☐ **1.** "I may develop hyperthyroidism because of my high blood pressure."
- ☐ **2.** "I need close monitoring because I may have a small-for-gestational-age infant."
- ☐ **3.** "It's possible that I will have excess amniotic fluid and may need a cesarean section."
- ☐ **4.** "I may develop placenta accreta, so I need to keep my clinic appointments."

35. After reinforcing the danger signs to report with a gravida 2 client at 32 weeks' gestation with an elevated blood pressure, which client statements would demonstrate her understanding of when to call the physician's office? Select all that apply.

☐ **1.** "If I get up in the morning and feel dizzy, even if the dizziness goes away."

☐ **2.** "If I see any bleeding, even if I have no pain."

☐ **3.** "If I have a pounding headache that doesn't go away."

☐ **4.** "If I notice the veins in my legs getting bigger."

☐ **5.** "If the leg cramps at night are waking me up."

☐ **6.** "If the baby seems to be more active than usual."

The Pregnant Client with Third-Trimester Bleeding

36. The nurse is caring for a 22-year-old G 2, P 2 client who has disseminated intravascular coagulation after delivering a dead fetus. Which of the following laboratory or assessment findings are the highest priority to report to the health care provider?

☐ **1.** Activated partial thromboplastin time (APTT) of 30 seconds.

☐ **2.** Hemoglobin of 11.5g/dl.

☐ **3.** Urinary output of 25 ml in the past hour.

☐ **4.** Platelets at 149,000/mm³.

37. A 24-year-old client, G 3, P 1, at 32 weeks' gestation, is admitted to the hospital because of vaginal bleeding. After reviewing the client's history, which of the following factors might lead the nurse to suspect abruptio placentae?

☐ **1.** Several hypotensive episodes.

☐ **2.** Previous low transverse cesarean delivery.

☐ **3.** One induced abortion.

☐ **4.** History of cocaine use.

38. When caring for a multigravid client admitted to the hospital with vaginal bleeding at 38 weeks' gestation, which of the following would the nurse anticipate administering intravenously if the client develops disseminated intravascular coagulation (DIC)?

☐ **1.** Ringer's lactate solution.

☐ **2.** Fresh frozen platelets.

☐ **3.** 5% dextrose solution.

☐ **4.** Warfarin sodium (Coumadin).

39. When assessing a 34-year-old multigravid client at 34 weeks' gestation experiencing moderate vaginal bleeding, which of the following would most likely alert the nurse that placenta previa is present?

☐ **1.** Painless vaginal bleeding.

☐ **2.** Uterine tetany.

☐ **3.** Intermittent pain with spotting.

☐ **4.** Dull lower back pain.

40. After giving instruction about the cause of the vaginal bleeding to a multigravid client at 36 weeks' gestation diagnosed with placenta previa, the nurse determines that the teaching has been effective when the client says that the bleeding results from which of the following?

☐ **1.** Diminished clotting factors.

☐ **2.** Exposure of maternal blood sinuses.

☐ **3.** Increased platelet levels.

☐ **4.** A large-for-gestational-age fetus.

41. During an interview, a multigravid client at 35 weeks' gestation who was admitted to the hospital with placenta previa and ordered to strict bed rest states, "My last baby was born 6 weeks early and had to stay in a special care nursery." Which of the following would the nurse formulate as the priority nursing diagnosis?

☐ **1.** *Risk for constipation* related to bed rest.

☐ **2.** *Interrupted family processes* related to hospitalization.

☐ **3.** *Anxiety* related to unknown outcome of client/fetus.

☐ **4.** *Impaired physical mobility* related to vaginal bleeding.

42. The physician orders whole blood replacement for a multigravid client with abruptio placentae. Before administering the intravenous blood product, which of the following should the nurse do first?

☐ **1.** Validate client information and the blood product with another nurse.

☐ **2.** Check the vital signs before transfusing over 5 to 6 hours.

☐ **3.** Ask the client if she has ever had any allergies.

☐ **4.** Administer 100 ml of 5% dextrose solution intravenously.

43. Following a cesarean delivery for abruptio placentae, a multigravid client tells the nurse, "I feel like such a failure. None of my other deliveries were like this." The nurse's response to the client is based on the understanding of which of the following?

☐ **1.** The client will most likely have postpartum blues.

☐ **2.** Maternal-infant bonding is likely to be difficult.

☐ **3.** The client's feeling of grief is a normal reaction.

☐ **4.** This type of delivery was necessary to save the client's life.

44. Epidural anesthesia is effective in controlling pain for cesarean and vaginal births and for tubal ligations after birth. Place an X over the highest point on the body locating the level of anesthesia expected for a cesarean birth.

45. Which of the following actions would the nurse anticipate as the highest priority when preparing for the admission of a multigravid client at 36 weeks' gestation with a probable diagnosis of abruptio placentae?
- ☐ **1.** Preparing the client for a vaginal examination.
- ☐ **2.** Obtaining a brief history from the client.
- ☐ **3.** Inserting a large-gauge intravenous catheter.
- ☐ **4.** Preparing the client for an ultrasound scan.

The Pregnant Client with Preterm Labor

46. The health care provider has determined that a preterm labor client at 34 weeks' gestation has no fetal fibronectin present. The nurse should expect which of the following outcomes in the next week?
- ☐ **1.** The client will develop preeclampsia.
- ☐ **2.** The fetus will develop mature lungs.
- ☐ **3.** The client will not likely develop preterm labor.
- ☐ **4.** The fetus will not develop gestational diabetes.

47. A nurse is discussing preterm labor in a prenatal class. After class, a client and her partner ask the nurse to identify again the nursing strategies to prevent preterm labor. The nurse knows the clients need further instruction when they state which of the following?
- ☐ **1.** "I need to stay hydrated all the time."
- ☐ **2.** "I need to avoid any infections."
- ☐ **3.** "I should include frequent rest breaks if we travel."
- ☐ **4.** "Changing to filter cigarettes is helpful."

48. A 31-year-old client, G 3, T 0, P 2, Ab 0, L 0, at 32 weeks' gestation, is admitted to the hospital with contractions of moderate intensity occurring every 3 to 4 minutes. The client, who has previously delivered two nonviable fetuses at 30 weeks' gestation, is crying on admission. The client asks, "What causes preterm labor?" After giving instruction about various risks for preterm labor, the nurse determines that additional explanation is needed when the client says that preterm labor is commonly associated with which of the following?
- ☐ **1.** Age older than 30 years.
- ☐ **2.** Polyhydramnios.
- ☐ **3.** Chronic hypertension.
- ☐ **4.** Multifetal gestation.

49. A multigravid client at 34 weeks' gestation is being treated with indomethacin (Indocin) to halt preterm labor. If the client should deliver a preterm infant, the nurse would notify the nursery personnel about this therapy because of the possibility for which of the following?
- ☐ **1.** Pulmonary hypertension.
- ☐ **2.** Respiratory distress syndrome (RDS).
- ☐ **3.** Hyperbilirubinemia.
- ☐ **4.** Cardiomyopathy.

50. A multigravid client at 34 weeks' gestation who is leaking amniotic fluid has just been hospitalized with a diagnosis of preterm labor. The client's contractions are 20 minutes apart, lasting 20 to 30 seconds. Her cervix is dilated at 2 cm. The client asks the nurse, "Why is God punishing me? I go to church every Sunday. What did I do wrong to cause this?" Which of the following would be the priority nursing diagnosis?
- ☐ **1.** *Risk for impaired parenting* related to hospitalization.
- ☐ **2.** *Spiritual distress* related to feelings of guilt and preterm labor.
- ☐ **3.** *Risk for infection* related to possible chorioamnionitis.
- ☐ **4.** *Disturbed body image* related to pregnancy and hospitalization.

51. The nurse is preparing to administer terbutaline (Brethine) to a multigravid client in preterm labor. Before administering this drug intravenously, the nurse should assess which of the following?
- ☐ **1.** Hematocrit.
- ☐ **2.** Weight gain.
- ☐ **3.** Urinary output.
- ☐ **4.** Heart rate.

52. In which of the following maternal locations would the nurse place the ultrasound transducer of the external electronic fetal heart rate monitor if a fetus at 34 weeks' gestation is in the left occipitoanterior (LOA) position?
- ☐ **1.** Near the symphysis pubis.
- ☐ **2.** Two inches above the umbilicus.
- ☐ **3.** Below the umbilicus on the left side.
- ☐ **4.** At the level of the umbilicus.

53. The physician orders betamethasone (Celestone) for a 34-year-old multigravid client at 32 weeks' gestation who is experiencing preterm labor. Previously, the client has experienced one infant death due to preterm birth at 28 weeks' gestation. The nurse explains that this drug is given for which of the following reasons?
- ☐ **1.** To enhance fetal lung maturity.
- ☐ **2.** To counter the effects of tocolytic therapy.
- ☐ **3.** To treat chorioamnionitis.
- ☐ **4.** To decrease neonatal production of surfactant.

54. A client at 28 weeks' gestation in premature labor was placed on ritodrine (Yutopar). To maintain the pregnancy, the physician orders the client to have 10 mg now, 10 mg in 2 hours, and then 20 mg every 4 hours while contractions persist, not to exceed the maximum daily oral dose of 120 mg. At what time will the client have reached the maximum dose if she begins taking the medication at 10:00 a.m. and follows the physician's order?

_____ a.m.

55. The nurse is caring for a multigravid client at 34 weeks' gestation diagnosed with preterm labor. The client has delivered two stillborn infants at 30 weeks' gestation. The client is scheduled for a sonogram before an amniocentesis. Which of the following would be a priority nursing diagnosis for the client?
- ☐ **1.** *Acute pain* related to abnormal uterine contractions.
- ☐ **2.** *Anxiety* related to diagnostic tests for fetal well-being.
- ☐ **3.** *Ineffective coping* related to hospitalization.
- ☐ **4.** *Deficient knowledge* related to consequences of preterm birth.

56. When preparing a multigravid client at 34 weeks' gestation experiencing preterm labor for the shake test performed on amniotic fluid, the nurse would instruct the client that this test is done to evaluate the maturity of which of the following fetal systems?
- ☐ **1.** Urinary.
- ☐ **2.** Gastrointestinal.
- ☐ **3.** Cardiovascular.
- ☐ **4.** Pulmonary.

The Pregnant Client with Premature Rupture of the Membranes

57. The nurse is planning care for a multigravid client hospitalized at 36 weeks' gestation with confirmed rupture of membranes and no evidence of labor. Which of the following would the nurse expect the physician to order?
- ☐ **1.** Frequent assessments of cervical dilation.
- ☐ **2.** Intravenous oxytocin administration.
- ☐ **3.** Vaginal culture for *Neisseria gonorrhoeae*.
- ☐ **4.** Sonogram for amniotic fluid volume index.

58. A multigravid client at 34 weeks' gestation visits the hospital because she suspects that her water has broken. After testing the leaking fluid with nitrazine paper, the nurse confirms that the client's membranes have ruptured when the paper turns which of the following colors?
- ☐ **1.** Yellow.
- ☐ **2.** Green.
- ☐ **3.** Blue.
- ☐ **4.** Red.

59. A primigravid client at 30 weeks' gestation has been admitted to the hospital with premature rupture of the membranes without contractions. Her cervix is 2 cm dilated and 50% effaced. Which of the following would be a priority assessment for this client?
- ☐ **1.** Red blood cell count.
- ☐ **2.** Degree of discomfort.
- ☐ **3.** Urinary output.
- ☐ **4.** Temperature.

60. A multigravid client at 34 weeks' gestation with premature rupture of the membranes tests positive for group B streptococcus. The client is having contractions every 4 to 6 minutes. Her vital signs are as follows: blood pressure, 120/80 mm Hg; temperature, 100° F (37.8° C); pulse, 100 bpm; respirations, 18 breaths/minute. Which of the following would the nurse expect the physician to order?
- ☐ **1.** Intravenous penicillin.
- ☐ **2.** Intravenous gentamicin sulfate (Garamycin).
- ☐ **3.** Intramuscular betamethasone (Celestone).
- ☐ **4.** Intramuscular cefaclor (Ceclor).

61. A primigravid client at 36 weeks' gestation with premature rupture of the membranes is to be discharged home on bed rest with follow-up by the home health nurse. After instruction about care while at home, which of the following client statements indicates effective teaching?
- ☐ **1.** "It is permissible to douche if the fluid irritates my vaginal area."
- ☐ **2.** "I can take either a tub bath or a shower when I feel like it."
- ☐ **3.** "I should limit my fluid intake to less than 1 quart daily."
- ☐ **4.** "I should contact the doctor if my temperature is 100.4° F or higher."

62. A primigravid client at 34 weeks' gestation is experiencing contractions every 3 to 4 minutes lasting for 35 seconds. Her cervix is 2 cm dilated and 50% effaced. While the nurse is assessing the client's vital signs, the client says, "I think my bag of water just broke." Which of the following would the nurse do first?
- ☐ **1.** Check the status of the fetal heart rate.
- ☐ **2.** Turn the client to her right side.
- ☐ **3.** Test the leaking fluid with nitrazine paper.
- ☐ **4.** Perform a sterile vaginal examination.

The Pregnant Client with Diabetes Mellitus

63. A client with gestational diabetes who is entering her third trimester is learning how to monitor her fetus's movements. After teaching the client about the kick count, the nurse should know the client needs further instruction if she makes which of the following statements?
- ☐ **1.** "The baby may be more active at different times of the day."
- ☐ **2.** "How I feel my baby move is different than my friend."
- ☐ **3.** "The baby should be moving less than 10 times in 3 hours."
- ☐ **4.** "The baby may not move at times because it is asleep."

64. A 27-year-old primigravid client with insulin-dependent diabetes at 34 weeks' gestation undergoes a nonstress test, the results of which are documented as reactive. The nurse tells the client that the test results indicate which of the following?
- ☐ **1.** A contraction stress test is necessary.
- ☐ **2.** The nonstress test should be repeated.
- ☐ **3.** Chorionic villus sampling is necessary.
- ☐ **4.** There is evidence of fetal well-being.

65. A primigravid client with insulin-dependent diabetes tells the nurse that the contraction stress test performed earlier in the day was suspicious. The nurse interprets this test result as indicating that the fetal heart rate pattern showed which of the following?
- ☐ **1.** Frequent late decelerations.
- ☐ **2.** Decreased fetal movement.
- ☐ **3.** Inconsistent late decelerations.
- ☐ **4.** Lack of fetal movement.

66. Which of the following statements about a fetal biophysical profile would be incorporated into the teaching plan for a primigravid client with insulin-dependent diabetes?
- ☐ **1.** It determines fetal lung maturity.
- ☐ **2.** It is noninvasive using real-time ultrasound.
- ☐ **3.** It will correlate with the newborn's Apgar score.
- ☐ **4.** It requires the client to have an empty bladder.

67. A 30-year-old multigravid client at 8 weeks' gestation has a history of insulin-dependent diabetes since age 20. When explaining about the importance of blood glucose control during pregnancy, which of the following should the nurse expect to occur regarding the client's insulin needs during the first trimester?
- ☐ **1.** They will increase.
- ☐ **2.** They will decrease.
- ☐ **3.** They will remain constant.
- ☐ **4.** They will be unpredictable.

68. The nurse explains the complications of pregnancy that occur with diabetes to a primigravid client at 10 weeks' gestation who has a 5-year history of insulin-dependent diabetes. Which of the following, if stated by the client as a complication, indicates the need for additional teaching?
- ☐ **1.** *Candida albicans* infection.
- ☐ **2.** Twin-to-twin transfer.
- ☐ **3.** Polyhydramnios.
- ☐ **4.** Preeclampsia.

69. When developing a teaching plan for a primigravid client with insulin-dependent diabetes about monitoring blood glucose control and insulin dosages at home, which of the following would the nurse expect to include as a desired target range for blood glucose levels?
- ☐ **1.** 40 to 60 mg/dl between 2:00 and 4:00 pm.
- ☐ **2.** 60 to 100 mg/dl before meals and bedtime snacks.
- ☐ **3.** 110 to 140 mg/dl before meals and bedtime snacks.
- ☐ **4.** 140 to 160 mg/dl 1 hour after meals.

70. When teaching a primigravid client with diabetes about common causes of hyperglycemia during pregnancy, which of the following would the nurse include?
- ☐ **1.** Fetal macrosomia.
- ☐ **2.** Obesity before conception.
- ☐ **3.** Maternal infection.
- ☐ **4.** Pregnancy-induced hypertension.

71. After teaching a diabetic primigravida about symptoms of hyperglycemia and hypoglycemia, the nurse determines that the client understands the instruction when she says that hyperglycemia may be manifested by which of the following?
- ☐ **1.** Dehydration.
- ☐ **2.** Pallor.
- ☐ **3.** Sweating.
- ☐ **4.** Nervousness.

72. At 38 weeks' gestation, a primigravid client with poorly controlled diabetes and severe preeclampsia is admitted for a cesarean delivery. The nurse explains to the client that delivery helps to prevent which of the following?
- ☐ **1.** Neonatal hyperbilirubinemia.
- ☐ **2.** Congenital anomalies.
- ☐ **3.** Perinatal asphyxia.
- ☐ **4.** Stillbirth.

73. A primigravid client with diabetes at 39 weeks' gestation is seen in the high-risk clinic. The physician estimates that the fetus weighs at least 4,500 g (10 lb). The client asks, "What causes the baby to be so large?" The nurse's response is based on the understanding that fetal macrosomia is usually related to which of the following?
- ☐ **1.** Family history of large infants.
- ☐ **2.** Fetal anomalies.
- ☐ **3.** Maternal hyperglycemia.
- ☐ **4.** Maternal hypertension.

74. With plans to breast-feed her neonate, a pregnant client with insulin-dependent diabetes asks the nurse about insulin needs during the postpartum period. Which of the following statements about postpartal insulin requirements for breast-feeding mothers would the nurse include in the explanation?
- ☐ **1.** They fall significantly in the immediate postpartum period.
- ☐ **2.** They remain the same as during the labor process.
- ☐ **3.** They usually increase in the immediate postpartum period.
- ☐ **4.** They need constant adjustment during the first 24 hours.

The Pregnant Client with Heart Disease

75. After instruction of a primigravid client at 8 weeks' gestation diagnosed with class I heart disease about self-care during pregnancy, which of the following client statements would indicate the need for additional teaching?
- ☐ **1.** "I should avoid being near people who have a cold."
- ☐ **2.** "I may be given antibiotics during my pregnancy."
- ☐ **3.** "I should reduce my intake of protein in my diet."
- ☐ **4.** "I should limit my salt intake at meals."

76. While caring for a primigravid client with class II heart disease at 28 weeks' gestation, the nurse would instruct the client to contact her physician immediately if the client experiences which of the following?
- ☐ **1.** Mild ankle edema.
- ☐ **2.** Emotional stress on the job.
- ☐ **3.** Weight gain of 1 lb in 1 week.
- ☐ **4.** Increased dyspnea at rest.

77. When developing the collaborative plan of care for a multigravid client at 10 weeks' gestation with a history of cardiac disease who was being treated with digitalis therapy before this pregnancy, which of the following would the nurse anticipate happening with the client's drug therapy regimen?
- ☐ **1.** Need for an increased dosage.
- ☐ **2.** Continuation of the same dosage.
- ☐ **3.** Switching to a different medication.
- ☐ **4.** Addition of a diuretic to the regimen.

78. Which of the following anticoagulants would the nurse expect to administer when caring for a primigravid client at 12 weeks' gestation who has class II cardiac disease due to mitral valve stenosis?
- ☐ **1.** Heparin.
- ☐ **2.** Warfarin (Coumadin).
- ☐ **3.** Enoxaparin (Lovenox).
- ☐ **4.** Ardeparin (Normiflo).

79. A primigravid client with class II heart disease who is visiting the clinic at 8 weeks' gestation tells the nurse that she has been maintaining a low-sodium, 1,800-calorie diet. Which of the following instructions should the nurse give the client?
- ☐ **1.** Avoid folic acid supplements to prevent megaloblastic anemia.
- ☐ **2.** Severely restrict sodium intake throughout the pregnancy.
- ☐ **3.** Take iron supplements with milk to enhance absorption.
- ☐ **4.** Increase caloric intake to 2,200 calories daily to promote fetal growth.

The Client with an Ectopic Pregnancy

80. On arrival at the emergency department, a client tells the nurse that she suspects that she may be pregnant but has been having a small amount of bleeding and has severe pain in the lower abdomen. The client's blood pressure is 70/50 mm Hg and her pulse rate is 120 bpm. The nurse notifies the physician immediately because which of the following is suspected?
- ☐ **1.** Ectopic pregnancy.
- ☐ **2.** Abruptio placentae.
- ☐ **3.** Gestational trophoblastic disease.
- ☐ **4.** Complete abortion.

81. A multigravid client seen in the emergency department complaining of sharp abdominal pain and vaginal spotting is diagnosed with an ectopic pregnancy. When explaining to the client and family members about an ectopic pregnancy, which of the following would the nurse include as the most common site of implantation?
- ☐ **1.** Fallopian tube.
- ☐ **2.** Intestine.
- ☐ **3.** Interstitial lining.
- ☐ **4.** Ovary.

82. A multigravid client at 8 weeks' gestation is admitted with a diagnosis of probable ectopic pregnancy. Which of the following would be the most appropriate nursing diagnosis for this client?
- ☐ **1.** *Fear* related to the outcome of possible surgery.
- ☐ **2.** *Ineffective coping* related to ectopic pregnancy.
- ☐ **3.** *Disturbed body image* related to surgical scarring.
- ☐ **4.** *Anticipatory grieving* related to the loss of the pregnancy.

83. Before surgery to remove an ectopic pregnancy and the fallopian tube, which of the following would alert the nurse to the possibility of tubal rupture?
- ☐ **1.** Amount of vaginal bleeding and discharge.
- ☐ **2.** Falling hematocrit and hemoglobin levels.
- ☐ **3.** Slow, bounding pulse rate of 80 bpm.
- ☐ **4.** Marked abdominal edema.

84. A multigravid client diagnosed with a probable ruptured ectopic pregnancy is scheduled for emergency surgery. In addition to monitoring the client's blood pressure before surgery, which of the following would the nurse assess?
- ☐ **1.** Uterine cramping.
- ☐ **2.** Abdominal distention.
- ☐ **3.** Hemoglobin and hematocrit.
- ☐ **4.** Pulse rate.

85. A 36-year-old multigravid client is admitted to the hospital with possible ruptured ectopic pregnancy. When obtaining the client's history, which of the following would be most important to identify as a predisposing factor?
- ☐ **1.** Urinary tract infection.
- ☐ **2.** Marijuana use during pregnancy.
- ☐ **3.** Episodes of pelvic inflammatory disease.
- ☐ **4.** Use of estrogen-progestin contraceptives.

86. After surgery to remove a ruptured fallopian tube, a multigravid client receives discharge instructions about potential complications to report to her physician. Which of the following, if stated by the client as a complication, indicates a need for additional teaching?
- ☐ **1.** Pain.
- ☐ **2.** Headache.
- ☐ **3.** Fever.
- ☐ **4.** Bleeding.

87. A multigravid client is admitted to the hospital with a diagnosis of ectopic pregnancy. The nurse anticipates that, because the client's fallopian tube has not yet ruptured, which of the following may be ordered?
- ☐ **1.** Progestin contraceptives (Hylutin).
- ☐ **2.** Medroxyprogesterone (Depo-Provera).
- ☐ **3.** Methotrexate.
- ☐ **4.** Dyphylline (Dilor).

The Pregnant Client with Hyperemesis Gravidarum

88. After instruction of a primigravid client at 8 weeks' gestation about measures to overcome early morning nausea and vomiting, which of the following client statements indicates the need for additional teaching?
- ☐ **1.** "I'll eat dry crackers or toast before arising in the morning."
- ☐ **2.** "I'll drink adequate fluids separate from my meals or snacks."
- ☐ **3.** "I'll eat two large meals daily with frequent protein snacks."
- ☐ **4.** "I'll snack on a small amount of carbohydrates throughout the day."

89. A multigravid client thought to be at 14 weeks' gestation reports that she is experiencing such severe morning sickness that "she has not been able to keep anything down for a week." The nurse should assess for signs and symptoms of which of the following?
- ☐ **1.** Hypercalcemia.
- ☐ **2.** Hypobilirubinemia.
- ☐ **3.** Hypokalemia.
- ☐ **4.** Hyperglycemia.

90. A multigravid client is admitted at 16 weeks' gestation with a diagnosis of hyperemesis gravidarum. The nurse should explain to the client that hyperemesis gravidarum is thought to be related to high levels of which of the following hormones?
- ☐ **1.** Progesterone.
- ☐ **2.** Estrogen.
- ☐ **3.** Somatotropin.
- ☐ **4.** Aldosterone.

91. The physician orders 1,000 ml of Ringer's lactate intravenously over an 8-hour period for a 29-year-old primigravid client at 16 weeks' gestation with hyperemesis gravidarum. The nurse would administer the intravenous infusion at which of the following rates?
- ☐ **1.** 60 ml per hour.
- ☐ **2.** 100 ml per hour.
- ☐ **3.** 125 ml per hour.
- ☐ **4.** 150 ml per hour.

92. A primigravid client admitted to the hospital with a diagnosis of hyperemesis gravidarum will be placed on nothing-by-mouth (NPO) status and receive intravenous therapy. Which of the following would the nurse most likely include when explaining to the client about oral intake of food and fluids?
- ☐ **1.** Withholding them indefinitely until acidosis is corrected.
- ☐ **2.** Giving them in small quantities whenever the client desires.
- ☐ **3.** Providing them as clear liquids after 24 hours if vomiting subsides.
- ☐ **4.** Withholding them until total parenteral nutrition replaces lost electrolytes.

The Client with a Hydatidiform Mole

93. A pregnant client at 15 weeks' gestation is admitted with dark brown vaginal bleeding and continuous nausea and vomiting. Her blood pressure is 142/98 mm Hg and fundal height is 19 cm. Based on these findings, the nurse determines that the client is most likely suffering from which obstetrical problem?
- ☐ **1.** Preeclampsia.
- ☐ **2.** Ectopic pregnancy.
- ☐ **3.** Hyperemesis gravidarum.
- ☐ **4.** Hydatidiform mole.

94. A 38-year-old client at about 14 weeks' gestation is admitted to the hospital with a diagnosis of complete hydatidiform mole. Soon after admission, the nurse would assess the client for signs and symptoms of which of the following?
- ☐ **1.** Pregnancy-induced hypertension.
- ☐ **2.** Gestational diabetes.
- ☐ **3.** Hypothyroidism.
- ☐ **4.** Polycythemia.

95. After a dilatation and curettage (D&C) to evacuate a molar pregnancy, assessing the client for signs and symptoms of which of the following would be most important?
☐ **1.** Urinary tract infection.
☐ **2.** Hemorrhage.
☐ **3.** Abdominal distention.
☐ **4.** Chorioamnionitis.

96. When preparing a multigravid client who has undergone evacuation of a hydatidiform mole for discharge, the nurse explains the need for follow-up care. The nurse determines that the client understands the instruction when she says that she is at risk for developing which of the following?
☐ **1.** Ectopic pregnancy.
☐ **2.** Choriocarcinoma.
☐ **3.** Multifetal pregnancies.
☐ **4.** Infertility.

97. After suction and evacuation of a complete hydatidiform mole, the 28-year-old multigravid client asks the nurse when she can become pregnant again. The nurse would advise the client not to become pregnant again for at least which of the following time spans?
☐ **1.** 6 months.
☐ **2.** 12 months.
☐ **3.** 18 months.
☐ **4.** 24 months.

The Pregnant Client with Miscellaneous Complications

98. The nurse is working with four clients on the obstetrical unit. Which client will be the highest priority for a cesarean section?
☐ **1.** Client at 40 weeks' gestation whose fetus weighs 8 lb by ultrasound estimate.
☐ **2.** Client at 37 weeks' gestation with fetus in ROP position.
☐ **3.** Client at 32 weeks' gestation with fetus in breech position.
☐ **4.** Client at 38 weeks' gestation with active herpes lesions.

99. A nurse notices that a client who has just delivered her infant is immediately short of breath, begins to cough, and suffers cardiac arrest. As the nurse immediately assesses and implements care for this client, what diagnosis should the nurse suspect?
☐ **1.** Heart failure.
☐ **2.** Preeclampsia.
☐ **3.** Septic shock.
☐ **4.** Amniotic fluid embolism.

100. A client in sickle cell crisis has been hospitalized during her pregnancy. Discharge instructions have been given in preparation for her return home. The nurse knows the client needs further teaching when she states which of the following?
☐ **1.** "I will need more frequent appointments during the remainder of the pregnancy."
☐ **2.** "Signs of any type of infection must be reported immediately."
☐ **3.** "At the earliest signs of a crisis, I need to seek treatment."
☐ **4.** "I have this disease because I don't eat enough food with iron."

101. A laboring client at −2 station has a spontaneous rupture of the membranes and a cord immediately protrudes from the vagina. The highest priority is which of the following?
☐ **1.** Place gentle pressure upward on the fetal head.
☐ **2.** Place the cord back into the vagina to keep it moist.
☐ **3.** Begin oxygen by face mask at 8 to 10 L/min.
☐ **4.** Turn the client on her left side.

102. A client has just had a cesarean section for a prolapsed cord. In reviewing the client's history, which of the following factors places a client at risk for cord prolapse? Select all that apply.
☐ **1.** −2 station.
☐ **2.** Low birth weight infant.
☐ **3.** Rupture of membranes.
☐ **4.** Breech presentation.
☐ **5.** Prior abortion.
☐ **6.** Low lying placenta.

103. A postpartum client is being discharged. Part of the discharge teaching involves identifying postpartum hemorrhage. The discharge instructions would include reporting which of the following?
☐ **1.** Bleeding that becomes lighter each day
☐ **2.** Clots the size of golf balls
☐ **3.** Saturating a pad in an hour
☐ **4.** Lochia that last longer than 1 week

104. A postpartum client is Rh-negative and has delivered an Rh-positive infant. The client is being educated concerning RhoGAM, which has been ordered. The nurse realizes the client understands the purpose of RhoGAM when she states:
☐ **1.** "RhoGAM will protect my next baby if it is Rh-negative."
☐ **2.** "RhoGAM will prevent antibody formation in my blood."
☐ **3.** "RhoGAM will be given to prevent German measles."
☐ **4.** "RhoGAM will be used to prevent bleeding in my newborn."

105. During a follow-up visit in the home setting, a client at 4 weeks postpartum tells the public health nurse that she can't cope any longer and is overwhelmed by her newborn. The baby has old formula on her clothes and under her neck. The mother does not remember when she last bathed the baby and states she does not want to care for the infant. When the baby cries, the mother walks away. The nurse should encourage the client and her husband to call her health care provider because she needs treatment for which of the following?
- ☐ **1.** Postpartum blues.
- ☐ **2.** Postpartum depression.
- ☐ **3.** Poor bonding.
- ☐ **4.** Infant abuse.

106. The nurse and a nursing assistant are caring for clients in a birthing center. Which of the following tasks should the nurse delegate to the nursing assistant? Select all that apply.
- ☐ **1.** Removing a Foley catheter from a preeclamptic client.
- ☐ **2.** Assisting an active labor client with breathing and relaxation.
- ☐ **3.** Ambulating a postcesarean client to the bathroom.
- ☐ **4.** Calculating hourly I.V. totals for a preterm labor client.
- ☐ **5.** Intake and output catheterization for culture and sensitivity.
- ☐ **6.** Calling a report of normal findings to the health care provider.
- ☐ **7.** Removing lunch trays and documenting lunch intake.

Correct Answers and Rationales

The letter in parentheses after each rationale identifies the client need addressed in the item, including management of care (M), safety and infection control (S), health promotion and maintenance (H), psychosocial adaptation (P), basic care and comfort (C), pharmacological and parenteral therapies (D), reduction of risk potential (R), and physiological adaptation (A).

The Pregnant Client with Preeclampsia or Eclampsia

1. 3. A preeclamptic client with +3 proteinuria and epigastric pain is at risk for seizing, which would jeopardize the mother and the fetus. Thus, this client would be the highest priority. The client at 13 weeks' gestation with nausea and vomiting is a concern because the presence of ketones indicates that her body does not have glucose to break down. However, this situation is a lower priority than the preeclamptic client or the insulin-dependent diabetic. The insulin-dependent diabetic is a high priority; however, fetal movement indicates that the fetus is alive but may be ill. As few as 4 fetal movements in 12 hours can be considered normal. (The client may need additional testing to further evaluate fetal well-being.) The primigravida who is at 17 weeks' gestation is too early in her pregnancy to experience fetal movement and would be the last person to be seen. (M)

2. 50

$$\frac{500 \text{ ml}}{20 \text{ g}} \times \frac{2g}{hr} = \frac{\overset{50}{\cancel{1,000}} \text{ g/ml}}{\underset{1}{\cancel{20}} \text{ g/hr}} = \frac{50 \text{ ml}}{1 \text{ hr}}$$

3. 3. The two major defining characteristics of preeclampsia are blood pressure elevation of 140/90 mm Hg or greater and proteinuria. Because the client's blood pressure meets the gestational hypertension criteria, the next nursing responsibility is to determine if she has protein in her urine. If she does not, then she may be having transient hypertension. The edema is within normal limits for someone at this gestational age, particularly because it is in the lower extremities. The preeclamptic client will have significant edema in the face and hands. Headaches are significant in pregnancy-induced hypertension but may have other etiologies. The client's blood glucose level has no bearing on a preeclampsia diagnosis. (A)

4. 4. The fetus is considered well if it moves more often than 3 times in one hour. Daily fetal movement counting is part of all high-risk assessments and is a noninvasive, inexpensive method of monitoring fetal well-being. The health care provider should be notified if there is a gradual slowing over time of fetal activity, if each day it takes longer for the fetus to move a minimum of 10 times, or if the fetus stops moving for 12 hours or longer. (R)

5. 1. *Risk for central nervous system injury* to the mother is the priority diagnosis. If the mother suffers central nervous system (CNS) damage, it will impact oxygenation and the entire health status of mother and fetus. Any physical injury or problem takes priority over psychosocial or social problems, such as *Anxiety*. Anxiety is a concern but can be addressed as other care takes place with client. Hepatic injury as a result of liver damage will impact perfusion of the mother and infant but would occur more slowly than CNS damage from a stroke or seizure. Fetal injury is a concern that will impact care but to a lesser degree than damage to the mother and infant. (A)

6. 3. Clients with increased risk for preeclampsia include primigravid clients younger than 20 years or older than 40 years, clients with five or more pregnancies, women of color, women with multifetal pregnancies, women with diabetes or heart disease, and women with hydramnios. A total weight gain of 20 lb at 32 weeks' gestation with a 1-lb weight gain in the last 2 weeks is within normal limits. Short stature is not associated with the development of preeclampsia. A trace amount of protein in the urine is common during pregnancy. However, protein amounts of 1+ or more may be a symptom of pregnancy-induced hypertension. (R)

7. **4.** A weight gain of 2 lb (0.9 kg) in the last week during the third trimester and mild peripheral edema are associated with mild preeclampsia. With severe preeclampsia, peripheral edema is extensive. Blood pressure readings of 160 mm Hg systolic and 100 mm Hg diastolic on two separate occasions and oliguria (urine output less than 400 ml in 24 hours) are signs of severe preeclampsia. Proteinuria, 3+ to 4+ or more than 5 g in a 24-hour sample, also indicates severe preeclampsia. Normal serum creatinine levels range from 0.5 to 1.1 ml/dl. A serum creatinine concentration of 1.4 ml/dl is greatly elevated, indicating severe preeclampsia. (A)

8. **3.** Because the client has peripheral edema with preeclampsia, the most appropriate nursing diagnosis is *Deficient fluid volume* related to fluid shift from intravascular to extravascular space. The scenario supplies no data to suggest noncompliance. If the client refused to remain on bed rest, then *Noncompliance* would be the priority diagnosis. The scenario also supplies no data to suggest delayed growth and development. If the client exhibited regression to an immature stage or childlike behaviors such as thumb-sucking, then *Delayed growth and development* would be an appropriate diagnosis. The client may be experiencing social isolation related to the prolonged bed rest, but there is no evidence of situational low self-esteem. Evidence of low self-esteem would include a disheveled appearance or statements by the client such as "I look so awful" or "I'm really fat." (A)

9. **4.** The diagnosis of mild preeclampsia is further confirmed if the client exhibits mild edema in the hands, fingers, or face resulting from fluid retention. A pounding headache after reading may indicate that a more severe form of preeclampsia is developing. A history of a urinary tract infection is not related to preeclampsia unless the client develops diabetes with renal impairment. Frequent voiding in large amounts is not related to preeclampsia. Women in the third trimester of pregnancy commonly void frequently in large amounts because of increased fluid intake and pressure of the uterus on the bladder. (A)

10. **3.** The client with mild preeclampsia is commonly treated at home with activity restriction. Bed rest for most of the day with the client lying in the left lateral recumbent position is recommended. This position helps to decrease pressure on the vena cava, thus increasing venous return, circulatory volume, and renal and placental perfusion. A decrease in angiotensin II improves renal blood flow, lowers blood pressure, and increases diuresis. Typically, the client is monitored with home visits twice a week. The client usually returns to the clinic every 2 weeks until 36 weeks' gestation. After that time, clinic visits occur at least every week or more often, if needed. The client's diet needs to be well balanced, with ample protein intake. Fiber intake may need to be increased to prevent complications from prolonged bed rest, such as constipation. If magnesium sulfate is necessary, as in severe preeclampsia, the drug is usually administered intravenously, and the client

is carefully monitored in the hospital setting because of the possible risk of seizure activity. (A)

11. **1.** Congenital anomalies such as hydrocephalus are not associated with preeclampsia. Conditions such as stillbirth, prematurity, abruptio placentae, intrauterine growth retardation, and poor placental perfusion are associated with preeclampsia. Abruptio placentae occurs because of severe vasoconstriction. Intrauterine growth retardation is possible owing to poor placental perfusion. Poor placental perfusion results from increased vasoconstriction. (A)

12. **3.** Numerous methods have been proposed to record the maternal perceptions of fetal movement or "kick counts." A commonly used method is the Cardiff count-to-10 method. The client begins counting fetal movements at a specified time (e.g., 8:00 a.m.) and notes the time when the 10th movement is felt. If the client does not feel at least 6 movements in a 1-hour period, she should notify the health care provider. The fetus typically moves an average of 1 to 2 times every 10 minutes or 10 to 12 times per hour. A 30- or 45-minute period is not enough time to evaluate fetal movement accurately. The client should monitor fetal movements more frequently than 1 time per week. One hour of monitoring each day is adequate. (R)

13. **3.** For clients with mild preeclampsia, a regular diet with ample protein and calories is recommended. If the client experiences constipation, she should increase the fiber in her diet, such as by eating raw fruits and vegetables, and increase fluid intake. A high-residue diet is not a nutritional need in preeclampsia. Sodium and fluid intake should not be restricted or increased. A high-protein diet is unnecessary. (C)

14. **4.** Iron deficiency can lead to anemia, but this has not been linked to preeclampsia. Although the exact cause of preeclampsia is not yet known, several theories have been proposed. Conditions that make a client more susceptible to preeclampsia include multifetal pregnancy, impaired vascular invasion of the uterine lining, genetic predisposition, diabetes mellitus, age older than 35 years, hydramnios, and low socioeconomic status. Calcium deficiency also has been implicated by some researchers. Multifetal pregnancy (e.g., twins) is associated with preeclampsia. This is related to an increased incidence of hydramnios, which is common in multifetal pregnancies. Diabetes mellitus is associated with preeclampsia; this is related to increased vasoconstriction, which is common in diabetes. Preeclampsia occurs more frequently in clients who are older than 35 years; this is thought by some researchers to be related to underlying hypertension. (A)

15. **1.** Severe headache, visual disturbances such as blurred vision, and epigastric pain are associated with the development of severe preeclampsia and possibly eclampsia. These danger signs and symptoms must be reported immediately. Severe headache and visual disturbances are related to severe vasoconstriction and a severe increase in blood pressure. Epigastric pain is related to hepatic dysfunction. Ankle edema is common during the third trimester. However, facial edema is associated with increased fluid retention and the progression from mild to severe preeclampsia. Increased energy levels are not associated with a progression of the client's preeclampsia or the development of complications. In fact, some women report an "energy spurt" before the onset of labor. Mild backache is a common discomfort of pregnancy, unrelated to a progression of the client's preeclampsia. It also may be associated with bed rest when the mattress is not firm. Some multiparous women have reported a mild backache as a sign of impending labor. (R)

16. **2.** A client with preeclampsia complaining of a continuous headache for 2 days should be seen by a health care provider immediately. Continuous headache, drowsiness, and mental confusion indicate poor cerebral perfusion and are symptoms of severe preeclampsia. Immediate care is recommended because these symptoms may lead to eclampsia or seizures if left untreated. Advising the client to take two acetaminophen tablets would be inappropriate and may lead to further complications if the client is not evaluated and treated. Although the application of cool compresses may ease the pain temporarily, this would delay treatment. Aspirin with codeine may temporarily relieve the client's headache. However, this delays immediate treatment, which is crucial. Additionally, pregnant women are advised not to take aspirin at this time because it may cause clotting problems in the neonate. Codeine generally is not prescribed. (R)

17. **2.** Signs of severe preeclampsia include blood pressure of 160/110 mm Hg or greater measured at two different times at least 6 hours apart, severe blurring of vision or seeing spots in front of the eyes, oliguria, proteinuria of 5 g or greater in a 24-hour specimen, a serum creatinine concentration of 1.2 ml/dl, and a urine specific gravity of 1.04 or greater. A blood pressure of 138/94 mm Hg would suggest mild preeclampsia, as would proteinuria of less than 2 g in a 24-hour urine specimen. A weight gain of 1 lb per week in the third trimester is normal. However, a weight gain of 2 lb or more suggests severe preeclampsia. (A)

18. **4.** The client with severe preeclampsia may develop eclampsia, which is characterized by seizures. The client needs a darkened, quiet room and side rails with thick padding. This helps decrease the potential for injury should a seizure occur. Airways, a suction machine, and oxygen also should be available. If the client is to undergo induction of labor, oxytocin infusion solution can be obtained at a later time. Tongue blades are not necessary. However, the emergency cart should be placed nearby in case the client experiences a seizure. The ultrasound machine may be used at a later point to provide information about the fetus. In many hospitals, the client with severe preeclampsia is admitted to the labor area, where she and the fetus can be closely monitored. The safety of the client and her fetus is the priority. (A)

19. **3.** The client receiving magnesium sulfate intravenously is at risk for possible toxicity. The antidote for magnesium sulfate toxicity is calcium gluconate, which should be readily available at the client's bedside. Diazepam (Valium), used to treat anxiety, usually is not given to pregnant women. Hydralazine (Apresoline) would be used to treat hypertension, and phenytoin (Dilantin) would be used to treat seizures. (D)

20. **1.** Typical signs of hypermagnesemia include decreased deep tendon reflexes, sweating or a flushing of the skin, oliguria, decreased respirations, and lethargy progressing to coma as the toxicity increases. The nurse should check the client's patellar, biceps, and radial reflexes regularly during magnesium sulfate therapy. Cool skin temperature may result from peripheral vasodilation, but the opposite—flushing and sweating—are usually seen. A rapid pulse rate commonly occurs in hypomagnesemia. Tingling in the toes may suggest hypocalcemia, not hypermagnesemia. (A)

21. **2.** The only known cure for severe preeclampsia is delivery of the fetus. In severe cases, labor induction is initiated or a cesarean section is performed. However, some women remain hypertensive even after delivery. Early diagnosis and careful management are used to control the disease. Medical treatment for severe preeclampsia includes bed rest in a quiet, darkened room; a regular diet; restoration of fluid and electrolyte balance; sedation; and antihypertensive medications. Glucocorticoids such as betamethasone are used to enhance fetal lung maturity. Phenytoin may be used to control seizures in eclampsia; however, it is not a first-line drug, and it exerts no curative effect on the client's hypertension. Additionally, the drug usually is not prescribed for pregnant women because of the significant risk for fetal malformations. Although reduction of fluid retention may make the client more comfortable, thiazide diuretics can result in serious sodium and potassium depletion, hemorrhagic pancreatitis, and neonatal thrombocytopenia. (A)

22. **4.** The highest priority for a client with severe preeclampsia is to prevent seizures, thereby minimizing the possibility of adverse effects on the mother and fetus, and then to deliver the infant safely. Efforts to decrease edema, reduce blood pressure, increase urine output, limit kidney damage, and maintain sedation are desirable but are not as important as preventing seizures. It would take several days or weeks for the edema to be decreased. Sedation and decreased reflex excitability can occur with the administration of intravenous magnesium sulfate, which peaks in 30 minutes, much sooner than 48 hours. (A)

23. **3.** Magnesium sulfate, an anticonvulsant, acts as a central nervous system depressant by blocking peripheral neuromuscular transmissions and decreasing the amount of acetylcholine liberated. Although the drug relaxes smooth muscle and reduces vasoconstriction, it does not act as a peripheral vasodilator or a sedative-hypnotic. Other drugs, such as hydralazine (Apresoline), labetalol (Normodyne), or nifedipine (Procardia), may be used to control blood pressure in a client with severe preeclampsia. (D)

24. 1. A respiratory rate of 12 breaths/minute suggests potential respiratory depression, an adverse effect of magnesium sulfate therapy. The medication must be stopped and the physician should be notified immediately. A patellar reflex of +2 is normal. Absence of a patellar reflex suggests magnesium toxicity. A blood pressure reading of 160/88 mm Hg would be a common finding in a client with severe preeclampsia. Urinary output exceeding intake is not likely in a client receiving intravenous magnesium sulfate. Oliguria is more common. (D)

25. 1. The most appropriate nursing diagnosis at this time is *Risk for injury* related to possibility of further seizure activity. Unless the client's blood pressure can be brought under control, the risk of another seizure is high. The scenario provides no information to suggest *Deficient knowledge*. Questions about the causes or treatment would suggest a knowledge deficit. *Hypertensive crisis* is a medical diagnosis, not a nursing diagnosis. There is also no basis for a diagnosis of *Situational low self-esteem*. Client statements about her appearance or feeling depressed would suggest a self-esteem disturbance. (R)

26. 3. If a client begins to have a seizure, the first action by the nurse is to remain with the client and call for immediate assistance. The nurse needs to have some assistance in managing this client. After the seizure, the client needs intensive monitoring. An airway can be inserted, if appropriate, after the seizure ends. Noting the time the seizure begins and ends and turning the client to her left side should be done after assistance is obtained. (R)

27. 1. One of the most common adverse effects of the drug hydralazine (Apresoline) is tachycardia. Therefore, the nurse should assess the client's heart rate and pulse. Hydralazine acts to lower blood pressure by peripheral dilation without interfering with placental circulation. Bradypnea and polyuria are usually not associated with hydralazine use. Dysphagia is not a typical adverse effect of hydralazine. (D)

28. 4. These findings would be documented as 4+. 1+ indicates a diminished response; 2+ indicates a normal response; 3+ indicates a response that is brisker than average but not abnormal. Mild clonus is said to be present when there are two movements. (A)

29. 3. Epigastric pain or acute right upper quadrant pain is associated with the development of eclampsia and an impending seizure; this is thought to be related to liver ischemia. Decreased contraction intensity is unrelated to the severity of the preeclampsia. Typically, the client's temperature increases because of increased cerebral pressure. A decrease in temperature is unrelated to an impending seizure. Hyporeflexia is not associated with an impending seizure. Typically, the client would exhibit hyperreflexia. (A)

30. 4. After an eclamptic seizure, the client commonly falls into a deep sleep or coma. The nurse must continually monitor the client for signs of impending labor, because the client will not be able to verbalize that contractions are occurring. Oliguria is more common than polyuria after an eclamptic seizure. Facial flushing is not common unless it is caused by a reaction to a medication. Typically, the client remains hypertensive unless medications such as magnesium sulfate are administered. (A)

31. 1. After an eclamptic seizure, the client is at risk for abruptio placentae due to severe vasoconstriction resulting in hemorrhage into the decidua basalis. Abruptio placentae is manifested by a board-like abdomen and nonreassuring fetal heart rate tracing. Transverse lie or shoulder presentation, placenta accreta, and uterine atony are not related to eclampsia. Causes of a transverse lie may include relaxation of the abdominal wall secondary to grand multiparity, preterm fetus, placenta previa, abnormal uterus, contracted pelvis, and excessive amniotic fluid. Placenta accreta, a rare phenomenon, refers to a condition in which the placenta abnormally adheres to the uterine lining. Uterine atony, or relaxed uterus, may occur after delivery, leading to postpartum hemorrhage. (A)

32. 3. HELLP syndrome refers to a form of severe preeclampsia involving hemolysis, elevated liver enzymes, and low platelet count, also termed thrombocytopenia. This syndrome occurs in 4% to 12% of clients with severe preeclampsia. It is a serious syndrome with a maternal mortality rate as high as 24%. Hypofibrinogenemia is associated with HELLP syndrome because of vascular damage resulting from vasospasm. The increase in liver enzymes in HELLP is a result of obstruction of the hepatic blood flow by fibrin deposits. Hyponatremia may be a complication of HELLP, but it is not one of the underlying problems associated with this condition. (R)

The Pregnant Client with a Chronic Hypertensive Disorder

33. 1. Pregnancy is not the time for clients to begin a diet. Clients with chronic hypertension need to consume adequate calories to support fetal growth and development. They also need an adequate protein intake. Meat and beans are good sources of protein. Most pregnant women report that eating more frequent, smaller meals decreases heartburn resulting from the reflux of acidic secretions into the lower esophagus. Pregnant women need adequate hydration (fluids) and fiber to prevent constipation. (C)

34. 2. Women with chronic hypertension during pregnancy are at risk for complications such as preeclampsia (about 25%), abruptio placentae, and intrauterine growth retardation, resulting in a small-for-gestational-age infant. There is no association between chronic hypertension and hyperthyroidism. Pregnant women with chronic hypertension are not at an increased risk for hydramnios (polyhydramnios), an abnormally large amount of amniotic fluid.

Clients with diabetes and multiple gestations are at risk for this condition. Placenta accreta, a rare placental abnormality, refers to a condition in which the placenta abnormally adheres to the uterine lining. It is not associated with chronic hypertension. (R)

35. 2, 3, 6. Vaginal bleeding with or without pain could signify placenta previa or abruptio placentae. Continuous or pounding headache could indicate an elevated blood pressure, and change in the strength or frequency of fetal movements could indicate that the fetus is in distress. Orthostatic hypotension can occur during pregnancy and can be alleviated by rising slowly. Leg veins may increase in size due to additional pressure from the increasing uterine size, while leg cramps may also occur and can commonly be decreased with calcium supplements. (R)

The Pregnant Client with Third-Trimester Bleeding

36. 3. Urinary output of less than 30 ml/hour indicates renal compromise and would be the most important assessment finding to report to the health care provider. The APTT is within normal limits and the hemoglobin is lower than values for an adult female but within normal limits for a pregnant female. Although the platelet level is slightly low and may impact blood clotting, when compared to renal failure, it is less important. (M)

37. 4. Although the exact cause of abruptio placentae is unknown, possible contributing factors include excessive intrauterine pressure caused by hydramnios or multiple pregnancy, cocaine use, cigarette smoking, alcohol ingestion, trauma, increased maternal age and parity, and amniotomy. A history of hypertension is associated with an increased risk of abruptio placentae. A previous low transverse cesarean section delivery and a history of one induced abortion are associated with increased risk of placenta previa, not abruptio placentae. (A)

38. 2. Treatment of DIC includes treating the causative factor, replacing maternal coagulation factors, and supporting physiologic functions. Intravenous infusions of whole blood, fresh-frozen plasma, or platelets are used to replace depleted maternal coagulation factors. Although Ringer's lactate solution and 5% dextrose solution may be used as intravenous fluid replacement, the client needs blood component therapy. Therefore, normal saline must be used. Intravenous heparin, not warfarin sodium (Coumadin) may be administered to halt the clotting cascade. (A)

39. 1. The most common assessment finding associated with placenta previa is painless vaginal bleeding. With placenta previa, the placenta is abnormally implanted, covering a portion or all of the cervical os. Uterine tetany, intermittent pain with spotting, and dull lower back pain are not associated with placenta previa. Uterine tetany is associated with oxytocin administration. Intermittent pain with spotting commonly is associated with a spontaneous

abortion. Dull lower back pain is commonly associated with poor maternal posture or a urinary tract infection with renal involvement. (A)

40. 2. Bleeding precipitated by placenta previa results from exposure of the maternal sinuses when placental villi are torn from the uterine wall as the lower uterine segment contracts and dilates in the later weeks of pregnancy. The bleeding is not initiated because of diminished clotting factors. Diminished clotting factors are associated with DIC. Increased platelet levels would suggest an increased risk for clotting. A large-for-gestational-age fetus may be related to hereditary factors or diabetes. (A)

41. 3. The client's statement reflects concern for her present fetus based on her previous experience. Therefore, the priority diagnosis is *Anxiety*. This is further supported by the fact that the client is at only 35 weeks' gestation, and delivery at this time most likely would result in a preterm neonate. The client needs a supportive nurse who will allow her to express her feelings. The client may be at *Risk for constipation* after prolonged bed rest, but the priority at this time is the client's anxiety. There is no evidence presented to support a diagnosis of *Interrupted family processes*. Expression of concerns related to the family, such as "I'm worried about my other children," would suggest this diagnosis. A diagnosis of *Impaired physical mobility* is inappropriate because the client is still able to move about in bed. (P)

42. 1. When administering blood replacement therapy, extreme caution is needed. Before administering any blood product, the nurse should validate the client information and the blood product with another nurse to prevent administration of the wrong blood transfusion. Although baseline vital signs are necessary, she should initiate the infusion of blood slowly for the first 10 to 15 minutes. Then, if there is no evidence of a reaction, she should adjust the rate of infusion to ensure that the blood product is infused over 2 to 4 hours. The nurse can ask the client if she has ever had a reaction to a blood product, but a general question about allergies may not elicit the most complete response about any reactions to blood product administration. Blood transfusions are typically given with intravenous normal saline solution, not dextrose solutions. (D)

43. 3. Feelings of loss, grief, and guilt are normal after a cesarean section delivery, particularly if it was not planned. The nurse should support the client, listen with empathy, and allow the client time to grieve. The likelihood of the client experiencing postpartum blues is not known, and no evidence is presented. Although maternal-infant bonding may be delayed owing to neonatal complications or maternal pain and subsequent medications, it should not be difficult. Although the nurse is aware that that this type of delivery was necessary to save the client's life, using this as the basis for the response does not acknowledge the mother's feelings. (P)

44. Epidural anesthesia for a cesarean birth must be at the level of T4 to T6, approximately the nipple line. The level of anesthesia achieved via epidural anesthesia for a vaginal birth is T10 (approximately the hips). (D)

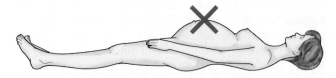

45. **3.** Abruptio placentae is a medical emergency because the degree of hypovolemic shock may be out of proportion to visible blood loss. On admission, the nurse should plan to first insert a large-gauge intravenous catheter for fluid replacement and oxygen by mask to decrease fetal anoxia. Vaginal examination usually is not performed on pregnant clients who are experiencing third-trimester bleeding due to abruptio placentae because it can result in damage to the placenta and further fetal anoxia. The client's history can be obtained once the client has been admitted and the intravenous line has been started. The goal is to get the fetus delivered, usually by emergency cesarean delivery. The nurse should also plan to monitor the client's vital signs and the fetal heart rate. Ultrasound is of limited use in the diagnosis of abruptio placentae. (R)

The Pregnant Client with Preterm Labor

46. **3.** The absence of fetal fibronectin in a vaginal swab between 22 and 37 weeks' gestation indicates there is less than 1% risk of developing preterm labor in the next week. Fetal fibronectin is an extra cellular protein normal found in fetal membranes and deciduas and has no correlation with preeclampsia, fetal lung maturation, or gestational diabetes. (R)

47. **4.** Smoking in any form is contraindicated in pregnancy, regardless of the type of filtering system used. Smoking is a major risk factor for preterm labor and decreased fetal weight. Dehydration is a risk factor for preterm labor as is prolonged standing and remaining in one position. Infection is thought to be a primary cause of preterm labor and the client would need to avoid contracting any type of infection. While taking trips, frequent emptying of the bladder prevents infection and ambulates the woman. (M)

48. **1.** Although the exact cause of preterm labor has not been determined, various risk factors are associated with this condition. Age younger than 19 or older than 40 years has been associated with preterm labor. Other factors associated with preterm labor include polyhydramnios, poor pregnancy weight gain, chronic hypertension, multifetal gestation, prior preterm delivery, cervical incompetence, reproductive tract infection, urinary tract infection, and renal disease. (R)

49. **1.** Indomethacin (Indocin) has been successfully used to halt preterm labor. However, if the client should deliver a preterm infant, the nurse would notify the nursery personnel about the tocolytic therapy because this drug can lead to premature closure of the fetal ductus arteriosus, resulting in pulmonary hypertension. Prematurity is associated with RDS because of the immaturity of the fetal lungs. RDS is not a result of indomethacin. Hyperbilirubinemia is more common in preterm infants. Use of indomethacin to halt preterm labor is not associated with cardiomyopathy in the infant. (D)

50. **2.** The priority nursing diagnosis at this time is *Spiritual distress* related to feelings of guilt. The client is visibly upset, asking why God is punishing her and what she did wrong to cause the preterm labor. The nurse needs to be supportive and allow the client to verbalize her feelings. The client may desire to speak to a member of the clergy. There is no evidence to suggest *Risk for impaired parenting.* Statements about poor mothering abilities or lack of family support would support this diagnosis. Although the client's amniotic fluid is leaking, this may cease with bed rest and other treatments for preterm labor. *Risk for infection* may be a priority later in the client's care. No evidence is suggested to support a diagnosis of *Disturbed body image.* Statements about the client's appearance or body would suggest this diagnosis. (H)

51. **4.** Tachycardia is a common adverse effect of terbutaline therapy. If the client's heart rate is 130 bpm or faster, the nurse should contact the physician before administering the medication. After the drug has been administered, the client should also be carefully monitored for dyspnea or other symptoms of pulmonary edema. Other adverse effects include premature ventricular contractions, increased stroke volume, increased systolic pressure with decreased diastolic pressure, palpitations, tremors, nausea and vomiting, and shortness of breath. Other adverse effects include hyperglycemia, metabolic acidosis, hypokalemia, and anemia. Terbutaline has no known effects on the client's hemoglobin or hematocrit levels, or on weight. However, the drug can cause nausea. Terbutaline may result in perspiration, but there are no known effects on urinary output. (D)

52. **3.** As the uterus contracts, the abdominal wall rises and, when external monitoring is used, presses against the transducer. This movement is transmitted into an electrical current, which is then recorded. With the fetus in the LOA position, the cardiotransducer should be placed below the umbilicus on the side where the fetal back is located and uterine displacement during contractions is greatest. If the fetal back is near the symphysis pubis, the fetus is presenting as a transverse lie. If the fetus is in a breech position, the fetal back may be at or above the umbilicus. (R)

53. **1.** Betamethasone therapy is indicated when the fetal lungs are immature. The fetus must be between 28 and 34 weeks' gestation and delivery must be delayed for

24 to 48 hours for the drug to achieve a therapeutic effect. Antibiotics would be used to treat chorioamnionitis. Betamethasone is not an antagonist for tocolytic therapy. It increases, not decreases, the production of neonatal surfactant. (D)

54. 8

If 10 mg were administered at 10:00 a.m. and 12:00 p.m. and then 20 mg were administered at 4:00 p.m., 8:00 p.m., 10:00 p.m., 12:00 a.m., 4:00 a.m., and 8:00 a.m., the dose at 8:00 a.m. reached the maximum oral dose of 120 mg/day. (D)

55. **2.** For this client, who has experienced two still-births, the most appropriate diagnosis is *Anxiety* related to diagnostic tests for fetal well-being. With most antepartal diagnostic tests, pain is absent or minimal. Information to support the diagnoses of *Ineffective coping* or *Deficient knowledge* is lacking. (R)

56. **4.** The shake test helps determine the maturity of the fetal pulmonary system. The test is based on the fact that surfactant foams when mixed with ethanol. The more stable the foam, the more mature the fetal pulmonary system. Although the shake test is inexpensive and provides rapid results, problems have been noted with its reliability. Therefore, the lecithin-sphingomyelin ratio is usually determined in conjunction with the shake test. (R)

The Pregnant Client with Premature Rupture of the Membranes

57. **3.** Because an intrauterine infection may occur when membranes have ruptured, vaginal cultures for *N. gonorrhoeae*, group B streptococcus, and chlamydia are usually taken. Prophylactic antibiotics may be prescribed to reduce the risk of infection in the newborn. Frequent vaginal examinations should be avoided because they can further increase the client's risk for infection. Intravenous oxytocin to initiate labor may be used if an infection occurs. Bed rest can sometimes prolong the pregnancy and prevent a preterm birth. A sonogram may be used to validate rupture of the membranes with an amniotic fluid index. However, it is not needed if the physician has confirmed the rupture. (R)

58. **3.** If the client's membranes have ruptured, the nitrazine paper will turn blue, an alkaline reaction. False positives may occur when the nitrazine paper is exposed to blood or semen. The definitive test for rupture of membranes is fern testing, where amniotic fluid is allowed to dry on a slide and then viewed under a microscope. Dried amniotic fluid will form a fern pattern. No other fluid forms this type of pattern. (R)

59. **4.** Premature rupture of the membranes is commonly associated with chorioamnionitis, or an infection. A priority assessment for the nurse to make is to document the client's temperature every 2 to 4 hours. Temperature elevation may indicate an infection. Lethargy and an elevated white blood cell count also indicate an infection. The red blood cell count would provide information related to anemia, not infection. The client is not in labor. Therefore, assessing the degree of discomfort is not a priority at this time. Urinary output is not a reliable indicator of an infection such as chorioamnionitis. (R)

60. **1.** Because group B streptococcus is a gram-positive bacteria, the physician probably will order intravenous penicillin to treat the mother's infection and prevent fetal infection. Gentamicin sulfate, which acts on gram-negative bacteria, would be inappropriate. Administering a corticosteroid, such as betamethasone, is inappropriate because the premature rupture of the membranes enhances fetal lung maturity. The lack of amniotic fluid causes early maturation of lung tissue. Cefaclor, which is available only in the oral form, is used for upper and lower respiratory tract infections and urinary tract infections by gram-negative staphylococci. (D)

61. **4.** Because of the client's increased risk for infection, successful teaching is indicated when the client states that she will contact the doctor if her temperature is 100.4° F (38° C) or greater. The client should be instructed to monitor her temperature twice daily. The client should refrain from coitus, douching, and tub bathing, which can increase the potential for infection. Showering is permitted because water in the shower doesn't enter the vagina and increase the risk of infection. A fluid intake of at least 2 L daily is recommended to prevent potential urinary tract infection. (R)

62. **1.** The priority is to determine whether a prolapsed cord has occurred as a result of the spontaneous rupture of membranes. The nurse's first action should be to check the status of the fetal heart rate. Complications of premature rupture of the membranes include a prolapsed cord or increased pressure on the fetal umbilical cord inhibiting fetal nutrient supply. Variable decelerations or fetal bradycardia may be seen on the external fetal monitor. The cord also may be visible. Turning the client to her right side is not necessary. If the cord does prolapse, the client should be placed in a knee-to-chest or Trendelenburg position. Checking the fluid with nitrazine paper and vaginal examination are appropriate once the status of the fetus has been evaluated. (R)

The Pregnant Client with Diabetes Mellitus

63. **3.** Feeling 4 kicks in 30 minutes or feeling 10 or more kicks in 3 hours are norms. Fetuses are more active at various times of the day particularly after a mother has eaten (when the blood glucose level is high) and in the evening. Each individual perceives their fetus to move differently. Fetuses do sleep several times per day for about 30 minutes each time. (S)

64. 4. The nonstress test is considered reactive when two or more fetal heart rate accelerations of at least 15 bpm occur (from a baseline fetal heart rate of 120 to 160 bpm), along with fetal movement, during a 10- to 20-minute period. A reactive nonstress test indicates fetal heart rate accelerations and well-being. There is no indication for further evaluation (such as a contraction stress test). However, contraction stress tests are commonly scheduled for pregnant clients with insulin-dependent diabetes in the latter part of pregnancy and are repeated periodically until delivery. Chorionic villus sampling is usually performed early in the pregnancy to detect fetal abnormalities. (R)

65. 3. A contraction stress test is used to evaluate fetal well-being during a simulated labor. A suspicious contraction stress test indicates inconsistent late deceleration patterns requiring further evaluation. A negative contraction stress test indicates no late decelerations and is the desired outcome. A positive contraction stress test indicates fetal compromise with frequent late decelerations. Fetal movements are one of the parameters of a biophysical profile and are detected with nonstress testing. Decreased or absent fetal movements may indicate central nervous system dysfunction or prematurity. Lack of fetal movement or decreased fetal movement is not associated with contraction stress testing. (R)

66. 2. The fetal biophysical profile, a noninvasive test using real-time ultrasound, assesses five parameters: fetal heart rate reactivity, fetal breathing movements, gross fetal body movements, fetal tone, and amniotic fluid volume. Fetal heart rate reactivity is determined by a nonstress test; the other four parameters are determined by ultrasound scanning. The results are available as soon as the test is completed and interpreted. The lecithin-sphingomyelin ratio is used to determine fetal lung maturity. Although the fetal biophysical profile is useful in predicting which fetuses may be at greater risk for compromise, there is no correlation with the newborn's Apgar score. The biophysical score is sometimes referred to as the fetal Apgar score. A score of 8 to 10 indicates fetal well-being. Use of an ultrasound requires the mother to have a full bladder. (D)

67. 2. During the first trimester, it is not unusual for insulin needs to decrease, commonly as a result of nausea and vomiting. Progressive insulin resistance is characteristic of pregnancy, particularly in the second half of pregnancy. It is not unusual for insulin needs to increase by as much as four times the nonpregnant dose after about the 24th week of gestation. This resistance is caused by the production of human placental lactogen, also called *human chorionic somatotropin*, by the placenta and by other hormones, such as estrogen and progesterone, which are insulin antagonists. (D)

68. 2. Clients who are pregnant and have diabetes are not at greater risk for multifetal pregnancy and subsequent twin-to-twin transfer unless they have undergone fertility treatments. The pregnant diabetic client is at higher risk for complications such as infection, polyhydramnios, ketoacidosis, and preeclampsia, compared with the pregnant nondiabetic client. (R)

69. 2. The goal is to maintain blood plasma glucose levels at 60 to 100 mg/dl before meals and bedtime snacks. A range of 40 to 60 mg/dl indicates hypoglycemia. A range of 110 to 140 mg/dl suggests hyperglycemia. A range of 140 to 160 mg/dl 1 hour after meals suggests hyperglycemia. The target range 1 hour after meals is 100 to 120 mg/dl. (D)

70. 3. Maternal infection is the most common cause of maternal hyperglycemia and can lead to ketoacidosis, coma, and death. The client should notify the physician immediately if she experiences symptoms of an infection. Fetal macrosomia, obesity before conception, and pregnancy-induced hypertension are not associated with maternal hyperglycemia during pregnancy. (A)

71. 1. Dehydration, polyuria, fatigue, flushed hot skin, dry mouth, and drowsiness are manifestations of hyperglycemia. Hyperglycemia is a medical emergency and requires immediate action to prevent maternal and fetal mortality. Pallor, sweating, and nervousness are early signs of hypoglycemia, not hyperglycemia. (R)

72. 4. Stillbirths caused by placental insufficiency occur with increased frequency in women with diabetes and severe preeclampsia. Clients with poorly controlled diabetes may experience unanticipated stillbirth as a result of premature aging of the placenta. Therefore, labor is commonly induced in these clients before term. If induction of labor fails, a cesarean delivery is necessary. Induction and cesarean delivery do not prevent neonatal hyperbilirubinemia, congenital anomalies, or perinatal asphyxia. (R)

73. 3. Maternal hyperglycemia and poor control of the mother's diabetes mellitus have been implicated in fetal macrosomia. When the mother is hyperglycemic, large amounts of amino acids, free fatty acids, and glucose are transferred to the fetus. Although maternal insulin does not cross the placenta, the fetal pancreas responds by hypertrophy of the islet cells of the pancreas. The islet cells produce large amounts of insulin, which acts as a growth hormone. A family history of large infants usually is not the reason for large-for-gestational-age fetuses in diabetic mothers. Maternal hypertension is associated with small-for-gestational-age fetuses because of vasoconstriction of the maternal and placental blood vessels. (A)

74. **1.** Insulin needs fall significantly for the first 24 hours postpartum because the client has usually been on nothing-by-mouth status for a period of time during labor and the labor process has used maternal glycogen stores. If the client breast-feeds, lower blood glucose levels decrease the insulin requirements. With insulin resistance gone, the client commonly needs little or no insulin during the immediate postpartum period. Although the need for insulin decreases during the intrapartum period, the insulin requirements fall further during the first 24 hours postpartum. After the first 24 hours postpartum, insulin requirements may fluctuate markedly, needing adjustment during the next few days as the mother's body returns to a nonpregnant state. (D)

The Pregnant Client with Heart Disease

75. **3.** The client needs a diet that is adequate in protein and calories to prevent anemia, which can place additional strain on the cardiac system, further compromising the client's cardiac status. The client should avoid contact with people who have infections because of the increased risk for developing endocarditis. The client may need antibiotics during the pregnancy to prevent endocarditis. Limiting sodium intake can help to prevent excessive expansion of blood volume and decrease cardiac workload. (R)

76. **4.** Increased dyspnea at rest must be reported immediately because it may be indicative of increasing congestive heart failure. Mild ankle edema in the third trimester is a common finding. However, generalized or pitting edema, suggesting increasing congestive heart failure, must be reported immediately. Emotional stress on the job increases cardiac demand. However, it needs to be reported only if the client experiences symptoms, such as palpitations or irregular heart rate, indicating heart failure related to the increased stress. Weight gain of 1 lb per week is a normal finding during the third trimester. (R)

77. **2.** Unless the client has cardiac decompensation during the pregnancy, she will most likely be able to continue taking the same dose of medication. The client may be prescribed prophylactic antibiotics, particularly if she has had rheumatic fever. The medication would be switched only if digitalis toxicity occurs. A diuretic is added only if congestive heart failure is not controlled by sodium and activity restrictions. (M)

78. **1.** Although there is no completely safe anticoagulant therapy during pregnancy, heparin is typically the drug of choice. Warfarin (Coumadin), a pregnancy category D drug, can cause fetal malformations. Enoxaparin (Lovenox) is not typically prescribed because it can result in thrombocytopenia. Ardeparin (Normiflo) also can cause fetal malformations. (D)

79. **4.** The client can continue a low-sodium diet but should increase the caloric intake to 2,200 calories daily to provide adequate nutrients to support fetal growth and development. Folic acid supplements, a standard component of care, are used to prevent folic acid deficiency, which is associated with megaloblastic anemia during pregnancy. Severe restriction of sodium intake is not recommended because sodium is necessary to maintain fluid volume. Iron supplements should be taken with acidic foods and fluids (e.g., citrus juices) for maximum absorption. Milk decreases the absorption of iron. (R)

The Client with an Ectopic Pregnancy

80. **1.** The client's signs and symptoms indicate a probable ectopic pregnancy, which can be confirmed by ultrasound examination or by culdocentesis. The physician is notified immediately because hypovolemic shock may develop without external bleeding. Once the fallopian tube ruptures, blood will enter the pelvic cavity, resulting in shock. Abruptio placentae would be manifested by a board-like uterus in the third trimester. Gestational trophoblastic disease would be suspected if the client exhibited no fetal heart rate and symptoms of pregnancy-induced hypertension before 20 weeks' gestation. A client with a complete abortion would exhibit a normal pulse and blood pressure with scant vaginal bleeding. (A)

81. **1.** An ectopic pregnancy is defined as any gestation located outside the uterus. About 95% of ectopic pregnancies occur in the fallopian tube. Ectopic pregnancies are the second most common cause of bleeding early in pregnancy; they are commonly associated with pelvic inflammatory disease and scars from tubal surgery. An intestinal implantation is extremely rare, occurring in fewer than 1% of ectopic pregnancies. Interstitial implantation occurs in fewer than 3% of ectopic pregnancies. Ovarian implantation is extremely rare, occurring in fewer than 1% of ectopic pregnancies. (A)

82. **4.** The most appropriate nursing diagnosis for this client is *Anticipatory grieving* related to the loss of the pregnancy. Most women form an emotional attachment to the fetus during the first trimester of pregnancy. This is a crisis for the client, and she needs emotional support. More information, such as a client's expression of being afraid, is needed to support a nursing diagnosis of *Fear* related to surgery. Demonstration of inappropriate behaviors (e.g., screaming or yelling) would be needed to support a nursing diagnosis of *Ineffective coping*. A statement such as "I don't want any scars on my body" would be needed to support a nursing diagnosis of *Disturbed body image*. (P)

83. **2.** Falling hematocrit and hemoglobin levels indicate shock, which occurs if the tube ruptures. Other common symptoms of tubal rupture include severe knife-like lower quadrant abdominal pain and referred shoulder pain. The amount of vaginal bleeding that is evident is a poor estimate of actual blood loss. Slight vaginal bleeding, commonly described as *spotting*, is common. A rapid, thready pulse, a symptom of shock, is more common with tubal rupture than a slow, bounding pulse. Abdominal edema is a late sign of a tubal rupture in ectopic pregnancy. (R)

84. **4.** Fallopian tube rupture is an emergency situation because of extensive bleeding into the peritoneal cavity. Shock soon develops if precautionary measures are not taken. The nurse readying a client for surgery should be especially careful to monitor blood pressure and pulse rate for signs of impending shock. The nurse should be prepared to administer fluids, blood, or plasma expanders as necessary through an intravenous line that should already be in place. Because the fertilized ovum has implanted outside the uterus, uterine cramping is unlikely. However, abdominal tenderness or knife-like pain may occur. Abdominal fullness may be present, but abdominal distention is rare unless peritonitis has developed. Although the hemoglobin and hematocrit may be checked routinely before surgery, the laboratory results may not truly reflect the presence or degree of acute hemorrhage. (R)

85. **3.** Anything that causes a narrowing or constriction in the fallopian tubes so that a fertilized ovum cannot be properly transported to the uterus for implantation predisposes an ectopic pregnancy. Pelvic inflammatory disease is the most common cause of constricted or narrow tubes. Developmental defects are other possible causes. Ectopic pregnancy is not related to urinary tract infections. Use of marijuana during pregnancy is not associated with ectopic pregnancy, but its use can result in cognitive reduction if the mother's use during pregnancy is extensive. Progestin-only contraceptives and intrauterine devices have been associated with ectopic pregnancy. (A)

86. **2.** The client should not experience a headache or dizziness. Symptoms that the client should report include pain (caused by stretching of the tube), temperature elevation (suggesting infection), and bleeding (suggesting hemorrhage). The client should also be instructed that infertility may occur as a result of the removal of one fallopian tube. (R)

87. **3.** Because the fallopian tube has not yet ruptured, methotrexate may be given, followed by leucovorin. This chemotherapeutic agent attacks the fast-growing zygote and trophoblast cells. RU-486 is also effective. A hysterosalpingogram is usually performed after chemotherapy to determine whether the tube is still patent. Progestin-only contraceptives and medroxyprogesterone are ineffective in clearing the fallopian tube. Dyphylline is a bronchodilator and is not used. (D)

The Pregnant Client with Hyperemesis Gravidarum

88. **3.** The client needs further instructions when she says she should eat two meals a day with frequent protein snacks to decrease nausea and vomiting. The client should eat more frequent, smaller meals, with frequent carbohydrate snacks to decrease nausea and vomiting. Eating dry crackers or toast before arising, consuming fluids separately from meals, and avoiding greasy or spicy foods may also help to decrease nausea and vomiting. (C)

89. **3.** Gastrointestinal secretion losses from excessive vomiting, diarrhea, and excessive perspiration can result in hypokalemia, hyponatremia, decreased chloride levels, metabolic alkalosis, and eventual acidosis if precautionary measures are not taken. Ketones may be present in the urine. Dehydration can lead to poor maternal and fetal outcomes. Persistent vomiting can lead to hypocalcemia, not hypercalcemia. Hyperbilirubinemia, not hypobilirubinemia, is typical in clients with hyperemesis. Persistent vomiting may affect liver function and subsequently the excretion of bilirubin from the body. Hypoglycemia, not hyperglycemia, may occur as a result of decreased intake of food and fluids, decreased metabolism of nutrients, and excessive vomiting. (R)

90. **2.** Although the cause of hyperemesis is still unclear, it is thought to be related to high estrogen and human chorionic gonadotropin levels or to trophoblastic activity or gonadotrophin production. Hyperemesis is also associated with infectious conditions, such as hepatitis or encephalitis, intestinal obstruction, peptic ulcer, and hydatidiform mole. Progesterone is a relaxant used during pregnancy and would not stimulate vomiting. Somatotropin is a growth hormone used in children. Aldosterone is a male hormone. (A)

91. **3.** 1,000 ml divided by 8 hours equals 125 ml per hour. (D)

92. **3.** Usually the client remains NPO for at least 24 hours with intravenous therapy. Total parenteral nutrition is started only if other measures fail. If the client is not vomiting after 24 hours, she may be offered clear liquids. If she tolerates liquids, then dry toast, crackers, or cereal may be given every 2 to 3 hours. The client should be given a choice of foods. The temperature of the foods and fluids should be appropriate (i.e., hot foods served hot and cold foods served cold). (A)

The Client with a Hydatidiform Mole

93. 4. The symptoms all support hydatidiform mole. Elevated blood pressure at this point in the pregnancy could indicate chronic hypertension as well as hydatidiform mole. The fundal height is higher than it typically would be at 15 weeks' gestation. The dark brown vaginal bleeding in isolation can indicate an abortion. The continuous nausea and vomiting is abnormal at this point in the pregnancy and can be a result of the high levels of progesterone from a molar pregnancy. When all signs and symptoms are reviewed in relationship to one another, they support the diagnosis of hydatidiform mole. Preeclampsia usually begins after 24 weeks and does not have the same signs and symptoms, other than an increase in blood pressure. Ectopic pregnancy signs and symptoms include pain on one side or the other (bleeding, syncope, referred shoulder pain), which are not seen in this client. The listed signs and symptoms are not indicative of hyperemesis gravidarum. (A)

94. 1. Hydatidiform mole is suspected when the following are present: pregnancy-induced hypertension before the 24th week of gestation, brownish or prune-colored vaginal bleeding, anemia, absence of fetal heart tones, passage of hydropic vessels, uterine enlargement greater than expected for gestational age, and increased human chorionic gonadotrophin levels. Gestational diabetes is related to an increased risk of preeclampsia and urinary tract infections, but it is not associated with hydatidiform mole. Hyperthyroidism, not hypothyroidism, occurs occasionally with hydatidiform mole. If it does occur, it can be a serious complication, possibly life-threatening to the mother and fetus from cardiac problems. Polycythemia is not associated with hydatidiform mole. Rather, anemia from blood loss is associated with molar pregnancies. (R)

95. 2. After D&C to evacuate a molar pregnancy, the nurse should assess the client's vital signs and monitor for signs of hemorrhage, because the surgical procedure may have traumatized the uterine lining, leading to hemorrhage. Urinary tract infections, not common after evacuation of a molar pregnancy, are most commonly related to urinary catheterization. Typically, urinary catheters are not used during evacuation of a molar pregnancy. The client should not experience abdominal distention, because the contents of the uterus have been removed. Chorioamnionitis is an inflammation of the amniotic fluid membranes. With complete mole, no embryonic or fetal tissue or membranes are present. (R)

96. 2. A client who has had a hydatidiform mole removed should have regular checkups to rule out the presence of choriocarcinoma, which may complicate the client's clinical picture. The client's human chorionic gonadotropin (hCG) levels are monitored for 1 year. During this time, she should be advised not to become pregnant because this would be reflected in rising hCG levels. Ectopic or multifetal pregnancy is not associated with hydatidiform mole. Women who have molar pregnancies have fertility rates similar to the general population. (R)

97. 2. A client who has experienced a molar pregnancy is at risk for development of choriocarcinoma and requires close monitoring of human chorionic gonadotropin (hCG) levels. Pregnancy would interfere with monitoring these levels. High hCG titers are common for up to 7 weeks after the evacuation of the mole, but then these levels gradually begin to decline. Clients should have a pelvic examination and a blood test for hCG titers every month for 6 months and then every 2 months for 1 year. Gradually declining hCG levels suggest no complications. Increasing levels are indicative of a malignancy and should be treated with methotrexate. If after 1 year the hCG levels are negative, the client is theoretically free of the risk of a malignancy developing and could plan another pregnancy. (R)

The Pregnant Client with Miscellaneous Complications

98. 4. Herpes simplex virus can be transmitted to the infant during a vaginal delivery. The neonatal effects of herpes are severe enough that a cesarean birth is warranted if active lesions—primary or secondary—are present. A client with a primary infection during pregnancy sheds the virus for up to 3 months after the lesion has healed. The client carrying an infant weighing 8 lb will be given a trial of labor before a cesarean. The client with a fetus in the right occiput posterior position will have a slow labor with increased back pain but can deliver vaginally. The fetus in a breech position still has many weeks to change positions before being at term. At 7 months' gestation, the breech position is not a concern. (A)

99. 4. These signs and symptoms all indicate amniotic fluid embolism, also called *anaphylactoid syndrome*. In this disorder, amniotic fluid enters the maternal circulation and is transported to the mother's lungs. Particulate matter in the fluid, such as vernix and meconium, obstruct the vessels in the pulmonary system. The mortality rate is around 50% if implementation of care is not immediate. In cardiac disease, cardiac arrest may occur but other signs and symptoms are typically noticeable prior to heart failure. There are no symptoms of preeclampsia (high blood pressure, proteinuria) seen with this client. There is no evidence of infection leading to septic shock. (A)

100. 4. Sickle cell disease is an autosomal recessive disorder requiring both parents to have a sickle cell trait to pass the disease to a child. Deoxygenated hemoglobin cells assume a sickle shape and obstruct tissues. Tissue obstruction causes hypoxia to the area (vasoocclusion) and results in pain, called *sickle cell crisis*. This type of anemia is an inherited disorder; it is not caused by lack of iron in the diet. Self-monitoring for any type of infections or sickle cell crisis and increased frequency of antenatal care visits are part of the teaching plan of care. (A)

101. **1.** The nurse should place her hand on the fetal head and provide gentle upward pressure to relieve the compression on the cord. Doing so allows oxygen to continue flowing to the fetus. The cord should never be placed back into the vagina because doing so may further compress it. Administering oxygen is an appropriate measure but will not serve a useful purpose until the pressure is relieved on the cord, enabling perfusion to the infant. Turning the client to her left side facilitates better perfusion to the mother but, until the compression on the cord is relieved, the increased oxygen will not serve its purpose. Placing the client in a Trendelenburg or knee-chest position would be position changes to increase perfusion to the infant by relieving cord compression. (M)

102. **1, 2, 3, 4.** Having the fetus at a negative station places the client at risk for a cord prolapse. With a negative station, there is room between the fetal head and the maternal pelvis for the cord to slip through. A small infant is more mobile within the uterus and the cord can rest between the fetus and the inside of the uterus or below the fetal head. With a large infant, the head is usually in a vertex presentation and occludes the lower portion of the uterus, preventing the cord from slipping by. When membranes rupture, the cord can be swept through with the amniotic fluid. In a breech presentation, the fetal head is in the fundus and smaller portions of the fetus settle into the lower portion of the uterus, allowing the cord to lie beside the fetus. Prior abortion and a low lying placenta have no correlation to cord prolapse. (A)

103. **3.** A postpartum client who saturates a pad in an hour or less at any time in the postpartum period is considered to be hemorrhaging. As the normal postpartum client heals, bleeding changes from red to pink to off-white. It also decreases in amount each day. Passing blood clots the size of a fist or larger is a reportable problem. Lochia varies in how long it lasts and is considered normal up to 6 weeks postpartum. (H)

104. **2.** RhoGAM is given to new mothers who are Rh-negative and not previously sensitized and who have delivered an Rh-positive infant. RhoGAM must be given within 72 hours of the delivery of the infant because antibody formation begins at that time. The vaccine is used only when the mother delivered an Rh-positive infant—not an Rh-negative infant. RhoGAM does not prevent German measles and is not given to a newborn. (D)

105. **2.** The client is experiencing and verbalizing signs of postpartum depression, which usually appears at about 4 weeks postpartum but can occur at any time within the first year after birth. It is more severe and lasts longer than postpartum blues, also called "baby blues." Baby blues are the mildest form of depression and are seen in the later part of the first week after birth. Symptoms usually disappear shortly. Depression may last several years and is disabling to the woman. Poor bonding may be seen at any time but commonly becomes evident as the mother begins interacting with the infant shortly after birth. Infant abuse may take the form of neglect or injuries to the infant. A depressed mother is at risk for injuring or abusing her infant. (R)

106. **2, 3, 7.** The nursing assistant could assist the client with breathing and relaxation, and ambulate the postcesarean client to the bathroom. Removing lunch trays and adding the intake to the input and output sheet is a nursing assistant responsibility. Removing a Foley catheter would also involve assessment of bladder status and totaling the intake and output and would be a nursing responsibility. Calculating the hourly I.V. totals for a preterm labor client would involve assessments that require nursing expertise. In-and-out catheterization, a sterile procedure, and calling reports to health care providers, which requires gathering and analysis of data, are responsibilities of the nurse. (M)

The Birth Experience

- The Primigravid Client in Labor
- The Multigravid Client in Labor
- The Labor Experience
- The Intrapartal Client with Risk Factors
- Correct Answers and Rationales

The Primigravid Client in Labor

1. The physician orders intermittent fetal heart rate monitoring for a 20-year-old obese primigravid client at 40 weeks' gestation who is admitted to the birthing center in the first stage of labor. The nurse would monitor the client's fetal heart rate pattern at which of the following intervals?
- ☐ **1.** Every 15 minutes during the latent phase.
- ☐ **2.** Every 30 minutes during the active phase.
- ☐ **3.** Every 60 minutes during the initial phase.
- ☐ **4.** Every 2 hours during the transition phase.

2. Assessment reveals that the fetus of a primigravid client is at +1 station. The nurse interprets this finding as indicating that the fetal presenting part is positioned at which of the following?
- ☐ **1.** 1 cm above the ischial spines.
- ☐ **2.** 1 cm below the ischial spines.
- ☐ **3.** 1 cm above the ischial tuberosities.
- ☐ **4.** 1 cm below the sacral promontory.

3. Assessment of a primigravid client in active labor who has had no analgesia or anesthesia reveals complete cervical effacement, dilation of 8 cm, and the fetus at 0 station. Which of the following behaviors would the nurse anticipate that the client will exhibit during this phase of labor?
- ☐ **1.** Excitement.
- ☐ **2.** Loss of control.
- ☐ **3.** Numbness of the legs.
- ☐ **4.** Feelings of relief.

4. While caring for a moderately obese primigravid client in active labor at term, the nurse would expect to monitor the client for signs of which of the following?
- ☐ **1.** Hypotonic reflexes.
- ☐ **2.** Increased uterine resting tone.
- ☐ **3.** Soft tissue dystocia.
- ☐ **4.** Increased fear and anxiety.

5. The nurse is caring for a primigravid client in active labor at 42 weeks' gestation. The client has had no analgesia or anesthesia and has been in the second stage of labor for 2½ hours. The nurse determines that the client may be exhibiting symptoms of which of the following?
- ☐ **1.** Cephalopelvic disproportion.
- ☐ **2.** Twin gestation.
- ☐ **3.** Anencephaly.
- ☐ **4.** Breech presentation.

6. The physician has ordered prostaglandin gel to be administered vaginally to a newly admitted primigravid client. Which of the following would indicate to the nurse that the client has had a therapeutic response to the medication?
- ☐ **1.** Resting period of 2 minutes between contractions.
- ☐ **2.** Normal patellar and elbow reflexes for the past 2 hours.
- ☐ **3.** Softening of the cervix and beginning effacement.
- ☐ **4.** Leaking of clear amniotic fluid in small amounts.

7. A primigravid client is admitted as an outpatient for an external cephalic version. For which of the following would the nurse assess the client as a possible contraindication for the procedure?
- ☐ **1.** Multiple gestation.
- ☐ **2.** Breech presentation.
- ☐ **3.** Maternal Rh-negative blood type.
- ☐ **4.** History of gestational diabetes.

8. A primigravida is admitted to the labor suite with ruptured membranes and contractions occurring every 2 to 3 minutes and lasting 45 seconds. After 6 hours of labor, the client's contractions are now every 7 to 10 minutes, lasting 30 seconds. Which of the following would the nurse anticipate that the physician will order?
- ☐ **1.** Morphine sulfate.
- ☐ **2.** Oxytocin (Pitocin).
- ☐ **3.** Nalbuphine (Nubain).
- ☐ **4.** Ampicillin.

9. A primigravid client in the second stage of labor feels the urge to push. The client has had no analgesia or anesthesia. Anatomically, which of the following would be the best position for the client to assume?
- ☐ **1.** Dorsal recumbent.
- ☐ **2.** Lithotomy.
- ☐ **3.** Hands and knees.
- ☐ **4.** Squatting.

10. A 21-year-old primigravid client at 40 weeks' gestation is admitted to the hospital in active labor. The client's cervix is 8 cm and completely effaced at 0 station. During the transition phase of labor, which of the following would the nurse identify as a priority nursing diagnosis?
- ☐ **1.** *Impaired urinary elimination* related to nothing-by-mouth status.
- ☐ **2.** *Risk for injury* related to hyperventilation and dizziness.
- ☐ **3.** *Ineffective coping* related to lack of confidence.
- ☐ **4.** *Pain* related to increasing frequency and intensity of uterine contractions.

11. A 24-year-old primigravid client who delivers a viable term neonate is ordered to receive oxytocin intravenously after delivery of the placenta. Which of the following signs would indicate to the nurse that the placenta is about to be delivered?
- ☐ **1.** The cord lengthens outside the vagina.
- ☐ **2.** There is decreased vaginal bleeding.
- ☐ **3.** The uterus cannot be palpated.
- ☐ **4.** Uterus changes to discoid shape.

12. A primiparous client, who has just delivered a healthy term neonate after 12 hours of labor, holds and looks at her neonate and begins to cry. The nurse correctly interprets this behavior as a sign of which of the following?
- ☐ **1.** Disappointment in the baby's gender.
- ☐ **2.** Grief over the ending of the pregnancy.
- ☐ **3.** A normal response to the birth.
- ☐ **4.** Indication of postpartum "blues."

13. The cervix of a 15-year-old primigravid client admitted to the labor area is 2 cm dilated and 50% effaced. Her membranes are intact, and contractions are occurring every 5 to 6 minutes. Which of the following should the nurse recommend first after the client is admitted?
- ☐ **1.** Resting in the right lateral recumbent position.
- ☐ **2.** Lying in the left lateral recumbent position.
- ☐ **3.** Walking around in the hallway until she gets tired.
- ☐ **4.** Sitting in a comfortable chair for a period of time.

14. Which of the following would the nurse include in the teaching plan for a 16-year-old primigravid client in early labor concerning active relaxation techniques to help her cope with pain?
- ☐ **1.** Relaxing uninvolved body muscles during uterine contractions.
- ☐ **2.** Practicing being in a deep, meditative, sleeplike state.
- ☐ **3.** Focusing on an object in the room during the contractions.
- ☐ **4.** Breathing rapidly and deeply between contractions.

15. A primigravid client in early labor asks the nurse what effleurage means. The nurse explains that effleurage is a type of massage involving which of the following?
- ☐ **1.** Deep kneading of superficial muscles.
- ☐ **2.** Secure grasping of muscular tissues.
- ☐ **3.** Light stroking of the skin surface.
- ☐ **4.** Prolonged pressure on specific sites.

16. A 24-year-old primigravid client in active labor requests use of the jet hydrotherapy tub to aid in pain relief. The nurse bases the response on the understanding that this therapy is commonly contraindicated for clients with which of the following?
- ☐ **1.** Ruptured membranes.
- ☐ **2.** Multifetal gestation.
- ☐ **3.** Diabetes mellitus.
- ☐ **4.** Hypotonic labor patterns.

17. A primigravid client admitted to the labor area in early labor tells the nurse that her brother was born with cystic fibrosis. When teaching the client about this disorder, the nurse understands that this disorder is considered as which of the following?
- ☐ **1.** X-linked recessive.
- ☐ **2.** X-linked dominant.
- ☐ **3.** Autosomal recessive.
- ☐ **4.** Autosomal dominant.

18. The physician orders an amniocentesis for a primigravid client at 37 weeks' gestation in early labor to determine fetal lung maturity. The nurse expects the fluid sample to be tested for which of the following?
- ☐ **1.** Amount of bilirubin present.
- ☐ **2.** Presence of red blood cells.
- ☐ **3.** Barr body determination.
- ☐ **4.** Lecithin-sphingomyelin (L/S) ratio.

19. Assessment of a 15-year-old primigravid client at term in active labor reveals cervical dilation at 7 cm with complete effacement. Because the client is only 15 years old, which of the following would the nurse assess the client for during labor?
- ☐ **1.** Uterine inversion.
- ☐ **2.** Cephalopelvic disproportion (CPD).
- ☐ **3.** Rapid third stage of labor.
- ☐ **4.** Decreased ability to push.

20. The nurse is working on a busy labor and delivery unit with other nurses and a licensed practical nurse. Which of the following labor clients would the nurse assign to the licensed practical nurse?
☐ **1.** A G 4, P 3 client with a history of gestational diabetes.
☐ **2.** A G 3, P 1, Ab 1 client at 35 weeks' gestation.
☐ **3.** A G 1, P 0 client with leaking green amniotic fluid.
☐ **4.** A G 2, P 1 client with a history of hyperemesis gravidarum.

21. A 19-year-old primigravid client at 38 weeks' gestation is admitted to the hospital in active labor that began 8 hours ago. When the client's cervix is 7 cm dilated and the presenting part is at +1 station, the client tells the nurse, "I need to push!" Which of the following would the nurse do next?
☐ **1.** Use the McDonald procedure to widen the pelvic opening.
☐ **2.** Increase the rate of oxygen and intravenous fluids.
☐ **3.** Instruct the client to use a pant-blow pattern of breathing.
☐ **4.** Tell the client to push only when absolutely necessary.

22. Which of the following would be the priority when caring for a primigravid client whose cervix is dilated at 8 cm when the fetus is at 1+ station and the client has had no analgesia or anesthesia?
☐ **1.** Giving frequent sips of water.
☐ **2.** Applying extra blankets for warmth.
☐ **3.** Providing frequent perineal cleansing.
☐ **4.** Offering encouragement and support.

23. To determine whether a primigravid client in labor with a fetus in the left occipitoanterior (LOA) position is completely dilated, the nurse performs a vaginal examination. During the examination the nurse would expect to palpate which of the following cranial sutures?
☐ **1.** Sagittal.
☐ **2.** Lambdoidal.
☐ **3.** Coronal.
☐ **4.** Frontal.

24. After a lengthy labor process, a primigravid client delivers a healthy newborn boy with a moderate amount of skull molding. Which of the following would the nurse include when explaining to the parents about this condition?
☐ **1.** It is typically seen with breech deliveries.
☐ **2.** It usually lasts a day or two before resolving.
☐ **3.** It is unusual when the brow is the presenting part.
☐ **4.** Surgical intervention may be necessary to alleviate pressure.

25. A primiparous client has just delivered her baby. The physician has informed the labor nurse that he believes the uterus has inverted. Which signs or symptoms would help to confirm this diagnosis? Select all that apply.
☐ **1.** Hypotension.
☐ **2.** Gush of blood from the vagina.
☐ **3.** Intense, severe, tearing type of abdominal pain.
☐ **4.** Uterus is hard and in a constant state of contraction.
☐ **5.** Inability to palpate the uterus.
☐ **6.** Diaphoresis.

26. After delivery of a viable neonate, a 20-year-old primiparous client comments to her mother and the nurse about the baby. Which of the following comments would the nurse interpret as a possible sign of potential maternal-infant bonding problems?
☐ **1.** "He's got my funny-looking ears!"
☐ **2.** "I think my mother should give him the first feeding."
☐ **3.** "He's a lot bigger than I expected him to be."
☐ **4.** "I want to buy him a blue outfit to wear when we get home."

27. Assessment of a 23-year-old primigravid client at term who is admitted to the birthing unit in active labor reveals that her cervix is 4 cm dilated and 100% effaced. Contractions are occurring every 4 minutes. When developing the teaching plan about the gate-control theory of pain, which of the following statements would the nurse expect to include?
☐ **1.** Input from the large sensory fibers opens the gate.
☐ **2.** Labor pain is a matter of individual perception.
☐ **3.** Slow abdominal breathing can open the gate.
☐ **4.** The gating mechanism is in the spinal cord.

28. The nurse explains to a newly admitted primigravid client in active labor that, according to the gate-control theory of pain, a closed gate means that the client should experience which of the following?
☐ **1.** No pain.
☐ **2.** Sharp pain.
☐ **3.** Light pain.
☐ **4.** Moderate pain.

29. The cervix of a primigravid client in active labor who received epidural anesthesia 4 hours ago is now completely dilated, and the client is ready to begin pushing. Before the client begins to push, which of the following would the nurse assess?
☐ **1.** Fetal heart rate variability.
☐ **2.** Cervical dilation again.
☐ **3.** Status of membranes.
☐ **4.** Bladder status.

30. For the past 8 hours, a 20-year-old primigravid client in active labor with intact membranes has been experiencing regular contractions. The fetal heart rate is 136 bpm with good variability. After determining that the client is still in the latent phase of labor, for which of the following would the nurse expect to observe the client closely?
☐ **1.** Exhaustion.
☐ **2.** Chills and fever.
☐ **3.** Fluid overload.
☐ **4.** Meconium-stained fluid.

31. A primigravid client whose cervix is 7 cm dilated with the fetus at 0 station and in a left occipitoposterior (LOP) position requests pain relief for severe back pain. In developing the plan of care for this client, the nurse would anticipate which of the following?
☐ **1.** Providing firm pressure to the client's sacral area.
☐ **2.** Preparing the client for a cesarean delivery.
☐ **3.** Preparing the client for a precipitate delivery.
☐ **4.** Maintaining the client in a left side-lying position.

32. A primigravid client in active labor has had no anesthesia. The client's cervix is 7 cm dilated, and she is starting to feel considerable discomfort during contractions. The nurse suggests that the client change from slow chest breathing to which of the following?
☐ **1.** Rapid, shallow chest breathing.
☐ **2.** Deep chest breathing.
☐ **3.** Rapid pant-blow breathing.
☐ **4.** Slow abdominal breathing.

33. A 16-year-old primigravid client, with a history of attending one prenatal visit, is admitted to the hospital in active labor at 37 weeks' gestation. Her cervix is 7 cm dilated with the presenting part at 0 station. She enters the labor unit appearing anxious and hyperventilating. Because of the hyperventilation, the nurse would assess the client for symptoms of which of the following?
☐ **1.** Metabolic alkalosis.
☐ **2.** Metabolic acidosis.
☐ **3.** Respiratory alkalosis.
☐ **4.** Respiratory acidosis.

34. The physician orders scalp stimulation of the fetal head for a primigravid client in active labor. When explaining to the client about this procedure, which of the following would the nurse include as the purpose?
☐ **1.** Assessment of the fetal hematocrit level.
☐ **2.** Increase in the strength of the contractions.
☐ **3.** Increase in the fetal heart rate and variability.
☐ **4.** Assessment of fetal position.

35. The nurse is caring for a primigravid client in active labor who has had two fetal blood samplings to check for fetal hypoxia. The nurse determines that the fetus is showing signs of acidosis when the scalp blood pH is below which of the following?
☐ **1.** 7.5.
☐ **2.** 7.4.
☐ **3.** 7.3.
☐ **4.** 7.2.

36. Assessment of a primigravid client reveals cervical dilation at 8 cm and complete effacement. The client complains of severe back pain during this phase of labor. The nurse explains that the client's severe back pain is most likely caused by the fetal occiput being in a position that is identified as which of the following?
☐ **1.** Breech.
☐ **2.** Transverse.
☐ **3.** Posterior.
☐ **4.** Anterior.

37. The nurse assesses a primiparous client in labor for 20 hours. The nurse identifies late decelerations on the monitor and initiates standard procedures for the labor client with this wave pattern. Which interventions should the nurse perform? Select all that apply.
☐ **1.** Administering oxygen via mask to the client.
☐ **2.** Questioning the client about the effectiveness of pain relief.
☐ **3.** Placing the client on her side.
☐ **4.** Readjusting the monitor to a more comfortable position.
☐ **5.** Applying an internal fetal monitor to help identify the cause of the decelerations.

38. When performing Leopold's maneuvers on a primigravid client, the nurse is palpating the uterus as shown below. Which of the following maneuvers is the nurse performing?
☐ **1.** First maneuver.
☐ **2.** Second maneuver.
☐ **3.** Third maneuver.
☐ **4.** Fourth maneuver.

39. Before placing the fetal monitoring device on a primigravid client's fundus, the nurse performs Leopold's maneuvers. When performing the third maneuver, the nurse explains that this maneuver is done for which of the following reasons?
- ☐ **1.** To determine whether the fetal presenting part is engaged.
- ☐ **2.** To locate the fetal cephalic prominence.
- ☐ **3.** To distinguish between a breech and a cephalic presentation.
- ☐ **4.** To locate the position of the fetal arms and legs.

40. A primigravid client in active labor with a fetus in LOP position complains of severe back pressure. Which of the following would be the priority nursing diagnosis for this client?
- ☐ **1.** *Anxiety* related to fear of maternal-fetal outcomes.
- ☐ **2.** *Ineffective coping* related to lack of experience in labor.
- ☐ **3.** *Urinary retention* related to prolonged labor process.
- ☐ **4.** *Pain* related to occipitoposterior position and prolonged fetal descent.

41. One-half hour after vaginal delivery of a term neonate, the nurse palpates the fundus of a primigravid client, noting several large clots and a small trickle of bright red vaginal bleeding. The client's blood pressure is 136/92 mm Hg. Which of the following would the nurse do next?
- ☐ **1.** Continue to monitor the client's fundus every 15 minutes.
- ☐ **2.** Ask the physician for an order for methylergonovine (Methergine).
- ☐ **3.** Immediately notify the physician of the client's symptoms.
- ☐ **4.** Change the client's perineal pads every 15 minutes.

The Multigravid Client in Labor

42. A multigravida in active labor is 7 cm dilated. The fetal heart rate baseline is 130 bpm with moderate variability. The client begins to have variable decelerations to 100 to 110 bpm. What should the nurse do next?
- ☐ **1.** Perform a vaginal examination.
- ☐ **2.** Notify the physician of the decelerations.
- ☐ **3.** Reposition the client and continue to evaluate the tracing.
- ☐ **4.** Administer oxygen via mask at 2 L/minute.

43. A nurse is preparing a change-of-shift report and has been caring for a multigravid client with a normally progressing labor. Which of the following information should be part of this report? Select all that apply.
- ☐ **1.** Interpretation of the fetal monitor strip.
- ☐ **2.** Analgesia or anesthesia being used.
- ☐ **3.** Anticipated method of birth control.
- ☐ **4.** Amount of vaginal bleeding or discharge.
- ☐ **5.** Support persons with the client.
- ☐ **6.** Prior delivery history.

44. A multigravid client is admitted at 4-cm dilation and requesting pain medication. The nurse gives the client Nubain 15 mg and Phenergan 25 mg slow I.V. push. Within five minutes, the client tells the nurse she feels like she needs to have a bowel movement. Which intervention by the nurse would be the priority?
- ☐ **1.** Have naloxone hydrochloride (Narcan) available in the delivery room.
- ☐ **2.** Complete a vaginal examination to determine dilation, effacement, and station.
- ☐ **3.** Prepare for delivery.
- ☐ **4.** Document the client's relief due to pain medication.

45. A multigravid laboring client has an extensive documented history of drug addiction. Her last reported usage was 5 hours ago. She is 2 cm dilated with contractions every 3 minutes of moderate intensity. The physician orders nalbuphine (Nubain) 15 mg slow I.V. push for pain relief followed by an epidural when the client is 4 cm dilated. Within 10 minutes of receiving the nalbuphine, the client states she thinks she is going to have her baby now. Of the following drugs available at the time of the delivery, which should the nurse avoid using with this client in this situation?
- ☐ **1.** 1% lidocaine (Xylocaine).
- ☐ **2.** Naloxone hydrochloride (Narcan).
- ☐ **3.** Local anesthetic.
- ☐ **4.** Pudendal block.

46. A 31-year-old multigravid client at 39 weeks' gestation admitted to the hospital in active labor is receiving intravenous lactated Ringer's solution and a continuous epidural anesthetic. During the first hour after administration of the anesthetic, the nurse would monitor the client for which of the following?
- ☐ **1.** Hypotension.
- ☐ **2.** Diaphoresis.
- ☐ **3.** Headache.
- ☐ **4.** Tremors.

47. A 30-year-old G 3, P 2 is being monitored internally. She is being induced with I.V. oxytocin (Pitocin) because she is overdue. The nurse notes the pattern below. The client is wedged to her side while lying in bed and is approximately 6 cm dilated and 100% effaced. What is the first nursing intervention?

☐ **1.** Continue to observe.
☐ **2.** Anticipate rupture of the membranes.
☐ **3.** Prepare for fetal oximetry.
☐ **4.** Discontinue the Pitocin infusion.

48. The nurse, while shopping in a local department store, hears a multiparous woman say loudly, "I think the baby's coming." After asking someone to call 911, the nurse assists the client to deliver a term neonate. While waiting for the ambulance, the nurse suggests that the mother initiate breast-feeding, primarily for which of the following reasons?

☐ **1.** To begin the parental-infant bonding process.
☐ **2.** To prevent neonatal hypothermia.
☐ **3.** To provide glucose to the neonate.
☐ **4.** To contract the mother's uterus.

49. Approximately 15 minutes after delivery of a viable term neonate, a multiparous client complains of a chill. Which of the following would the nurse do next?

☐ **1.** Assess the client's pulse rate.
☐ **2.** Decrease the rate of intravenous fluids.
☐ **3.** Provide the client with a warm blanket.
☐ **4.** Assess the amount of blood loss.

50. The physician plans to perform an amniotomy on a multiparous client admitted to the labor area at 41 weeks' gestation for labor induction. After the amniotomy, which of the following would the nurse expect do first?

☐ **1.** Monitor the client's contraction pattern.
☐ **2.** Assess the fetal heart rate (FHR) for 1 full minute.
☐ **3.** Assess the client's temperature and pulse.
☐ **4.** Document the color of the amniotic fluid.

51. Which of the following nursing diagnoses would the nurse identify as the priority after delivery for a multiparous client who received an epidural anesthetic?

☐ **1.** *Pain* related to episiotomy and exhaustive pushing efforts.
☐ **2.** *Anxiety* related to inability to move legs and toes.
☐ **3.** *Risk for injury* related to epidural anesthesia.
☐ **4.** *Excess fluid volume* overload related to labor process and intravenous fluids.

52. Which of the following would the nurse expect as a common finding for a multiparous client delivering a viable neonate at 41 weeks' gestation with the aid of a vacuum extractor?

☐ **1.** Caput succedaneum.
☐ **2.** Cephalohematoma.
☐ **3.** Maternal lacerations.
☐ **4.** Neonatal intracranial hemorrhage.

53. The nurse is assessing fetal presentation in a multiparous client. The illustration below indicates which of the following types of presentation?

☐ **1.** Frank breech.
☐ **2.** Complete breech.
☐ **3.** Footling breech.
☐ **4.** Vertex.

54. Two hours ago, a multigravid client was admitted in active labor with her cervix dilated at 5 cm and completely effaced and the fetus at 0 station. Currently, the client is experiencing nausea and vomiting, a slight chill with perspiration beads on her lip, and extreme irritability. Which of the following actions would be most appropriate at this time?

☐ **1.** Warm the temperature of the room by a few degrees.
☐ **2.** Increase the rate of intravenous fluid administration.
☐ **3.** Obtain an order for an intramuscular antiemetic medication.
☐ **4.** Assess the client's cervical dilation and station.

55. When assessing the frequency of contractions of a multiparous client in active labor admitted to the birthing area, the nurse should assess the interval between which of the following?

☐ **1.** Acme of one contraction to the beginning of the next contraction.
☐ **2.** Beginning of one contraction to the end of the next contraction.
☐ **3.** End of one contraction to the end of the next contraction.
☐ **4.** Beginning of one contraction to the beginning of the next contraction.

56. While a client is being admitted to the birthing unit she states, "My water broke last night, but my labor started two hours ago." Which of the following assessment findings would be cause for concern? Select all that apply.

☐ **1.** Maternal vital signs: T. 99.5, HR 80, R 24, BP 130/80 mm Hg.

☐ **2.** Blood and mucus on perineal pad.

☐ **3.** Baseline fetal heart rate of 140 with a range between 110 and 160 with contractions.

☐ **4.** Peripad stained with green fluid.

☐ **5.** The client states, "This baby wants out—he keeps kicking me."

57. While the nurse is caring for a multiparous client in active labor at 36 weeks' gestation, the client tells the nurse, "I think my water just broke." Which of the following would the nurse do first?

☐ **1.** Turn the client to the right side.

☐ **2.** Assess the color, amount, and odor of the fluid.

☐ **3.** Assess the fetal heart rate pattern.

☐ **4.** Check the client's cervical dilation.

58. The nurse has obtained a urine specimen from a G 6, P 5 client admitted to the labor unit. The woman asks to go to the bathroom and reports that she feels she has to move her bowels. Which actions would be appropriate? Select all that apply.

☐ **1.** Assisting her to the bathroom.

☐ **2.** Applying an external fetal monitor to obtain fetal heart rate.

☐ **3.** Assessing her stage of labor.

☐ **4.** Asking if she had back labor pains like this with any of her other deliveries.

☐ **5.** Allowing her support person to take her to the bathroom to maintain privacy.

☐ **6.** Checking the degree of fetal descent.

59. A multigravid client admitted to the labor area is scheduled for a cesarean delivery under spinal anesthesia. After instructions by the anesthesiologist, the nurse determines that the client has understood the instructions when she says which of the following?

☐ **1.** "The medication will be administered while I am in a side-lying position."

☐ **2.** "The anesthetic may cause a severe headache which is treatable."

☐ **3.** "My blood pressure may increase if I lie down too soon after the injection."

☐ **4.** "I can expect immediate anesthesia that can be reversed very easily."

60. When developing the plan of care for a multiparous client in active labor who receives an epidural anesthetic, which of the following would the nurse anticipate that the physician will order if the client develops moderate hypotension?

☐ **1.** Ephedrine sulfate.

☐ **2.** Epinephrine (Adrenalin Chloride).

☐ **3.** Methylergonovine (Methergine).

☐ **4.** Atropine sulfate.

61. The physician determines that the fetus of a multiparous client in active labor is in distress, necessitating a cesarean delivery with general anesthesia. Before the cesarean delivery, the anesthesiologist orders cimetidine (Tagamet) 300 mg PO. The nurse prepares to administer this drug based on the understanding that it reduces which of the following?

☐ **1.** Incidence of bronchospasm.

☐ **2.** Oral and respiratory secretions.

☐ **3.** Acid level of the stomach contents.

☐ **4.** Incidence of postoperative gastric ulcer.

62. The nurse prepares a client for lumbar epidural anesthesia. Before anesthesia administration, the nurse instructs the client to assume which of the following positions?

☐ **1.** Lithotomy.

☐ **2.** Side-lying.

☐ **3.** Knee-to-chest.

☐ **4.** Prone.

63. The nurse is assessing the perineal changes of a multigravid client in the second stage of labor. The illustration below represents which of the following perineal changes?

☐ **1.** Anterior-posterior slit.

☐ **2.** Oval opening.

☐ **3.** Circular shape.

☐ **4.** Crowning.

64. After suctioning to clear the airway of a term neonate who appears in good condition after spontaneous vaginal delivery, which of the following would the nurse do next?

☐ **1.** Place the infant in a radiant warmer.

☐ **2.** Instill erythromycin in the eyes.

☐ **3.** Obtain the neonate's weight.

☐ **4.** Put identification bracelets on each wrist.

The Labor Experience

65. A client is admitted at 30 weeks' gestation with contractions every 3 minutes. Her cervix is 1 to 2 cm dilated and 75% effaced. Following a 4-g bolus dose, I.V. magnesium sulfate is infusing at 2 g/hour. How will the nurse know the medication is having the intended effect?
- ☐ 1. Contractions will increase in frequency, leading to delivery.
- ☐ 2. The client will maintain a respiratory rate greater than 12 breaths per minute.
- ☐ 3. Contractions will decrease in frequency, intensity, and duration.
- ☐ 4. The client will maintain blood pressure readings of 120/80 mm Hg.

66. A client at 33 weeks' gestation is admitted in preterm labor. She is given betamethasone (Celestone) 12 mg I.M. q 24 hours × 2. What is the expected outcome of this drug therapy?
- ☐ 1. The contractions will end within 24 hours.
- ☐ 2. The client will deliver a neonate without respiratory distress.
- ☐ 3. The client will deliver a full-term neonate.
- ☐ 4. The neonate will be delivered with mature lungs.

67. A full-term client is admitted for an induction of labor. The health care provider has assigned a Bishop score of 10. Which drug would the nurse anticipate administering to this client?
- ☐ 1. Oxytocin (Pitocin) 10 units in 500 ml D_5W.
- ☐ 2. Prostaglandin gel (Prepidil) 0.5 mg.
- ☐ 3. Misoprostol (Cytotec) 50 mcg P.O.
- ☐ 4. Dinoprostone (Cervidil) 10 mg.

68. A full-term client is admitted for induction of labor. When admitted, her cervix is 25/0. The initial goal is cervical ripening prior to labor induction. Which drug will prepare her cervix for induction?
- ☐ 1. Nalbuphine (Nubain).
- ☐ 2. Oxytocin (Pitocin).
- ☐ 3. Dinoprostone (Cervidil).
- ☐ 4. Betamethasone (Celestone).

69. The nurse is explaining the medication options available for pain relief during labor. The nurse realizes the client needs further teaching when the client states which of the following?
- ☐ 1. "Nubain (nalbuphine) and Phenergan (promethazine) will give relief from pain and nausea during early labor."
- ☐ 2. "I can have an epidural as soon as I start contracting."
- ☐ 3. "If I have a cesarean, I can have an epidural."
- ☐ 4. "If I have an emergency cesarean, I may be put to sleep for the delivery."

70. The health care provider has performed an amniotomy on a laboring client. Which of the following details must be included in the documentation of this procedure? Select all that apply.
- ☐ 1. Time of rupture.
- ☐ 2. Color and clarity of fluid.
- ☐ 3. Fetal heart rate (FHR) and pattern before and after the procedure.
- ☐ 4. Size of amnio-hook used during the procedure.
- ☐ 5. Odor and amount of fluid.

71. Following an epidural and placement of internal monitors, a client's labor is augmented. Contractions are lasting greater than 90 seconds and occurring every 1½ minutes. The uterine resting tone is greater than 20 mm mercury with a nonreassuring fetal heart rate and pattern. Which of the following actions should the nurse take first?
- ☐ 1. Notify the health care provider.
- ☐ 2. Turn off the oxytocin (Pitocin) infusion.
- ☐ 3. Turn the client to her left side.
- ☐ 4. Increase the maintenance I.V. fluids.

72. A client is induced with oxytocin (Pitocin). The fetal heart rate is showing accelerations lasting 15 seconds and exceeding the baseline with fetal movement. What action associated with this finding should the nurse take?
- ☐ 1. Turn the client to her left side.
- ☐ 2. Administer oxygen via facemask at 10 to 12 L/minute.
- ☐ 3. Notify the health care provider of the situation.
- ☐ 4. Document fetal well-being.

73. As a nurse begins her shift on the obstetrical unit, there are several new admissions. The client with which of the following conditions would be a candidate for induction?
- ☐ 1. Pregnancy-induced hypertension (PIH).
- ☐ 2. Active herpes.
- ☐ 3. Face presentation.
- ☐ 4. Fetus with late decelerations.

74. A nurse and an LPN are working in the labor and delivery unit. Of the following assessments and interventions that must be done immediately, which should the nurse assign to the LPN?
- ☐ 1. Complete an initial assessment on a client.
- ☐ 2. Increase the oxytocin (Pitocin) rate on a laboring client.
- ☐ 3. Perform a straight catheterization for protein analysis.
- ☐ 4. Assess a laboring client for a change in labor pattern.

75. A nurse and a nursing assistant are caring for clients in a labor and delivery unit. Which task should the registered nurse assign to the nursing assistant?
- ☐ 1. Perform a fundal check on a 2-day postpartum client.
- ☐ 2. Remove a fetal monitor and assist a client to the bathroom.
- ☐ 3. Give ibuprofen 800 mg by mouth to a newly delivered client.
- ☐ 4. Teach a new mother how to bottle-feed her infant.

76. A laboring client smiles pleasantly at the nurse when asked simple questions. The client speaks no English and the interpreter is busy with an emergency situation. At her last vaginal examination, the client was 5 cm dilated, 100% effaced, and at 0 station. While working with this client, which of the following responses indicates to the nurse that the client may be approaching delivery?
- ☐ 1. The fetal monitor strip shows late decelerations.
- ☐ 2. The client begins to speak to her family in her native language.
- ☐ 3. The fetal monitor strip shows early decelerations.
- ☐ 4. The client's facial expressions become animated.

The Intrapartal Client with Risk Factors

77. A client is admitted with a suspected abruptio placentae. The nurse would anticipate the client to have which of the following signs and symptoms? Select all that apply.
- ☐ 1. Bleeding that is concealed or apparent.
- ☐ 2. Abdominal rigidity.
- ☐ 3. Painful abdomen.
- ☐ 4. Painless bleeding.
- ☐ 5. Large placenta.
- ☐ 6. Bleeding that stops spontaneously.

78. A multigravid client is in active labor with twins at 38 weeks' gestation. The nurse should monitor the client closely for symptoms of which of the following?
- ☐ 1. Pregnancy-induced hypertension.
- ☐ 2. Urinary tract infection.
- ☐ 3. Chorioamnionitis.
- ☐ 4. Precipitous delivery.

79. A 39-year-old multigravid client at 39 weeks' gestation admitted to the hospital in active labor has been diagnosed with class II heart disease. To ensure cardiac emptying and adequate oxygenation during labor, the nurse plans to encourage the client to do which of the following?
- ☐ 1. Breathe slowly after each contraction.
- ☐ 2. Avoid the use of analgesics for the labor pain.
- ☐ 3. Remain in a side-lying position with the head elevated.
- ☐ 4. Request local anesthesia for vaginal delivery.

80. When developing the plan of care for a multigravid client with class III heart disease, which of the following areas should the nurse expect to assess frequently?
- ☐ 1. Dehydration.
- ☐ 2. Nausea and vomiting.
- ☐ 3. Iron-deficiency anemia.
- ☐ 4. Tachycardia.

81. A multigravid client in active labor has been diagnosed with class II heart disease and has had a prosthetic valve replacement. When developing the plan of care for this client, the nurse should anticipate that the physician most likely will order which of the following medications?
- ☐ 1. Anticoagulants.
- ☐ 2. Antibiotics.
- ☐ 3. Diuretics.
- ☐ 4. Folic acid supplements.

82. A primigravid client at 39 weeks' gestation is admitted to the hospital for induction of labor. The physician has ordered prostaglandin E_2 gel (Dinoprostone) for the client. Before administering prostaglandin E_2 gel to the client, which of the following should the nurse do first?
- ☐ 1. Assess the frequency of uterine contractions.
- ☐ 2. Place the client in a side-lying position.
- ☐ 3. Determine whether the membranes have ruptured.
- ☐ 4. Prepare the client for an amniotomy.

83. A multigravid client at 39 weeks' gestation diagnosed with insulin-dependent diabetes is admitted for induction of labor with oxytocin (Pitocin). Which of the following should the nurse include in the teaching plan as a possible disadvantage of this procedure?
- ☐ 1. Urinary frequency.
- ☐ 2. Maternal hypoglycemia.
- ☐ 3. Preterm birth.
- ☐ 4. Neonatal jaundice.

84. Which of the following nursing diagnoses would be the priority for a multigravid diabetic client at 38 weeks' gestation who is scheduled for labor induction with oxytocin (Pitocin)?
- ☐ 1. *Risk for deficient fluid volume* related to oxytocin infusion.
- ☐ 2. *Pain* related to prolonged labor and uterine ischemia.
- ☐ 3. *Fear* related to possible need for cesarean delivery.
- ☐ 4. *Risk for injury, maternal or fetal,* related to potential uterine hyperstimulation.

85. A multigravid client is receiving oxytocin (Pitocin) augmentation. When the client's cervix is dilated to 6 cm, her membranes rupture spontaneously with meconium-stained amniotic fluid. Which of the following actions should the nurse do next?
- ☐ 1. Increase the rate of the oxytocin infusion.
- ☐ 2. Turn the client to a knee-to-chest position.
- ☐ 3. Assess cervical dilation and effacement.
- ☐ 4. Monitor the fetal heart rate continuously.

86. A multigravid client in active labor at 39 weeks' gestation has a history of smoking one to two packs of cigarettes daily. For which of the following should the nurse be alert when assessing the client's neonate?
- ☐ **1.** Hyperirritability.
- ☐ **2.** Hyperbilirubinemia.
- ☐ **3.** Low birth weight.
- ☐ **4.** Hypocalcemia.

87. A primigravid client who has had a prolonged labor but now is completely dilated has received epidural anesthesia. Which of the following should the nurse expect to include in the teaching plan about pushing?
- ☐ **1.** The client needs to push for at least 1 to 3 minutes.
- ☐ **2.** Pushing is most effective when the client holds her breath.
- ☐ **3.** The client should be urged to push with an open glottis.
- ☐ **4.** Pushing is limited to times when she feels the urge.

88. The physician determines that outlet forceps are needed to assist in the delivery of a primigravid client in active labor with a large-for-gestational-size fetus. The nurse reinforces the physician's explanation for using forceps based on the understanding about which of the following concerning the location of the fetal skull?
- ☐ **1.** It is engaged past the inlet.
- ☐ **2.** It is at +1 station.
- ☐ **3.** It is visible at the perineal floor.
- ☐ **4.** It has reached the level of the ischial spines.

89. The physician orders an amnioinfusion for a primigravid client at term who is diagnosed with oligohydramnios. Which of the following should the nurse include in the client's teaching plan about the purpose of this procedure?
- ☐ **1.** To decrease the frequency and severity of variable decelerations.
- ☐ **2.** To minimize the possibility of fetal metabolic alkalosis.
- ☐ **3.** To increase the fetal heart rate accelerations during a contraction.
- ☐ **4.** To raise the amniotic fluid index to more than 15 cm.

90. A primigravid client at 37 weeks' gestation who has been diagnosed with pregnancy-induced hypertension is to be admitted to the labor and delivery area. Which of the following client care rooms should the nurse determine to be most appropriate for this client?
- ☐ **1.** A brightly lit private room at the end of the hall from the nurses' station.
- ☐ **2.** A semiprivate room midway down the hall from the nurses' station.
- ☐ **3.** A private room with many windows that is near the operating room.
- ☐ **4.** A darkened private room as close to the nurses' station as possible.

91. A multigravid client is admitted to the labor area from the emergency room. At the time of admission, the fetal head is crowning, and the client yells, "The baby's coming!" To help the client remain calm and cooperative during the imminent delivery, which of the following responses by the nurse is most appropriate?
- ☐ **1.** "You're right, the baby is coming, so just relax."
- ☐ **2.** "Please don't push because you'll tear your cervix."
- ☐ **3.** "Your doctor will be here as soon as possible."
- ☐ **4.** "I'll explain what's happening to guide you as we go along."

92. The nurse is caring for a multigravid client who speaks little English. As the nurse enters the client's room, the nurse observes the client squatting on the bed and the fetal head crowning. After calling for assistance and helping the client lie down, which of the following actions should the nurse do next?
- ☐ **1.** Tell the client to push between contractions.
- ☐ **2.** Provide gentle support to the fetal head.
- ☐ **3.** Apply gentle upward traction on the neonate's anterior shoulder.
- ☐ **4.** Massage the perineum to stretch the perineal tissues.

93. During the first hour after a precipitous delivery, the nurse should monitor a multiparous client for signs and symptoms of which of the following?
- ☐ **1.** Postpartum "blues."
- ☐ **2.** Uterine atony.
- ☐ **3.** Intrauterine infection.
- ☐ **4.** Urinary tract infection.

94. A multigravid client in labor at 38 weeks' gestation has been diagnosed with Rh sensitization and probable fetal hydrops and anemia. When the nurse observes the fetal heart rate pattern on the monitor, which of the following patterns is most likely?
- ☐ **1.** Early deceleration pattern.
- ☐ **2.** Sinusoidal pattern.
- ☐ **3.** Variable deceleration pattern.
- ☐ **4.** Late deceleration pattern.

95. The physician orders oxytocin to be added to the intravenous fluids of a 30-year-old multigravid client at 37 weeks' gestation with twins after vaginal delivery. The nurse anticipates administering the oxytocin after delivery of which of the following?
- ☐ **1.** First placenta.
- ☐ **2.** First twin.
- ☐ **3.** Second placenta.
- ☐ **4.** Second twin.

96. The nurse in the labor and delivery area receives a telephone call from the emergency room announcing that a multigravid client in active labor is being transferred to the labor area. The client has had no prenatal care. When the client arrives by stretcher, she says, "I think the baby's coming . . . Help!" The fetal skull is crowning. Which of the following should be a priority assessment for the nurse to make?

- ☐ 1. Estimated date of delivery.
- ☐ 2. Amniotic fluid status.
- ☐ 3. Gravida and parity.
- ☐ 4. Prenatal history.

97. A multiparous client delivers dizygotic twins at 37 weeks' gestation. The twin neonates require additional hospitalization after the client is discharged. In planning the family's care, an appropriate goal for the nurse to formulate is that, while the twins are hospitalized, the parents will do which of the following?

- ☐ 1. Discuss how they will cope with twin infants at home.
- ☐ 2. Participate in care of the twins as much as possible.
- ☐ 3. Take turns providing 24-hour observation of the twins.
- ☐ 4. Identify complications that may occur as the twins develop.

98. A primigravid client at 41 weeks' gestation is admitted to the hospital's labor and delivery unit in active labor. After 25 hours of labor with membranes ruptured for 24 hours, the client delivers a healthy neonate vaginally with a midline episiotomy. Which of the following nursing diagnoses should the nurse identify as the priority for the client?

- ☐ 1. *Activity intolerance* related to difficult labor process.
- ☐ 2. *Sleep deprivation* related to prolonged labor.
- ☐ 3. *Situational low self-esteem* related to lengthy labor process.
- ☐ 4. *Risk for infection* related to birth trauma and prolonged ruptured membranes.

99. The nurse is caring for a primiparous client and her neonate immediately after delivery. The neonate was born at 41 weeks' gestation and weighs 4,082 g (9 lb). Assessing for signs and symptoms of which of the following conditions should be a priority in this neonate?

- ☐ 1. Anemia.
- ☐ 2. Hypoglycemia.
- ☐ 3. Delayed meconium.
- ☐ 4. Elevated bilirubin.

100. A multigravid client in active labor at term is diagnosed with polyhydramnios. The physician has instructed the client about possible neonatal complications related to the polyhydramnios. The nurse determines that the client has understood the instructions when the client states that polyhydramnios is associated with which of the following in the fetus or neonate?

- ☐ 1. Renal dysfunction.
- ☐ 2. Intrauterine growth retardation.
- ☐ 3. Pulmonary hypoplasia.
- ☐ 4. Gastrointestinal disorders.

101. A primigravid client at 39 weeks' gestation is admitted to the hospital in active labor. On admission, the client's cervix is 6 cm dilated. After 2 hours of active labor, the client's cervix is still dilated at 6 cm with 100% effacement at 21 station. Contractions are 3 to 5 minutes apart, lasting 45 seconds, and of moderate intensity. The nurse determines that the client is most likely experiencing which of the following?

- ☐ 1. Cephalopelvic disproportion.
- ☐ 2. Prolonged latent phase.
- ☐ 3. Prolonged transitional phase.
- ☐ 4. Hypotonic contraction pattern.

102. The physician who elects to perform a cesarean delivery on a primigravid client for fetal distress has informed the client of possible risks during the procedure. When the nurse asks the client to sign the consent form, the client's husband says, "I'll sign it for her. She's too upset by what is happening to make this decision." Which of the following actions would be most appropriate?

- ☐ 1. Ask the client if this is acceptable to her.
- ☐ 2. Have the client and her husband both sign the consent form.
- ☐ 3. Ask the client to sign the consent form.
- ☐ 4. Ask the doctor to witness the consent form.

103. A multigravid client at term is admitted to the hospital for a trial labor and possible vaginal birth. She has a history of previous cesarean delivery because of fetal distress. When the client is 4 cm dilated, she receives nalbuphine (Nubain) intravenously. While monitoring the fetal heart rate, the nurse observes minimal variability and a rate of 120 bpm. The nurse should explain to the client that the decreased variability is most likely caused by which of the following?

- ☐ 1. Maternal fatigue.
- ☐ 2. Fetal malposition.
- ☐ 3. Small-for-gestational-age fetus.
- ☐ 4. Effects of analgesic medication.

104. The nurse is caring for a primipara in active labor when the fetus develops severe bradycardia with late decelerations, and an emergency cesarean delivery is performed with the client under general anesthesia. After the delivery, the client tells the nurse, "I feel terrible. This is exactly what I didn't want to happen!" Which of the following would be a priority nursing diagnosis for this client?
- ☐ **1.** *Interrupted family processes* related to cesarean delivery.
- ☐ **2.** *Anxiety* related to incisional scar and neonatal outcome.
- ☐ **3.** *Pain* related to surgical incision and uterine cramping.
- ☐ **4.** *Situational low self-esteem* related to inability to deliver vaginally.

105. During a scheduled cesarean delivery of a primigravid client with a fetus at 39 weeks' gestation in a breech presentation, a neonatologist is present in the operating room. The nurse explains to the client that the neonatologist is present because neonates born by cesarean delivery tend to have an increased incidence of which of the following?
- ☐ **1.** Congenital anomalies.
- ☐ **2.** Pulmonary hypertension.
- ☐ **3.** Meconium aspiration syndrome.
- ☐ **4.** Respiratory distress syndrome.

106. A 28-year-old multigravid client at 28 weeks' gestation diagnosed with acute pyelonephritis is receiving intravenous fluids and antibiotics. After teaching the client about the rationale for the aggressive therapy, the nurse determines that the client needs further instruction when she says that acute pyelonephritis can lead to which of the following?
- ☐ **1.** Preterm labor.
- ☐ **2.** Maternal sepsis.
- ☐ **3.** Intrauterine growth retardation.
- ☐ **4.** Congenital fetal anomalies.

107. A primigravid client at 38 weeks' gestation is admitted to the labor suite in active labor. The client's physical assessment reveals a chlamydial infection. The nurse explains that if the infection is left untreated, the neonate may develop which of the following?
- ☐ **1.** Conjunctivitis.
- ☐ **2.** Heart disease.
- ☐ **3.** Harlequin sign.
- ☐ **4.** Brain damage.

108. A 34-year-old primigravid client at 39 weeks' gestation admitted to the hospital in active labor has type B Rh-negative blood. The nurse should instruct the client that if the neonate is Rh positive, the client will receive an Rh immune globulin (RHIG) injection for which of the following reasons?
- ☐ **1.** To prevent Rh-positive sensitization with the next pregnancy.
- ☐ **2.** To provide active antibody protection for this pregnancy.
- ☐ **3.** To decrease the amount of Rh-negative sensitization for the next pregnancy.
- ☐ **4.** To destroy fetal Rh-positive cells during the next pregnancy.

109. A 16-year-old primigravid client admitted at 38 weeks' gestation with severe pregnancy-induced hypertension is given intravenous magnesium sulfate and lactated Ringer's solution. Which of the following assessments should the nurse expect?
- ☐ **1.** Urinary output every 8 hours.
- ☐ **2.** Deep tendon reflexes every 4 hours.
- ☐ **3.** Respiratory rate every hour.
- ☐ **4.** Blood pressure every 6 hours.

110. The labor and delivery room nurse has received a telephone call from the emergency room indicating that a multigravid client in early labor and diagnosed with probable placenta previa will be arriving soon. In preparation for the client's arrival, the nurse anticipates that the physician will order which of the following?
- ☐ **1.** Whole blood replacement.
- ☐ **2.** Continuous blood pressure monitoring.
- ☐ **3.** Internal fetal heart rate monitoring.
- ☐ **4.** An immediate cesarean delivery.

111. During admission, a multigravida in early active labor acts somewhat euphoric and tells the nurse that she smoked some crack cocaine before coming to the hospital. In addition to fetal heart rate assessment, the nurse should monitor the client for symptoms of which of the following?
- ☐ **1.** Placenta previa.
- ☐ **2.** Ruptured uterus.
- ☐ **3.** Maternal hypotension.
- ☐ **4.** Abruptio placentae.

112. A primigravid client in early labor tells the nurse that she was exposed to rubella at about 14 weeks' gestation. After delivery, the nurse should assess the neonate for which of the following?
- ☐ **1.** Hydrocephaly.
- ☐ **2.** Cardiac disorders.
- ☐ **3.** Renal disorders.
- ☐ **4.** Bulging fontanels.

113. A primigravid client in early labor with abruptio placentae develops disseminated intravascular coagulation (DIC). Which of the following should the nurse expect the physician to order?
- ☐ 1. Magnesium sulfate.
- ☐ 2. Warfarin sodium (Coumadin).
- ☐ 3. Fresh-frozen platelets.
- ☐ 4. Meperidine hydrochloride (Demerol).

114. A multigravid client diagnosed with chronic hypertension is now in early labor at 34 weeks' gestation. The physician has ordered intravenous terbutaline (Brethine) 5 µg/minute, with the dose increased every 10 minutes until a maximum dosage of 80 µg/minute is achieved. The nurse determines that the medication has had a therapeutic effect when which of the following is observed?
- ☐ 1. Increase in fetal heart rate accelerations.
- ☐ 2. Decrease in the frequency and number of contractions.
- ☐ 3. Increased variability of the fetal heart rate.
- ☐ 4. Decrease in the maternal pulse rate.

115. A primigravid client who was successfully treated for preterm labor at 30 weeks' gestation had a history of mild hyperthyroidism before becoming pregnant. The nurse should instruct the client to do which of the following?
- ☐ 1. Continue taking low-dose oral propylthiouracil (PTU) as ordered.
- ☐ 2. Discontinue taking the methimazole (Tapazole) until after delivery.
- ☐ 3. Consider breast-feeding the neonate after the delivery.
- ☐ 4. Contact the physician if bradycardia occurs.

116. A primigravid client at 37 weeks' gestation has been hospitalized for several days with severe pregnancy-induced hypertension. While caring for the client, the nurse observes that the client is beginning to have a seizure. Which of the following actions should the nurse do first?
- ☐ 1. Pad the side rails of the client's bed.
- ☐ 2. Turn the client to the right side.
- ☐ 3. Insert a padded tongue blade into the client's mouth.
- ☐ 4. Call for immediate assistance in the client's room.

117. While assessing a primigravid client admitted at 36 weeks' gestation, the nurse observes multiple bruises on the client's face, neck, and abdomen. When asked about the bruises, the client admits that her boyfriend beats her now and then and says, "I want to leave him because I'm afraid he will hurt the baby." Which of the following actions is the nurse's most appropriate response?
- ☐ 1. Tell the client to leave the boyfriend immediately.
- ☐ 2. Ask the client when she last felt the baby move.
- ☐ 3. Refer the client to a social worker for possible options.
- ☐ 4. Report the incident to the unit nursing supervisor.

118. A multigravid client in active labor at term suddenly sits up and says, "I can't breathe! My chest hurts really bad!" The client's skin begins to turn a dusky gray color. After calling for assistance, which of the following should the nurse do next?
- ☐ 1. Administer oxygen by face mask.
- ☐ 2. Begin cardiopulmonary resuscitation.
- ☐ 3. Administer intravenous oxytocin.
- ☐ 4. Obtain an order for intravenous fibrinogen.

Correct Answers and Rationales

The letter in parentheses after each rationale identifies the client need addressed in the item, including management of care (M), safety and infection control (S), health promotion and maintenance (H), psychosocial adaptation (P), basic care and comfort (C), pharmacological and parenteral therapies (D), reduction of risk potential (R), and physiological adaptation (A).

The Primigravid Client in Labor

1. 2. Labor is categorized into three phases: latent, active, and transition. During the active stage of labor, intermittent fetal monitoring is performed every 30 minutes to detect changes in fetal heart rate such as bradycardia, tachycardia, or decelerations. If complications develop, more frequent or continuous electronic fetal monitoring may be needed. During the latent phase, intermittent monitoring is usually performed every 2 hours because contractions during this time are usually less frequent. During the transition phase, intermittent monitoring is performed every 5 to 15 minutes because the client is getting closer to delivery of the baby. There is no initial phase of labor. (R)

2. 2. The ischial spines are used as landmarks to determine the descent of the fetal presenting part. The station +1 means that the presenting part is 1 cm below the level of the ischial spines. The station –1 means that the presenting part is 1 cm above the level of the ischial spines. The ischial tuberosities and sacral promontory are not used to determine the fetal station. (R)

3. 2. Assessment findings indicate that the client is in the transition phase of labor. During this phase, it is not unusual for clients to exhibit a loss of control or irritability. Leg tremors, nausea, vomiting, and an urge to bear down also are common. Excitement is associated with the latent phase of labor. Numbness of the legs may occur when epidural anesthesia has been given; however, it is rare when no anesthesia is given. Feelings of relief generally occur during the second stage, when the client begins bearing-down efforts. (H)

4. 3. The obese pregnant client is more susceptible to soft tissue dystocia, which can impede the progress of labor. Symptoms of soft tissue dystocia would include an arrest of labor, prolonged labor, or an arrest of descent of the fetus. Hypotonic reflexes are associated with magnesium sulfate therapy, and increased uterine resting tone is associated with hypertonic labor patterns in early labor, not with obesity and pregnancy. Increased fear and anxiety are also not associated with obesity. However, they may be associated with a primigravid client who does not know what to expect during labor. (R)

5. 1. Cephalopelvic disproportion (CPD) may occur in clients with diabetes, multiparity, or postdate pregnancies. A prolonged second stage and arrest of descent are signs of CPD. Twin gestations are typically suspected by an oversized uterus and can be confirmed with ultrasound. Anencephaly would not contribute to a prolonged second stage. However, hydrocephaly can complicate delivery because the enlarged fetal skull can prevent descent. Breech presentation would be suspected by palpation of the buttocks or feet during a vaginal examination and can be confirmed by ultrasound visualization of the presenting part. (R)

6. 3. Prostaglandin gel may be used for cervical ripening before the induction of labor with oxytocin. It is usually administered by catheter or suppository, or by vaginal insertion. Two to three doses are usually needed to begin the softening process. Common adverse effects include nausea, vomiting, fever, and diarrhea. Continuous fetal heart rate monitoring and close monitoring of maternal vital signs are necessary to detect subtle changes or adverse effects. Prostaglandin gel usually does not initiate contractions; therefore, the rest period between contractions will be greater than 2 minutes. There is no need to assess reflexes based on prostaglandin use. Leaking of amniotic fluid is not caused by the use of this gel. (D)

7. 1. External cephalic version is the turning of the fetus from a breech position to the vertex position to prevent the need for a cesarean delivery. Gentle pressure is used to rotate the fetus in a forward direction to a cephalic lie. Contraindications to the procedure include multiple gestation because of the potential for fetal injury or uterine injury, severe oligohydramnios (decreased amniotic fluid), contraindications to a vaginal birth (e.g., cephalopelvic disproportion), and unexplained third trimester bleeding. If the mother has Rh-negative blood type, the procedure can be performed and Rh immunoglobulin should be administered in case minimal bleeding occurs. A history of gestational diabetes is not a contraindication unless the fetus is large for gestational age and the client has cephalopelvic disproportion. (R)

8. 2. Augmentation of labor with oxytocin (Pitocin) is needed when labor contractions begin spontaneously but then become weak, irregular, or ineffective (hypotonic) and assistance is needed to strengthen them. This condition is commonly caused by the administration of analgesia or anesthesia early in the labor process. Morphine

sulfate analgesia is administered to clients who are experiencing hypertonic contractions to allow the client to rest. Nubain is an analgesic and may result in further hypotonic contractions. Ampicillin is an antibiotic; there is no justification for administration of an antibiotic at this time. (D)

9. 4. Anatomically, the best position for the client to assume is the squatting position because this enhances pelvic diameters and allows gravity to assist in the expulsion stage of labor. This position also provides for natural pressure anesthesia as the fetal presenting part presses on the stretched perineum. If the client is extremely fatigued from a lengthy labor process, she may prefer the dorsal recumbent position. However, this position is not considered the best position anatomically. The lithotomy position may be ineffective and uncomfortable for a client who is ready to push. The hands and knees position may help to alleviate some back pain. However, this position can cause discomfort to the arms and wrists and is tiring over a long period of time. (H)

10. 4. During transition, contractions are increasing in frequency, duration, and intensity. The most appropriate nursing diagnosis is *Pain* related to strength and duration of the contractions. Insufficient information is provided in the scenario to support the other listed nursing diagnoses. *Impaired urinary elimination* would be appropriate if the client had a full bladder and was unable to void. *Risk for injury* might apply if the client were completely out of control or thrashing around in the bed. *Ineffective coping* might apply if the client said, "I can't do this" or something similar. (H)

11. 1. The most reliable sign that the placenta has detached from the uterine wall is lengthening of the cord outside the vagina. Other signs include a sudden gush of (rather than a decrease in) vaginal blood. Usually, when placenta detachment occurs, the uterus becomes more firm and changes in shape from discoid to globular. This process takes about 5 minutes. If the placenta does not separate, manual removal may be necessary to prevent postpartum hemorrhage. (H)

12. 3. Childbirth is a very emotional experience. An expression of happiness with tears is a normal reaction. Cultural factors, exhaustion, and anxieties over the new role can all affect maternal responses, so the nurse must be sensitive to the client's emotional expressions. There is no evidence to suggest that the mother is disappointed in the baby's gender, grieving over the end of the pregnancy, or a candidate for postpartum "blues." However, approximately 80% of postpartum clients experience transient postpartum blues several days after delivery. (H)

13. 3. Most authorities suggest that a woman in an early stage of labor should be allowed to walk if she wishes as long as no complications are present. Birthing centers and single-room maternity units allow women considerable latitude without much supervision at this stage of labor. Gravity and walking can assist the process of labor in some clients. If the client becomes tired, she can rest in bed in the left lateral recumbent position or sit in a comfortable chair. Resting in the left lateral recumbent position improves circulation to the fetus. (H)

14. **1.** Childbirth educators use various techniques and methods to prepare parents for labor and delivery. Active relaxation involves relaxing uninvolved muscle groups while contracting a specific group and using chest breathing techniques to lift the diaphragm off the contracting uterus. A deep, meditative, sleeplike state is a form of passive relaxation. Focusing on an object in the room is part of Lamaze technique for distraction. Breathing rapidly and deeply can lead to hyperventilation and is not recommended. (H)

15. **3.** Light stroking of the skin, or *effleurage,* is commonly used with the Lamaze method of childbirth preparation. Light abdominal massage with just enough pressure to avoid tickling is thought to displace the pain sensation during a contraction. Deep kneading and secure grasping are typically associated with relaxation massages to relieve stress. Prolonged pressure on specific sites is associated with acupressure. (H)

16. **1.** Some physicians do not allow clients with ruptured membranes to use a hot tub or jet hydrotherapy tub during labor for fear of infections. The temperature of the water should be between 98° and 100° F (36.7° to 37.8° C) to prevent hyperthermia. Jet hydrotherapy is not contraindicated for clients with multifetal gestation, diabetes mellitus, or hypotonic labor patterns. (R)

17. **3.** Cystic fibrosis and other inborn errors of metabolism are inherited as autosomal recessive traits. Such diseases do not occur unless there are two genes for the disease present. If one of the parents does not have the gene, the child will not have the disease. X-linked recessive genes can result in hemophilia A or color blindness. X-linked recessive genes are present only on the X chromosome and are typically manifested in the male child. X-linked dominant genes, which are located on and transmitted only by the female sex chromosome, can result in hypophosphatemia, an inborn error of metabolism marked by abnormally low serum alkaline phosphatase activity and excretion of phosphoethanolamine in the urine. This disorder is manifested as rickets in infants and children. Autosomal dominant gene disorders can result in muscular dystrophy, Marfan's syndrome, and osteogenesis imperfecta (brittle bone disease). Typically, a dominant gene for the disease trait is present along with a corresponding healthy recessive gene. (H)

18. **4.** To determine fetal lung maturity, the sample of amniotic fluid will be tested for the L/S ratio. When fetal lungs are mature, the ratio should be 2:1. Bilirubin indicates hemolysis and, if present in the fluid, suggests Rh disease. Red blood cells should not appear in the amniotic fluid because their presence suggests fetal bleeding. Barr body determination is a chromosome analysis of the sex chromosomes that is sometimes used when a child is born with ambiguous genitalia. (H)

19. **2.** Adolescent pregnancy carries an increased risk of pregnancy-induced hypertension, iron-deficiency anemia, and CPD. CPD is a concern because maturation of the skeletal bones (including the pelvis) is commonly not complete in adolescents. Adolescent labor does not differ from labor in the older woman if no CPD is present. A prolonged first stage of labor and poor fetal descent may indicate that CPD exists. Uterine inversion, a rapid third stage of labor, or decreased ability to push may occur regardless of the client's age. (R)

20. **4.** Delegation of duties and clients to ancillary personnel is commonly the responsibility of the registered nurse. The client who is a G 2, P 1 with a history of hyperemesis gravidarum is the client with the least potential for labor complications. Hyperemesis gravidarum typically occurs and is treated in the first or second trimester of pregnancy and should be resolved by this point in the pregnancy. A G 4, P 3 client with a history of gestational diabetes may have cephalopelvic disproportion due to a large-for-gestational-age fetus requiring a cesarean section delivery. The G 3, P 1, Ab 1 client is preterm at 35 weeks' gestation and may require an intensive care neonatal team. In a G 1, P 0 client, leaking green amniotic fluid indicates that there has been fetal distress. (M)

21. **3.** Pushing during the first stage of labor, when the urge is felt but the cervix is not completely dilated, may produce cervical swelling, making labor more difficult. The client should be encouraged to use a pant-blow (or blow-blow) pattern of breathing to help overcome the urge to push. The McDonald procedure is used for cervical cerclage for an incompetent cervix and is inappropriate here. Increasing the rate of oxygen and intravenous fluids will not alleviate the pressure that the client is feeling. The client should not push even if she feels the urge to do so because this may result in cervical edema at 7 cm dilation. (H)

22. **4.** The client is in the transition phase of the first stage of labor. During this phase, the client needs encouragement and support because this is a difficult and painful time, when contractions are especially strong. Usually, the client finds it difficult to maintain self control. Everything else seems secondary to her as she progresses into the second stage of labor and delivery. Although ice chips may be given, typically the client does not desire sips of water. Labor is hard work. Generally, the client is perspiring and does not desire additional warmth. Frequent perineal cleansing is not necessary unless there is excessive amniotic fluid leaking. (H)

23. **1.** The sagittal suture is the most readily felt during a vaginal examination. When the fetus is in the LOA position, the occiput faces the mother's left. The lambdoid suture is on the side of the skull. The coronal suture is a horizontal suture across the front portion of the fetal skull that forms the anterior fontanel. It may be felt with a brow presentation. The frontal suture may be felt with a brow or face presentation. (H)

24. **2.** Molding occurs with vaginal deliveries and is commonly seen in newborns. This is especially true with primigravid clients experiencing a lengthy labor process. Parents need to be reassured that it is not permanent and that it typically lasts a day or two before resolving. Molding rarely is present if the fetus is in a breech or brow presentation. Surgical intervention is not necessary. (H)

25. **1, 2, 5, 6.** Uterine inversion is indicated by a sudden gush of blood from the vagina leading to decreased blood pressure, and an inability to palpate the uterus since it may be in or protruding from the vagina and any signs of blood loss such as diaphoresis, paleness, or dizziness could be observed at this time. Intense pain and a hard contracting uterus are not associated with uterine inversion. (R)

26. **2.** Avoidance, hostility, or low-key (passive) behavior toward the baby may be a cue to potential bonding problems. The nurse should encourage the client to give the baby the first feeding to begin the bonding process. Expressions of disappointment with the baby's gender may also signal problems with maternal-infant bonding. Comparing the baby's features to her own indicates identification of the neonate as belonging to her, suggesting bonding with neonate. Comparing the actual neonate with the "fantasized neonate" is a normal maternal reaction. Wanting to buy a blue outfit indicates an interest in and connection with the neonate and is a sign of bonding. (R)

27. **4.** According to the gate-control theory of pain perception, when the endings of small peripheral nerve fibers detect a stimulus, they transmit it to cells in the dorsal horn of the spinal cord. These impulses pass through a network of cells in the spinal cord called the substantia gelatinosa, and a synapse occurs that returns the transmission to the peripheral site through a motor nerve. The impulse is then transmitted through the spinal cord to the brain, where the impulse is perceived as pain. Gate-control mechanisms in the spinal cord are capable of halting these impulses (closing the gate), so that pain is not perceived. Input from the large sensory fibers closes the gate. Telling the client that labor pain is a matter of individual perception is not helpful and does not explain the gate-control theory. Deep chest breathing or other breathing techniques can help to keep the "gate" closed, not open. (H)

28. **1.** According to the gate-control theory of pain, a closed gate means that the client should feel no pain. The gate-control theory of pain refers to the gate-control mechanisms in the substantia gelatinosa that are capable of halting an impulse at the level of the spinal cord so the impulse is never perceived at the brain level as pain (i.e., a process similar to keeping a gate closed). (H)

29. **4.** The bladder status should be monitored throughout the labor process, but especially before the client begins pushing. A full bladder can impede the progress of labor and slow fetal descent. Because she has had an epidural anesthetic, it is most likely that the client is receiving intravenous fluids, contributing to a full bladder. The client also does not feel the urge to void because of the anesthetic. Although it is important to monitor membrane status and fetal heart rate variability throughout labor, this does not affect the client's ability to push. There is no need to recheck cervical dilation because increasing the frequency of examinations can increase the client's risk for infection. (R)

30. **1.** The normal length of the latent stage of labor in a primigravid client is 6 hours. If the client is having prolonged labor, the nurse should monitor the client for signs of exhaustion as well as dehydration. Hypotonic contractions, which are painful but ineffective, may be occurring. Oxytocin augmentation may be necessary. Chills and fever are manifestations of an infection and are not associated with a prolonged latent phase of labor. Fluid overload can occur from rapid infusion of intravenous fluids administered if the client is experiencing hemorrhage or shock. It is not associated with prolonged latent phase. The client's membranes are intact, so it would be difficult to assess meconium staining of the fluid. Meconium-stained fluid is associated with fetal distress, and this fetus appears to be in a healthy state, as evidenced by a fetal heart rate within normal range and good variability. (R)

31. **1.** The client who has back pain during labor experiences marked discomfort because the fetus is in an LOP position. This pain is much greater than when the fetus is in the anterior position because the fetal head impinges on the sacrum in the course of rotating to the anterior position. Application of firm pressure to the sacral area can help alleviate the pain. Complaints of severe back pain during labor do not typically require a cesarean delivery. The physician may elect to do an episiotomy, but it is not necessarily required. It is unlikely that a primigravid client with a fetus in an LOP position will have a precipitous delivery; rather, labor is usually more prolonged. A hands-and-knees position or a right side-lying position may help to rotate the fetal head and thus alleviate some of the back pain. (H)

32. **1.** The psychoprophylaxis method of childbirth suggests using slow chest breathing until it becomes ineffective during labor contractions, then switching to shallow chest breathing (mostly at the sternum) during the peak of a contraction. The rate is 50 to 70 breaths per minute. Deep chest breathing is appropriate for the early phase of labor, in which the client exhibits less frequent contractions. When transition nears, a rapid pant-blow pattern of breathing is used. Slow abdominal breathing is very difficult for clients in labor. (H)

33. **3.** The carbon dioxide insufficiency that occurs during hyperventilation will lead to respiratory alkalosis. Symptoms include confusion, unconsciousness, elevated plasma pH (greater than 7.45), and elevated urine pH (above 7). The nurse should try to calm the client and, if the hyperventilation persists, should ask the client to breathe into a paper bag. Metabolic alkalosis is associated with vomiting when a large amount of hydrochloric acid is lost. Metabolic acidosis is associated with loss of sodium ions through diarrhea. Respiratory acidosis is associated with shallow breathing and an inability to expire completely. (R)

34. **3.** Fetal scalp stimulation is commonly ordered when there is decreased fetal heart rate variability. Pressure is applied with the fingers to the fetal scalp through the dilated cervix. This should cause a tactile response in the fetus and increase the fetal heart rate and variability. However, if the fetus is in distress and becoming acidotic, fetal heart rate acceleration will not occur. The fetal hematocrit level can be measured by fetal blood sampling. Scalp stimulation does not increase the strength of the contractions. However, it can increase fetal heart rate and variability. Fetal position is assessed by identifying skull landmarks (sutures) during a vaginal examination. (R)

35. **4.** If the fetus is hypoxic, the pH will fall below 7.2 and be indicative of fetal distress. This finding typically requires immediate vaginal or cesarean delivery. A scalp pH reading of 7.21 to 7.25 should be repeated again in 30 minutes for assessment of hypoxia and acidosis. (A)

36. **3.** When a client complains of severe back pain during labor, the fetus is most likely in an occipitoposterior position. This means that the fetal head presses against the client's sacrum, causing marked discomfort during contractions. These sensations may be so intense that the client requests medication for relief of the back pain rather than the contractions. Breech presentation and transverse lie are usually known prior to 8-cm dilation and a cesarean section is performed. Fetal occiput anterior position does not increase the pain felt during labor. (H)

37. **1, 3, 5.** Decelerations alert the nurse that the fetus is experiencing decreased blood flow from the placenta. Administering oxygen will increase tissue perfusion. Placing the mother on her side will increase placental perfusion and decrease cord compression. Using an internal fetal monitor would help in identifying the possible underlying cause of the decelerations, such as metabolic acidosis. Assessing for pain relief and readjusting the monitor would have no effect on correcting the late decelerations. (R)

38. **3.** The third maneuver involves grasping the lower portion of the abdomen just above the symphysis pubis between the thumb and index finger. This maneuver determines whether the fetal presenting part is engaged. The first maneuver involves facing the woman's head and using the tips of the fingers to palpate the uterine fundus. This maneuver is used to identify the part of the fetus that lies over the inlet to the pelvis. The second maneuver involves placing the palms of each hand on either side of the abdomen to locate the back of the fetus. The fourth maneuver involves placing fingers on both sides of the uterus and pressing downward and inward in the direction of the birth canal. This maneuver is done to determine fetal atti-

tude and degree of extension and should only be done if the fetus is in the cephalic presentation. (A)

39. **1.** Leopold's maneuvers are performed to determine the presentation and position of the fetus. The third maneuver determines whether the fetal presenting part is engaged in the maternal pelvis. The first maneuver distinguishes between a breech and a cephalic presentation through palpation of the top of the fundus. The second maneuver locates the fetal back, arms, and legs. The fetal heart rate monitoring device should be placed near the fetal skull and back for optimal fetal heart rate monitoring. The fourth maneuver is done to locate the fetal cephalic prominence if the fetus is in a cephalic position. (H)

40. **4.** The priority nursing diagnosis at this time is *Pain* related to LOP position and prolonged fetal descent. When the fetus is in this position, the fetal head presses against the client's sacrum, causing marked discomfort during contractions. Labor is usually longer and more uncomfortable when the fetus remains in an occipitoposterior position. *Anxiety* would be an appropriate nursing diagnosis if the client had stated that she was nervous, apprehensive, afraid, fearful, or restless. *Ineffective coping* would be appropriate if the client exhibited a loss of control, screaming, crying, or thrashing around in the bed. *Urinary retention* might be a related nursing diagnosis; however, if the nurse is vigilant in assessment of the client's bladder status, the client should void at least every 2 hours or have a catheterization performed. A full bladder can impair fetal descent and prolong labor. (H)

41. **3.** Small clots that are expressed during fundal examination in the immediate postpartum period are normal; however, large clots are indicative of retained placental tissue. A small trickle of bright red vaginal bleeding may indicate a laceration. The nurse should notify the physician immediately of these findings, because uterine atony may occur and the laceration, if present, needs to be repaired to prevent further blood loss. Continuing to monitor the client every 15 minutes is the standard of care for a postpartum client. Taking no action would indicate that the nurse thinks passage of clots and trickling of bright red blood is a normal situation, which it is not. Methylergonovine is a powerful drug that contracts the uterus, but it usually is not administered to a client with a blood pressure of 136/92 mm Hg because of its hypertensive effects. Changing the perineal pads every 15 minutes is not helpful if the client is experiencing a hemorrhage. (H)

The Multigravid Client in Labor

42. **3.** The cause of variable decelerations is cord compression, which may be relieved by moving the client to one side or another. If the client is already on the left side, changing the client to the right side is appropriate. Performing a vaginal examination will let the nurse know how far dilated the client is but will not relieve the cord compression. If the decelerations are not relieved by position changes, oxygen should be initiated but the rate should be

8 to 10 L/minute. Notifying the physician should occur if turning the client and administering oxygen do not relieve the decelerations. (M)

43. **1, 2, 4, 5, 6.** Knowledge of how the fetus is tolerating contractions as well as the frequency, intensity, and duration of contractions, as indicated on the fetal monitor strip, are extremely important. The type of analgesia or anesthesia being used, the client's response, and her pain rating should be included as well. The amount of vaginal bleeding indicates whether this labor is in the normal range. Vaginal discharge indicates if membranes are ruptured and the color, odor, and amount of amniotic fluid. The support persons with the client are an integral part of the labor process and greatly influence how she manages labor emotionally and, commonly, physically. A complete change-of-shift report would include the client's name, age, gravida and parity, current and prior illnesses that may influence this hospitalization, prior labor and delivery history if applicable, last vaginal examination time and findings, vaginal bleeding, support persons with client, current I.V.s and other medications being used, and pertinent laboratory test results. Future plan for birth control would be the least important information to be given to the next shift because it will not impact the labor care plan. (A)

44. **2.** The feeling of needing to have a bowel movement is commonly caused by pressure on the receptors low in the perineum when the fetal head is creating pressure on them. This feeling usually indicates advances in fetal station and that the client may be close to delivery. The nurse should respond initially to the client's signs and symptoms by checking to validate current effacement, dilation, and station. If the fetus is ready to be delivered, having the room ready for the delivery and having naloxone hydrochloride (Narcan) available are important. Narcan completely or partially reverses the effects of natural and synthetic opioids, including respiratory depression. Documenting pain relief takes time away from the vaginal examination, preparing for delivery, and obtaining Narcan. The delivery may be occurring rapidly. Being prepared for the delivery is a higher priority than documentation for this client. (S)

45. **2.** Naloxone hydrochloride (Narcan) would not be used in a client who has a history of drug addiction. Narcan would abruptly withdraw this woman from the drug she is addicted to as well as the Nubain. The withdrawal would occur within a few minutes of injection and, if severe enough, could jeopardize the mother and fetus. Xylocaine is a local anesthetic and numbs, rather than decreases the effects of Narcan. The local anesthetic and the pudendal block are both appropriate for this delivery but are used to numb the maternal perineum for delivery. (D)

46. **1.** When a client receives an epidural anesthetic, sympathetic nerves are blocked along with the pain nerves, possibly resulting in vasodilation and hypotension. Other adverse effects include bladder distention, pro-

longed second stage of labor, nausea and vomiting, pruritus, and delayed respiratory depression for up to 24 hours after administration. Diaphoresis and tremors are not usually associated with the administration of epidural anesthesia. Headache, a common adverse effect of many drugs, also is not associated with administration of epidural anesthesia. (D)

47. **4.** The fetal monitor strip shows late decelerations. The first intervention would be to turn off the Pitocin because the medication is causing the contractions. The stress caused by the contractions demonstrates that the fetus is not being perfused during the entire contraction (as shown by the late decelerations). There is no time to continue to observe in this situation; intervention is a priority. The client is attached to an internal fetal monitor, which would be possible only if her membranes had already ruptured. If the fetus continues to experience stress, fetal oximetry may be initiated. (A)

48. **4.** After an emergency delivery, the nurse suggests that the mother begin breast-feeding to contract the uterus. Breast-feeding stimulates the natural production of oxytocin. In a multiparous client, uterine atony is a potential complication because of the stretching of the uterine fibers following each subsequent pregnancy. Although breast-feeding does help to begin the parental-infant bonding process, this is not the primary reason for the nurse to suggest breast-feeding. Prevention of neonatal hypothermia is accomplished by placing blankets on both the neonate and the mother. Although colostrum in breast milk provides the neonate with nutrients and immunoglobulins, the primary reason for breast-feeding is to stimulate the natural production of oxytocin to contract the uterus. (R)

49. **3.** A chill shortly after delivery is a common, normal occurrence. Warm blankets can help provide comfort for the client. It has been suggested that the shivering response is caused by a difference between internal and external body temperatures. A different theory proposes that the woman is reacting to fetal cells that have entered the maternal bloodstream through the placental site. Assessing the client's pulse rate will provide no further information about the chill. Decreasing the I.V. rate will not influence the length of time the client trembles. Assessing blood loss is a standard of care at this point postpartum but has no correlation to the chill. (H)

50. **2.** After an amniotomy, the nurse should plan to first assess the FHR for 1 full minute. One of the complications of amniotomy is cord compression and/or prolapsed cord, and a FHR of 100 bpm or less should be promptly reported to the physician. A cord prolapse requires prompt delivery by cesarean section. The client's contraction pattern should be monitored once labor has been established. The client's temperature, pulse, and respirations should be assessed every 2 to 4 hours after rupture of the membranes to detect an infection. The nurse should document the color, quantity, and odor of the amniotic fluid, but this can be done after the FHR is assessed and a reassuring pattern is present. (H)

51. 3. The most appropriate diagnosis at this time is *Risk for injury* related to the effects of the epidural anesthesia because the client may have no sensation in her lower abdomen and legs for several hours postpartum. Care should be taken to avoid injury, and ambulation should be delayed until sensation has returned. No information is presented in the scenario to suggest *Pain* due to episiotomy and exhaustive pushing. Multiparous clients commonly have shortened labors and may not require an episiotomy. If the client did have an episiotomy and the epidural anesthetic has worn off, then this nursing diagnosis would be appropriate. *Anxiety* would apply if the client expressed feelings of anxiety or nervousness because of a problem with moving her legs or toes. *Excess fluid volume* would apply if the client received excessive amounts of intravenous fluid or complained of oliguria, an early sign of pulmonary edema. (D)

52. 1. Caput succedaneum is common after the use of a vacuum extractor to assist the client's expulsion efforts. This edema may persist up to 7 days. Vacuum extraction is not associated with cephalohematoma. Maternal lacerations may occur, but they are more common when forceps are used. Neonatal intracranial hemorrhage is a risk with both vacuum extraction and forceps deliveries, but it is not a common finding. (H)

53. 1. Breech presentations account for 5% of all births and the most common is frank breech. In frank breech, there is flexion of the fetal thighs and extension of the knees. The feet rest at the side of the fetal head. In complete breech, there is flexion of the fetal thighs and knees; the fetus appears to be squatting. Footling breech occurs when there is an extension of the fetal knees and one or both feet protrude through the cervix. Vertex presentation occurs in 95% of deliveries with the head is engaged in the pelvis. (A)

54. 4. The nurse should assess the client's cervical dilation and station, because the client's symptoms are indicative of the transition phase of labor. Multiparous clients can proceed 5 to 9 cm per hour during the active phase of labor. Warming the temperature of the room is not helpful because the client will soon be ready to begin expulsive pushing. Increasing the intravenous fluid rate is not warranted unless the client is experiencing dehydration. Administration of an antiemetic at this point in labor is not warranted and may result in neonatal depression should a rapid delivery occur. (H)

55. 4. To assess the frequency of the client's contractions, the nurse should assess the interval from the beginning of one contraction to the beginning of the next contraction. The duration of a contraction is the interval between the beginning and the end of a contraction. The acme identifies the peak of a contraction. (H)

56. 3, 4, 5. The range of fetal heart rate fluctuating too high and low could indicate fetal distress. The green peripad fluid indicates meconium, which could be associated with fetal distress. Increased fetal activity during labor may also indicate distress. The maternal vital signs noted and a perineal pad with blood and mucus are normal findings. (R)

57. 3. After spontaneous rupture of the amniotic fluid, the gushing fluid may carry the umbilical cord out of the birth canal. Sudden deceleration of the fetal heart rate commonly signifies cord compression and/or prolapse of the cord, which would require immediate delivery. This client is particularly at risk because the fetus is preterm and the fetal head may not be engaged. Turning the client to the right side is not a priority action. However, changing the client's position would be appropriate if variable decelerations are present. The nurse should assess the color, amount, and odor of the fluid, but this can be done once the fetal heart rate is assessed and no problems are detected. Cervical dilation should be checked but only after the fetal heart rate pattern is assessed. (R)

58. 3, 6. The pressure from the fetus descending into the birth canal can cause the client to feel she needs to move her bowels and could be near delivery. Failure to assess the stage of labor and degree of fetal descent before allowing the client to go to the bathroom may lead to progression of labor and could result in a delivery in the bathroom. Applying a fetal monitor may reassure the nurse that the fetus is doing well; however, it does not help to determine if the fetus is ready for delivery, which is the higher priority in this situation. Regardless of the client's prior experience with back labor pain, the fetal head moving lower into the birth canal causes pressure in the lower back area similar to the feeling of pressure with a bowel movement. (S)

59. 2. Spinal anesthesia is used less commonly today because of preference for epidural block anesthesia. One of the adverse effects of spinal anesthesia is a "spinal headache" caused by leakage of spinal fluid from the needle insertion. This can be treated by applying a cool cloth to the forehead, keeping the client in a flat position, or using a blood patch that can clot and seal off any further leakage of fluid. Spinal anesthesia is administered with the client in a sitting position. Another adverse effect of spinal anesthesia is hypotension caused by vasodilation. General anesthesia provides immediate anesthesia, whereas the full effects of spinal anesthesia may not be felt for 20 to 30 minutes. General anesthesia can be discontinued quickly when the anesthesiologist administers oxygen instead of nitrous oxide. Epidural anesthesia may take 1 to 2 hours to wear off. (D)

60. 1. The drug of choice when hypotension occurs as a result of epidural anesthesia is ephedrine sulfate because it provides a quick reversal of the vasodilator effects of the anesthesia. Epinephrine is typically used to treat anaphylactic shock. Methylergonovine is a vasoconstrictor that is used for severe postpartum hemorrhage. Atropine sulfate is used to dry the oral and respiratory secretions and may be used during operative procedures. (D)

61. 3. Cimetidine (Tagamet) is ordered by some anesthesiologists who will be giving a general anesthetic to reduce the level of acid in the stomach contents, altering the pH to reduce the risk of complications should aspiration of vomitus occur. Aspiration of vomitus is the fifth most common cause of maternal mortality. Most anesthesiologists insert an endotracheal tube to reduce the incidence of aspiration. Isoproterenol (Isuprel) is used to decrease the incidence of bronchospasm. Atropine sulfate is administered to dry oral and nasal secretions. Although cimetidine is useful for gastric ulcer therapy, gastric ulcers are not a common effect associated with operative deliveries. (D)

62. 2. Lumbar epidural anesthesia is usually administered with the client in a sitting or a left side-lying position with shoulders parallel and legs slightly flexed. These positions expose the vertebrae to the anesthesiologist. Paracervical and local anesthetics are usually administered with the client in the lithotomy position. The knee-to-chest and prone positions are not used for anesthesia administration. (D)

63. 2. Anterior-posterior slit occurs as the perineum flattens and is followed by an oval opening. As labor progresses, the perineum takes on a circular shape. Crowning occurs when the fetal head is visible. (A)

64. 1. A neonate in good condition needs to be kept warm. This reduces cold stress and potential respiratory problems. Cold stress causes the neonate to burn much-needed brown fat. The infant can be evaluated under a radiant warmer or wrapped in dry, warm blankets on the mother's abdomen. Instilling erythromycin ointment, weighing the neonate, and applying identification bracelets can be done once the neonate has been placed under a radiant warmer and the temperature has stabilized. (H)

The Labor Experience

65. 3. The expected outcome of magnesium sulfate administration is suppression of the contractions because the client is in preterm labor. Magnesium sulfate is a smooth muscle relaxant used to slow and stop contractions. Having contractions that lead to delivery is not the intended effect of this drug when used for preterm labor. Respirations lower than 12 breaths/minute may indicate magnesium sulfate toxicity. Another use of magnesium sulfate is to treat preeclampsia by preventing seizures and, secondarily, lowering maternal blood pressure. However, in this scenario, preterm labor—not preeclampsia—is being treated. (D)

66. 4. Betamethasone is a corticosteroid that induces the production of surfactant. The pulmonary maturation that results causes the fetal lungs to mature more rapidly than normal. Because the lungs are mature, the risk of respiratory distress in the neonate is lowered but not eliminated. Betamethasone also decreases the surface tension within the alveoli. Betamethasone has no influence on contractions or carrying the fetus to full term. (D)

67. 1. A Bishop score evaluates cervical readiness for labor based on five factors: cervical softness, cervical effacement, dilation, fetal position, and station. A Bishop score of 5 or greater in a multipara or a score of 8 or greater in a primipara indicate that a vaginal birth is likely to result from the induction process. The nurse should expect that labor will be induced using Pitocin because the Bishop score indicates that the client is 60% to 70% effaced, 3 to 4 cm dilated, and in an anterior position. The cervix is soft and the presenting part is at a –1 to 0 position. Prepidil, Cytotec, and Cervidil are all cervical ripening agents and the doses are accurate; however, cervical ripening has already taken place. (D)

68. 3. Cervical ripening, or creating a cervix that is soft, anterior, and dilated to 2 to 3 cm, must occur before the cervix can efface and dilate with oxytocin (Pitocin). Drugs to accomplish this goal include dinoprostone (Cervidil), misoprostol (Cytotec), and prostaglandin E2 (PGE2). Nubain is a narcotic analgesic used in early labor and has no influence on the cervix. Betamethasone (Celestone) is a corticosteroid given to mature fetal lungs. (D)

69. 2. Typically, a client will be able to have an epidural when she is 3 to 4 cm dilated or the active phase of labor has been established. Waiting until the cervix is dilated to this point ensures that the client is in labor and the epidural is less likely to halt labor contractions. Nubain and Phenergan are used to provide relief until the client is about 7 cm dilated. If given after this time, narcotics may cause neonatal respiratory depression in the neonate. The majority of clients have an epidural or spinal for a cesarean section. The only time general anesthesia is used is for an emergency cesarean section. (D)

70. 1, 2, 3, 5. The time of rupture; color, odor, amount, and clarity of amniotic fluid; and FHR and pattern before and after the procedure are all information that must be documented on the client's record. There is only one size for an amnio-hook. (M)

71. 2. The client is experiencing uterine hyperstimulation from the oxytocin (Pitocin). The first intervention should be to stop the oxytocin infusion, which may be the cause of the long, frequent contractions, elevated resting tone, and nonreassuring fetal heart patterns. Only after turning off the oxytocin, should the nurse turn the client to her left side to better perfuse the mother and fetus. Then she should increase the maintenance I.V. fluids to allow available oxygen to be carried to the mother and fetus. When all other interventions are initiated, she should notify the health care provider. (M)

72. 4. Accelerations that are episodic and occur during fetal movement demonstrate fetal well-being. Turning the client to the left side, applying oxygen by face mask and notifying the health care provider are interventions used for late and variable decelerations indicating the fetus is not tolerating the induction process well. (A)

73. **1.** The client with PIH would be a candidate for the induction process because ending the pregnancy is the only way to cure PIH. A client with active herpes would be a candidate for a cesarean section to prevent the fetus from contracting the virus while passing through the birth canal. The woman with a face presentation will not be able to deliver vaginally due to the extended position of the neck. The client whose fetus exhibits late decelerations without oxytocin (Pitocin) would be at greater risk for fetal distress with use of this drug. Late decelerations indicate the fetus does not have enough placental reserves to remain oxygenated during the entire contraction. This client may require a cesarean section. (M)

74. **3.** The straight catheterization is within the scope of practice of a licensed practical nurse. An initial or continuing assessment is the responsibility of the registered nurse. Assessment must be complete before increasing the I.V. rate of Pitocin. The assessment and the increase in Pitocin rate are responsibilities for the nurse. (M)

75. **2.** Removing a fetal monitor from a client and assisting her to the bathroom are within the realm of practice of a nursing assistant. Performing a fundal check is an assessment, which is a responsibility of a registered nurse. A nursing assistant is not permitted to administer medication by any route. Education is also part of the professional nursing role. Although a nursing assistant can assist a mother with bottle feeding, the formal patient education must be completed and validated by the nurse. (M)

76. **3.** When the fetal head is compressed, early decelerations are seen as a vagal response occurs and the fetal heart rate decelerates and inversely mirrors the contraction. This response commonly occurs when the client is 9 to 10 cm dilated or pushing. If communication cannot be facilitated, early decelerations are one indicator that delivery may be approaching. Late decelerations may occur at this time but indicate uteroplacental insufficiency rather than imminent birth. At any time during the labor process, the client may communicate with her family in her native language. The client's facial expressions may change at any point during labor and cannot be used as an indicator of imminent delivery. (A)

The Intrapartal Client with Risk Factors

77. **1, 2, 3.** With abruptio placentae, bleeding may occur vaginally, may be obstructed by the fetal head, or it may be hidden behind a portion of the placenta. Abdominal rigidity occurs, particularly with a concealed hemorrhage because the girth and fundal height increase. Abdominal pain is one of the classic symptoms of abruption. The pain may be intermittent, as in labor contractions, or continuous. The placenta with abruption is not larger than a normal placenta and the bleeding does not end spontaneously. (A)

78. **1.** Clients who are pregnant with two (or more) fetuses are at greater risk for pregnancy-induced hypertension, hydramnios, placenta previa, preterm labor, and anemia. During delivery, occasionally the placenta of the second twin separates before that twin is delivered, causing profound bleeding. Urinary tract infections and chorioamnionitis are not more common in clients with multifetal gestation compared with women with single-fetus pregnancies. Although multiparous women frequently deliver more quickly than a nullipara does, precipitous delivery is not more common with twin gestations. (R)

79. **3.** The multigravid client with class II heart disease has a slight limitation of physical activity and may become fatigued with ordinary physical activity. A side-lying or semi-Fowler's position with the head elevated helps to ensure cardiac emptying and adequate oxygenation. In addition, oxygen by mask, analgesics and sedatives, diuretics, prophylactic antibiotics, and digitalis may be warranted. Although breathing slowly during a contraction may assist with oxygenation, it would have no effect on cardiac emptying. It is essential that the laboring woman with cardiac disease be relieved of discomfort and anxiety. Effective intrapartum pain relief with analgesia and epidural anesthesia may reduce cardiac workload as much as 20%. Local anesthetics are effective only during the second stage of labor. (R)

80. **4.** Assessing for signs and symptoms associated with cardiac decompensation is the priority. Class III heart disease during pregnancy has a 25% to 50% mortality. These clients are markedly compromised, with marked limitation of physical activity. They frequently experience fatigue, palpitations, dyspnea, or anginal pain. A pulse rate greater than 100 bpm or a respiratory rate greater than 25 breaths/minute may indicate cardiac decompensation that could result in cardiac arrest. Additional symptoms include dyspnea, peripheral edema, orthopnea, tachypnea, rales, and hemoptysis. (R)

81. **2.** Clients who have been diagnosed with class II heart disease and prosthetic valve replacement are most likely to have an order for antibiotic medications to prevent the development of bacterial endocarditis and bacteremia. Clients with valvular heart disease have a high susceptibility to subacute bacterial endocarditis. Anticoagulant therapy is usually discontinued during labor and delivery because of the potential for hemorrhage. Diuretic medications are generally not prescribed for clients with class I or class II heart disease. Diuretics usually are not necessary and may result in potassium depletion. Folic acid supplements are usually prescribed for clients with megaloblastic anemia. Folic acid is also included in many prenatal vitamins and can help to prevent neural tube defects in the fetus. (D)

82. **1.** Before administering prostaglandin E2 gel, the nurse would assess the frequency and duration of any uterine contractions first, because prostaglandin E2 gel is contraindicated if the client is having contractions. If there are no contractions, the client should be placed in a semi-Fowler's position to allow for vaginal insertion of the gel. Although determining whether the client's membranes have ruptured is part of the assessment of any client in labor, it is not specifically related to the administration of prostaglandin E2 gel. If the membranes remain intact, an amniotomy may be performed once the client begins to dilate and the fetal head is engaged. However, it is not necessary for the nurse to prepare the client for this procedure at this time. (D)

83. **4.** One of the potential disadvantages of oxytocin induction is neonatal jaundice or hyperbilirubinemia. Oxytocin decreases the elimination of bilirubin from the neonate. Other adverse effects include maternal hypertension and frontal headache, which disappear when the drug is discontinued. The drug has antidiuretic properties that can lead to maternal water intoxication. Dangerous effects of this powerful drug include uterine hyperstimulation or tetanic contractions, which can result in abruptio placentae and uterine rupture. Urinary frequency, maternal hypoglycemia, and preterm birth are not associated with oxytocin administration. Ultrasound procedures are used to estimate gestational age to prevent preterm delivery. Clients who are diabetic commonly deliver before term because the placenta begins to deteriorate, which can result in stillbirth. (D)

84. **4.** The highest priority nursing diagnosis for the client at this time is *Risk for injury, maternal or fetal* related to uterine hyperstimulation. Diabetic mothers have a higher incidence of pregnancy-induced hypertension, polyhydramnios, preterm birth, and larger-than-average fetuses and commonly have decreased placental perfusion. Infants of diabetic mothers may have polycythemia, congenital anomalies, and respiratory distress. Because of its antidiuretic properties, oxytocin infusion poses a risk of fluid overload, not fluid deficit. There is no information to support the diagnosis of *Pain* related to prolonged labor. For multigravid clients, labor is commonly shorter than for primigravidas. A labor duration longer than 12 hours would indicate a prolonged labor. There is no indication that the client will require cesarean delivery at this time. (D)

85. **4.** A common sign of fetal distress related to an inadequate transfer of oxygen to the fetus is meconium-stained fluid. Because the fetus has suffered hypoxia, close fetal heart rate monitoring is necessary. In addition, all clients are monitored continuously after rupture of membranes for fetal distress caused by cord prolapse. If there are increasing signs of fetal distress (e.g., late decelerations), the physician should be notified immediately. A cesarean delivery may be performed for fetal distress. Increasing the rate of the oxytocin infusion could lead to further fetal distress. Turning the client to the left side, rather than a knee-chest position, improves placental perfusion. The physician may wish to determine the extent of cervical dilation to make a decision about whether a cesarean delivery is warranted, but continuous fetal heart rate monitoring is essential to determine fetal status. (R)

86. **3.** Neonates born to mothers who smoke tend to have lower-than-average birth weights. Neonates born to mothers who smoke also are at higher risk for stillbirth, sudden infant death syndrome, bronchitis, allergies, delayed growth and development, and polycythemia. Maternal smoking is not related to higher neonatal hyperirritability, hyperbilirubinemia, or hypocalcemia. Rather, cocaine use during pregnancy is associated with neonatal hyperirritability and withdrawal symptoms. Hyperbilirubinemia is associated with Rh or ABO incompatibility or the administration of intravenous oxytocin during labor. Approximately 50% of neonates born to mothers with insulin-dependent diabetes experience hypocalcemia during the first 3 days of life. (H)

87. **3.** The client should be urged to push with an open glottis to prevent the Valsalva maneuver. Pushing with a closed glottis increases intrathoracic pressure, preventing venous return. Blood pressure also falls, and cardiac output decreases. Pushing for at least 1 to 3 minutes is too long; prolonged pushing can lead to reduced blood flow and fatigue. Pushing for the duration of the contraction is sufficient. Pushing while holding the breath results in the Valsalva maneuver. Because the client has had an epidural anesthetic, she may not feel the urge to push and may need coaching during the pushing phase. (D)

88. **3.** The American College of Obstetricians and Gynecologists has classified forceps applications into three categories: outlet, low, or middle. When the fetal skull is on the perineum with the scalp visible at the perineal floor or vaginal opening, this is considered outlet forceps application. When the head is higher in the pelvis but engaged and its greatest diameter has passed the inlet, the operation is termed midforceps. Midforceps deliveries are not recommended because they are extremely dangerous for the mother and fetus because of the possibility of uterine rupture. If the head is not engaged, at −1 station, this is termed high forceps. High forceps deliveries also are exceedingly dangerous for both the mother and fetus because of the possibility of uterine rupture and are not recommended. Cesarean delivery is preferred in these situations. The fetal head at station +2 or lower is termed low forceps. (R)

89. **1.** Oligohydramnios, or a decrease in the volume of amniotic fluid, is associated with variable fetal heart rate decelerations due to cord compression. Maintenance of an adequate amniotic fluid volume during labor provides protective cushioning of the umbilical cord and minimizes cord compression. Cord compression can result in fetal metabolic acidosis, not alkalosis. Amnioinfusion is used to minimize cord compression, not to increase the fetal heart rate accelerations during a contraction. The goal is to maintain the amniotic fluid index at 8 cm. This can be determined by ultrasound. (R)

90. **4.** A primigravid client diagnosed with pregnancy-induced hypertension has the potential for developing seizures (eclampsia). This client should be in a room with the least amount of stimulation possible to reduce the risk of seizures and as close to the nurses' station as possible in case the client requires immediate assistance. Bright lighting and sunshine can be a stimulant, possibly increasing the risk of seizures, as can being in a semiprivate room with roommate, visitors, conversation, and noise. (M)

91. **4.** The client is experiencing a precipitous delivery. The nurse should remain calm during a precipitous delivery. Explaining to the client what is happening as the birth progresses and how she can assist is likely to help her remain calm and cooperative. Maintaining eye contact is also beneficial. Telling the client that she is right and to just relax is inappropriate because the client may not be able to relax because of the strong urge to push the fetus out of the birth canal. Telling the client not to push because she may tear the cervix can instill fear, not cooperation. Saying that the physician will be there soon may not be an accurate statement and is not reassuring if the client is concerned about the delivery. (P)

92. **2.** During a precipitous delivery, after calling for assistance and helping the client lie down, the nurse should provide support to the fetal head to prevent it from coming out. It is not appropriate to tell the client to push between contractions because this may lead to lacerations. The shoulder should be delivered by applying downward traction until the anterior shoulder appears fully at the introitus, then upward pressure to lift out the other shoulder. Priority should be given to safe delivery of the infant over protecting the perineum by massage. (R)

93. **2.** Because delivery occurs so rapidly and the fetus is propelled quickly through the birth canal, the major complication of a precipitous delivery is a boggy fundus, or uterine atony. The neonate should be put to the breast, if the mother permits, to allow for the release of natural oxytocin. In a hospital setting, the physician will probably order administration of oxytocin. The nurse should gently massage the fundus to ensure that it is firm. There is no relationship between a precipitous delivery and postpartum "blues" or intrauterine infection. Postpartum "blues" usually does not occur until about 3 days postpartum, and symptoms of postpartum infection usually occur after the first 24 hours. There is no relationship between a precipitous delivery and urinary tract infection even though the delivery has been accomplished under clean rather than sterile technique. Symptoms of urinary tract infection typically begin on the first or second postpartum day. (R)

94. **2.** The fetal heart rate of a multipara diagnosed with Rh sensitization and probable fetal hydrops and anemia will most likely demonstrate a sinusoidal pattern that resembles a sine wave. It has been hypothesized that this pattern reflects an absence of autonomic nervous control over the fetal heart rate resulting from severe hypoxia. This client will most likely require a cesarean delivery to improve the fetal outcome. Early decelerations are associated with head compression; variable decelerations are associated with cord compression; and late decelerations are associated with poor placental perfusion. (R)

95. **3.** Oxytocin, given postpartum to contract the uterus, should be administered after both twins and both placentas have been delivered. If oxytocin is given any earlier—after the first twin, after the first placenta, or after the second twin—the uterus will contract and make delivery of the placenta or placentas difficult. (D)

96. **1.** A priority assessment for the nurse to make is to determine the estimated date of delivery or probable gestational age of the fetus. If the gestation is less than 37 weeks, the neonatal team should be called to begin resuscitative efforts if needed. Amniotic fluid status is not important at this point, because if the fetal skull is crowning, delivery is imminent. Determination of gravida and parity is part of the normal nursing history, but the priority is the status of the fetus and safe delivery. Prenatal history is part of the nursing assessment, but this information is not especially relevant until the fetus is safely delivered and has been given immediate care. (H)

97. **2.** It is important that the parents be allowed to touch, hold, and participate in care of the twins whenever they desire. Ideally, this will be on a daily basis, to promote parent-infant bonding. It is not appropriate to discuss how the couple will cope with twin infants at home until they are ready to take the infants home. They are too overwhelmed at this point and are focused on the well-being of their infants while hospitalized. Having the couple visit the twins to provide care on a 24-hour basis is not warranted. Identifying complications that may occur is not appropriate. If complications arise, the parents should be well informed and given opportunities for discussion related to the care provided. (P)

98. **4.** The priority diagnosis is *Risk for infection* related to birth trauma and prolonged ruptured membranes. Infection can be a serious postpartum complication. Although the client may be fatigued, she should not be experiencing activity intolerance. Clients with heart disease may experience activity intolerance due to excessive cardiac workload. Although the client may be experiencing sleep deprivation, most clients are alert and awake after delivery of a newborn. *Situational low self-esteem* is not a priority diagnosis. Clients who undergo a cesarean delivery commonly feel a sense of failure because of not delivering vaginally, but this is not the case for this client. (R)

99. **2.** Postmature neonates commonly have difficulty maintaining adequate glucose reserves and usually develop hypoglycemia soon after birth. Other common problems include meconium aspiration syndrome, polycythemia, congenital anomalies, seizure activity, and cold stress. These complications result primarily from a combination of advanced gestational age, placental insufficiency, and continued exposure to amniotic fluid. Delayed meconium is not associated with post-term gestation. Hyperbilirubinemia occurs in term neonates as well as post-term neonates, but unless there is an Rh incompatibility it does not develop until after the first 24 hours of life. (R)

100. **4.** Polyhydramnios is an abnormally large amount of amniotic fluid in the uterus. The client has understood the instructions when the client states that polyhydramnios is associated with gastrointestinal disorders (e.g., tracheoesophageal fistula). Polyhydramnios is also associated with maternal illnesses such as diabetes and anemia. Other fetal/neonatal disorders associated with this condition include congenital anomalies of the central nervous system (e.g., anencephaly), upper gastrointestinal obstruction, and macrosomia. Polyhydramnios can lead to preterm labor, premature rupture of the membranes, and cord prolapse. Renal dysfunction and intrauterine growth retardation are associated with oligohydramnios, not polyhydramnios. Pulmonary hypoplasia (poorly developed lungs) is associated with prolonged oligohydramnios. (R)

101. **1.** If a client has been in active labor and there is no change in cervical dilation after 2 hours, the nurse should suspect cephalopelvic disproportion. This may be caused by an inadequate pelvis size of the mother or by a large-for-gestational-age fetus. The physician should be notified about the client's lack of progress. If the fetus cannot descend, a cesarean delivery is warranted. The client is not experiencing a prolonged latent phase (0 to 3 cm dilation), because her cervix is dilated to 6 cm. She has not reached the transitional phase, characterized by a cervical dilation of 8 to 10 cm. With a hypotonic labor pattern, contractions are painful but far apart and not very intense. This client's contractions are of moderate intensity. (R)

102. **3.** Preparation for cesarean delivery is similar to preparation for any abdominal surgery. The client must give informed consent. Another person may not sign for the client unless the client is unable to sign the form. If this is the case, only certain designated people can do so legally. The husband does not need to sign the form unless his wife is unable to do so. In an emergency, surgery may be performed without a written consent if it is done to save the life of the mother or the child, or both. (M)

103. **4.** Decreased variability may be seen in various conditions. However, it is most commonly caused by analgesic administration. Other factors that can cause decreased variability include anesthesia, deep fetal sleep, anencephaly, prematurity, hypoxia, tachycardia, brain damage, and arrhythmias. Maternal fatigue, fetal malposition, and small-for-gestational-age fetus are not commonly associated with decreased variability. (H)

104. **4.** It is not unusual for clients who undergo an emergency cesarean delivery to express thoughts of failure. Pain, hemorrhage, and anxiety may all occur, but the priority diagnosis at this time is *Situational low self-esteem*. In this situation, the nurse should be supportive and should allow the client to verbalize any feelings of failure, guilt, or anger. Nursing care should include reviewing the events that occurred and clearing up any questions or misconceptions. (P)

105. **4.** Respiratory distress syndrome is more common in neonates delivered by cesarean section than in those delivered vaginally. During a vaginal delivery, pressure is exerted on the fetal chest, which aids in the fetal inhalation and exhalation of air and lung expansion. This pressure is not exerted on the fetus with a cesarean delivery. Congenital anomalies are not more common with cesarean delivery. Pulmonary hypertension occurs more commonly in infants with meconium aspiration syndrome, congenital diaphragmatic hernia, respiratory distress syndrome, or neonatal sepsis, not with cesarean delivery. Meconium aspiration syndrome occurs more commonly with vaginal delivery, post-term neonate, and prolonged labor, not with cesarean delivery. (H)

106. **4.** Congenital anomalies are not related to maternal urinary tract infections. A multigravid client with acute pyelonephritis is susceptible to preterm labor, premature rupture of the membranes, maternal sepsis, intrauterine growth retardation, and fetal loss. The most common organism responsible for the urinary tract infection is *Escherichia coli*. (R)

107. **1.** Conjunctivitis is a common complication of neonates who are born to mothers with untreated chlamydial infection. Neonatal pneumonia is another condition associated with chlamydial infection of the mother. Untreated chlamydial infection is not associated with heart disease or brain damage. Exposure to rubella may lead to neonatal heart defects, and brain damage may occur as a result of prolonged shoulder dystocia or difficulty delivering the fetal head during a vaginal breech delivery. Occasionally, because of immature circulation, a neonate who has been lying on his or her side appears red on one side of the body. This "harlequin sign" is transient and is of no clinical significance. Presence of a harlequin sign is unrelated to untreated chlamydial infection. (R)

108. **1.** The purpose of the RHIG is to provide passive antibody immunity and prevent Rh-positive sensitization with the next pregnancy. It should be given within 72 hours after delivery of an Rh-positive neonate. Clients who are Rh-negative and conceive an Rh-negative fetus do not need antibody protection. Rh-positive cells contribute to sensitization, not Rh-negative cells. The RHIG does not cross the placenta and destroy fetal Rh-positive cells. (R)

109. **3.** Because magnesium sulfate is a central nervous system depressant, the nurse should plan to assess the client's respiratory rate every hour. If the respiratory rate is less than 12 breaths/minute, the client may be experiencing magnesium sulfate overdose. Urinary output via an indwelling catheter should be assessed hourly and should be at least 30 ml/hour. Deep tendon reflexes and blood pressure should also be assessed every hour. At some institutions continuous electronic blood pressure monitoring will be performed. (D)

110. **2.** For a client diagnosed with probable placenta previa, hypovolemic shock is a complication. Continuous blood pressure monitoring with an electronic cuff is the priority assessment after the client's admission. Once the client is admitted, an ultrasound examination will be performed to determine the placement of the placenta. Whole blood replacement is not warranted at this time. However, it may be necessary if the client demonstrates signs and symptoms of hemorrhage or shock. Internal fetal heart rate monitoring is contraindicated because the monitoring device may puncture the placenta and place both the mother and fetus in jeopardy. An immediate cesarean delivery is not necessary until there has been an assessment of the amount of bleeding and the location of the placenta previa. (R)

111. **4.** Dramatic vasoconstriction occurs as a result of sniffing crack cocaine. This can lead to increased respiratory and cardiac rates and hypertension. It can severely compromise placental circulation, resulting in abruptio placentae and preterm labor and delivery. Infants of these women can experience intracranial hemorrhage and withdrawal symptoms of tremulousness, irritability, and rigidity. Placenta previa, ruptured uterus, and maternal hypotension are not associated with cocaine use. Placenta previa may be associated with grand multiparity. Ruptured uterus may be associated with a large-for-gestational-age fetus. (R)

112. **2.** Pregnant women who become infected with the rubella virus early in pregnancy risk having a neonate born with rubella syndrome. The symptoms include thrombocytopenia, cataracts, cardiac disorders, deafness, microcephaly, and motor and cognitive impairment. The most extensive neonatal effects occur when the mother is exposed during the first 2 to 6 weeks and up to 12 weeks' gestation, when critical organs are forming. Bulging fontanels are associated with increased intracranial pressure and meningitis, which can occur as the result of a b-hemolytic streptococcal infection. (R)

113. **3.** To stop the process of DIC, the underlying insult that began the phenomenon must be halted. Treatment includes fresh-frozen platelets or blood administration. The physician also may order heparin before the administration of blood products to restore the normal clotting mechanism. Immediate delivery of the fetus is essential. Magnesium sulfate is given for pregnancy-induced hypertension or preterm labor. Heparin, not warfarin sodium (Coumadin), is used to treat DIC. Meperidine hydrochloride (Demerol) is used for pain relief. (D)

114. **2.** The nurse determines that the medication has had a therapeutic effect when a decrease in the frequency and number of contractions is noted. Terbutaline (Brethine) is a tocolytic that is used to halt the preterm labor process. This medication is administered as a "piggyback" to the regular intravenous fluids. Adverse effects include tachycardia. It should not be given if the client's pulse rate is greater than 120 bpm. (D)

115. **1.** Although thioamides such as propylthiouracil and methimazole are considered teratogenic to the fetus and can lead to congenital hyperthyroidism (goiter) in the neonate, they still represent the treatment of choice. The client should be regulated on the lowest possible dose. Hyperthyroidism is associated with preterm labor and a low-birth-weight infant, so the client should contact the physician or health care provider if the contractions begin again. The client should not be urged to breast-feed, because medications such as propylthiouracil and methimazole are secreted in breast milk. Tachycardia (not bradycardia) is associated with thyroid storm, a medical emergency, and should be reported to the physician. (D)

116. **4.** The first action by the nurse should be to call for immediate assistance in the client's room, because this is an emergency. Throughout the seizure, the nurse should note the time and length of the seizure and continue to monitor the status of both client and fetus. The side rails should have been padded at the time of the client's admission to the hospital as part of seizure precautions. The client should be turned to her left side to improve placental perfusion. Inserting a tongue blade is not recommended because it can further obstruct the airway or cause injury to the client's teeth. (S)

117. **3.** In an abusive situation, the client's safety is the priority. The nurse should refer the client to a social worker who can provide the client with options such as a safe shelter. Commonly clients who are battered feel powerless and fear that the batterer will kill them. As a result, they remain in the abusive situation. Telling the client to leave the boyfriend immediately is not helpful and reflects the values of the nurse. Although asking about fetal movement is important and is part of a routine assessment, a sonogram can be performed to confirm fetal well-being. The referral is more important at this time. Although it may be part of the unit's policies and procedures to report any incidents such as this one to the unit supervisor, the client's immediate need for safety must be addressed first. (M)

118. **1.** The client's symptoms are indicative of amniotic fluid embolism, which is a medical emergency. After calling for assistance, the first action should be to administer oxygen by face mask or cannula to ensure adequate oxygenation of mother and fetus. If the client needs cardiopulmonary resuscitation, this can be started once oxygen has been administered. If the client survives, disseminated intravascular coagulation will probably develop, and the client will need intravenous fibrinogen and heparin. Oxytocin, a vasoconstrictor, is not warranted for amniotic fluid embolism. (A)

Postpartal Care

The Postpartal Client with a Vaginal Birth

1. A client is in the first hour of her recovery after a vaginal delivery. During an assessment, the lochia is moderate, bright red, and is trickling from the vagina. The nurse locates the fundus at the umbilicus; it is firm and midline with no palpable bladder. The client's vital signs remain at their baseline. Based on this information, the nurse would implement which of the following actions?
- [ ] **1.** Increase the I.V. rate.
- [ ] **2.** Recheck the admission hematocrit and hemoglobin levels.
- [ ] **3.** Report the findings to the health care provider.
- [ ] **4.** Document the findings as normal.

2. The nurse is caring for a G 3, T 3, P 0, Ab 0, L 3 woman who is one day postpartum following a vaginal delivery. Which assessment of the client indicates a need for further assessment?
- [ ] **1.** Increased hematocrit and hemoglobin.
- [ ] **2.** White blood cell (WBC) count of 15,000.
- [ ] **3.** Pulse of 60.
- [ ] **4.** Temperature of 100.8° F.

3. The nurse is caring for a postpartum client who delivered vaginally 4 hours ago and has not voided since delivery. Feeling has returned to her perineal area, and she has ambulated to the bathroom and attempted to void twice. She has ice on her edematous perineum. Her uterus is 3 fingerbreadths above the umbilicus, to the right of midline, and firm only with massage. What would be the priority nursing action(s)?
- [ ] **1.** Evaluate the client with a bladder scan.
- [ ] **2.** Insert a Foley catheter.
- [ ] **3.** Medicate the client with a nonsteroidal anti-inflammatory drug (NSAID).
- [ ] **4.** Massage the fundus until it is firm and perform a one-time catheterization on the client.

4. A client delivered vaginally two hours ago and has a third-degree laceration. There is ice in place on her perineum. However, her perineum is slightly edematous and the client is complaining of pain rated 6 on a scale of 1 to 10. Which nursing intervention would be the most appropriate at this time?
- [ ] **1.** Begin sitz baths.
- [ ] **2.** Administer pain medication per order.
- [ ] **3.** Replace ice packs to the perineum.
- [ ] **4.** Initiate anesthetic sprays to the perineum.

5. A client is in the fourth stage of labor. Which set of interventions is the highest priority at this time?
- [ ] **1.** Assessment of the ability to push with contractions, hydration, and emotional stability.
- [ ] **2.** Assessment of maternal vital signs, fetal heart tones, and the contraction pattern.
- [ ] **3.** Assessment of maternal vital signs, the fundus, the bladder, and lochia.
- [ ] **4.** Assessment of maternal emotional status, infant bonding, and feeding preferences.

6. A primigravid client delivered vaginally 2 hours ago with no complications. As the nurse plans care for this postpartum client, which postpartum goal would have the highest priority?
- [ ] **1.** By discharge, the family will bond with the neonate.
- [ ] **2.** The client will demonstrate self-care and infant care by the end of the shift.
- [ ] **3.** The client will state instructions for discharge during the first postpartum day.
- [ ] **4.** By the end of the shift, the client will describe a safe home environment.

7. In response to the nurse's question about how she is feeling, a postpartum client states that she is fine. She then begins talking to the baby, checking the diaper, and asking infant care questions. The nurse determines the client is in which postpartal phase of psychological adaptation?
- [ ] **1.** Taking in.
- [ ] **2.** Taking on.
- [ ] **3.** Taking hold.
- [ ] **4.** Letting go.

8. A client has admitted use of cocaine prior to beginning labor. After the infant is born, the nurse should anticipate the need to include which of the following actions in the infant's plan of care?
☐ **1.** Urine toxicology screening.
☐ **2.** Notifying hospital security.
☐ **3.** Limiting contact with visitors.
☐ **4.** Contacting local law enforcement.

9. The nurse is evaluating the client who delivered vaginally 2 hours ago and is experiencing postpartum pain rated 8 on scale of 1 to 10. The client is a G 4, P 4, breast-feeding mother who would like medication to decrease the pain in her uterus. Which of the medications listed on the orders sheet would be the most appropriate analgesic for this client?
☐ **1.** Aspirin 1,000 mg P.O. q 4 to 6 hr p.r.n.
☐ **2.** Ibuprofen 800 mg P.O. q 6 to 8 hr p.r.n.
☐ **3.** Colace 100 mg P.O. b.i.d.
☐ **4.** Vicodin 1 to 2 tabs P.O. q 4 to 6 hr p.r.n.

10. At which of the following locations would the nurse expect to palpate the fundus of a primiparous client immediately after delivery of a neonate?
☐ **1.** Halfway between the umbilicus and the symphysis pubis.
☐ **2.** At the level of the umbilicus.
☐ **3.** Just below the level of the umbilicus.
☐ **4.** Above the level of the umbilicus.

11. When instilling erythromycin ointment into the eyes of a neonate 1 hour old, the nurse would explain to the parents that the medication is used to prevent which of the following?
☐ **1.** Chorioretinitis from cytomegalovirus.
☐ **2.** Blindness secondary to gonorrhea.
☐ **3.** Cataracts from beta-hemolytic streptococcus.
☐ **4.** Strabismus resulting from neonatal maturation.

12. The physician orders an intramuscular injection of phytonadione (AquaMEPHYTON) for a term neonate. The nurse explains to the mother that this medication is used to prevent which of the following?
☐ **1.** Hypoglycemia.
☐ **2.** Hyperbilirubinemia.
☐ **3.** Hemorrhage.
☐ **4.** Polycythemia.

13. When developing the plan of care for a primiparous client during the first 12 hours after vaginal delivery, which of the following concerns of the client should be the nurse's primary focus of care?
☐ **1.** The neonate.
☐ **2.** The family.
☐ **3.** The client's own comfort.
☐ **4.** The client's significant other.

14. The nurse assesses a swollen ecchymosed area to the right of an episiotomy on a primiparous client 6 hours after a vaginal delivery. Which of the following actions should the nurse do next?
☐ **1.** Apply an ice pack to the perineal area.
☐ **2.** Assess the client's temperature.
☐ **3.** Have the client take a warm sitz bath.
☐ **4.** Contact the physician for orders for an antibiotic.

15. Two hours after vaginally delivering a viable male neonate under epidural anesthesia, the client with a midline episiotomy ambulates to the bathroom to void. After voiding, the nurse assesses the client's bladder, finding it distended. The nurse interprets this finding based on the understanding that the client's bladder distention is most likely caused by which of the following?
☐ **1.** Prolonged first stage of labor.
☐ **2.** Urinary tract infection.
☐ **3.** Pressure of the uterus on the bladder.
☐ **4.** Edema in the lower urinary tract area.

16. A primiparous client who is bottle-feeding her neonate at 12 hours after birth asks the nurse, "When will my menstrual cycle return?" Which of the following responses by the nurse would be most appropriate?
☐ **1.** "Your menstrual cycle will return in 3 to 4 weeks."
☐ **2.** "It will probably be 6 to 10 weeks before it starts again."
☐ **3.** "You can expect your menses to start in 12 to 14 weeks."
☐ **4.** "Your menses will return in 16 to 18 weeks."

17. While the nurse is preparing to assist the primiparous client to the bathroom to void 6 hours after a vaginal delivery under epidural anesthesia, the client says that she feels dizzy when sitting up on the side of the bed. The nurse explains that this is most likely caused by which of the following?
☐ **1.** Effects of the anesthetic during labor.
☐ **2.** Hemorrhage during the delivery process.
☐ **3.** Effects of analgesics used during labor.
☐ **4.** Decreased blood volume in the vascular system.

18. The nurse delegates the care of a multiparous client who delivered a viable term neonate vaginally 30 hours ago and is preparing to be discharged to a licensed practical nurse (LPN). The nurse expects to be notified by the LPN if the client exhibits which of the following?
☐ **1.** Pulse rate of 100 bpm.
☐ **2.** Oral temperature of 99° F (36.8° C).
☐ **3.** Excessive perspiration during the assessment.
☐ **4.** Frequent voiding in large amounts.

19. Which of the following would be a priority nursing diagnosis for a primiparous client 4 hours after a low forceps vaginal delivery with a midline episiotomy and prolonged labor under epidural anesthesia who required catheterization during labor and once during the delivery?

☐ **1.** *Risk for infection* related to prolonged labor and catheterization.

☐ **2.** *Disturbed body image* related to midline episiotomy.

☐ **3.** *Risk for imbalanced fluid volume* related to prolonged labor and anesthesia.

☐ **4.** *Urinary retention* related to trauma of delivery.

20. The nurse enlists the aid of an interpreter when caring for a primiparous client from Mexico who speaks very little English and delivered a viable term neonate 8 hours ago. When developing the postpartum dietary plan of care for the client, the nurse would encourage the client's intake of which of the following?

☐ **1.** Tomatoes.

☐ **2.** Potatoes.

☐ **3.** Corn products.

☐ **4.** Meat products.

21. Three hours postpartum, a primiparous client's fundus is firm and midline. On perineal inspection, the nurse observes a small, constant trickle of blood. Which of the following conditions should the nurse suspect?

☐ **1.** Retained placental tissue.

☐ **2.** Uterine inversion.

☐ **3.** Bladder distention.

☐ **4.** Perineal lacerations.

22. While making a home visit to a postpartum client on day 11, the nurse would anticipate that the client's lochia would be which of the following colors?

☐ **1.** Dark red.

☐ **2.** Pink.

☐ **3.** Brown.

☐ **4.** White.

23. After instructing a primiparous client about episiotomy care, which of the following client statements indicates successful teaching?

☐ **1.** "I'll use hot, sudsy water to clean the episiotomy area."

☐ **2.** "I wipe the area from front to back using a blotting motion."

☐ **3.** "Before bedtime, I'll use a cold water sitz bath."

☐ **4.** "I can use ice packs for 3 to 4 days after delivery."

24. After explaining the procedure for using a portable sitz bath to a primiparous client who delivered 30 hours ago, which of the following would the nurse do next?

☐ **1.** Fill the collecting bag with water at a temperature of 107° F (41.25° C).

☐ **2.** Spray the perineal area with the ordered analgesic spray.

☐ **3.** Wash hands and don clean gloves for the procedure.

☐ **4.** Assess the client's perineum for swelling and redness.

25. A primiparous client, 20 hours after delivery, asks the nurse about starting postpartum exercises. Which of the following would be most appropriate to include in the nurse's instructions?

☐ **1.** Start in a sitting position, then lie back, and return to a sitting position, repeating this five times.

☐ **2.** Assume a prone position, then do push-ups by using the arms to lift the upper body.

☐ **3.** Flex the knees while supine, then inhale deeply and exhale while contracting the abdominal muscles.

☐ **4.** Flex the knees while supine, then bring chin to chest while exhaling and reach for the knees by lifting the head and shoulders while inhaling.

26. A multiparous client whose fundus is firm and midline at the umbilicus 8 hours after a vaginal delivery tells the nurse that when she ambulated to the bathroom after sleeping for 4 hours, her dark red lochia seemed heavier. Which of the following would the nurse include when explaining to the client about the increased lochia on ambulation?

☐ **1.** Her bleeding needs to be reported to the physician immediately.

☐ **2.** The increased lochia occurs from lochia pooling in the vaginal vault.

☐ **3.** The increase in lochia may be an early sign of postpartum hemorrhage.

☐ **4.** This increase in lochia usually indicates retained placental fragments.

27. Four hours after delivering a viable neonate by spontaneous vaginal delivery under epidural anesthesia, the client states she needs to urinate. Which of the following would the nurse anticipate doing next?

☐ **1.** Catheterize the client to obtain an accurate measurement.

☐ **2.** Palpate the bladder to determine distention.

☐ **3.** Assess the fundus to see if it is at the midline.

☐ **4.** Measure the first two voidings and record the amount.

28. A primiparous client who delivered vaginally 8 hours ago desires to take a shower. The nurse anticipates remaining nearby the client to assess for which of the following?

☐ **1.** Fatigue.
☐ **2.** Fainting.
☐ **3.** Diuresis.
☐ **4.** Hygiene needs.

29. A primiparous client who delivered 12 hours ago under epidural anesthesia with a midline episiotomy tells the nurse that she is experiencing a great deal of discomfort when she sits in a chair with the baby. Which of the following instructions would be most appropriate?

☐ **1.** "Ask for some pain medication before you sit down."
☐ **2.** "Squeeze your buttock muscles together before sitting down."
☐ **3.** "Keep a relaxed posture before sitting down with your full weight."
☐ **4.** "Ask the physician for some analgesic cream or spray."

30. Which of the following would the nurse include in the primiparous client's discharge teaching plan about measures to provide visual stimulation for the neonate?

☐ **1.** Maintain eye contact while talking to the baby.
☐ **2.** Paint the baby's room in bright colors accented with teddy bears.
☐ **3.** Use brightly colored animals and cartoon figures on the wall.
☐ **4.** Move a brightly colored rattle in front of the baby's eyes.

31. A primiparous client has just delivered a healthy male infant. The client and her husband are Muslim and the husband begins chanting a song in Arabic while holding the neonate. The nurse interprets the father's actions as indicative of which of the following?

☐ **1.** Thanking Allah for giving him a male heir.
☐ **2.** Singing to his son from the Koran in praise of Allah.
☐ **3.** Expressing appreciation that his wife and son are healthy.
☐ **4.** Performing a ritual similar to baptism in other religions.

32. An adolescent primiparous client 24 hours postpartum asks the nurse how often she can hold her baby without "spoiling" him. Which of the following responses would be most appropriate?

☐ **1.** "Hold him when he is fussy or crying."
☐ **2.** "Hold him as much as you want to hold him."
☐ **3.** "Try to hold him infrequently to avoid overstimulation."
☐ **4.** "You can hold him periodically throughout the day."

33. The nurse on the night shift finds a multiparous client, 8 hours postpartum, drenched in perspiration. The client's temperature is 99° F (36.8° C), the pulse is 68 bpm, and the blood pressure is 120/80 mm Hg. Which of the following nursing diagnoses would be most appropriate?

☐ **1.** *Risk for infection* (postpartum) related to birth trauma.
☐ **2.** *Ineffective thermoregulation* related to hormonal changes.
☐ **3.** *Ineffective tissue perfusion: Renal* related to the status of multiparity.
☐ **4.** *Excess fluid volume* related to normal postpartal diuresis.

34. On the first postpartum day, the primiparous client complains of perineal pain that was unrelieved by ibuprofen 800 mg given 2 hours ago. The nurse would assess for which of the following?

☐ **1.** Puerperal infection.
☐ **2.** Vaginal lacerations.
☐ **3.** History of drug abuse.
☐ **4.** Perineal hematoma.

35. The nurse assigns an individual who is an unlicensed assistive personnel to care for a client who is one day postpartum. Which of the following would be appropriate to delegate to this person? Select all that apply.

☐ **1.** Changing the perineal pad and reporting the drainage.
☐ **2.** Assisting the mother to latch the infant onto the breast.
☐ **3.** Checking the location of the fundus prior to ambulating the client.
☐ **4.** Reinforcing good hygiene while assisting the client with washing the perineum.
☐ **5.** Discussing postpartum depression with the client who is found crying.
☐ **6.** Assisting the client with ambulation shortly after delivery.

36. While the nurse is caring for a primiparous client on the first postpartum day, the client asks, "How is that woman doing who lost her baby from prematurity? We were in labor together." Which of the following responses by the nurse would be most appropriate?

☐ **1.** Ignore the client's question and continue with morning care.
☐ **2.** Tell the client "I'm not sure how the other woman is doing today."
☐ **3.** Tell the client "I need to ask the woman's permission before discussing her well-being."
☐ **4.** Explain to the client that "Nurses are not allowed to discuss other clients on the unit."

37. A newly delivered primiparous client asks the nurse, "Can my baby see?" Which of the following statements about neonatal vision should the nurse include in the explanation?
- ☐ **1.** Neonates primarily focus on moving objects.
- ☐ **2.** They can see objects up to 12 inches away.
- ☐ **3.** Usually they see clearly by about 2 days after birth.
- ☐ **4.** Neonates primarily distinguish light from dark.

38. While assessing the fundus of a multiparous client 36 hours after delivery of a term neonate, the nurse notes a separation of the abdominal muscles. Which of the following should the nurse anticipate?
- ☐ **1.** A surgical repair at 6 weeks postpartum.
- ☐ **2.** Limited activity and bed rest until resolution occurs.
- ☐ **3.** Resolution on its own with the right posture and diet.
- ☐ **4.** Exercises involving head and shoulder raising in a lying position.

39. A postpartum client delivered 6 hours ago without anesthesia and just voided 100 ml. The nurse palpates the fundus 2 fingerbreadths above the umbilicus and off to the right side. What should the nurse do first?
- ☐ **1.** Administer ibuprofen (Motrin).
- ☐ **2.** Reassess in 1 hour.
- ☐ **3.** Catheterize the client.
- ☐ **4.** Administer an I.V. bolus of 500 ml to rehydrate per policy.

40. While the nurse is assessing the fundus of a multiparous client who delivered 24 hours ago, the client asks, "What can I do to get rid of these stretch marks?" Which of the following responses would be most appropriate?
- ☐ **1.** "As long as you don't get pregnant again, the marks will disappear completely."
- ☐ **2.** "They usually fade to a silvery-white color over a period of time."
- ☐ **3.** "You'll need to use a specially prescribed cream to help them disappear."
- ☐ **4.** "If you lose the weight you gained during pregnancy, the marks will fade to a pale pink."

41. A primiparous client who delivered a viable neonate 8 hours ago tells the nurse that she gained 26 lb during pregnancy and asks how long it will take to return to her normal prepregnant weight. Which of the following would the nurse include as the usual time frame for returning to prepregnant weight?
- ☐ **1.** 4 weeks.
- ☐ **2.** 6 weeks.
- ☐ **3.** 8 weeks.
- ☐ **4.** 12 weeks.

42. An adolescent primiparous client at 24 hours postpartum tells the nurse that she and her baby will be living with her boyfriend's parents so that she can finish high school and go on to college. The client's boyfriend and parents have been supportive of the client and neonate. Which of the following would be an appropriate nursing diagnosis at this time?
- ☐ **1.** *Anxiety* related to return to high school and peer pressure.
- ☐ **2.** *Ineffective coping* related to inability to view motherhood realistically.
- ☐ **3.** *Readiness for enhanced family coping*, related to the addition of a new family member.
- ☐ **4.** *Deficient knowledge* related to the financial and emotional costs of childrearing.

43. A primiparous client who delivered a viable term neonate vaginally 48 hours ago has a midline episiotomy and repair of a third-degree laceration. When preparing the client for discharge, which of the following assessments would be most important?
- ☐ **1.** Constipation.
- ☐ **2.** Diarrhea.
- ☐ **3.** Excessive bleeding.
- ☐ **4.** Rectal fistulas.

44. In preparation for discharge, the nurse discusses sexual issues with a primiparous client who had a routine vaginal delivery with a midline episiotomy. Which of the following would the nurse include as the most appropriate time for resuming sexual intercourse?
- ☐ **1.** In 6 weeks when the episiotomy is completely healed.
- ☐ **2.** After a postpartum check by the health care provider.
- ☐ **3.** Whenever the client is feeling amorous and desirable.
- ☐ **4.** When lochia flow and episiotomy pain have stopped.

45. The physician orders docusate sodium (Colace) 100 mg at bedtime for a primiparous client after vaginal delivery of a term neonate after a midline episiotomy. The nurse explains that this medication is used for which of the following reasons?
- ☐ **1.** Analgesia for episiotomy pain.
- ☐ **2.** Contraction of the uterus.
- ☐ **3.** Softening of the stool.
- ☐ **4.** Aid in sleeping.

46. While caring for a multiparous client 4 hours after vaginal delivery of a term neonate, the nurse notes that the mother's temperature is 99.8° F (37.2° C), the pulse is 66 bpm, and the respirations are 18 breaths/minute. Her fundus is firm, midline, and at the level of the umbilicus. Which of the following actions would be most appropriate?
- ☐ **1.** Continue to monitor the client's vital signs.
- ☐ **2.** Assess the client's lochia for large clots.
- ☐ **3.** Notify the client's physician about the findings.
- ☐ **4.** Offer the mother an ice pack for her forehead.

47. While assessing the episiotomy site of a primiparous client on the first postpartum day, the nurse observes a fairly large hemorrhoid at the client's rectum. After instructing the client about measures to relieve hemorrhoid discomfort, which of the following client statements indicates the need for additional teaching?
- ☐ **1.** "I should try to gently manually replace the hemorrhoid."
- ☐ **2.** "Analgesic sprays and witch hazel pads can relieve the pain."
- ☐ **3.** "I should lie on my back as much as possible to relieve the pain."
- ☐ **4.** "I should drink lots of water and eat foods that have a lot of roughage."

48. A primiparous client is on a regular diet 24 hours postpartum. She is from Guatemala and speaks little English. The client's mother asks the nurse if she can bring her daughter some "special foods from home." The nurse responds, based on the understanding about which of the following?
- ☐ **1.** Foods from home are generally discouraged on the postpartum unit.
- ☐ **2.** The mother can bring the daughter any foods that she desires.
- ☐ **3.** This is permissible as long as the foods are nutritious and high in iron.
- ☐ **4.** The client's physician needs to give permission for the foods.

49. A primiparous client, 48 hours after a vaginal delivery, is to be discharged with a prescription for vitamins with iron because she is anemic. To maximize absorption of the iron, the nurse instructs the client to take the medication with which of the following?
- ☐ **1.** Orange juice.
- ☐ **2.** Herbal tea.
- ☐ **3.** Milk.
- ☐ **4.** Grape juice.

50. The nurse is caring for a multiparous client after vaginal delivery of a set of male twins 2 hours ago. Which of the following would the nurse encourage the mother and husband to do?
- ☐ **1.** Bottle-feed the twins to prevent exhaustion and fatigue.
- ☐ **2.** Plan for each parent to spend equal amounts of time with each twin.
- ☐ **3.** Avoid assistance from other family members until attachment occurs.
- ☐ **4.** Relate to each twin individually to enhance the attachment process.

51. Twelve hours after a vaginal delivery with epidural anesthesia, the nurse palpates the fundus of a primiparous client and finds it to be firm, above the umbilicus, and deviated to the right. Which of the following would the nurse do next?
- ☐ **1.** Document this as a normal finding in the client's record.
- ☐ **2.** Contact the physician for an order for methylergonovine.
- ☐ **3.** Encourage the client to ambulate to the bathroom and void.
- ☐ **4.** Gently massage the fundus to expel the clots.

52. A nurse is discussing discharge instructions with a client. Which of the following statements indicate that the client understands the resources and information available if needed after discharge? Select all that apply.
- ☐ **1.** "I know to wait 2 weeks before I start my birth control pills."
- ☐ **2.** "I have the hospital phone number if I have any questions."
- ☐ **3.** "If I have any breathing problems, chest pain, or pounding fast heart rate, I will seek medical assistance."
- ☐ **4.** "My mother is coming to help for a month so I will be fine."
- ☐ **5.** "I know if I get fever or chills or change in lochia to call the physician."
- ☐ **6.** "I will continue my prenatal vitamins until my postpartum checkup or longer."

The Postpartal Client Who Breast-Feeds

53. The nurse is reviewing discharge instructions with a postpartum breast-feeding client who is going home. She has chosen medroxyprogesterone (Depo-Provera) as birth control. Which statement by the client identifies that she needs further instruction concerning birth control?
- ☐ **1.** "I will wait for my 6-week check up to get my first Depo-Provera shot."
- ☐ **2.** "Depo-Provera injections last for 90 days."
- ☐ **3.** "My milk supply should be well established before using Depo-Provera."
- ☐ **4.** "You will give me my first Depo-Provera shot before I leave today."

54. A postpartum primiparous client is having difficulty breast-feeding her infant. The infant latches on to the breast but the mother's nipples are extremely sore during and after each feeding. The client needs further instruction about breast-feeding when she states:
- ☐ 1. "The baby needs to have as much of the nipple and areola in his mouth as possible to prevent sore and cracked nipples."
- ☐ 2. "I can put breast milk on my nipples to heal the sore areas."
- ☐ 3. "As long as some of my nipple is in the baby's mouth, the baby will receive enough milk."
- ☐ 4. "Feeding the baby for a half-hour on each side will not make my breasts sore. "

55. The nurse is caring for a primipara who delivered her baby yesterday and has chosen to breast-feed her neonate. Which assessment finding is considered unusual for the client at this point postpartum?
- ☐ 1. Milk production.
- ☐ 2. Diaphoresis.
- ☐ 3. Constipation.
- ☐ 4. Diuresis.

56. The nurse is caring for several mother-baby couplets. In planning the care for each of the couplets, which mother would the nurse expect to have the most severe afterbirth pains?
- ☐ 1. G 4, P 1 client who is breast-feeding her infant.
- ☐ 2. G 3, P 3 client who is breast-feeding her infant.
- ☐ 3. G 2, P 2 cesarean client who is bottle-feeding her infant.
- ☐ 4. G 3, P 3 client who is bottle-feeding her infant.

57. A breast-feeding client is seen at home by the visiting nurse 10 days after a vaginal delivery. The client is complaining of a warm, red, painful breast; a temperature of 100° F; and flulike symptoms. What should the nurse do?
- ☐ 1. Encourage the client to breast-feed her infant using the unaffected breast.
- ☐ 2. Refer the woman to her primary health care provider.
- ☐ 3. Inform the client that she needs to discontinue breast-feeding.
- ☐ 4. Instruct the woman to apply warm compresses to the affected breast.

58. A diabetic postpartum client plans to breast-feed. The nurse determines that the client's understanding of breast-feeding instructions is sufficient when she states:
- ☐ 1. "Insulin will be transferred to the baby through breast milk."
- ☐ 2. "Breast-feeding is not recommended for diabetic mothers."
- ☐ 3. "Breast milk from diabetic mothers contains few antibodies."
- ☐ 4. "Breast-feeding will assist in lowering maternal blood glucose."

59. A primiparous client who delivered a viable neonate 48 hours ago experienced a third-degree laceration. In preparation for discharge, the nurse instructs the client, who is breast-feeding her neonate, about perineal care. Which of the following client statements indicates the need for further instructions?
- ☐ 1. "I can take acetaminophen every 3 to 4 hours or ibuprofen every 6 to 8 hours for the discomfort."
- ☐ 2. "Warm sitz baths three or four times a day for 20 minutes can offer relief."
- ☐ 3. "I should try to prevent constipation by drinking plenty of fluids."
- ☐ 4. "I can take an aspirin with codeine every 4 hours for the discomfort."

60. During the home visit, a breast-feeding client asks the nurse what contraception method she and her husband should use until she has her 6-week postpartal examination. Which of the following would be most appropriate for the nurse to suggest?
- ☐ 1. Condom with spermicide.
- ☐ 2. Oral contraceptives.
- ☐ 3. Rhythm method.
- ☐ 4. Abstinence.

61. A primiparous client who is beginning to breast-feed her neonate asks the nurse, "Is it important for my baby to get colostrum?" When instructing the client, the nurse would explain that colostrum provides the neonate with which of the following?
- ☐ 1. More fat than breast milk.
- ☐ 2. Vitamin K, which the neonate lacks.
- ☐ 3. Delayed meconium passage.
- ☐ 4. Passive immunity from maternal antibodies.

62. Which of the following forms the basis for the teaching plan about avoiding medication use unless prescribed for a primiparous client who is breast-feeding?
- ☐ 1. Breast milk quality and richness are decreased.
- ☐ 2. The mother's motivation to breast-feed is diminished.
- ☐ 3. Medications may be excreted in breast milk to the nursing neonate.
- ☐ 4. Medications interfere with the mother's let-down reflex.

63. A breast-feeding primiparous client with a midline episiotomy is prescribed ibuprofen 200 mg orally. The nurse instructs the client to take the medication at which of the following times?
- ☐ 1. Before going to bed.
- ☐ 2. Midway between feedings.
- ☐ 3. Immediately after a feeding.
- ☐ 4. When providing supplemental formula.

64. Which of the following would the nurse include in the teaching plan for a primiparous client about the frequency of breast-feeding the neonate during the first few days?

☐ **1.** Feeding the neonate whenever he or she cries.

☐ **2.** Restricting feedings to 1 to 2 minutes per side.

☐ **3.** Feeding the neonate for at least 10 minutes per side.

☐ **4.** Maintaining feeding for 20 to 30 minutes per side.

65. A multiparous client, 28 hours after cesarean delivery, who is breast-feeding complains of severe cramps or afterpains. The nurse explains that these are caused by which of the following?

☐ **1.** Flatulence accumulation after a cesarean delivery.

☐ **2.** Healing of the abdominal incision after cesarean delivery.

☐ **3.** Adverse effects of the medications administered after delivery.

☐ **4.** Release of oxytocin during the breast-feeding session.

66. After the nurse counsels a primiparous client who is breast-feeding her neonate about diet and nutritional needs during the lactation period, which of the following client statements indicates a need for additional teaching?

☐ **1.** "I need to increase my intake of vitamin D."

☐ **2.** "I should drink at least five glasses of fluid daily."

☐ **3.** "I need to get an extra 500 calories per day."

☐ **4.** "I need to make sure I have enough calcium in my diet."

67. The client is breast-feeding and asks the nurse about nutrition and diet. Which of the following statements by the client indicate understanding of dietary needs to promote successful breast-feeding? Select all that apply.

☐ **1.** "I need to increase the number of meals I eat from three to five each day."

☐ **2.** "I have to add about 500 more calories to my diet while I breast-feed."

☐ **3.** "I need at least two servings of protein, like meat or eggs, with each meal."

☐ **4.** "I need to double my fluids from my normal three to six glasses each day."

☐ **5.** "I can include fats in my diet now."

☐ **6.** "I can eat more cheese and drink orange juice with calcium to increase my calcium intake."

68. A breast-feeding primiparous client asks the nurse how breast milk differs from cow's milk. The nurse responds by saying that breast milk is higher in which of the following?

☐ **1.** Fat.

☐ **2.** Iron.

☐ **3.** Sodium.

☐ **4.** Calcium.

69. While assisting a primiparous client with her first breast-feeding session, which of the following actions would the nurse instruct the mother to do to stimulate the neonate to open the mouth and grasp the nipple?

☐ **1.** Pull down gently on the neonate's chin and insert the nipple.

☐ **2.** Squeeze both of the neonate's cheeks simultaneously.

☐ **3.** Place the nipple into the neonate's mouth on top of the tongue.

☐ **4.** Brush the neonate's lips lightly with the nipple.

70. A 25-year-old primiparous client who delivered a viable neonate 2 hours ago has decided to breast-feed her neonate. Which of the following instructions should the nurse address as the highest priority in the teaching plan about preventing nipple soreness?

☐ **1.** Keeping plastic liners in the brassiere to keep the nipple drier.

☐ **2.** Placing as much of the areola as possible into the baby's mouth.

☐ **3.** Smoothly pulling the nipple out of the mouth after 10 minutes.

☐ **4.** Removing any remaining milk left on the nipple with a soft washcloth.

71. Which of the following client statements indicates effective teaching about burping a breast-fed neonate?

☐ **1.** "Breast-fed babies who are burped frequently will take more on each breast."

☐ **2.** "If I supplement the baby with formula, I will rarely have to burp him."

☐ **3.** "I'll breast-feed my baby every 3 hours so I won't have to burp him."

☐ **4.** "When I switch to the other breast, I'll burp the baby."

72. After the nurse teaches a primiparous client planning to return to work in 6 weeks about storing breast milk, which of the following client statements indicates the need for further teaching?

☐ **1.** "I can let the milk sit out in a bottle for up to 10 hours."

☐ **2.** "I'll be sure to label the milk with the date, time, and amount."

☐ **3.** "I can safely store the milk for 3 days in the refrigerator."

☐ **4.** "I can keep the milk in a deep-freeze in clean glass bottles for up to 1 year."

73. During a home visit on the fourth postpartum day, a primiparous client tells the nurse that she is aware of a "let-down sensation" in her breasts and asks what causes it. The nurse explains that the let-down sensation is stimulated by which of the following?

☐ **1.** Adrenalin.

☐ **2.** Estrogen.

☐ **3.** Prolactin.

☐ **4.** Oxytocin.

74. A 19-year-old primiparous client delivered a viable male neonate 2 hours ago. She has decided to breast-feed, and her 22-year-old husband supports her decision. The neonate has a strong sucking reflex. Which of the following would be a priority nursing diagnosis?
- [ ] **1.** *Ineffective role performance* related to time involved in breast-feeding.
- [ ] **2.** *Risk for impaired skin integrity* related to neonate's sucking needs.
- [ ] **3.** *Deficient knowledge* related to inexperience with breast-feeding.
- [ ] **4.** *Fear* related to lack of motivation about breast-feeding.

75. During a home visit on the fourth postpartum day, a primiparous client tells the nurse that she has been experiencing breast engorgement. To relieve engorgement, the nurse teaches the client that before nursing her baby, the client should do which of the following?
- [ ] **1.** Apply an ice cube to the nipples.
- [ ] **2.** Rub her nipples gently with lanolin cream.
- [ ] **3.** Express a small amount of breast milk.
- [ ] **4.** Offer the neonate a small amount of formula.

76. A breast-feeding primiparous client who delivered 8 hours ago asks the nurse, "How will I know that my baby is getting enough to eat?" Which of the following guidelines should the nurse include in the teaching plan as evidence of adequate intake?
- [ ] **1.** Six to eight wet diapers by the fifth day.
- [ ] **2.** Three to four transitional stools on the fourth day.
- [ ] **3.** Ability to fall asleep easily after feeding on the first day.
- [ ] **4.** Regain of lost birth weight by the third day.

77. Which of the following should the nurse include in the teaching plan for a primiparous client who asks about weaning her neonate?
- [ ] **1.** "Wait until you have breast-fed for at least 4 months."
- [ ] **2.** "Eliminate the baby's favorite feeding times first."
- [ ] **3.** "Plan to omit the daytime feedings last."
- [ ] **4.** "Gradually eliminate one feeding at a time."

78. Two weeks after a breast-feeding primiparous client is discharged, she calls the birthing center and says that she is afraid she is "losing my breast milk. The baby had been nursing every 4 hours, but now she's crying to be fed every 2 hours." The nurse interprets the neonate's behavior as most likely caused by which of the following?
- [ ] **1.** Lack of adequate intake to meet maternal nutritional needs.
- [ ] **2.** The mother's fears about the baby's weight gain.
- [ ] **3.** Preventing the neonate from sucking long enough with each feeding.
- [ ] **4.** The neonate's temporary growth spurt, which requires more feedings.

79. During a home visit to a breast-feeding primiparous client at 1 week postpartum, the client tells the nurse that her nipples have become sore and cracked from the feedings. Which of the following would the nurse instruct the client to do?
- [ ] **1.** Wipe off any lanolin creams from the nipple before each feeding.
- [ ] **2.** Position the baby with the entire areola in the baby's mouth.
- [ ] **3.** Feed the baby less often for the next several days.
- [ ] **4.** Use a mild soap while in the shower to prevent an infection.

The Postpartal Client Who Bottle-Feeds

80. A bottle-feeding client is being seen for her postpartum check up 6 weeks after a vaginal delivery of a normal, full-term infant. Which client findings would indicate a problem at this time postpartum?
- [ ] **1.** Firm fundus at the symphysis.
- [ ] **2.** White, thick vaginal discharge.
- [ ] **3.** Striae that are silver in color.
- [ ] **4.** Soft breasts without milk.

81. A client delivered two days ago and has been given instructions on breast care for bottle-feeding mothers. Which of the following statements indicates that the nurse must reinforce the instructions to the client?
- [ ] **1.** "I will wear a sports bra or a well fitting bra for several days."
- [ ] **2.** "When showering, I'll direct water onto my shoulders."
- [ ] **3.** "I will only use only water to clean my nipples."
- [ ] **4.** "I will use a breast pump to remove any milk that may appear."

82. A newly graduated nurse is giving a shift report about a client in labor. Which of the following information is the lowest priority to include to complete the report at the change of shift?
- [ ] **1.** Gravida, term, preterm, abortion, living.
- [ ] **2.** Cervical effacement, dilation, station.
- [ ] **3.** Support person with the client.
- [ ] **4.** Bottle- or breast-feeding preference.

83. A 24-year-old primipara who has delivered a healthy neonate in the hospital's birthing center plans to bottle-feed her neonate. When developing the nutritional teaching plan for the mother about the neonate's daily calorie allotment, the nurse should determine that the number of calories required by the neonate each day per pound of body weight is which of the following?
- [ ] **1.** 30 to 35.
- [ ] **2.** 40 to 45.
- [ ] **3.** 50 to 55.
- [ ] **4.** 60 to 65.

84. A primiparous client with a neonate who is 36 hours old asks the nurse, "Why does my baby spit up a small amount of formula after feeding?" The nurse explains that the regurgitation is thought to result from which of the following?
- [ ] **1.** An immature cardiac sphincter.
- [ ] **2.** A defect in the gastrointestinal system.
- [ ] **3.** Burping the infant too frequently.
- [ ] **4.** Moving the infant during the feeding.

85. A primiparous client who will be bottle-feeding her neonate asks, "What is the best position for the baby after feeding?" Which of the following positions should the nurse recommend as best to aid digestion?
- [ ] **1.** Supine position.
- [ ] **2.** On the left side.
- [ ] **3.** Prone without a pillow.
- [ ] **4.** Sitting on mom's lap for 20 minutes.

86. A primiparous client who is bottle-feeding her neonate asks, "When should I start giving the baby solid foods?" The nurse instructs the client to introduce solid foods no sooner than at which age?
- [ ] **1.** 2 months.
- [ ] **2.** 6 months.
- [ ] **3.** 8 months.
- [ ] **4.** 10 months.

87. After instructing a primiparous client who is bottle-feeding about burping, which of the following client statements indicates that the client needs further teaching?
- [ ] **1.** "I'll burp him after 15 minutes of feeding him formula."
- [ ] **2.** "After he takes one-half ounce of formula, I'll burp him."
- [ ] **3.** "I'll burp him while he is in an upright position."
- [ ] **4.** "I'll gently pat his back to get him to burp."

88. When teaching a primiparous client about the growth and development of the neonate, which of the following should the nurse include as the usual age at which most babies are able to drink from a cup independently?
- [ ] **1.** 5 to 7 months.
- [ ] **2.** 8 to 10 months.
- [ ] **3.** 12 to 14 months.
- [ ] **4.** 15 to 16 months.

89. When preparing for discharge a 15-year-old primipara who is bottle-feeding her neonate, the nurse instructs the client not to "prop" the bottle while feeding the neonate because this can lead to which of the following?
- [ ] **1.** Overfeeding and obesity.
- [ ] **2.** Aspiration of the formula.
- [ ] **3.** Tooth decay in the formative months.
- [ ] **4.** Sudden infant death syndrome (SIDS).

The Postpartal Client with a Cesarean Birth

90. The nurse is assessing a cesarean section client who delivered 12 hours ago. Findings include a distended abdomen with faint bowel sounds × 1 quadrant, fundus firm at umbilicus, lochia scant, rubra, and pain rated 4 on a scale of 1 to 10. The I.V. and Foley catheter have been discontinued and the client was medicated 3 hours ago for pain. When planning care for this client, what should the nurse identify as the highest priority intervention?
- [ ] **1.** Medicate the client.
- [ ] **2.** Incentive spirometry.
- [ ] **3.** Ambulate the client.
- [ ] **4.** Encourage caring for infant.

91. Carboprost (Hemabate) was injected into the uterus of a client to treat uterine atony during a cesarean section. In preparing to care for this client postpartum, the nurse should anticipate the client may experience which of the following common adverse effects of the medication?
- [ ] **1.** Vertigo and confusion.
- [ ] **2.** Nausea and diarrhea.
- [ ] **3.** Restlessness and increased vaginal bleeding.
- [ ] **4.** Headache and hypertension.

92. A 30-year-old woman, G 4, P 4, has delivered a healthy term female neonate by cesarean delivery due to a nonreassuring fetal heart rate tracing. At 2 hours postpartum, the nurse assesses the client's retention catheter and observes that the client's urine is slightly red tinged. Which of the following would the nurse do next?
- [ ] **1.** Continue to monitor the client's input and output.
- [ ] **2.** Palpate the client's fundus gently every 15 minutes.
- [ ] **3.** Assess the placement of the retention catheter.
- [ ] **4.** Contact the client's physician for further orders.

93. While changing the neonate's diaper, the client asks the nurse about some red-tinged drainage from the neonate's vagina. Which of the following responses would be most appropriate?
- [ ] **1.** "It's of no concern because it is such a small amount."
- [ ] **2.** "The cause is usually related to swallowing blood during the delivery."
- [ ] **3.** "Sometimes baby girls have this from hormones received from the mother."
- [ ] **4.** "This vaginal spotting is caused by hemorrhagic disease of the newborn."

94. Four hours after cesarean delivery of a neonate weighing 4,000 g (8 lb, 13 oz), the primiparous client asks, "If I get pregnant again, will I need to have a cesarean?" When responding to the client, which of the following would the nurse need to keep in mind about vaginal birth after cesarean delivery (VBAC)?
- [ ] **1.** VBAC may be possible if the client has not had a classic uterine incision.
- [ ] **2.** A history of rapid labor is a necessary criterion for VBAC.
- [ ] **3.** A low transverse incision contraindicates the possibility for VBAC.
- [ ] **4.** VBAC is not possible because the neonate was large for gestational age.

95. A client who had a cesarean delivery 24 hours ago complains of pain from abdominal distention. The client has been on nothing-by-mouth status for the past 36 hours. Which of the following actions would be most appropriate?
- [ ] **1.** Offer the client a carbonated beverage twice daily.
- [ ] **2.** Tell the client to use a straw when drinking fluids.
- [ ] **3.** Limit the client to a soft diet until more bowel sounds exist.
- [ ] **4.** Encourage ambulation in the hallway.

96. A primiparous client who underwent a cesarean delivery 30 minutes ago is a candidate for Rho(D) immune globulin (RhoGAM). The nurse anticipates administering this ordered medication within which of the following time frames after delivery?
- [ ] **1.** 8 hours.
- [ ] **2.** 24 hours.
- [ ] **3.** 72 hours.
- [ ] **4.** 96 hours.

97. While the nurse is caring for a primiparous client with cephalopelvic disproportion 4 hours after a cesarean delivery, the client requests assistance in breast-feeding. To promote maximum maternal comfort, which of the following would be most appropriate for the nurse to suggest?
- [ ] **1.** Football hold.
- [ ] **2.** Scissors hold.
- [ ] **3.** Cross-cradle hold.
- [ ] **4.** Cradle hold.

The Postpartal Client with Complications

98. Which of the following would be most appropriate for the nurse to do after assessing a multiparous client at 24 hours postpartum who demonstrates a positive Homan's sign with discomfort?
- [ ] **1.** Place a cold pack on the client's perineal area.
- [ ] **2.** Place the client in a semi-Fowler's position.
- [ ] **3.** Notify the client's physician immediately.
- [ ] **4.** Ask the client to ambulate around the room.

99. Prophylactic heparin therapy is ordered to treat thrombophlebitis in a multiparous client who delivered 24 hours ago. After instructing the client about the medication, the nurse determines that the client understands the instructions when she states which of the following as the purpose of the drug?
- [ ] **1.** To thin the blood clots.
- [ ] **2.** To increase the lochial flow.
- [ ] **3.** To increase the perspiration for diuresis.
- [ ] **4.** To prevent further blood clot formation.

100. While caring for a primipara diagnosed with deep vein thrombosis at 48 hours postpartum who is receiving treatment with bed rest and intravenous heparin therapy, the nurse would contact the client's physician immediately if the client exhibited which of the following?
- [ ] **1.** Pain in her calf.
- [ ] **2.** Dyspnea.
- [ ] **3.** Hypertension.
- [ ] **4.** Bradycardia.

101. A primiparous client 3 days postpartum is to be discharged on heparin therapy. After teaching her about possible adverse effects of heparin therapy, the nurse determines that the client needs further instruction when she states that the adverse effects include which of the following?
- [ ] **1.** Epistaxis.
- [ ] **2.** Bleeding gums.
- [ ] **3.** Slow pulse.
- [ ] **4.** Petechiae.

102. After being treated with heparin therapy for thrombophlebitis, a multiparous client who delivered 4 days ago is to be discharged on oral warfarin (Coumadin). After teaching the client about the medication and possible effects, which of the following client statements indicates successful teaching?
- [ ] **1.** "I can take two aspirin if I get uterine cramps."
- [ ] **2.** "Protamine sulfate should be available if I need it."
- [ ] **3.** "I should use a soft toothbrush to brush my teeth."
- [ ] **4.** "I can drink an occasional glass of wine if I desire."

103. A nurse is discussing basic principles of asepsis and infection control standards to the unit. This new nurse shows a clear understanding of the highest priority intervention in preventing infection through which statement?
- [ ] **1.** "I must use barrier isolation."
- [ ] **2.** "I must wear a gown and gloves."
- [ ] **3.** "I must use individual client care equipment."
- [ ] **4.** "I must practice frequent hand washing."

104. A postpartum multiparous client diagnosed with endometritis is to receive intravenous antibiotic therapy with ampicillin sodium (Polycillin). Before administering this drug, the nurse must do which of the following?
- [ ] **1.** Ask the client if she has any drug allergies.
- [ ] **2.** Assess the client's pulse rate.
- [ ] **3.** Place the client in a side-lying position.
- [ ] **4.** Check the client's perineal pad.

105. Which of the following would be most important for the nurse to encourage in a primiparous client diagnosed with endometritis who is receiving intravenous antibiotic therapy?
- [ ] **1.** Ambulate to the bathroom frequently.
- [ ] **2.** Discontinue breast-feeding temporarily.
- [ ] **3.** Maintain bed rest in Fowler's position.
- [ ] **4.** Restrict visitors to prevent contamination.

106. Which of the following measures would the nurse expect to include in the teaching plan for a multiparous client who delivered 24 hours ago and is receiving intravenous antibiotic therapy for cystitis?
- [ ] **1.** Limiting fluid intake to 1 L daily to prevent overload.
- [ ] **2.** Emptying the bladder every 2 to 4 hours while awake.
- [ ] **3.** Washing the perineum with povidone iodine (Betadine) after voiding.
- [ ] **4.** Avoiding the intake of acidic fruit juices until the treatment is discontinued.

107. The nurse is caring for a primiparous client who is diagnosed with cystitis on the second postpartum day. The client has been requesting medication for back pain every 3 to 4 hours. Which of the following would be an appropriate nursing diagnosis for the client at this time?
- [ ] **1.** *Fear* related to intravenous therapy and outcome.
- [ ] **2.** *Ineffective coping* related to prolonged hospitalization.
- [ ] **3.** *Ineffective role performance* related to prolonged bed rest.
- [ ] **4.** *Pain* related to dysuria and urinary frequency.

108. A primiparous client diagnosed with cystitis at 48 hours postpartum who is receiving intravenous ampicillin asks the nurse, "Can I still continue to breast-feed my baby?" Which of the following responses by the nurse would be most appropriate?
- [ ] **1.** "You can continue to breast-feed as long as you want to do so."
- [ ] **2.** "Alternate your breast-feeding with formula feeding to help you rest."
- [ ] **3.** "You'll need to discontinue breast-feeding until the antibiotic therapy is stopped."
- [ ] **4.** "You'll need to modify your technique by manually pumping your breasts."

109. Four days after a vaginal delivery, the client visits the clinic complaining of excessive lochia rubra with clots. The physician orders methylergonovine maleate (Methergine), 0.2 mg intramuscularly. Before administering this drug, which of the following would the nurse need to assess?
- [ ] **1.** Blood pressure.
- [ ] **2.** Pulse rate.
- [ ] **3.** Breath sounds.
- [ ] **4.** Bowel sounds.

110. During the first hour after delivery, assessment of a multiparous client who delivered a neonate weighing 4,593 g (10 lb, 2 oz) by cesarean delivery reveals a soft fundus with excessive lochia rubra. Which of the following would the nurse expect to include in the client's plan of care?
- [ ] **1.** Administration of intravenous oxytocin.
- [ ] **2.** Placement of the client in a side-lying position.
- [ ] **3.** Rigorous fundal massage every 5 minutes.
- [ ] **4.** Preparation for an emergency hysteromyomectomy.

111. A primiparous client who was diagnosed with hydramnios and breech presentation while in early labor is diagnosed with early postpartum hemorrhage at 1 hour after a cesarean delivery. The client asks, "Why am I bleeding so much?" The nurse responds based on the understanding that the most likely cause of uterine atony in this client is which of the following?
- [ ] **1.** Trauma during labor and delivery.
- [ ] **2.** Moderate fundal massage after delivery.
- [ ] **3.** Lengthy and prolonged second stage of labor.
- [ ] **4.** Overdistention of the uterus from hydramnios.

112. Thirty-six hours after a vaginal delivery, a multiparous client is diagnosed with endometritis due to b-hemolytic streptococcus. When assessing the client, which of the following would the nurse expect to find?
- [ ] **1.** Profuse amounts of lochia.
- [ ] **2.** Abdominal distention.
- [ ] **3.** Nausea and vomiting.
- [ ] **4.** Odorless vaginal discharge.

113. A multiparous client visits the urgent care center 5 days after a vaginal delivery experiencing persistent lochia rubra in a moderate to heavy amount. The client asks the nurse, "Why am I continuing to bleed like this?" The nurse should instruct the client that this type of postpartum bleeding is usually caused by which of the following?
- [ ] **1.** Uterine atony.
- [ ] **2.** Cervical lacerations.
- [ ] **3.** Vaginal lacerations.
- [ ] **4.** Retained placental fragments.

114. A 26-year-old primiparous client is seen in the urgent care clinic 2 weeks after delivering a viable female neonate. The client, who is breast-feeding, is diagnosed with infectious mastitis of the right breast. The client asks the nurse, "Can I continue breast-feeding?" Which of the following responses would be most appropriate?
- [ ] **1.** "You can continue to breast-feed, feeding your baby more frequently."
- [ ] **2.** "You can continue once your symptoms begin to decrease."
- [ ] **3.** "You must discontinue breast-feeding until antibiotic therapy is completed."
- [ ] **4.** "You must stop breast-feeding because the breast is contaminated."

115. A primiparous client who had a vaginal delivery 1 hour ago voices anxiety because she has a nephew with Down syndrome. After teaching the client about Down syndrome, which of the following client statements indicates the need for additional teaching?

☐ 1. "Down syndrome is an abnormality that can result from a missing chromosome."

☐ 2. "Down syndrome usually results in some degree of mental retardation."

☐ 3. "There are several methods available to determine whether my baby has Down syndrome."

☐ 4. "Older mothers are more likely to have a baby with chromosomal abnormalities."

116. A 15-year-old unmarried primiparous client is being cared for in the hospital's birthing center after vaginal delivery of a viable neonate. The neonate is being placed for adoption through a social service agency. Four hours postpartum, the client asks if she can feed her baby. Which of the following responses would be most appropriate?

☐ 1. "I'll bring the baby to you for feeding."

☐ 2. "I think we should ask your physician if this is a good idea."

☐ 3. "It's not a good idea for you to have any contact with the baby."

☐ 4. "I'll check with the social worker to see if the adopting parents will permit this."

117. After teaching a primiparous client about treatment and self-care of infectious mastitis of the right breast, the nurse determines that the client needs further instruction when she states which of the following?

☐ 1. "I can apply localized heat to the infected area."

☐ 2. "I should increase my fluid intake to 2,000 ml per day."

☐ 3. "I'll need to take antibiotics for 7 to 10 days before I am cured."

☐ 4. "I should begin breast-feeding on the right side to decrease the pain."

118. During a home visit to a primiparous client who delivered vaginally 14 days ago, the client says, "I've been crying a lot the last few days. I just feel so awful. I am a rotten mother. I just don't have any energy. Plus, my husband just got laid off from his job." The nurse observes that the client's appearance is disheveled. Which of the following would be the nurse's best response?

☐ 1. "These feelings commonly indicate symptoms of postpartum blues and are normal. They'll go away in a few days."

☐ 2. "I think you're probably overreacting to the labor and delivery process. You're doing the best you can as a mother."

☐ 3. "It's not unusual for some mothers to feel depressed after the birth of a baby. I think I should contact your doctor."

☐ 4. "This may be a symptom of a serious mental illness. I think you should probably go to the hospital."

Correct Answers and Rationales

The letter in parentheses after each rationale identifies the client need addressed in the item, including management of care (M), safety and infection control (S), health promotion and maintenance (H), psychosocial adaptation (P), basic care and comfort (C), pharmacological and parenteral therapies (D), reduction of risk potential (R), and physiological adaptation (A).

The Postpartal Client with a Vaginal Birth

1. 3. At any point in the postpartum period, the lochia should be dark in color, rather than bright red. The volume should not be great enough to trickle or run from the vagina. The information provided states the fundus is firm, midline, and at the umbilicus, which are the expected outcomes at this point postpartum. These findings would indicate to the nurse that the bleeding is not coming from the uterus or from uterine atony. The bladder is not palpable, which indicates the that the bleeding is not related to a full bladder, which is further validated by the fundus being at the umbilicus. The most likely etiology is cervical or vaginal lacerations or tears. The nurse is unable to do anything to stop this type of bleeding and must notify the health care provider. Increasing the I.V. rate will not decrease the amount or type of vaginal bleeding. Rechecking the hematocrit and hemoglobin will only provide background information for the nurse and identify the beginning levels for this mother, rather than where she is now. It will do nothing to stop the bleeding. The bleeding level and color is not normal and documenting such findings as normal is incorrect. (M)

2. 4. Within the first 24 hours postpartum, the maternal temperature may increase to 100.4° F, a normal postpartum finding attributed to dehydration. A temperature higher than 100.4° F after the first 24 hours indicates a potential for infection. Hemoconcentration is a normal finding postpartum due to the remobilization and rapid loss of excess body fluids. WBC count is normally elevated as a response to the inflammation, pain, and stress of the birthing process. A pulse rate of 60 bpm is normal at this period and results from an increased cardiac output (mobilization of excess extracellular fluid into the vascular bed, decreased pressure from the uterus on vessels, blood flow back to the heart from the uterus returning to the central circulation) and alteration in stroke volume. (A)

3. 4. Uterine massage enables immediate contraction of the uterus to prevent bleeding. In-and-out catheterization relieves bladder distention, eliminates displacement, firms the uterus, and prevents uterine bleeding. A bladder scan is not necessary because the nurse is able to palpate the full bladder. The positioning of the uterus indicates a full bladder. An indwelling urinary catheter is not necessary because most clients spontaneously void within 12 hours. The use of an NSAID will help reduce the inflammation that may be present but its action is not immediate and the status of the fundus needs more immediate interventions because of the risk of postpartum hemorrhage associated with a full bladder. (M)

4. **2.** Pain medication is the first strategy to initiate at this pain level. When trauma has occurred to any area, the usual intervention is ice for the first 24 hours and heat after the first 24 hours. Sitz baths are initiated at the conclusion of ice therapy. Ice has already been initiated and will prevent further edema to the rectal sphincter and perineum and continue to reduce some of the pain. Anesthetic sprays can also be utilized for the perineal area when pain is involved but would not lower the pain to a level that the client considers tolerable. (A)

5. **3.** Stage four is the first 2 to 4 hours postpartum. At this time, the nurse should frequently assess maternal vital signs, the fundus, bladder status, and lochia. The vital signs indicate the ability of the client to transition from pregnancy to postpartum and the physical status of the mother. The maternal fundus should remain firm, midline, and at the umbilicus or lower. A bladder that is distended may displace the normally firm uterus and cause hemorrhage. The lochia is assessed for color, odor, and amount postpartum. Assessment of the mother's ability to push, hydration, emotional stability, contraction patterns, and fetal heart tones is important in stages one and two. Maternal vital signs will be assessed during all stages of labor. Maternal emotional status and infant bonding and feeding preferences are lower priorities than the physical well-being of the mother. (R)

6. **2.** Educating the client about caring for herself and her infant are the two highest priority goals. Following delivery, all mothers, especially the primigravida, require instructions regarding self-care and infant care. Learning needs should be assessed in order to meet the specific needs of each client. Bonding is significant, but is only one aspect of the needs of this client and the bonding process would have been implemented immediately postpartum, rather than waiting 2 hours. Planning the discharge occurs after the initial education has taken place for mother and infant and the nurse is aware of any need for referrals. Safety is an aspect of education taught continuously by the nurse and should include maternal as well as newborn safety. (M)

7. **3.** The client is in the taking hold phase with a demonstrated focus on the neonate and learning about and fulfilling infant care and needs. The taking in phase is the first period after delivery where there is emphasis on reviewing and reliving the labor and delivery process, concern with self and needing to be mothered. Eating and sleep are high priorities during this phase. Taking on is not a phase of postpartum psychological adaptation. Letting go is the process beginning about 6 weeks postpartum when the mother may be preparing to go back to work.

During this time, she can have other individuals assume care of the infant and begins the separation process. (P)

8. **1.** A urine toxicology screening will be collected to document that the infant has been exposed to illegal drug use. This documentation will be the basis for legal action for the protection of this infant. If the infant tests positive for cocaine, the legal system will be activated to provide and ensure protective custody for this child. Hospital security would not become involved unless the mother is obtaining or using drugs on hospital premises. The mother and infant have the same privileges as any hospitalized clients unless the safety of the infant is jeopardized, thus limiting contact with visitors would not be appropriate. Local law enforcement agencies would be contacted only if the mother initiates use of the drugs on hospital premises and such contact would be made through the hospital security system. (A)

9. **4.** Acetaminophen and hydrocodone (Vicodin) would be the drug of choice for this situation because the pain level is so high. Aspirin is not usually used because of the bleeding risk associated with its use. Although ibuprofen would typically be a good choice because it inhibits the prostaglandin synthesis associated with a multiparous client breast-feeding, the pain level is too high for this drug to have an acceptable effect. Docusate (Colace) is used as a stool softener postpartum but does not provide pain relief. (D)

10. **1.** Immediately after delivery of the placenta, the nurse would expect to palpate the fundus halfway between the umbilicus and the symphysis pubis. Within 2 hours postpartum, the fundus should be palpated at the level of the umbilicus. The fundus remains at this level or may rise slightly above the umbilicus for approximately 12 hours. After the first 12 hours, the fundus should decrease one fingerbreadth (1 cm) per day in size. By the ninth or tenth day, the fundus usually is no longer palpable. (H)

11. **2.** The instillation of erythromycin into the neonate's eyes provides prophylaxis for ophthalmia neonatorum, or neonatal blindness caused by gonorrhea in the mother. Erythromycin is also effective in the prevention of infection and conjunctivitis from *Chlamydia trachomatis*. The medication may result in redness of the neonate's eyes, but this redness will eventually disappear. Erythromycin ointment is not effective in treating neonatal chorioretinitis from cytomegalovirus. No effective treatment is available for a mother with cytomegalovirus. Erythromycin ointment is not effective in preventing cataracts. Additionally, neonatal infection with beta-hemolytic streptococcus results in pneumonia, bacterial meningitis, or death. Cataracts in the neonate may be congenital or may result from maternal exposure to rubella. Erythromycin ointment is also not effective for preventing and treating strabismus (crossed eyes). Infants may exhibit intermittent strabismus until 6 months of age. (D)

12. **3.** Phytonadione (vitamin K or AquaMEPHYTON) acts as a preventive measure against neonatal hemorrhagic disease. At birth, the neonate does not have the intestinal flora to produce vitamin K, which is necessary for coagulation. Hypoglycemia is prevented and treated by feeding the infant. Hyperbilirubinemia severity can be decreased by early feeding and passage of meconium to excrete the bilirubin. Hyperbilirubinemia is treated with phototherapy. Polycythemia may occur in neonates who are large for gestational age or post-term. Clamping of the umbilical cord before pulsations cease reduces the incidence of polycythemia. Generally, polycythemia is not treated unless it is extremely severe. (D)

13. **3.** The first 12 hours after delivery are part of the taking-in phase of maternal postpartum adjustment, which typically lasts from 1 to 3 days. During the taking-in phase, the client is primarily concerned with her own needs. After the first 1 to 3 days postpartum, the client is in the taking-hold phase and can focus more on the needs of the neonate. Although the family is an important unit of care and the significant other is important for the mother's emotional support, during the taking-in phase the mother is focused on herself. (H)

14. **1.** The client has a hematoma. During the first 24 hours postpartum, ice packs can be applied to the perineal area to reduce swelling and discomfort. Ice packs usually are not effective after the first 24 hours. Although vital signs, including temperature, are important assessments, taking the client's temperature is unrelated to the hematoma and would provide no additional information about swelling. After 24 hours, the client may obtain more relief by taking a warm sitz bath. This moist heat is an effective way to increase circulation to the perineum and provide comfort. Usually, hematomas resolve without further treatment within 6 weeks. Additionally, the nurse should measure the hematoma to provide a baseline for subsequent measurements and should notify the physician of its presence. An antibiotic is not warranted at this point because the client is not exhibiting any signs or symptoms of infection. (H)

15. **4.** Urinary retention soon after delivery is usually caused by edema and trauma of the lower urinary tract; this commonly results in difficulty with initiating voiding. Hyperemia of the bladder mucosa also commonly occurs. The combination of hyperemia and edema predisposes to decreased sensation to void, overdistention of the bladder, and incomplete bladder emptying. A prolonged first stage of labor can contribute to exhaustion and uterine atony, not urinary retention. If the client had a urinary tract infection, she would exhibit symptoms such as dysuria and a burning sensation. After delivery, the uterus is contracting, which leads to less pressure on the bladder. Pressure of the uterus on the bladder occurs during labor. (H)

16. **2.** For clients who are bottle-feeding, the menstrual flow should return in 6 to 10 weeks, after a rise in the production of follicle-stimulating hormone by the pituitary gland. Nonlactating mothers rarely ovulate before 4 to 6 weeks postpartum. Therefore, 3 to 4 weeks is too early for the menstrual cycle to resume. For women who are breast-feeding, the menstrual flow may not return for 3 to 4 months (12 to 16 weeks) or, in some women, for the entire period of lactation, because ovulation is suppressed. (H)

17. **4.** The client's dizziness is most likely caused by orthostatic hypotension secondary to the decreased volume of blood in the vascular system resulting from the physiologic changes occurring in the mother after delivery. The client is experiencing dizziness because not enough blood volume is available to perfuse the brain. The nurse should first allow the client to "dangle" on the side of the bed for a few minutes before attempting to ambulate. By 6 hours postpartum, the effects of the anesthesia should be worn off completely. Typically, the effects of epidural anesthesia wear off by 1 to 2 hours postpartum, and the effects of local anesthesia usually disappear by 1 hour. The client scenario provides no information to indicate that the client experienced any postpartum hemorrhage. Normal blood loss during delivery should not exceed 500 ml. (H)

18. **1.** During the first week postpartum, the client's pulse rate should be slow, with an average of 60 to 70 bpm. A pulse of 100 bpm warrants further investigation to rule out a possible infectious process or postpartum hemorrhage. An oral temperature of 99° F (36.8° C) is within normal limits. Excessive perspiration and frequent voiding in large amounts are caused by the normal diuresis that occurs as the body returns to its prepregnant state. (M)

19. **4.** The priority nursing diagnosis at this time is *Urinary retention* related to the trauma of delivery, particularly since forceps, which may result in trauma, were used during the delivery. The client is at some risk for infection, specifically urinary tract infection, from the repeated need for catheterization. However, this is not a priority at this time. With proper technique and adequate cleanliness and hygiene, infection can be prevented. *Disturbed body image* related to the episiotomy is not a priority at this time. The client may be feeling some discomfort from the episiotomy. There is no indication that the client is experiencing a risk for fluid volume imbalance related to the prolonged labor and anesthesia. Most likely, the client would be receiving intravenous fluid replacement. (H)

20. **4.** Because the diet of Hispanic Americans from Mexico and Central America commonly includes beans, corn products, tomatoes, chili peppers, potatoes, milk, cheeses, and eggs, the nurse needs to encourage an intake of meats, dark green leafy vegetables, and other high-protein products that are rich in iron. Doing so helps to compensate for the significant blood loss and subsequent iron loss that occurs during the postpartum period. Additionally, fresh fruits, meats, and green leafy vegetables may be scarce, possibly resulting in deficiencies of vitamin A, vitamin D, and iron. Tomatoes are high in vitamin C, potatoes are good sources of carbohydrates and vitamin C, and corn products are high in thiamine, but these are not rich sources of iron. (H)

21. 4. A small, constant trickle of blood and a firm fundus are usually indicative of a vaginal tear or cervical laceration. If the client had retained placental tissue, the fundus would fail to contract fully (uterine atony), exhibiting as a soft or boggy fundus. Also, vaginal bleeding would be evident. Uterine inversion occurs when the uterus is displaced outside of the vagina and is obvious on inspection. Bladder distention may result in uterine atony because the pressure of the bladder displaces the fundus, preventing it from fully contracting. In this case the fundus would be soft, possibly boggy, and displaced from midline. (R)

22. 4. On about the eleventh postpartum day, the lochia should be lochia alba, clear or white in color. Lochia rubra, which is dark red to red, may persist for the first 2 to 3 days postpartum. From day 3 to about day 10, lochia serosa, which is pink or brown, is normal. (H)

23. 2. The nurse should instruct the client to cleanse the perineal area with warm water and to wipe from front to back with a blotting motion. Warm water is soothing to the tender tissue, and wiping from front to back reduces the risk of contamination. Hot, sudsy water may increase the client's discomfort and may even burn the client in a very tender area. After the first 24 hours, warm water sitz baths taken three or four times a day for 20 minutes can help increase circulation to the area. Ice packs are helpful for the first 24 hours. (H)

24. 3. After explaining the procedure to the client, the nurse should wash hands and don clean gloves for the procedure. Washing the hands prevents the spread of infection. Standard precautions are necessary to protect both the client and the nurse. The temperature of the water should be between 100° and 105° F (37.4° and 40° C) to prevent burns. Spraying the perineal area with the ordered analgesic spray is done after the sitz bath to provide the greatest pain relief. Assessing the client's perineum for swelling and redness is part of the nursing assessment and needs to be done after hand washing and donning clean gloves. Also, the assessment would be done before the nurse explains the procedure. (S)

25. 3. After an uncomplicated delivery, postpartum exercises may begin on the first postpartum day with exercises to strengthen the abdominal muscles. These are done in the supine position with the knees flexed, inhaling deeply while allowing the abdomen to expand and then exhaling while contracting the abdominal muscles. Exercises such as sit-ups (sitting, then lying back, and returning to a sitting position) and push-ups or exercises involving reaching for the knees are ordinarily too strenuous for the first postpartum day. Sit-ups may be done later in the postpartum period, after approximately 3 to 6 weeks. (H)

26. 2. Lochia can be expected to increase when the client first ambulates. Lochia tends to pool in the uterus and vagina when the client is recumbent and flows out when the client arises. If the client had reported that her lochia was bright red, the nurse would suspect bleeding. In this situation, the client would be put back in bed and the physician would be notified. Early postpartum hemorrhage occurs during the first 24 hours, but typically the fundus is soft or "boggy." The client's fundus here is firm and midline. Late postpartal hemorrhage, occurring after the first 24 hours, is usually caused by retained placental fragments or abnormal involution of the placental site. (H)

27. 4. After delivery, the nurse should plan to measure the client's first two voidings and record the amount to make sure that the client is emptying the bladder. Frequent voidings of less than 150 ml suggest that the client is experiencing urinary retention. In addition, if urinary retention is occurring, the bladder may be palpable and the fundus may be displaced from midline. The client does not need to be catheterized unless there is evidence of urinary retention. Palpation of the bladder before voiding is unnecessary. However, if the client has difficulty voiding or exhibits signs of urinary retention, then bladder palpation is indicated. The fundus can be displaced by a full bladder and should be assessed after the client voids. (H)

28. 2. Clients sometimes feel faint or dizzy when taking a shower for the first time after delivery because of the sudden change in blood volume in the body. Primarily for this reason, the nurse remains nearby while the client takes her first shower after delivery. If the client becomes dizzy or expresses symptoms of feeling faint, the nurse should get the client back to bed as soon as possible. If the client faints while in the shower, the nurse should cover the client to protect her privacy, stay with the client, and call for assistance. Fatigue postpartum is common and will precede taking a shower. Diuresis is a normal physiologic response during the postpartum period and not associated with showering. Hygiene needs also precede the shower. (S)

29. 2. The nurse should instruct the client to squeeze or contract the muscles of the buttocks together before sitting down in the chair; this contracts the pelvic floor muscles, which reduces the tension on the tender perineal area. Then the client should put her full weight slowly down on the chair. Pain medication may only be ordered for every 3 to 4 hours, so the client may not be able to receive pain medication every time she desires to sit in the chair. The episiotomy pain usually fades by the fifth or sixth postpartum day. Maintaining a relaxed posture before sitting does not contract the pelvic floor muscles. Most physicians order an analgesic cream or spray when a client has an episiotomy, but they provide only temporary relief. (H)

30. 1. Neonates like to look at eyes, and eye-to-eye contact is a highly effective way to provide visual stimulation. The parent's eyes are circular, move from side to side, and become larger and smaller. Neonates have been observed to fix on them. In general, neonates prefer circular objects of darkness against a white background. Sharp black and white images of geometric figures are appropriate. Use of bright colors on the walls and moving a colorful rattle do not provide as much visual stimulation as eye-to-eye contact with talking. Brightly colored animals and cartoon figures are more appropriate at approximately 1 year of age. (H)

31. 2. The father is praying to Allah because of the Muslim belief that the first sounds a child hears should be from the Koran in praise of and supplication to Allah. Although male children are revered in this culture, this practice is performed by Muslims whether the child is male or female. The father's actions are unrelated to his wife and son's being healthy. The nurse should allow the practice because doing so demonstrates cultural sensitivity and builds a trusting relationship with the family. The Muslim faith does not have a baptism rite whereby the child becomes a member of the faith. (H)

32. 2. According to Erikson, infants are in the trust versus mistrust stage. Holding, talking to, singing to, and patting neonates helps them develop trust in caregivers. Tactile stimulation is important and should be encouraged. Holding neonates often is unlikely to spoil them because they are totally dependent on other human beings to meet their needs. Being held makes infants feel loved and cared for and should be encouraged. The mother can hold the neonate as often as she wants, not just when the baby is crying or fussy. Overstimulation typically does not result from holding an infant. (H)

33. 4. Excessive perspiration and diuresis is common during the puerperium as the body attempts to return to its prepregnant state. The most appropriate nursing diagnosis is *Excess fluid volume* related to normal postpartal diuresis. A temperature of 99° F (37.2° C) is normal during the first 24 hours postpartum. Foul-smelling lochia and a temperature higher than 100.4° F (38° C) would suggest an infection. Although hormonal shifts occur during the postpartum period, the client's diaphoresis is related to diuresis, not to a problem with thermoregulation caused by hormonal changes. No evidence is presented to suggest altered renal tissue perfusion related to the client's multiparity status. Clients with renal disease or renal failure may exhibit painful urination, flank pain, or lack of urinary output. (H)

34. 4. If the client continues to complain of perineal pain after an analgesic medication has been given, the nurse should inspect the client's perineum for a hematoma, because this is the usual cause of such discomfort. Ibuprofen is a nonsteroidal anti-inflammatory medication used to relieve mild pain. Pain from a perineal hematoma can be moderate to severe, possibly requiring a stronger analgesic, such as acetaminophen with codeine (Tylenol with Codeine). Ice applied to the perineum during the first 24 hours postpartum may decrease the severity of hematoma formation. Application of warm heat, such as a sitz bath three times daily for 20 minutes, also can help to relieve the discomfort when implemented after the first 24 hours. Typically hematomas resolve themselves within 6 weeks. A puerperal infection would be indicated if the client's temperature were 100.4° F (41° C) or higher. Also, lochia most likely would be foul smelling. A continuous trickle of lochia rubra would suggest a possible vaginal laceration. No evidence is presented to suggest a history of drug abuse. (R)

35. 1, 4, 6. Delegating care to unlicensed assistive personnel requires that the nurse knows which tasks are within their capability. Changing the perineal pad and reporting drainage, reinforcing hygiene with perineal care, and assisting with ambulation are within the individual's capacity. Unlicensed assistive personnel should never be asked to complete any assessments, such as checking fundal location or performing skilled procedures on a client. In addition, it would be above the scope for unlicensed assistive personnel to assist the mother with latching on and discussing postpartum depression with the client. State boards of nursing list the procedures and tasks that unlicensed assistive personnel can complete when directed. (M).

36. 4. The Health Information Portability and Accountability Act (HIPAA) regulations and ethical decision making require that the nurse maintain confidentiality at all times. The nurse's best response is to explain to the client that nurses are not allowed to discuss other clients on the unit. Ignoring the client's question is inappropriate because doing so would interfere with the development of a trusting nurse-client relationship. Confidentiality must be maintained at all times. Telling the client that the nurse isn't sure may imply that the nurse will find out and then tell the client about the other woman. Asking the other woman's permission to discuss her with another client is inappropriate because confidentiality must be maintained at all times. (M)

37. **2.** The neonate has immature oculomotor coordination, an inability to accommodate for distance, and poorly developed eyes, visual nerves, and brain. However, the normal neonate can see objects clearly within a range of 9 to 12 inches, whether or not they are moving. Visual acuity at birth is 20/100 to 20/150, but it improves rapidly during infancy and toddlerhood. Newborns can distinguish colors as well as light from dark. (H)

38. **4.** The client is experiencing diastasis recti, a separation of the longitudinal muscles (recti) of the abdomen that is usually palpable on the third postpartum day. An exercise involving raising the head and shoulders about 8 inches with the client lying on her back with knees bent and hands crossed over the abdomen is preferred. This exercise helps to pull the abdominal muscles together and the client gradually works up to performing this exercise 50 times per day. However, until the diastasis has closed, the client should avoid exercises that rotate the trunk, twist the hips, or bend the trunk to one side, because further separation may occur. The condition does not need a surgical repair, and limited activity and bed rest are not necessary. Correct posture and adequate diet assist the body to return to its prepregnancy state more quickly but do not resolve the separation of abdominal muscles. (R)

39. ~~1.~~ ³ A uterine fundus located off to one side and above the level of the umbilicus is commonly the result of a full bladder. Although the client had voided, the client may be experiencing urinary retention with overflow. If anesthesia has been used for delivery, the inability to void may be related to the lingering effects of anesthesia; however, that is not the case here. Physicians commonly write a one-time order for catheterization. After which, typically, enough edema has subsided making it easier and less painful for the client to void and completely empty her bladder. Administering ibuprofen would have no effect on the uterine fundus. Waiting to reassess in 1 hour could be detrimental since the client's distended bladder is interfering with uterine involution, predisposing her to possible hemorrhage. Administering a bolus of fluid would be inappropriate because it would only add to the client's full bladder. (R)

40. **2.** Stretch marks, or *striae gravidarum,* are caused by stretching of the tissues, particularly over the abdomen. After delivery, the tissues atrophy, leaving silver scars. These skin pigmentations will not disappear completely. The striae gravidarum may reappear as pink streaks if the client becomes pregnant again. Special creams are not warranted because they are not helpful and may be expensive. Weight loss does not make the marks disappear. Striae gravidarum tend to run in families. (H)

41. **2.** In most cases, unless complications develop or the client has gained excessive weight during the antepartal period, she can expect to return to her prepregnant weight by 6 weeks. Many clients lose 14 to 20 lb by 2 weeks postpartum, primarily because of the birth of the fetus, the placenta, and fluid losses. Diet and exercise can help the client return to her prepregnant weight. (H)

42. **3.** The most appropriate nursing diagnosis based on the information provided is *Readiness for enhanced family coping,* related to the addition of a new family member. Based on the scenario, the client has the support of the boyfriend and his parents. A nursing diagnosis of *Anxiety* would be appropriate if the client verbalized anxious thoughts or feelings or worries about the situation. A nursing diagnosis of *Ineffective coping* would be appropriate if the client showed little interest in the neonate or in mothering behaviors. A nursing diagnosis of *Deficient knowledge* would be appropriate if the client expressed concerns about the financial and emotional costs of child rearing or questions about caring for the child. (P)

43. **1.** The client with a third-degree laceration should be assessed for constipation, because a third-degree laceration extends into a portion of the anal sphincter. Constipation, not diarrhea, is more likely because this condition is extremely painful, possibly causing the client to be reluctant to have a bowel movement. The laceration has been sutured and should not be bleeding at 48 hours postpartum. Rectal fistulas may develop at a later time, but not at 48 hours postpartum. (R)

44. **4.** For most clients, sexual intercourse can be resumed when the lochia has stopped flowing and episiotomy pain has ceased, usually about 3 weeks postpartum. Sexual intercourse may be painful until the episiotomy has healed. The client also needs instructions about the possibility that pregnancy may occur before the return of the client's menstrual flow. The postpartum check by the health care provider typically occurs 4 to 6 weeks after delivery and most women have already had intercourse by this time. Typically, new mothers are exhausted and may not feel amorous or desirable for quite a while. In addition, the mother's physiologic responses may be diminished because of low hormonal levels, adjustments to the maternal role, and fatigue due to lack of rest and sleep. (H)

45. **3.** Docusate sodium (Colace) is a stool softener, used to assist in bowel elimination. The client is at risk for constipation because of decreased food and fluid intake and pain from the episiotomy. Numerous analgesics, such as ibuprofen (Motrin) or acetaminophen (Tylenol), could be used to treat episiotomy pain, helping the client achieve comfort and thus fall asleep. Oxytocin is used to contract the uterus. (D)

46. **1.** The nurse needs to continue to monitor the client's vital signs. During the first 24 hours postpartum it is normal for the mother to have a slight temperature elevation because of dehydration. A temperature of 100.4° F (38° C) that persists after the first 24 hours may indicate an infection. Bradycardia during the first week postpartum is normal because of decreased blood volume, diuresis, and diaphoresis. The client's respiratory rate is within normal limits. Large clots are indicative of hemorrhage. However, the client's vital signs are within normal limits and her fundus is firm and midline. Therefore, large clots and possible hemorrhage can be ruled out. The physician does not need to be notified at this time. An ice pack is not necessary because the client's temperature is within normal limits. (H)

47. **3.** The client needs more teaching when she states, "I should lie on my back as much as possible to relieve the pain." Instead, the client should lie in the Sims position as much as possible to aid venous return to the rectal area and to reduce discomfort. Gentle manual replacement of the hemorrhoid is an appropriate measure to help relieve the discomfort and prevent enlargement. Analgesic sprays and witch hazel pads are helpful in reducing the discomfort of hemorrhoids. Drinking lots of water and eating roughage aid in bowel elimination, minimizing the risk of straining and subsequent hemorrhoidal development or enlargement. (C)

48. **2.** On most postpartum units, clients on regular diets are allowed to eat whatever kinds of food they desire. Generally, foods from home are not discouraged. The nurse does not need to obtain the physician's permission. Although it is preferred, the foods do not necessarily have to be high in iron. In many Latino cultures, there is a belief in the "hot-cold" theory of disease; certain foods (hot) are preferred during the postpartum period, and other foods (cold) are avoided. Therefore, the nurse should allow the mother to bring her daughter "special foods from home." Doing so demonstrates cultural sensitivity and aids in developing a trusting relationship. (C)

49. **1.** Iron is best absorbed in an acid environment or with vitamin C. For maximum iron absorption, the client should take the medication with orange juice or a vitamin C supplement. Herbal tea has no effect on iron absorption. Milk decreases iron absorption. Grape juice is not acidic and therefore would have no effect on iron absorption. (D)

50. **4.** It is believed that the process of attachment is structured so that the parents become attached to only one infant at a time. Therefore, the nurse should encourage the parents to relate to each twin individually, rather than as a unit, to enhance the attachment process. Mothers of twins are usually able to breast-feed successfully because the milk supply increases on demand. However, possible fatigue and exhaustion require that the mother rest whenever possible. It would be highly unlikely and unrealistic that each parent would be able to spend equal amounts of time with both twins. Other responsibilities, such as employment, may prevent this. The parents should try to engage assistance from family and friends, because caring for twins or other multiple births (e.g., triplets) can be exhausting for the family. (P)

51. **3.** At 12 hours postpartum, the fundus normally should be in the midline and at the level of the umbilicus. When the fundus is firm yet above the umbilicus, and deviated to the right rather than in the midline, the client's bladder is most likely distended. The client should be encouraged to ambulate to the bathroom and attempt to void, because a full bladder can prevent normal involution. A firm but deviated fundus above the level of the umbilicus is not a normal finding and if voiding does not return it to midline, it should be reported to the physician. Methylergonovine (Methergine) is used to treat uterine atony. This client's fundus is firm, not boggy or soft, which would suggest atony. Gentle massage is not necessary because there is no evidence of atony or clots. (R)

52. **2, 3, 5, 6.** The nurse is responsible for providing discharge instructions that include signs and symptoms that need to be reported to the physician as well as resources and follow-up for home care if needed. Phone numbers and health practices to promote healing, such as the use of prenatal vitamins, are also essential pieces of information. The use of birth control pills needs to be discussed with the physician. A progesterone-only pill is used if the client is breast-feeding. Oral contraceptives should be initiated according to the physician's advice. Although the client's mother may be helpful, the client's statement that she will be fine because her mother is coming indicates that she is unaware or ignoring information about valuable information and resources. (R)

The Postpartal Client Who Breast-Feeds

53. **4.** Depo-Provera is a progestin contraceptive that can reduce the initial production of breast milk. It is given to a breast-feeding woman when she returns for the 6-week postpartum check up. By this time, the milk supply is well established and will remain at that level. Depo-Provera is effective as a contraceptive for 90 days. Clients who are bottle-feeding may be given Depo-Provera prior to discharge from the hospital. (D)

54. **3.** As much of the mother's nipple and areola need to be in the infant's mouth in order to establish a latch that does not cause nipple cracks or fissures. Having the nipple and the areola deep in the infant's mouth decreases the stress on the end of the nipple, therefore decreasing pain, cracking and fissures. Breast milk has been found to heal nipples when placed on the nipple at the completion of a feeding. The length of time the baby feeds on each nipple is not a factor as long as the nipple is correctly placed in the infant's mouth. (H)

55. 1. New mothers usually begin to produce milk at about the third day postpartum and colostrum is produced until that time. For clients who have breast-fed another infant during pregnancy, having milk shortly after delivery is not unusual. Diaphoresis and diuresis are considered normal during this time as the body excretes the additional fluids that are no longer needed after the pregnancy. Constipation may continue for several days as a result of progesterone remaining in the system, the consummation of iron, and trauma to the perineum. (A)

56. 2. The major reasons for afterbirth pains are breast-feeding, high parity, overdistended uterus during pregnancy, and a uterus filled with blood clots. Physiologically, afterbirth pains are caused by intermittent contraction and relaxation of the uterus. These contractions are stronger in multigravidas in order to maintain a contracted uterus. The release of oxytocin when breast-feeding also stimulates uterine contractions. There is no data to suggest any of these clients has had an overdistended uterus or currently has clots within the uterus. The G 3, P 3 client who is breast-feeding has the highest parity of the clients listed, which—in addition to breast-feeding—places her most at risk for afterbirth pains. The G 2, P 2 postcesarean client may have cramping but it should be less than the G 3, P 3 client. The G 3, P 3 client who is bottle-feeding would be at risk for afterbirth pains because she has delivered several children, but her choice to bottle-feed reduces her risk of pain. (A)

57. 2. The client is exhibiting signs and symptoms of a breast infection (mastitis). The nurse should instruct her to contact her health care provider, who will likely order a prescription for antibiotics. She should continue to breast-feed the infant from both breasts. Frequent breast-feeding is encouraged rather than discontinuing the process for anyone having a breast infection. Applying warm compresses may relieve pain. However, the underlying infection indicated by the elevated temperature indicates that additional treatment with antibiotics will be needed. (M)

58. 4. Breast-feeding consumes maternal calories and requires energy which increases the maternal basal metabolic rate and assists in lowering the maternal blood glucose level. Insulin is not transferred to the infant through breast milk. Breast-feeding is recommended for diabetic mothers because it does lower blood glucose levels. The number of antibodies in breast milk is not altered by maternal diabetes. (A)

59. 4. Postpartum clients who are breast-feeding need to be cautioned about taking various medications, many of which can be passed to the infant via breast milk. Aspirin and codeine products should be avoided because the drug can increase bleeding or cause sleepiness in the infant. Medications such as ibuprofen or acetaminophen can be used to help to relieve the discomfort without causing any apparent harm to the neonate. Warm sitz baths three to four times a day for 20 minutes can be helpful in relieving the client's discomfort. Application of moist heat is soothing and increases perineal circulation. Increased fluid (and fiber) intake promotes bowel elimination, thus preventing constipation, which can increase the client's discomfort. (H)

60. 1. If not contraindicated for moral, cultural, or religious reasons, a condom with spermicide is commonly recommended for contraception after delivery until the client's 6-week postpartal examination. This method has no effect on the neonate who is breast-feeding. Oral contraceptives containing estrogen are not advised for women who are breast-feeding because the hormones decrease the production of breast milk. Women who are not breast-feeding may use oral contraceptive agents. The rhythm method is not effective because the client is unlikely to be able to determine when ovulation has occurred until her menstrual cycle returns. Although breast-feeding is not considered an effective form of contraception, breast-feeding usually delays the return of both ovulation and menstruation. The length of the delay varies with the duration of lactation and the frequency of breast-feeding. While abstinence is one form of birth control and safe while breast-feeding, it may not be acceptable to this couple who is asking about a method that will allow them to resume sexual relations. (H)

61. 4. Colostrum is a thin, watery, yellow fluid composed of protein, sugar, fat, water, minerals, vitamins, and maternal antibodies (e.g., immunoglobulin A). It is important for the neonate to receive colostrum for passive immunity. Colostrum is lower in fat and lactose than mature breast milk. Colostrum does not contain vitamin K. The neonate will produce vitamin K once a feeding pattern is established. Colostrum may speed, rather than delay, the passage of meconium. (H)

62. 3. Various medications can be excreted in the breast milk and affect the nursing neonate. The client should avoid all nonprescribed medications (such as acetaminophen) unless approved by the physician. Medications typically do not affect the quality of the mother's breast milk. Medications usually do not interfere with or diminish the mother's motivation to breast-feed, nor do they interfere with the mother's let-down reflex. (H)

63. 3. Taking ibuprofen 200 mg orally immediately after breast-feeding helps minimize the neonate's exposure to the drug because drugs are most highly concentrated in the body soon after they are taken. Most mothers breast-feed on demand or every 2 to 3 hours, so the effects of the ibuprofen should be decreased by the next breast-feeding session. Taking the medication before going to bed is inappropriate because, although the mother may go to bed at a certain time, the neonate may wish to breast-feed soon after the mother goes to bed. If the mother takes the medication midway between feedings, then its peak action may occur midway between feedings. Breast milk is sufficient for the neonate's nutritional needs. Most breast-feeding mothers should not be encouraged to provide supplemental feedings to the infant because this may result in nipple confusion. (D)

64. **3.** During the first few days postpartum, the mother should be encouraged to nurse frequently. Breast-feeding for at least 10 minutes per side is recommended for the let-down reflex to begin. Feeding the infant whenever the infant cries is not appropriate and can lead to maternal exhaustion. Feeding for 1 to 2 minutes per side is insufficient for the let-down reflex. Also, this short period of time prevents the neonate from latching on and obtaining the needed nutrition. Initially, feeding for 10 minutes per side is sufficient until the infant becomes more comfortable with breast-feeding. Then the mother can increase the breast-feeding time gradually to 20 to 30 minutes. (H)

65. **4.** Breast-feeding stimulates oxytocin secretion, which causes the uterine muscles to contract. These contractions account for the discomfort associated with afterpains. Flatulence may occur after a cesarean delivery. However, the mother typically would complain of abdominal distention and a bloating feeling, not a "cramplike" feeling. Stretching of the tissues or healing may cause slight tenderness or itching, not cramping feelings of discomfort. Medications such as mild analgesics or stool softeners, commonly administered postpartum, typically do not cause cramping. (H)

66. **2.** For the breast-feeding client, drinking at least 8 to 10 glasses of fluid a day is recommended. Breast-feeding women need an increased intake of vitamin D for calcium absorption. A breast-feeding woman requires an extra 500 calories per day above the recommended nonpregnancy intake to produce quality breast milk. Breast-feeding women need adequate calcium for blood clotting and strong bones and teeth. (C)

67. **2, 3, 4, 5, 6.** To maintain adequate milk supply, lactating women need to increase their calories by 500. They also need to increase protein (to 7 servings daily), fluid (4 to 5 glasses of milk plus 2 additional glasses), fat (from sparing use prepregnancy to 5 daily servings), and calcium intake (1,000 to 1,200 mg daily). (H)

68. **1.** Breast milk has a higher fat content than cow's milk. Thirty percent to 55% of the calories in breast milk are from fat. Breast milk contains less iron than cow's milk does. However, the iron absorption from breast milk is greater in the neonate than with cow's milk. Breast milk contains less sodium and calcium than cow's milk. (C)

69. **4.** Lightly brushing the neonate's lips with the nipple causes the neonate to open the mouth and begin sucking. The neonate should be taught to open the mouth and grasp the nipple on his or her own. The neonate should not be forced to nurse. (H)

70. **2.** Several methods can be used to prevent nipple soreness. Placing as much of the areola as possible into the neonate's mouth is one method. This action prevents compression of the nipple between the neonate's gums, which can cause nipple soreness. Other methods include changing position with each feeding, avoiding breast engorgement, nursing more frequently, and feeding on demand. Plastic liners are not helpful because they prevent air circulation, thus promoting nipple soreness. Instead, air drying is recommended. Pulling the baby's mouth out smoothly after only 10 minutes may prevent the baby from getting the entire feeding and increases nipple soreness. Any breast milk remaining on the nipples should not be wiped off, because the milk has healing properties. (H)

71. **4.** Breast-fed neonates do not swallow as much air as bottle-fed neonates, but they still need to be burped. Good times to burp the neonate are when the mother switches from one breast to the other and at the end of the breast-feeding session. Neonates do not eat more if they are burped frequently. Breast-feeding mothers are advised not to supplement the feedings with formula because this may cause nipple confusion and decrease milk production. If supplements are given, the baby still needs to be burped. Neonates who are fed every 3 hours still need to be burped. (H)

72. **3.** Stored breast milk can be safely kept in the refrigerator for up to 7 days or in a deep-freeze at 0° F (−18° C) for 12 months. Breast milk should be stored in glass containers because immunoglobulin tends to stick to plastic bottles. Breast milk can remain without refrigeration or loss of nutrients for up to 10 hours. The containers should be labeled with date, time, and amount to prevent inadvertent administration of spoiled milk. Frozen breast milk should be thawed in the refrigerator for a few hours, placed under warm tap water, then shaken. (H)

73. **4.** Oxytocin stimulates the let-down reflex when milk is carried to the nipples. A lactating mother can experience the let-down reflex suddenly when she hears her baby cry or when she anticipates a feeding. Some mothers have reported feeling the let-down reflex just by thinking about the baby. Adrenalin may increase if the mother is excited, but this hormone has no direct influence on breast-feeding. Estrogen influences development of female secondary sex characteristics and controls menstruation. Prolactin stimulates milk production. (H)

74. **3.** The most appropriate initial nursing diagnosis for this client is *Deficient knowledge* related to inexperience with breast-feeding. This is the client's first baby and first experience with breast-feeding. Also, as a young adult, the client needs guidance and education. *Ineffective role performance* would be indicated if the client had expressed concern about her role changes. *Risk for impaired skin integrity* is not a priority at this time. With education and knowledge about proper positioning, the client's skin and nipple area should remain intact. Although this is the client's first experience with breast-feeding, there is no evidence that the client is fearful. The client also has the support of her husband. (H)

75. **3.** Expressing a little milk before nursing, massaging the breasts gently, or taking a warm shower before feeding also may help to improve milk flow. Although various measures such as ice, heat, and massage may be tried to relieve breast engorgement, prevention of breast engorgement by frequent feedings is the method of choice. Applying ice to the nipples does not relieve breast engorgement. However, it may temporarily relieve the discomfort associated with breast engorgement. Using lanolin on the nipples does not relieve breast engorgement and is unnecessary. Use of lanolin may cause sensitivity and irritation. Having frequent breast-feeding sessions, rather than offering the neonate a small amount of formula, is the method of choice for preventing and relieving breast engorgement. In addition, offering the neonate small amounts of formula may result in nipple confusion. (H)

76. **1.** The nurse should instruct the client that the baby is getting enough to eat when there are six to eight wet diapers by the fifth day of age. Other signs include good suckling sounds during feeding, dripping breast milk at the mouth, and quiet rest or sleep after the feeding. By the fourth day of age, the infant should have soft yellow stools, not transitional (greenish) stools. Falling asleep easily after feeding on the first day is not a good indicator because most infants are sleepy during the first 24 hours. Most infants regain their lost birth weight in 7 to 10 days after birth. An infant who has gained weight during the first well-baby checkup (usually at 2 weeks) is getting sufficient breast milk at feedings. (H)

77. **4.** The client should wean the infant gradually, eliminating one feeding at a time. The baby can be weaned to a bottle (formula) anytime the mother desires; she does not have to breast-feed for 4 months. Most infants (and mothers) develop a "favorite feeding time," so this feeding session should be eliminated last. The client may wish to begin weaning with daytime feedings when the infant is busy. (H)

78. **4.** Neonates normally increase breast-feeding during periods of rapid growth (growth spurts). These can be expected at age 10 to 14 days, 5 to 6 weeks, 2.5 to 3 months, and 4.5 to 6 months. Each growth spurt is usually followed by a regular feeding pattern. Lack of adequate intake to meet maternal nutritional needs is not associated with the neonate's desire for more frequent breast-feeding sessions. However, an intake of adequate calories is necessary to produce quality breast milk. The mother's fears about weight gain and preventing the neonate from sucking long enough are not associated with the desire for more frequent breast-feeding sessions. (H)

79. **2.** Even if the nipples are sore and cracked, the mother should position the baby with the entire areola in the baby's mouth so that the nipple is not compressed between the baby's gums during feeding. The best method is to prevent cracked nipples before they occur. This can be done by feeding frequently and using proper positioning. Warm, moist tea bags can soothe cracked nipples because of tannic acid in the tea. Creams on the nipples should be avoided; wiping off any lanolin creams from the nipple before each feeding can cause further soreness. Feeding the baby less often for the next few days will cause engorgement (and possible neonatal weight loss), leading to additional problems. Soap use while in the shower should be avoided to prevent drying and removal of protective oils. (R)

The Postpartal Client Who Bottle-Feeds

80. **1.** By 4 to 6 weeks postpartum, the fundus should be deep in the pelvis and the size of a nonpregnant uterus. Subinvolution, caused by infection or retained placental fragments, is a problem associated with a uterus that is larger than expected at this time. Normal expectations include a white, thick vaginal discharge, striae that are beginning to fade to silver, and breasts that are soft without evidence of milk production (in a bottle-feeding mother). (A)

81. **4.** The use of a breast pump to remove milk is contraindicated in bottle-feeding mothers. Nipple and breast stimulation and emptying of the breasts produce milk, rather than eliminate milk production. The bottle-feeding client is discouraged from stimulating the breasts in any way. A sports bra that is well fitting provides support and decreases stimulation. (Binders are not suggested.) Having the water in a shower land on the shoulders of the mother rather than the breasts also decreases stimulation. Only water is necessary to clean nipples when breast or bottle-feeding. (C)

82. **4.** The bottle- or breast-feeding preference is the least important information to be reported to the oncoming shift. The bottle- or breast-feeding plans will be important after delivery as many mothers breast-feed within an hour after delivery. The client's obstetrical history is a higher priority because it provides information about previous birthing experience. Information on cervical effacement, dilation, and station indicates the current state of labor and is essential for planning continuity of care for this client. Nurses on the incoming shift should also know the extent of support the client will need and who is currently providing that support. (A)

83. **3.** As a general rule, most neonates require 50 to 55 calories per pound of body weight, or about 117 calories per kilogram of weight, each day. If the neonate receives less than this amount, malnutrition may occur. More than this amount can lead to obesity. (C)

84.   1. Initial regurgitation in the neonate during the first 12 to 24 hours may be caused by excessive mucus and gastric irritation from foreign substances in the stomach. After the first 24 hours, regurgitation is thought to be caused by the neonate's immature cardiac sphincter. It represents an overflow of stomach contents and is probably a result of feeding the neonate too fast or too much. A defect in the gastrointestinal system usually results in more severe symptoms. A small amount of regurgitation is normal, but vomiting or forceful fluid expulsion is not. Burping the infant often during a feeding can decrease the amount of air in the stomach from swallowing. However, burping too often can lead the neonate to become tired or fussy. Moving the infant usually does not result in regurgitation. (H)

85.   1. To aid digestion, the neonate should be placed in a supine position or on the right side propped with a small blanket roll after a feeding. Placing the neonate on the right side promotes gastric emptying and digestion. Placing the neonate in a prone position has been associated with sudden infant death syndrome. Although the mother may desire to hold the infant in her lap after feeding, this is not necessary for the neonate's digestion. (H)

86.   2. Pediatricians recommend that infants be given either breast milk or formula until at least 6 months of age because of the neonate's difficulty digesting solid foods. Giving solid foods too early can lead to food allergies. Because chewing movements do not begin until 7 to 9 months of age, foods requiring chewing should be delayed until this time. (H)

87.   1. The client needs further instruction when she says burping should be done after 15 minutes of formula feeding. The entire feeding should take only 15 to 20 minutes, and the neonate should be burped before that time. During initial feedings, the burping should be done after each half-ounce of formula with the neonate in an upright position, patting the neonate gently on the back. (H)

88.   2. Most babies are developmentally ready to drink independently from a cup by the age of 8 to 10 months. If the child has not mastered drinking from a cup by this time, there may be a problem with motor development that requires further investigation. (H)

89.   2. Bottle "propping" is not recommended because it can lead to aspiration, delayed bonding, feelings of mistrust (Erikson), and possible otitis media. The neonate will not be overfed during bottle propping but may suck too quickly, possibly resulting in aspiration of the formula. Putting the neonate to bed with a bottle can lead to tooth decay later in the formative years, but an infant cannot hold the bottle. The cause of SIDS has not been determined. However, it is associated with placing the infant in a prone position after eating. (R)

The Postpartal Client with a Cesarean Birth

90.   3. The client should have more active bowel sounds by this time postpartum. Ambulation will encourage passing flatus and begin peristaltic action in the gastrointestinal track. Medicating the client should be evaluated prior to ambulating but it is probably too soon because the last dose was only 3 hours ago and her pain assessment rating is fairly low. Pain medications should not have codeine as a component as it decreases peristaltic activity. Incentive spirometry or asking the client to turn, cough and deep breathe are appropriate to encourage good oxygen exchange in the lungs prior to ambulation, and walking can be used concurrently with these intervention. Participating in infant care is another way to encourage the mother to move about but the primary goal would be to have her walk on the unit, a more purposeful activity. (A)

91.   2. Hemabate is an oxytocic prostaglandin that causes uterine contraction in women who are bleeding heavily. Nausea, vomiting, diarrhea, and fever are common adverse effects of prostaglandin administration. Vertigo and confusion are not associated with this drug. Vaginal bleeding may occur with inadequate amounts of Hemabate if the client continues to bleed. Restlessness may result if inadequate amounts of Hemabate are used and the woman continues to bleed and goes into shock. If too large a dose is given, the client may experience headache and hypertension because Hemabate does contract smooth muscles. (D)

92.   4. Slightly red-tinged urine may indicate that the bladder was accidentally cut during the cesarean delivery. The nurse should notify the physician as soon as possible about the urine color. Continuing to monitor the client's input and output should be done after the physician is contacted. Palpating the fundus every 15 minutes is not necessary unless the client's fundus becomes soft or "boggy." Assessment of the retention catheter is a normal part of the elimination assessment by the nurse, but displacement is not the cause of the red-tinged urine. (R)

93.   3. The most appropriate response would be to explain that the vaginal spotting in female neonates is associated with hormones received from the mother. Estrogen is believed to cause slight vaginal bleeding or spotting in the female neonate. The condition disappears spontaneously, so there is no need for concern. Telling the mother that it is of no concern does not allay the mother's worry. The vaginal spotting is related to hormones received from the mother, not to swallowing blood during the delivery or hemorrhagic disease of the neonate. Anemia is associated with hemorrhagic disease. (H)

94. **1.** VBAC can be attempted if the client has not had a classic uterine incision. This type of incision carries a danger of uterine rupture. A physician must be available, and a cesarean delivery must be possible within 30 minutes. A history of rapid labor is not a criterion for VBAC. A low transverse incision is not a contraindication for VBAC. A classic (vertical) incision is a contraindication because the client has a greater possibility for uterine rupture. Estimated fetal weight greater than 4000 g by itself is not a contraindication if the mother is not diabetic. (H)

95. **4.** Abdominal distention, a major source of discomfort for the postoperative client, is best relieved by having the client ambulate more frequently. Ambulation stimulates circulation and peristalsis, thereby promoting the passage of flatus. Carbonated beverages contribute to additional gas formation, as can drinking through a straw, and should be avoided. The client can progress from full liquids to soft foods and then to a regular diet, once bowel sounds are present. The client does not need to limit her diet to soft foods, but she may wish to avoid foods that increase intestinal gas, such as beans or brussel sprouts. (C)

96. **3.** For maximum effectiveness, RhoGAM should be administered within 72 hours postpartum. Most Rh-negative clients also receive RhoGAM during the prenatal period at 28 weeks' gestation and then again after delivery. The drug is given to Rh-negative mothers who have a negative Coombs test and deliver Rh-positive neonates. If there is doubt about the fetus's blood type after pregnancy is terminated, the mother should receive the medication. (D)

97. **1.** After a cesarean delivery, most mothers have the greatest comfort when the neonate is positioned in the football hold with the mother in a semi-Fowler position, supporting the neonate's head in her hand and resting the neonate's body on pillows alongside her hip. This position prevents pressure on the uterine incision yet allows the neonate easy access to the mother's breast. The scissors hold, where the mother places her hand well back on the breast to prevent touching the areola and interfering with the neonate's mouth placement, is used by the mother to hold the breast and support it during breast-feeding. The cross-cradle hold is done when the mother holds the neonate's head in the hand opposite from the breast on which the neonate will feed and the mother's arm supports the neonate's body across her lap. This position can be uncomfortable because of the pressure placed on the client's incision line. For the cradle hold, the mother cradles the infant alongside the arm at the breast on which the neonate will feed. This position also can be uncomfortable because of the pressure placed on the incision line. (C)

The Postpartal Client with Complications

98. **3.** A positive Homan's sign, discomfort behind the knee or in the upper calf area on dorsiflexion of the foot, may be indicative of thrombophlebitis. Other signs include edema and redness at the site and may be more reliable as an indicator of thrombophlebitis. The nurse should notify the physician immediately and ask the client to remain in bed to minimize the risk for pulmonary embolus, a serious consequence of thrombophlebitis should a clot dislodge. The Homan sign is observed on the client's legs, so placing an ice pack on the perineal area is inappropriate. However, ice to the perineum would be useful for episiotomy pain and swelling. The client does not need to be positioned in a semi-Fowler's position but should remain on bed rest to prevent dislodgement of a potential clot. (R)

99. **4.** Heparin therapy is ordered to prevent further clot formation by inhibiting further thrombus and clot formation. Heparin, an anticoagulant, does not make blood clots thinner. An adverse effect of heparin therapy during the puerperium is increased lochia flow, so the nurse must be observant for symptoms of hemorrhage, such as heavy lochial flow. Heparin does not increase diaphoresis, which is normal for the postpartum client. (D)

100. **2.** A major complication of deep vein thrombosis is pulmonary embolism. Signs and symptoms, which may occur suddenly and require immediate treatment, include dyspnea, severe chest pain, apprehension, cough (possibly accompanied by hemoptysis), tachycardia, fever, hypotension, diaphoresis, pallor, shortness of breath, and friction rub. Pain in the calf is common with a diagnosis of deep vein thrombosis. Hypotension, not hypertension, would suggest a possible pulmonary embolism. It also could suggest possible hemorrhage secondary to intravenous heparin therapy. Bradycardia for the first 7 days in the postpartum period is normal. (R)

101. **3.** A slow pulse (bradycardia) is normal for the first 7 days postpartum as the body begins to adjust to the decrease in blood volume and return to the prepregnant state. Adverse effects of heparin therapy suggesting prolonged bleeding include hematuria, epistaxis, increased lochial flow, and bleeding gums. Typically, tachycardia, not bradycardia, would be associated with hemorrhage. Petechiae indicate bleeding under the skin or in subcutaneous tissue. (R)

102. **3.** Successful teaching is demonstrated when the client says, "I should use a soft toothbrush to brush my teeth." Heparin therapy can cause the gums to bleed, so a soft toothbrush should be used to minimize this adverse effect. Use of aspirin and other nonsteroidal anti-inflammatory medications should be avoided because of the increased risk for possible hemorrhage. Protamine sulfate is the antidote for heparin therapy. Vitamin K is the antidote for warfarin excess. Alcohol can inhibit the metabolism of oral anticoagulants and should be avoided. (D)

103. **4.** Frequent hand washing is the highest priority intervention. The nurse can emphasize, monitor, and ensure this strategy for all who come in contact with a client. The use of gowns and gloves are appropriate for specific situations only. Individual client care equipment is a nursing responsibility but commonly depends on multiple factors related to budgeting within the hospital system and is not directly under the control of the nurse. (R)

104. **1.** Before administering ampicillin sodium (Polycillin) intravenously, the nurse must ask the client if she has any drug allergies, especially to penicillin. Antibiotic therapy can cause adverse effects, such as rash or even anaphylaxis. If the client is allergic to penicillin, the physician should be notified and ampicillin should not be given. Checking the client's pulse rate or placing her in a side-lying position and are not necessary. Assessing the amount of lochia by checking the perineal pad is important for all postpartum clients but is not necessary before antibiotic therapy. (D)

105. **3.** The nurse should encourage the client to maintain Fowler's position, which promotes comfort and facilitates drainage. Endometritis can make the client feel extremely uncomfortable and fatigued, so ambulation during intravenous therapy is not as important at this time. The client does not need to discontinue breast-feeding, although she may become quite fatigued and need assistance in caring for the neonate. Typically, breast-feeding would be discontinued only if the mother lacks the necessary energy. The institution's policy regarding visitors is to be followed. However, visitors do not need to be restricted to prevent contamination because the client is not considered to be contagious. The nurse should maintain the client's need for privacy and rest and should respect the client's wishes related to visitors. (R)

106. **2.** The client diagnosed with cystitis needs to void every 2 to 4 hours while awake to keep her bladder empty. In addition, she should maintain adequate fluid intake; 3,000 ml per day is recommended. Intake of acidic fruit juices (e.g., cranberry, apricot) is recommended because of their association with reducing the risk for infection. The client should wear cotton underwear and avoid tight-fitting slacks. She does not need to wash with povidone iodine (Betadine) after voiding. Plain warm water is sufficient to keep the perineal area clean. (C)

107. **4.** Because the client has been requesting medication for back pain every 3 to 4 hours, the priority nursing diagnosis at this time is *Pain* related to dysuria and urinary frequency. There are no data to suggest *Fear* as a diagnosis, which would be evidenced by expression of feelings such as, "I'm afraid of needles." There are no data to suggest *Ineffective coping* as a diagnosis. This diagnosis would be appropriate if the client expressed concerns about her children or husband and their abilities related to functioning at home while the client is hospitalized. *Ineffective role performance* would be appropriate if the client expresses an inability to perform her normal roles at home. (A)

108. **1.** The client can continue to breast-feed as often as she desires. Continuation of breast-feeding is limited only by the client's discomfort or malaise. Antibiotics for treatment are chosen carefully so that they avoid affecting the neonate through breast milk. Drugs such as sulfonamides, nitrofurantoin, and cephalosporins usually are not prescribed for breast-feeding mothers. Manual pumping of the breasts is not necessary. (H)

109. **1.** Methylergonovine maleate (Methergine) can cause hypertension, so the nurse should assess the client's blood pressure before and after administration. This drug should not be administered to clients who are hypertensive. Assessing pulse, respiration, and temperature is important for all postpartum clients to provide evidence of possible complications, such as infection. Tachycardia and diminished breath sounds are associated with pulmonary embolism, but these signs are not specific to methylergonovine (Methergine) administration. Assessing breath sounds would be important for a client who has had pregnancy-induced hypertension and received magnesium sulfate before delivery. However, by the fourth postpartum day, the effects of magnesium sulfate should have disappeared. Bowel sounds should be assessed after an operative delivery to determine whether peristalsis has begun so that the client can begin to drink clear liquids or eat soft foods. (D)

110. **1.** The client is exhibiting signs of early postpartal hemorrhage, defined as blood loss greater than 500 ml in the first 24 hours postpartum. Rapid intravenous oxytocin infusion of 40 to 80 units in 1,000 ml of normal saline, oxygen therapy, and gentle fundal massage to contract the uterus are usually effective. If bleeding persists, the nurse should inspect the cervix and vagina for lacerations. Intramuscular or intravenous methylergonovine may be administered, but this drug elevates the blood pressure. Other pharmacologic interventions include prostaglandin (Hemabate, Prostin, $PGF_{2\alpha}$) I.M. and misoprostol (Cytotec) rectally or vaginally. Severe uncontrolled hemorrhage may require bimanual uterine compression, a dilation and curettage to remove any retained placental tissue, or a hysterectomy to prevent maternal death from hemorrhage. The client should be placed in the supine position to allow evaluation of the fundus. The side-lying position is not helpful in controlling postpartum hemorrhage. Vigorous fundal massage every 5 minutes is unnecessary. In addition, it can be very painful for the mother. Rather, gentle massage along with oxytocin administration is used to stimulate the uterus to contract. A hysteromyomectomy is used to remove fibroid tumors. With massive hemorrhage, a hysterectomy (removal of the uterus) may be necessary to control the bleeding. (H)

111. **4.** The most likely cause of this client's uterine atony is overdistention of the uterus caused by the hydramnios. As a result, the stretched uterine musculature contracts less vigorously. Besides hydramnios, a large infant, bleeding from abruptio placentae or placenta previa, and rapid labor and delivery can also contribute to uterine atony during the postpartum period. Trauma during labor and delivery is not a likely cause. In addition, no evidence of excessive trauma was described in the scenario. Moderate fundal massage helps to contract the uterus, not contribute to uterine atony. Although a lengthy or prolonged labor can contribute to uterine atony, this client had a cesarean delivery for breech presentation. Therefore, it is unlikely that she had a long labor. (A)

112. 4. Scant and odorless vaginal discharge is associated with endometritis due to b-hemolytic streptococcus. The client also will exhibit "sawtooth" temperature spikes between 101° and 104° F (38.3° to 40° C), tachycardia, and chills. The classic symptom of foul-smelling lochia is not associated with this type of endometritis. Profuse and foul-smelling lochia is associated with classic endometritis from pathogens such as chlamydia or staphylococcus, not group B hemolytic streptococcus. Abdominal distention is associated with parametritis as the pelvic cellulitis advances and spreads, causing severe pain and distention. Nausea and vomiting are associated with parametritis resulting from an abscess and advancing pelvic cellulitis. (R)

113. 4. The most likely cause of delayed postpartum hemorrhage is retained placental fragments. The client may be scheduled for a dilatation and curettage to remove remaining placental fragments. Uterine atony, cervical lacerations, and vaginal lacerations are commonly associated with early, not late, postpartum hemorrhage. (H)

114. 1. The client being treated for infectious mastitis should continue to breast-feed often, or at least every 2 to 3 hours. Treatment also includes bed rest, increased fluid intake, local heat application, analgesics, and antibiotic therapy. Continually emptying the breasts decreases the risk of engorgement or breast abscess. The client should not discontinue breast-feeding unless she chooses to do so. The client may continue breast-feeding while receiving antibiotic therapy. Generally, the breast milk is not contaminated by the offending organism and is safe for the neonate. (A)

115. 1. Down syndrome is a genetic abnormality that is caused by an extra chromosome that results in mental retardation. The degree of mental retardation is difficult to predict in a neonate, although most children born with Down syndrome have some degree of mental retardation. Various methods can be used to determine whether a neonate has Down syndrome, which is commonly manifested by hypotonia, poor Moro reflex, flat facial profile, upslanting palpebral fissures, epicanthal folds, and hyperflexible joints. Genetic studies can be indicative of this disorder. Mothers older than 35 years of age are at a higher risk for having a child with Down syndrome. However, chromosomal abnormalities can occur regardless of the mother's age. (R)

116. 1. After birth, the client should make the decision about how much she would like to participate in the neonate's care. Seeing and caring for the neonate commonly facilitates the grief process. The nurse should be nonjudgmental and should allow the client any opportunity to see, hold, and care for the neonate. The physician does not need to be contacted about the client's desire to see the baby, which is a normal reaction. The social worker and the adoptive parents do not need to give the client permission to feed the baby. (H)

117. 4. The client needs further instruction when she says that she should begin feeding on the right (painful) breast to decrease the pain. Starting the feeding on the unaffected (left) breast can stimulate the milk ejection reflex in the right breast and thereby decrease the pain. Frequent nursing or pumping is recommended to empty the breast. For some mothers, mastitis is so painful that they choose to discontinue breast-feeding, so these mothers need a great deal of support. Applying heat to the infected area before starting to feed is appropriate because heat stimulates circulation and promotes comfort. Increasing fluid intake is advised to ensure adequate hydration. Antibiotics need to be taken until all medication has been used, usually 7 to 10 days to ensure eradication of the infection. (R)

118. 3. The client is probably experiencing postpartum depression, and the doctor should be contacted. Postpartum depression is usually treated with psychotherapy, social support groups, and antidepressant medications. Contributing factors include hormonal fluctuations, a history of depression, and environmental factors (e.g., job loss). An estimated 50% to 70% of women experience some degree of postpartum "blues," but these feelings of sadness disappear within 1 to 2 weeks after birth. However, the client is voicing more than just sadness. Telling her that she is overreacting is not helpful and may make her feel even less worthy. She is not exhibiting symptoms of a serious mental illness (loss of contact with reality) and does not need hospitalization. (H)

The Neonatal Client

- Neonatal Care
- Physical Assessment of the Neonatal Client
- The Preterm Neonate
- The Post-term Neonate
- The Neonate with Risk Factors
- Correct Answers and Rationales

Neonatal Care

1. A neonate is delivered by primary cesarean section at 36 weeks' gestation. The temperature in the delivery room is 70° F. To prevent heat loss from convection, which action should the nurse take?
- ☐ 1. Dry the neonate quickly after delivery.
- ☐ 2. Keep the neonate away from air conditioning vents.
- ☐ 3. Place the neonate away from outside windows.
- ☐ 4. Prewarm the bed.

2. The physician orders ampicillin 100 mg/kg/dose for a newly admitted neonate. The neonate weighs 1,350 g. How many milligrams should the nurse administer?

_____ mg

3. A neonate delivered at 30 weeks' gestation and weighing 2,000 g is admitted to the neonatal intensive care unit. What nursing measure will decrease insensible water loss in a neonate?
- ☐ 1. Bathing the baby as soon after birth as possible.
- ☐ 2. Use of eye patches with phototherapy.
- ☐ 3. Use of humidity in the incubator.
- ☐ 4. Use of a radiant warmer.

4. A neonate delivered at 37 weeks' gestation has been admitted to the neonatal intensive care unit for respiratory distress. The physician has ordered an I.V. for fluid support. To increase safety prior to hanging new I.V. fluids for a neonate, the nurse should:
- ☐ 1. Check the neonate's weight.
- ☐ 2. Determine if the neonate has adequate urine output.
- ☐ 3. Determine the neonate's glucose level.
- ☐ 4. Double-check the fluids and physician's order with another nurse.

5. A septic preterm neonate's I.V. was removed due to infiltration. While restarting the I.V., the nurse should carefully assess the neonate for:
- ☐ 1. Fever.
- ☐ 2. Hyperkalemia.
- ☐ 3. Hypoglycemia.
- ☐ 4. Tachycardia.

6. The physician is calling in an order for ampicillin for a neonate. The nurse should do which of the following? Select all that apply.
- ☐ 1. Write down the order.
- ☐ 2. Ask the physician to come to the hospital and write the order on the chart.
- ☐ 3. Repeat the order to the physician over the telephone.
- ☐ 4. Ask the physician to confirm that the order is correct.
- ☐ 5. Ask the nursing supervisor to cosign the telephone order as transcribed by the nurse.
- ☐ 6. Ask the nursing assistant to speak to the physician to take the order.

7. A nurse is administering indomethacin to a neonate. To ensure that she has identified the neonate correctly, the nurse should do which of the following? Select all that apply.
- ☐ 1. Ask the parents to confirm that this is their baby.
- ☐ 2. Ask another nurse to confirm that this is the neonate for whom the medication has been prescribed.
- ☐ 3. Check the neonate's identification band against the medical record number.
- ☐ 4. Verify the date of birth from the medical record with the date of birth on the client's identification band.
- ☐ 5. Compare the number on the crib with the number on the client's identification band.

8. The nurse makes a home visit to a 3-day-old full-term neonate who weighed 3,912 g (8 lb, 10 oz) at birth. Today the neonate, who is being bottle-fed, weighs 3,572 g (7 lb, 14 oz). Which of the following instructions would the nurse most likely give to the mother?
- ☐ 1. Continue feeding every 3 to 4 hours since the weight loss is normal.
- ☐ 2. Contact the physician if the weight loss continues over the next few days.
- ☐ 3. Switch to a soy-based formula because the current one seems inadequate.
- ☐ 4. Change to a higher-calorie formula to prevent further weight loss.

9. Commercial formulas contain 20 calories per ounce. A 1-day-old infant's weight in the morning was 8 lb and he was fed 45 ml at 2 a.m., 5:30 a.m., 8 a.m., 11 a.m., 2 p.m., 4:30 p.m., 8 p.m., and 10:30 p.m. What is the total amount of calories the infant received today?

_____ calories

10. A viable female neonate delivered vaginally at term has Apgar scores of 9 at 1 minute and 10 at 5 minutes after birth. Immediately postpartum, the nurse keeps the infant under a radiant warmer away from the cooling ducts in the room to prevent heat loss by which of the following mechanisms?
- ☐ **1.** Evaporation.
- ☐ **2.** Convection.
- ☐ **3.** Conduction.
- ☐ **4.** Radiation.

11. After explaining to the mother of a male neonate scheduled to receive an injection of vitamin K soon after birth about the rationale for the medication, which of the following statements by the mother indicates successful teaching?
- ☐ **1.** "My baby doesn't have the normal bacteria in his intestines to produce this vitamin."
- ☐ **2.** "My baby is at a high risk for a problem involving his blood's ability to clot."
- ☐ **3.** "The red blood cells my baby formed during pregnancy are destroying the vitamin K."
- ☐ **4.** "My baby's liver is not able to produce enough of this vitamin so soon after birth."

12. When developing the teaching plan for a new mother about the neonate's need for sensory and visual stimulation, information about which of the following as the most highly developed sense in the neonate would the nurse expect to include?
- ☐ **1.** Taste.
- ☐ **2.** Hearing.
- ☐ **3.** Touch.
- ☐ **4.** Vision.

13. While making a home visit to a primiparous client and her 3-day-old son, the nurse observes the mother changing the baby's disposable diaper. Before putting the clean diaper on the neonate, the mother begins to apply baby powder to the neonate's buttocks. Which of the following statements about baby powder would the nurse relate to the mother?
- ☐ **1.** It may cause pneumonia to develop.
- ☐ **2.** It helps prevent diaper rash.
- ☐ **3.** It keeps the diaper from adhering to the skin.
- ☐ **4.** It can result in allergies later in life.

14. After teaching a new mother about the care of her neonate after circumcision with a Gomco clamp, which of the following statements by the mother would indicate to the nurse that the mother needs additional instructions?
- ☐ **1.** "The petroleum gauze may fall off into the diaper."
- ☐ **2.** "A few drops of blood oozing from the site is normal."
- ☐ **3.** "I'll leave the gauze in place for 24 hours."
- ☐ **4.** "I'll remove any yellowish crusting gently with water."

15. After completing discharge instructions for a primiparous client who is bottle-feeding her term neonate, the nurse determines that the mother understands the instructions when the mother says that she should contact the pediatrician if the neonate exhibits which of the following?
- ☐ **1.** Ability to fall asleep easily after each feeding.
- ☐ **2.** Spitting up of a tablespoon of formula after feeding.
- ☐ **3.** Passage of a liquid stool with a watery ring.
- ☐ **4.** Production of one to two light brown stools daily.

16. The nurse instructs a primiparous client about bottle-feeding her neonate. Which of the following demonstrates that the mother has understood the nurse's instructions?
- ☐ **1.** Placing the neonate on his back after the feeding.
- ☐ **2.** Bubbling the baby after 1 oz of formula.
- ☐ **3.** Putting three-fourths of the bottle nipple into the baby's mouth.
- ☐ **4.** Pointing the nipple toward the neonate's palate.

17. When caring for a term neonate during the first hour after birth, the nurse expects to assess the neonate's blood glucose level, obtaining the blood sample from the neonate's foot near which of the following areas?
- ☐ **1.** Lateral aspect of the heel.
- ☐ **2.** Middle of the heel.
- ☐ **3.** Middle of the foot.
- ☐ **4.** Base of the toes.

18. After circumcision with a Plastibell, the nurse instructs the neonate's mother to cleanse the circumcision site with which of the following?
- ☐ **1.** Antibacterial soap.
- ☐ **2.** Warm water.
- ☐ **3.** Povidone-iodine (Betadine) solution.
- ☐ **4.** Diluted hydrogen peroxide.

19. Approximately 90 minutes after birth, the nurse encourages the mother of a term neonate to do which of the following?
- ☐ **1.** Feed the neonate.
- ☐ **2.** Allow the neonate to sleep.
- ☐ **3.** Get to know the neonate.
- ☐ **4.** Change the neonate's diaper.

Physical Assessment of the Neonatal Client

20. A full-term neonate is admitted to the normal newborn nursery. The nurse notes a Moro reflex. What should the nurse do next?
- ☐ **1.** Call a code.
- ☐ **2.** Identify this reflex as a normal finding.
- ☐ **3.** Place the neonate on seizure precautions.
- ☐ **4.** Start supplemental oxygen.

21. After the delivery of a neonate, a quick assessment is completed. The neonate is found to be apneic. After quickly drying the neonate, what should the nurse do next?
- ☐ **1.** Assign the first Apgar score.
- ☐ **2.** Place the head in a "sniff" position.
- ☐ **3.** Administer oxygen.
- ☐ **4.** Start cardiac compressions.

22. A 6-lb, 8-oz neonate was delivered vaginally at 38 weeks' gestation. At 5 minutes of life, the neonate has the following signs: heart rate 110, intermittent grunting with respiratory rate of 70, flaccid tone, no response to stimulus, overall pale white in color. The Apgar score is:
- ☐ **1.** 2.
- ☐ **2.** 3.
- ☐ **3.** 4.
- ☐ **4.** 6.

23. A neonate has a large amount of secretions. After vigorously suctioning the neonate, the nurse should assess for what possible result?
- ☐ **1.** Bradycardia.
- ☐ **2.** Rapid eye movement.
- ☐ **3.** Seizures.
- ☐ **4.** Tachycardia.

24. When reviewing the prenatal history for a newly delivered neonate, the nurse notes that the mother has neurofibromatosis. Which of the following conditions should the nurse expect?
- ☐ **1.** Acrocyanosis.
- ☐ **2.** Café au lait spots.
- ☐ **3.** Port wine nevus.
- ☐ **4.** Strawberry hemangiomas.

25. A 24-hour-old, full-term neonate is showing signs of possible sepsis in a septic work-up. The nurse is assisting the physician with a lumbar puncture on this neonate. What should the nurse do to assist in this procedure? Select all that apply.
- ☐ **1.** Administer the I.V. antibiotic.
- ☐ **2.** Hold the neonate steady in the correct position.
- ☐ **3.** Ensure a patent airway.
- ☐ **4.** Maintain a sterile field.
- ☐ **5.** Obtain a serum glucose level.

26. After a vaginal delivery of a term neonate, the nurse observes that the neonate has one artery and one vein in the umbilical cord. The nurse notifies the pediatrician based on the analysis that this may be indicative of which of the following?
- ☐ **1.** Respiratory anomalies.
- ☐ **2.** Musculoskeletal anomalies.
- ☐ **3.** Cardiovascular anomalies.
- ☐ **4.** Facial anomalies.

27. While assessing a male neonate about 12 hours old after a vaginal delivery, the nurse notes a swelling on the neonate's scalp that crosses the suture line. The nurse should expect that this finding is most likely caused by which of the following?
- ☐ **1.** Cephalohematoma.
- ☐ **2.** Caput succedaneum.
- ☐ **3.** Cranial edema.
- ☐ **4.** Craniotabes.

28. Shortly after birth, the nurse measures the circumference of a term neonate's head and chest. When the two measurements are compared, which of the following would the nurse expect to find about the head circumference?
- ☐ **1.** Equal to the chest circumference.
- ☐ **2.** Approximately 2 cm larger than the chest.
- ☐ **3.** About 3 cm smaller than the chest.
- ☐ **4.** Approximately 4 cm larger than the chest.

29. After explaining to a primiparous client about the causes of her neonate's cranial molding, which of the following statements by the mother indicates the need for further instruction?
- ☐ **1.** "The molding was caused by an overlapping of the baby's cranial bones during my labor."
- ☐ **2.** "The amount of molding is related to the amount and length of pressure on the head."
- ☐ **3.** "The molding will usually disappear in a couple of days."
- ☐ **4.** "Brain damage may occur if the molding doesn't resolve quickly."

30. Initial assessment of a term female neonate about 4 hours old reveals a normal anterior fontanel. The nurse documents its shape as which of the following?
- ☐ **1.** Oval.
- ☐ **2.** Square.
- ☐ **3.** Diamond shaped.
- ☐ **4.** Triangular.

31. Which of the following observations would the nurse expect when assessing the gestational age of a neonate delivered at term?
- ☐ **1.** Ear lying flat against the head.
- ☐ **2.** Absence of rugae in the scrotum.
- ☐ **3.** Sole creases covering the entire foot.
- ☐ **4.** Square window sign angle of 90 degrees.

32. While performing a complete assessment of a term neonate, which of the following findings would alert the nurse to notify the pediatrician?
☐ 1. Red reflex in the eyes.
☐ 2. Expiratory grunt.
☐ 3. Respiratory rate of 45 breaths/minute.
☐ 4. Prominent xiphoid process.

33. After instructing a mother about normal reflexes of term neonates, the nurse determines that the mother understands the instructions when she describes the tonic neck reflex as occurring when the neonate does which of the following?
☐ 1. Steps briskly when held upright near a firm, hard surface.
☐ 2. Pulls both arms and does not move the chin beyond the point of the elbows.
☐ 3. Turns head to the left, extends left extremities, and flexes right extremities.
☐ 4. Extends and abducts the arms and legs with the toes fanning open.

34. A primiparous client expresses concern, asking the nurse why her neonate's eyes are crossed. Which of the following would the nurse include when teaching the mother about neonatal strabismus?
☐ 1. The neonate's eyes are unable to focus on light at this time.
☐ 2. Neonates commonly lack eye muscle coordination.
☐ 3. Congenital cataracts may be present.
☐ 4. The neonate is able to fixate on distant objects immediately.

35. While performing a physical assessment on a term neonate shortly after birth, which of the following would cause the nurse to notify the pediatrician?
☐ 1. Deep creases across the soles of the feet.
☐ 2. Frequent sneezing during the assessment.
☐ 3. Single crease on each of the palms.
☐ 4. Absence of lanugo on the skin.

36. Metabolic screening of an infant revealed a high phenylketonuria (PKU) level. Which of the following statements by the infant's mother indicates understanding of the disease and its management? Select all that apply.
☐ 1. "My baby can't have milk-based formulas."
☐ 2. "My baby will grow out of this by the age of 2."
☐ 3. "This is a hereditary disease, so any future children will have it, too."
☐ 4. "My baby will eventually become retarded because of this disease."
☐ 5. "We have to follow a strict phenylalanine diet."
☐ 6. "A dietitian can help me plan a diet that keeps a safe phenylalanine level but lets my baby grow."

37. Assessment of a term neonate at 2 hours after birth reveals a heart rate of 110 bpm, periods of apnea approximately 25 to 30 seconds in length, and mild cyanosis around the mouth. The nurse notifies the pediatrician based on the interpretation that these findings may lead to which condition?
☐ 1. Respiratory arrest.
☐ 2. Bronchial pneumonia.
☐ 3. Intraventricular hemorrhage.
☐ 4. Epiglottitis.

38. A new mother asks, "When will the soft spot near the front of my baby's head close?" Which of the following ages should the nurse relate when responding to the mother about closure of the anterior fontanel?
☐ 1. 2 to 3 months.
☐ 2. 6 to 8 months.
☐ 3. 9 to 10 months.
☐ 4. 12 to 18 months.

39. Which of the following assessment findings in a term neonate would cause the nurse to notify the pediatrician?
☐ 1. Absence of tears.
☐ 2. Unequally sized corneas.
☐ 3. Pupillary constriction to bright light.
☐ 4. Red circle on pupils with ophthalmoscopic examination.

40. At 24 hours of age, assessment of the neonate reveals the following: eyes closed, skin pink, no sign of eye movements, heart rate of 120 bpm, and respiratory rate of 35 breaths/minute. The nurse interprets these findings as indicating that this neonate is most likely experiencing which of the following?
☐ 1. Drug withdrawal.
☐ 2. First period of reactivity.
☐ 3. A state of deep sleep.
☐ 4. Respiratory distress.

41. While assessing a male neonate whose mother desires him to be circumcised, the nurse observes that the neonate's urinary meatus appears to be located on the ventral surface of the penis. The physician is notified because the nurse suspects which of the following?
☐ 1. Phimosis.
☐ 2. Hydrocele.
☐ 3. Epispadias.
☐ 4. Hypospadias.

The Preterm Neonate

42. The nurse is discussing kangaroo care with the parents of a premature neonate. The nurse should tell the parents that the advantages of kangaroo care include which of the following? Select all that apply.
☐ 1. Facilitate a positive bonding experience.
☐ 2. Increased IQ.
☐ 3. Physiologic stability.
☐ 4. Shorten length of stay in the neonatal intensive care unit.
☐ 5. Time to grow.

43. A neonate at 37 weeks' gestation is delivered by cesarean delivery because of placenta previa. Which of the following would the circulating nurse do first as soon as the neonate is delivered?
☐ **1.** Stimulate the neonate to cry vigorously.
☐ **2.** Aspirate mucus from the mouth with a bulb syringe.
☐ **3.** Begin resuscitation procedures with a bag and mask.
☐ **4.** Hold the neonate upright for the mother to view.

44. After a vaginal delivery, a preterm neonate is to receive oxygen via mask. While administering the oxygen, the nurse would place the neonate in which of the following positions?
☐ **1.** Left side, with the neck slightly flexed.
☐ **2.** Back, with the head turned to the left side.
☐ **3.** Abdomen, with the head down.
☐ **4.** Back, with the neck slightly extended.

45. Which of the following actions should the nurse take when performing external cardiac massage on a neonate born at 28 weeks' gestation?
☐ **1.** Alternate cardiac massage with ventilation.
☐ **2.** Compress the sternum with the palm of the hand.
☐ **3.** Compress the chest 70 to 80 times per minute.
☐ **4.** Displace the chest wall half the depth of the anterior-posterior diameter of the chest.

46. A preterm neonate who has been stabilized is placed in a radiant warmer and is receiving oxygen via an oxygen hood. While administering oxygen in this manner, the nurse should do which of the following?
☐ **1.** Humidify the air being delivered.
☐ **2.** Cover the neonate's scalp with a warm cap.
☐ **3.** Record the neonate's temperature every 3 to 4 minutes.
☐ **4.** Assess the neonate's blood glucose level.

47. Two hours ago, a neonate at 38 weeks' gestation and weighing 3,175 g (7 lb) was born to a primiparous client who tested positive for beta-hemolytic *Streptococcus.* Which of the following would alert the nurse to notify the pediatrician?
☐ **1.** Alkalosis.
☐ **2.** Increased muscle tone.
☐ **3.** Temperature instability.
☐ **4.** Positive Babinski's reflex.

48. Which of the following would the nurse suspect when assessment of a 2-day-old neonate delivered at 34 weeks' gestation reveals absent apical pulse left of the midclavicular line, cyanosis, grunting, and diminished breath sounds?
☐ **1.** Diaphragmatic hernia.
☐ **2.** Pneumothorax.
☐ **3.** Coarctation of the aorta.
☐ **4.** Bacterial pneumonia.

49. Twenty-four hours after cesarean delivery, a neonate at 30 weeks' gestation is diagnosed with respiratory distress syndrome (RDS). When explaining to the parents about the cause of this syndrome, the nurse should include a discussion about an alteration in the body's secretion of which of the following?
☐ **1.** Somatotropin.
☐ **2.** Surfactant.
☐ **3.** Testosterone.
☐ **4.** Progesterone.

50. When caring for a neonate born at 30 weeks' gestation who is in an isolette and receiving continuous oxygen, which of the following would the nurse use as the best method to determine the effectiveness of this treatment?
☐ **1.** Evidence of cyanosis on mouth, hands, and feet.
☐ **2.** Continuous pulse rate monitoring.
☐ **3.** Arterial blood gas levels.
☐ **4.** Percentage of oxygen delivered.

51. A viable male neonate delivered to a 28-year-old multiparous client by cesarean delivery because of placenta previa is diagnosed with respiratory distress syndrome (RDS). Which of the following would the nurse explain as the factor placing the neonate at the greatest risk for this syndrome?
☐ **1.** Mother's development of placenta previa.
☐ **2.** Neonate delivered preterm.
☐ **3.** Mother receiving analgesia 4 hours before delivery.
☐ **4.** Neonate with sluggish respiratory efforts after delivery.

52. While the nurse is caring for a neonate at 32 weeks' gestation in an isolette with continuous oxygen administration, the neonate's mother asks why the neonate's oxygen is humidified. Which of the following would be the nurse's best response?
☐ **1.** "The humidity promotes expansion of the neonate's immature lungs."
☐ **2.** "The humidity helps to prevent viral or bacterial pneumonia."
☐ **3.** "Oxygen is drying to the mucous membranes unless it is humidified."
☐ **4.** "Circulation to the baby's heart is improved with humidified oxygen."

53. A preterm neonate admitted to the neonatal intensive care unit at about 30 weeks' gestation is placed in an oxygenated isolette. The neonate's mother tells the nurse that she was planning to breast-feed the neonate. Which of the following instructions about breast-feeding would be most appropriate?
- ☐ 1. Breast-feeding is not recommended because the neonate needs increased fat in the diet.
- ☐ 2. Once the neonate no longer needs oxygen and continuous monitoring, breast-feeding can be done.
- ☐ 3. Breast-feeding is contraindicated because the neonate needs a high-calorie formula every 2 hours.
- ☐ 4. Gavage feedings using breast milk can be given until the neonate can coordinate sucking and swallowing.

54. Which of the following best identifies the reason for assessing a neonate weighing 1,500 g at 32 weeks' gestation for retinopathy of prematurity (ROP)?
- ☐ 1. The neonate is at risk because of multiple factors.
- ☐ 2. Oxygen is being administered at a level of 21%.
- ☐ 3. The neonate was alkalotic immediately after birth.
- ☐ 4. Phototherapy is likely to be ordered by the pediatrician.

55. Which of the following would lead the nurse to suspect retinopathy of prematurity (ROP) when assessing a neonate at 32 weeks' gestation who weighs 2,000 g?
- ☐ 1. Sunken orbital sockets.
- ☐ 2. Strabismus.
- ☐ 3. Reaction to bright light.
- ☐ 4. Constricted retinal vessels.

56. Which of the following subjects should the nurse include when teaching the mother of a neonate diagnosed with retinopathy of prematurity (ROP) about possible treatment for complications?
- ☐ 1. Laser therapy.
- ☐ 2. Cromolyn sodium (Intal) eye drops.
- ☐ 3. Frequent testing for glaucoma.
- ☐ 4. Corneal transplants.

57. Which of the following nursing diagnoses would be the priority for a neonate admitted to the neonatal intensive care nursery at 28 weeks' gestation weighing 1,474 g (3 lb, 4 oz)?
- ☐ 1. *Risk for impaired skin integrity* related to gestational age.
- ☐ 2. *Imbalanced nutrition: Less than body requirements* related to preterm gestational age.
- ☐ 3. *Impaired gas exchange* related to immature pulmonary vasculature.
- ☐ 4. *Risk for delayed development* related to prematurity.

58. Three days after admission of a neonate delivered at 30 weeks' gestation, the neonatologist plans to assess the neonate for periventricular-intraventricular hemorrhage (PIVH). The nurse would plan to assist the neonatologist by preparing the neonate for which of the following?
- ☐ 1. Computed tomography scan.
- ☐ 2. Arterial blood specimen collection.
- ☐ 3. Radiographs of the skull.
- ☐ 4. Complete blood count specimen collection.

59. Which of the following would the nurse expect to assess in a neonate delivered at 28 weeks' gestation who is diagnosed with intraventricular hemorrhage (IVH)?
- ☐ 1. Increased muscle tone.
- ☐ 2. Hyperbilirubinemia.
- ☐ 3. Bulging fontanels.
- ☐ 4. Hyperactivity.

60. An infant born premature at 34 weeks is receiving gavage feedings. The client holding her infant asks why the nurse places a pacifier in the infant's mouth during these feedings. The nurse replies that the pacifier helps in what ways? Select all that apply.
- ☐ 1. Teaches the infant to suck and swallow.
- ☐ 2. Provides oral stimulation.
- ☐ 3. Keeps oral mucus membranes moist while the tube is in place.
- ☐ 4. Reminds the infant how to suck.
- ☐ 5. Stimulates secretions that help gastric emptying.

61. While caring for a neonate delivered at 32 weeks' gestation, the nurse assesses the neonate daily for symptoms of necrotizing enterocolitis (NEC). Which of the following would alert the nurse to notify the neonatologist?
- ☐ 1. The presence of 1 ml of gastric residual before a gavage feeding.
- ☐ 2. Jaundice appearing on the face and chest.
- ☐ 3. An increase in bowel peristalsis.
- ☐ 4. Abdominal distention.

62. Which of the following statements by the mother of a neonate diagnosed with bronchopulmonary dysplasia (BPD) indicates effective teaching?
- ☐ 1. "BPD is an acute disease that can be treated with antibiotics."
- ☐ 2. "My baby may require permanent assisted ventilation."
- ☐ 3. "Bronchodilators can cure my baby's condition."
- ☐ 4. "My baby may have seizures later on in life because of this condition."

63. A neonate delivered at 34 weeks' gestation is diagnosed with a pneumothorax. Which of the following would the nurse expect the neonatologist to order?
- ☐ 1. Placement of the neonate on a ventilator.
- ☐ 2. Administration of bronchodilators through the nares.
- ☐ 3. Suctioning of the neonate's nares with wall suction.
- ☐ 4. Insertion of a chest tube into the neonate.

64. Which of the following would alert the nurse to suspect that a neonate delivered at 34 weeks' gestation who is currently in an isolette with humidified oxygen and receiving intravenous fluids has developed overhydration?
☐ **1.** Hypernatremia.
☐ **2.** Polycythemia.
☐ **3.** Hypoproteinemia.
☐ **4.** Increased urine specific gravity.

65. A newborn weighing 6½ lb is to be given naloxone hydrochloride (Narcan) due to respiratory depression as a result of a narcotic given to the mother shortly before delivery. The drug is to be given 0.01 mg/kg into the umbilical vein. The vial is marked 0.4 mg/ml. How many milligrams would the newborn receive? Round to two decimals.

_____ mg

The Post-Term Neonate

66. A neonate born by cesarean delivery at 42 weeks' gestation, weighing 4.1 kg (9 lb, 1 oz), with Apgar scores of 8 at 1 minute and 9 at 5 minutes after birth, develops an increased respiratory rate and tremors of the hands and feet 2 hours postpartum. Which of the following nursing diagnoses would be the priority?
☐ **1.** *Ineffective airway clearance* related to post-term gestational age.
☐ **2.** *Hyperthermia* related to large size and use of a radiant warmer.
☐ **3.** *Decreased cardiac output* related to difficult delivery.
☐ **4.** *Imbalanced nutrition: Less than body requirements* related to depleted glycogen stores.

67. At a home visit, the nurse assesses a neonate delivered vaginally at 41 weeks' gestation 5 days ago, noting the following findings: frequent hiccups; loose, watery stool in diaper; red rash on face; and dry, peeling skin. Which of these findings warrants further assessment?
☐ **1.** Frequent hiccups.
☐ **2.** Loose, watery stool in diaper.
☐ **3.** Pink papular vesicles on the face.
☐ **4.** Dry, peeling skin.

68. When performing an initial assessment of a post-term male neonate weighing 4,000 g (9 lb) who was admitted to the observation nursery after a vaginal delivery with low forceps, the nurse detects Ortolani's sign. Which of the following actions should the nurse do next?
☐ **1.** Determine the length of the mother's labor.
☐ **2.** Notify the pediatrician immediately.
☐ **3.** Keep the neonate under the radiant warmer for 2 hours.
☐ **4.** Obtain a blood sample to check for hypoglycemia.

69. A neonate is admitted to the neonatal intensive care unit for observation with a diagnosis of probable meconium aspiration syndrome (MAS). The neonate weighs 10 lb, 4 oz (4,650 g) and is at 41 weeks' gestation. Which of the following nursing diagnoses would be the priority for this neonate?
☐ **1.** *Impaired skin integrity* related to post-term status.
☐ **2.** *Imbalanced nutrition: More than body requirements* related to large size.
☐ **3.** *Risk for impaired parent-infant-child attachment* related to transfer to the intensive care unit.
☐ **4.** *Impaired gas exchange* related to the effects of respiratory distress.

70. When developing the initial plan of care for a neonate who was born at 41 weeks' gestation, was diagnosed with meconium aspiration syndrome (MAS), and requires mechanical ventilation, which of the following would the nurse include?
☐ **1.** Care of an umbilical arterial line.
☐ **2.** Frequent ultrasound scans.
☐ **3.** Orogastric feedings as soon as possible.
☐ **4.** Assessment for symptoms of hyperglycemia.

71. A post-term neonate diagnosed with persistent pulmonary hypertension is prescribed intravenous tolazoline (Priscoline). Which of the following would the nurse need to monitor while administering this drug?
☐ **1.** Feeding behaviors.
☐ **2.** Temperature.
☐ **3.** Skin color.
☐ **4.** Blood pressure.

The Neonate with Risk Factors

72. A nurse is attempting to resuscitate a neonate. After following the Neonatal Resuscitation Program guidelines, 30 seconds of chest compressions have been completed. The neonate's heart rate remains less than 60 bpm. Epinephrine is given. What is the expected outcome for a neonate who has received epinephrine during resuscitation?
☐ **1.** Increased urine output.
☐ **2.** A normal heart rate.
☐ **3.** Pain relief.
☐ **4.** Sedation.

73. A mother is visiting her neonate in the neonatal intensive care unit. Her baby is fussy and the mother wants to know what to do. In order to quiet a sick neonate, which of the following can the nurse teach the mother to do?
☐ **1.** Bring in toys for distraction.
☐ **2.** Place a musical mobile over the crib.
☐ **3.** Stroke the neonate's back.
☐ **4.** Use constant, gentle touch.

74. A neonate delivered at 40 weeks' gestation admitted to the nursery is found to be hypoglycemic. At 4 hours of age, the neonate appears pale and his pulse oximeter is reading 75%. The nurse should:
- ☐ **1.** Increase the I.V. rate.
- ☐ **2.** Provide supplemental oxygen.
- ☐ **3.** Record the finding on the chart and repeat the reading in 30 minutes.
- ☐ **4.** Wrap the neonate to increase body temperature.

75. A neonate born at 29 weeks' gestation received nasal continuous positive airway pressure. The neonate is receiving oxygen at 1 L/minute via nasal cannula at a fraction of inspired oxygen (FiO_2) of 0.23. The pulse oximetry reading is 70% saturation. In which order of priority should the nurse take these actions?

1. Increase the FiO_2.
2. Make sure the pulse oximeter is correlating to the heart rate.
3. Assess the neonate for color.
4. Assess the neonate for respiratory effort.

76. A neonate with heart failure is being discharged home. In teaching the parents about the neonate's nutritional needs, the nurse should explain that:
- ☐ **1.** Fluids should be restricted.
- ☐ **2.** Decreased activity level should reduce the need for additional calories.
- ☐ **3.** The formula should be low in sodium.
- ☐ **4.** The neonate may need a formula with higher calories per fluid ounce.

77. During an assessment of a neonate born at 33 weeks' gestation, a nurse finds and reports a heart murmur. An echocardiogram reveals patent ductus arteriosis, for which the neonate received indomethacin. An expected outcome after the administration of indomethacin to a neonate with patent ductus arteriosis is:
- ☐ **1.** Closure of a patent ductus arteriosus.
- ☐ **2.** Decreased bleeding time.
- ☐ **3.** Increased gastrointestinal function.
- ☐ **4.** Increased renal output.

78. A preterm neonate is unable to breast- or bottle-feed. The physician writes an order to feed the neonate via nasogastric (NG) tube. When choosing an NG feeding tube for a neonate, the nurse should base the tube size on the neonate's:
- ☐ **1.** Disease process.
- ☐ **2.** Gestational age.
- ☐ **3.** Length.
- ☐ **4.** Weight.

79. A nurse is reviewing a client's maternal prenatal record and notes that the mother used narcotics during her pregnancy. A primary nursing intervention when caring for a drug-exposed neonate is to:
- ☐ **1.** Assess vital signs including blood pressure every hour.
- ☐ **2.** Minimize environmental stimuli.
- ☐ **3.** Place the infant in a well-lighted area for observation.
- ☐ **4.** Provide stimulation to increase adaptation to the environment.

80. The nurse is receiving over the telephone a laboratory results report of a neonate's blood glucose level. The nurse should:
- ☐ **1.** Write down the results, read back the results to the caller from the laboratory, and receive confirmation from the caller that the nurse understands the results.
- ☐ **2.** Repeat the results to the caller from the laboratory, write the results on scrap paper first, and then transfer the results to the chart.
- ☐ **3.** Indicate to the caller that the nurse cannot receive verbal results from laboratory tests for neonates, and ask the laboratory to bring the written results to the nursery.
- ☐ **4.** Request that the laboratory send the results by e-mail to transfer to the client's electronic record.

81. A multiparous client who has a neonate diagnosed with hemolytic disease of the newborn asks the nurse why the neonate has developed this problem. Which of the following responses by the nurse would be most appropriate?
- ☐ **1.** "You are Rh-positive and the neonate's father is Rh-negative."
- ☐ **2.** "You and the neonate's father are both Rh-negative."
- ☐ **3.** "You are Rh-negative and the neonate's father is Rh-positive."
- ☐ **4.** "The fetus is Rh-negative and you are Rh-positive."

82. After teaching the multiparous mother about hemolytic disease of the newborn and Rh sensitization, the nurse determines that the client understands why she was not sensitized during her other pregnancy when she says which of the following?
- ☐ **1.** "My other baby had a different father."
- ☐ **2.** "Like most women, I have immunity against the Rh factor."
- ☐ **3.** "Antibodies are not usually formed until after exposure to an antigen."
- ☐ **4.** "My blood couldn't neutralize antibodies formed from my first pregnancy."

83. After teaching a multiparous client about the effects of hemolysis due to Rh sensitization on the neonate at delivery, the nurse determines that the client needs further instruction when the mother reports that the neonate may have which of the following?
- ☐ **1.** Cardiac decompensation.
- ☐ **2.** Polycythemia.
- ☐ **3.** Anemia.
- ☐ **4.** Splenic enlargement.

84. After delivery, a direct Coombs test is performed on the umbilical cord blood of a neonate with Rh-positive blood born to a mother with Rh-negative blood. The nurse explains to the client that this test is done to detect which of the following?
- ☐ **1.** Degree of anemia in the neonate.
- ☐ **2.** Electrolyte imbalances in the neonate.
- ☐ **3.** Antibodies coating the neonate's red blood cells.
- ☐ **4.** Antigens coating the neonate's red blood cells.

85. After teaching the mother of a neonate with erythroblastosis fetalis who is to receive an exchange transfusion, which of the following, if stated by the mother as the purpose of the transfusion, indicates effective teaching?
- ☐ **1.** To replenish the neonate's leukocytes.
- ☐ **2.** To restore the fluid and electrolyte balance.
- ☐ **3.** To correct the neonate's anemia.
- ☐ **4.** To replace Rh-negative blood with Rh-positive blood.

86. The nurse explains to the mother of a neonate diagnosed with erythroblastosis fetalis that the exchange transfusion is necessary to prevent damage primarily to which of the following organs in the neonate?
- ☐ **1.** Kidneys.
- ☐ **2.** Brain.
- ☐ **3.** Lungs.
- ☐ **4.** Liver.

87. The nurse determines that a newborn is hypoglycemic based on which of the following findings? Select all that apply.
- ☐ **1.** Glucometer reading of 40 mg/dl.
- ☐ **2.** Family history of insulin-dependent diabetes.
- ☐ **3.** Internal fetal monitor tracing.
- ☐ **4.** Irregular respirations, tremors, and hypothermia.
- ☐ **5.** Large for gestational age.

88. A neonate whose mother has insulin-dependent diabetes weighs 4,564 g (10 lb, 1 oz), is large for gestational age, and is admitted to the neonatal intensive care unit. Which of the following would be a priority nursing diagnosis for this neonate?
- ☐ **1.** *Hyperthermia* related to large-for-gestational-age size.
- ☐ **2.** *Impaired skin integrity* related to maternal diabetes.
- ☐ **3.** *Risk for disproportionate growth* related to excessive birth weight.
- ☐ **4.** *Imbalanced nutrition: Less than body requirements* related to increased glucose metabolism.

89. The nurse is caring for an infant of an insulin-dependent diabetic primiparous client. When the mother visits the neonate at 1 hour after birth, the nurse explains to the mother that the neonate is being closely monitored for symptoms of hypoglycemia because of which of the following?
- ☐ **1.** Increased use of glucose stores during a difficult labor and delivery process.
- ☐ **2.** Interrupted supply of maternal glucose and continued high neonatal insulin production.
- ☐ **3.** A normal response that occurs during transition from intrauterine to extrauterine life.
- ☐ **4.** Increased pancreatic enzyme production caused by decreased glucose stores.

90. When caring for the neonate of a diabetic mother weighing 4,564 g (10 lb, 1 oz) who was delivered vaginally, the nurse would assess the neonate for fracture of which of the following?
- ☐ **1.** Clavicle.
- ☐ **2.** Skull.
- ☐ **3.** Wrist.
- ☐ **4.** Rib cage.

91. While caring for a neonate of a diabetic mother soon after delivery, after the neonate has received treatment for hypoglycemia, the nurse observes that the neonate's blood glucose level is 60 mg/dl but the neonate is still exhibiting jitteriness and tremors. The nurse notifies the physician because these symptoms may indicate which of the following?
- ☐ **1.** Phenylketonuria.
- ☐ **2.** Biliary duct obstruction.
- ☐ **3.** Hypermagnesemia.
- ☐ **4.** Hypocalcemia.

92. The nurse is caring for a neonate weighing 4,536 g (10 lb) who was born via cesarean delivery 1 hour ago. The mother is a class B insulin-dependent diabetic primipara. She asks the nurse, "Why is my baby in the neonatal intensive care unit?" The nurse bases her response on the understanding that neonates of class B diabetic mothers commonly develop which of the following conditions?
- ☐ **1.** Anemia.
- ☐ **2.** Persistent pulmonary hypertension.
- ☐ **3.** Hemolytic disease.
- ☐ **4.** Hypoglycemia.

93. While assessing a neonate weighing 3,175 g (7 lb) who was born at 39 weeks' gestation to a primiparous client who admits to cocaine use during pregnancy, which of the following would alert the nurse to possible cocaine withdrawal?
☐ **1.** Bradycardia.
☐ **2.** High-pitched cry.
☐ **3.** Sluggishness.
☐ **4.** Hypocalcemia.

94. After teaching a primiparous client who used cocaine during pregnancy about possible gastrointestinal signs and symptoms in her neonate, which of the following, if stated by the mother as common, indicates effective teaching?
☐ **1.** Hypotonia.
☐ **2.** Constipation.
☐ **3.** Vomiting.
☐ **4.** Abdominal distention.

95. When teaching a primiparous client who used cocaine during pregnancy how to comfort her fussy neonate, which of the following would the nurse suggest?
☐ **1.** Tightly swaddling the neonate.
☐ **2.** Feeding the neonate extra, high-calorie formula.
☐ **3.** Keeping the neonate in a brightly lit environment.
☐ **4.** Minimizing touching of the neonate (touching only when the neonate is crying).

96. A neonate born at 38 weeks' gestation is admitted to the neonatal nursery for observation. The neonate's mother, who is positive for human immunodeficiency virus (HIV) infection, has received no prenatal care. The mother asks the nurse if her neonate is positive for HIV. The nurse tells the mother which of the following?
☐ **1.** "More than 50% of neonates born to mothers who are positive for HIV will be positive at 18 months of age."
☐ **2.** "An enlarged liver at birth generally means the neonate is HIV positive."
☐ **3.** "A complete blood count analysis is the primary method for determining whether the neonate is HIV positive."
☐ **4.** "Most neonates are asymptomatic at birth and usually test positive for the HIV antibody at this time."

97. When caring for a multiparous client who is human immunodeficiency virus (HIV)–positive and asking to breast-feed her neonate as soon as possible, which of the following instructions about breast milk should the nurse include in the teaching plan?
☐ **1.** It may help prevent the spread of the HIV virus.
☐ **2.** It contains antibodies that can protect the neonate from HIV.
☐ **3.** It can be beneficial for the bonding process.
☐ **4.** It has been found to contain the retrovirus HIV.

98. While caring for the neonate of a human immunodeficiency virus–positive mother, the nurse prepares to administer an ordered hepatitis B intramuscular injection at 4 hours after birth. Which of the following actions should the nurse do first?
☐ **1.** Bathe the neonate with an antibacterial soap.
☐ **2.** Place the neonate under a radiant warmer.
☐ **3.** Wash the injection site with povidone-iodine (Betadine) solution.
☐ **4.** Apply clean gloves before administering the medication.

99. A male neonate born at 38 weeks' gestation by cesarean delivery after prolonged rupture of the membranes and a maternal oral temperature of 102° F (38.8° C) is being observed for signs and symptoms of infection. Which of the following would alert the nurse to notify the physician?
☐ **1.** Leukocytosis.
☐ **2.** Apical heart rate of 132 bpm.
☐ **3.** Behavioral changes.
☐ **4.** Warm, moist skin.

100. The nurse is caring for a neonate shortly after birth when the neonate is diagnosed with sepsis and is to be treated with intravenous antibiotics. Which of the following will the nurse need to instruct the parents to do because of the neonate's infection?
☐ **1.** Use caution near the isolation incubator and equipment.
☐ **2.** Visit but do not touch the neonate.
☐ **3.** Wash their hands thoroughly before touching the neonate.
☐ **4.** Wear a mask when holding the neonate.

101. A female neonate delivered vaginally at term with a cleft lip and cleft palate is admitted to the regular nursery. Which of the following actions should the nurse do the first time that the parents visit the neonate in the nursery?
☐ **1.** Explain the surgical interventions that will be performed.
☐ **2.** Stress that this defect is not life-threatening.
☐ **3.** Emphasize the neonate's normal characteristics.
☐ **4.** Reassure the parents about the success rate of the surgery.

102. After teaching the parents of a neonate born with a cleft lip and cleft palate about appropriate feeding techniques, the nurse determines that the mother needs further instruction when the mother says which of the following?
☐ **1.** "I should clean her mouth with soapy water after feeding."
☐ **2.** "I should feed her in an upright position."
☐ **3.** "I need to remember to burp her often."
☐ **4.** "I may need to use a special nipple for feeding."

103. Which of the following diagnoses should the nurse identify as a priority nursing diagnosis for a neonate diagnosed with a cleft palate at 1 hour postpartum?
- ☐ 1. *Activity intolerance* related to respiratory distress syndrome.
- ☐ 2. *Risk for infection* related to potential aspiration during feedings.
- ☐ 3. *Compromised family coping* related to congenital malformation of the neonate.
- ☐ 4. *Impaired skin integrity* related to frequent treatments and feedings.

104. A male neonate born at 36 weeks' gestation is admitted to the neonatal intensive care nursery with a diagnosis of probable fetal alcohol syndrome (FAS). The mother visits the nursery soon after the neonate is admitted. Which of the following instructions should the nurse expect to include when developing the teaching plan for the mother about FAS?
- ☐ 1. Withdrawal symptoms usually do not occur until 7 days postpartum.
- ☐ 2. Large-for-gestational-age size is common with this condition.
- ☐ 3. Facial deformities associated with FAS can be corrected by plastic surgery.
- ☐ 4. Symptoms of withdrawal include tremors, sleeplessness, and seizures.

105. Which of the following characteristics should the nurse teach the mother about her neonate diagnosed with fetal alcohol syndrome (FAS)?
- ☐ 1. Neonates are commonly listless and lethargic.
- ☐ 2. The IQ scores are usually average.
- ☐ 3. Hyperactivity and speech disorders are common.
- ☐ 4. The mortality rate is 70% unless treated.

106. Which of the following nursing diagnoses would be the priority for a neonate with fetal alcohol syndrome (FAS) admitted to the special care nursery soon after birth?
- ☐ 1. *Delayed growth and development* related to poor parenting abilities of the mother.
- ☐ 2. *Imbalanced nutrition: Less than body requirements* related to hyperirritability.
- ☐ 3. *Impaired swallowing* related to FAS.
- ☐ 4. *Risk for trauma* related to immature parenting methods.

107. When developing the plan of care for a neonate diagnosed with gastroschisis, which of the following actions should the nurse expect to do first?
- ☐ 1. Weigh the neonate.
- ☐ 2. Insert an orogastric tube.
- ☐ 3. Prepare for immediate blood transfusion.
- ☐ 4. Cover the abdomen with a moistened sterile gauze.

108. The father of a neonate diagnosed with gastroschisis tells the nurse that his wife had planned on breast-feeding the neonate. Which of the following should the nurse include in the preoperative teaching plan about feeding the neonate?
- ☐ 1. The neonate will remain on nothing-by-mouth (NPO) status until after surgery.
- ☐ 2. An iron-fortified formula will be given before surgery.
- ☐ 3. The neonate will need total parenteral nutrition for nourishment.
- ☐ 4. The mother may breast-feed the neonate before surgery.

109. The nurse is providing care for a neonate who is to undergo gastroschisis surgery. What should the priorities be? Select all that apply.
- ☐ 1. Prevention of hypothermia.
- ☐ 2. Maintenance of fluid and electrolyte balance.
- ☐ 3. Provision of time for parental bonding.
- ☐ 4. Prevention of infection.
- ☐ 5. Providing developmental care.

110. While caring for a male neonate diagnosed with gastroschisis, the nurse observes that the parents seem hesitant to touch the neonate because of his appearance. The nurse determines that the parents are most likely experiencing which of the following stages of grief?
- ☐ 1. Denial.
- ☐ 2. Shock.
- ☐ 3. Bargaining.
- ☐ 4. Anger.

111. Which of the following instructions should the nurse give to the parents of a neonate diagnosed with hyperbilirubinemia who is receiving phototherapy?
- ☐ 1. Keep the neonate's eyes completely covered.
- ☐ 2. Use a regular diaper on the neonate.
- ☐ 3. Offer feedings every 4 hours.
- ☐ 4. Check the oral temperature every 8 hours.

112. While caring for a term neonate who has been receiving phototherapy for 8 hours, the nurse notifies the pediatrician if which of the following is noted?
- ☐ 1. Bronze-colored skin.
- ☐ 2. Maculopapular chest rash.
- ☐ 3. Urine specific gravity of 1.018.
- ☐ 4. Absent Moro reflex.

113. The nurse is caring for a neonate at 38 weeks' gestation when the nurse observes marked peristaltic waves on the neonate's abdomen. After this observation, the neonate exhibits projectile vomiting. The nurse notifies the pediatrician because these signs are indicative of which of the following?
- ☐ 1. Esophageal atresia.
- ☐ 2. Pyloric stenosis.
- ☐ 3. Diaphragmatic hernia.
- ☐ 4. Hiatal hernia.

114. The nurse is caring for a term neonate who is diagnosed with patent ductus arteriosus. While performing a physical assessment of the neonate, the nurse anticipates that the neonate will exhibit which of the following?
☐ **1.** Decreased cardiac output with faint peripheral pulses.
☐ **2.** Profound cyanosis over most of the body.
☐ **3.** Loud cardiac murmurs through systole and diastole.
☐ **4.** Harsh systolic murmurs with a palpable thrill.

115. Assessment of a term neonate at 8 hours after birth reveals tachypnea, dyspnea, sternal retractions, diminished femoral pulses, poor lower body perfusion, and cyanosis of the lower body and extremities, with a pink upper body. The nurse notifies the pediatrician based on the interpretation that these symptoms are associated with which of the following?
☐ **1.** Coarctation of the aorta.
☐ **2.** Atrioventricular septal defect.
☐ **3.** Pulmonary atresia.
☐ **4.** Transposition of the great arteries.

116. The nurse is caring for a 2-day-old neonate in the recovery room 30 minutes after surgical correction for the cardiac defect, transposition of the great vessels. Which of the following would alert the nurse to notify the physician?
☐ **1.** Oxygen saturation of 90%.
☐ **2.** Pale pink extremities.
☐ **3.** Warm, dry skin.
☐ **4.** Femoral pulse of 90 bpm.

117. A term neonate at 2 hours of life is diagnosed with tricuspid atresia. The nurse anticipates that the pediatrician will order which of the following medications intravenously?
☐ **1.** Indomethacin (Indocin).
☐ **2.** Digoxin (Lanoxin).
☐ **3.** Prostaglandin E (PGE1 [Prostin VR Pediatric]).
☐ **4.** Hydrochlorothiazide (HydroDIURIL).

118. After the physician explains the prognosis and medical management for atrial septal defect to a primiparous client whose 2-day-old female neonate was diagnosed with this condition, the nurse determines that the mother needs further instructions when she says which of the following?
☐ **1.** "As my child grows, she may have increased fatigue and difficulty breathing."
☐ **2.** "My child may need to have antibiotics if she develops an infection."
☐ **3.** "This condition occurs more commonly in females than in males."
☐ **4.** "About half of the children born with this defect heal spontaneously."

Correct Answers and Rationales

The letter in parentheses after each rationale identifies the client need addressed in the item, including management of care (M), safety and infection control (S), health promotion and maintenance (H), psychosocial adaptation (P), basic care and comfort (C), pharmacological and parenteral therapies (D), reduction of risk potential (R), and physiological adaptation (A).

The Neonatal Client

1. 2. The neonate should be kept away from drafts, such as from air conditioning vents, which may cause heat loss by convection. Evaporation is the one of the most common mechanisms by which the neonate will lose heat, such as when the moisture on the newly delivered neonate's body is converted to vapor. Radiation is heat loss between solid objects that are not in contact with one another such as walls and windows. Conduction is when heat is transferred between solid objects in contact with one another, such as when a neonate comes in contact with a cold mattress or scale. (R)

2. 135

The recommended dose of ampicillin for a neonate is 100 mg/kg/dose. First, determine the neonate's weight in kilograms, and then multiply the kilograms by 100 mg. The nurse should use this formula:

$$1,000 \text{ g} = 1 \text{ kg}$$

$$1,350 \text{ g} = 1.35 \text{ kg}$$

$$100 \text{ mg} \times 1.35 \text{ kg} = 135 \text{ mg/kg}$$

(D)

3. 3. Adding humidity to the incubator adds moisture to the ambient air, which helps to decrease the insensible water loss. Bathing and the use of eye patches has no impact on insensible water loss. The use of a radiant warmer will increase the insensible water loss by drawing moisture out of the skin. (R)

4. 4. Safe practice and error reduction can be increased by double-checking orders and medications before administration. Knowing the neonate's weight, urinary output, and glucose level is an important part of understanding the potential needs of the neonate; however, double-checking orders and interventions is the most important step to increase safety. (S)

5. 3. Neonates that are septic use glucose at an increased rate. During the time the I.V. is not infusing, the neonate is using the limited glucose stores available to a preterm neonate and may deplete them. Hypoglycemia is too little glucose in the blood; without the constant infusion of I.V. glucose, hypoglycemia will result. Fevers and hyperkalemia are not related to glucose levels. Tachycardia is the result of untreated hypoglycemia. (R)

6. **1, 3, 4.** The nurse should write down the order, read the order back to the physician, and receive confirmation from the physician that the order is correct as understood by the nurse. It is not necessary for the physician to come to the hospital to write the order on the chart, or to have the nursing supervisor cosign the telephone order. To ensure client safety when obtaining telephone orders, the order must be received by a registered nurse. (S)

7. **3, 4.** The nurse should use at least two sources of identification prior to administering medication to any client, such as the medical record number and the client's date of birth. It is not safe practice to ask the parent or a nurse to verify the correct client. It is also not safe to use the room number or crib number as a source of identification because clients' locations in the hospital change frequently. (S)

8. **1.** This 3-day-old neonate's weight loss falls within a normal range, and therefore no action is needed at this time. Full-term neonates tend to lose 5% to 10% of their birth weight during the first few days after birth, most likely because of minimal nutritional intake. With bottle-feeding, the neonate's intake varies from one feeding to another. Additionally, the neonate experiences a loss of extracellular fluid. Typically, neonates regain any weight loss by 7 to 10 days of life. If the weight loss continues after that time, the physician should be called. (H)

9. **240**

$$45 \text{ ml} = 1\frac{1}{2} \text{ oz}$$

$$1\frac{1}{2} \text{ oz} \times 8 \text{ feedings} = 12$$

$$12 \times 20 \text{ calories/oz} = 240 \text{ calories}$$

(C)

10. **2.** Keeping the neonate away from drafts and cooling ducts prevents heat loss by convection (flow of heat from the body surface to the cooler surrounding air). The neonate also loses heat through evaporation (conversion of a liquid to a vapor, as when a wet surface, such as the neonate's skin, is exposed to air); conduction (transfer of body heat to a cooler solid object in contact with the baby, as when the neonate comes in direct contact with a cold surface such as a scale or a cold stethoscope); and radiation (transfer of heat to cooler solid objects that are not in direct contact with the baby, as when the neonate is placed near a cold window surface or air conditioner). (H)

11. **1.** To begin vitamin K synthesis, which occurs in the intestines, food and normal intestinal flora are needed. However, at birth, the neonate's intestines are sterile. Therefore, vitamin K is administered via injection to prevent a vitamin K deficiency that may result in a bleeding tendency. When administered, vitamin K promotes formation in the liver of clotting factors II, VII, IX, and X. Neonates are not normally susceptible to clotting disorders, unless they are diagnosed with hemophilia or demonstrate a deficiency of or a problem with clotting factors. Hemolysis of fetal red blood cells does not destroy vitamin K. Hemolysis may be caused by Rh or ABO incompatibility, which leads to anemia and necessitates an exchange transfusion. Vitamin K synthesis occurs in the intestines, not the liver. (D)

12. **3.** Currently, the sense of touch is believed to be the most highly developed sense at birth. It is probably for this reason that neonates respond well to touch. Auditory sense typically is relatively immature in the neonate, as evidenced by the neonate's selective response to the human voice. By 4 months, the neonate should turn his eyes and head toward a sound coming from behind. Visual sense tends to be relatively immature. At birth, visual acuity is estimated at approximately 20/100 to 20/150, but it improves rapidly during infancy and toddlerhood. Taste is well developed, with a preference toward glucose; however, touch is more developed at birth. (H)

13. **1.** The nurse should inform the mother that baby powder can enter the neonate's lungs and result in pneumonia secondary to aspiration of the particles. The best prevention for diaper rash is frequent diaper changing and keeping the neonate's skin dry. The new disposable diapers have moisture-collecting materials and generally do not adhere to the skin unless the diaper becomes saturated. Typically, allergies are not associated with the use of baby powder in neonates. (R)

14. **4.** The mother needs further instruction when she says that a yellowish crust should be removed with water. The yellowish crust is normal and indicates scar formation at the site. It should not be removed, because to do so might cause increased bleeding. The petroleum gauze prevents the diaper from sticking to the circumcision site, and it may fall off in the diaper. If this occurs, the mother should not attempt to replace it but should simply apply plain petroleum jelly to the site. The gauze should be left in place for 24 hours, and the mother should continue to apply petroleum jelly with each diaper change for 48 hours after the procedure. A few drops of oozing blood is normal, but if the amount is greater than a few drops the mother should apply pressure and contact the physician. Any bleeding after the first day should be reported. (R)

15. **3.** The mother demonstrates understanding of the discharge instructions when she says that she should contact the pediatrician if the baby has a liquid stool with a watery ring, because this indicates diarrhea. Infants can become dehydrated very quickly, and frequent diarrhea can result in dehydration. Normally, babies fall asleep easily after a feeding because they are satisfied and content. Spitting up a tablespoon of formula is normal. However, projectile or forceful vomiting in larger amounts should be reported. Bottle-fed infants typically pass one to two light brown stools each day. (R)

16. **1.** Placing the neonate on his back after the feeding is recommended to minimize the risk for sudden infant death syndrome (SIDS). Placing the neonate on the abdomen after feeding has been associated with SIDS. The mother should bubble or burp the baby after ½ oz of formula has been taken and then again when the baby is finished. Waiting until the baby has eaten 1 oz of formula can lead to regurgitation. The entire nipple should be placed on top of the baby's tongue and into the mouth to prevent excessive air from being swallowed. The nipple is pointed directly into the mouth, not toward the neonate's palate, to provide adequate sucking. (R)

17. 1. In a neonate, the lateral aspect of the heel is the most appropriate site for obtaining a blood specimen. Using this area prevents damage to the calcaneus bone, which is located in the middle of the heel. The middle of the heel is to be avoided because of the increased risk for damaging the calcaneus bone located there. The middle of the foot contains the medial plantar nerve and the medial plantar artery, which could be injured if this site is selected. Using the base of the toes as the site for specimen collection would cause a great deal of discomfort for the neonate; therefore, it is not the preferred site. (R)

18. 2. After circumcision with a Plastibell, the most commonly recommended procedure is to clean the circumcision site with warm water with each diaper change. Other treatments are necessary only if complications, such as an infection, develop. Antibacterial soap or diluted hydrogen peroxide may cause pain and is not recommended. Povidone-iodine solution may cause stinging and burning, and therefore its use is not recommended. (H)

19. 2. As part of the neonate's physiologic adaptation to birth, at 90 minutes after birth the neonate typically is in the rest or sleep phase. During this time, the heart and respiratory rates slow and the neonate sleeps, unresponsive to stimuli. At this time, the mother should rest and allow the neonate to sleep. Feedings should be given during the first period of reactivity, considered the first 30 minutes after birth. During this period, the neonate's respirations and heart rate are elevated. Getting to know the neonate typically occurs within the first hour after birth and then when the neonate is awake and during feedings. Changing the neonate's diaper can occur at any time, but at 90 minutes after birth the neonate is usually in a deep sleep, unresponsive, and probably hasn't passed any meconium. (H)

Physical Assessment of the Neonatal Client

20. 2. The Moro reflex is a normal reflex of a neonate and requires no intervention. Calling a code, placing the neonate on seizure precautions, and starting supplemental oxygen are not necessary for a normally occurring reflex. (C)

21. 2. When resuscitating the neonate, the principle of airway-breathing-circulation (ABCs) must be followed. Positioning the neonate on the back with the neck slightly extended in the "sniffing" position will open the airway, allowing oxygen to get to the neonate's lungs. Apgar scores are an evaluation of the neonate's status at 1 and 5 minutes

of life. Waiting to open the airway until after assigning an Apgar score would be a waste of valuable time. If the airway is not patent, oxygen cannot be delivered. Cardiac compression must be accompanied by adequate oxygenation. (A)

22. 3. The neonate has a heart rate greater than 100, which earns him 2 points. His respiratory rate of 70 is equivalent to a 2 on the scale. His flaccid muscle tone is equal to 0 on the scale. The lack of response to stimulus also equals 0, as does his overall pale white color. Thus, the total score equals 4. (C)

23. 1. As a result of vigorous suctioning the nurse must watch for bradycardia due to potential vagus nerve stimulation. Rapid eye movement is not associated with vagus nerve stimulation. Vagal stimulation will not cause seizures or tachycardia. (R)

24. 2. There is a correlation between café au lait spots and the development of neurofibromatosis. Acrocyanosis is a normal finding of bluish hands and feet as a result of poor capillary perfusion. Port wine nevus and strawberry hemangiomas are a collection of dilated capillaries and are not associated with any other disease process. (R)

25. 2, 3, 4. Holding the neonate steady and in the proper position will help ensure a safe and accurate lumbar puncture. The neonate is usually held in a "C" position to open the spaces between the vertebral column. This position puts the neonate at risk for airway obstruction. Thus, ensuring the patency of the airway is the first priority, and the nurse should observe the neonate for adequate ventilation. Maintaining a sterile field is important to avoid infection in the neonate. It is not necessary to administer antibiotics or obtain a serum glucose level during the procedure. (S)

26. 3. Normally, the umbilical cord has two umbilical arteries and one vein. When a neonate is born with only one artery and one vein, the nurse should notify the pediatrician for further evaluation of cardiac anomalies. Other common congenital problems associated with a missing artery include renal anomalies, central nervous system lesions, tracheoesophageal fistulas, trisomy 13, and trisomy 18. Respiratory anomalies are associated with dyspnea and respiratory distress; musculoskeletal anomalies include fractures or dislocated hip; and facial anomalies are associated with fetal alcohol syndrome or Down syndrome, not a missing umbilical artery. (R)

27. 2. Caused by pressure on the head during labor, caput succedaneum is an edematous area over the place where the scalp was encircled by the cervix, possibly crossing the suture line. It usually results from a difficult and long labor or from vacuum extraction. Caput succedaneum is usually reabsorbed within 12 hours to a few days after birth. Cephalohematoma is caused by blood between the bone and the periosteum. Because bleeding is under the periosteum, it cannot cross the suture line, whereas a caput succedaneum can. A cephalohematoma may take as long as a few weeks or months to disappear. Cranial edema is swelling of the brain tissue. Separation of suture lines and bulging fontanelles would be noted in this condition. *Craniotabes* refers to a reduction in mineralization of the skull with abnormal softness of the bones. (H)

28. 2. Normally at birth, the neonate's head circumference is approximately 2 cm larger than the chest circumference. The average normal head circumference is 13 to 14 inches (33 to 35 cm); average normal chest circumference is 12.5 to 14 inches (31 to 35 cm). A head circumference that is equal to or smaller than the chest circumference may indicate microcephaly; a head that is larger than normal may indicate hydrocephalus. The presence of any of these conditions warrants further evaluation. (H)

29. 4. The mother needs further instruction if she says the molding can result in brain damage. Brain damage is highly unlikely. Molding occurs during vaginal delivery when the cranial bones tend to override or overlap as the head accommodates to the size of the mother's birth canal. The amount and duration of pressure on the head influence the degree of molding. Molding usually disappears in a few days without any special attention. (H)

30. 3. The anterior fontanel is normally diamond-shaped, approximately 2 to 3 cm wide and 3 to 4 cm long. This allows for brain growth during the early months of life. The posterior fontanel is small and triangular. (H)

31. 3. Sole creases covering the entire foot are indicative of a term neonate. If the neonate's ear is lying flat against the head, the neonate is most likely preterm. An absence of rugae in the scrotum typically suggests a preterm neonate. A square window sign angle of 0 degrees occurs in neonates of 40 to 42 weeks' gestation. A 90-degree square window angle suggests an immature neonate of approximately 28 to 30 weeks' gestation. (H)

32. 2. An expiratory grunt is significant and should be reported promptly, because it may indicate respiratory distress and the need for further intervention such as oxygen or resuscitation efforts. The presence of a red reflex in the eyes is normal. An absent red reflex may indicate congenital cataracts. A respiratory rate of 45 breaths/minute and a prominent xiphoid process are normal findings in a term neonate. (R)

33. 3. The tonic neck reflex, also called the fencing position, is present when the neonate turns the head to the left side, extends the left extremities, and flexes the right extremities. This reflex disappears in a matter of months as the neonatal nervous system matures. The stepping reflex is demonstrated when the infant is held upright near a hard, firm surface. The prone crawl reflex is demonstrated when the infant pulls both arms but does not move the chin beyond the elbows. When the infant extends and abducts the arms and legs with the toes fanning open, this is a normal Babinski reflex. (H)

34. 2. Convergent strabismus is common during infancy until about age 6 months because of poor oculomotor coordination. The neonate has peripheral vision and can fixate on close objects for short periods. The neonate can also perceive colors, shapes, and faces. Neonates can focus on light and should blink or close their eyes in response to light. However, this is not associated with strabismus. An absent red reflex or white areas over the pupils, not strabismus, may indicate congenital cataracts. Most neonates cannot focus well or accommodate for distance immediately after birth. (H)

35. 3. A single crease across the palm (simian crease) is most commonly associated with chromosomal abnormalities, notably Down syndrome. Deep creases across the soles of the feet is a normal finding in a term neonate. Frequent sneezing in a term neonate is normal. This occurs because the neonate is a nose breather and sneezing helps to clear the nares. An absence of lanugo on the skin of a term neonate is a normal finding. (R)

36. 1, 5, 6. Phenylketonuria, an inherited autosomal recessive disorder, involves the body's inability to metabolize the amino acid phenylalanine. A diet low in phenylalanine must be followed. Such foods as meats, eggs, and milk are high in phenylalanine. Assistance from a dietitian is commonly necessary to keep phenylalanine levels low and to provide the essential amino acids necessary for cell function and tissue growth. With autosomal recessive disorders, future children will have a 25% chance of having the disease, a 50% chance of carrying the disease, and a 35% chance of being free of the disease. If a diet low in phenylalanine is followed until brain growth is complete (sometime in adolescence), the child should achieve normal intelligence. (H)

37. 1. Periods of apnea lasting longer than 20 seconds, mild cyanosis, and a heart rate of 110 bpm (bradycardia) are associated with a potentially life-threatening event and subsequent respiratory arrest. The neonate needs further evaluation by the pediatrician. Pneumonia is associated with tachycardia, anorexia, malaise, cyanosis, diminished breath sounds, and crackles. Intraventricular hemorrhage is associated with prematurity. Assessment findings include bulging fontanels and seizures. Epiglottitis is a bacterial form of croup. Assessment findings include inspiratory stridor, cough, and irritability. It occurs most commonly in children age 3 to 7 years. (R)

38. 4. Normally, the anterior fontanel closes between ages 12 and 18 months. Premature closure (craniostenosis or premature synostosis) prevents proper growth and expansion of the brain, resulting in mental retardation. The posterior fontanel typically closes by ages 2 to 3 months. (H)

39. 2. Corneas of unequal size should be reported because this may indicate congenital glaucoma. An absence of tears is common because the neonate's lacrimal glands are not yet functioning. The neonate's pupils normally constrict when a bright light is focused on them. The finding implies that light perception and visual acuity are present, as they should be after birth. A red circle on the pupils is seen when an ophthalmoscope's light shines onto the retina and is a normal finding. Called the red reflex, this indicates that the light is shining onto the retina. (R)

40. **3.** At 24 hours of age, the neonate is probably in a state of deep sleep, as evidenced by the closed eyes, lack of eye movements, normal skin color, and normal heart rate and respiratory rate. Jitteriness, a high-pitched cry, and tremors are associated with drug withdrawal. The first period of reactivity occurs in the first 30 minutes after birth, evidenced by alertness, sucking sounds, and rapid heart rate and respiratory rate. There is no evidence to suggest respiratory distress because the neonate's respiratory rate of 35 breaths/minute is normal. (H)

41. **4.** The condition in which the urinary meatus is located on the ventral surface of the penis, termed hypospadias, occurs in 1 of every 500 male infants. Circumcision is delayed until the condition is corrected surgically, usually between 6 and 12 months of age. Phimosis is an inability to retract the prepuce at an age when it should be retractable or by age 3 years. Phimosis may necessitate circumcision or surgical intervention. Hydrocele is a painless swelling of the scrotum that is common in neonates. It is not a contraindication for circumcision. Epispadias occurs when the urinary meatus is located on the dorsal surface of the penis. It is extremely rare and is commonly associated with bladder extrophy. (R)

The Preterm Neonate

42. **1, 3, 4.** Kangaroo care is skin-to-skin holding of a neonate by one of the parents. Research has shown increased bonding, physiologic stability, and decreased length of stay for neonates who experience this method of holding. Research has not shown an increase in IQ as a developmental outcome. Kangaroo care has not been shown to cause the neonate to gain weight quickly. The experience is usually limited to 1 to 2 hours, 2 to 3 times per day. (H)

43. **2.** The first step after cesarean delivery is to aspirate mucus from the neonate's mouth. If this is not done, the neonate will aspirate mucus when beginning to breathe. A patent airway is most important. Once mucus has been aspirated, the neonate may be stimulated to cry if necessary. If, once the airway has been established, the neonate does not begin breathing efforts on his or her own, then resuscitation may be necessary. Although the mother will want to see the neonate, holding the neonate upright is inappropriate because the neonate's head should be kept lower than the rest of the body to aid in the expulsion of mucus or other fluids. (H)

44. **4.** When receiving oxygen by mask, the neonate is placed on the back with the neck slightly extended, in the "sniffing" or neutral position. This position optimizes lung expansion and places the upper respiratory tract in the best position for receiving oxygen. Placing a small rolled towel under the neonate's shoulders helps to extend the neck properly without overextending it. Once stabilized and transferred to an isolette in the intensive care unit, the neonate can be positioned in the prone position, which allows for lung expansion in the oxygenated environment. Placing the neonate on the left side does not allow for maximum lung expansion. Also, slightly flexing the neck interferes with opening the airway. Placing the neonate on the back with the head turned to the left side does not allow for lung expansion. Placing the neonate on the abdomen interferes with proper positioning of the oxygen mask. (D)

45. **1.** Cardiac massage should be alternated with ventilation to ensure breathing and circulation. Two fingers, not the palm of the hand, are used to compress a neonate's sternum. The chest is compressed 100 to 120 times per minute. The proper technique recommended by the American Heart Association and the American Academy of Pediatrics is to use enough pressure to depress the sternum to a depth of approximately one-third of the anterior-posterior diameter of the chest. (A)

46. **1.** Whenever oxygen is administered, it should be humidified to prevent drying of the nasal passages and mucous membranes. Because the neonate is under a radiant warmer, a stocking cap is not necessary. Temperature, continuously monitored by a skin probe attached to the radiant warmer, is recorded every 30 to 60 minutes initially. Although the oxygen concentration in the hood requires close monitoring and measurement of blood gases, checking the blood glucose level is not necessary. (D)

47. **3.** The neonate is at high risk for sepsis due to exposure to the mother's infection. Temperature instability in a neonate at 38 weeks' gestation is an early sign of sepsis. Other signs include tachycardia, decreased muscle tone, acidosis, apnea, respiratory distress, hypotension, poor feeding behaviors, vomiting, and diarrhea. Late signs of infection include jaundice, seizures, enlarged liver and spleen, respiratory failure, and shock. Alkalosis is not typically seen in neonates who develop sepsis. Acidosis and respiratory distress may develop unless treatment such as antibiotics is started. A positive Babinski's reflex is a normal finding and does not need to be reported. (R)

48. **2.** With an absent apical pulse left of the midclavicular line accompanied by cyanosis, grunting, and diminished breath sounds, the neonate is most likely experiencing pneumothorax. Pneumothorax occurs when alveoli are overdistended and subsequently the lung collapses, compressing the heart and lung and compromising the venous return to the right side of the heart. This condition can be confirmed by X-ray or ultrasound studies. Diaphragmatic hernia is associated with respiratory distress soon after birth, not typically 2 days later. Bowel sounds also may be auscultated in the chest. Coarctation of the aorta is associated with poor lower body perfusion exhibited as cyanosis, metabolic acidosis, and congestive heart failure. Assessment findings include absent or diminished femoral pulses, increased brachial pulses, and a late systolic murmur. Commonly, bacterial pneumonia is associated with fever, diminished breath sounds, and crackles. (R)

49. **2.** RDS, previously called hyaline membrane disease, is a developmental condition involving a decrease in lung surfactant leading to improper expansion of the lung alveoli. Surfactant contains a group of surface-active phospholipids, of which one component—lecithin—is the most critical for alveolar stability. Surfactant production peaks at about 35 weeks' gestation. This syndrome primarily attacks preterm neonates, although it can also affect term and post-term neonates. Altered somatotropin secretion is associated with growth disorders such as gigantism or dwarfism. Altered testosterone secretion is associated with masculinization. Altered progesterone secretion is associated with spontaneous abortion during pregnancy. (A)

50. **3.** The best way to determine the adequacy of oxygen therapy is to monitor the neonate's arterial blood gas values. These results quantitatively measure oxygen and carbon dioxide tensions. Cyanosis, a late sign, can validate laboratory findings, but without laboratory results it is not a reliable indicator of the effectiveness of oxygen therapy. Likewise, pulse rate does not serve as a good index because there is poor correlation between it and extreme hyperoxia. The percentage of oxygen received is not a good indicator of the arterial blood gas level of oxygen. Even with high levels of oxygen, the preterm neonate may continue to have poor perfusion because of immature development of the heart and lungs. The percentage delivered is based on the analysis of the neonate's arterial blood gases. (R)

51. **2.** RDS is a developmental condition that primarily affects preterm infants before 35 weeks' gestation because of inadequate lung development from deficient surfactant production. The development of placenta previa has little correlation with the development of RDS. Although excessive analgesia can depress the neonate's respiratory condition if it is given shortly before birth, the scenario presents no information that this has occurred. The neonate's sluggish respiratory activity postpartum is not the likely cause of RDS but may be a sign that the neonate has the condition. (R)

52. **3.** Oxygen should be humidified before administration to help prevent drying of the mucous membranes in the respiratory tract. Drying impedes the normal functioning of cilia in the respiratory tract and predisposes to mucous membrane irritation. Humidification of oxygen does not promote expansion of the immature lungs. Expansion is promoted by placing the infant in a prone position or providing the preterm infant with surfactant medication. Humidified oxygen does not prevent viral or bacterial pneumonia. In fact, in some nurseries, *Staphylococcus aureus* has been detected in moist environments and on the hands and nails of staff members, predisposing the neonate to pneumonia. Humidified oxygen does not improve blood circulation in the cardiac system. (D)

53. **4.** Many intensive care units that care for high-risk neonates recommend that the mother pump her breasts, store the milk, and bring it to the unit so the neonate can be fed with it, even if the neonate is being fed by gavage. As soon as the neonate has developed a coordinated suck-and-swallow reflex, breast-feeding can begin. Secretory immunoglobulin A, found in breast milk, is an important immunoglobulin that can provide immunity to the mucosal surfaces of the gastrointestinal tract. It can protect the neonate from enteric infections, such as those caused by *Escherichia coli* and *Shigella* species. Some studies have also shown that breast-fed preterm neonates maintain transcutaneous oxygen pressure and body temperature better than bottle-fed neonates. There is some evidence that breast milk can decrease the incidence of necrotizing enterocolitis. The preterm neonate does not need additional fat in the diet. However, some neonates may need an increased caloric intake. In such cases, breast milk can be fortified with an additive to provide additional calories. Neonates who are receiving oxygen can breast-feed. During feedings, supplemental oxygen can be delivered by nasal cannula. (H)

54. **1.** ROP, previously called retrolental fibroplasia, is associated with multiple risk factors, including high arterial blood oxygen levels, prematurity, and very low birth weight (less than 1,500 g). In the early acute stages of ROP, the neonate's immature retinal vessels constrict. If vasoconstriction is sustained, vascular closure follows, and irreversible capillary endothelial damage occurs. Normal room air is at 21%. Acidosis, not alkalosis, is commonly seen in preterm neonates, but this is not related to the development of ROP. Phototherapy is not related to the development of ROP. However, during phototherapy, the neonate's eyes should be constantly covered to prevent damage from the lights. (R)

55. **4.** Constricted retinal vessels may indicate the degree of ROP. In ROP, immature blood vessels in the retina constrict and become permanently occluded. New vessels proliferate to reestablish circulation. If the new vessels extend into the vitreous humor of the eye, hemorrhage can occur, resulting in scarring and retinal detachment. Sunken orbital sockets would be suggestive of dehydration, not ROP. Strabismus ("crossed eyes") is common in all neonates because of poor oculomotor coordination. A reaction to bright light is a normal finding. (R)

56. **1.** Because the retina may become detached with ROP, laser therapy has been used successfully in some medical centers to treat ROP. Cromolyn sodium (Intal) is used to treat seasonal allergies. ROP is not associated with glaucoma, so frequent testing is not necessary. Because the vessels of the eye are affected, not the corneas, corneal transplantation is not used. (A)

57. **3.** The priority nursing diagnosis for a preterm neonate is *Impaired gas exchange* related to immature pulmonary vasculature. Respiratory distress syndrome is a primary problem for preterm neonates and a particular problem for neonates of 28 weeks' gestation because of the lack of surfactant in the lungs. *Risk for impaired skin integrity* related to gestational age is not a priority at this time. Preterm infants are at risk for delayed development but plans to promote growth and development can be made once the neonate is stabilized. Preterm infants do suffer from imbalanced nutrition (less than body requirements). However, the nurse will first ensure adequate respirations and gas exchange, and then make plans to improve the nutritional status by administering oral and I.V. fluids, as ordered, according to the neonate's needs. (H)

58. **1.** Neonates who weigh less than 1,500 g or are born at less than 34 weeks' gestation are susceptible to PIVH. Computed tomography scanning or ultrasound scanning can confirm the diagnosis. The spinal fluid will show an increased number of red blood cells. Arterial blood gas specimen collection is done to evaluate the neonate's oxygen saturation level. Skull radiographs are not commonly used because of the danger of radiation. Additionally, computed tomography scans have replaced the use of skull X-ray films because they can provide more definitive results. Complete blood count specimen collection is usually performed to determine the hemoglobin, hematocrit, and white blood cell count. The results are not specific for PIVH. (R)

59. **3.** A common finding of IVH is a bulging fontanel. The most common site of hemorrhage is the periventricular subependymal germinal matrix, where there is a rich blood supply and where the capillary walls are thin and fragile. Rapid volume expansion, hypercarbia, and hypoglycemia contribute to the development of IVH. Other common manifestations include neurologic signs such as hypotonia, lethargy, temperature instability, nystagmus, apnea, bradycardia, decreased hematocrit, and increasing hypoxia. Seizures also may occur. Hyperbilirubinemia refers to an increase in bilirubin in the blood and is not associated with IVH. (A)

60. **2, 4, 5.** Nonnutritive sucking has been seen in infants as early as 28 weeks and ultrasound examinations have shown thumb sucking in utero even earlier. Nonnutritive sucking provides oral stimulation and allows the baby to maintain the sucking reflex needed for breast- or bottle-feedings later. It does not teach the infant how to suck and swallow. Sucking is thought to help with gastric emptying by stimulating secretions of GI peptides. Moisture of the mucus membranes is an indication of adequate hydration, and nonnutritive sucking will not have an effect. (C)

61. **4.** Indications of NEC include abdominal distention with gastric retention and vomiting. Other signs may include lethargy, irritability, positive blood culture in stool, absent or diminished bowel sounds, apnea, diarrhea, metabolic acidosis, and unstable temperature. A gastric residual of 1 ml is not significant. Jaundice of the face and chest is associated with the neonate's immature liver function and increased bilirubin, not NEC. Typically with NEC,

the neonate would exhibit absent or diminished bowel sounds, not increased peristalsis. (A)

62. **2.** BPD is a chronic illness that may require prolonged hospitalization and permanent assisted ventilation. The disease typically occurs in compromised very-low-birth-weight neonates who require oxygen therapy and assisted ventilation for treatment of respiratory distress syndrome. The cause is multifactorial, and the disease has four stages. The neonate's activities may be limited by the disease. Antibiotics may be ordered, and bronchodilators may be used, but these medications will not cure the chronic disease state. Seizure activity is associated with periventricular-intraventricular hemorrhage, not BPD. (A)

63. **4.** Pneumothorax is an accumulation of air in the thoracic cavity between the parietal and visceral pleurae. A life-threatening situation, it requires immediate removal of the accumulated air. Initially, the air is aspirated with a syringe attached to an 18-G catheter or a 23-G butterfly drain inserted into the second or third intercostal space at the midclavicular line with the neonate in a supine position. Complete resolution of pneumothorax requires a size 10F chest tube connected to continuous negative pressure. The neonate does not need to be placed on a ventilator unless there is evidence of severe respiratory distress. The goal of treatment is to reinflate the collapsed lung. Administering bronchodilators through the nares or suctioning the neonate's nares would do nothing to aid in lung reinflation. (A)

64. **3.** Decreased protein or hypoproteinemia is a sign of overhydration, which can lead to patent ductus arteriosus or congestive heart failure. Bulging fontanels, decreased serum sodium, decreased urine specific gravity, and decreased hematocrit are other signs of overhydration. Hypernatremia (increased serum sodium concentration) or increased urine specific gravity would suggest dehydration, not overhydration. Polycythemia evidenced by an elevated hematocrit would suggest hypoxia or congenital heart disorder. (R)

65. **0.03**

$$6\tfrac{1}{2}\ \text{lb} \div 2.2 = 2.95\ \text{kg}$$

$$2.95\ \text{kg} \times 0.01\ \text{mg} = 0.029\ \text{mg, rounded to } 0.03\ \text{mg}$$

(D)

The Post-Term Neonate

66. **4.** Increased respiratory rate and tremors are indicative of hypoglycemia, which commonly affects the post-term neonate because of depleted glycogen stores. Therefore, *Imbalanced nutrition: Less than body* requirements is the priority nursing diagnosis. There is no indication that the neonate has ineffective airway clearance, which would be evidenced by excessive amounts of mucus or visualization of meconium on the vocal cords. Lethargy, not tremors, would suggest infection or hyperthermia.

Furthermore, the post-term neonate typically has difficulty maintaining temperature, resulting in hypothermia, not hyperthermia. Decreased cardiac output is not indicated, particularly because the neonate was delivered by cesarean delivery, which is not considered a difficult delivery. (H)

67. **2.** A loose, watery stool in the diaper is indicative of diarrhea and needs immediate attention. The infant may become severely dehydrated quickly because of the higher percentage of water content per body weight in the neonate, compared with the adult. Frequent hiccups are considered normal in a neonate and do not warrant additional investigation. Pink papular vesicles (*erythema toxicum*) on the face are considered normal in a neonate and disappear without treatment. Dry, peeling skin is normal in a post-term neonate. (H)

68. **2.** Ortolani's maneuver involves flexing the neonate's knees and hips at right angles and bringing the sides of the knees down to the surface of the examining table. A characteristic click or "clunk," felt or heard, represents a positive Ortolani's sign, suggesting a possible hip dislocation. The nurse should notify the physician promptly because treatment is needed, while maintaining the dislocated hip in a position of flexion and abduction. Determining the length of the mother's labor provides no useful information related to the nurse's finding. Keeping the infant under the radiant warmer is necessary only if the neonate's temperature is low or unstable. Checking for hypoglycemia is not indicated at this time, unless the neonate is exhibiting jitteriness. (R)

69. **4.** The priority nursing diagnosis for the neonate with probable MAS is *Impaired gas exchange* related to the effects of respiratory distress. Obstruction of the airways may be complete or partial. Meconium aspiration may lead to pneumonia or pneumothorax. Establishing adequate respirations is the primary goal. *Impaired skin integrity* related to post-term status is a concern, but establishing and maintaining an airway and gas exchange is always the priority. Although nutrition may be altered, oxygenation takes priority over nutrition. If the parents do not express interest or concern for the neonate, then *Risk for impaired parent-infant-child attachment* may be appropriate once the airway is established. (A)

70. **1.** Care of an umbilical arterial line would be included in the neonate's plan of care because an umbilical arterial line is commonly inserted to monitor arterial blood pressures, blood pH, blood gases, and infusion of intravenous fluids, blood, or medications. Frequent ultrasound scans are not indicated at this time. However, chest radiographs may be used to detect lung densities, because pneumonia is a major complication of this disorder. Orogastric feeding may not be feasible while the health care team focuses on interventions to establish adequate oxygenation. The neonate with MAS commonly experiences hypoglycemia, not hyperglycemia. Hypoglycemia occurs because of depletion of glucose stores related to hypothermia. (A)

71. **4.** Tolazoline (Priscoline) can cause profound hypotension. Therefore, the nurse should monitor the neonate's blood pressure when giving this drug. Adverse effects of the medication include petechiae, dark stools, bleeding, and diarrhea. Plasma expanders are commonly used with tolazoline to prevent dramatic changes in blood pressure. Feeding behaviors, temperature, and skin color are routine assessments for all neonates, unrelated to the use of tolazoline. (D)

The Neonate with Risk Factors

72. **2.** Epinephrine is given for severe bradycardia and hypotension. An expected outcome would be an increased heart rate to a normal range. Epinephrine decreases renal blood flow, so a decrease in urine output would be expected. Epinephrine also stimulates alpha- and beta-adrenergic receptors, which do not offer pain relief or sedation. (D)

73. **4.** Neonates that are sick do not have the physical resources or energy to respond to all elements of the environment. The use of a constant touch provides comfort and only requires one response to a stimulus. To comfort a sick neonate, the care provider applies gentle, constant physical support or touch. Toys for distraction are not developmentally appropriate for a neonate. Sick neonates react to any stimulus; in responding, the sick neonate may have increased energy demands and increased oxygen requirements. A musical mobile may be too much audio stimulation and thus increases energy and oxygen demands. Repetitive touching with a hand going off and on the neonate, as with stroking or patting, requires the neonate to respond to every touch, thus increasing energy and oxygen demands. (C)

74. **2.** Recommended pulse oximetry reading in a full-term neonate is 95% to 100%. The saturation reading of only 75% is an indication that the neonate is not adequately oxygenating in room air. Providing supplemental oxygen will increase the neonate's oxygen saturation. Increasing the I.V. rate will not improve the oxygen saturation. Documenting the finding and taking no action is not appropriate with a saturation of 75%. Wrapping and increasing the body temperature of the neonate may increase the saturation reading only if it is inaccurate due to cold extremities. Caution must be used because overheating a neonate can be harmful. (R)

75.

4.	Assess the neonate for respiratory effort.

3.	Assess the neonate for color.

2.	Make sure the pulse oximeter is correlating to the heart rate.

1.	Increase the F_{IO_2}.

Assessment of the neonate is the most important priority and should be completed first. Respiratory effort must be assessed first to determine if the neonate is breathing. Once breathing is established, assessment of color is next. Then verification of proper equipment function is necessary. The last measure is to increase the F_{IO_2} due to the potential harmful effects of oxygen. Oxygen should be viewed as a drug and its use evaluated carefully. Increasing the F_{IO_2} should be done only when indicated; possible causes of low saturation readings must be evaluated first. (R)

76. 4. Neonates with heart failure may need calorie-dense formula to provide extra calories for growth. Fluids should not be restricted because the nutritional requirements are based on calories per ounce of formula. Decreasing fluid intake will decrease calories needed for growth. These neonates may have limited energy due to their heart condition but have a high caloric need to stimulate proper growth and development. The sodium level should be at a normal level to ensure adequate fluid and electrolyte balance unless prescribed by the physician. (H)

77. 1. The indication for the use of indomethacin is to close a patent ductus arteriosus. Adverse effects include decreased renal blood flow, platelet dysfunction with coagulation defects, decreased GI motility, and an increase in necrotizing enterocolitis. Thus, increased bleeding time, decreased gastrointestinal function, and decreased renal output would be expected outcomes after the administration of indomethacin. (D)

78. 4. The size of the nasogastric (NG) feeding tube is based on the neonate's weight. A larger feeding tube can be inserted into a heavier neonate. The disease process plays no role in the size of the feeding tube used. The neonate's weight and size can vary widely; thus, there is no standard tube size for any gestational age. Length will determine the depth at which the NG tube is placed in the stomach, not the size of the tube. (C)

79. 2. A quiet environment with decreased stimulation is the best treatment for a drug-exposed neonate. The drug-exposed neonate has limited ability to deal with stress and cope with stimuli. Assessing vital signs with blood pressure every hour will disturb the neonate's rest periods and cause increased physical and psychological demands. Placement in a well-lighted or stimulating environment is overwhelming for the neonate and will increase the neonate's stress level. (A)

80. 1. To ensure client safety, the nurse should first write the results on the chart, then read them back to the caller and wait for the caller to confirm that the nurse has understood the results. Using a scrap paper increases the risk of losing the results as well as transcription errors. The nurse may receive results by telephone, and while electronic transfer to the client's electronic record is appropriate, the nurse can also accept the telephone results if the laboratory has called the results to the nursery. Sending client information via e-mail is unacceptable due to potential security and privacy issues. (S)

81. 3. Hemolytic disease of the newborn is associated with Rh problems. Hemolytic disease of the newborn occurs most commonly when the mother is Rh-negative and the father is Rh-positive. About 13% of white Americans, 7% to 8% of African Americans, and 1% of Asian Americans are Rh-negative. Rh-positive cells enter the mother's Rh-negative bloodstream, and antibodies to the Rh-positive cells are produced. In a subsequent pregnancy, the antibodies cross the placenta to the Rh-positive fetus and begin the destruction of Rh-positive cells through hemolysis. This results in severe fetal anemia. (A)

82. 3. The problem of Rh sensitivity arises when the mother's blood develops antibodies after fetal red blood cells enter the maternal circulation. In cases of Rh sensitivity, this usually does not occur until after the first pregnancy. Hence, hemolytic disease of the newborn is rare in a primiparous client. A mismatched blood transfusion in the past or an unrecognized spontaneous abortion could also result in hemolytic disease because the transfusion or abortion would have the same effects on the client. The statement about the other baby having a different father may be true. However, if both fathers were Rh-positive, then sensitization could occur. Most women do not have immunity against the antibodies formed when Rh-positive cells enter the mother's bloodstream. Antibodies are not neutralized by the mother's system. (R)

83. 2. The Rh-sensitized neonate generally does not have problems related to polycythemia. Therefore, the client needs additional teaching. In general, moderate to severe Rh sensitization can cause anemia, enlarged spleen, and cardiac decompensation. Cardiac decompensation (as in heart failure) occurs because of severe anemia. Anemia is caused by the destruction of red blood cells by antibodies as the severity of hemolytic disease of the neonate increases. Splenic enlargement is caused by the excessive destruction of fetal red blood cells. (A)

84. 3. A direct Coombs test is done on umbilical cord blood to detect antibodies coating the neonate's red blood cells. Hematocrit is used to detect anemia. Sodium, potassium, and chloride are used to detect electrolyte imbalances. Antigens on the neonate's red blood cells are proteins that help determine the neonate's blood type. (R)

85. 3. An exchange transfusion is done to reduce the blood concentration of bilirubin and correct the anemia. The exchange transfusion does not replenish the white blood cells or restore the fluid and electrolyte balance. The neonate's Rh-positive blood is replaced by Rh-negative blood. (R)

86. 2. The organ most susceptible to damage from uncontrolled hemolytic disease is the brain. Bilirubin levels increase as the red blood cells are destroyed. Bilirubin crosses the blood-brain barrier and damages the cells of the central nervous system. This condition, called kernicterus, is potentially fatal. Although the kidneys, lungs, and liver may be affected by increased bilirubin levels, the brain will sustain the most life-threatening injury. (R)

87. **1, 4.** A glucometer reading of 40 mg/dl (or less) and irregular respirations, tremors, and hypothermia are indicative of hypoglycemia. Internal fetal monitors detect the strength of contractions and the fetal heart rate. An infant of an insulin-dependent mother and a large-for-gestational-age infant are at greater risk of developing hypoglycemia and need to be observed carefully but these findings are not definitive for the diagnosis of hypoglycemia. (A)

88. **4.** A priority nursing diagnosis is *Imbalanced nutrition: Less than body requirements* related to increased glucose metabolism. The increased glucose metabolism is a result of the hyperinsulinemia. Maternal hyperglycemia is accompanied by fetal hyperglycemia. On delivery, the neonate is no longer dependent on maternal glucose, and a hypoglycemic state soon develops. Hyperthermia is not a priority at this time; large-for-gestational-age neonates tend to become hypothermic as they deplete their glucose stores. *Impaired skin integrity* and *Risk for disproportionate growth* are important nursing diagnoses; however, glucose stabilization to protect the central nervous system is the priority. (H)

89. **2.** Glucose crosses the placenta, but insulin does not. Hence, a high maternal blood glucose level causes a high fetal blood glucose level. This causes the fetal pancreas to secrete more insulin. At birth, the neonate loses the maternal glucose source but continues to produce much insulin, which commonly causes a drop in blood glucose levels (hypoglycemia), usually at 30 to 60 minutes postpartum. Most neonates do not develop hypoglycemia if their mothers are not insulin dependent unless they are preterm. Therefore, hypoglycemia is not a normal response as the neonate transitions to extrauterine life. (R)

90. **1.** Infants born to diabetic mothers tend to be larger than average, and this neonate weighs 10 lb, 1 oz (4,564 g). The most common fractures are those of the clavicle and long bones, such as the femur. In a neonate, the skull bones are not fused and move to allow for vaginal delivery, so skull fracture is rarely seen. Wrist and rib cages are rarely fractured. (R)

91. **4.** Tremors occurring after therapy for hypoglycemia are clinical signs of hypocalcemia. At term, diabetic women tend to have higher calcium levels, which can cause secondary hypoparathyroidism in their neonates. Other factors that can contribute to hypocalcemia in neonates include hypophosphatemia from tissue metabolism, vitamin D antagonism from increased cortisol levels, and decreased serum magnesium levels. Neonates with phenylketonuria will have a musty odor to their urine. The neonate with biliary duct obstruction will show signs of jaundice. Hypotonia and flaccidity are signs of hypermagnesemia. (R)

92. **4.** Hypoglycemia is caused by the rapid depletion of glucose stores. In addition, neonates born to class B diabetic women are about seven times more likely to suffer from respiratory distress syndrome than neonates born to nondiabetic women. This neonate should be closely monitored for symptoms of hypoglycemia and respiratory distress. Neonates of diabetic mothers commonly have polycythemia, not anemia. Anemia and hemolytic disease are associated with erythroblastosis fetalis. Persistent pulmonary hypertension is associated with meconium aspiration syndrome. (R)

93. **2.** Manifestations of cocaine withdrawal in the neonate include a shrill, high-pitched cry; tachycardia; muscle rigidity; irritability; restlessness; fist-sucking; and an exaggerated startle reflex. These signs usually appear within 72 hours and persist for several days. These neonates are difficult to console, have poor feeding behaviors, and have diarrhea. Bradycardia is associated with preterm neonates. Sluggishness and lethargy are associated with neonates whose mothers received analgesia shortly before delivery. Hypocalcemia occurs most commonly in infants of diabetic mothers, premature infants, and low-birth-weight infants. (R)

94. **3.** Neonates experiencing cocaine withdrawal have gastrointestinal problems similar to those of adults withdrawing from cocaine. The neonates exhibit poor sucking, vomiting, drooling, diarrhea, regurgitation, and anorexia. In addition, they are difficult to console and difficult to feed. Because of these problems, the neonate withdrawing from cocaine needs to be monitored carefully to prevent dehydration. Neonates with cocaine exposure experience hypertonia, not hypotonia, due to increased central nervous system irritability. Diarrhea, not constipation, is seen in these neonates. Abdominal distention is associated with necrotizing enterocolitis, not cocaine withdrawal. (R)

95. **1.** A neonate undergoing cocaine withdrawal is irritable, often restless, difficult to console, and often in need of increased activity. It is commonly helpful to swaddle the neonate tightly with a blanket, offer a pacifier, and cuddle and rock the neonate. Offering extra nourishment is not advised because overfeeding tends to increase gastrointestinal problems such as vomiting, regurgitation, and diarrhea. Environmental stimuli such as bright lights and loud noises should be kept to a minimum to decrease agitation. Minimizing touching of the neonate to only when he or she is crying will not aid the bonding process between mother and neonate. Frequent holding and touching are permissible. (R)

96. **4.** Although most neonates are asymptomatic, they do test positive for HIV at birth because of the mother's antibodies. It may take several months before an accurate diagnosis can be made. It is estimated that 20% to 40% of all HIV-positive mothers deliver HIV-positive infants. With appropriate drug intervention to the mother during pregnancy, 95% of these neonates can be born unaffected. An enlarged liver at birth is associated with erythroblastosis fetalis, not HIV infection. Virologic testing, such as deoxyribonucleic acid polymerase chain reaction, viral culture, or ribonucleic acid plasma assay, can diagnose HIV infection by 6 months of age and commonly in the first month. (R)

97. **4.** Breast milk has been found to contain the retrovirus HIV. In general, mothers are discouraged from breast-feeding if they are HIV positive because of the risk of possible transmission of the virus if the neonate is HIV negative. Breast milk does contain some immunoglobulins, but it does not protect the neonate from HIV infection. (H)

98. **4.** As part of standard precautions, the nurse should don a pair of clean gloves. Additionally, the site is cleaned thoroughly with an alcohol swab before the skin is injected. Sterile gloves are not necessary. Bathing the neonate is not necessary before giving the injection. Some research suggests that bathing removes the neonate's protective skin oils. Placing the neonate under the radiant warmer is not necessary unless the neonate's temperature is subnormal. The neonate's temperature has usually stabilized by 4 hours of age. Washing the injection site with povidone-iodine before giving the injection is not necessary because of the risk for possible allergy to iodine preparations. (S)

99. **3.** Symptoms of infection in a neonate include subtle behavioral changes, such as lethargy and irritability, and color changes such as pallor or cyanosis. Other symptoms include temperature instability, poor feeding, gastrointestinal disorders, hyperbilirubinemia, and apnea. Leukocytosis, an elevated white blood cell count possibly as high as 30,000 cells/mm³ or more, may be normal during the first 24 hours. An apical heart rate of 132 bpm is normal. Warm, moist skin is not a typical sign of infection in neonates. Typically, temperature instability is common. The neonate's temperature is low and the skin is cool and dry. (H)

100. **3.** The parents of a neonate with an infection should be allowed to participate in daily care as long as they use good handwashing technique. This includes touching and holding the neonate. The parents must be careful around medical equipment to ensure proper function and around the intravenous site so that it is not dislodged. Restricting parental visits has not been shown to have any effect on the infection rate and may have detrimental effects on the neonate's psychological development. Normally, the neonate does not need to be isolated. It is not necessary for the parents to wear a mask while holding the neonate. The neonate is not contagious and is receiving treatment for the infection. (S)

101. **3.** On the initial visit, the parents may be shocked, fearful, and anxious. Nursing care should include spending time with the parents to allow them to express their emotions. The nurse should initially emphasize the neonate's normal characteristics. After the parents have had sufficient time to adjust to the neonate's special needs, surgical interventions can be discussed. Telling the parents that this is not a life-threatening defect or that everything will be all right after the surgery is not helpful. Doing so discounts their feelings. Reassuring the parents about the success rate of the surgery can be done once the parents have had time to adjust to the neonate and express their emotions. (P)

102. **1.** After feeding, the mouth should be cleaned with sterile water, not soapy water, to reduce the risk for aspiration. The cleft lip should be cleaned with sterile water to prevent crusting before surgical repair. The neonate needs to be fed in an upright position to prevent aspiration. The neonate with a cleft lip and palate commonly swallows large amounts of air during feeding. Therefore, the neonate needs to be burped frequently to help eliminate the air and decrease the risk for regurgitation. The neonate with a cleft lip and palate should be fed with a special soft nipple that fills the cleft and facilitates sucking. (R)

103. **2.** One hour after birth, the priority nursing diagnosis for the neonate with a cleft palate is *Risk for infection* related to potential aspiration. Feeding difficulties are the primary problem before surgical repair. Activity intolerance may occur, but this is not a primary problem and there is no evidence of the neonate's having been diagnosed with respiratory distress syndrome. There is no evidence presented to suggest compromised family coping. However, this nursing diagnosis may be appropriate later on since the infant may require frequent health care follow-up visits and surgeries. Impaired skin integrity is not a problem for this neonate, who is allowed to engage in normal activity without restraint before surgery. After surgery the infant may have restraints to prevent damage to the suture line, thus requiring frequent position changes. (R)

104. **4.** The long-term prognosis for neonates with FAS is poor. Symptoms of withdrawal include tremors, sleeplessness, seizures, abdominal distention, hyperactivity, and inconsolable crying. Symptoms of withdrawal commonly occur within 6 to 12 hours or, at the latest, within the first 3 days of life. The neonate with FAS is usually growth deficient at birth. Most neonates with FAS are mildly to severely mentally retarded. The facial deformities, such as short palpebral fissures, epicanthal folds, broad nasal bridge, flattened midfacies, and short, upturned nose are not easily corrected with plastic surgery. (R)

105. **3.** Central nervous system disorders are common in neonates with FAS. Speech and language disorders and hyperactivity are common manifestations of central nervous system dysfunction. Mild to severe mental retardation and feeding problems also are common. Delayed growth and development is expected. These neonates feed poorly and commonly have persistent vomiting until age 6 to 7 months. These neonates do not have a 70% mortality rate, and there is no treatment for FAS. (R)

106. **2.** The priority nursing diagnosis for the neonate with FAS is *Imbalanced nutrition: Less than body requirements* related to hyperirritability. The neonate's hyperirritability interferes with the ability to ingest adequate nutrients. There are no data to suggest that growth and development will be altered because of poor parenting abilities, although the mother's alcohol use may continue once the neonate arrives home. If it does, then this does become a potential problem. The neonate has poor feeding behaviors, but this is caused by exaggerated mouthing behaviors and hyperirritability, not impaired swallowing. Although the neonate may be at an increased risk for abuse and neglect if the mother's alcohol use continues once at home, the priority at this time is the neonate's nutritional status. (R)

107. **4.** Gastroschisis is a rare anomaly characterized by the evisceration of abdominal contents through a full-thickness defect in the abdominal wall. The nurse should first protect the abdominal contents with a sterile gauze moistened with sterile saline. Immediate surgery is required. Weighing the neonate is not a priority at this time, but it may need to be done before surgery to determine the appropriate amount of anesthesia. An orogastric tube is not necessary because the infant will not be fed before surgery. An immediate blood transfusion is not needed at this time. (R)

108. **1.** The parents need to know that the neonate will be kept on NPO status and will receive intravenous therapy before surgery. After surgery, feeding will depend on the neonate's condition. Total parenteral nutrition may be ordered after surgery, but not before. Breast-feeding may be started after surgery if the neonate's condition is stable. The mother can pump the breasts until that time. (R)

109. **1, 2, 4.** The major goals for the neonate include preventing hypothermia, maintaining fluid and electrolyte balance, and preventing infection. The neonate needs immediate surgery, so bonding is not a priority at this time. Developmental care is important and should be addressed after the closure of the abdominal wall defect. (R)

110. **2.** The physical appearance of the anomaly and the life-threatening nature of the disorder may result in shock to the parents. The parents may hesitate to form a bond with the neonate because of the guarded prognosis. Denial would be evidenced if the parents acted as if nothing were wrong. Bargaining would be evidenced by parental statements involving "if-then" phrasing, such as, "If the surgery is successful, I will go to church every Sunday." Anger would be evidenced if the parents attempted to blame someone, such as health care personnel, for the neonate's condition. (P)

111. **1.** To prevent eye damage from phototherapy, the eyes must remain covered at all times while under the lights. The eye patches can be removed when the neonate is held out of the lights by the parents for feeding. Instead of a regular diaper, a "string" diaper or disposable face mask may be used to help contain loose stools, while allowing maximum skin exposure. Feeding formula or breast milk every 2 to 3 hours is recommended to prevent hypoglycemia and to encourage gastrointestinal motility. Because the phototherapy lights can overheat the neonate, the temperature should be checked by the axillary route every 2 to 4 hours. (R)

112. **4.** An absent Moro reflex, lethargy, opisthotonos, and seizures are symptoms of bilirubin encephalopathy, which, although rare, can be life-threatening. Bronze discoloration of the skin and maculopapular chest rash are normal and are caused by the phototherapy. They will disappear once the phototherapy is discontinued. A urine specific gravity of 1.001 to 1.020 is normal in term neonates. (R)

113. **2.** Marked visible peristaltic waves in the abdomen and projectile vomiting are signs of pyloric stenosis. If the condition progresses without surgical intervention, the neonate will become dehydrated and develop metabolic alkalosis. Signs of esophageal atresia include coughing and regurgitation with feedings. Diaphragmatic hernia, a life-threatening event in which the abdominal contents herniate into the thoracic cavity, may be evidenced by breath sounds being heard over the abdomen and significant respiratory distress with cyanosis. Signs of hiatal hernia include vomiting, failure to thrive, and short periods of apnea. (R)

114. **3.** With a patent ductus arteriosus, a cardiac defect marked by a failure of the patent ductus arteriosus to close completely at birth, blood from the aorta flows into the pulmonary arteries to be reoxygenated in the lungs and returned to the left atrium and ventricle. The effect of this altered circulation includes increased workload on the left side of the heart and increased pulmonary vascular congestion. Term infants are commonly asymptomatic, but a loud, machinery-like murmur may be heard throughout systole and diastole. This murmur may be accompanied by a suprasternal thrill, and the heart may be enlarged. Decreased cardiac output with faint peripheral pulses, poor peripheral perfusion, feeding difficulties, and severe congestive heart failure are symptoms associated with severe aortic stenosis. With this defect, the aortic valve is thickened and rigid, leading to decreased cardiac output and reduced myocardial blood flow. Profound cyanosis over most of the body, fatigue on exertion, feeding difficulties, and chronic hypoxemia are associated with tetralogy of Fallot. With this defect, malalignment of the ventricular system results in nonrestricted ventral septal defects, pulmonic stenosis, overriding of the aorta, and hypertrophy of the left ventricle. The heart appears boot shaped. A harsh systolic murmur with a palpable thrill is associated with truncus arteriosus. It is marked by incomplete division of the great vessel. This is caused by a ventral septal defect. Bounding pulses and a widening pulse pressure may also be present. (R)

115. **1.** Coarctation of the aorta accounts for 5% to 7% of congenital heart disease. There is localized constriction of the aorta, at or near the insertion site of the ductus arteriosus, that increases afterload and decreases cardiac output. The infant with coarctation of the aorta presents with symptoms of poor lower body perfusion, metabolic acidosis, and congestive heart failure. Cyanosis is present in the lower part of the body because of decreased cardiac output. The child with a partial atrioventricular septal defect may be asymptomatic at birth. The symptoms in a child with a complete defect depend on the pulmonary artery pressure. If the pressure is high, the child will experience cyanosis on exertion; if it is low, congestive heart failure, manifested by tachypnea, dyspnea, and sternal retractions, may be present. The child with pulmonary atresia has profound (complete) cyanosis. On auscultation, the second heart sound is heard as a single sound. This is caused by failure of the pulmonary valve to develop and is accompanied by hypoplastic development of the pulmonary artery and right ventricle. Transposition of the great arteries is associated with complete cyanosis during the first few hours of life. These infants demonstrate hypoxemia with a minimal response to oxygen. In this defect, the pulmonary and systemic systems exist in parallel. Systemic blood (unoxygenated) travels to the right atrium and right ventricle, then into the aorta. Pulmonary venous blood (oxygenated) recirculates through the left side of the heart and through the lungs. (R)

116. **4.** The normal pulse rate in a neonate is 120 to 160 bpm. Therefore, a femoral pulse rate of 90 bpm is too low. Diminished peripheral pulses, coolness and mottling of the extremities, delayed capillary refill, hypotension, and decreased urine output are indicative of low cardiac output and poor perfusion. The neonate may be experiencing a complication of the surgery, such as blood loss or leaking of fluid into the interstitial space. The surgeon should be notified immediately to correct the diminished pulse, through either medications or transfusions. An oxygen saturation between 85% and 100% is considered normal. The surgeon does not need to be notified unless the oxygen saturation falls below 85%. Pale pink extremities are considered a normal finding. If mottling or cyanosis develops, the surgeon should be notified immediately. Warm, dry skin is also a normal finding. If the skin becomes cool or appears cyanotic, the surgeon should be notified. (R)

117. **3.** Continuous PGE1 infusion is necessary for the infant diagnosed with tricuspid atresia to reestablish pulmonary blood flow. This medication maintains a patent ductus arteriosus, which is necessary for the oxygenation of the neonate before surgical intervention. Absence of the tricuspid valve forces all of the blood entering the right atrium to be shunted through the foramen ovale into the left atrium, bypassing the lungs. Oxygenation takes place by retrograde blood flow through a persistent patent ductus arteriosus. Indomethacin (Indocin) is used to allow ductal closure when a patent ductus arteriosus is present in the neonate. It is a prostaglandin inhibitor that promotes ductal closure. Digoxin (Lanoxin) is used for children diagnosed with patent ductus arteriosus or atrioventricular septal defects. This medication helps to control the symptoms of congestive heart failure associated with these defects. Hydrochlorothiazide (HydroDIURIL) is used for children diagnosed with patent ductus arteriosus, ventricular septal defects, or atrioventricular septal defects. This medication helps to control the symptoms of congestive heart failure associated with these defects. (D)

118. **4.** A child with atrial septal defect will be monitored by a cardiologist. Nonsurgical closure may be attempted via cardiac catheterization. Surgical closure, using either a prosthetic patch or sutures, is performed on an elective basis early in childhood. Children diagnosed with this disorder do not have spontaneous healing or closure. About 20% to 60% of children born with a ventricular septal defect, an abnormal opening between the right and left ventricles, have spontaneous closure. Atrial septal defect accounts for approximately 10% of all congenital heart disease and is seen in more female than male neonates. This lesion consists of an abnormal opening between the atria. Ostium secundum, a defect located in the middle of the atrial septum, is the most common type seen. As the child grows, she may experience fatigue and dyspnea on exertion. A large defect may result in congestive heart failure if the lesion is unrepaired. Bacterial endocarditis prophylaxis with antibiotics may be ordered if the child develops an infection. (R)

2

The Nursing Care of Children

TEST 1

Health Promotion

- Health Promotion of the Infant and Family
- Health Promotion of the Toddler and Family
- Health Promotion of the Preschooler and Family
- Health Promotion of the School-Age Child and Family
- Health Promotion of the Adolescent and Family
- Common Childhood and Adolescent Health Problems
- Correct Answers and Rationales

Health Promotion of the Infant and Family

1. Which of the following is appropriate language development for an 8-month-old? The child should be:
- ☐ **1.** Saying "dada" and "mama" specifically ("dada" to father and "mama" to mother).
- ☐ **2.** Saying three other words besides "mama" and "dada."
- ☐ **3.** Saying "dada" and "mama" nonspecifically.
- ☐ **4.** Saying "ball" when parents point to a ball.

2. The nurse should refer the parents of an 8-month-old child to a health care provider if the child is unable to:
- ☐ **1.** Stand momentarily without holding onto furniture.
- ☐ **2.** Stand alone well for long periods of time.
- ☐ **3.** Stoop to recover an object.
- ☐ **4.** Sit without support for long periods of time.

3. The nurse is teaching the parents of an 8-month-old about what the child should eat. The nurse should include which of the following points in the teaching plan?
- ☐ **1.** Items from all four food groups should be introduced to the infant by the time the child is 10 months old.
- ☐ **2.** Solid foods should not be introduced until the infant is 10 months old.
- ☐ **3.** Iron deficiency rarely develops before 12 months of age, so iron-fortified cereals should not be introduced until the infant is 12 months old.
- ☐ **4.** The infant's diet can be changed from formula to whole milk when the infant is 12 months old.

4. A 10-month-old looks for objects that have been removed from his view. The nurse should instruct the parents that:
- ☐ **1.** Neuromuscular development enables the child to reach out and grasp objects.
- ☐ **2.** The child's curiosity has increased.
- ☐ **3.** The child understands the permanence of objects even though the child cannot see them.
- ☐ **4.** The child is now able to transfer objects from hand to hand.

5. Which of the following structures should be closed by the time the child is 2 months old?
- ☐ **1.** A.
- ☐ **2.** B.
- ☐ **3.** C.
- ☐ **4.** D.

6. The nurse is discharging from the hospital an 8-month-old who weighs 15 lb. The parents have put the child in the back seat of the car with the car seat facing the front seat. The nurse should:
- ☐ **1.** Ask the parents to wait while the nurse obtains the correct car seat.
- ☐ **2.** Complete the discharge with the child sitting facing the front seat.
- ☐ **3.** Give the parents a manual on proper car seat placement.
- ☐ **4.** Show the parents proper placement of the car seat facing the back seat.

7. A mother who brings her 4-month-old infant to the clinic for a regular checkup is concerned that her infant is not developing appropriately. When assessing the infant, which of the following should the nurse expect to find?
- ☐ **1.** Sitting up with support.
- ☐ **2.** Finger-to-thumb grasping.
- ☐ **3.** Reaching for a toy.
- ☐ **4.** Saying "mama" or "dada."

8. In addition to immunizing for diphtheria, tetanus, and acellular pertussis (DTaP) during the first 6 months of life, the nurse should administer which of the following immunizations?
- ☐ **1.** Mumps.
- ☐ **2.** Measles.
- ☐ **3.** Tuberculosis.
- ☐ **4.** Hepatitis B.

9. The parents of a 9-month-old bring the infant to the clinic for a regular checkup. The infant has received no immunizations. Which of the following would be appropriate for the nurse to administer at this visit?
- ☐ **1.** Diphtheria, tetanus, and acellular pertussis (DTaP); *Haemophilus influenzae* type B (Hib); inactivated poliomyelitis vaccine (IPV); and purified protein derivative (PPD).
- ☐ **2.** DTaP; Hib; oral polio vaccine (OPV); and measles, mumps, and rubella (MMR).
- ☐ **3.** PPD, MMR, hepatitis B (hepB), and OPV.
- ☐ **4.** HepB, IPV, Hib, and varicella.

10. The mother of a 1-month-old infant states that she is curious as to whether her infant is developing normally. Which of the following developmental milestones should the nurse expect the infant to perform?
- ☐ **1.** Smiling and laughing out loud.
- ☐ **2.** Rolling from back to side.
- ☐ **3.** Holding a rattle briefly.
- ☐ **4.** Turning the head from side to side.

11. The mother of a 6-month-old states that she has started her infant on 2% milk. Which of the following should be the nurse's best response?
- ☐ **1.** "Your baby will probably be fine with this milk."
- ☐ **2.** "The baby should be switched to whole milk."
- ☐ **3.** "You need to keep the infant on formula."
- ☐ **4.** "You need to switch to formula right now."

12. The nurse notes that an infant stares at an object placed in her hand and takes it to her mouth, coos and gurgles when talked to, and sustains part of her own weight when held in a standing position. The nurse correctly interprets these findings as characteristic of an infant at which of the following ages?
- ☐ **1.** 2 months.
- ☐ **2.** 4 months.
- ☐ **3.** 7 months.
- ☐ **4.** 9 months.

13. An 8-month-old infant is seen in the well-child clinic for a routine checkup. The nurse should expect the infant to be able to do which of the following? Select all that apply.
- ☐ **1.** Say "mama" and "dada" with specific meaning.
- ☐ **2.** Feed self with a spoon.
- ☐ **3.** Play peek-a-boo.
- ☐ **4.** Walk independently.
- ☐ **5.** Stack two blocks.
- ☐ **6.** Transfer object from hand to hand.

14. A parent seems concerned about the fact that the infant's soft spot is still open. Which of the following should the nurse include when explaining about the usual age for closure of the soft spot near the front of the infant's head?
- ☐ **1.** 2 to 4 months.
- ☐ **2.** 5 to 8 months.
- ☐ **3.** 9 to 11 months.
- ☐ **4.** 12 to 18 months.

15. A mother states that she thinks her 9-month-old "is developing slowly." When assessing the infant's development, the nurse is also concerned because the infant should be demonstrating which of the following characteristics?
- ☐ **1.** Vocalizing single syllables.
- ☐ **2.** Standing alone.
- ☐ **3.** Building a tower of two cubes.
- ☐ **4.** Drinking from a cup with little spilling.

Health Promotion of the Toddler and Family

16. A 2-year-old tells his mother he is afraid to go to sleep because "the monsters will get him." The nurse should tell his mother to:
- ☐ **1.** Allow him to sleep with his parents in their bed whenever he is afraid.
- ☐ **2.** Increase his activity before he goes to bed, so he eventually falls asleep from being tired.
- ☐ **3.** Read a story to him before bedtime and allow him to have a cuddly animal or a blanket.
- ☐ **4.** Allow him to stay up an hour later with the family until he falls asleep.

17. A 2-year-old always puts his teddy bear at the head of his bed before he goes to sleep. The parents ask the nurse if this behavior is normal. The nurse should explain to the parents that toddlers use ritualistic patterns to:
- ☐ **1.** Establish a sense of identity.
- ☐ **2.** Establish control over adults in their environment.
- ☐ **3.** Establish sequenced patterns of learning behavior.
- ☐ **4.** Establish a sense of security.

18. Which development is necessary for toilet training readiness for a 2-year-old? Select all that apply.
- ☐ **1.** Adequate neuromuscular development for sphincter control.
- ☐ **2.** Appropriate chronological age.
- ☐ **3.** Ability to communicate the need to use the toilet.
- ☐ **4.** Desire to please the parents.
- ☐ **5.** Ability to play with other 2-year-olds.

19. A mother of a toilet-trained 3-year-old expresses concern over her child's bedwetting while hospitalized. The most appropriate response for the nurse to make is to tell the mother:
- ☐ **1.** "He was too immature to be toilet trained. In a few months he should be old enough."
- ☐ **2.** "Children are afraid in the hospital and frequently wet their bed."
- ☐ **3.** "It's very common for children to regress when they're in the hospital."
- ☐ **4.** "This is normal. He probably received too much fluid the night before."

20. A nurse working in the nursery identifies a goal for a mother of a newborn to demonstrate positive attachment behaviors upon discharge. Which intervention would be least effective in accomplishing this goal?
- ☐ **1.** Provide opportunities for the mother to hold and examine the newborn.
- ☐ **2.** Engage the mother in the newborn's care.
- ☐ **3.** Create an environment that fosters privacy for the mother and newborn.
- ☐ **4.** Identify strategies to prevent difficulties in parenting.

21. A mother brings her 18-month-old to the clinic because the child "eats ashes, crayons, and paper." Which of the following information about the toddler should the nurse assess first?
- ☐ **1.** Evidence of eruption of large teeth.
- ☐ **2.** Amount of attention from the mother.
- ☐ **3.** Any changes in the home environment.
- ☐ **4.** Intake of a soft, low-roughage diet.

22. When assessing a 2-year-old child brought by his mother to the clinic for a routine checkup, which of the following should the nurse expect the child to be able to do?
- ☐ **1.** Ride a tricycle.
- ☐ **2.** Tie his shoelaces.
- ☐ **3.** Kick a ball forward.
- ☐ **4.** Use blunt scissors.

23. A 2-year-old child brought to the clinic by her parents is uncooperative when the nurse tries to look in her ears. Which of the following should the nurse try first?
- ☐ **1.** Ask another nurse to assist.
- ☐ **2.** Allow a parent to assist.
- ☐ **3.** Wait until the child calms down.
- ☐ **4.** Restrain the child's arms.

24. When observing the parent instilling prescribed ear drops ordered twice a day for a toddler, the nurse decides that the teaching about positioning of the pinna for instillation of the drops is effective when the parent pulls the toddler's pinna in which of the following directions?
- ☐ **1.** Up and forward.
- ☐ **2.** Up and backward.
- ☐ **3.** Down and forward.
- ☐ **4.** Down and backward.

25. The mother asks the nurse for advice about discipline for her 18-month-old. Which of the following should the nurse suggest that the mother use first?
- ☐ **1.** Structured interactions.
- ☐ **2.** Spanking.
- ☐ **3.** Reasoning.
- ☐ **4.** Time out.

26. When assessing for pain in a toddler, which of the following methods should be the most appropriate?
- ☐ **1.** Ask the child about the pain.
- ☐ **2.** Observe the child for restlessness.
- ☐ **3.** Use a numeric pain scale.
- ☐ **4.** Assess for changes in vital signs.

27. When planning a 15-month-old toddler's daily diet with the parents, which of the following amounts of milk should the nurse include?
- ☐ **1.** ½ to 1 cup.
- ☐ **2.** 2 to 3 cups.
- ☐ **3.** 3 to 4 cups.
- ☐ **4.** 4 to 5 cups.

Health Promotion of the Preschooler and Family

28. To encourage autonomy in a 4-year-old, the nurse should instruct the mother to:
- ☐ **1.** Discourage the child's choice of clothing.
- ☐ **2.** Button the child's coat and blouse.
- ☐ **3.** Praise the child's attempts to dress herself.
- ☐ **4.** Tell the child when the combination of clothes is not appropriate.

29. The mother of a 4-year-old expresses concern that her child may be hyperactive. She describes the child as always in motion, constantly dropping and spilling things. Which of the following actions would be most appropriate at this time?

- ☐ **1.** Determine whether there have been any changes at home.
- ☐ **2.** Explain that this is not unusual behavior.
- ☐ **3.** Explore the possibility that the child is being abused.
- ☐ **4.** Suggest that the child be seen by a pediatric neurologist.

30. The mother of a preschooler reports that her child creates a scene every night at bedtime. The nurse and the mother decide that the best course of action would be to do which of the following?

- ☐ **1.** Allow the child to stay up later one or two nights a week.
- ☐ **2.** Establish a set bedtime and follow a routine.
- ☐ **3.** Encourage active play before bedtime.
- ☐ **4.** Give the child a cookie if bedtime is pleasant.

31. The parents of a preschooler ask the nurse how to handle their child's temper tantrums. Which of the following should the nurse include in the teaching plan? Select all that apply.

- ☐ **1.** Putting the child in "time-out."
- ☐ **2.** Telling the child to go to his bedroom.
- ☐ **3.** Ignoring the child.
- ☐ **4.** Putting the child to bed.
- ☐ **5.** Spanking the child.
- ☐ **6.** Trying to reason with the child.

32. After teaching a group of parents of preschoolers attending a well-child clinic about oral hygiene and tooth brushing, the nurse determines that the teaching has been successful when the parents state that children can begin to brush their teeth without help at which of the following ages?

- ☐ **1.** 3 years.
- ☐ **2.** 5 years.
- ☐ **3.** 7 years.
- ☐ **4.** 9 years.

33. After having a blood sample drawn, a 5-year-old child insists that the site be covered with an adhesive bandage strip. When the mother tries to remove the bandage before leaving the office, the child screams that all the blood will come out. The nurse interprets this behavior as indicating a fear of which of the following?

- ☐ **1.** Injury.
- ☐ **2.** Compromised body integrity.
- ☐ **3.** Pain.
- ☐ **4.** Loss of control.

34. A mother is concerned because her 5-year-old son seems prone to minor accidents such as skinning his elbows and knees and falling off his scooter. The nurse explains to the mother that childhood accidents are more likely to occur in which of the following situations?

- ☐ **1.** The child is the sole child in the family.
- ☐ **2.** The family has limited formal education.
- ☐ **3.** The family is experiencing changes.
- ☐ **4.** The child and family live in the suburbs.

35. When developing the teaching plan about illness for the mother of a preschooler, which of the following should the nurse include about how a preschooler perceives illness?

- ☐ **1.** A necessary part of life.
- ☐ **2.** A test of self-worth.
- ☐ **3.** A punishment for wrongdoing.
- ☐ **4.** The will of God.

Health Promotion of the School-Age Child and Family

36. A nurse is assessing the growth and development of a 10-year-old. What is the expected behavior of this child?

- ☐ **1.** Enjoys physical demonstrations of affection.
- ☐ **2.** Is selfish and insensitive to the welfare of others.
- ☐ **3.** Is uncooperative in play and school.
- ☐ **4.** Has a strong sense of justice and fair play.

37. The nurse asks a 9-year-old child and her mother about the child's best friend to assess which of the following about the child?

- ☐ **1.** Language development.
- ☐ **2.** Motor development.
- ☐ **3.** Neurologic development.
- ☐ **4.** Social development.

38. A 10-year-old child proudly tells the nurse that brushing and flossing her teeth is her responsibility. The nurse interprets this statement as indicating which of the following about the child?

- ☐ **1.** She is too young to be given this responsibility.
- ☐ **2.** She is most likely capable of this responsibility.
- ☐ **3.** She should have assumed this responsibility much sooner.
- ☐ **4.** She is probably just exaggerating the responsibility.

39. The mother tells the nurse that her 8-year-old child is continually telling jokes and riddles to the point of driving the other family members crazy. The nurse should explain this behavior is a sign of what?

- ☐ **1.** Inadequate parental attention.
- ☐ **2.** Mastery of language ambiguities.
- ☐ **3.** Inappropriate peer influence.
- ☐ **4.** Excessive television watching.

40. The mother asks the nurse about her 9-year-old child's apparent need for between-meal snacks, especially after school. When developing a sound nutritional plan for the child with the mother, which of the following should the nurse need to keep in mind?
- ☐ **1.** The child does not need to eat between-meal snacks.
- ☐ **2.** The child should eat the snacks the mother thinks are appropriate.
- ☐ **3.** The child should help with preparing his or her own snacks.
- ☐ **4.** The child will instinctively select nutritional snacks.

41. A nurse compares a child's height and weight with standard growth charts and finds the child to be in the 50th percentile for height and in the 45th percentile for weight. The nurse interprets these findings as indicating that the child is:
- ☐ **1.** Average height and weight.
- ☐ **2.** Overweight for height.
- ☐ **3.** Underweight for height.
- ☐ **4.** Abnormal in height.

Health Promotion of the Adolescent and Family

42. The nurse is teaching an adolescent with asthma how to use an inhaler. In which order should the nurse instruct the client to follow the steps?

1. Inhale through an open mouth.

2. Breathe out through the mouth.

3. Hold the breath for 5 to 10 seconds.

4. Press the canister to release the medication.

43. Initiation of which of the following immunizations is recommended prior to the adolescent entering college?
- ☐ **1.** Diphtheria, tetanus, and acellular pertussis (DTaP).
- ☐ **2.** Varicella.
- ☐ **3.** Meningococcal.
- ☐ **4.** Pneumococcal conjugate vaccine (PCV).

44. The school nurse develops a plan with an adolescent to provide relief of dysmenorrhea to aid in her development of which of the following?
- ☐ **1.** Positive peer relations.
- ☐ **2.** Positive self-identity.
- ☐ **3.** A sense of autonomy.
- ☐ **4.** A sense of independence.

45. An adolescent tells the school nurse that she would like to use tampons during her period. Which of the following would be most appropriate for the nurse to do?
- ☐ **1.** Assess her usual menstrual flow pattern.
- ☐ **2.** Determine whether she is sexually active.
- ☐ **3.** Provide information about preventing toxic shock syndrome.
- ☐ **4.** Refer her to a specialist in adolescent gynecology.

46. The school nurse is invited to attend a meeting with several parents who express frustration with the amount of time their adolescents spend in front of the mirror and the length of time it takes them to get dressed. The nurse explains that this behavior indicates:
- ☐ **1.** An abnormal narcissism.
- ☐ **2.** A method of procrastination.
- ☐ **3.** A way of testing the parents' limit-setting.
- ☐ **4.** A result of developing self-concept.

47. Several high-school seniors are referred to the school nurse because of suspected alcohol misuse. When the nurse assesses the situation, what would be most important to determine?
- ☐ **1.** What they know about the legal implications of drinking.
- ☐ **2.** The type of alcohol they usually drink.
- ☐ **3.** The reasons they choose to use alcohol.
- ☐ **4.** When and with whom they use alcohol.

Common Childhood and Adolescent Health Problems

48. Which of the following actions initiated by the parents of an 8-month-old indicates they need further teaching about preventing childhood accidents?
- ☐ **1.** Placing a fire screen in front of the fireplace.
- ☐ **2.** Placing a car seat in a front-seat, front-facing position.
- ☐ **3.** Inspecting toys for loose parts.
- ☐ **4.** Placing toxic substances out of reach or in a locked cabinet.

49. The mother of a 2-year-old is concerned because the child's right eye seems to turn in toward his nose when he is tired. The nurse should:
- ☐ 1. Assure the mother that this is a normal event when the child is tired.
- ☐ 2. Advise the mother to continue to watch his eyes closely and if the problem persists to call the clinic.
- ☐ 3. Test the child with the cover-uncover test and refer the mother and child to an ophthalmologist if the test is abnormal.
- ☐ 4. Explain to the mother that the child will probably outgrow the weakness and she need not be concerned.

50. A nurse is assessing the growth and development of a 14-year-old boy. He reports that his 13-year-old sister is 2 inches taller than he is. The nurse should advise the boy that the growth spurt in adolescent boys, compared with the growth spurt of adolescent girls:
- ☐ 1. Occurs at the same time.
- ☐ 2. Occurs 2 years earlier.
- ☐ 3. Occurs 2 years later.
- ☐ 4. Occurs 1 year earlier.

51. Parents of a 15-year-old state that he is moody and rude. The nurse should advise his parents to:
- ☐ 1. Restrict his activities.
- ☐ 2. Discuss their feelings with their child.
- ☐ 3. Obtain family counseling.
- ☐ 4. Talk to other parents of adolescents.

52. A parent asks the nurse about head lice (pediculosis capitis) infestation during a visit to the clinic. Which of the following symptoms should the nurse tell the parent is most common in a child infected with head lice?
- ☐ 1. Itching of the scalp.
- ☐ 2. Scaling of the scalp.
- ☐ 3. Serous weeping on the scalp surface.
- ☐ 4. Pinpoint hemorrhagic spots on the scalp surface.

53. A parent asks, "Can I get head lice too?" The nurse indicates that adults can also be infested with head lice but that pediculosis is more common among school children, primarily for which of the following reasons?
- ☐ 1. An immunity to pediculosis usually is established by adulthood.
- ☐ 2. School-age children tend to be more neglectful of frequent handwashing.
- ☐ 3. Pediculosis usually is spread by close contact with infested children.
- ☐ 4. The skin of adults is more capable of resisting the invasion of lice.

54. After teaching the parents about the cause of ringworm of the scalp (tinea capitis), which of the following, if stated by the father, indicates successful teaching?
- ☐ 1. "It results from overexposure to the sun."
- ☐ 2. "It's caused by infestation with a mite."
- ☐ 3. "It's a fungal infection of the scalp."
- ☐ 4. "It's an allergic reaction."

55. Griseofulvin (Grisactin) was ordered to treat a child's ringworm of the scalp. The nurse instructs the parents to use the medication for several weeks for which of the following reasons?
- ☐ 1. A sensitivity to the drug is less likely if it is used over a period of time.
- ☐ 2. Fewer side effects occur as the body slowly adjusts to a new substance over time.
- ☐ 3. Fewer allergic reactions occur if the drug is maintained at the same level long-term.
- ☐ 4. The growth of the causative organism into new cells is prevented with long-term use.

56. A mother asks the nurse, "How did my children get pinworms?" The nurse explains that pinworms are most commonly spread by which of the following when contaminated?
- ☐ 1. Food.
- ☐ 2. Hands.
- ☐ 3. Animals.
- ☐ 4. Toilet seats.

57. A mother tells the nurse that one of her children has chickenpox and asks what she should do to care for that child. When teaching the mother, which of the following would be most important to prevent?
- ☐ 1. Acid-base imbalance.
- ☐ 2. Malnutrition.
- ☐ 3. Skin infection.
- ☐ 4. Respiratory infection.

58. A mother calls the clinic to talk to the nurse. The mother states that a physician described her daughter as having 20/60 vision and she asks the nurse what this means. The nurse responds based on the interpretation that the child is experiencing which of the following?
- ☐ 1. A loss of approximately one-third of her visual acuity.
- ☐ 2. Ability to see at 60 feet what she should see at 20 feet.
- ☐ 3. Ability to see at 20 feet what she should see at 60 feet.
- ☐ 4. Visual acuity three times better than average.

59. After teaching a group of parents about temper tantrums, the nurse knows the teaching has been effective when one of the parents states which of the following?
- ☐ 1. "I will ignore the temper tantrum."
- ☐ 2. "I should pick up the child during the tantrum."
- ☐ 3. "I'll talk to my daughter during the tantrum."
- ☐ 4. "I should put my child in time out."

60. The nurse discusses the eating habits of school-age children with their parents, explaining that these habits are most influenced by which of the following?
- ☐ 1. Food preferences of their peers.
- ☐ 2. Smell and appearance of foods offered.
- ☐ 3. Examples provided by parents at mealtimes.
- ☐ 4. Parental encouragement to eat nutritious foods.

61. When discussing the onset of adolescence with parents, the nurse explains that it occurs at which of the following times?
- ☐ **1.** Same age for both boys and girls.
- ☐ **2.** 1 to 2 years earlier in boys than in girls.
- ☐ **3.** 1 to 2 years earlier in girls than in boys.
- ☐ **4.** 3 to 4 years later in boys than in girls.

62. A mother has heard that several children have been diagnosed with mononucleosis. She asks the nurse what precautions should be taken to prevent this from occurring in her child. Which of the following should the nurse advise the mother to do?
- ☐ **1.** Take no particular precautionary measures.
- ☐ **2.** Sterilize the child's eating utensils before they are reused.
- ☐ **3.** Wash the child's linens separately in hot, soapy water.
- ☐ **4.** Wear masks when providing direct personal care.

63. A father asks the nurse how he would know if his child had developed mononucleosis. The nurse explains that in addition to fatigue, which of the following would be most common?
- ☐ **1.** Liver tenderness.
- ☐ **2.** Enlarged lymph glands.
- ☐ **3.** Persistent nonproductive cough.
- ☐ **4.** A blush-like generalized skin rash.

64. A parent asks why it is recommended that the second dose of the measles, mumps, and rubella (MMR) vaccine be given at 4 to 6 years of age? The nurse should explain to the parent that the second dose is given at this age for what reason?
- ☐ **1.** If the child reaches puberty and becomes pregnant when receiving the vaccine, the risks to the fetus are high.
- ☐ **2.** The chance of contracting the disease is much lower at this age.
- ☐ **3.** The dangers associated with a strong reaction to the vaccine are increased at this age.
- ☐ **4.** A serious complication from the vaccine is swelling of the joints.

Correct Answers and Rationales

The letter in parentheses after each rationale identifies the client need addressed in the item, including management of care (M), safety and infection control (S), health promotion and maintenance (H), psychosocial adaptation (P), basic care and comfort (C), pharmacological and parenteral therapies (D), reduction of risk potential (R), and physiological adaptation (A).

Health Promotion of the Infant and Family

1. 3. It is important for the nurse to assist parents in assessing speech development in their child so that developmental delays can be identified early. According to the Denver Developmental Screening Examination, at 8 months of age, the child should say "mama" and "dada" nonspecifically and imitate speech sounds. A child cannot say "dada" or "mama" specifically or use more than three words until they are about 12 months of age. A child cannot respond to specific commands or point to objects when requested until about 17 months of age. (H)

2. 4. According to the Denver Developmental Screening Examination, a child of 8 months should sit without support for long periods of time. An 8-month-old child does not have the ability to stand without hanging on to a stationary object for support. His muscles are not developed enough to support all his weight without assistance. His balance has not developed to the point that he can stand and stoop over to reach an object. (H)

3. 4. Infants should be kept on formula or breast milk until 1 year of age. The protein in cow's milk is harder to digest than that found in formula. The infant cannot digest fats well, so some foods from the four food groups are not necessary in his diet during infancy. Solids are introduced into the infant's diet around 4 to 6 months, after the extrusion reflex has diminished and when the child will accept new textures. Iron deficiency develops in term infants between 4 to 6 months when the prenatal iron stores are depleted. Fortified cereals can be added to the infant's diet at 4 to 6 months to prevent iron deficiency anemia. (H)

4. 3. Understanding object permanence means that the child is aware of the existence of objects that are covered or displaced. Neuromuscular development, curiosity, and the ability to transfer objects are not associated with the principle of object permanence. Although, at 10 months, neuromuscular development is sufficient to grasp objects and a child's curiosity has increased, neither are related to the thought process involved in object permanence. (H)

5. 3. The posterior fontanel should be closed by age 2 months. The anterior fontanel and sagittal and frontal sutures should be closed by age 18 months. (H)

6. 4. The proper placement for a car seat for a child less than 20 lb and younger than 1 year is in the back seat, facing the rear of the car. Demonstrating proper car seat placement and explaining the reason for this position reinforces correct car seat positioning and may motivate the parents to continue this practice the next time they place the child in a vehicle. The car seat is not in question and does not need to be replaced. Keeping the child in an improperly installed car seat while the nurse continues the discharge only reinforces incorrect placement of the car seat. The parents are not likely to read a manual, especially since the child is 8 months old already and they have probably been placing the child in this position since birth. (S)

7. 1. Typically, a 4-month-old infant should be able to sit with support from a person holding the infant lightly in the area of the hips or lower chest. Fine pincer grasp, finger-to-thumb grasp, usually develops at about 9 months of age. Typically, an infant can reach for a toy at about 8 months of age. Saying recognizable syllables like "mama" or "dada" occurs at about 7 months of age. (H)

8. 4. According to the guidelines developed by the American Academy of Pediatrics for immunization of children (Report of the Committee on Infectious Diseases, 2006), a series of three injections of DTaP and a series of three injections of *Haemophilus influenzae* type B (Hib) vaccine are recommended during the first year of life. In addition, the infant should receive three immunizations for hepatitis B. Poliomyelitis protection is administered twice during the first year, unless the disease is prevalent in the area where the child lives, in which case another dose may be given. Measles, mumps, and rubella vaccine and Hib vaccine are recommended when the child is between 12 and 15 months of age. An immunization for tuberculosis is not used. However, infants are tested for tuberculosis with the purified protein derivative test, which is not administered until the infant is at least age 9 months. (H)

9. 1. The American Academy of Pediatrics recommends that infants who are delayed in receiving their immunizations or have not started their series by 9 months of age begin with DTaP, Hib, IPV, and PPD. OPV is not used because cases of polio have been reported with use of the vaccine. MMR and varicella vaccines are not administered until 12 months of age. (H)

10. 4. A 1-month-old infant usually is able to lift the head and turn it from side to side when lying prone. The full-term infant with no abnormalities or complications probably has been able to do this since birth. Smiling and laughing aloud are expected behaviors for a 2- to 3-month-old infant. Rolling from the back to the side is a characteristic behavior of a 4-month-old infant. Holding a rattle for a brief time is characteristic behavior of a 4-month old infant. (H)

11. 2. The mother has already changed the infant from formula to cow's milk, so she probably will not change the infant back to formula. Therefore, the best the nurse can hope for is that the mother will switch to whole milk. Because cow's milk causes microscopic blood loss in the intestine, it is best for the infant to remain on formula until 1 year of age and then be switched to whole milk, which has a higher fat content than 2% milk. The fat is needed for brain growth. (H)

12. 2. Holding the head erect when sitting, staring at an object placed in the hand, taking the object to the mouth, cooing and gurgling, and sustaining part of her body weight when in a standing position are behaviors characteristic of a 4-month old infant. A 2-month-old typically vocalizes, follows objects to the midline, and smiles. A 7-month-old typically is able to sit without support, turns toward the voice, and transfers object from hand to hand. Usually, a 9-month-old can crawl, stand while holding on, and initiate speech sounds. (H)

13. 3, 6. Typical abilities demonstrated by 8-month-old infants include playing peek-a-boo and transferring objects from one hand to another. The ability to say "dada" and "mama" is more typical of 10-month-old infants. Infants usually are at least 12 months old when they achieve the ability to walk independently. Infants who are 15 months old commonly can feed themselves with a spoon and stack two blocks. (H)

14. 4. The anterior fontanel, the soft spot near the front of the infant's head, usually closes between age 12 and 18 months. The small posterior fontanel usually closes by 6 to 8 weeks of age. (H)

15. 1. Normally, a 9-month-old infant should have been voicing single syllables since 6 months of age. Absence of this finding would be a cause for concern. An infant usually is able to stand alone at about 10 months of age. An infant usually is able to build a tower of 2 cubes at about 15 months of age. An infant usually is able to drink from a cup with little spilling at about 15 months of age. (H)

Health Promotion of the Toddler and Family

16. 3. Behavior problems related to sleep and rest are common in young children. Consistent rituals around bedtime help to create an easier transition from waking to sleep. Allowing a child to sleep with his parents commonly creates more problems for the family and child and does not alleviate the problem or foster autonomy. Increasing activity before bedtime does not alleviate the separation anxiety in the toddler and causes further anxiety. Allowing him to stay up later than his normal time for bed will increase his anxiety, make it more difficult for him to fall asleep, and do nothing to lessen his fear. (P)

17. 4. Toddlers establish ritualistic patterns to feel secure, despite inconsistencies in their environment. Establishing a sense of identity is the developmental task of the adolescent. The toddler's developmental task is to use rituals and routines to help in making autonomy easier to accomplish. Ritualistic patterns do involve patterns of behavior but they are not utilized to develop learning behaviors. (P)

18. 1, 3, 4. Readiness for toilet training is based on neurological, psychological, and physical developmental readiness. The nurse can introduce concepts of readiness for toilet training and encourage parents to look for adaptive and psychomotor signs such as the ability to walk well, balance, climb, sit in a chair, dress oneself, please the parent, and communicate awareness of the need to urinate or defecate. Chronological age is not an indicator for toilet training. Two-year-olds engage in parallel play, which is not an indicator of readiness for toilet training. (H)

19. **3.** A child will regress to a behavior used in an earlier stage of development in order to cope with a perceived threatening situation. Readiness for toilet training should be based on neurological, physical, and psychological development, not the age of the child. Children are afraid of hospitalization but the bedwetting is a compensatory mechanism done to regress to a previous stage of development that is more comfortable and secure for the child. Telling the mother that bedwetting is related to fluid intake does not provide an adequate explanation for the underlying regression to an earlier stage of development. (P)

20. **4.** Identifying ways to prevent difficulties in parenting would be helpful in reducing the incidence of child abuse and reducing the stress of child rearing. However, it would not help to develop positive attachment behaviors. Providing opportunities for the mother to hold and examine the newborn and help with care helps establish a positive emotional bond between the mother and newborn. Providing time for the mother to be alone with the infant further allows the mother and newborn to bond. (P)

21. **3.** A craving to eat nonfood substances is known as pica. Toddlers use oral gratification as a means to cope with anxiety. Therefore, the nurse should first assess whether the child is experiencing any change in the home environment that could cause anxiety. Teething or the eruption of large teeth and the amount of attention from the mother are unlikely causes of pica. Nutritional deficiencies, especially iron deficiency, were once thought to cause pica, but research has not substantiated this theory. A soft, low-roughage diet is an unlikely cause. (A)

22. **3.** A 2-year-old child usually can kick a ball forward. Riding a tricycle is characteristic of a 3-year-old child. Tying shoelaces is a behavior to be expected of a 5-year-old child. Using blunt scissors is characteristic of a 3-year-old child. (H)

23. **2.** Parents can be asked to assist when their child becomes uncooperative during a procedure. Most commonly, the child's difficulty in cooperating is caused by fear. In most situations, the child will feel more secure with a parent present. Other methods, such as asking another nurse to assist or waiting until the child calms down, may be necessary, but obtaining a parent's assistance is the recommended first action. Restraints should be used only as a last resort, after all other attempts have been made to encourage cooperation. (H)

24. **4.** In a child younger than 3 years of age, the pinna is pulled back and down, because the auditory canals are almost straight in children. In an adult, the pinna is pulled up and backward because the auditory canals are directed inward, forward, and down. (D)

25. **4.** Time out is the most appropriate discipline for toddlers. It helps to remove them from the situation and allows them to regain control. Structuring interactions with 3-year-olds helps minimize unacceptable behavior. This approach involves setting clear and reasonable rules and calling attention to unacceptable behavior as soon as it occurs. Physical punishment, such as spanking, does cause a dramatic decrease in a behavior but has serious negative effects. However, slapping a child's hand is effective when the child refuses to listen to verbal commands. Reasoning is more appropriate for older children, such as preschoolers and those older, especially when moral issues are involved. Unfortunately, reasoning combined with scolding often takes the form of shame or criticism and children take such remarks seriously, believing that they are "bad." (H)

26. **2.** Toddlers usually express pain through such behaviors as restlessness, facial grimaces, irritability, and crying. It is not particularly helpful to ask toddlers about pain. In most instances, they would be unable to understand or describe the nature and location of their pain because of their lack of verbal and cognitive skills. However, preschool and older children have the verbal and cognitive skills to be able to respond appropriately. Numeric pain scales are more appropriate for children who are of school age or older. Changes in vital signs do occur as a result of pain, but behavioral changes usually are noticed first. (A)

27. **2.** Toddlers around the age of 15 months need 2 to 3 cups of milk per day to supply necessary nutrients such as calcium. A daily intake of more than 3 cups of milk may interfere with the ingestion of other necessary nutrients. (H)

Health Promotion of the Preschooler and Family

28. **3.** At age 4, the child should be learning to dress without supervision. A child will feel more autonomous if allowed to try to take on tasks herself. Such attempts should be encouraged to increase self-esteem. Allowing choices encourages the child's capacity to control her behavior. Continued dependency may cause the child to doubt her own abilities. Telling the child that a combination of clothes is not appropriate may cause the child to doubt her abilities. Feelings of guilt can develop from not being able to accomplish what the child feels the adult expects of her. (H)

29. **2.** Preschool-age children have been described as powerhouses of gross motor activity who seem to have endless energy. A limitation of their motor ability is that in moving as quickly as they do, they are not always able to judge distances, nor are they able to estimate the amount of strength and balance needed for activities. As a result, they have frequent mishaps. This level of activity typically is not associated with changes at home. However, if the behavior intensifies, a referral to a pediatric neurologist would be appropriate. Children who have been abused usually demonstrate withdrawn behaviors, not endless energy. (H)

30. **2.** Bedtime is often a problem with preschoolers. Recommendations for reducing conflicts at bedtime include establishing a set bedtime; having a dependable routine, such as story reading; and conveying the expectation that the child will comply. Allowing the child to stay up late one or two nights interferes with establishing the needed bedtime rituals. Excitement, such as active play, just before bedtime should be avoided because it stimulates the child, making it difficult for the child to calm down and prepare for sleep. Using food such as a cookie as a reward if bedtime is pleasant should be avoided because it places too much importance on food. Other rewards, such as stickers, could be used as an alternative. (H)

31. **1, 3.** Some parents find that putting the child in time-out until control is regained is very effective. Others find that ignoring the behaviors works just as well with their child. Both suggestions are appropriate to include in the teaching plan. Sending the child to his bedroom means the child is being punished for having a tantrum. Spanking the child is never an option. Attempting to reason with a child having a temper tantrum does not work because the child is out of control. A more appropriate time to discuss it with the child is when the child regains control. (H)

32. **3.** Children younger than 7 years of age do not have the manual dexterity needed for tooth brushing. Therefore, parents need to help with this task until that time. (H)

33. **2.** The preschool-age child does not have an accurate concept of skin integrity and can view medical and surgical treatments as hostile invasions that can destroy or damage the body. The child does not understand that exsanguination will not occur from an injection site. Fear of pain would be manifested if the child thought that bodily harm would occur. If the child thought that he would urinate in his pants, then he would be demonstrating a fear of loss of control. (H)

34. **3.** Family changes and stresses (e.g., moving, having company, taking vacations, adding new members) can distract parental attention and contribute to accidents. Because only children tend to receive more attention than children with siblings, the risk for accidents would be less. The parents' limited formal education is unrelated to a child's risk for accidents. Families living in the suburbs usually are more affluent and therefore better able to afford to maintain a home that is less conducive to accidents. (H)

35. **3.** Preschool-age children may view illness as punishment for their fantasies. At this age children do not have the cognitive ability to separate fantasies from reality and may expect to be punished for their "evil thoughts." Viewing illness as a necessary part of life requires a higher level of cognition than preschoolers possess. This view is seen in children of middle school age and older. Perceiving illness as a test of self-worth or as the will of God is more characteristic of adults. (H)

Health Promotion of the School-Age Child and Family

36. **4.** School-age children are concerned about justice and fair play. They become upset when they think someone is not playing fair. Physical affection makes them embarrassed and uncomfortable. They are concerned about others and are cooperative in play and school. (H)

37. **4.** During the school-age years, a child learns to socialize with children of the same age. Therefore, the nurse is assessing the child's social development. The "best friend" stage, which occurs at about 9 or 10 years of age, is very important in providing a foundation for self-esteem and later relationships. Language development is best assessed by having the child read and participate in conversations. Motor development usually is assessed with a neurologic examination. Neurologic development is assessed by testing deep tendon reflexes and having the child tandem walk and perform visual-perceptual activities. (H)

38. **2.** Children are capable of mastering the skills required for flossing when they reach 9 years of age. At this age, many children are able to assume responsibility for personal hygiene. She is not too young to assume this responsibility and she should not have been expected to assume this responsibility much earlier. It is not likely that she is exaggerating; this is an expected behavior at this age. (H)

39. **2.** School-age children delight in riddles and jokes. Mastery of the ambiguities of language and of sentence structure allows the school-age child to manipulate words, and telling riddles and jokes is a way of practicing this skill. Children who suffer from inadequate attention from parents tend to demonstrate abnormal behavior. Peer influence is less important to school-age children, and while the child may learn the joke from a friend, he is telling the joke to master language. Watching television does not influence the extent of joke telling. (H)

40. **3.** Snacks are necessary for school-age children because of their high energy level. School-age children are in a stage of cognitive development in which they can learn to categorize or classify and can also learn cause and effect. By preparing their own snacks, children can learn the basics of nutrition (such as what carbohydrates are and what happens when they are eaten). The mother and child should make the decision about appropriate foods together. School-age children learn to make decisions based on information, not instinct. Some knowledge of nutrition is needed to make appropriate choices. (H)

41. **1.** The values of height and weight percentiles are usually similar for an individual child. Measurements between the 5th and 95th percentiles are considered normal. Marked discrepancies identify overweight or underweight children. (H)

Health Promotion of the Adolescent and Family

42.

2.	Breathe out through the mouth.
1.	Inhale through an open mouth.
4.	Press the canister to release the medication.
3.	Hold the breath for 5 to 10 seconds.

When dispensing medication from an inhaler, the client should first breathe out through the mouth. Next the client inhales through an open mouth and then presses the canister to dispense the medication while continuing to inhale and holds the breath for 5 to 10 seconds. The client can then exhale and breathe normally. (D)

43. 3. Meningococcal vaccine should be administered before the adolescent enters college because outbreaks of this type of meningitis are likely when people live in close association, such as in college dorms. DTaP, varicella, and PCV are given as boosters or initial doses before the child enters preschool or kindergarten. (H)

44. 2. Relieving dysmenorrhea in adolescence is crucial for the female's development of positive self-identity, of which positive body image and sexual identity are important components. Menstruation should not be viewed as painful and debilitating. Positive peer relations and a sense of independence would develop with a positive self-identity. Sense of autonomy, according to Erikson, is the developmental task of toddlers that, if successfully mastered, leads to a sense of self-control. (A)

45. 3. The nurse should provide the adolescent with information about toxic shock syndrome because of the identified relationship between tampon use and the syndrome's development. Additionally, about 95% of cases of toxic shock syndrome occur during menses. Most adolescent females can use tampons safely if they change them frequently. Using tampons is not related to menstrual flow or sexual activity. There is no need to refer the girl to a gynecologist; a nurse can provide health teaching about tampon use. (R)

46. 4. An adolescent's body is undergoing rapid changes. Adolescence is a time of integrating these rapidly occurring physical changes into the self-concept to achieve the developmental task of a positive self-identity. Thus, most adolescents spend much time worrying about their personal appearance. This behavior is not abnormal narcissism, a method of procrastination, or a way of testing the parents' limits. (H)

47. 3. Information about why adolescents choose to use alcohol or other drugs can be used to determine whether they are becoming responsible users or problem users. The senior students likely know the legal implica-

tions of drinking, and the nurse will establish a more effective relationship with the students by understanding motivations for use. The type of alcohol and when and with whom they are using it are not the first data to obtain when assessing the situation. (H)

Common Childhood and Adolescent Health Problems

48. 2. The recommended safety-seat arrangement for infants up to 20 lb and less than 1 year old is rear-facing with shoulder restraints. The middle of the back seat is considered the safest area of the car. Burns are a major cause of childhood accidents, and using fire screens in front of fireplaces can help prevent children from getting too close to a fire in a fireplace. Toys that contain loose parts or plastic eyes that can be swallowed or aspirated by small children should be avoided. Parents should inspect all toys for these parts before giving one to a child. Poisonings are most commonly caused by improper storage of a toxic substance. Keeping toxic substances in a child-proof container in a locked cabinet and continually observing the child's activities can prevent most poisonings. (S)

49. 3. Strabismus is diagnosed through observation and use of the corneal light reflex test. The cover-uncover test will reveal movement of the affected eye when the unaffected eye is covered, indicating abnormal fixation of the affected eye. The child should be referred to an ophthalmologist as soon as possible so that the correct vision in the affected eye can be restored. It is never normal for one eye to turn inward or outward even if the child is tired. If this condition is not corrected early, blindness can result in the unaffected eye due to the brain suppressing the double vision. Thus, telling the mother to watch the child and call later with concerns is not an appropriate response. The child will not grow out of this type of condition and may need surgery, an eye patch, daily exercises, or a combination of these interventions. (H)

50. 3. Adolescent boys lag about 2 years behind adolescent girls in growth. Most girls are 1 to 2 inches taller than boys at the beginning of adolescence but tend to stop growing approximately 2 to 3 years after menarche with the closure of the epiphyseal lines of the long bones. (H)

51. 2. Parents need to discuss with their adolescent how they perceive his behavior and how they feel about it. Moodiness is characteristic of adolescents. The adolescent may have a reason for or not be aware of his behavior. Restricting the adolescent's activities will not change his mood or the way he responds to others. It may increase his unacceptable responses. Counseling may not be needed at this time if the parents are open to communicating and listening to the adolescent. Talking to other parents may be of some help, but what is helpful to others may not be helpful to their child. (H)

52. 1. The most common characteristic of head lice infestation (pediculosis capitis) is severe itching. The head is the most common site of lice infestation. If the child scratches, scaling may occur. Itching also occurs when lice infest other parts of the body. Scratch marks are almost always found when lice are present. Weeping on the scalp surface may be an indication of an infection or other dermatologic condition. Hemorrhagic spots are not a symptom of head lice, but may be caused by scratch marks. (A)

53. 3. Lice are spread by close personal contact and by contact with infested clothing, bed and bathroom linens, and combs and brushes. Lice are more common in school-age children than in adults because of the close contact in school and the common practice of sharing possessions. Lice are not commonly spread by hand contact. There is no immunity conferred by having head lice. Adults can have head lice, particularly if they come in close contact with their children's infested clothing or linens. (A)

54. 3. Ringworm of the scalp is caused by a fungus of the dermatophyte group of the species. Overexposure to the sun would result in sunburn. Mites, such as chiggers or ticks, produce bites on the skin, resulting in inflammation. An allergic reaction commonly is manifested by hives, rash, or anaphylaxis. (A)

55. 4. Griseofulvin is an antifungal agent that acts by binding to the keratin that is deposited in the skin, hair, and nails as they grow. This keratin is then resistant to the fungus. But as the keratin is normally shed, the fungus enters new, uninfected cells unless drug therapy continues. Long-term administration of griseofulvin does not prevent sensitivity or allergic reactions. As the body adjusts to a new substance over time, side effects are variable and do not necessarily decrease. (D)

56. 2. The adult pinworm emerges from the rectum and colon at night onto the perianal area to lay its eggs. Itching and scratching introduces the eggs to the hands, from where they can easily reinfect the child or infect others. Nightclothes and bed linens can be sources of infection. The eggs can also be transmitted by dust in the home. Although transmission through contaminated food and water supplies is possible, it is rare. Contaminated animals can spread histoplasmosis and salmonella. The spread of infections by toilet seats has not been supported by research. (A)

57. 3. The care of a child with chickenpox focuses primarily on preventing infection in the lesions. The lesions cause severe itching, and organisms are ordinarily introduced into the lesion through scratching. Acid-base imbalance rarely occurs with chickenpox. Malnutrition is a chronic problem associated with the ingestion of an inadequate diet over a long period. It is not associated with chickenpox. Secondary infection in the lesions, not the respiratory tract, is most common. (A)

58. 3. A child with 20/60 vision sees at 20 feet what those with 20/20 vision see at 60 feet. A visual acuity of 20/200 is considered to be the boundary of legal blindness. (A)

59. 1. Children who have temper tantrums should be ignored as long as they are safe. They should not receive either positive or negative reinforcement to avoid perpetuating the behavior. Temper tantrums are a toddler's way of achieving independence. (H)

60. 3. Although children may be influenced by their peers and smell and appearance of foods may be important, children are most likely to be influenced by the example and atmosphere provided by their parents. Coaxing and badgering a child to eat most likely will aggravate poor eating habits. (H)

61. 3. Girls experience the onset of adolescence about 1 to 2 years earlier than boys. The reason for this is not understood. (H)

62. 1. The cause of infectious mononucleosis is thought to be the Epstein-Barr virus. No precautionary measures are recommended for clients with mononucleosis. The virus is believed to be spread only by direct intimate contact. (A)

63. 2. Mononucleosis usually has an insidious onset, with fatigue and the inability to maintain usual activity levels as the most common symptoms. The lymph nodes are typically enlarged, and the spleen also may be enlarged. Fever and a sore throat often accompany mononucleosis. A persistent nonproductive cough can follow an upper respiratory tract infection. A blush-like generalized skin rash is more characteristic of rubella. (A)

64. 1. After receiving the MMR vaccine, the person develops a mild form of the disease, stimulating the body to develop an immunity. Administration to a pregnant adolescent early in pregnancy puts the fetus at risk for deformity or spontaneous abortion. Some authorities recommend withholding the immunization for rubella until after puberty because a woman does not always know when she is pregnant and a fetus could be placed in jeopardy. However, the risk of contracting the disease is not lower at this age. There is no difference in the reaction to the vaccine at this age or in an older child. Swelling of the joints is a rare complication of the rubella vaccine. (D)

The Child with Respiratory Health Problems

The Client with Tonsillitis

1. Postoperative nursing care of a 7-year-old child who has had a tonsillectomy includes frequent blood pressure monitoring. Proper cuff size is:
- ☐ **1.** No less than half and no more than two-thirds of the extremity being measured.
- ☐ **2.** No less than one-third and no more than two-thirds of the extremity being measured.
- ☐ **3.** 2½ times the diameter of the extremity being measured.
- ☐ **4.** Same size as the diameter of the extremity being measured.

2. Which of the following should the nurse identify as a priority nursing diagnosis when preparing the preoperative plan of care for a 4-year-old undergoing a tonsillectomy and adenoidectomy?
- ☐ **1.** *Anxiety* related to surgery.
- ☐ **2.** *Impaired parenting* related to surgery.
- ☐ **3.** *Pain* related to surgery.
- ☐ **4.** *Imbalanced nutrition: Less than body requirements* related to surgery.

3. The nurse identifies a nursing diagnosis of *Risk for perioperative-positioning injury* related to the surgical procedure for a school-age child scheduled for a tonsillectomy. Which of the following should be the most appropriate expected outcome for this nursing diagnosis?
- ☐ **1.** The child is able to tell about the surgery and recovery.
- ☐ **2.** The child remains on nothing-by-mouth (NPO) status for the designated preoperative period.
- ☐ **3.** The child and family demonstrate an understanding of the procedure.
- ☐ **4.** The child knows the parents will not leave.

4. After a tonsillectomy and adenoidectomy, which of the following findings should alert the nurse to suspect early hemorrhage in a 5-year-old child?
- ☐ **1.** Drooling of bright red secretions.
- ☐ **2.** Pulse rate of 95 bpm.
- ☐ **3.** Vomiting of 25 ml of dark brown emesis.
- ☐ **4.** Blood pressure of 95/56 mm Hg.

5. After teaching the parents of a preschooler who has undergone a tonsillectomy and adenoidectomy about appropriate foods to give the child after discharge, which of the following, if stated by the parents as appropriate foods, indicates successful teaching?
- ☐ **1.** Meat loaf and uncooked carrots.
- ☐ **2.** Pork and noodle casserole.
- ☐ **3.** Cream of chicken soup and orange sherbet.
- ☐ **4.** Hot dog and potato chips.

6. A nurse is teaching the parents of a preschooler about the possibility of postoperative hemorrhage after a tonsillectomy and adenoidectomy. The nurse should explain that the risk is greatest at which of the following times?
- ☐ **1.** 2 to 4 days after surgery.
- ☐ **2.** 5 to 7 days after surgery.
- ☐ **3.** 8 to 10 days after surgery.
- ☐ **4.** 11 to 13 days after surgery.

The Client with Otitis Media

7. An adolescent female is prescribed amoxicillin for an ear infection. The nurse should teach the adolescent about the risks associated with her concurrent use of:
- ☐ **1.** Antacids.
- ☐ **2.** Oral contraceptives.
- ☐ **3.** Multiple vitamins.
- ☐ **4.** Protein shakes.

8. A 2-year-old child returns to the clinic after completing a 10-day course of amoxicillin prescribed to relieve an infection in his right ear. After completing the medication, the child has become fussy and has a low-grade fever. On physical examination, his right tympanic membrane is bulging and he is tugging at his ear. The nurse should:
☐ 1. Suggest to the mother that a decongestant may help the child.
☐ 2. Tell the mother the health care provider will probably repeat the 10-day course of amoxicillin.
☐ 3. Suggest that the child should see an ear, nose, and throat specialist for myringotomy tubes.
☐ 4. Report the assessment to the health care provider with the probability that another antibiotic will be used for a 10-day course.

9. When determining the parents' compliance with treatment for their infant who has otitis media, which of the following measures should the nurse expect the parents to describe?
☐ 1. Cleaning the child's ear canals with hydrogen peroxide.
☐ 2. Administering continuous, low-dose antibiotic therapy.
☐ 3. Instilling ear drops regularly to prevent cerumen accumulation.
☐ 4. Holding the child upright when feeding with a bottle.

10. A toddler is scheduled to have tympanostomy tubes inserted. When approaching the toddler for the first time, which of the following should the nurse do?
☐ 1. Talk to the mother first so that the toddler can get used to the new person.
☐ 2. Hold the toddler so that the toddler becomes more comfortable.
☐ 3. Walk over and pick the toddler up right away so that the mother can relax.
☐ 4. Pick up the toddler and take the child to the play area so that the mother can rest.

11. After insertion of bilateral tympanostomy tubes in a toddler, which of the following instructions should the nurse include in the child's discharge plan for the parents?
☐ 1. Insert ear plugs into the canals when the child bathes.
☐ 2. Blow the nose forcibly during a cold.
☐ 3. Administer the prescribed antibiotic while the tubes are in place.
☐ 4. Disregard any drainage from the ear after 1 week.

The Client with Foreign Body Aspiration

12. A child brought to the emergency department by his parents is diagnosed with a foreign body aspiration. Which of the following nursing diagnoses should the nurse identify as the priority for this child?
☐ 1. *Ineffective airway clearance* related to foreign body aspiration.
☐ 2. *Risk for injury* related to foreign body aspiration.
☐ 3. *Impaired parenting* related to foreign body aspiration.
☐ 4. *Ineffective health maintenance* related to foreign body aspiration.

13. The mother asks the nurse why peanuts are one of the worst things a child can aspirate. Which of the following should the nurse include in the explanation as the main reason for the problem associated with aspirating peanuts?
☐ 1. They swell when wet.
☐ 2. They contain a fixed oil.
☐ 3. They decompose when wet.
☐ 4. They contain sodium.

14. After teaching the parents of a toddler about commonly aspirated foods, which of the following foods, if identified by the parents as easily aspirated, would indicate the need for additional teaching?
☐ 1. Popcorn.
☐ 2. Raw vegetables.
☐ 3. Round candy.
☐ 4. Crackers.

15. A toddler who has been treated for a foreign body aspiration begins to fuss and cry when the parents attempt to leave the hospital for an hour. The parents will be returning to take the toddler home. As the nurse tries to take the child out of the crib, the child pushes the nurse away. The nurse interprets this behavior as indicating separation anxiety involving which of the following?
☐ 1. Protest.
☐ 2. Despair.
☐ 3. Regression.
☐ 4. Detachment.

16. After teaching the parents of an 18-month-old who was treated for a foreign body obstruction about the three cardinal signs indicative of choking, the nurse determines that the teaching has been successful when the parents state that a child is choking when he or she cannot speak, turns blue, and does which of the following?
☐ 1. Vomits.
☐ 2. Gasps.
☐ 3. Gags.
☐ 4. Collapses.

The Client with Asthma

17. An 11-year-old is admitted for treatment of an asthma attack. Which of the following indicates immediate intervention is needed?
- ☐ **1.** Thin, copious mucous secretions.
- ☐ **2.** Productive cough.
- ☐ **3.** Intercostal retractions.
- ☐ **4.** Respiratory rate of 20 breaths/minute.

18. A 12-year-old client with asthma is receiving I.V. hydrocortisone, ampicillin, and theophylline. The client vomits after breakfast and lunch, and is very irritable. Her heart rate is 120 bpm. The nurse should:
- ☐ **1.** Increase the hydrocortisone to prevent potassium loss.
- ☐ **2.** Inform the primary health care provider that the child is having an allergic reaction to the ampicillin.
- ☐ **3.** Hold the next dose of theophylline and inform the physician of the client's vomiting and pulse rate.
- ☐ **4.** Administer oxygen to decrease the heart rate.

19. A 12-year-old with asthma wants to exercise. Which of the following activities should the nurse suggest to improve her breathing?
- ☐ **1.** Soccer.
- ☐ **2.** Swimming.
- ☐ **3.** Track.
- ☐ **4.** Gymnastics.

20. When preparing the teaching plan for the mother of a child with asthma, which of the following should the nurse include as signs to alert the mother that her child is having an asthma attack?
- ☐ **1.** Secretion of thin, copious mucus.
- ☐ **2.** Tight, productive cough.
- ☐ **3.** Wheezing on expiration.
- ☐ **4.** Temperature of 99.4° F (37.4° C).

21. Which assessment findings should lead the nurse to suspect that a toddler is experiencing respiratory distress? Select all that apply.
- ☐ **1.** Coughing.
- ☐ **2.** Respiratory rate of 35 breaths/minute.
- ☐ **3.** Heart rate of 95 bpm.
- ☐ **4.** Restlessness.
- ☐ **5.** Malaise.
- ☐ **6.** Diaphoresis.

22. A 10-year-old child who is 5′ 4″ (138 cm) tall with a history of asthma uses an inhaled bronchodilator only when needed. He takes no other medications routinely. His best peak expiratory flow rate is 270 L/minute. The child's current peak flow reading is 180 L/minute. The nurse interprets this reading as indicating which of the following?
- ☐ **1.** The child's asthma is under good control, so the routine treatment plan should continue.
- ☐ **2.** The child needs to start a short-acting inhaled beta$_2$-agonist medication.
- ☐ **3.** This is a medical emergency requiring a trip to the emergency department for treatment.
- ☐ **4.** The child needs to begin treatment with inhaled cromolyn sodium (Intal) for asthma control.

23. An adolescent complains of chest pain and goes to the school nurse. The nurse determines that the teenager has a history of asthma but has had no problems for years. Which of the following should the nurse do next?
- ☐ **1.** Call the adolescent's parent.
- ☐ **2.** Have the adolescent lie down for 30 minutes.
- ☐ **3.** Obtain a peak flow reading.
- ☐ **4.** Give two puffs of a short-acting bronchodilator.

24. A 7-year-old child with a history of asthma controlled without medications is referred to the school nurse by the teacher because of persistent coughing. Which of the following should the nurse do first?
- ☐ **1.** Obtain the child's heart rate.
- ☐ **2.** Give the child a nebulizer treatment.
- ☐ **3.** Call a parent to obtain more information.
- ☐ **4.** Have a parent come and pick up the child.

25. When developing a teaching plan for the mother of an asthmatic child concerning measures to reduce allergic triggers, which of the following suggestions should the nurse expect to include?
- ☐ **1.** Keep the humidity in the home between 50% and 60%.
- ☐ **2.** Have the child sleep in the bottom bunk bed.
- ☐ **3.** Use a scented room deodorizer to keep the room fresh.
- ☐ **4.** Vacuum the carpet once or twice a week.

26. After discussing asthma as a chronic condition, which of the following statements by the father of a child with asthma best reflects the family's positive adjustment to this aspect of the child's disease?
- ☐ **1.** "We try to keep him happy at all costs; otherwise, he has an asthma attack."
- ☐ **2.** "We keep our child away from other children to help cut down on infections."
- ☐ **3.** "Although our child's disease is serious, we try not to let it be the focus of our family."
- ☐ **4.** "I'm afraid that when my child gets older, he won't be able to care for himself like I do."

27. An 8-year-old child with asthma states, "I want to play some sports like my friends. What can I do?" The nurse responds to the child based on the understanding of which of the following?
☐ **1.** Physical activities are inappropriate for children with asthma.
☐ **2.** Children with asthma must be excluded from team sports.
☐ **3.** Vigorous physical exercise frequently precipitates an asthmatic episode.
☐ **4.** Most children with asthma can participate in sports if the asthma is controlled.

The Client with Cystic Fibrosis and Bronchopneumonia

28. A 9-month-old child with cystic fibrosis does not like taking pancreatic enzyme supplement with meals and snacks. The mother does not like to force the child to take the supplement. The most important reason for the child to take the pancreatic enzyme supplement with meals and snacks is:
☐ **1.** The child will become dehydrated if the supplement is not taken with meals and snacks.
☐ **2.** The child needs these pancreatic enzymes to help the digestive system absorb fats, carbohydrates, and proteins.
☐ **3.** The child needs the pancreatic enzymes to aid in liquefying mucus to keep the lungs clear.
☐ **4.** The child will experience severe diarrhea if the supplement is not taken as prescribed.

29. A client's diagnosis of cystic fibrosis was made 13 years ago, and he has since been hospitalized several times. On the latest admission, the client has labored respirations, fatigue, malnutrition, and failure to thrive. Which nursing actions are most important initially?
☐ **1.** Placing the client on bed rest and ordering a blood gas analysis.
☐ **2.** Ordering a high-calorie, high-protein, low-fat, vitamin-enriched diet and pancreatic granules.
☐ **3.** Applying an oximeter and initiating respiratory therapy.
☐ **4.** Inserting an I.V. line and initiating antibiotic therapy.

30. A nurse is planning a diet for a client with cystic fibrosis. Which of the following foods should not be included in the meal plan?
☐ **1.** Roasted chicken.
☐ **2.** Fried scallops.
☐ **3.** Milk shake.
☐ **4.** Egg omelet.

31. A child with cystic fibrosis is receiving gentamicin. Which of the following nursing actions is most important?
☐ **1.** Monitoring intake and output.
☐ **2.** Obtaining daily weights.
☐ **3.** Monitoring the client for indications of constipation.
☐ **4.** Obtaining stool samples for hemoccult testing.

32. A 12-year-old with cystic fibrosis is being treated in the hospital for pneumonia. The physician is calling in a telephone order for ampicillin. The nurse should do which of the following? Select all that apply.
☐ **1.** Ask the unit clerk to listen on the speaker phone with the nurse and write down the order.
☐ **2.** Ask the physician to come to the hospital and write the order on the chart.
☐ **3.** Repeat the order to the physician.
☐ **4.** Ask the physician to confirm that the order is correct as understood by the nurse.
☐ **5.** Ask the nursing supervisor to cosign the telephone order as transcribed by the nurse.

33. When developing the plan of care for a child with cystic fibrosis (CF) who is scheduled to receive postural drainage, the nurse should anticipate performing postural drainage at which of the following times?
☐ **1.** After meals.
☐ **2.** Before meals.
☐ **3.** After rest periods.
☐ **4.** Before inhalation treatments.

34. When teaching the parents of an older infant with cystic fibrosis (CF) about the type of diet the child should consume, which of the following would be most appropriate?
☐ **1.** Low-protein diet.
☐ **2.** High-fat diet.
☐ **3.** Low-carbohydrate diet.
☐ **4.** High-calorie diet.

35. At a follow-up appointment after being hospitalized, an adolescent with a history of cystic fibrosis (CF) describes his stools to the nurse. Which of the following descriptions should the nurse interpret as indicative of continued problems with malabsorption?
☐ **1.** Soft with little odor.
☐ **2.** Large and foul-smelling.
☐ **3.** Loose with bits of food.
☐ **4.** Hard with streaks of blood.

36. When developing a recreational therapy plan of care for a 3-year-old child hospitalized with pneumonia and cystic fibrosis, which of the following toys would be most supportive?
☐ **1.** 100-piece jigsaw puzzle.
☐ **2.** Child's favorite doll.
☐ **3.** Fuzzy stuffed animal.
☐ **4.** Scissors, paper, and paste.

37. Which of the following, if described by the parents of a child with cystic fibrosis (CF), indicates that the parents understand the underlying problem of the disease?
- [ ] **1.** An abnormality in the body's mucus-secreting glands.
- [ ] **2.** Formation of fibrous cysts in various body organs.
- [ ] **3.** Failure of the pancreatic ducts to develop properly.
- [ ] **4.** Reaction to the formation of antibodies against streptococcus.

38. Which of the following outcome criteria would the nurse develop for a child with cystic fibrosis who has a nursing diagnosis of *Ineffective airway clearance* related to increased pulmonary secretions and inability to expectorate?
- [ ] **1.** Respiratory rate and rhythm within expected range.
- [ ] **2.** Absence of chills and fever.
- [ ] **3.** Ability to engage in age-related activities.
- [ ] **4.** Ability to tolerate usual diet without vomiting.

39. A school-age child with cystic fibrosis asks the nurse what sports she can become involved in as she becomes older. Which of the following activities would be most appropriate for the nurse to suggest?
- [ ] **1.** Swimming.
- [ ] **2.** Track.
- [ ] **3.** Baseball.
- [ ] **4.** Javelin throwing.

The Client with Sudden Infant Death Syndrome

40. Which one of the following children is at most risk for sudden infant death syndrome (SIDS)?
- [ ] **1.** Infant who is 3 months old.
- [ ] **2.** 2-year-old who has apnea lasting up to 5 seconds.
- [ ] **3.** First-born child whose parents are in their early forties.
- [ ] **4.** 6-month-old who has had two bouts of pneumonia.

41. Parents bring their child to the emergency department because the child has stopped breathing. A nurse obtains a brief history of events occurring before and after the parents found the infant not breathing. Which of the following questions would be most appropriate for the nurse to ask the parents?
- [ ] **1.** "Was the infant sleeping while wrapped in a blanket?"
- [ ] **2.** "Was the infant lying on his stomach?"
- [ ] **3.** "What did the infant look like when you found him?"
- [ ] **4.** "When had you last checked on the infant?"

42. When planning a visit to the parents of an infant who died of sudden infant death syndrome (SIDS) at home, the community health nurse should expect to visit the parents at which of the following times?
- [ ] **1.** A few days after the funeral.
- [ ] **2.** Two weeks after the funeral.
- [ ] **3.** As soon as the parents are ready to talk.
- [ ] **4.** As soon after the infant's death as possible.

43. When developing the ongoing plan of care for the parents whose infant died of sudden infant death syndrome (SIDS) , the community health nurse should expect to accomplish which of the following on the second home visit?
- [ ] **1.** Allow the parents to express their feelings.
- [ ] **2.** Have the parents gain an understanding of the disease.
- [ ] **3.** Assess the impact of the infant's death on their other children.
- [ ] **4.** Deal with issues such as having other children.

The Client Who Requires Immediate Care and Cardiopulmonary Resuscitation

44. A child has just ingested about 10 adult-strength acetaminophen (Tylenol) pills. The mother brings the child to the emergency department. What should the nurse do? Place the interventions in the order of priority.

1. Administer activated charcoal.
2. Assess the airway.
3. Reassure the mother.
4. Check serum acetaminophen levels.

45. On finding a child who is not breathing, which of the following should the nurse do first?
- [ ] **1.** Clear the airway.
- [ ] **2.** Begin mouth-to-mouth resuscitation.
- [ ] **3.** Initiate oxygen therapy.
- [ ] **4.** Start chest compressions.

46. Which of the following breathing rates should the nurse use when performing rescue breathing during cardiopulmonary resuscitation for a 5-year-old?
- [ ] **1.** 10 breaths/minute.
- [ ] **2.** 12 breaths/minute.
- [ ] **3.** 15 breaths/minute.
- [ ] **4.** 20 breaths/minute.

47. At which of the following rates should the nurse deliver external chest compressions to a 5-year-old child who is pulseless?
☐ **1.** 60 compressions/minute.
☐ **2.** 80 compressions/minute.
☐ **3.** 100 compressions/minute.
☐ **4.** 120 compressions/minute.

48. As part of a health education program, the nurse teaches a group of parents of preschoolers how to perform chest compressions during cardiopulmonary resuscitation. The nurse determines that the teaching has been effective when the parents state that the child's chest should be compressed to which of the following depths?
☐ **1.** 1 to 1.5 inches.
☐ **2.** 1.5 to 2 inches.
☐ **3.** One-quarter to one-third the depth of the chest.
☐ **4.** One-third to one-half the depth of the chest.

49. When performing cardiopulmonary resuscitation (CPR), which of the following assessments should indicate to the nurse that external chest compressions are effective?
☐ **1.** Mottling of the skin.
☐ **2.** Pupillary dilation.
☐ **3.** Palpable pulse.
☐ **4.** Cool, dry skin.

50. A nurse walks into the room just as a 10-month-old infant places an object in his mouth and starts to choke. After opening the infant's mouth, which of the following should the nurse do next to clear the airway?
☐ **1.** Use blind finger sweeps.
☐ **2.** Deliver back slaps and chest thrusts.
☐ **3.** Apply four subdiaphragmatic abdominal thrusts.
☐ **4.** Attempt to visualize the object.

51. When preparing to deliver back slaps to an infant who is choking on a foreign body, in which of the following positions should the nurse position the infant?
☐ **1.** Head down and lower than the trunk.
☐ **2.** Head up and raised above the trunk.
☐ **3.** Head to one side and even with the trunk lower than the head.
☐ **4.** Head parallel to the nurse and supported at the buttocks.

52. When teaching the parents of an infant how to perform back slaps to dislodge a foreign body, which of the following should the nurse tell the parents to use to deliver the blows?
☐ **1.** Palm of the hand.
☐ **2.** Heel of the hand.
☐ **3.** Fingertips.
☐ **4.** Entire hand.

53. While the nurse is delivering abdominal thrusts to a 6-year old who is choking on a foreign body, the child begins to cry. Which of the following should the nurse do next?
☐ **1.** Tap or gently shake the shoulders.
☐ **2.** Deliver back slaps.
☐ **3.** Perform a blind finger sweep of the mouth.
☐ **4.** Observe the child closely.

The Client with Croup

54. A three-year-old is brought into the emergency department in her mother's arms. The child's mouth is open and she is drooling and lethargic. Her mother states that she became ill suddenly within the past 2 hours. What should the nurse do first?
☐ **1.** Draw blood cultures for complete blood count.
☐ **2.** Start an intravenous line.
☐ **3.** Inspect the child's throat with a tongue blade.
☐ **4.** Maintain the child in an undisturbed, upright position.

55. The father of a 16-month-old child calls the clinic because the child has a low-grade fever, cold symptoms, and a hoarse cough. Which of the following should the nurse suggest that the father do?
☐ **1.** Offer extra fluids frequently.
☐ **2.** Bring the child to the clinic immediately.
☐ **3.** Count the child's respiratory rate.
☐ **4.** Use a hot air vaporizer.

56. A 21-month-old child admitted with the diagnosis of croup now has a respiratory rate of 48 breaths/minute, a heart rate of 120 bpm, and a temperature of 100.8° F (38.2° C) rectally. The nurse is having difficulty calming the child. Which of the following should the nurse do next?
☐ **1.** Administer acetaminophen (Tylenol).
☐ **2.** Notify the physician immediately.
☐ **3.** Allow the toddler to continue to cry.
☐ **4.** Offer clear fluids every few minutes.

The Client with Bronchiolitis or Pharyngitis

57. A child has viral pharyngitis. The nurse should advise the parents to do which of the following? Select all that apply.
☐ **1.** Use a cool mist vaporizer.
☐ **2.** Offer a soft-to-liquid diet.
☐ **3.** Administer amoxicillin.
☐ **4.** Administer acetaminophen.
☐ **5.** Place the child on secretion precautions.

58. A father brings his 3-month-old infant to the clinic, reporting that the infant has a cold, is having trouble breathing, and "just doesn't seem to be acting right." Which of the following actions should the nurse do first?
☐ **1.** Check the infant's heart rate.
☐ **2.** Weigh the infant.
☐ **3.** Assess the infant's oxygen saturation.
☐ **4.** Obtain more information from the father.

59. While the nurse is working in a homeless shelter, assessment of a 6-month-old infant reveals a respiratory rate of 52 breaths/minute, retractions, and wheezing. The mother states that her infant was doing fine until yesterday. Which of the following actions would be most appropriate?
☐ **1.** Administer a nebulizer treatment.
☐ **2.** Send the infant for a chest radiograph.
☐ **3.** Refer the infant to the emergency department.
☐ **4.** Provide teaching about cold care to the mother.

60. An infant is being treated at home for bronchiolitis. Which of the following should the nurse teach the parent about home care? Select all that apply.
☐ **1.** Offering small amounts of fluids frequently.
☐ **2.** Allowing the infant to sleep prone.
☐ **3.** Calling the clinic if the infant vomits.
☐ **4.** Writing down how much the infant drinks.
☐ **5.** Performing chest physiotherapy every 4 hours.
☐ **6.** Watching for difficulty breathing.

61. In preparation for discharge, the nurse teaches the mother of an infant diagnosed with bronchiolitis about the condition and its treatment. Which of the following statements by the mother indicates successful teaching?
☐ **1.** "I need to be sure to take my child's temperature every day."
☐ **2.** "I hope I don't get a cold from my child."
☐ **3.** "Next time my child gets a cold I need to listen to the chest."
☐ **4.** "I need to wash my hands more often."

Correct Answers and Rationales

The letter in parentheses after each rationale identifies the client need addressed in the item, including management of care (M), safety and infection control (S), health promotion and maintenance (H), psychosocial adaptation (P), basic care and comfort (C), pharmacological and parenteral therapies (D), reduction of risk potential (R), and physiological adaptation (A).

The Client with Tonsillitis

1. 1. Proper blood pressure cuff size is important for accurate readings. It should not be less than half or more than two-thirds the length of the extremity being mea-sured. A cuff less than half the length of the extremity being measured would falsely elevate the blood pressure. A cuff 2½ times the size or the same size of the extremity would be too large and cause a false-low reading. (C)

2. 1. A 4-year-old child is aware of what is happening and would be anxious in a new environment when not sure of what may happen or what is expected. The parents also would be anxious about how the child will tolerate the surgery and any complications that may occur. The child will pick up on the parents' anxiety. There are no data provided to support the nursing diagnosis of *Impaired parenting*. During the preoperative period, the child is not in any pain. However, pain may be a priority in the postoperative period. Even though the child will be put on nothing-by-mouth status preoperatively, intravenous fluids will be initiated once surgery begins, minimizing the risk of harm or problems. (H)

3. 2. The most appropriate outcome for a nursing diagnosis of *Risk for perioperative-positioning injury* related to the surgical procedure would be that the child remains NPO for the designated period of time before surgery, thereby minimizing the risk of aspiration during the surgery. Ability to tell about the surgery and demonstrating an understanding of the procedure are appropriate outcomes for a nursing diagnosis of *Deficient knowledge*. Knowing that the parents will not leave is associated with a nursing diagnosis of *Anxiety* or *Fear* related to separation from support systems or an unfamiliar environment. (R)

4. 1. After a tonsillectomy and adenoidectomy, drooling bright red blood is considered an early sign of hemorrhage. Often, because of discomfort in the throat, children tend to avoid swallowing; instead, they drool. Frequent swallowing would also be an indication of hemorrhage because the child attempts to clear the airway of blood by swallowing. Secretions may be slightly blood-tinged because of a small amount of oozing after surgery. However, bright red secretions indicate bleeding. A pulse rate of 95 bpm is within the normal range for a 5-year-old child, as is a blood pressure of 95/56 mm Hg. A small amount of blood that is partially digested, and therefore dark brown, is often present in postoperative emesis. (R)

5. 3. For the first few days after a tonsillectomy and adenoidectomy, liquids and soft foods are best tolerated by the child while the throat is sore. Children typically do not chew their food thoroughly, and solid foods are to be avoided because they are difficult to swallow. Although meat loaf would be considered a soft food, uncooked carrots would not be. Pork is frequently difficult to chew. Foods that have sharp edges, such as potato chips, are contraindicated because they are hard to chew and may cause more throat discomfort. (C)

6. 3. The risk for hemorrhage is greatest about 1 week after surgery as tissue sloughing occurs during the healing process. (R)

The Client with Otitis Media

7. 2. When a person is taking amoxicillin as well as an oral contraceptive it renders the contraceptive less effective. Because pregnancy can occur in such a situation, the nurse should advise the client to use additional means of birth control during the time she is taking the antibiotic. There are no risks associated with the concurrent use of amoxicillin and antacids, vitamins, or food. (P)

8. 4. Treatment of otitis media involves antibiotic therapy for 10 days and then a follow-up check of the ears by the health care provider. If the infection is not cleared, the health care provider will restart the client on another antibiotic. The bulging tympanic membrane and continued pain suggest that an infection remains. A decongestant may help to drain the eustachian tubes, but it would not clear the infection. Repeating the same antibiotic that didn't clear the infection during the first course of treatment would probably not be helpful if taken for another 10 days. Myringotomy tubes are not indicated with just one ear infection. (H)

9. 4. Sitting or holding a child upright for formula feedings helps prevent pooling of formula in the pharyngeal area. When the vacuum in the middle ear opens into the pharyngeal cavity, formula (along with bacteria) is drawn into the middle ear. Cleaning the ear canals does not reduce the incidence of otitis media because the pathogenic bacteria are in the nasopharynx, not the external area of the ears. Continuous low-dose antibiotic therapy is used only in cases of recurrent otitis media, when the child finishes a course of antibiotics but then develops another ear infection a few days later. Although accumulation of cerumen makes it difficult to visualize the tympanic membrane, it does not promote inner ear infections. (H)

10. 1. Toddlers should be approached slowly, because they are wary of strangers and need time to get used to someone they do not know. The best approach is to ignore them initially and to focus on talking to the parents. The child will likely resist being held by a stranger, so the nurse should not pick up or hold the child until the child indicates a readiness to be approached or the mother indicates that it is okay. (H)

11. 1. Placing ear plugs in the ears will prevent contaminated bathwater from entering the middle ear through the tympanostomy tube and causing an infection. Blowing the nose forcibly during a cold causes organisms to ascend through the eustachian tube, possibly leading to otitis media. It is not necessary to administer antibiotics continuously to a child with a tympanostomy tube. Antibiotics are appropriate only when an ear infection is present. Drainage from the ear may be a sign of middle ear infection and should be reported to the health care provider. (R)

The Client with Foreign Body Aspiration

12. 1. The child with a foreign body aspiration is experiencing an airway obstruction and requires immediate intervention to ensure adequate ventilation. Therefore, the priority is *Ineffective airway clearance. Risk for injury* related to foreign body aspiration may be important once the child's airway patency has been established. *Impaired parenting* related to foreign body aspiration requires obtaining additional data about how the aspiration occurred. Data are not sufficient to suggest a diagnosis of *Ineffective health maintenance.* Even if this diagnosis is confirmed, it is not the immediate priority. (A)

13. 1. Peanuts swell and become soft when moistened with bronchial secretions, making them difficult to remove. Although peanuts contain a fixed oil that can cause lipoid pneumonia, begin to decompose when wet, and contain sodium, these factors do not make them particularly dangerous when aspirated. (H)

14. 4. Crackers, because they crumble and easily dissolve, are not commonly aspirated. Because children commonly eat popcorn hulls or pieces that have not popped, popcorn can be easily aspirated. Toddlers frequently do not chew their food well, making raw vegetables a commonly aspirated food. Round candy is often difficult to chew and comes in large pieces, making it easily aspirated. (H)

15. 1. Young children have specific reactions to separation and hospitalization. In the protest stage, the toddler physically and verbally attacks anyone who attempts to provide care. Here, the child is fussing and crying and visibly pushes the nurse away. In the despair stage, the toddler becomes withdrawn and obviously depressed (for example, not engaging in play activities and sleeping more than usual). Regression is a return to a developmentally earlier phase because of stress or crisis (for example, a toddler who could feed himself before this event is not doing so now). Denial or detachment occurs if the toddler's stay in the hospital without the parent is prolonged because the toddler settles in to the hospital life and denies the parents' existence (for example, not reacting when the parents come to visit). (P)

16. 4. The three cardinal signs indicating that a child is truly choking and requires immediate life-saving interventions include inability to speak, blue color (cyanosis), and collapse. Vomiting does not occur while a child is unable to breathe. Once the object is dislodged, however, vomiting may occur. Gasping, a sudden intake of air, indicates that the child is still able to inhale. When a child is choking, air is not being exchanged, so gagging will not occur. (R)

The Client with Asthma

17. 3. Intercostal retractions indicate an increase in respiratory effort, which is a sign of respiratory distress. During an asthma attack, secretions are thick, the cough is tight, and respiration is difficult (and shortness of breath may occur). If mucous secretions are copious but thin, the client can expectorate them, which indicates an improvement in the condition. If the cough is productive it means the bronchospasms and the inflammation have been resolved to the extent that the mucus can be expectorated. A respiratory rate of 20 breaths/minute would be considered normal and no intervention would be needed. (A)

18. 3. A toxic level of theophylline can cause vomiting, irritability, headache, and tachycardia. The therapeutic level of theophylline is 10 to 20 mcg/ml. Increasing the hydrocortisone would result in a decreased serum potassium and an increase in serum sodium. Rash, urticaria, respiratory distress, and hypotension—not vomiting and tachycardia—are the characteristic manifestations of an allergic reaction to ampicillin. Although the child's heart rate could indicate hypoxia, none of the other signs indicate a need for oxygen. (P)

19. 2. Swimming is appropriate for this child because it requires controlled breathing, assists in maintaining cardiac health, enhances skeletal muscle strength, and promotes ventilation and perfusion. Stop-and-start activities, such as soccer, track, and gymnastics, commonly trigger symptoms in asthmatic clients. (H)

20. 3. The child who is experiencing an asthma attack typically demonstrates wheezing on expiration initially. This results from air moving through narrowed airways secondary to bronchoconstriction. The child's expiratory phase is normally longer than the inspiratory phase. Expiration is passive as the diaphragm relaxes. During an asthma attack, secretions are thick and are not usually expelled until the bronchioles are more relaxed. At the beginning of an asthma attack the cough will be tight but not productive. Fever is not always present unless there is an infection that may have triggered the attack. (A)

21. 2, 4, 6. The early signs of respiratory distress include restlessness, tachypnea, tachycardia, and diaphoresis. Coughing and malaise typically do not indicate respiratory distress. A heart rate of 95 bpm is normal for a toddler. Other signs and symptoms include hypertension, nasal flaring, expiratory grunting, wheezing, and intercostal retractions. (R)

22. 2. The peak flow of 180 L/minute is in the yellow zone, or 50% to 80% of the child's personal best. This means that the child's asthma is not well controlled, thereby necessitating the use of a short-acting beta$_2$-agonist medication to relieve the bronchospasm. A peak flow reading greater than 80% of the child's personal best (in this case, 220 L/minute or better) would indicate that the child's asthma is in the green zone or under good control. A peak flow reading in the red zone, or less than 50% of the child's personal best (135 L/minute or less), would require notification of the health care provider or a trip to the emergency department. Cromolyn sodium (Intal) is not used for short-term treatment of acute bronchospasm. It is used as part of a long-term therapy regimen to help desensitize mast cells and thereby help to prevent symptoms. (R)

23. 3. Complaints of chest pain in children and adolescents are rarely cardiac. With a history of asthma, the most likely cause of the chest pain is related to the asthma. Therefore, the nurse should check the adolescent's peak flow reading to evaluate the status of the air flow. Calling the adolescent's parent would be appropriate, but this would be done after the nurse obtains the peak flow reading and additional assessment data. Having the adolescent lie down may be an option, but more data need to be collected to help establish a possible cause. Because the adolescent has not experienced any asthma problems for a long time, it would be inappropriate for the nurse to administer a short-acting bronchodilator at this time. (R)

24. 3. Because persistent coughing may indicate an asthma attack and a 7-year-old child would be able to provide only minimal history information, it would be important to obtain information from the parent. Although determining the child's heart rate is an important part of the assessment, it would be done after the history is obtained. More information needs to be obtained before giving the child a nebulizer treatment. Although it may be necessary for the parent to come and pick up the child, a thorough assessment including history information should be obtained first. (R)

25. 1. To help reduce allergic triggers in the home, the nurse should recommend that the humidity level be kept between 50% and 60%. Doing so keeps the air moist and comfortable for breathing. When air is dry, the risk for respiratory infections increase. Too high a level of humidity increases the risk for mold growth. Typically, the child with asthma should sleep in the top bunk bed to minimize the risk of exposure to dust mites. The risk of exposure to dust mites increases when the child sleeps in the bottom bunk bed because dust mites fall from the top bed, settling in the bottom bed. Scented sprays should be avoided because they may trigger an asthmatic episode. Ideally, carpeting should be avoided in the home if the child has asthma. However, if it is present, carpeting in the child's room should be vacuumed often, possibly daily, to remove dust mites and dust particles. (R)

26. 3. Positive adjustment to a chronic condition requires placing the child's illness in its proper perspective. Children with asthma need to be treated as normally as possible within the scope of the limitations imposed by the illness. They also need to learn how to manage exacerbations and then resume as normal a life as possible. Trying to keep the child happy at all costs is inappropriate and can lead to the child's never learning how to accept responsibility for behavior and get along with others. Although minimizing the child's risk for exposure to infections is important, the child needs to be with his or her peers to ensure appropriate growth and development. Children with a chronic illness need to be involved in their care so that they can learn to manage it. Some parents tend to overprotect their child with a chronic illness. This overprotectiveness may cause a child to have an exaggerated feeling of importance or later, as an adolescent, to rebel against the overprotectiveness and the parents. (P)

27. 4. Physical activities are beneficial to asthmatic children, physically and psychosocially. Most children with asthma can engage in school and sports activities that are geared to the child's condition and within the limits imposed by the disease. The coach and other team members need to be aware of the child's condition and know what to do in case an attack occurs. Those children who have exercise-induced asthma usually use a short-acting bronchodilator before exercising. (H)

The Client with Cystic Fibrosis and Bronchopneumonia

28. 2. The child must take the pancreatic enzyme supplement with meals and snacks to help absorb nutrients so he can grow and develop normally. In cystic fibrosis, the normally liquid mucus is tenacious and blocks three digestive enzymes from entering the duodenum and digesting essential nutrients. Without the supplemental pancreatic enzyme, the child will have voluminous, foul, fatty stools due to the undigested nutrients and may experience developmental delays due to malnutrition. Dehydration is not a problem related to cystic fibrosis. The pancreatic enzymes have no effect on the viscosity of the tenacious mucus. Diarrhea is not caused by failing to take the pancreatic enzyme supplement. (D)

29. 3. Clients with cystic fibrosis commonly die from respiratory problems. The mucus in the lungs is tenacious and difficult to expel, leading to lung infections and interference with oxygen and carbon dioxide exchange. The client will likely need supplemental oxygen and respiratory treatments to maintain adequate gas exchange, as identified by the oximeter reading. The child will be on bed rest due to respiratory distress. However, although blood gases will probably be ordered, the oximeter readings will be used to determine oxygen deficit and are, therefore, more of a priority. A diet high in calories, proteins, and vitamins with pancreatic granules added to all foods ingested will increase nutrient absorption, and help the malnutrition; however, this intervention is not the priority at this time. Inserting an I.V. to administer antibiotics is important, and can be done after ensuring adequate respiratory function. (A)

30. 2. Fried scallops are high in fat, and fats are difficult for a client with cystic fibrosis to digest; scallops are also not commonly preferred by most children. Clients with cystic fibrosis commonly lack calories and protein because their bodies do not absorb nutrients. Nutrients are not absorbed because tenacious mucus blocks key diges-

tive enzymes from entering the digestive system. Thus, a diet rich in proteins and carbohydrates is essential for these clients. Roasted chicken and an egg omelet are high in protein and help with growth and development. The milk shake is high in carbohydrate and protein. (H)

31. 1. Monitoring intake and output is the most important nursing action when administering an aminoglycoside, such as gentamicin, because a decrease in output is an early sign of renal damage. Daily weight monitoring is not indicated when the client is receiving an aminoglycoside. Constipation and bleeding are not adverse effects of aminoglycosides. (D)

32. 3, 4. To ensure client safety in obtaining telephone orders, the order must be received by a registered nurse. The nurse should write the order, read the order back to the physician, and receive confirmation from the physician that the order is correct. It is not necessary to ask the unit clerk to listen to the order, to require the physician to come to the hospital to write the order on the chart, or to have the nursing supervisor cosign the telephone order. (S)

33. 2. Postural drainage, which aids in mobilizing the thick, tenacious secretions commonly associated with CF, is usually performed before meals to avoid the possibility of vomiting or regurgitating food. Although the child with CF needs frequent rest periods, this is not an important factor in scheduling postural drainage. However, the nurse would not want to interrupt the child's rest period to perform the treatment. Inhalation treatments are usually given before postural drainage to help loosen secretions. (R)

34. 4. CF affects the exocrine glands. Mucus is thick and tenacious, sticking to the walls of the pancreatic and bile ducts and eventually causing obstruction. Because of the difficulty with digestion and absorption, a high-calorie, high-protein, high-carbohydrate, moderate-fat diet is indicated. (A)

35. 2. In children with CF, poor digestion and absorption of foods, especially fats, results in frequent bowel movements that are bulky, large, and foul-smelling. The stools also contain abnormally large quantities of fat, which is called *steatorrhea*. An adolescent experiencing good control of the disease would describe soft stools with little odor. Stool described as loose with bits of food indicates diarrhea. Stool described as hard with streaks of blood may indicate constipation. (A)

36. 2. The child's favorite doll would be a good choice of toys. The doll provides support and is familiar to the child. Although a 3-year-old may enjoy puzzles, a 100-piece jigsaw puzzle is too complicated for an ill 3-year-old child. In view of the child's lung pathology, a fuzzy stuffed animal would not be advised because of its potential as a reservoir for dust and bacteria, possibly predisposing the child to additional respiratory problems. Scissors, paper, and paste are not appropriate for a 3-year-old unless the child is supervised closely. (H)

37. 1. CF is characterized by a dysfunction in the body's mucus-producing exocrine glands. The mucus secretions are thick and sticky rather than thin and slippery. The mucus obstructs the bronchi, bronchioles, and pancreatic ducts. Mucus plugs in the pancreatic ducts can prevent pancreatic digestive enzymes from reaching the small intestine, resulting in poor digestion and poor absorption of various food nutrients. Fibrous cysts do not form in various organs. Cystic fibrosis is an autosomal recessive inherited disorder and does not involve any reaction to the formation of antibodies against streptococcus. (A)

38. 1. After treatment, the client outcome would be that respiratory status would be within normal limits, as evidenced by a respiratory rate and rhythm within expected range. Absence of chills and fever, although related to an underlying problem causing the respiratory problem (for example, the infection), do not specifically relate to the respiratory problem of ineffective airway clearance. The child's ability to engage in age-related activities may provide some evidence of improved respiratory status. However, this outcome criterion is more directly related to a nursing diagnosis of *Activity intolerance*. Although the child's ability to tolerate his or her usual diet may indirectly relate to respiratory function, this outcome is more specifically related to a nursing diagnosis of *Imbalanced nutrition: Less than body requirements*, which may or may not be related to the child's respiratory status. (A)

39. 1. Swimming would be the most appropriate suggestion because it coordinates breathing and movement of all muscle groups and can be done on an individual basis or as a team sport. Because track events, baseball, and javelin throwing usually are performed outdoors, the child would be breathing in large amounts of dust and dirt, which would be irritating to her mucous membranes and pulmonary system. The strenuous activity and increased energy expenditure associated with track events, in conjunction with the dust and possible heat, would play a role in placing the child at risk for an upper respiratory tract infection and compromising her respiratory function. (H)

The Client with Sudden Infant Death Syndrome

40. 1. The highest incidence of SIDS occurs in infants between ages 2 and 4 months. About 90% of SIDS occurs before the age of 6 months. Apnea lasting longer than 20 seconds has also been associated with a higher incidence of SIDS. SIDS occurs with higher frequency in families where a child in the family has already died of SIDS, but the age of the parents has not been shown to contribute to SIDS. A respiratory infection such as pneumonia has not been shown to cause a higher incidence of SIDS. (H)

41. 3. Because this is an especially disturbing and upsetting time for the parents, they must be approached in a sensitive manner. Asking what the infant looked like when found allows the parents to verbalize what they saw and felt, thereby helping to minimize their feelings of guilt without implying any blame, neglect, wrongdoing, or abuse. Asking if the child was wrapped in a blanket or lying on his stomach, or when the parents last checked on the infant, implies that the parents did something wrong or failed in their care of the infant, thus blaming them for the event. (A)

42. 4. The community health nurse should visit as soon after the death as possible, because the parents may need help to deal with the sudden, unexpected death of their infant. Parents often have a great deal of guilt in these situations and need to express their feelings to someone who can provide counseling. (P)

43. 1. The goal of the second home visit is to help the parents express their feelings more openly. Many parents are reluctant to express their grief and need help. The goal of the first visit is to help the parents understand the disease and what happened. The first visit also provides time to help the parents understand that they are not to blame. Although it is important to assess the impact of SIDS on siblings, this is not the primary goal for the second visit. However, the nurse must be flexible in case problems involving this area arise. Typically, parents are unable to deal with decisions such as having other children during the second visit because they are grieving for the child that they lost. This topic may be discussed later in the course of care. (P)

The Client Who Requires Immediate Care and Cardiopulmonary Resuscitation

44.

2.	Assess the airway.

1.	Administer activated charcoal.

3.	Reassure the mother.

4.	Check serum acetaminophen levels.

Immediate care of the child who has ingested acetaminophen is to ensure airway, breathing, and circulation. Next, the nurse should administer activated charcoal. Acetylcysteine (Mucomyst) may also be used as an antidote. When the child is stable, the nurse should reassure the mother. The serum acetaminophen level should be obtained 4 hours after ingestion. (S)

45. 1. When breathlessness is determined, the priority nursing action is to clear the airway. This action alone may reestablish spontaneous respiration. If the client does not begin breathing, mouth-to-mouth resuscitation is initiated. Oxygen therapy would not be initiated at this time, because the child is not breathing. Also, administering oxygen therapy would interfere with providing mouth-to-mouth resuscitation. Chest compressions are begun only after the client is determined to be pulseless. (A)

46. **1.** Rescue breaths should be delivered slowly at a volume that makes the chest rise and fall. For a 5-year-old child, the rate is 10 breaths per minute. If the nurse is also administering chest compressions, the rate is 2 breaths for every 15 compressions. (A)

47. **3.** For a 5-year-old child, external chest compressions should be delivered at a rate of 100 times per minute. This rate approximates the resting minimum pulse, which allows for adequate brain perfusion. A rate of 120 times per minute is too fast. Rates of 60 times and 80 times per minute are not frequent enough. (A)

48. **4.** For preschoolers ages 3 to 5 years, the chest is compressed one-third to one-half of its depth. This depth forces blood out of the heart and into the vital organs (lungs and brain). Deeper compressions could damage the liver, lungs, or other underlying structures. Shallower compressions would not provide adequate circulation to the vital organs. (A)

49. **3.** With CPR, effectiveness of external chest compressions is indicated by palpable peripheral pulses, the disappearance of mottling and cyanosis, the return of pupils to normal size, and warm, dry skin. To determine whether the victim of cardiopulmonary arrest has resumed spontaneous breathing and circulation, chest compressions must be stopped for 5 seconds at the end of the first minute and every few minutes thereafter. (A)

50. **2.** The nurse should use mechanical force—back slaps and chest thrusts—in an attempt to dislodge the object. Blind finger sweeps are not appropriate in infants and children because the foreign body may be pushed back into the airway. Subdiaphragmatic abdominal thrusts are not used for infants age 1 year or younger because of the risk of injury to abdominal organs. If the object is not visible when opening the mouth, time is wasted in looking for it. Action is required to dislodge the object as quickly as possible. (R)

51. **1.** To deliver back slaps, the nurse should place the infant face down, straddled over the nurse's arm, with the head lower than the trunk and the head supported. This position, together with the back slaps, facilitates dislodgment and removal of a foreign object and minimizes aspiration if vomiting occurs. Placing the infant with the head up and raised above the trunk would not aid in dislodging and removing the foreign object. In addition, this position places the infant at risk for aspiration should vomiting occur. Placing the head to one side may minimize the risk of aspiration. However, it would not help with removal of an object that is dislodged by the back slaps. Placing the infant with the head parallel to the nurse and supported at the buttocks is more appropriate for burping the infant. (A)

52. **2.** Back slaps are delivered rapidly and forcefully with the heel of the hand between the infant's shoulder blades. Slowly delivered back slaps are less likely to dislodge the object. Using the heel of the hand allows more force to be applied than when using the palm or the whole hand, increasing the likelihood of loosening the object. The fingertips would be used to deliver chest compressions to an infant younger than 1 year of age. (A)

53. **4.** Crying indicates that the airway obstruction has been relieved. No additional thrusts are needed. However, the child needs to be observed closely for complications, including respiratory distress. Tapping or shaking the shoulders is used initially to determine unresponsiveness in someone who appears unconscious. Delivering chest or back slaps could jeopardize the child's now-patent airway. Because the obstruction has been relieved, there is no need to sweep the child's mouth. Additionally, blind finger sweeps are contraindicated because the object may be pushed further back, possibly causing a complete airway obstruction. (A)

The Client with Croup

54. **4.** This child is in severe respiratory distress with the potential for complete airway obstruction. The nurse should refrain from disturbing the child at this time to avoid irritating the epiglottis and causing it to completely obstruct the child's airway. The child may be intubated or undergo a tracheotomy. However, initially, the child should be kept as calm as possible with as little disruption as possible. Any attempt to restrain the child, draw blood, insert an I.V., or examine her throat could result in total airway obstruction. (A)

55. **1.** The toddler is exhibiting cold symptoms. A hoarse cough may be part of the upper respiratory tract infection. The best suggestion is to have the father offer the child additional fluids at frequent intervals to help keep secretions loose and membranes moist. There is no evidence presented to suggest that the child needs to be brought to the clinic immediately. Although having the father count the child's respiratory rate may provide some additional information, it may lead the father to suspect that something is seriously wrong, possibly leading to undue anxiety. A hot air vaporizer is not recommended. However, a cool mist vaporizer would cause vasoconstriction of the respiratory passages, making it easier for the child to breathe and loosening secretions. (A)

56. **2.** The nurse may be having difficulty calming the child because the child is experiencing increasing respiratory distress. The normal respiratory rate for a 21-month-old is 25 to 30 breaths/minute. The child's respiratory rate is 48 breaths/minute. Therefore the physician needs to be notified immediately. Typically, acetaminophen is not given to a child unless the temperature is 101° F (38.6° C) or higher. Letting the toddler cry is inappropriate with croup because crying increases respiratory distress. Offering fluids every few minutes to a toddler experiencing increasing respiratory distress would do little, if anything, to calm the child. Also, the child would have difficulty coordinating breathing and swallowing, possibly increasing the risk of aspiration. (A)

The Client with Bronchiolitis or Pharyngitis

57. **1, 2, 4.** Viral pharyngitis is treated with symptomatic, supportive therapy. Treatment includes use of a cool mist vaporizer, feeding a soft or liquid diet, and administration of acetaminophen for comfort. Viral infections do not respond to antibiotic administration. The child does not need to be on secretion precautions because viral pharyngitis is not contagious. (P)

58. **3.** In an infant with these symptoms, the first action by the nurse would be to obtain an oxygen saturation reading to determine how well the infant is oxygenating, which is valuable information for an infant with trouble breathing. Because the father probably can provide no other information, checking the heart rate would be the second action done by the nurse. Then the nurse would obtain the infant's weight. (R)

59. **3.** Based on the assessment findings of increased respiratory rate, retractions, and wheezing, this infant needs further evaluation, which could be obtained in an emergency department. Without a definitive diagnosis, administering a nebulizer treatment would be outside the nurse's scope of practice unless there was an order for such a treatment. Sending the infant for a radiograph may not be in the nurse's scope of practice. The findings need to be reported to a physician who can then determine whether or not a chest radiograph is warranted. The infant is exhibiting signs and symptoms of respiratory distress and is too ill to send out with just instructions on cold care for the mother. (A)

60. **1, 6.** An infant with bronchiolitis will have increased respirations and will tire more quickly, so it is best and easiest for the infant to take fluids more often in smaller amounts. The parents also would be instructed to watch for signs of increased difficulty breathing, which signal possible complications. Healthy infants and even those with bronchiolitis should sleep in the supine position. Calling the clinic for an episode of vomiting would not be necessary. However, the parents would be instructed to call if the infant cannot keep down any fluids for a period of more than 4 hours. Parents would not need to record how much the infant drinks. Chest physiotherapy is not indicated because it does not help and further irritates the infant. (C)

61. **4.** Handwashing is the best way to prevent respiratory illnesses and the spread of disease. Bronchiolitis, a viral infection primarily affecting the bronchioles, causes swelling and mucus accumulation of the lumina and subsequent hyperinflation of the lung with air trapping. It is transmitted primarily by direct contact with respiratory secretions as a result of eye-to-hand or nose-to-hand contact or from contaminated fomites. Therefore, handwashing minimizes the risk for transmission. Taking the child's temperature is not appropriate in most cases. As long as the child is getting better, taking the temperature will not be helpful. The mother's statement that she hopes she doesn't get a cold from her child does not indicate understanding of what to do after discharge. For most parents, listening to the child's chest would not be helpful because the parents would not know what they were listening for. Rather, watching for an increased respiratory rate, fever, or evidence of poor eating or drinking would be more helpful in alerting the parent to potential illness. (A)

The Child with Cardiovascular and Hematologic Health Problems

- The Client Undergoing a Cardiac Catheterization
- The Client with a Congenital Heart Defect
- The Client with Rheumatic Fever
- The Client with Kawasaki Disease
- The Client with Sickle Cell Anemia
- The Client with Iron Deficiency Anemia
- The Client with Hemophilia
- The Client with Leukemia
- Correct Answers and Rationales

The Client Undergoing a Cardiac Catheterization

1. Which of the following nursing diagnoses should the nurse identify as the priority for a 4-year-old child diagnosed with a ventricular septal defect who will be undergoing a cardiac catheterization?
- [ ] **1.** *Pain* related to the structural defect.
- [ ] **2.** *Deficient knowledge (parental)* related to cardiac catheterization.
- [ ] **3.** *Risk for infection* related to decreased oxygenation.
- [ ] **4.** *Decreased cardiac output* related to the structural defect.

2. When developing the plan of care for a 3-year-old child diagnosed with ventricular septal defect, the nurse should include actions that foster the development of which of the following psychosocial tasks according to Erikson?
- [ ] **1.** Autonomy versus shame and doubt.
- [ ] **2.** Identity versus role diffusion.
- [ ] **3.** Initiative versus guilt.
- [ ] **4.** Industry versus inferiority.

3. When teaching the parents of a child with a ventricular septal defect who is scheduled for a cardiac catheterization, the nurse explains that this procedure involves the use of which of the following?
- [ ] **1.** Ultra-high-frequency sound waves.
- [ ] **2.** Catheter placed in the right femoral vein.
- [ ] **3.** Cutdown procedure to place a catheter.
- [ ] **4.** General anesthesia.

4. When developing the discharge teaching plan for the parents of a child who has undergone a cardiac catheterization for ventricular septal defect, which of the following should the nurse expect to include?
- [ ] **1.** Restriction of the child's activities for the next 3 weeks.
- [ ] **2.** Use of sponge baths until the stitches are removed.
- [ ] **3.** Use of prophylactic antibiotics before receiving any dental work.
- [ ] **4.** Maintenance of a pressure dressing until a return visit with the physician.

The Client with a Congenital Heart Defect

5. An 18-month-old with a congential heart defect is to receive digoxin twice a day. The nurse should instruct the parents about which of the following?
- [ ] **1.** Digoxin enables the heart to pump more effectively with a slower and more regular rhythm.
- [ ] **2.** Signs of toxicity include loss of appetite, vomiting, increased pulse, and visual disturbances.
- [ ] **3.** Digoxin is absorbed better if taken with meals.
- [ ] **4.** If the child vomits within 15 minutes of administration, the dosage should be repeated.

6. Twelve hours after cardiac surgery on a 3-year-old, which of the following indicates a nursing intervention is required?
- [ ] **1.** Urinary output of 1 ml/kg of body weight per hour.
- [ ] **2.** Strong peripheral pulses in all four extremities.
- [ ] **3.** Fluctuation of fluid in the collection chamber of the chest drainage system.
- [ ] **4.** Alterations in level of consciousness, cool extremities, and mottling of the skin.

7. The nurse is transferring a child who has had open heart surgery from the pediatric intensive care unit to the pediatric unit. The child's blood pressure has been fluctuating but has been stable during the last two hours. The nurse from the pediatric intensive care unit should include which of the following information in the report to the nurse on the pediatric unit? Select all that apply.

☐ **1.** Medications being used.
☐ **2.** Current vital signs.
☐ **3.** Potential for blood pressure to drop.
☐ **4.** Drip rate for the intravenous infusion.
☐ **5.** Time of the most recent dose of pain medication.

8. A child diagnosed with tetralogy of Fallot becomes upset, crying and thrashing around when a blood specimen is obtained. The child's color becomes blue and the respiratory rate increases to 44 breaths/minute. Which of the following actions should the nurse do first?

☐ **1.** Obtain an order for sedation for the child.
☐ **2.** Assess for an irregular heart rate and rhythm.
☐ **3.** Explain to the child that it will only hurt for a short time.
☐ **4.** Place the child in a knee-to-chest position.

9. When teaching a preschool-age child how to perform coughing and deep-breathing exercises before corrective surgery for tetralogy of Fallot, which of the following teaching and learning principles should the nurse address first?

☐ **1.** Organizing information to be taught in a logical sequence.
☐ **2.** Arranging to use actual equipment for demonstrations.
☐ **3.** Building the teaching on the child's current level of knowledge.
☐ **4.** Presenting the information in order from simplest to most complex.

10. When planning care for a child before corrective surgery for tetralogy of Fallot, which of the following would the nurse identify as the priority nursing diagnosis?

☐ **1.** *Ineffective coping* related to upcoming surgery and complications.
☐ **2.** *Pain* related to surgical incision required to correct the defect.
☐ **3.** *Deficient knowledge* related to upcoming surgery and postoperative events.
☐ **4.** *Impaired gas exchange* related to structural cardiac defect.

11. When assessing a child after heart surgery to correct tetralogy of Fallot, which of the following should alert the nurse to suspect a low cardiac output?

☐ **1.** Bounding pulses and mottled skin.
☐ **2.** Altered level of consciousness and thready pulse.
☐ **3.** Capillary refill of 2 seconds and blood pressure of 96/67 mm Hg.
☐ **4.** Extremities warm to the touch and pale skin.

12. When developing the teaching plan for the parents of a child who has had open heart surgery to repair tetralogy of Fallot with a patch, which of the following should the nurse expect to include?

☐ **1.** Antibiotic therapy administration before any invasive procedures.
☐ **2.** Intake of at least 10 glasses of water per day before the next appointment.
☐ **3.** Need for frequent nap and rest periods for the first 4 weeks at home.
☐ **4.** Restriction of ingestion of bananas and citrus fruits.

13. Which of the following should the nurse expect to include in the plan of care for a child diagnosed with tetralogy of Fallot who has undergone corrective surgery?

☐ **1.** 2 to 3 g of sodium in the diet each day.
☐ **2.** Physical activity restrictions.
☐ **3.** Visits limited to a selected few.
☐ **4.** Assignment to an isolation room.

14. After surgery to correct tetralogy of Fallot, the child's parents express concern to the nurse that their 4-year-old child wants to be held more frequently than usual. The nurse interprets the child's behavioral response to stress as which of the following?

☐ **1.** Repression.
☐ **2.** Depression.
☐ **3.** Regression.
☐ **4.** Discomfort.

15. The mother of a child diagnosed with tetralogy of Fallot who is hospitalized tells the nurse that the child's 3-year-old sibling has become quiet and shy and demonstrates more than the usual amount of sexual curiosity since her other child has been hospitalized. The nurse responds to the mother based on the interpretation that these behaviors reflect which of the following?

☐ **1.** Usual behavior for a 3-year-old.
☐ **2.** Need for more attention.
☐ **3.** Exposure to a sexual experience.
☐ **4.** Indication of depression.

The Client with Rheumatic Fever

16. A 13-year-old has been admitted with a diagnosis of rheumatic fever and is on bed rest. He complains of a sore throat. His joints are painful and swollen. He has a red rash on his trunk and is experiencing aimless movements of his extremities. Use the chart below to determine what the nurse should do first.

☐ **1.** Report the heart rate to the physician.
☐ **2.** Apply lotion to the rash.
☐ **3.** Splint the joints to relieve the pain.
☐ **4.** Request an order for medication to treat the elevated temperature.

VITAL SIGNS

Time	8:00 am	12:00 noon
Temperature 104.0 / 102.2 / 100.4 / 98.6 / 96.8 / 95.0 / 93.2		
Respirations 30 / 25 / 20 / 15 / 10 / 5		
Apical heart rate 160 / 150 / 140 / 130 / 120 / 110 / 100 / 90		
Blood pressure 150 / 140 / 130 / 120 / 110 / 100 / 90 / 80		

17. A nurse is planning care for a 12-year-old with rheumatic fever. The nurse should teach the parents to:

☐ **1.** Observe the child closely.
☐ **2.** Allow the child to participate in activities that will not tire him.
☐ **3.** Provide for adequate periods of rest between activities.
☐ **4.** Encourage someone in the family to be with the child 24 hours a day.

18. A 12-year-old with rheumatic fever has a history of long-term aspirin use. Which of the following statements by the child indicates to the nurse that she should assess the child further?

☐ **1.** "I hear ringing in my ears."
☐ **2.** "Is it alright to put lotion on my itchy skin?"
☐ **3.** "My stomach hurts after I take those."
☐ **4.** "These pills make me cough."

19. Which of the following should the nurse expect to include in the plan of care for a child who is diagnosed with rheumatic fever and carditis and admitted to the hospital?

☐ **1.** Ensuring continuous parental presence at the child's bedside.
☐ **2.** Providing the child with periods of rest.
☐ **3.** Encouraging participation in age-appropriate activities.
☐ **4.** Advising the child to eat as much as possible.

20. Which of the following outcomes indicates that the activity restriction necessary for a 7-year-old child with rheumatic fever during the acute phase has been effective?

☐ **1.** Joints demonstrate absence of permanent injury.
☐ **2.** The resting heart rate is between 60 and 100 bpm.
☐ **3.** The child exhibits a decrease in chorea movements.
☐ **4.** The subcutaneous nodules over the joints are no longer palpable.

21. Which of the following initial physical findings would indicate the development of carditis in a child with rheumatic fever?

☐ **1.** Heart murmur.
☐ **2.** Low blood pressure.
☐ **3.** Irregular pulse.
☐ **4.** Anterior chest wall pain.

22. The physician orders pulse assessment several times through the night for a child with rheumatic fever who has a daytime heart rate of 120 bpm. The nurse explains to the mother that the primary reason for obtaining a sleeping pulse rate is to ensure that the elevation in the child's pulse rate is unrelated to which of the following?

☐ **1.** Morning dose of digitalis.
☐ **2.** Normal activity during waking hours.
☐ **3.** Warmer environment during the day than at night.
☐ **4.** Variations in pulse rates obtained during day and evening hours.

23. Which of following should the nurse perform to help alleviate a child's joint pain associated with rheumatic fever?

☐ **1.** Maintaining the joints in an extended position.
☐ **2.** Applying gentle traction to the child's affected joints.
☐ **3.** Supporting proper alignment with rolled pillows.
☐ **4.** Using a bed cradle to avoid the weight of bed linens on joints.

The Client with Kawasaki Disease

24. When developing the plan of care for a newly admitted 2-year-old child with the diagnosis of Kawasaki disease, which of the following should be the priority?
- [ ] 1. Taking vital signs every 6 hours.
- [ ] 2. Monitoring intake and output every hour.
- [ ] 3. Minimizing skin discomfort.
- [ ] 4. Providing passive range-of-motion exercises.

25. A child with Kawasaki disease is receiving low dose aspirin. The mother calls the clinic and states that the child has been exposed to influenza. Which recommendations should the nurse make? Select all that apply.
- [ ] 1. Increase fluid intake.
- [ ] 2. Stop the aspirin.
- [ ] 3. Keep the child home from school.
- [ ] 4. Watch for fever.
- [ ] 5. Weigh the child daily.

26. A 16-month-old child diagnosed with Kawasaki disease (KD) is very irritable, refuses to eat, and exhibits peeling skin on the hands and feet. Which of the following should the nurse interpret as the priority?
- [ ] 1. Applying lotion to the hands and feet.
- [ ] 2. Offering foods the toddler likes.
- [ ] 3. Placing the toddler in a quiet environment.
- [ ] 4. Encouraging the parents to get some rest.

27. Which of the following should the nurse include when completing discharge instructions for the parents of a 12-month-old child diagnosed with Kawasaki disease (KD) and being discharged to home?
- [ ] 1. Offer the child extra fluids every 2 hours for 2 weeks.
- [ ] 2. Take the child's temperature daily for several days.
- [ ] 3. Check the child's blood pressure daily until the follow-up appointment.
- [ ] 4. Call the physician if the irritability lasts for 2 more weeks.

The Client with Sickle Cell Anemia

28. A 14-year-old girl with sickle cell disease has her fourth hospitalization for sickle cell crisis. Her family is planning a ski vacation in the mountains. The nurse should:
- [ ] 1. Encourage them to go on the trip.
- [ ] 2. Go on the trip, but find a sitter for the 14-year-old.
- [ ] 3. Suggest the trip be postponed until next year.
- [ ] 4. Explain that the high altitude may cause a crisis.

29. The nurse is teaching the parents of a child with sickle cell disease. To instruct them on how to prevent sickle cell crisis, she should include which instruction?
- [ ] 1. Restrict the child's fluid intake to less than 1 quart per day.
- [ ] 2. Drink at least 2 quarts of fluids per day.
- [ ] 3. Stay away from other teenagers.
- [ ] 4. Avoid physical activity.

30. The nurse explains to the parents of a 1-year-old child admitted to the hospital in sickle cell crisis that the local tissue damage the child has on admission is caused by which of the following?
- [ ] 1. Autoimmune reaction complicated by hypoxia.
- [ ] 2. Lack of oxygen in the red blood cells.
- [ ] 3. Obstruction to circulation.
- [ ] 4. Elevated serum bilirubin concentration.

31. The mother asks the nurse why her child's hemoglobin was normal at birth but now the child has S hemoglobin. Which of the following responses by the nurse would be most appropriate?
- [ ] 1. "The placenta bars passage of the hemoglobin S from the mother to the fetus."
- [ ] 2. "The red bone marrow does not begin to produce hemoglobin S until several months after birth."
- [ ] 3. "Antibodies transmitted from you to the fetus provide the newborn with temporary immunity."
- [ ] 4. "The newborn has a high concentration of fetal hemoglobin in the blood for some time after birth."

32. Which of the following should the nurse identify as the priority nursing diagnosis during a toddler's vasoocclusive sickle cell crisis?
- [ ] 1. *Ineffective coping* related to presence of a life-threatening disease.
- [ ] 2. *Decreased cardiac output* related to abnormal hemoglobin formation.
- [ ] 3. *Pain* related to tissue anoxia.
- [ ] 4. *Excess fluid volume* related to infection.

The Client with Iron Deficiency Anemia

33. Which of the following actions indicates that the parents of a 12-month-old with iron deficiency anemia understand how to administer iron supplements? Select all that apply.
- [ ] 1. They administer iron supplements in combination with fruit juice.
- [ ] 2. They administer iron supplements with meals.
- [ ] 3. They report dark stools.
- [ ] 4. They brush the child's teeth after administering the iron supplements.
- [ ] 5. They decrease dietary intake of foods fortified with iron.

34. A mother asks the nurse if her child's iron deficiency anemia is related to the child's frequent infections. The nurse responds based on the understanding of which of the following?
- [ ] 1. Little is known about iron deficiency anemia and its relationship to infection in children.
- [ ] 2. Children with iron deficiency anemia are more susceptible to infection than are other children.
- [ ] 3. Children with iron deficiency anemia are less susceptible to infection than are other children.
- [ ] 4. Children with iron deficiency anemia are equally as susceptible to infection as are other children.

35. Which statements by the mother of a toddler should lead the nurse to suspect that the child is at risk for iron deficiency anemia? Select all that apply.
☐ 1. "He drinks over three cups of milk per day."
☐ 2. "I can't keep enough apple juice in the house; he must drink over 10 oz per day."
☐ 3. "He refuses to eat more than two different kinds of vegetables."
☐ 4. "He doesn't like meat, but he will eat small amounts of it."
☐ 5. "He sleeps 12 hours every night and takes a 2-hour nap."

36. Which of the following foods should the nurse encourage the mother to offer to her child with iron deficiency anemia?
☐ 1. Rice cereal, whole milk, and yellow vegetables.
☐ 2. Potato, peas, and chicken.
☐ 3. Macaroni, cheese, and ham.
☐ 4. Pudding, green vegetables, and rice.

The Client with Hemophilia

37. The physician has ordered several laboratory tests to help diagnose an infant's bleeding disorder. Which of the following tests, if abnormal, should the nurse interpret as most likely to indicate hemophilia?
☐ 1. Bleeding time.
☐ 2. Tourniquet test.
☐ 3. Clot retraction test.
☐ 4. Partial thromboplastin time (PTT).

38. A diagnosis of hemophilia A is confirmed in an infant. Which of the following instructions should the nurse provide the parents as the infant becomes more mobile and starts to crawl?
☐ 1. Administer one-half of a children's aspirin for a temperature higher than 101° F (38.3° C).
☐ 2. Sew thick padding into the elbows and knees of the child's clothing.
☐ 3. Check the color of the child's urine every day.
☐ 4. Expect the eruption of the primary teeth to produce moderate to severe bleeding.

39. Which of the following assessments in a child with hemophilia should lead the nurse to suspect early hemarthrosis?
☐ 1. Child's reluctance to move a body part.
☐ 2. Cool, pale, clammy extremity.
☐ 3. Ecchymosis formation around a joint.
☐ 4. Instability of a long bone on passive movement.

40. Because of the risks associated with administration of factor VIII concentrate, the nurse should teach the child's family to recognize and report which of the following?
☐ 1. Yellowing of the skin.
☐ 2. Constipation.
☐ 3. Abdominal distention.
☐ 4. Puffiness around the eyes.

41. The mother tells the nurse she will be afraid to allow her child with hemophilia to participate in sports because of the danger of injury and bleeding. After explaining that physical fitness is important for children with hemophilia, which of the following activities should the nurse suggest as ideal?
☐ 1. Snow skiing.
☐ 2. Swimming.
☐ 3. Basketball.
☐ 4. Gymnastics.

The Client with Leukemia

42. A 15-year-old has been admitted to the hospital with the diagnosis of acute lymphocytic leukemia. Which of the following signs and symptoms require the most immediate nursing intervention?
☐ 1. Fatigue and anorexia.
☐ 2. Fever and petechiae.
☐ 3. Swollen neck lymph glands and lethargy.
☐ 4. Enlarged liver and spleen.

43. A 12-year-old with leukemia is receiving cyclophosphamide (Cytoxan). The nurse should assess for the adverse effect of:
☐ 1. Photosensitivity.
☐ 2. Ataxia.
☐ 3. Cystitis.
☐ 4. Cardiac arrhythmias.

44. After teaching the parents of a child newly diagnosed with leukemia about the disease, which of the following descriptions given by the mother best indicates that she understands the nature of leukemia?
☐ 1. "The disease is an infection resulting in increased white blood cell production."
☐ 2. "The disease is a type of cancer characterized by an increase in immature white blood cells."
☐ 3. "The disease is an inflammation associated with enlargement of the lymph nodes."
☐ 4. "The disease is an allergic disorder involving increased circulating antibodies in the blood."

45. Laboratory findings indicate that a child with leukemia is also anemic. The nurse interprets this finding as most likely resulting from which of the following?
☐ 1. Inadequate dietary folic acid intake.
☐ 2. Decreased red blood cell production.
☐ 3. Increased destruction of red blood cells by lymphocytes.
☐ 4. Progressive replacement of bone marrow with scar tissue.

46. Which of the following statements should the nurse use to describe to the parents why their child with leukemia is at risk for infections?
☐ **1.** "Play activities are too strenuous."
☐ **2.** "Vitamin C intake is reduced over a period of time."
☐ **3.** "The number of red blood cells is inadequate for carrying oxygen."
☐ **4.** "Immature white blood cells are incapable of handling an infectious process."

47. Which of the following beverages should the nurse plan to give a child with leukemia if nausea should occur?
☐ **1.** Orange juice.
☐ **2.** Weak tea.
☐ **3.** Plain water.
☐ **4.** A carbonated beverage.

48. Which of the following medication orders to help relieve discomfort in a child with leukemia should the nurse question?
☐ **1.** Acetaminophen (Tylenol).
☐ **2.** Acetaminophen with codeine (Tylenol with Codeine).
☐ **3.** Ibuprofen (Motrin).
☐ **4.** Propoxyphene hydrochloride (Darvon).

49. After teaching a child with leukemia scheduled for a bone marrow aspiration about the procedure, the nurse determines that the teaching has been successful when the child identifies which of the following as the puncture site?
☐ **1.** Right lateral side of the right wrist.
☐ **2.** Middle of the chest.
☐ **3.** Distal end of the thigh.
☐ **4.** Back of the hipbone.

50. Which of the following nursing diagnoses should the nurse identify as the priority when dealing with a child newly diagnosed with leukemia and the child's family?
☐ **1.** *Risk for injury* related to malignant process.
☐ **2.** *Pain* related to treatment modalities.
☐ **3.** *Imbalanced nutrition: Less than body requirements* related to loss of appetite.
☐ **4.** *Anticipatory grieving* related to diagnosis and potential loss of child.

51. The nurse and parents are planning for the discharge of a child with leukemia who is receiving dactinomycin (actinomycin D) and vincristine (Oncovin). Which of the following should the nurse expect to teach the parents to do?
☐ **1.** Encourage increased fluid intake.
☐ **2.** Keep the child out of the sun.
☐ **3.** Monitor the child's heart rate.
☐ **4.** Observe the child for drowsiness.

52. After doing well for a period of time, a child with leukemia develops an overwhelming infection. The child's death is imminent. Which of the following statements offers the nurse the best guide in making plans to assist the parents in dealing with their child's imminent death?
☐ **1.** Knowing that the prognosis is poor helps prepare relatives for the death of children.
☐ **2.** Relatives are especially grieved when a child does well at first but then declines rapidly.
☐ **3.** Trust in health care personnel is most often destroyed by a death that is considered untimely.
☐ **4.** It is more difficult for relatives to accept the death of an older child than that of a toddler.

53. A 12-year-old with leukemia will be taking vincristine. The nurse should encourage the child to eat what kind of diet?
☐ **1.** High-residue.
☐ **2.** Low-residue.
☐ **3.** Low-fat.
☐ **4.** High-calorie.

54. A 10-year-old with leukemia is taking immunosuppressive drugs. The child should:
☐ **1.** Continue with her immunizations.
☐ **2.** Not receive any live attenuated vaccines.
☐ **3.** Receive vitamin and mineral supplements.
☐ **4.** Stay away from her peers.

55. A nurse is teaching the family of an 8-year-old boy with acute lymphocytic leukemia about appropriate activities. Which of the following activities should the nurse recommend?
☐ **1.** Home schooling.
☐ **2.** Restriction from participating in athletic activities.
☐ **3.** Avoiding trips to the shopping mall.
☐ **4.** Being treated as "normal" as much as possible.

Correct Answers and Rationales

The letter in parentheses after each rationale identifies the client need addressed in the item, including management of care (M), safety and infection control (S), health promotion and maintenance (H), psychosocial adaptation (P), basic care and comfort (C), pharmacological and parenteral therapies (D), reduction of risk potential (R), and physiological adaptation (A).

The Client Undergoing a Cardiac Catheterization

1. 2. Before the procedure, the child and family would need to know what cardiac catheterization is, what to expect, why it is being performed, and what care will be provided both before and after the procedure. *Deficient knowledge*, not *Decreased cardiac output*, is the priority. *Pain* might be a priority nursing diagnosis after the catheterization because the procedure is invasive. A 4-year-old child with a ventricular septal defect would not be at risk for infection related to decreased oxygenation. With this condition, blood flow increases through the pulmonary system, allowing the blood to become oxygenated before going on to the systemic circulation. (R)

2. 3. Erikson maintained that the chief psychosocial task of the preschool period is acquiring a sense of initiative. The child's activities center around energetic learning and seeking accomplishment and satisfaction in these activities. The conflict of guilt arises when the child oversteps the limits of abilities and behaves or acts inappropriately. Autonomy versus shame and doubt is the psychosocial task of toddlers. Identity versus role diffusion is the psychosocial task of early adolescents. Industry versus inferiority is the psychosocial task of school-age children. (H)

3. 2. In children, cardiac catheterization usually involves a right-sided approach because septal defects permit entry into the left side of the heart. The catheter is usually inserted into the femoral vein through a percutaneous puncture. Echocardiography involves the use of ultra-high-frequency sound waves. A cutdown procedure is rarely used. The catheterization is usually performed under local, not general, anesthesia with sedation. (R)

4. 3. Prophylactic antibiotics are suggested for children with heart defects before dental work is done to reduce the risk of bacterial infection. Typically, activities are not restricted after a cardiac catheterization. A percutaneous approach is used to insert the catheter, so stitches are not necessary. Showering or bathing is allowed as usual. The pressure dressing will be removed before the child is discharged. (R)

The Client with a Congenital Heart Defect

5. 1. Digoxin's effect is to slow the rate of the electrical conduction through the heart and increase the strength of the heart's contraction. Signs of toxicity include anorexia and decreased heart rate. Digoxin should be taken 1 hour before meals or 2 hours after meals in order to obtain better absorption of the drug. If the child vomits within 15 minutes of administration, the dose should not be repeated because it is not known how much of the medication has been absorbed. (P)

6. 4. Clinical signs of low cardiac output and poor tissue perfusion include pale, cool extremities; cyanosis or mottled skin; delayed capillary refill; weak, thready pulses; oliguria; and alterations in level of consciousness. An adequate urinary output for a child over 1 year should be 1 ml/kg/hour. Adequate urinary output is one indication of adequate cardiac output. Strong peripheral pulses indicate there is adequate circulation to the extremities and is one indication of adequate cardiac output. Drainage from the chest tubes should show fluctuation in the drainage compartment of the Pleur-Evac system. The fluid level normally fluctuates as proof that the apparatus is airtight. On about the third postoperative day, the fluctuation ceases indicating the lungs have fully expanded. (A)

7. 1, 2, 3, 4, 5. The report made when nurses are "handing off" a client from one nursing unit to another must include information about the condition of the client, potential for changes in the client's condition, current medications, and care and services received. (S)

8. 4. The child is experiencing a tet or hypoxic episode. Therefore the nurse should place the child in a knee-to-chest position. Flexing the legs reduces venous flow of blood from the lower extremities and reduces the volume of blood being shunted through the interventricular septal defect and the overriding aorta in the child with tetralogy of Fallot. As a result, the blood then entering the systemic circulation has a higher oxygen content, and dyspnea is reduced. Flexing the legs also increases vascular resistance and pressure in the left ventricle. An infant often assumes a knee-to-chest position in the crib, or the mother learns to put the infant over her shoulder while holding the child in a knee-to-chest position to relieve dyspnea. If this position is ineffective, then the child may need a sedative. Once the child is in the position, the nurse may assess for an irregular heart rate and rhythm. Explaining to the child that it will only hurt for a short time does nothing to alleviate the hypoxia. (A)

9. 3. Before developing any teaching program for a child, the nurse's first step is to assess the child to determine what is already known. Most older preschool children have some understanding of a condition present since birth. However, the child's interest will soon be lost if familiar material is repeated too often. The nurse can then organize the information in a sequence, because there are several steps to be demonstrated. These exercises do not require the use of equipment. The nurse should judge the amount and complexity of the information to be provided, based on the child's current knowledge and response to teaching. (A)

10. 3. When planning care for a child with tetralogy of Fallot who is to undergo corrective surgery, *Deficient knowledge* would be the priority nursing diagnosis. The child and parents would need to be prepared for what occurs before and after surgery. *Pain* would be a priority nursing diagnosis after surgery. However, pain management would be addressed in the preoperative period, with teaching to correct the knowledge deficit. The child with tetralogy of Fallot has experienced cyanosis from birth. Therefore, *Impaired gas exchange* would not be a priority diagnosis. (A)

11. 2. With a low cardiac output and subsequent poor tissue perfusion, signs and symptoms would include pale, cool extremities; cyanosis; weak, thready pulses; delayed capillary refill; and decrease in level of consciousness. (A)

12. **1.** Children who have undergone open heart surgery to repair tetralogy of Fallot with a patch as part of the correction are at risk for infections, specifically subacute bacterial endocarditis (SBE). Therefore the parents need instruction about SBE precautions, including the need for antibiotic therapy administration before any invasive procedure. Having the child drink a large amount of fluid before a follow-up appointment is not necessary. Also, too great a fluid intake could possibly lead to overload, increasing the workload of the heart. Children gear their rest schedule to their activities. Therefore, frequent rest and nap periods are not necessary. No evidence is provided to indicate that the child has a high serum potassium concentration that would necessitate the restriction of foods high in potassium, such as bananas and citrus fruits. (A)

13. **1.** Because of the hemodynamic changes that occur with open heart surgical repair, particularly with septal defects, transient congestive heart failure may develop. Therefore, the child's sodium intake typically is restricted to 2 to 3 g/day. Activity restrictions are inappropriate. Typically, the child is encouraged to walk in the halls of the unit. Visitors are not restricted unless the pediatric unit has restrictive visiting policies. The child can be placed in a room with other children who are not contagious. Placement in an isolation room is not warranted. After correction of the defect, the risk for infection in the child is the same as that for any postoperative client. (A)

14. **3.** The child's behavior suggests *regression*, defined as the act of moving backward. In psychology, the term is used to describe a person who reverts to an earlier stage of behavior or emotion. *Repression* is a defense mechanism by which an unacceptable or painful experience is put out of the conscious mind. For example, months later, the child does not recall having the surgery or being hospitalized. *Depression* is characterized by feelings of sadness, gloom, and dispiritedness, manifested by behaviors such as crying or whining. *Discomfort* is a negative feeling state often evidenced by squirming. (P)

15. **2.** The central psychosocial task for the preschool-age child is to develop a sense of initiative versus guilt, according to Erikson's theory. Any environmental change may affect a child. In this situation, the sibling is probably feeling less attention from the mother and is attempting to resolve the conflict with inappropriate behavior. Three-year-old children are usually active and outgoing; this behavior represents a change. Data are not sufficient to conclude that the child has been exposed to a sexual experience. Symptoms of depression include withdrawal and fatigue. (H)

The Client with Rheumatic Fever

16. **1.** The child's heart rate of 150 bpm is significantly above its rate at the time of his admission. The nurse must notify the physician. The increase in heart rate may indicate carditis, a possible complication of rheumatic fever

that can cause serious and life-long effects on the heart. The physician will intervene with medication and cardiac monitoring. While lotion may soothe the itching, the most important action for the nurse is to notify the physician of the increased heart rate. Splinting will not help the inflammation that is causing the painful joints. The painful joints migrate and will subside with time. The temperature is not elevated at this time, and does not require intervention. (A)

17. **3.** The nurse should teach the parents to provide for sufficient periods of rest to decrease the client's cardiac workload. The client's condition does not warrant close observation unless cardiac complications develop. The child's activity level will be based on the results of the sedimentation rate, c-reactive protein, heart rate, and cardiac function. The family does not need to be with the client 24 hours a day unless carditis develops and his condition deteriorates. (C)

18. **1.** Tinnitus is an adverse effect of prolonged aspirin use, and the child should be examined for hearing loss. Itchy skin commonly accompanies the rash typically associated with rheumatic fever and applying lotion would be appropriate. Aspirin taken on an empty stomach commonly causes abdominal discomfort. Coughing after ingesting aspirin can be caused by inadequate fluids during administration. (H)

19. **2.** The nurse should encourage and plan to provide periods of rest for the child with rheumatic fever and carditis to allow the heart to rest. The parents should be made to feel that they can come and go as they need to. The child is not in critical condition, so the parents do not need to be present at the child's bedside continuously. The child should be allowed to participate in nonstrenuous activities that avoid overtaxing the heart, thus allowing the heart time to rest. There is no reason to encourage the child to eat as much as possible; in fact, overeating should be discouraged because it taxes the heart muscle. (A)

20. **2.** During the acute phase of rheumatic fever, the heart is inflamed and every effort is made to reduce the work of the heart. Bedrest with limited activity is necessary to prevent heart failure. Therefore, the most reliable indicator that activity restriction has been effective is a resting heart rate between 60 and 100 bpm, normal for a 7-year-old child. No permanent damage to the joints occurs with rheumatic fever. The chorea movements associated with rheumatic fever are self-limited and usually disappear in 1 to 3 months. They are unrelated to activity restrictions. Subcutaneous nodules that occur over joint surfaces also resolve over time with no treatment. Therefore, they are not appropriate for evaluating the effectiveness of activity restrictions. (A)

21. **1.** In rheumatic fever, the connective tissue of the heart becomes inflamed, leading to carditis. The most common signs of carditis are heart murmurs, tachycardia during rest, cardiac enlargement, and changes in the electrical conductivity of the heart. Heart murmurs are present in about 75% of all clients during the first week of carditis and in 85% of clients by the third week. Signs of carditis do not include hypotension or chest pain. The client may have a rapid pulse, but it is usually not irregular. (A)

22. 2. An above-average pulse rate that is out of proportion to the degree of activity is an early sign of cardiac failure in a client with rheumatic fever. The sleeping pulse is used to determine whether mild tachycardia continues during sleep (inactivity) or whether it is the result of daytime activity. The environmental temperature would need to be quite warm before it could influence the heart rate. Digitalis lowers the heart rate, so the heart rate would be decreased during the daytime. (R)

23. 4. For a child with arthritis associated with rheumatic fever, the joints are usually so tender that even the weight of bed linens can cause pain. Use of a bed cradle is recommended to help remove the weight of the linens on painful joints. Joints need to be maintained in good alignment, not positioned in extension, to ensure that they remain functional. Applying gentle traction to the joints is not recommended because traction is usually used to relieve muscle spasms, not typically associated with rheumatic fever. Supporting the body in good alignment and changing the client's position are recommended, but these measures are not likely to relieve pain. (R)

The Client with Kawasaki Disease

24. 2. Cardiac status must be monitored carefully in the initial phase of KD because the child is at high risk for congestive heart failure (CHF). Therefore, the nurse needs to assess the child frequently for signs of CHF, which would include respiratory distress and decreased urine output. Vital signs would be obtained more often than every 6 hours because of the risk of CHF. Although minimizing skin discomfort would be important, it is does not take priority over monitoring the child's hourly intake and output. Passive range-of-motion exercises would be done if the child develops arthritis. (A)

25. 2, 4. Aspirin needs to be stopped because of its possible link to Reye's syndrome. Additionally, the parents need to watch for signs and symptoms of influenza. Children with influenza frequently present with fever, cold symptoms, and gastrointestinal symptoms. Increasing the child's fluid intake and weighing the child daily are not needed at this time because the child is not ill. Keeping the child home from school is not necessary, because the child is not ill and has already been exposed. (R)

26. 3. One of the characteristics of children with KD is irritability. They are often inconsolable. Placing the child in a quiet environment may help quiet the child and reduce the workload of the heart. Although peeling of the skin occurs with KD, the child's irritability takes priority over applying lotion to the hands and feet. Children with KD usually are not hungry and do not eat well regardless of what is served. There is no indication that the parents need rest.

Additionally, in this situation, the child takes priority over the parents. (A)

27. 2. The child's temperature should be taken daily for several days after discharge, because recurrent fever may develop. Offering the child fluids every 2 hours is not necessary. Doing so increases the child's risk for CHF. Checking the child's blood pressure at home usually is not included as part of the discharge instructions because, by the time of discharge, the child is considered stable and the risk for cardiac problems is minimal. Most children with KD recover fully. Irritability may last for 2 months after discharge. (A)

The Client with Sickle Cell Anemia

28. 4. High altitude causes deoxygenation, which might precipitate a crisis. In clients with sickle cell anemia, cells sickle when the client experiences any situation where increased demand for oxygen is needed, such as in an infection or dehydration, or when low oxygen concentration is experienced, such as in high altitudes or deep sea diving. Crises can commonly be prevented by maintaining hydration. It would be unsafe to encourage the family, or to say nothing about taking the client to high altitude areas, but giving the parents adequate information will allow them to make an appropriate decision. Postponing the trip or leaving the child at home does not address the immediate concern for the child's health. (H)

29. 2. Increasing fluid intake and being well hydrated will help prevent cell stasis in the small vessels. Restricting fluids causes stasis of red blood cells and promotes obstruction and increases the chance of sickling with hypoxia and pain to the part that is involved. Clients with sickle cell disease should stay away from others who have infections. When the spleen of a client who has sickle cell disease has become fibrotic and nonfunctional, the client is more susceptible to infections. Clients with sickle cell disease should not avoid physical activity as long as the client stays well hydrated. (H)

30. 3. Characteristic sickle cells tend to cause "log jams" in capillaries. This results in poor circulation to local tissues, leading to ischemia and necrosis. The basic defect in sickle cell disease is an abnormality in the structure of the red blood cells. The erythrocytes are sickle-shaped, rough in texture, and rigid. Sickle cell disease is an inherited disease, not an autoimmune reaction. Elevated serum bilirubin concentrations are associated with jaundice, not sickle cell disease. (A)

31. 4. Sickle cell disease is an inherited disease that is present at birth. However, 60% to 80% of a newborn's hemoglobin is fetal hemoglobin, which has a structure different from that of hemoglobin S or hemoglobin A. Sickle cell symptoms usually occur about 4 months after birth, when hemoglobin S begins to replace the fetal hemoglobin. The gene for sickle cell disease is transmitted at the time of conception, not passed through the placenta. Some hemoglobin S is produced by the fetus near term. The fetus produces all its own hemoglobin from the earliest production in the first trimester. Passive immunity conferred by maternal antibodies is not related to sickle cell disease, but this transmission of antibodies is important to protect the infant from various infections during early infancy. (A)

32. 3. For the child in sickle cell crisis, *Pain* is the priority nursing diagnosis because the sickled cells clump and obstruct the blood vessels, leading to occlusion and subsequent tissue ischemia. Although *Ineffective coping* may be important, it is not the priority. *Decreased cardiac output* is not a problem with this type of vasoocclusive crisis. Typically, a sickle cell crisis can be precipitated by a fluid volume deficit or dehydration. (A)

The Client with Iron Deficiency Anemia

33. 1, 4. Parent teaching concerning a child with iron deficiency anemia should include directions about giving iron combined with fruit juice, in divided doses, between meals, and with a dropper for a 12-month-old or through a straw for older toddlers. Iron stains teeth; so brushing the teeth and administering liquid iron through a dropper or straw are necessary to prevent staining the teeth. Iron should not be given with milk, antacids, or tea and should be administered on an empty stomach. Iron will cause the stool to become black or green, which is normal and does not need to be reported. However, light-colored stools indicate the iron is not being absorbed and should be reported. (P)

34. 2. Children with iron deficiency anemia are more susceptible to infection because of marked decreases in bone marrow functioning with microcytosis. (A)

35. 1, 2. Toddlers should have between two and three cups of milk per day and 8 oz of juice per day. If they have more than that, then they are probably not eating enough other foods, including iron-rich foods that have the needed nutrients. Food preferences vary among children. It is acceptable for the child to refuse foods as long as the diet is balanced and contains adequate calories. The child is obtaining a normal amount of sleep. (C)

36. 2. Potatoes, peas, chicken, green vegetables, and rice cereal contain significant amounts of iron and therefore would be recommended. Milk and yellow vegetables are not good iron sources. Rice by itself also is not a good source of iron. Macaroni, cheese, and ham are not high in iron. While pudding (made with fortified milk) and green vegetables contain some iron, the better diet has protein and iron from the chicken and potato. (A)

The Client with Hemophilia

37. 4. PTT measures the activity of thromboplastin, which is dependent on intrinsic clotting factors. In hemophilia, the intrinsic clotting factor VIII (antihemophilic factor) is deficient, resulting in a prolonged PTT. Bleeding time reflects platelet function; the tourniquet test measures vasoconstriction and platelet function; and the clot retraction test measures capillary fragility. All of these are unaffected in people with hemophilia. (R)

38. 2. As the hemophilic infant begins to acquire motor skills, the risk of bleeding increases because of falls and bumps. Such injuries can be minimized by padding vulnerable joints. Aspirin is contraindicated because of its antiplatelet properties, which increase the infant's risk for bleeding. Because genitourinary bleeding is not a typical problem in children with hemophilia, urine testing is not indicated. Although some bleeding may occur with tooth eruption, it does not normally cause moderate to severe bleeding episodes in children with hemophilia. (S)

39. 1. Bleeding into the joints in the child with hemophilia leads to pain and tenderness, resulting in restricted movement. Therefore, an early sign of hemarthrosis would be the child's reluctance to move a body part. If the bleeding into the joint continues, the area becomes hot, swollen, and immobile—not cool, pale, and clammy. Ecchymosis formation around a joint would be difficult to assess. Instability of a long bone on passive movement is not associated with joint hemarthrosis. (A)

40. 1. Because factor VIII concentrate is derived from large pools of human plasma, the risk of hepatitis is always present. Clinical manifestations of hepatitis include yellowing of the skin, mucous membranes, and sclera. Use of factor VIII concentrate is not associated with constipation, abdominal distention, or puffiness around the eyes. (D)

41. 2. Swimming is an ideal activity for a child with hemophilia because it is a noncontact sport. Many noncontact sports and physical activities that do not place excessive strain on joints are also appropriate. Such activities strengthen the muscles surrounding joints and help control bleeding in these areas. Noncontact sports also enhance general mental and physical well-being. Falls and subsequent injury to the child may occur with snow skiing. Basketball is a contact sport and therefore increases the child's risk for injury. Gymnastics is a very strenuous sport. Gymnasts frequently have muscle and joint injuries that result in bleeding episodes. (H)

The Client with Leukemia

42. 2. Fever and petechiae associated with acute lymphocytic leukemia indicate a suppression of normal white blood cells and thrombocytes by the bone marrow and put the client at risk for other infections and bleeding. The nurse should initiate infection control and safety precautions to reduce these risks. Fatigue is a common symptom of leukemia due to red blood cell suppression. Although the client should be told about the need for rest and meal planning, such teaching is not the priority intervention. Swollen glands and lethargy may be uncomfortable but they do not require immediate intervention. An enlarged liver and spleen do require safety precautions that prevent injury to the abdomen; however, these precautions are not the priority. (R)

43. 3. Cystitis is a potential adverse effect of cyclophosphamide. The client should be monitored for pain on urination. Photosensitivity, ataxia, and cardiac arrhythmias are not adverse effects associated with cyclophosphamide. (D)

44. 2. Leukemia is a neoplastic, or cancerous, disorder of blood-forming tissues that is characterized by a proliferation of immature white blood cells. Leukemia is not an infection, inflammation, or allergic disorder. (A)

45. 2. The anemia seen in children with leukemia is caused by the bone marrow's overproduction of immature white blood cells at the expense of producing red blood cells and platelets. In this client, anemia is not caused by an inadequate intake of iron but, rather, by insufficient red blood cells. The anemia is not caused by destruction of red blood cells by lymphocytes or by the replacement of bone marrow with scar tissue. (R)

46. 4. In leukemia, the number of normal white blood cells that are capable of fighting an infection is decreased. Although there is an increased number of immature white blood cells, they are unable to combat infection. Therefore, a child with leukemia is subject to infection. The major morbidity and mortality factor associated with leukemia is infection resulting from the presence of granulocytopenia. While increased activity may cause fatigue, it does not put the child at risk for infection. Vitamin C intake should not decrease if the child has adequate dietary intake. Decreased red blood cells are not directly caused by infection. (R)

47. 4. Carbonated beverages ordinarily are the best tolerated when a child feels nauseated. Many children find cola drinks especially easy to tolerate, but noncola beverages are also recommended. Orange juice usually is not tolerated well because of its high acid content. Tea may also be too acidic and many children do not like tea. Water does not relieve nausea. (R)

48. 3. Ibuprofen prolongs bleeding time and is contraindicated in clients with leukemia. Non-narcotic drugs other than ibuprofen or aspirin, such as acetaminophen (Tylenol), may be prescribed to control pain. Narcotic analgesics, such as acetaminophen with codeine or propoxyphene hydrochloride, may be required when pain is severe. (D)

49. 4. Although bone marrow specimens may be obtained from various sites, the most commonly used site in children is the posterior iliac crest, the back of the hip-bone. This area is close to the body's surface but removed from vital organs. The area is large, so specimens can easily be obtained. For infants, the proximal tibia and the posterior iliac crest are used. The middle of the chest or sternum is the usual site for bone marrow aspiration in an adult. The wrist, chest, and thigh are not sites from which to obtain bone marrow specimens. (R)

50. 4. Most commonly, the newly diagnosed child and parents are overwhelmed when first informed of the diagnosis. The family and child go through the beginning stages of grieving in anticipation of what may occur. The priority nursing diagnosis initially would be *Anticipatory grieving*. While the child may be at risk for injury or have a loss of appetite, the priority nursing diagnosis and care centers around the diagnosis of leukemia. (P)

51. 1. Dactinomycin and vincristine both cause nausea and vomiting. Oral fluids are encouraged, and antiemetics are given to prevent dehydration. Avoiding sun exposure is not necessary because photosensitivity is not associated with these drugs. Heart rate changes and drowsiness also are not associated with either of these two drugs. (D)

52. 2. It has been found that parents are more grieved when optimism is followed by defeat. The nurse should recognize this when planning various ways to help the parents of a dying child. It is not necessarily true that knowing about a poor prognosis for years helps prepare parents for a child's death. Death is still a shock when it occurs. Trust in health care personnel is not necessarily destroyed when a death is untimely if the family views the personnel as having done all that was possible. It is not more difficult for parents to accept the death of an older child than that of a younger child. (P)

53. 1. Vincristine may cause constipation, so the client should be encouraged to eat a high-residue (fiber) diet. The other diets do not help with constipation that can occur while receiving vincristine. (A)

54. 2. Children who are immunosuppressed should not receive any live attenuated vaccines. Clients who are immunosuppressed and are given live attenuated vaccines such as measles, mumps, rubella and oral polio vaccine can develop severe forms of the diseases for which they are being immunized, which can result in death. Inactivated vaccines may be given if necessary, but the client is not able to adequately produce needed antibodies and it is recommended that immunizations be delayed for 3 months after the immunosuppressive drugs have be discontinued. Vitamin and mineral supplements are not normally given in conjunction with immunosuppressive drugs. When the client is immunosuppressed, the client should avoid only persons who have an infection. (H)

55. 4. Any child with a chronic illness should be treated as normally as possible. Unless the child has severe bone marrow depression, he should be allowed to go to school with others and can go to the mall. If the child is in remission, athletic activities are allowed. (H)

The Child with Health Problems of the Upper Gastrointestinal Tract

The Client with Cleft Lip and Palate

1. What is the priority order for immediate nursing care following surgery for a child born with cleft lip?

| 1. Maintaining a clear and adequate airway. |

| 2. Maintaining sufficient fluid and caloric intake. |

| 3. Providing emotional comfort to the child. |

| 4. Applying elbow restraints. |

| 5. Teaching the parents proper feeding methods. |

| |

| |

| |

| |

| |

2. When developing the plan of care for an infant with a cleft lip before corrective surgery is performed, which of the following should be a priority?
- ☐ **1.** Maintaining skin integrity in the oral cavity.
- ☐ **2.** Using techniques to minimize crying.
- ☐ **3.** Altering the usual method of feeding.
- ☐ **4.** Preventing the infant from putting fingers in the mouth.

3. Which of the following measures would be most effective in helping the infant with a cleft lip and palate to retain oral feedings?
- ☐ **1.** Burp the infant at frequent intervals.
- ☐ **2.** Feed the infant small amounts at one time.
- ☐ **3.** Place the end of the nipple far to the back of the infant's tongue.
- ☐ **4.** Maintain the infant in a lying position while feeding.

4. When teaching the mother of an infant who has undergone surgical repair of a cleft lip how to care for the suture line, the nurse demonstrates how to remove formula and drainage. Which of the following solutions should the nurse use?
- ☐ **1.** Mouthwash.
- ☐ **2.** Povidone-iodine (Betadine) solution.
- ☐ **3.** A mild antiseptic solution.
- ☐ **4.** Half-strength hydrogen peroxide.

5. After teaching the parent of an infant who has had a surgical repair for a cleft lip about the use of elbow restraints at home, the nurse determines that the teaching has been successful when the parent states which of the following?
- ☐ **1.** "We will keep the restraints on continuously except when checking the skin under them for redness."
- ☐ **2.** "We will keep the restraints on during the day while he is awake, but take them off when we put him to bed at night."
- ☐ **3.** "After we get home, we won't have to use the restraints because our child does not suck on his hands or fingers."
- ☐ **4.** "We will be sure to keep the restraints on all the time until we come to see the physician for a follow-up visit."

6. The parent of an infant with a cleft lip and palate asks the nurse when the infant's cleft palate will be repaired. The nurse responds by stating that the first repair of a cleft palate is usually done at which of the following times?
☐ **1.** Before the eruption of teeth.
☐ **2.** When the child weighs approximately 10 kg (22 lb).
☐ **3.** Before the development of speech.
☐ **4.** After the child learns to drink from a cup.

7. On the second postoperative day after repair of a cleft palate, which of the following should the nurse expect as most appropriate to use with a toddler?
☐ **1.** Cup.
☐ **2.** Straw.
☐ **3.** Rubber-tipped syringe.
☐ **4.** Large-holed nipple.

8. Immediately on return to the nursing unit after surgical repair of a cleft palate, in which of the following positions should the nurse place the child?
☐ **1.** On the back with the head in a position of comfort.
☐ **2.** In low Fowler's position with the head turned to the side.
☐ **3.** Lying on the abdomen with the head turned to the side.
☐ **4.** In reverse Trendelenburg with the head tilted forward.

The Client with Tracheoesophageal Fistula

9. The nurse notices that a 1-day-old girl is having an increased number of drooling and choking episodes with excessive amounts of mucus and cyanotic episodes, especially after feeding. Which disorder does the nurse suspect?
☐ **1.** Gastroesophageal reflux.
☐ **2.** A tracheoesophageal fistula (TEF).
☐ **3.** Bronchopulmonary dysplasia.
☐ **4.** Hydrocephalus.

10. The parents of a child with a tracheoesophageal fistula express feelings of guilt about their baby's anomaly. Which of the following approaches by the nurse would best support the parents?
☐ **1.** Helping the parents accept their feelings as a normal reaction.
☐ **2.** Explaining that the parents did nothing to cause the newborn's defect.
☐ **3.** Encouraging the parents to concentrate on planning their baby's care.
☐ **4.** Urging the parents to visit their newborn as often as possible.

11. After teaching the parents of a neonate diagnosed with a tracheoesophageal fistula (TEF) about this anomaly, the nurse determines that the teaching was successful when the father describes the condition as which of the following?
☐ **1.** "The muscle below the stomach is too tight, causing the baby to vomit forcefully."
☐ **2.** "There is a blind upper pouch and an opening from the esophagus into the airway."
☐ **3.** "The lower bowel is lacking certain nerves to allow normal function."
☐ **4.** "A part of the bowel is on the outside without anything covering it."

12. Which of the following nursing diagnoses should the nurse identify as a priority for the infant with a tracheoesophageal fistula (TEF) ?
☐ **1.** *Impaired parenting* related to newborn's illness.
☐ **2.** *Risk for injury* related to increased potential for aspiration.
☐ **3.** *Ineffective breathing pattern* related to a weak diaphragm.
☐ **4.** *Imbalanced nutrition: less than body requirements* related to poor sucking ability.

13. Which of the following would indicate that an infant with a tracheoesophageal fistula (TEF) needs suctioning?
☐ **1.** Brassy cough.
☐ **2.** Substernal retractions.
☐ **3.** Decreased activity level.
☐ **4.** Increased respiratory rate.

14. When administering gastrostomy feedings to an infant after surgery to correct a tracheoesophageal fistula (TEF) , which of the following would be most appropriate to prevent air from entering the stomach once the syringe barrel is attached to the gastrostomy tube?
☐ **1.** Unclamp the tube after pouring the complete amount of formula to be administered into the syringe barrel.
☐ **2.** Pour all of the formula to be administered into the syringe barrel after opening the clamp.
☐ **3.** Maintain a continuous flow of formula down the side of the syringe barrel once the clamp is opened.
☐ **4.** Allow a small amount of formula to enter the stomach before pouring more formula into the syringe barrel.

15. After surgery to repair a tracheoesophageal fistula, an infant receives gastrostomy tube feedings. After feeding the infant by this method, the nurse cradles and rocks the infant for about 15 minutes, primarily to help accomplish which of the following?
☐ **1.** Promote intestinal peristalsis.
☐ **2.** Prevent regurgitation of formula.
☐ **3.** Relieve pressure on the surgical site.
☐ **4.** Associate eating with a pleasurable experience.

16. A newborn who had a surgical repair of a tracheo-esophageal fistula (TEF) is started on oral feedings. Which of the following should the nurse include in the teaching plan for the mother about oral feedings?
☐ **1.** They are better tolerated when small, frequent feedings are offered.
☐ **2.** They should be offered on a feeding schedule to help the infant accept the feedings more readily.
☐ **3.** They are best accepted by the infant when offered by the same nurse or by the infant's mother.
☐ **4.** They are best planned in conjunction with observations of the infant's behavior.

The Client with an Anorectal Anomaly

17. A newborn with the diagnosis of imperforate anus is to be scheduled for a radiographic examination. The nurse explains to the parents that this examination is done to determine the distance between the anal dimple and which of the following?
☐ **1.** Perineum.
☐ **2.** Closed end of the rectum.
☐ **3.** Colon.
☐ **4.** Rectovesical pouch.

18. Which of the following might the nurse assess in a newborn diagnosed with an anorectal malformation? Select all that apply.
☐ **1.** Abdominal distension.
☐ **2.** Loose stools.
☐ **3.** Vomiting.
☐ **4.** Meconium in the urine.
☐ **5.** Meconium stools.

19. While caring for a neonate with an imperforate anus, the nurse assesses the neonate's urine output for which of the following?
☐ **1.** Meconium.
☐ **2.** Blood.
☐ **3.** Bile.
☐ **4.** Acetone.

20. After teaching the mother of a neonate who has successfully undergone surgery to repair a low anorectal anomaly, the mother indicates that she understands her child's prognosis when she states which of the following?
☐ **1.** "My child will need to wear protective pads until puberty."
☐ **2.** "My child will need extra fluids to prevent constipation."
☐ **3.** "My child will probably always need a high-fiber diet."
☐ **4.** "My child has a good chance of being potty trained."

21. When the infant returns to the unit after imperforate anus repair, the nurse should place the infant in which of the following positions?
☐ **1.** On the abdomen, with legs pulled up under the body.
☐ **2.** On the back, with legs extended straight out.
☐ **3.** Lying on the side with the hips elevated.
☐ **4.** Lying on the back in a position of comfort.

22. The father of a neonate scheduled for gastrointestinal surgery asks the nurse how newborns respond to painful stimuli. Which of the following should be the nurse's best response?
☐ **1.** "Newborns cry and cannot be distracted to stop crying."
☐ **2.** "When faced with a pain, newborns try to roll away from it."
☐ **3.** "Newborns typically move their whole body in response to pain."
☐ **4.** "Pain causes the newborn to withdraw the affected part."

23. When developing the plan of care for a neonate who was diagnosed with an anorectal malformation and who subsequently underwent surgery, which of the following would be most helpful in facilitating parent–infant bonding?
☐ **1.** Explaining to the parents that they can visit at any time.
☐ **2.** Encouraging the parents to hold their infant.
☐ **3.** Asking the parents to help monitor the infant's intake and output.
☐ **4.** Helping the parents plan for their infant's discharge.

The Client with Pyloric Stenosis

24. A 4-week-old infant admitted with the diagnosis of hypertrophic pyloric stenosis presents with a history of vomiting. The nurse should anticipate that the infant's vomitus would contain gastric contents and which of the following?
☐ **1.** Bile and streaks of blood.
☐ **2.** Mucus and bile.
☐ **3.** Mucus and streaks of blood.
☐ **4.** Stool and bile.

25. An infant is admitted to the pediatric unit with a diagnosis of hypertrophic pyloric stenosis after vomiting for several days. Which of the following nursing diagnoses should be the priority?
☐ **1.** *Deficient fluid volume* related to prolonged vomiting.
☐ **2.** *Ineffective airway clearance* related to impaired swallowing.
☐ **3.** *Imbalanced nutrition: Less than body requirements* related to prolonged vomiting.
☐ **4.** *Bowel incontinence* related to abdominal pain.

26. When an infant with pyloric stenosis is admitted to the hospital, which of the following should the nurse do first?
☐ **1.** Weigh the infant.
☐ **2.** Begin an intravenous infusion.
☐ **3.** Switch the infant to an oral electrolyte solution.
☐ **4.** Orient the mother to the hospital unit.

27. After teaching the mother of an infant with pyloric stenosis about the disease, which of the following, if stated by the mother as a cause, indicates effective teaching?
☐ **1.** "An enlarged muscle below the stomach sphincter."
☐ **2.** "A telescoping of the large bowel into the smaller bowel."
☐ **3.** "A result of giving the baby more formula than is necessary."
☐ **4.** "A result of my baby taking the formula too quickly."

28. Fluid replacement therapy is ordered for an infant diagnosed with pyloric stenosis. In addition to dextrose, water, and sodium chloride, which of the following should the nurse anticipate the physician to order as an additive to the intravenous solution?
☐ **1.** Calcium chloride.
☐ **2.** Bicarbonate chloride.
☐ **3.** Potassium chloride.
☐ **4.** Magnesium chloride.

29. When developing the plan of care for an infant with pyloric stenosis, the nurse identifies a nursing diagnosis of *Deficient fluid volume* related to prolonged vomiting. Which of the following parameters should the nurse expect to use when evaluating the client outcome?
☐ **1.** Abdominal distention.
☐ **2.** Weight loss.
☐ **3.** Vomiting.
☐ **4.** Respiratory effort.

30. After undergoing surgical correction of pyloric stenosis, an infant is returned to the room in stable condition. While standing by the crib, the mother says, "Perhaps if I had brought my baby to the hospital sooner, the surgery could have been avoided." Which of the following should be the nurse's best response?
☐ **1.** "Surgery is the most effective treatment for pyloric stenosis."
☐ **2.** "Try not to worry; your baby will be fine."
☐ **3.** "Do you feel that this problem indicates that you are not a good mother?"
☐ **4.** "Do you think that earlier hospitalization could have avoided surgery?"

31. After surgery to correct pyloric stenosis, the nurse instructs the parents about the postoperative feeding schedule for their infant. The parents exhibit understanding of these instructions when they state that they can start feeding the child within which of the following time frames?
☐ **1.** 6 hours.
☐ **2.** 8 hours.
☐ **3.** 10 hours.
☐ **4.** 12 hours.

32. Immediately after the first oral feeding after corrective surgery for pyloric stenosis, a 4-week-old infant is fussy and restless. Which of the following actions would be most appropriate at this time?
☐ **1.** Encourage the parents to hold the infant.
☐ **2.** Hang a mobile over the infant's crib.
☐ **3.** Give the infant more to eat.
☐ **4.** Give the infant a pacifier to suck on.

33. Which of the following behaviors exhibited by the parents of an infant with pyloric stenosis should the nurse correctly interpret as a positive indication of parental coping?
☐ **1.** Telling the nurse that they have to get away for a while.
☐ **2.** Discussing the infant's care realistically.
☐ **3.** Repeatedly asking if their child is normal.
☐ **4.** Exhibiting fear that they will disturb the infant.

The Client with Intussusception

34. When assessing a 4-month-old infant diagnosed with possible intussusception, the nurse should expect the mother to relate which of the following about the infant's crying and episodes of pain?
☐ **1.** Constant accompanied by leg extension.
☐ **2.** Intermittent with knees drawn to the chest.
☐ **3.** Shrill during ingestion of solids.
☐ **4.** Intermittent while being held in the mother's arms.

35. When obtaining the nursing history from the mother of an infant with suspected intussusception, which of the following questions would be most helpful?
☐ **1.** "What do the stools look like?"
☐ **2.** "When was the last time your child urinated?"
☐ **3.** "Is your child eating normally?"
☐ **4.** "Has your child had any episodes of vomiting?"

36. A nasogastric tube inserted during surgery to correct an infant's intussusception is no longer freely removing gastric secretions. Which of the following should the nurse do next?
☐ 1. Aspirate the tube with a syringe.
☐ 2. Irrigate the tube with distilled water.
☐ 3. Increase the level of suction.
☐ 4. Rotate the tube.

37. Which of the following assessments should be the priority for an infant who has had surgery to correct an intussusception and is now at risk for development of a paralytic ileus postoperatively?
☐ 1. Measurement of urine specific gravity.
☐ 2. Auscultation of bowel sounds.
☐ 3. Inspection of the first stool passed.
☐ 4. Measurement of gastric output.

38. An infant is to be discharged after surgery for intussusception. Which of the following would the nurse expect to include in the discharge teaching plan for the mother?
☐ 1. The infant will experience a change in the normal home routine.
☐ 2. The infant can return to the prehospital routine immediately.
☐ 3. The infant needs to ingest more calories at home than what was consumed in the hospital.
☐ 4. The infant will continue to experience abdominal cramping for a few days.

The Client with Inguinal Hernia

39. When assessing an infant with suspected inguinal hernia, which of the following findings would be most significant?
☐ 1. The inguinal swelling is reddened, and the abdomen is distended.
☐ 2. The infant is irritable, and a thickened spermatic cord is palpable.
☐ 3. The inguinal swelling can be reduced, and the infant has a stool in the diaper.
☐ 4. The infant's diaper is wet with urine, and the abdomen is nontender.

40. The physician is able to reduce an infant's hernia and schedules the infant for a herniorrhaphy in 2 days. The mother asks the nurse why the surgery is not performed now. Which of the following responses indicates that the nurse understands the rationale for delaying the surgery?
☐ 1. "Delaying the surgery ensures that your infant will receive the proper preoperative preparation."
☐ 2. "We need to make sure that your infant receives nothing by mouth for at least 24 hours before the surgery."
☐ 3. "Waiting these 2 days helps to allow any edema and inflammation in the area to subside."
☐ 4. "Your infant needs to wear a truss for at least 24 hours before any surgery can be attempted."

41. Preoperatively, the nurse develops a plan to prepare a 7-month-old infant psychologically for a scheduled herniorrhaphy the next day. Which of the following should the nurse expect to implement to accomplish this goal?
☐ 1. Explaining the preoperative and postoperative procedures to the mother.
☐ 2. Having the mother stay with the infant.
☐ 3. Making sure the infant's favorite toy is available.
☐ 4. Allowing the infant to play with surgical equipment.

42. Which of the following instructions should the nurse expect to include in the discharge teaching plan for the parent of an infant who has had an inguinal herniorrhaphy?
☐ 1. Change diapers as soon as they become soiled.
☐ 2. Apply an abdominal binder.
☐ 3. Keep the incision covered with a sterile dressing.
☐ 4. Restrain the infant's hands.

43. A mother asks, "How should I bathe my baby now that he's had surgery for his inguinal hernia?" Which of the following instructions should the nurse give the mother?
☐ 1. "Clean his face and diaper area for 2 weeks."
☐ 2. "Use sterile sponges to cleanse the inguinal incision."
☐ 3. "Give him a sponge bath daily for 1 week."
☐ 4. "Give the infant full tub baths every day."

44. A male adolescent who underwent repair of an inguinal hernia earlier today and is getting ready to go home receives instructions about resuming physical activities. Which of the following statements would indicate that he has understood the instructions?
☐ 1. "I can start riding my bike next week."
☐ 2. "I have to skip physical education classes for 2 weeks."
☐ 3. "I can start wrestling again in 3 weeks."
☐ 4. "I can return to my weight-lifting class in 2 weeks."

The Client with Hirschsprung's Disease

45. During physical assessment of a 4-month-old infant with Hirschsprung's disease, the nurse should most likely note which of the following?
☐ **1.** Scaphoid-shaped abdomen.
☐ **2.** Weight less than expected for height and age.
☐ **3.** Cyanosis of the fingers and toes.
☐ **4.** Hyperactive deep tendon reflexes.

46. An infant diagnosed with Hirschsprung's disease is scheduled to receive a temporary colostomy. When initially discussing the diagnosis and treatment with the parents, which of the following would be most appropriate?
☐ **1.** Assessing the adequacy of their coping skills.
☐ **2.** Reassuring them that their child will be fine.
☐ **3.** Encouraging them to ask questions.
☐ **4.** Giving them printed material on the procedure.

47. After teaching the parents of an infant diagnosed with Hirschsprung's disease, the nurse determines that the parents understand the diagnosis when the father states which of the following?
☐ **1.** "There is no rectal opening for stool to pass."
☐ **2.** "There is a tube between the trachea and esophagus."
☐ **3.** "The nerves at the end of the large colon are missing."
☐ **4.** "The muscle below the stomach is too tight."

48. When developing the preoperative plan of care for an infant with Hirschsprung's disease, which of the following should the nurse expect to include?
☐ **1.** Administering a tap water enema.
☐ **2.** Inserting a gastrostomy tube.
☐ **3.** Restricting oral intake to clear liquids.
☐ **4.** Using povidone-iodine solution to prepare the perineum.

49. The nurse is showing the parent of a child with Hirschsprung's disease where the aganglionic area is located. Identify the area the nurse should point out as being aganglionic.

50. An infant diagnosed with Hirschsprung's disease undergoes surgery with the creation of a temporary colostomy. Which of the following statements by the mother about her child's colostomy indicates the need for further teaching?
☐ **1.** "My child should be able to care for the colostomy by the time he's 8 years old."
☐ **2.** "The colostomy will give the intestine time to shrink to its normal size."
☐ **3.** "The colostomy may include two separate abdominal openings."
☐ **4.** "Right after the procedure, the stoma will appear small and purple."

51. When teaching the mother of an infant who has received a temporary colostomy for treatment of Hirschsprung's disease about how the stoma should normally appear, which of the following descriptions about the stoma's appearance should the nurse include in the teaching?
☐ **1.** Becoming dark brown in 2 months.
☐ **2.** Staying deep red in color.
☐ **3.** Changing to several shades of pink.
☐ **4.** Turning almost purple in color.

52. When teaching the parent of an infant with Hirschsprung's disease who received a temporary colostomy about the types of foods the infant will be able to eat, which of the following would the nurse recommend?
☐ **1.** High-fiber diet.
☐ **2.** Low-fat diet.
☐ **3.** High-residue diet.
☐ **4.** Regular diet.

53. Eight hours ago, an infant with Hirschsprung's disease had surgery to create a colostomy. Which of the following findings should alert the nurse to notify the physician immediately?
☐ **1.** A 3-cm increase in abdominal circumference.
☐ **2.** Periods of occasional fussiness.
☐ **3.** Absence of bowel sounds since surgery.
☐ **4.** Evidence of the infant's returning appetite.

54. An infant with Hirschsprung's disease is to be discharged 1 or 2 days after surgery to create a colostomy. After teaching the infant's parents about the overall effects of their infant's surgery, the nurse determines that the teaching has been effective when the parents state which of the following?
☐ **1.** "His abdomen will be large for awhile."
☐ **2.** "When he's ready, toilet training may be difficult."
☐ **3.** "We need to limit his intake of dairy products."
☐ **4.** "We will give him vitamin supplements until he is an adolescent."

The Client with Diarrhea, Gastroenteritis, or Dehydration

55. A mother brings her 3-month-old child into the emergency department. The child is listless with dry mucous membranes, tenting of the skin on the forehead, a depressed fontanel, and a history of vomiting and diarrhea for the last 36 hours. In what order of priority should the nurse intervene?

| 1. Obtain vital signs and weight. |
| 2. Insert an I.V. and infuse fluids as ordered. |
| 3. Apply a urine collection bag. |
| 4. Draw blood for laboratory tests. |

| |
| |
| |
| |

56. A child is admitted with a tentative diagnosis of shigella. The nurse should do which of the following? Select all that apply.
☐ 1. Assess the child for nausea and vomiting.
☐ 2. Collect a stool specimen for white blood cells (WBCs).
☐ 3. Place the child on strict isolation.
☐ 4. Monitor the child for signs and symptoms of dehydration.
☐ 5. Initiate an intake and output record.

57. Which of the following would most likely alert the nurse to the possibility that a preschooler is experiencing moderate dehydration?
☐ 1. Deep, rapid respirations.
☐ 2. Diaphoresis.
☐ 3. Absence of tear formation.
☐ 4. Decreased urine specific gravity.

58. Which of the following would be an important assessment finding for an 8-month-old infant admitted with severe diarrhea?
☐ 1. Absent bowel sounds.
☐ 2. Pale yellow urine.
☐ 3. Normal skin elasticity.
☐ 4. Depressed anterior fontanel.

59. Which of the following would be the best activity for the nurse to include in the plan of care for an infant experiencing severe diarrhea?
☐ 1. Monitoring the total 8-hour formula intake.
☐ 2. Weighing the infant each day.
☐ 3. Checking the anterior fontanel every shift.
☐ 4. Monitoring abdominal skin turgor every shift.

60. The physician orders an intravenous infusion of 5% dextrose in 0.25 normal saline to be infused at 2 ml/kg/hour in an infant who weighs 9 lb. How many milliliters per hour of the solution should the nurse infuse? Round to one decimal.

_____ ml/hour

61. Which of the following would be most appropriate for the nurse to teach the mother of a 6-month-old infant hospitalized with severe diarrhea to help her comfort her infant who is fussy?
☐ 1. Offering a pacifier.
☐ 2. Placing a mobile above the crib.
☐ 3. Sitting at crib side talking to the infant.
☐ 4. Turning the television on to cartoons.

62. Which of the following nursing diagnoses would be appropriate for the nurse to identify as a priority diagnosis for an infant just admitted to the hospital with a diagnosis of gastroenteritis?
☐ 1. *Pain* related to repeated episodes of vomiting.
☐ 2. *Deficient fluid volume* related to excessive losses from severe diarrhea.
☐ 3. *Impaired parenting* related to infant's loss of fluid.
☐ 4. *Impaired urinary elimination* related to increased fluid intake feeding pattern.

63. Which of the following should the nurse use to determine achievement of the expected outcome for an infant with severe diarrhea and a nursing diagnosis of *Deficient fluid volume* related to passage of profuse amounts of watery diarrhea?
☐ 1. Moist mucous membranes.
☐ 2. Passage of a soft, formed stool.
☐ 3. Absence of diarrhea for a 4-hour period.
☐ 4. Ability to tolerate intravenous fluids well.

64. Which of the following should the nurse include when teaching the father of an infant just admitted with gastroenteritis about initial treatment for his infant?
☐ 1. The infant will receive no liquids by mouth.
☐ 2. Intravenous antibiotics will be started.
☐ 3. The infant will be placed in a mist tent.
☐ 4. An iron-fortified formula will be used.

65. The nurse teaches the father of an infant hospitalized with gastroenteritis about the next step of the treatment plan once the infant's condition has been controlled. The nurse should determine that the father understands when he explains that which of the following will occur with his infant?
☐ **1.** The infant will receive clear liquids for a period of time.
☐ **2.** Formula and juice will be offered.
☐ **3.** Blood will be drawn daily to test for anemia.
☐ **4.** The infant will be allowed to go to the playroom.

66. The mother of a toddler who has just been admitted with severe dehydration secondary to gastroenteritis says that she cannot stay with her child because she has to take care of her other children at home. Which of the responses by the nurse would be most appropriate?
☐ **1.** "You really shouldn't leave right now. Your child is very sick."
☐ **2.** "I understand, but feel free to visit or call anytime to see how your child is doing."
☐ **3.** "It really isn't necessary to stay with your child. We'll take very good care of him."
☐ **4.** "Can you find someone to stay with your children? Your child needs you here."

67. A child is admitted to the pediatric unit with the diagnosis of severe gastroenteritis. Which of the following would be most appropriate for the nurse to do?
☐ **1.** Institute standard precautions.
☐ **2.** Place the child in a semiprivate room.
☐ **3.** Use regular eating utensils.
☐ **4.** Single-bag all linens.

68. A 9-month-old is admitted because of dehydration. How should the nurse go about accurately monitoring fluid intake and output? Select all that apply.
☐ **1.** Weighing and recording all wet diapers.
☐ **2.** Obtaining a urine specific gravity measure.
☐ **3.** Obtaining an accurate daily weight.
☐ **4.** Restricting fluids prior to weighing the child.
☐ **5.** Obtaining an accurate stool count.

69. The physician orders intravenous fluid replacement therapy with potassium chloride to be added for a child with severe gastroenteritis. Before adding the potassium chloride to the intravenous fluid, which of the following assessments would be most important?
☐ **1.** Ability to void.
☐ **2.** Passage of stool today.
☐ **3.** Baseline electrocardiogram.
☐ **4.** Serum calcium level.

70. Which of the following would first alert the nurse to suspect that a child with severe gastroenteritis who has been receiving intravenous therapy for the past several hours may be developing circulatory overload?
☐ **1.** A drop in blood pressure.
☐ **2.** Change to slow, deep respirations.
☐ **3.** Auscultation of moist crackles.
☐ **4.** Marked increase in urine output.

71. The stool culture of a child with profuse diarrhea reveals *Salmonella* bacilli. After teaching the mother about the course of *Salmonella enteritidis,* which of the following statements by the mother indicates effective teaching?
☐ **1.** "Some people become carriers and stay infectious for a long time."
☐ **2.** "After the acute stage passes, the organism is usually not present in the stool."
☐ **3.** "Although the organism may be alive indefinitely, in time it will be of no danger to anyone."
☐ **4.** "If my child continues to have the organism in the stool, an antitoxin can help destroy the organism."

72. A child is started on a soft diet after having been on clear liquids following an episode of severe gastroenteritis. When helping the mother choose foods for her child, which of the following foods would be most appropriate?
☐ **1.** Muffins and eggs.
☐ **2.** Bananas and rice cereal.
☐ **3.** Bran cereal and a bagel.
☐ **4.** Pancakes and sausage.

73. A child undergoes rehydration therapy after having diarrhea and dehydration. A nurse is teaching the child's parents about dietary management. The nurse understands that the teaching plan has been successful when the parents tell the nurse that they will follow which type of diet?
☐ **1.** Regular.
☐ **2.** Clear liquid.
☐ **3.** Full liquid.
☐ **4.** Soft.

74. When assessing a child diagnosed with diarrhea due to *Salmonella,* for which of the following possible sources should the nurse be alert during history taking?
☐ **1.** Nonrefrigerated custard.
☐ **2.** A pet canary.
☐ **3.** Undercooked eggs.
☐ **4.** Unwashed fruit.

75. On a home visit following discharge from the hospital after treatment for severe gastroenteritis, the mother tells the nurse that her toddler answers "No!" and is difficult to manage. After discussing this further with the mother, the nurse explains that the child's behavior is most probably the result of which of the following?
- ☐ 1. Beginning leadership skills.
- ☐ 2. Inherited personality trait.
- ☐ 3. Expression of individuality.
- ☐ 4. Usual lack of interest in everything.

76. The mother of a toddler hospitalized for episodes of diarrhea reports that when her toddler cannot have things the way she wants, she throws her legs and arms around, screams, and cries. The mother says, "I don't know what to do!" After teaching the mother about ways to manage this behavior, which of the following statements indicates that the nurse's teaching was successful?
- ☐ 1. "Next time she screams and throws her legs, I'll ignore the behavior."
- ☐ 2. "I'll allow her to have what she wants once in a while."
- ☐ 3. "I'll explain why she cannot have what she wants."
- ☐ 4. "When she behaves like this, I'll tell her that she is being a bad girl."

77. The mother of a potty-trained toddler who was admitted to the hospital for severe gastroenteritis and subsequent dehydration and is now at home asks the nurse why the child still wets the bed. Which of the following should be the nurse's best response?
- ☐ 1. "Hospitalization is a traumatic experience for children. Regression is common and it takes time for them to return to their former behavior."
- ☐ 2. "The stress of hospitalization is hard for many children, but usually they have no problems when they return home."
- ☐ 3. "After returning home from being hospitalized, children still feel they should be the center of attention."
- ☐ 4. "Children do not feel comfortable in their home surroundings once they return home from being hospitalized."

The Client with Appendicitis

78. A child is admitted with a diagnosis of possible appendicitis. The child is in acute pain. Which of the following nursing interventions would be appropriate prior to surgery to decrease pain? Select all that apply.
- ☐ 1. Offer an ice pack.
- ☐ 2. Apply a heating pad.
- ☐ 3. Encourage the child to assume a position of comfort.
- ☐ 4. Limit the child's activity.
- ☐ 5. Request an order for a cathartic.

79. A 7-year-old child is experiencing pain after an appendectomy. Which data collection tool should the nurse use to assess the pain?
- ☐ 1. Visual analog scale.
- ☐ 2. Short Form McGill Questionnaire.
- ☐ 3. Numerical pain scale.
- ☐ 4. FACES Pain Rating Scale.

80. A 7-year-old has had an appendectomy on November 12. He has had pain for the last 24 hours. There is an order to administer Tylenol with Codeine every 3 to 4 hours as needed. The nurse is beginning the shift and the child is requesting pain medication. The nurse reviews the chart below for pain history. Based on the information in the chart, what should the nurse do next?
- ☐ 1. Administer the Tylenol with Codeine.
- ☐ 2. Distract the child by giving him breakfast.
- ☐ 3. Instruct the child to take deep breaths and blow his pain away.
- ☐ 4. Assess the child again in 1 hour.

NURSES PROGRESS NOTES

Date	Time	Progress Notes
11/12/07	03:00 pm	Tylenol with Codeine given PO. FACES pain scale changed from 5 to 2 within 15 minutes
11/12/07	06:00 pm	Tylenol with Codeine given PO. FACES pain scale changed from 5 to 2
11/12/07	09:30 pm	Tylenol with Codeine given PO. FACES pain scale changed from 5 to 2
11/13/07	01:00 am	Tylenol with Codeine given PO. FACES pain scale changed from 4 to 1
11/13/07	07:00 am	Client rates pain on FACES pain scale as 4

81. When obtaining the initial health history from a 10-year-old child with abdominal pain and suspected appendicitis, which of the following questions would be most helpful in eliciting data to help support the diagnosis?
- [ ] **1.** "Where did the pain start?"
- [ ] **2.** "What did you do for the pain?"
- [ ] **3.** "How often do you have a bowel movement?"
- [ ] **4.** "Is the pain continuous, or does it let up?"

82. When developing the plan of care for a school-age child with a suspected diagnosis of appendicitis who is complaining of severe abdominal pain, which of the following measures should the nurse expect to include in the child's plan of care?
- [ ] **1.** Application of a heating pad.
- [ ] **2.** Insertion of a rectal tube.
- [ ] **3.** Application of an ice bag.
- [ ] **4.** Administration of an intravenous narcotic.

83. Which of the following assessment findings should alert the nurse to suspect appendicitis in a male adolescent complaining of severe abdominal pain?
- [ ] **1.** Abdomen appears slightly rounded.
- [ ] **2.** Bowel sounds are heard twice in 2 minutes.
- [ ] **3.** All four abdominal quadrants reveal tympany.
- [ ] **4.** The client demonstrates a cremasteric reflex.

84. An adolescent male client scheduled for an emergency appendectomy is to be transferred directly from the emergency room to the operating room. Which of the following statements by the client should the nurse interpret as most significant?
- [ ] **1.** "All of a sudden it doesn't hurt at all."
- [ ] **2.** "The pain is centered around my navel."
- [ ] **3.** "I feel like I'm going to throw up."
- [ ] **4.** "It hurts when you press on my stomach."

85. Which of the following should be the priority assessment for an adolescent on return to the nursing unit after an appendectomy?
- [ ] **1.** The dressing on the surgical site.
- [ ] **2.** Intravenous fluid infusion site.
- [ ] **3.** Nasogastric (NG) tube function.
- [ ] **4.** Amount of pain.

86. An adolescent who has had an appendectomy and developed peritonitis complains of nausea. Which of the following should the nurse do first?
- [ ] **1.** Administer an antiemetic.
- [ ] **2.** Irrigate the nasogastric (NG) tube.
- [ ] **3.** Notify the surgeon.
- [ ] **4.** Take the blood pressure.

87. When developing the postoperative plan of care for an adolescent who has undergone an appendectomy for a ruptured appendix, in which of the following positions should the nurse expect to place the client during the early postoperative period?
- [ ] **1.** The semi-Fowler's position.
- [ ] **2.** Supine.
- [ ] **3.** Lithotomy position.
- [ ] **4.** Prone.

88. Which of the following should a nurse expect to hear from an adolescent who has just returned to her room after an appendectomy?
- [ ] **1.** "I'll need plastic surgery for this scar."
- [ ] **2.** "I'm worried about the size of my scar."
- [ ] **3.** "I don't want to have any pain."
- [ ] **4.** "What will my boyfriend say about the scar?"

89. Which of the following client actions should the nurse judge to be a healthy coping behavior for a male adolescent after an appendectomy?
- [ ] **1.** Insisting on wearing a T-shirt and gym shorts rather than pajamas.
- [ ] **2.** Avoiding interactions with other adolescents on the nursing unit.
- [ ] **3.** Refusing to fill out the menu, and allowing the nurse to do so.
- [ ] **4.** Not taking telephone calls from friends so he can rest.

90. When teaching an adolescent scheduled for an appendectomy about what to expect, which of the following approaches would be most effective?
- [ ] **1.** Providing the primary essential information.
- [ ] **2.** Offering advice and opinions as needed.
- [ ] **3.** Using diagrams when explaining procedures.
- [ ] **4.** Using age-appropriate jargon with explanations.

Correct Answers and Rationales

The letter in parentheses after each rationale identifies the client need addressed in the item, including management of care (M), safety and infection control (S), health promotion and maintenance (H), psychosocial adaptation (P), basic care and comfort (C), pharmacological and parenteral therapies (D), reduction of risk potential (R), and physiological adaptation (A).

The Client with Cleft Lip and Palate

1.

1. Maintaining a clear and adequate airway.
4. Applying elbow restraints.
2. Maintaining sufficient fluid and caloric intake.
3. Providing emotional comfort to the child.
5. Teaching the parents proper feeding methods.

The nurse should first ensure that the child has a patent airway, because swelling and secretions following surgery can block the airway. Next, the nurse should restrain the infant's arms to keep him from rubbing with his hands or fingers on the incision line, which could cause scarring and damage to the incision. The child will need adequate nourishment and fluids as soon as he recovers from anesthesia. The nurse must comfort the child, and try to prevent him from crying as much as possible, because crying puts a strain on the suture line and can cause scarring. The nurse should involve the parents in the child's care and feeding as soon as possible after she has assessed the child's ability to safely ingest his feedings. (A)

2. 3. Before corrective surgery for a cleft lip, the infant needs to consume formula. Methods for feeding may need to be adjusted to fit the infant's needs, because the infant with a cleft lip experiences a decreased ability to suck, which interferes with the infant's ability to compress the nipple. A special feeder may be used to feed the infant to ensure adequate caloric intake. Problems with infection and skin integrity in the mouth are uncommon because the areas of the defect are not open areas. Although crying may cause the infant to swallow more air because of the defect, crying poses no harm to the infant. There is no need to keep the infant's fingers out of the mouth preoperatively. The fingers will not harm the defect or cause an infection. (R)

3. 1. An infant with a cleft lip and palate typically swallows large amounts of air while being fed and therefore should be burped frequently. The soft palate defect allows air to be drawn into the pharynx with each swallow of formula. The stomach becomes distended with air, and regurgitation, possibly with aspiration, is likely if the infant is not burped frequently. Feeding frequently, even in small amounts, would not prevent swallowing of large amounts of air. A nipple placed in the back of the mouth is likely to cause the infant to gag and aspirate. Holding the infant in a lying position during feedings can also lead to regurgitation and aspiration of formula. The infant should be fed in an upright position. (A)

4. 4. Half-strength hydrogen peroxide is recommended for cleaning the suture line after cleft lip repair. The bubbling action of the hydrogen peroxide is effective for removing debris. Normal saline also may be used. Mouthwashes frequently contain alcohol, which can be irritating. Also, mouthwashes are not as effective in removing debris as half-strength peroxide solutions are. Povidone-iodine solution is not used because the iodine contained in the solution can be absorbed through the skin, leading to toxicity. A mild antiseptic solution has some antibacterial properties but is ineffective in removing suture-line debris. (A)

5. 1. To keep the infant from disturbing the suture line by placing fingers or other objects in the mouth, either intentionally or accidentally, the restraints should be in place at all times. They should be removed for a short period, however, so that the underlying skin can be checked for any redness or breakdown. While the restraints are removed, the parents should be instructed to manually restrain the hands and arms. (R)

6. 3. The optimal time for cleft palate repair depends on many factors. However, it is best done before speech develops and the child learns faulty speech habits as a result of the defect, usually before 12 to 15 months of age. Tooth eruption usually begins at about 6 months of age. The child should weigh about 10 kg (22 lb) at 6 months, but the important consideration is to schedule surgery before speech patterns begin to develop. An infant may learn to start drinking from a cup as early as 6 to 7 months of age, possibly up to the first birthday. (A)

7. 1. A cup is the preferred drinking or eating utensil after repair of a cleft palate. At the age when repair is done, the child is ordinarily able to drink from a cup. Use of a cup avoids having to place a utensil in the mouth, which would increase the potential for injury to the suture lines. (A)

8. 3. Immediately after a surgical repair of a cleft palate, the child is placed on the abdomen with the head turned to the side to lessen the chance of aspiration by allowing secretions to drain out. Positioning the child on the back places the child at risk for aspiration should any regurgitation or vomiting occur, even in low Fowler's position with the head to the side or in reverse Trendelenburg position with the head tilted forward. (A)

The Client with Tracheoesophageal Fistula

9. 2. Assessment of the infant with a TEF includes excessive salivation, choking, coughing, and sneezing at birth and cyanosis from laryngospasm, especially after feedings. Gastroesophageal reflux would cause vomiting after feedings with possible signs of aspiration. Bronchopulmonary dysplasia would cause respiratory difficulty, tachypnea, and cyanosis with decreased oxygen saturation. Hydrocephalus would cause signs and symptoms of increased intracranial pressure, such as vomiting, a bulging fontanel, lethargy or irritability, and an enlarged head circumference. (H)

10. 1. The parents of children born with defects often have feelings of guilt and ask what they might have done to cause the condition or how they might have avoided it. It is important to allow parents to express their feelings and to accept these feelings as normal reactions. Explaining that the parents are not at fault would not be appropriate until they have dealt with their feelings of guilt. Encouraging long-term planning generally is of little benefit to parents who are emotionally distraught. Additionally, the parents may interpret this as ignoring their feelings and confirming that they played a role in causing their child's anomaly. Urging the parents to visit their infant as often as possible would generally be of little help and could appear to the parents as though they are being "talked out" of their feelings. (P)

11. 2. Although a TEF can include several different structural anomalies, the most common type involves a blind upper pouch and a fistula from the esophagus into the trachea. Other types include a blind pouch at the end of the esophagus with no connection to the trachea and a normal trachea and esophagus with an opening that connects them. A tightened muscle below the stomach and projectile vomiting of normal amounts of formula are characteristic of pyloric stenosis. Aganglionic megacolon is a lack of autonomic parasympathetic ganglion cells in a portion of the lower intestine. Gastroschisis occurs when the bowel herniates through a defect in the abdominal wall and no membrane covers the exposed bowel. (A)

12. 2. Because the blind pouch associated with a TEF fills quickly with fluids, the child is at high risk for aspiration. Therefore, the priority nursing diagnosis would be *Risk for injury*. Children with TEF frequently develop aspiration pneumonia. Prevention of aspiration by suctioning or positioning is essential. *Impaired parenting* may occur any time there is an infant with an obvious defect. Parents often have difficulty accepting that their child is not perfect. If the infant did aspirate, then *Ineffective breathing pattern* would be appropriate. However, care focuses on preventing aspiration. Infants with TEF do not experience poor sucking as a result of the defect. Poor sucking ability may be related to something else, such as prematurity. Therefore, *Imbalanced nutrition* would not be an accurate diagnosis. (A)

13. 2. With a TEF, overflow of secretions into the larynx leads to laryngospasm. This obstruction to inspiration stimulates the strong contraction of accessory muscles of the thorax to assist the diaphragm in breathing. This produces substernal retractions. The laryngospasm that occurs with a TEF resolves quickly when secretions are removed from the oropharynx area. A brassy cough is related to a relatively constant laryngeal narrowing, usually caused by edema. It is not an indication of the need to suction. A decreased activity level and an increased respiratory rate in an infant with a TEF are usually the result of hypoxia, a relatively long-term and constant phenomenon in infants with a TEF. (A)

14. 1. The best way to prevent air from entering the stomach when feeding an infant through a gastrostomy tube is to open the clamp after all the formula has been placed in the syringe barrel. Doing so prevents air from mixing with the formula and thus being introduced into the stomach. Pouring all the formula into the barrel after opening the clamp, maintaining a continuous flow of formula down the side of the barrel after unclamping the tube, and allowing a small amount of formula to enter the stomach before adding more formula to the barrel permit air to enter the stomach. (R)

15. 4. The nurse can help meet the psychological needs of an infant being fed through a gastrostomy tube by rocking the infant after a feeding. The infant soon learns to associate eating with a pleasurable experience and learns to trust the caregiver. Rocking the infant will not promote peristalsis or prevent regurgitation. Holding the baby will not relieve pressure on the surgical site. However, holding the child right after feeding promotes comfort and pleasure. (P)

16. 4. When initiating oral feedings after surgical repair of a TEF, it is best to follow a plan of care in conjunction with observation of the infant's needs and behavior. When the infant's needs and behavior are overlooked, plans are likely to be unsatisfactory and are more likely to meet the nurse's needs rather than the infant's needs. After a surgical procedure, infants initially tolerate small amounts of fluids offered more frequently better than larger amounts offered less often. Smaller amounts cause less bloating as the infant becomes used to feeding again. Although infants accept feedings more readily from their mother or from someone who feeds the infant repeatedly, the priority is to meet the infant's nutritional needs based on the infant's behavior. (C)

The Client with an Anorectal Anomaly

17. 2. For the child with an imperforate anus, the purpose of the radiographic examination is to ascertain the distance between the anal dimple and the closed end of the rectum. (R)

18. 1, 3, 4. Anorectal malformations present with lack of stool or evidence of meconium in the urine through a fistula. Meconium is not found in the stool. Because stool does not pass, abdominal distension and vomiting occur. (A)

19. 1. Passage of meconium in the urine is a sign of rectourinary fistula, in which the rectum and bladder communicate. Blood in the urine would suggest an infection. Bile is not found in the urine. Acetone in the urine would indicate excessive fat catabolism. (A)

20. 4. Children who undergo surgical correction for low anorectal anomalies as infants usually are continent. Fecal continence can be expected after successful correction of anal membrane atresia. Therefore, this child probably has a good chance of being potty trained and will not need to wear protective pads. Extra fluids and a high-fiber diet are not required to prevent constipation. Children with high anorectal anomalies may or may not achieve continence. (A)

21. 3. After surgical repair for an imperforate anus, the infant should be positioned either supine with the legs suspended at a 90-degree angle or on either side with the hips elevated to prevent pressure on the perineum. A neonate who is placed on the abdomen pulls the legs up under the body, which puts tension on the perineum, as does positioning the neonate on the back with the legs extended straight out. (A)

22. 3. The neonate responds to pain with total body movement and brief, loud crying that ceases with distraction. After age 6 months, an infant reacts to pain with intense physical resistance and tries to escape by rolling away. A toddler reacts to pain by withdrawing the affected part. (H)

23. 2. Encouraging the parents to hold their neonate promotes parent–infant attachment. Parent–infant bonding is based on a relationship that begins when the parent first touches the infant. Both the parents and the infant have predictable steps that they go through in this process. Explaining that the parents can visit at any time promotes bonding only if they do visit with, talk to, and hold the newborn. Asking the parents to help monitor intake and output at this time may be too anxiety-producing, thus interfering with bonding. Helping the parents plan for the infant's discharge involves them in the newborn's care and is important. However, it is not the first step in the development of bonding. (P)

The Client with Pyloric Stenosis

24. 3. The vomitus of an infant with hypertrophic pyloric stenosis contains gastric contents, mucus, and streaks of blood. The vomitus does not contain bile or stool because the pyloric constriction is proximal to the ampulla of Vater. (A)

25. 1. Infants with pyloric stenosis usually have some degree of dehydration because of vomiting of the stomach contents. Therefore, a priority nursing diagnosis would be *Deficient fluid volume* related to prolonged vomiting. A nursing priority would be to restore fluid and electrolyte balance. Pyloric stenosis involves the pyloric valve distal to the stomach, not the respiratory tract. In addition, swallowing is not impaired with pyloric stenosis. Even though vomiting occurs, a normal infant should be able to protect the airway. Therefore, *Ineffective airway clearance* would be inappropriate. *Imbalanced nutrition: Less than body requirements* could be applicable but would not be the priority diagnosis. *Bowel incontinence* and abdominal pain are not typically associated with pyloric stenosis. (A)

26. 1. Unless the infant is in hypovolemic shock, obtaining a baseline weight is an important first action because the weight is used to calculate the child's fluid and electrolyte needs. The intravenous fluid rate and the amounts of electrolytes to be added to the fluid are based on the infant's weight. The weight also helps determine the infant's degree of dehydration. The intravenous infusion is initiated once the weight has been obtained. The child with pyloric stenosis typically experiences vomiting and is at risk for fluid volume deficit and metabolic acidosis. As a result, oral food and fluids are withheld and the infant is allowed nothing by mouth. Fluid replacement is given intravenously. Orientation can wait until treatment is under way. (A)

27. 1. Pyloric stenosis involves hypertrophy of the pylorus muscle distal to the stomach and obstruction of the gastric outlet resulting in vomiting, metabolic acidosis, and dehydration. Telescoping of the bowel is called intussusception. Overfeeding, feeding too quickly, or underfeeding is not associated with pyloric stenosis. (A)

28. 3. The child with pyloric stenosis experiences vomiting. The major electrolyte lost during vomiting is potassium. Infants with pyloric stenosis typically have low or low-normal serum potassium levels. Therefore, potassium chloride would be added to the intravenous solution. Vomiting also causes loss of hydrochloric acid, leading to metabolic alkalosis. Therefore, bicarbonate replacement would not be indicated. Typically, magnesium and calcium levels in the child with pyloric stenosis are within normal limits. (D)

29. 2. For the client with a nursing diagnosis of *Deficient fluid volume* related to vomiting, the outcome would focus on restoration of fluid balance. Typically, the nurse would evaluate the client for evidence of dehydration. Parameters would include assessment of the client's weight for loss or decreased skin turgor. Abdominal distention is caused by the stenosis and is not relieved until the child has surgery. The child may have increased respiratory effort due to abdominal distention; however, to evaluate the outcome related to fluid deficit, the nurse should weigh the infant. The nurse should record the amount of emesis, but evaluation of the outcome is accomplished by weighing the infant. (A)

30. 4. Restating or rephrasing a mother's response provides the opportunity for clarification and validation. It also helps to focus on what the mother is saying and address her concerns and feelings. Although surgery is the most effective treatment for pyloric stenosis, stating this ignores the mother's feelings and does not give her an opportunity to express them. Telling the mother not to worry also ignores the mother's feelings. Additionally, this type of statement gives the mother premature reassurance, which may turn out to be false. Asking the mother if she thinks the problem indicates that she is not a good mother implies such an idea. It does not allow her to express her concerns and feelings and therefore is not a therapeutic response. (P)

31. 1. Clear liquids containing glucose and electrolytes are usually prescribed 4 to 6 hours after surgery. If vomiting does not occur, formula or breast milk then can be gradually substituted for clear liquids until the infant is taking normal feedings. (A)

32. 4. Giving the infant a pacifier would help meet non-nutritive sucking needs and ensure oral gratification. Additionally, sucking aids in calming the infant. Holding the infant to decrease fussiness and restlessness is more effective in an older infant. Also, the reason for the infant's fussiness needs to be explored. Hanging a mobile over the crib frequently does not decrease fussiness. After surgery to correct pyloric stenosis, feeding the infant more formula would lead to vomiting, putting additional stress on the operative site. (R)

33. 2. The parents' ability to verbalize the infant's care realistically indicates that they are working through their fears and concerns. This behavior demonstrates an understanding of the infant's condition and needs. Without further data, the fact that the parents have to get away could be interpreted as ineffective coping, possibly suggesting that they are unable to handle the situation. Continuing to ask about the child's general condition even after answers have been given does not suggest effective coping. The parents are demonstrating that they are unsure of themselves as parents or are hoping for positive information. Exhibiting fear that they will disturb the infant does not suggest effective coping. This behavior indicates that they are uncertain or lack knowledge about infants. (P)

The Client with Intussusception

34. 2. The infant with intussusception experiences acute episodes of colic-like abdominal pain. Typically, the infant screams and draws the knees to the chest. Between these episodes of acute abdominal pain, the infant appears comfortable and normal. Feeding does not precipitate episodes of pain. Additionally, a 4-month-old infant typically would not be ingesting solid foods. Pain exhibited by crying that occurs when the infant is placed in a reclining position, as in the mother's arms, is not associated with intussusception. This type of cry may indicate that the infant wants attention, wants to be held, or needs to have a diaper change. (A)

35. 1. For the infant with intussusception, stools characteristically have the appearance of currant jelly because of the intestinal inflammation and hemorrhage resulting from intestinal obstruction. These stools occur later in the course of the disease process. Questions that focus on urination, vomiting, and food intake do not elicit information about the effects of intussusception. (A)

36. 1. The first action is to check the placement of the tube to ensure that it is in the correct position. To check tube position, the nurse should aspirate the tube with a syringe. A return of gastric contents indicates that the end of the tube is in the stomach. Another method is to inject a small amount of air while auscultating with a stethoscope over the epigastric area. The tube is irrigated with normal saline, not distilled water, and only after the position of the tube is confirmed. The suction level should not be increased, because doing so could damage the mucosa. Rotating the tube could irritate or traumatize the nasal mucosa. (R)

37. 2. Development of a paralytic ileus postoperatively is a functional obstruction of the bowel. Bowel sounds initially may be hyperactive, but then they diminish and cease. Measurement of urine specific gravity provides information about fluid and electrolyte status. The first stool and the amount of gastric output provide information about the return of gastric function. (A)

38. **1.** Infants who have had an interruption in their normal routine and experiences, such as hospitalization and surgery, typically manifest behavior changes when discharged. The infant's normal routine has been significantly altered, so it will take time to reestablish another routine. Calorie requirements at home will continue to be the same as those in the hospital. The infant does not need more calories at home. The surgical procedure corrected the problems, so the infant should not continue to have abdominal cramping. (A)

The Client with Inguinal Hernia

39. **1.** Abdominal distention and a redness of the inguinal swelling are significant findings. Their presence in conjunction with area tenderness and inability to reduce the hernia indicate an incarcerated hernia. An incarcerated hernia can lead to strangulation, necrosis, and gangrene of the bowel. Other findings associated with strangulation include irritability, anorexia, and difficulty in defecation. Irritability is nonspecific and could be caused by various factors. A palpable, thickened spermatic cord on the affected side is diagnostic of inguinal hernia and would be an expected finding. A wet diaper indicates that urine is being excreted, a finding unrelated to inguinal hernia. (A)

40. **3.** If nonoperative reduction is successful, delaying surgery for 2 to 3 days allows the edema and inflammation in the inguinal area to subside. Thus, the area to be operated will appear more normal, helping to decrease the risk of complications. The preoperative preparation for a herniorrhaphy is minimal and is not the reason for delaying the surgery. Typically, the infant is fed until a few hours before surgery to prevent dehydration. Trusses do not prevent incarceration, and there is no reason to use a truss preoperatively. (A)

41. **2.** The best way to prepare a 7-month-old infant psychologically for surgery is to have the primary caretaker stay with the child. Infants in the second 6 months of life commonly develop separation anxiety. Therefore, the priority in this case is to support the child by having the parent present. Teaching the mother what to expect may decrease her anxiety; this is important because infants sense anxiety and distress in parents, but the priority in this case is to have the parent present. Actual play and acting out life experiences are appropriate for preschool-age children. Allowing an infant to play with surgical equipment would be inappropriate and dangerous. (P)

42. **1.** Changing a diaper as soon as it becomes soiled helps prevent wound infection, the most common complication after inguinal hernia repair in an infant secondary to possible wound contamination with urine and stool. Because the surgical wound is unlikely to separate, an abdominal binder is unnecessary. The incision may or may not be covered with a dressing. If a dressing is not used, the physician may apply a topical spray to protect the wound. Restraining the infant's hands is unnecessary if the diaper is applied snugly. The infant would be unable to get the hands into the diaper close to the surgical site. (S)

43. **3.** The incision must be kept as clean and dry as possible. Therefore, daily sponge baths are given for about 1 week postoperatively. Cleaning the infant's face and diaper area should occur at least daily and continuously, not limited to a 2-week period. Because this type of surgery results in a wound that heals through primary intention, the skin will heal and cover the wound in 2 to 3 days. Therefore, it is not necessary to use sterile gauze to cleanse the incision; clean technique is acceptable. Because the incision must be kept as clean and dry, full tub baths are inappropriate. (R)

44. **3.** Because of possible stress on the suture line, physical activities such as bicycle riding, physical education classes, weight-lifting, and wrestling are contraindicated for about 3 weeks. (C)

The Client with Hirschsprung's Disease

45. **2.** Infants with Hirschsprung's disease typically display failure to thrive, with poor weight gain due to malabsorption of nutrients. Therefore, the nurse would expect to see a child who weighs less than that which is expected for height and age. A distended, rather than a scaphoid-shaped, abdomen would be noted. Cyanosis of fingers and toes is associated with congenital heart disease. Hyperactive deep tendon reflexes are associated with upper motor neuron problems, such as cerebral palsy. (A)

46. **3.** By encouraging parents to ask questions during information-sharing sessions, the nurse can clarify misconceptions and determine the parents' understanding of information. A better understanding of what is happening allows the parents to feel some control over the situation. Assessing the adequacy of the parents' coping skills is important but secondary to encouraging them to express their concerns. The questions they ask and their interactions with the nurse may provide clues to the adequacy of their coping skills. The nurse should never give false reassurance to parents. At this point, there is no way for the nurse to know whether the child will be fine. Written materials are appropriate for augmenting the nurse's verbal communication. However, these are secondary to encouraging questions. (P)

47. **3.** The primary defect in Hirschsprung's disease is an absence of autonomic parasympathetic ganglion cells in the distal portion of the colon. Thus, the nerves at the end of the large colon are missing. Absence of a rectal opening refers to an imperforate anus. A tube between the trachea and esophagus refers to a tracheoesophageal fistula. Presence of a tight muscle below the stomach refers to pyloric stenosis. (A)

48. 3. Before intestinal surgery, dietary intake is limited to clear liquids for 24 to 48 hours. A clear liquid diet meets the child's fluid needs and avoids the formation of fecal material in the intestine. Typically, repeated saline enemas, not tap water enemas, are given to empty the bowel. Soapsuds enemas are contraindicated for infants, as are tap water enemas. A nasogastric tube may be inserted for gastric decompression. Insertion of a gastrostomy tube is outside the scope of nursing practice. Because the perineal area is not involved in the surgery, it does not need to be prepared. (A)

49. In most instances, the absence of ganglionic innervation occurs in the lower portion of the sigmoid colon just above the anus. (A)

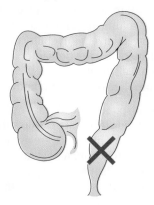

50. 2. The goal of surgery is to remove the aganglionic bowel and to improve functioning of the internal sphincter. A temporary loop or double-barreled colostomy is usually created to rest the bowel. This enables the normal distal bowel to regain its original tone and size. Final corrective surgery is done when the child is age 6 to 12 months or weighs about 10 kg. The colostomy probably will be reversed before the child is old enough to be responsible for its care. In the immediate postoperative period, a new stoma is swollen and erythematous. (A)

51. 2. Typically, the stoma should remain deep red in color as long as the infant has the colostomy. A dark-red to purplish color may indicate impaired circulation to the stoma. (A)

52. 4. A regular diet would be recommended for the child with a colostomy; no special diet is needed. High-fiber foods, such as fruits and vegetables, should be minimized because they increase the bulk in the stool. Fat is necessary for brain growth in the first year of life. A high-residue diet would result in bulkier stools and increased gas production, which will collect in the colostomy bag. Therefore, a high-residue diet is not indicated. (C)

53. 1. Abdominal circumference is measured to monitor for abdominal distention. An increase of 3 cm in 8 hours would require notification of the physician; it would indicate a substantial degree of abdominal distention, possibly from fluid or gas accumulation. Normally, after surgery, an infant experiences occasional periods of fussi-ness. However, as long as the infant is able to be quiet by himself or with the aid of a pacifier, the physician does not need to be contacted. Absence of bowel sounds would be expected after surgery because of the effects of anesthesia. It takes approximately 48 hours for gastric motility to resume. Even if the infant displays evidence that he is hungry, fluids will not be offered until bowel sounds are heard, indicating a functioning gastrointestinal tract. (R)

54. 2. Toilet-training is commonly more difficult for children who have undergone surgery for Hirschsprung's disease than it is for other children. This is because of the trauma to the area and the associated psychological implications. Abdominal distention is an early sign of infection and therefore the parents need to report it to the physician. Typically, dietary restrictions are not required. Usually the infant is placed on an age-appropriate diet. Vitamin supplementation is not necessary if the infant's dietary intake is adequate. (A)

The Client with Diarrhea, Gastroenteritis, or Dehydration

55.

1. Obtain vital signs and weight.
3. Apply a urine collection bag.
2. Insert an I.V. and infuse fluids as ordered.
4. Draw blood for laboratory tests.

The nurse should first obtain vital signs and evaluate the child for signs of shock or cardiac arrhythmias. The weight can also be obtained at this time to estimate the amount of fluid lost. The nurse should next apply the urine collection bag. As soon as possible after these steps, the nurse should insert an I.V. to replace lost fluids, electrolytes, and sugar to reduce the incidence of metabolic acidosis created by the lack of calorie intake and the loss of electrolytes. Blood should be drawn to assess the severity of electrolyte imbalance and other possible causes for the diarrhea and vomiting. (A)

56. 1, 2, 4, 5. Shigella is caused by the *Shigella* organism. Clinical manifestations of shigella include fever, nausea and vomiting, some cramping, headache, seizures, rectal prolapse, and loose, watery stools containing pus, mucus, and blood. The nurse should assess the child for these symptoms on an ongoing basis. Shigella is spread via direct contact with the organism, which is found in the stool. A stool specimen will show increased numbers of WBCs, blood, and mucus. Vomiting and loose stools can result in severe dehydration and electrolyte imbalance. Thus, the nurse should record intake, output, and daily weights. There is no need for strict isolation; masks are not needed as shigella is not transmitted by airborne methods. (A)

57. **3.** The absence of tears is typically found when moderate dehydration is observed as the body attempts to conserve fluids. Other typical findings associated with moderate dehydration include a dry mouth, sunken eyes, poor skin turgor, and an increased pulse rate. Deep, rapid respirations are associated with severe dehydration. Decreased perspiration, not diaphoresis, would be seen with moderate dehydration. The specific gravity of urine increases with decreased output in the presence of dehydration. (R)

58. **4.** An infant with severe diarrhea will experience some degree of dehydration. In an 8-month-old child, the anterior fontanel has not closed. Therefore, a depressed anterior fontanel would be an important finding. Additionally, the infant would exhibit dry mucous membranes, lethargy, hyperactive bowel sounds, dark urine, and sunken eyeballs. Skin turgor would be decreased or delayed (e.g., slow to return when pinched). (R)

59. **2.** Because an infant experiencing severe diarrhea is at high risk for *Deficient fluid volume*, the nurse needs to evaluate the infant's fluid balance status by weighing the infant at least every day. Body weight is the best indicator of hydration status because a higher proportion of an infant's body weight is water, compared with an adult. Initially, the infant with severe diarrhea is not allowed liquids but is given fluids intravenously. Therefore, monitoring the oral intake of formula is inappropriate. Although checking the anterior fontanel for depression or bulging provides information about hydration status, this method is not considered the best indicator of the infant's fluid balance. Monitoring skin turgor can provide information about fluid volume status. The abdomen is commonly used to assess skin turgor in an infant because it is a large surface area and can be accessed quickly. However, weight is the best indicator of fluid balance. (A)

60. **8.2**

$$2.2 \text{ lb/kg} = 9 \text{ lb}/X \text{ kg}$$

$$X = 9 \div 2.2$$

$$X = 4.09 \text{ kg, rounded to } 4.1 \text{ kg}$$

$$4.1 \text{ kg} \times 2 \text{ ml/kg} = 8.2 \text{ ml/hour}$$

(D)

61. **1.** Typically, an infant hospitalized with severe diarrhea receives fluid replacement intravenously rather than orally. Oral fluids and food are usually withheld. Although activities such as placing a mobile over the crib, speaking to the infant, or turning on the television may provide distraction for or help in calming the infant, a fussy infant receiving nothing by mouth is usually best comforted by providing a pacifier to satisfy sucking needs. (H)

62. **2.** Given this infant's history of gastroenteritis, the priority nursing diagnosis would be *Deficient fluid volume*. With gastroenteritis, vomiting and diarrhea occur, leading to the loss of fluids. This loss of fluids is problematic in infants because a higher proportion of their body weight is water. *Pain* is not a priority nursing diagnosis, although the nurse should continue to assess the infant for pain. There are no data to indicate impaired parenting. *Impaired urinary elimination* is related to the infant's fluid volume deficit resulting from vomiting and diarrhea associated with gastroenteritis. If the infant's fluid volume deficit is not corrected, then this nursing diagnosis may become the priority. (A)

63. **1.** The outcome of moist mucous membranes indicates adequate hydration and fluid balance, showing that the problem of fluid volume deficit has been corrected. Although a normal bowel movement, ability to tolerate intravenous fluids, and an increasing time interval between bowel movements are all positive signs, they do not specifically address the problem of deficient fluid volume. (A)

64. **1.** Children hospitalized with gastroenteritis are usually not allowed fluids by mouth to allow the gastrointestinal tract time to rest. Antibiotics are not indicated unless there is a bacterial infection. A mist tent would be used to treat respiratory disorders, not gastroenteritis. Once the infant is allowed oral intake, clear fluids are used initially. (H)

65. **1.** The usual way to treat an infant hospitalized with gastroenteritis is to keep the infant nothing-by-mouth status to rest the gastrointestinal tract. The resulting fluid volume deficit is treated with intravenous fluids. When the infant's condition is controlled (for example, when vomiting subsides), clear liquids are then started slowly. Formula and juice will be started once the infant's vomiting has subsided and the infant has demonstrated the ability to tolerate clear liquids for a period of time. In this situation, there is no need to test the infant's blood every day for anemia. Most likely, the infant's serum electrolyte levels would be monitored closely. Typically, an infant is placed in a private room because gastroenteritis is most commonly caused by a virus that is easily transmitted to others. (A)

66. **2.** The nurse's best course of action would be to support the mother. This is best done by conveying understanding and encouraging the mother to visit or call. Telling the mother that she shouldn't leave and that the child is very sick is critical and insensitive. Additionally, it implies guilt should the mother leave. Commenting that the child does not need anyone is not appropriate or true. Toddlers, in particular, need family members present because of the stresses associated with hospitalization. They experience separation anxiety, a normal aspect of development, and need constancy in their environment. Asking the mother to find someone else to stay with her children is inappropriate. The children at home also need the support of the mother and/or other family members to minimize the disruptions in family life resulting from the toddler's hospitalization and to maintain consistency. (P)

67. 1. For the child with severe gastroenteritis, diarrhea is a problem; it exposes all persons caring for the child to possibly infectious body fluids. Subsequently, any other clients being cared for by these individuals are also at risk. Therefore, the nurse would institute standard precautions, including good handwashing and use of appropriate personal protective equipment (gowns, gloves, eye protection) to minimize the risk for exposure. Typically, the child with severe gastroenteritis is placed in a private room until the causative organism is determined, to prevent transmission and protect others, including clients, families, and staff, from acquiring the infection. Because gastroenteritis is usually viral in origin and highly contagious, disposable eating utensils would be used to prevent transmission. For the child with gastroenteritis, double-bagging all linens is appropriate to prevent possible transmission from contaminated linens. (S)

68. 1, 2, 3, 5. Accurate intake and output recording includes noting all intake, including I.V. fluids; noting output, such as emesis and stool; weighing diapers; measuring weight daily; measuring urine specific gravity; monitoring serum electrolytes; and monitoring for signs of dehydration. Children who are dehydrated must receive sufficient fluid intake. Restricting fluids just prior to weighing the child will not alter the accuracy of the weight, and the nurse should continue to encourage fluids for this dehydrated child. (M)

69. 1. Potassium chloride is readily excreted in the urine. Before adding potassium chloride to the intravenous fluid, the nurse should ascertain whether the child can void; if not, potassium chloride may build up in the serum and cause hyperkalemia. An electrocardiogram could be done during intravenous potassium replacement therapy to evaluate for these changes. Having a stool daily is important but, because potassium is primarily excreted in the urine, the child's ability to void must be verified. Serum calcium levels do not indicate the child's ability to tolerate potassium replacement. (D)

70. 3. An early sign of circulatory overload is moist rales or crackles heard when auscultating over the chest wall. Elevated blood pressure, engorged neck veins, a wide variation between fluid intake and output (with a higher intake than output), shortness of breath, increased respiratory rate, dyspnea, and cyanosis occur later. (R)

71. 1. After having *Salmonella enteritidis,* some clients become chronic carriers of the causative organism and remain infectious for a long time as the organism continues to be shed from the body. During this time, the child is still considered infectious. No antitoxin is available to treat or prevent *Salmonella* infections. (A)

72. 2. After clear liquids, the foods of choice are soft foods. These foods should be easily digested and low in fat. Additionally, the foods should be non-bulk-forming. Bananas and rice cereal are low in fat and easy to digest. Muffins and eggs, as well as sausage and pancakes, are typically high in fat and would be avoided. Although a bagel is low in fat, bran cereal is high in fiber and would be avoided because it may cause more diarrhea. (C)

73. 1. Dietary management following rehydration for diarrhea and mild dehydration would include offering the child a regular diet. Following rehydration, there is no need for the child to be on a special diet, such as a clear liquid, full liquid, or soft diet. (C)

74. 3. Diarrhea related to *Salmonella* bacilli is commonly spread by raw or undercooked fowl and eggs, pet turtles, and kittens. Food poisoning caused by *Staphylococcus* species is commonly spread by inadequately cooked or refrigerated custards, cream fillings, or mayonnaise. Psittacosis, a respiratory illness, may be spread by canaries. Contaminated, unwashed fruit is associated with typhoid fever (caused by *Salmonella typhi*), a disorder rarely seen in the United States. (A)

75. 3. The "no" behavior demonstrated by a toddler is typical of this age group as the child attempts to be self-assertive as an individual. The negativism does not demonstrate an inherited personality trait or disinterest. Rather, it reflects the developmental task of establishing autonomy. The toddler is attempting to exert control over the environment. It is too early to assess leadership qualities in a toddler. (H)

76. 1. The child is demonstrating behavior associated with temper tantrums, which are relatively frequent normal occurrences during toddlerhood as the child attempts to develop a sense of autonomy. The development of autonomy requires opportunities for the child to make decisions and express individuality. Ignoring the outbursts is probably the best strategy. Doing so avoids rewarding the behavior and helps the child to learn limits, promoting the development of self-control. However, the mother should intervene in a temper tantrum if the child is likely to injure herself. Allowing the child to have what she wants occasionally would typically add to the problems associated with temper tantrums, because doing so rewards the behavior and prevents the child from developing self-control. Toddlers do not possess the capacity to understand explanations about behavior. Expressing disappointment in the child's behavior or telling her that she is being a bad girl reinforces feelings of guilt and shame, thus interfering the child's ability to develop a sense of autonomy. (H)

77. 1. Hospitalization is a traumatic time for a child, and it takes some time to readjust to the home environment. The child may regress at home for a period until she feels comfortable. Children normally do not dislike their home environment; in fact, they usually are eager to get home to familiar surroundings where they feel safe. (H)

The Client with Appendicitis

78. 1, 3, 4. Cold is a vasoconstrictor and supplies some degree of anesthesia. The child is usually more comfortable on his side with his legs flexed to take the strain off the inflamed appendix. Limiting the child's activity puts less stress on the inflamed appendix and lessens the discomfort. Heat increases circulation to an area, causing more engorgement and pain and, possibly, rupture of the appendix. Heat is contraindicated in any situation where rupture or perforation is a possibility. A cathartic is contraindicated when appendicitis is suspected. Increasing peristalsis can cause the appendix to rupture. (A)

79. 4. The nurse should use the FACES Pain Rating Scale for children or cognitively impaired clients so that the client can use a picture to identify the pain. The visual analog and numerical scales are used with adults. The Short Form McGill Questionnaire allows the client to give simple descriptions of pain by sensation and perception, which is inappropriate for a child. (C)

80. 1. The nurse should administer the Tylenol with Codeine as the client indicates he is having pain. Although the child reports less severe pain, he is still experiencing pain. The nurse will also want the child to have less pain because he will need to be more active during the day. Assessing the child later will likely cause the pain to have increased and be more difficult to manage. While distraction is appropriate for short-term pain, such as from a needle-stick or pain that the child might be able to manage himself, postoperative pain should be relieved with medication. (C)

81. 1. The most helpful question would be to determine the location of the pain when it started. The pain associated with appendicitis usually begins in the periumbilical area, then progresses to the right lower quadrant. After the nurse has determined the location of the pain, asking about what was done for the pain would be appropriate. Asking about the child's usual bowel movement pattern is a general question unrelated to child's condition. Children with appendicitis may have diarrhea or constipation. Additionally, knowledge about the child's usual pattern would not be a priority because the child with appendicitis typically is not hospitalized long enough to reestablish the normal pattern. Although the characteristics of the pain are important, asking if the pain is continuous or intermittent is vague and general because the pain could be associated with numerous conditions. With appendicitis, the client's pain may begin as intermittent, but it eventually becomes continuous. (A)

82. 3. Application of an ice bag may help to relieve pain by decreasing circulation to the area. A heating pad is contraindicated because heat may increase circulation to the appendix, possibly leading to rupture. Rectal tubes are contraindicated because they stimulate bowel motility and can exacerbate abdominal pain. Also, they would be ineffective because accumulation of gas in the lower bowel is not likely to be the cause of the child's discomfort. Because narcotics can mask the child's symptoms, such as pain and discomfort, and they also decrease bowel motility, they are not given until after a definitive diagnosis has been made. (A)

83. 2. Manifestations of appendicitis include decreased or absent bowel sounds. Normally, bowel sounds are heard every 10 to 30 seconds. Therefore, bowel sounds heard twice in 2 minutes suggests appendicitis. Normally, the contour of the male adolescent abdomen is flat to slightly rounded, and tympany is typically heard when auscultating over most of the abdomen. A cremasteric reflex is normal for male adolescents. (A)

84. 1. Sudden relief of pain in a client with appendicitis may indicate that the appendix has ruptured. Rupture relieves the pressure within the appendix but spreads the infection to the peritoneal cavity. Periumbilical pain (pain centered around the navel), vomiting, and abdominal tenderness on palpation are common findings associated with appendicitis. (A)

85. 1. The priority assessment after an appendectomy would be the dressing over the surgical site to determine whether there is any drainage or bleeding. The surgical dressing should be clean, dry, and intact. Once the dressing has been assessed, the nurse would assess the intravenous infusion site, assess the NG tube to be sure it is functioning, and finally, determine the degree of pain the client is experiencing. (A)

86. 2. After an appendectomy, the client who develops peritonitis typically has an NG tube in place. When a client complains of nausea, the nurse would first check to ensure that the NG tube is functioning correctly, because the client's nausea may be related to a blockage of the NG tube. If the tube is clogged, it can be irrigated with normal saline. An antiemetic may be given, but only after the nurse has determined that the NG tube is functioning properly. Postoperative orders usually include an antiemetic. Typically, the nurse would notify the surgeon if the client did not obtain relief from irrigation of the NG tube or administration of an ordered antiemetic. Although taking the client's blood pressure is an important postoperative nursing activity, it is unrelated to relieving the client's nausea. (A)

87. **1.** After an appendectomy for a ruptured appendix, assuming the semi-Fowler's or a right side-lying position helps localize the infection. These positions promote drainage from the peritoneal cavity and decrease the incidence of subdiaphragmatic abscess. (A)

88. **2.** Adolescents are concerned about the immediate state and functioning of their bodies. The adolescent needs to know whether any changes (e.g., illness, trauma, surgery) will alter her lifestyle or interfere with her quest for physical perfection. Having a scar may be devastating to the adolescent. The need for plastic surgery cannot be determined at this point. The adolescent has just returned from surgery and has yet to see the scar. Healing has yet to occur. Typically scars become smaller and fade over time. The desire for no pain is unrealistic. Although adolescents are worried about pain and how they will respond, they typically are discharged within 24 hours after an appendectomy with pain well controlled by oral analgesics. The immediate concern of adolescents is the state and functioning of their bodies. After concerns about themselves, then adolescents are concerned about their peer group and their responses. Although the boyfriend's response will matter, this concern would be more common later in the course of the adolescent's recovery. (H)

89. **1.** Adolescents struggle for independence and identity, needing to feel in control of situations and to conform with peers. Control and conformity are often manifested in appearance, including clothing, and this carries over into the hospital experience. The adolescent feels best when he is able to look and act as he normally does—for example, wearing a T-shirt and gym shorts. Adolescents normally want to interact with peers and commonly seek every opportunity to do so. Avoiding other adolescents on the nursing unit or not taking phone calls from friends might suggest ineffective coping behavior. Refusing to fill out the menu and allowing the nurse to do so demonstrates dependent behavior, not a healthy coping mechanism. (P)

90. **3.** Adolescents can comprehend scientific rationale and complexity. They appreciate detailed descriptions and explanations using charts, diagrams, and models. Adolescents want to know more than the essential information. They have questions and want to know what to expect. They dislike lectures and unsolicited advice and opinions. They need to feel that they have some control, fostered by allowing the adolescent to participate in the conversation rather than be lectured to or given advice. Participation helps to foster decision-making skills. Jargon is a means to establish the identity of the peer group. An adult's use of adolescent jargon may be viewed as false or dishonest. (H)

TEST 5

The Child with Health Problems Involving Ingestion, Nutrition, or Diet

- ■ The Client with Toxic Substance Ingestion
- ■ The Client with Lead Poisoning
- ■ The Client with Celiac Disease
- ■ The Client with Phenylketonuria
- ■ The Client with Colic
- ■ The Client with Obesity
- ■ The Client with Food Sensitivity
- ■ The Client with Failure to Thrive
- ■ Correct Answers and Rationales

The Client with Toxic Substance Ingestion

1. While conducting a medication inventory, the emergency department nurse of a pediatric hospital checks to ensure that syrup of ipecac is readily available. This action is based on the nurse's knowledge that this drug is used primarily to accomplish which of the following?
- ☐ **1.** Induce vomiting.
- ☐ **2.** Promote diuresis.
- ☐ **3.** Control seizure activity.
- ☐ **4.** Stimulate the heart.

2. A toddler is brought to the emergency room after ingesting an undetermined amount of drain cleaner. The nurse should expect to assist with which of the following first?
- ☐ **1.** Administering an emetic.
- ☐ **2.** Performing a tracheostomy.
- ☐ **3.** Performing gastric lavage.
- ☐ **4.** Inserting an indwelling urinary (Foley) catheter.

3. After the acute stage following an ingestion of drain cleaner by a child, the nurse should be alert for the development of which of the following as a likely complication?
- ☐ **1.** Tracheal stenosis.
- ☐ **2.** Tracheal varices.
- ☐ **3.** Esophageal strictures.
- ☐ **4.** Esophageal diverticula.

4. A child comes to the emergency department with a history of ingesting a large amount of acetaminophen. For which of the following problems should the nurse assess?
- ☐ **1.** Hypertension.
- ☐ **2.** Frequent urination.
- ☐ **3.** Right upper quadrant pain.
- ☐ **4.** Headache.

5. When developing the plan of care for a toddler who has taken an acetaminophen overdose, which of the following should the nurse expect to include as part of the initial treatment?
- ☐ **1.** Frequent blood level determinations.
- ☐ **2.** Gastric lavage.
- ☐ **3.** Tracheostomy.
- ☐ **4.** Electrocardiogram.

6. While assessing a preschooler brought by her parents to the emergency department after ingestion of kerosene, the nurse should be alert for which of the following?
- ☐ **1.** Uremia.
- ☐ **2.** Hepatitis.
- ☐ **3.** Carditis.
- ☐ **4.** Pneumonitis.

The Client with Lead Poisoning

7. Which of the following statements by the mother of an 18-month-old child should indicate to the nurse that the child needs laboratory testing for lead levels?
- ☐ **1.** "My child does not always wash after playing outside."
- ☐ **2.** "My child drinks 2 cups of milk every day."
- ☐ **3.** "My child has more temper tantrums than other kids."
- ☐ **4.** "My child is smaller than other kids of the same age."

8. A child's blood lead concentration is 17 mg/dl, and it has been higher than 10 mg/dl for several months. What should the nurse anticipate will happen?
- ☐ **1.** Need for follow-up in 3 months.
- ☐ **2.** Immediate initiation of chelation therapy.
- ☐ **3.** Investigation of the child's environment.
- ☐ **4.** Prompt admission to the hospital.

200

9. When teaching the mother of a toddler diagnosed with lead poisoning, which of the following should the nurse include as the most serious complication if the condition goes untreated?
☐ 1. Cirrhosis of the liver.
☐ 2. Stunted growth rate.
☐ 3. Neurologic deficits.
☐ 4. Heart failure.

10. When teaching a mother about measures to prevent lead poisoning in her children, which of the following preventive measures should the nurse include as the most effective?
☐ 1. Condemning of old housing developments.
☐ 2. Educating the public on common sources of lead.
☐ 3. Educating the public on the importance of good nutrition.
☐ 4. Keeping pregnant women out of old homes that are being remodeled.

11. Which of the following is the nurse's *best* response to a mother who asks about the outcome for her child with lead poisoning?
☐ 1. "Many children suffer brain damage from lead poisoning."
☐ 2. "Many of its effects require the child to receive special schooling."
☐ 3. "Most children with lead poisoning experience problems with the law."
☐ 4. "Most effects of lead poisoning are reversible if diagnosed early."

The Client with Celiac Disease

12. Which of the following statements by a mother about her child would suggest to the nurse that the child has celiac disease?
☐ 1. "His urine is so dark in color."
☐ 2. "His stools are large and smelly."
☐ 3. "His belly is so small."
☐ 4. "He is so short."

13. During assessment of a child with celiac disease, the nurse should most likely note which of the following physical findings?
☐ 1. Enlarged liver.
☐ 2. Protuberant abdomen.
☐ 3. Tender inguinal lymph nodes.
☐ 4. Periorbital edema.

14. After teaching the mother of a child with celiac disease about dietary management, which of the following statements by the mother indicates successful teaching?
☐ 1. "I will feed my child foods that contain wheat products."
☐ 2. "I will be sure to give my child lots of milk."
☐ 3. "I will plan to feed my child foods that contain rice."
☐ 4. "I will be sure my child gets oatmeal every day."

15. After teaching the parents of a child with celiac disease about diet, which of the following, if stated by the parents to be avoided, indicates effective teaching? Select all that apply.
☐ 1. Chocolate candy.
☐ 2. Hot dogs.
☐ 3. Bologna on rye sandwich.
☐ 4. Corn tortillas.
☐ 5. White rice.

16. Which of the following foods would be appropriate for a 12-month-old child with celiac disease?
☐ 1. Cheerios.
☐ 2. Pancakes.
☐ 3. Rice Chex.
☐ 4. Waffles.

17. The mother of a child with celiac disease asks, "How long must he stay on this diet?" Which response by the nurse is best?
☐ 1. "Until the jejunal biopsy is normal."
☐ 2. "Until his stools appear normal."
☐ 3. "For the next 6 months."
☐ 4. "For the rest of his life."

The Client with Phenylketonuria

18. When preparing to obtain a neonatal screening test for phenylketonuria, the neonate must have received which of the following to ensure reliable results?
☐ 1. A feeding of an iron-rich formula.
☐ 2. Nothing by mouth for 4 hours before the test.
☐ 3. Cow's or breast milk for 24 hours before the test.
☐ 4. A loading dose of glucose water.

19. When developing the plan of care for a child diagnosed with phenylketonuria (PKU), which of the following goals should the nurse expect to include as an appropriate goal of care?
☐ 1. Meeting the child's nutritional needs for optimal growth.
☐ 2. Ensuring that the special diet is started at age 3 weeks.
☐ 3. Maintaining serum phenylalanine level higher than 12 mg/100 ml.
☐ 4. Maintaining serum phenylalanine level lower than 2 mg/100 ml.

20. When taking a diet history from the mother of a 7-year-old child with phenylketonuria, a report of an intake of which of the following foods should cause the nurse to become concerned?
☐ 1. Cola.
☐ 2. Carrots.
☐ 3. Orange juice.
☐ 4. Bananas.

21. Which foods would the nurse teach the parents of a child with phenylketonuria (PKU) to avoid? Select all that apply.
- [ ] **1.** Hamburger.
- [ ] **2.** Hot dog.
- [ ] **3.** Ice cream.
- [ ] **4.** Juice.
- [ ] **5.** Cereal.

22. When teaching the mother of a child diagnosed with phenylketonuria (PKU) about its transmission, the nurse should use knowledge of which of the following as the basis for the discussion?
- [ ] **1.** Chromosome translocation.
- [ ] **2.** Chromosome deletion.
- [ ] **3.** Autosomal recessive gene.
- [ ] **4.** X-linked recessive gene.

23. A newborn diagnosed with phenylketonuria (PKU) is placed on a milk substitute, Lofenalac. The mother asks the nurse how long her infant will be taking this. Which of the following responses would be most appropriate?
- [ ] **1.** "Until the infant is taking solid foods well."
- [ ] **2.** "Until the child has stopped growing."
- [ ] **3.** "Until the phenylalanine level remains below normal for 6 months."
- [ ] **4.** "Probably for a long time, but it's not definitely known."

24. Even though several teaching sessions have been documented in the client's health record, the mother asks the nurse again what caused her child's phenylketonuria (PKU). Which of the following statements would best reflect the nurse's interpretation of why the mother keeps asking for information that she has already received?
- [ ] **1.** Because the child's condition is chronic, parents commonly want very detailed explanations about the causes of and treatments for their child's disease.
- [ ] **2.** Parents of a chronically ill child commonly require a long time to work through the grieving process for their child's disease.
- [ ] **3.** Parents commonly test health workers' knowledge about the causes of and treatments for their child's disease.
- [ ] **4.** Parents commonly deal with their guilt about possibly causing their child's disease by asking challenging questions.

The Client with Colic

25. When performing the nursing history, which of the following would be most important for the nurse to obtain from the mother of an infant with suspected colic?
- [ ] **1.** The type of formula the infant is taking.
- [ ] **2.** The infant's crying pattern.
- [ ] **3.** The infant's sleep position.
- [ ] **4.** The position of the infant during burping.

26. The parents of a child with colic are asked to describe the infant's bowel movements. Which of the following descriptions should the nurse expect?
- [ ] **1.** Soft, yellow stools.
- [ ] **2.** Frequent watery stools.
- [ ] **3.** Ribbon-like stools.
- [ ] **4.** Foul-smelling stools.

27. The mother tells the nurse that the diagnosis of colic upsets her because she knows her infant will continue to have colicky pain. Which of the following responses by the nurse would be most appropriate?
- [ ] **1.** "I know that your baby's crying upsets you, but she needs your undivided attention for the next few months."
- [ ] **2.** "It can be difficult to listen to your baby cry so loud and so long, so try to make sure that you get some free time."
- [ ] **3.** "It's must be distressing to see your baby in pain, but at least she doesn't have an intestinal obstruction."
- [ ] **4.** "The next 3 months will be a difficult time for you, but your baby will outgrow the colic by this time."

28. The nurse judges that the mother has understood the teaching about care of an infant with colic when the nurse observes the mother doing which of the following?
- [ ] **1.** Holding the infant prone while feeding.
- [ ] **2.** Holding the infant in her lap to burp.
- [ ] **3.** Placing the infant prone after the feeding.
- [ ] **4.** Burping the infant during and after the feeding.

The Client with Obesity

29. A mother brings her 7-month-old infant to the well-baby clinic for a checkup. She is concerned that the infant is overweight. She feeds the infant formula that has 20 calories per ounce whenever the infant is hungry. The nurse should instruct the mother to:
- [ ] **1.** Give the infant 2% milk formula and add vitamins.
- [ ] **2.** Use skim milk because it is high in protein and lower in calories.
- [ ] **3.** Decrease the amount of formula feedings to 16 oz daily, and supplement with juice and water.
- [ ] **4.** Continue with the formula, keep a 3-day record of the infant's intake, and bring the infant back to the clinic for further evaluation.

30. Which of the following methods should the nurse use to provide the most accurate assessment of an adolescent's status regarding obesity?
- [ ] **1.** A food intake diary for 1 week.
- [ ] **2.** Body mass index.
- [ ] **3.** A 4-hour dietary history.
- [ ] **4.** Skinfold thickness measurements.

31. When counseling an obese adolescent, the nurse should advise the client that which complication is the most common?
- [ ] 1. Lifelong obesity.
- [ ] 2. Gastrointestinal problems.
- [ ] 3. Orthopedic problems.
- [ ] 4. Psychosocial problems.

32. When developing a teaching plan for the mother of an infant about introducing solid foods into the diet, which of the following measures should the nurse expect to include in the plan to help prevent obesity?
- [ ] 1. Decreasing the amount of formula or breast milk intake as solid food intake increases.
- [ ] 2. Introducing the infant to the taste of vegetables by mixing them with formula or breast milk.
- [ ] 3. Mixing cereal and fruit in a bottle when offering solid food for the first few times.
- [ ] 4. Using a large-bowled spoon for feeding solid foods during the first several months.

33. A pregnant mother who has brought her toddler to the clinic for a check-up asks the nurse how she can keep her next baby from becoming obese. The mother plans to bottle-feed her next child. Which information should the nurse include in the teaching plan to help the mother avoid overnourishing her infant?
- [ ] 1. Recognizing clues indicating that a baby is full.
- [ ] 2. Establishing a regular feeding schedule.
- [ ] 3. Supplementing feedings with sterile water.
- [ ] 4. Adding more water than directed when preparing formula.

The Client with Food Sensitivity

34. A father tells the nurse that he has heard of cow's milk allergy but knows nothing about cow's milk sensitivity. The nurse should explain this condition as:
- [ ] 1. Hereditary disorder of carbohydrate metabolism.
- [ ] 2. Adverse reaction to cow's milk protein.
- [ ] 3. Acquired lactose intolerance.
- [ ] 4. Existence of a lifelong allergy.

35. After teaching the parents of a child with lactose intolerance about the disorder, the nurse determines that the teaching was effective when hearing the mother describe the condition to a visitor as which of the following?
- [ ] 1. "The lack of an enzyme to break down lactose."
- [ ] 2. "An allergy to lactose found in milk."
- [ ] 3. "Inability to digest proteins completely."
- [ ] 4. "Inability to digest fats completely."

36. After teaching the mother of a 2-year-old child with lactose intolerance about which dairy products to include in the child's diet, which of the following if stated by the mother indicates effective teaching?
- [ ] 1. Ice cream.
- [ ] 2. Creamed soups.
- [ ] 3. Pudding.
- [ ] 4. Cheese.

37. The breast-feeding mother of a 1-month-old diagnosed with cow's milk sensitivity asks the nurse what she should do about feeding her infant. Which of the following recommendations would be most appropriate?
- [ ] 1. Continue to breast-feed but eliminate all milk products from your own diet.
- [ ] 2. Discontinue breast-feeding and start using a predigested formula.
- [ ] 3. Limit breast-feeding to once per day and begin feeding an iron-fortified formula.
- [ ] 4. Change to a soy-based formula exclusively and begin solid foods.

The Client with Failure to Thrive

38. The nurse is inserting a nasogastric tube in an infant to administer feedings. In the figure below, indicate the location for the correct placement of the distal end of the tube.

39. The nurse formulates the nursing diagnosis *Imbalanced Nutrition: Less than body requirements* related to negative feeding patterns for a 5-month old infant diagnosed with failure to thrive. To meet the short-term outcomes of the infant's plan of care, the nurse should expect to do which of the following?
- [ ] 1. Instruct the parents in proper feeding techniques.
- [ ] 2. Give infant formula that has 24 calories/ounce.
- [ ] 3. Provide consistent staff to care for the infant.
- [ ] 4. Allow the infant to sit in a high chair during feedings.

40. The health care team determines that the family of an infant with failure to thrive who is to be discharged will need follow-up care. Which of the following would be the *most* effective method of follow-up?
- [ ] 1. Daily phone calls from the hospital nurse.
- [ ] 2. Enrollment in community parenting classes.
- [ ] 3. Twice-weekly clinic appointments.
- [ ] 4. Weekly visits by a community health nurse.

Correct Answers and Rationales

The letter in parentheses after each rationale identifies the client need addressed in the item, including management of care (M), safety and infection control (S), health promotion and maintenance (H), psychosocial adaptation (P), basic care and comfort (C), pharmacological and parenteral therapies (D), reduction of risk potential (R), and physiological adaptation (A).

The Client with Toxic Substance Ingestion

1. 1. Syrup of ipecac is an emetic that exerts its action by stimulating the vomiting center directly and producing irritating effects on the stomach mucosa. It is given with one to two glasses of water or fruit juice. If the child does not vomit within 20 minutes after taking syrup of ipecac, a second dose may be administered. Diuretics such as furosemide (Lasix) would promote diuresis. Drugs such as phenobarbital, diazepam (Valium), or phenytoin (Dilantin) are used to control seizures. Drugs such as epinephrine may be used to stimulate the heart. (D)

2. 2. Drain cleaner almost always contains lye, which can burn the mouth, pharynx, and esophagus on ingestion. The nurse would be prepared to assist with a tracheostomy, which may be necessary because of swelling around the area of the larynx. An emetic is contraindicated because, as the substance burns on ingestion, so too would it burn when vomiting. Additionally, the mucosa becomes necrotic and vomiting could lead to perforations. Gastric lavage is contraindicated because the mucosa is burned from the ingestion of the caustic lye, causing necrosis. Gastric lavage also could lead to perforation of the necrotic mucosa. Insertion of an indwelling urinary (Foley) catheter would be indicated after the measures to remove the caustic substance have been started. (R)

3. 3. As the burn from the lye ingestion heals, scar tissue develops and can lead to esophageal strictures, a common complication of lye ingestion. Tracheal stenosis would occur if the child had vomited and aspirated. Tracheal varices do not commonly occur after the ingestion of lye or other substances. Although very rare, esophageal diverticula may occur. Diverticula are commonly found in the colon of adults. (A)

4. 3. After ingesting a large amount of acetaminophen, the child would complain of right upper quadrant pain due to hepatic damage from glutathione combining with the metabolite of acetaminophen being broken down. Hypertension is not associated with acetaminophen ingestion. Frequent urination occurs as a result of intravenous fluid administration, not acetaminophen ingestion. Headache is not an expected finding with acetaminophen overdose. (A)

5. 2. Initial management of a child who has ingested a large amount of acetaminophen would include inducing vomiting or performing gastric lavage with or without activated charcoal to aid in the removal of the substance. Frequent blood level determinations may be obtained during the follow-up phase, but they are not done as part of the initial treatment. Tracheostomy is not typically part of the initial treatment for acetaminophen overdose. However, it may be necessary later if respiratory distress develops. Acetaminophen primarily affects the liver, not the heart. Therefore, an electrocardiogram would not be considered part of the initial treatment plan. (R)

6. 4. Chemical pneumonitis is the most common complication of ingestion of hydrocarbons, such as in kerosene. The pneumonitis is caused by irritation from the hydrocarbons aspirated into the lungs. Uremia is the result of renal insufficiency, which causes nitrogenous waste products to build up in the blood rather than being excreted. Hepatitis is caused by a viral infection. Carditis in a preschooler may be the result of rheumatic fever. (A)

The Client with Lead Poisoning

7. 1. Eating with dirty hands, especially after playing outside, can lead to lead poisoning because lead is often present in soil surrounding homes. Also, children who eat lead-containing paint chips commonly develop lead poisoning. Drinking 2 cups of milk per day is less than that which is recommended for this age group, so more nutritional information would need to be obtained. Temper tantrums are characteristic of 18-month-old children as they try to assert themselves. Determining whether the child is smaller than other children the same age requires measuring height and weight and plotting them on growth charts. In addition, inadequate growth could be a result of numerous causes, such as genetics, chronic illness, or chronic drug use (for example, prednisone). (A)

8. 3. The child is considered to be at moderate risk, because the increased blood level concentration has persisted. When blood levels reach 20 to 44 mg/dl, an investigation of the child's environment will be initiated. The nurse should follow up sooner than 3 months, particularly if intervention is required following the investigation of the child's environment. Oral chelation therapy is started when blood lead levels reach 45 mg/dl. When the blood levels reach 70 mg/dl, the child is usually hospitalized for intravenous chelation therapy. (R)

9. 3. The most serious and irreversible consequence of lead poisoning is mental retardation due to neurologic changes. It can be expected if lead poisoning is long-standing and goes untreated. Lead poisoning also affects the hematologic and renal systems. Cirrhosis is the end stage of several chronic liver diseases, such as biliary atresia and hepatitis. Lead poisoning is not associated with stunted growth. Chronic illnesses, such as cystic fibrosis, cause slowing of the growth velocity. Heart failure is associated with congenital heart disease and rheumatic fever. (A)

10. 2. Public education about the sources of lead that could cause poisoning has been found to be the most effective measure to prevent lead poisoning. This includes recent efforts to alert the public to lead in certain types of window blinds. Condemning old housing developments has been ineffective because lead paint still exists in many other dwellings. Providing education about good nutrition, although important, is not an effective preventive measure. Pregnant women and children should not remain in an older home that is being remodeled because they may breathe in lead in the dust, but this is not the most effective preventive measure. (S)

11. 4. Most of the pathologic effects of lead poisoning are reversible as long as the problem is diagnosed early. The most serious effects are those on the central nervous system (for example, brain damage, mental retardation, behavior changes), not problems with the law. However, because of screening programs, many children with lead poisoning are diagnosed and treated early. As a result, little if any brain damage occurs that would require children to receive special schooling. (A)

The Client with Celiac Disease

12. 2. Celiac disease is a disorder involving intolerance to the protein gluten, which is found in wheat, rye, oats, and barley. The stools of a child with celiac disease are characteristically malodorous, pale, large (bulky), and soft (loose). Excessive flatus is common, and bouts of diarrhea may occur. Dark urine is commonly associated with concentrated urine, such as when a child has dehydration. The belly of a child with celiac disease, a malabsorption disorder, typically is protuberant. A small belly may be associated with a child who is thin. Short stature is not associated with this malabsorption disorder. (A)

13. 2. The intestines of a child with celiac disease fill with accumulated undigested food and flatus, causing the characteristic protuberant abdomen. Celiac disease is not usually associated with any liver dysfunction, including poor liver functioning leading to liver enlargement. Tender inguinal lymph nodes are often associated with an infection. Periorbital edema, swelling around the eyes, is associated with nephritis. (A)

14. 3. Damage to intestinal mucosa in celiac disease is caused by gliadin, a part of the protein found in wheat, rye, barley, and oats. Foods containing these grains must be eliminated entirely from the diet of children with celiac disease. Foods containing rice and corn are a good substitute. Although an adequate intake of milk is important for any child, children with celiac disease do not need an increased milk intake. (A)

15. 1, 2, 3. Children with celiac disease should avoid foods containing the protein gluten, which is found in wheat, oats, rye, and barley grains. Children are allowed to eat foods containing rice or corn. Labels need to be read carefully since these glutens are used as fillers in many food items including many types of chocolate candy and hot dogs. (R)

16. 3. The child with celiac disease should not eat foods containing wheat, oats, rye, or barley. Foods containing rice, such as Rice Chex cereal, or corn are appropriate. Because Cheerios are made from oats, this cereal should be avoided. Pancakes and waffles are made from flour that typically is derived from wheat and therefore should be avoided. (A)

17. 4. Most children with celiac disease have a lifelong sensitivity to gluten, which requires that they maintain some type of diet restriction for the rest of their lives. (A)

The Client with Phenylketonuria

18. 3. PKU is an autosomal recessive genetic disorder involving the absence of an enzyme needed to metabolize the essential amino acid, phenylalanine, to tyrosine. To ensure reliable results, the neonate must have ingested a diet high in phenylalanine, such as cow's or breast milk, for at least 24 hours. Testing of the neonate before that time, excessive vomiting, or poor intake can yield false-negative results. The infant does not need to be in a fasting state for 4 hours before the test. A loading dose of glucose water is not necessary. (R)

19. 1. The goal of care is to prevent mental retardation by adjusting the diet to meet the infant's nutritional needs for optimal growth. The diet needs to be started as soon as the infant is diagnosed, ideally within a few days of birth. Serum phenylalanine level should be maintained between 3 and 7 mg/100 ml. Significant brain damage usually occurs if the serum phenylalanine level exceeds 10 to 15 mg/100 ml. If the level drops below 2 mg/100 ml, the body begins to catabolize its protein stores, causing growth retardation. (A)

20. 1. Foods with low phenylalanine levels include vegetables, fruits, and juices. Foods high in phenylalanine include meats and dairy products, which must be restricted or eliminated. Colas contain more phenylalanine than the fruits listed. (A)

21. 1, 2, 3. Children with PKU lack an enzyme to metabolize phenylalanine and convert it to tyrosine. Treatment is dietary management to control the amount of phenylalanine ingested. Foods with low phenylalanine levels include fruits, most vegetables, and cereals. High-protein foods have high levels of phenylalanine and include meats and dairy products. (R)

22. 3. PKU is caused by an inborn error of metabolism. It is an autosomal recessive disorder that inhibits the conversion of phenylalanine to tyrosine. A form of Down syndrome, trisomy 21, is an example of a disorder caused by chromosomal translocation. Cri du chat is an example of a disorder caused by chromosomal deletion. Hemophilia A is an example of a disorder caused by an X-linked recessive gene. (A)

23. **4.** Although it is not known how long diet therapy must continue for children with PKU, many experts suggest continuing it indefinitely because of academic difficulties and lower intelligence quotients in older children who have stopped the restrictive diet. For women it is necessary to resume the diet before conception to lower the phenylalanine levels in the fetus and prevent complications. (A)

24. **2.** PKU is considered a chronic illness. Parents typically grieve about the loss of health in their child afflicted with a chronic disease. Many times, they repeat questions, as though trying to deny what is really happening. This type of behavior represents an attempt to integrate the experience and their feelings with their self-image as they pass through the grieving process. Asking for detailed explanations, testing the competence of health workers, and expressing impatience with health workers may explain the parents' behavior, but viewing the behavior as a part of the grieving process is the most plausible explanation. (P)

The Client with Colic

25. **2.** Information on the crying pattern of the infant is most helpful in confirming the diagnosis of colic. Typically the colic attack begins abruptly, with the infant crying loudly and continuously, possibly for hours. The attack may end when the child becomes exhausted. The child also may attain some relief after passing stool or flatus. Often, in an attempt to alleviate the infant's crying, parents try to feed the infant, resulting in overfeeding leading to discomfort and distention. Asking about the type of formula, sleep position, or position for burping will not provide sufficient information to confirm the diagnosis of colic. However, the nurse can obtain additional information after determining the nature of the crying pattern. (A)

26. **1.** Infants with colic usually pass normal stools, typically soft and yellowish. Frequent watery stools might indicate diarrhea. Ribbon-like stools are suggestive of a narrowing of the colon or rectum. Foul-smelling stools by themselves are related to diet. When other symptoms such as large size and protuberant abdomen are present, malabsorption may be possible. (A)

27. **2.** The nurse needs to provide the parents with support because of the infant's crying. The parents are stressed and need to be encouraged to get out of the house and arrange for some free time. Although infants need lots of attention and care for the first few months, they do not need the mother's undivided attention. Comparing colic with other problems is inappropriate. Parents have the right to be upset. Although colic usually disappears spontaneously by age 3 months, the nurse should not make any guarantees. (P)

28. **4.** Infants with colic should be burped frequently during and after the feeding. Much of the discomfort of colic appears to be associated with the presence of air in the stomach and intestines. Frequent burping helps to relieve the air. Infants with colic should be held fairly upright while being fed, to help air rise. The preferred position for burping the infant with colic is to hold the infant at the mother's shoulder so that the infant's abdomen lies on the shoulder. This position causes more pressure to be exerted on the infant's abdomen, leading to a more forceful burp. The child should be placed in an infant seat after feedings. (A)

The Client with Obesity

29. **4.** A 3-day diet history is the best way to accurately assess the child's intake. Children under age 1 year should not drink cow's milk because of the risk of allergy. Children over age 1 year should drink whole milk because skim milk and 2% milk do not contain all the essential fatty acids needed by young children. It is unknown at this time how much formula the child is actually taking, but an infant should not have more than 6 oz of juice per day and additional water is usually not necessary. If an infant is taking no more than 32 oz of formula per day and is eating some baby food and cereal, additional fluids and frequent feeding should not be necessary. (H)

30. **2.** The most accurate way to determine whether an adolescent has a problem with obesity is to calculate the body mass index (BMI). The BMI indicates a relationship between height and weight. Numbers obtained through calculation are then applied to a BMI table for interpretation. A food diary will provide information on what the adolescent is eating but does not provide information about obesity. A 4-hour diet history will not provide sufficient information about the client's typical eating patterns over time. Measuring skinfold thickness with skinfold calipers is a common method used to assess obesity. The skinfold thickness test, which determines the amount of subcutaneous fat, determines obesity more accurately than does a height and weight chart. However, it is not the most accurate method and is not routinely performed by nurses. (H)

31. **1.** The most common complication of adolescent obesity is its persistence into adulthood. The incidence of gastrointestinal and orthopedic problems, such as Legg-Calvé-Perthes disease and genu valgum (knock knees), is greater for obese adolescents; however, they are not the most common complication. Although psychosocial problems do occur, they are not the most common complication. (R)

32. 1. Decreasing the amount of formula given as the infant begins to take solids helps prevent excess caloric intake. Because the infant is receiving calories from the solid foods, the formula no longer needs to provide the infant's total caloric requirements. Mixing vegetables with formula or breast milk does not allow the child to become accustomed to new textures or tastes. Solid foods should be given with a spoon, not in a bottle. Using a bottle with food allows the infant to ingest more food than is needed. Also, the infant needs to learn to eat from a spoon. A small-bowled spoon is recommended for infants because infants have a tendency to push food out with the tongue. The small-bowled spoon helps in placing the food at the back of the infant's tongue when feeding. (C)

33. 1. Infants generally do not overeat unless they are urged to do so. Parents should watch for clues indicating that the infant is full—for example, stopping sucking and pushing the nipple out of the mouth. Bottle-feeding instead of breast-feeding is more likely to lead to excessive caloric intake. A demand schedule, rather than a regulated schedule, allows the infant to regulate intake according to individual needs. Normally, giving an infant a regular supplementation of water is unnecessary; the infant's sucking needs can be met by providing a pacifier. Adding more water to the formula than as directed decreases the caloric intake and also places the infant at risk for hyponatremia due to decreased sodium and increased water intake. (C)

The Client with Food Sensitivity

34. 2. Cow's milk sensitivity is an adverse local and systemic gastrointestinal reaction to cow's milk protein. This is the most common nutritional allergy in infants. Cow's milk sensitivity is not inherited. Lactose intolerance involves a deficiency of the enzyme lactase, which is needed for digestion of lactose. Almost all sensitive children can tolerate cow's milk by 2 years of age. (C)

35. 1. Lactose intolerance is not an allergy. Rather, it is caused by the lack of the digestive enzyme lactase. This enzyme, found in the intestines, is necessary for the digestion of lactose, the primary carbohydrate in cow's milk. Protein and fat digestion are not affected. (A)

36. 4. People who are lactose-intolerant usually are able to tolerate dairy products in which lactose has been fermented, such as yogurt, cheese, and buttermilk. Pudding, ice cream, and creamed soups contain lactose that has not been fermented. (A)

37. 1. Mothers of infants with a cow's milk allergy can continue to breast-feed if they eliminate cow's milk from their diet. It is important to encourage mothers to continue to breast-feed because breast milk is usually the least allergenic and most easily digested food for an infant. In addition, the infant is able to obtain protein through the mother's milk. If the mother stops breast-feeding, then a predigested protein hydrolysate formula would be the first choice. An iron-fortified formula is a cow's milk-based formula. A soy-based formula is not used because approximately 20% of infants with cow's milk sensitivity are also sensitive to soy. Solid foods are not introduced until the infant is 4 to 6 months of age. (C)

The Client with Failure to Thrive

38. The nasogastric tube should reside in the stomach. The site placement can be verified by inserting 3 to 5 ml of air in the tube and auscultating the infant's abdomen for the sound of air. The nurse should then aspirate the injected air and a small amount of stomach contents and then test the contents for acidity. (S)

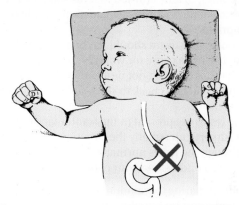

39. 3. In the short-term care of this infant, it is important that the same person feed the infant at each meal and that this person be able to assess for negative feeding patterns and replace them with positive patterns. Once the infant is gaining weight and shows progress in the feeding patterns, the parents can be instructed in proper feeding techniques. This is a long-term outcome of nursing care. Because there is no organic reason for the failure to thrive, it should not be necessary to increase the formula calorie content from 20 to 24 calories/ounce. A 5-month-old infant is too young to be expected to sit in a high chair for feedings and should still be bottle-fed. (A)

40. 4. The most effective follow-up care would occur in the home environment. The community health nurse can be supportive of the parents and will be able to observe parent-infant interactions in a natural environment. The community health nurse can evaluate the infant's progress in gaining weight, offer suggestions to the parents, and help the family solve problems as they arise. (A)

The Child with Health Problems of the Urinary System

The Client with Cryptorchidism

1. A father brings his 4-week-old son to the clinic for a checkup, stating that he is afraid that his son's testicle is missing. Which of the following explanations would be *most* appropriate?
- ☐ 1. "Although the testes should have descended by now, it is not a cause for worry."
- ☐ 2. "The testes often do not descend until age 6 months, but let's check to see whether the testes are present."
- ☐ 3. "The testes are present in the scrotal sac at birth, but surgery can remedy the situation."
- ☐ 4. "Although the testes normally descend by 1 year of age, I can understand your concern."

2. While preparing to examine a 6-week-old infant's scrotal sac and testes for possible undescended testes, which of the following would be *most* important for the nurse to do?
- ☐ 1. Check the diaper for recent urination.
- ☐ 2. Give the infant a pacifier.
- ☐ 3. Ensure that the room is kept warm.
- ☐ 4. Tap lightly on the left inguinal ring.

3. While the nurse is examining the infant for presence of testes, the father paces around the room shaking his head. Which of the following would be the most appropriate response by the nurse?
- ☐ 1. "I'm sure everything will work out for the best, and he'll be fine."
- ☐ 2. "You seem upset; please tell me how you're feeling."
- ☐ 3. "Don't worry; his testes will probably descend on their own."
- ☐ 4. "Would you like to talk with a parent of a child who has the same problem?"

4. When assessing an infant with an undescended testis, the nurse should be alert for which of the following?
- ☐ 1. Abnormal lower extremity reflexes.
- ☐ 2. A history of frequent emesis.
- ☐ 3. A bulging in the inguinal area.
- ☐ 4. Poor weight gain.

5. When developing the plan of care for an infant with an undescended testis, the nurse should expect to include which of the following as a nonsurgical treatment method?
- ☐ 1. A trial of human chorionic gonadotrophic hormone.
- ☐ 2. A trial of adrenocorticotropic hormone.
- ☐ 3. Frequent stimulation of the cremasteric reflex.
- ☐ 4. Use of several warm baths each day.

6. When developing the preoperative teaching plan for a 14-month-old child with an undescended testis who is scheduled to have surgery, which of the following methods should the nurse anticipate using?
- ☐ 1. Telling the child that his penis and scrotum will be "fixed."
- ☐ 2. Explaining to the parents how the defect will be corrected.
- ☐ 3. Telling the child that he will not see any incisions after surgery.
- ☐ 4. Using an anatomically correct doll to show the child what will be "fixed."

7. An adolescent with a history of surgical repair for an undescended testis comes to the clinic for a sports physical. Anticipatory guidance for the parents and adolescent should focus on which of the following as *most* important?
- ☐ 1. The adolescent's sterility.
- ☐ 2. The adolescent's future plans.
- ☐ 3. Technique for monthly testicular self-examinations.
- ☐ 4. Need for a lot of psychological support.

The Client with Hydrocele

8. When explaining to the parents of a child with a hydrocele about the possible cause of the condition, the nurse bases this explanation on the interpretation that a hydrocele is most likely the result of which condition?
☐ **1.** Blockage in the inguinal canal that allows fluid to accumulate in epididymis and ductus deferens.
☐ **2.** Failure of the upper part of the processus vaginalis to atrophy, allowing accumulation of fluid in the testicle and the peritoneal cavity.
☐ **3.** A patent processus vaginalis that results in the collection of fluid along the spermatic cord or tunica vaginalis of the testicle.
☐ **4.** An obliterated processus vaginalis that allows fluid to accumulate in the scrotal sac.

9. During a clinic visit, the mother of an infant with hydrocele states that the infant's scrotum is smaller now than when he was born. After teaching the mother about the infant's condition, which of the following statements by the mother indicates that the teaching has been effective?
☐ **1.** "I guess keeping his bottom up has helped."
☐ **2.** "Massaging his groin area is working."
☐ **3.** "It seems like the fluid is being reabsorbed."
☐ **4.** "Keeping him quiet and in an infant seat has helped."

10. Shortly after an infant is returned to his room following hydrocele repair, the infant's mother tells the nurse that the child's scrotum looks swollen and bruised. Which of the following responses by the nurse would be *most* appropriate?
☐ **1.** "Let me see if the doctor has ordered aspirin for him. If he did, I'll get it right away."
☐ **2.** "Why don't you wait in his room? Then you can ask me any questions when I get there."
☐ **3.** "What you are describing is unusual after this type of surgery. I'll let the doctor know."
☐ **4.** "This is normal after this type of surgery. Let's look at it together just to be sure."

The Client with Hypospadias

11. The parents of a neonate with hypospadias and chordee wish to have him circumcised. Which of the following rationales should the nurse incorporate into the discussion with the parents concerning the recommendation to delay circumcision?
☐ **1.** The associated chordee is difficult to remove during circumcision.
☐ **2.** The foreskin is used to repair the deformity surgically.
☐ **3.** The meatus can become stenosed, leading to urinary obstruction.
☐ **4.** The infant is too small to have a circumcision.

12. The nurse is caring for an infant with hypospadias. Identify the area where the nurse would assess for this condition.

13. A 1-year-old child is scheduled for surgery to correct hypospadias and chordee. The nurse explains to the parents that this is the preferred time for surgical repair based on which of the following?
☐ **1.** At this age, the child will experience less pain.
☐ **2.** The child is too young to have developed castration anxiety.
☐ **3.** The child will not remember the surgical experience.
☐ **4.** The repair is easier to perform after the child is toilet trained.

14. After a surgical repair of a hypospadias, a 12-month-old child returns to the nursing unit with an intravenous line, a urethral catheter, and a suprapubic catheter in place. Which of the following explanations should the nurse give to the parents as the primary purpose for the suprapubic catheter?
☐ **1.** To ensure an accurate measurement of urine output.
☐ **2.** To provide an alternative urinary elimination route.
☐ **3.** To provide an entry port for bladder irrigation.
☐ **4.** To assess for blood clots in the urine.

15. After teaching the parents about the urethral catheter placed after surgical repair of their son's hypospadias, the nurse determines that the teaching was successful when the mother states that the catheter in her child's penis accomplishes which of the following?
☐ **1.** Decreases pain at the surgical site.
☐ **2.** Keeps the new urethra from closing.
☐ **3.** Measures his urine correctly.
☐ **4.** Prevents bladder spasms.

16. While assessing the penis of a child who has had surgery for repair of a hypospadias, the nurse observes the appearance of the penis. The nurse should report which aspect to the surgeon?
☐ **1.** Swollen.
☐ **2.** Dusky blue at the tip.
☐ **3.** Somewhat misshapen.
☐ **4.** Pink.

17. When developing the teaching plan for the parents of a 12-month-old infant with hypospadias and chordee repair, which of the following should the nurse expect to include as *most* important?
- ☐ **1.** Assisting the child to become familiar with his dressings so he will leave them alone.
- ☐ **2.** Encouraging the child to ambulate as soon as possible by using a favorite push toy.
- ☐ **3.** Forcing fluids to at least 2,500 ml/day by offering his favorite juices.
- ☐ **4.** Preventing the child from disrupting the catheters by using soft restraints.

18. The physician orders a urinalysis for a child who has undergone surgical repair of a hypospadias. Which of the following results should the nurse report to the physician?
- ☐ **1.** Urine specific gravity of 1.017.
- ☐ **2.** Ten red blood cells per high-powered field.
- ☐ **3.** Twenty-five white blood cells per high-powered field.
- ☐ **4.** Urine pH of 6.0.

The Client with Urinary Tract Infection

19. A recent history of which sign or symptom should alert the nurse to suspect a urinary tract infection in a 2-year-old child who is exhibiting fever and fussiness?
- ☐ **1.** Abdominal pain.
- ☐ **2.** Swollen lymph glands.
- ☐ **3.** Skin rash.
- ☐ **4.** Back pain.

20. A father of a child with a urinary tract infection calls the clinic and explains, "My wife and I are concerned because our child refuses to obey us concerning the preventions you told us about. Our child refuses to take the medication unless we buy a present. We don't want to use discipline because of the illness, but we're worried about the behavior." Which response by the nurse is best?
- ☐ **1.** "I sympathize with your difficulties, but just ignore the behavior for now."
- ☐ **2.** "I understand it's hard to discipline a child who is ill, but things need to be kept as normal as possible."
- ☐ **3.** "I understand that things are difficult for you right now, but your child is ill and deserves special treatment."
- ☐ **4.** "I understand your concern, but this type of behavior happens all the time; your child will get over it when feeling better."

21. A nurse is teaching the parents of a child diagnosed with a urinary tract infection secondary to vesicoureteral reflux. How should the nurse explain how the reflux contributes to the infection?
- ☐ **1.** It prevents complete emptying of the bladder.
- ☐ **2.** It causes urine backflow into the kidney.
- ☐ **3.** It results in painful bladder spasms.
- ☐ **4.** It causes painful urination.

The Client with Glomerulonephritis

22. A 15-year-old has been diagnosed with acute glomerulonephritis and has been in the hospital for 1 day. Which of the following findings requires immediate action?
- ☐ **1.** Large amount of generalized edema.
- ☐ **2.** Urine specific gravity of 1.030.
- ☐ **3.** Large amount of albumin in the urine.
- ☐ **4.** 24-hour output of 1,500 ml.

23. Which of the following meals would be most appropriate for a 15-year-old with glomerulonephritis with severe hypertension?
- ☐ **1.** Egg noodles, hamburger, canned peas, milk.
- ☐ **2.** Baked ham, baked potato, pear, canned carrots, milk.
- ☐ **3.** Baked chicken, rice, beans, orange juice.
- ☐ **4.** Hot dog on a bun, corn chips, pickle, cookie, milk.

24. A 10-year-old with glomerulonephritis complains of a headache and blurred vision. The nurse should immediately:
- ☐ **1.** Put the client to bed.
- ☐ **2.** Obtain the child's blood pressure.
- ☐ **3.** Notify the physician.
- ☐ **4.** Administer acetaminophen (Tylenol).

25. Which of the following questions should the nurse ask *first* when obtaining a history from the mother of a 10-year-old child with a fever, complaints of not feeling well, and swelling around the eyes?
- ☐ **1.** "Has the child had a sore throat recently?"
- ☐ **2.** "Is the child playing with friends as usual?"
- ☐ **3.** "Does the child urinate as much as usual?"
- ☐ **4.** "Is the urine pale in color?"

26. A school-age client admitted to the hospital because of decreased urine output and periorbital edema is diagnosed with acute poststreptococcal glomerulonephritis. Which of the following actions should receive the *highest* priority?
- ☐ **1.** Assessing vital signs every 4 hours.
- ☐ **2.** Monitoring intake and output every 12 hours.
- ☐ **3.** Obtaining daily weight measurements.
- ☐ **4.** Obtaining serum electrolyte levels daily.

27. When developing the plan of care for a school-age child with acute poststreptococcal glomerulonephritis who has a fluid restriction of 1,000 ml/day, which of the following fluids should the nurse consider as *most* appropriate for the client's condition and effective for preventing excessive thirst?
- [ ] 1. Diet cola.
- [ ] 2. Ice chips.
- [ ] 3. Lemonade.
- [ ] 4. Tap water.

28. During hospitalization, a 10-year-old child with acute poststreptococcal glomerulonephritis and oliguria asks for food from home. After teaching the mother and child about diet, the nurse determines that the teaching had been effective when the mother brings in which food?
- [ ] 1. Pizza and cola.
- [ ] 2. Hamburger and fries.
- [ ] 3. Ice cream sundae.
- [ ] 4. Strawberries and kiwi.

29. The nurse is planning interventions for the nursing diagnosis *Deficient diversional activity* for a school-age child. Which of the following activities should the nurse expect to include?
- [ ] 1. Playing a card game with someone the same age.
- [ ] 2. Putting together a puzzle with mother.
- [ ] 3. Playing video games with a 4-year-old.
- [ ] 4. Watching a movie with a younger brother.

30. A 10-year-old child hospitalized with acute poststreptococcal glomerulonephritis during the acute stage has elevated blood pressure and low urine output for 14 hours. Which step should the nurse do *next*?
- [ ] 1. Assess the child's neurologic status.
- [ ] 2. Encourage the child to drink more water.
- [ ] 3. Advise the child to eat a low-sodium breakfast.
- [ ] 4. Help the client to ambulate in the hallway.

31. When developing the discharge plan for a school-age child diagnosed with acute poststreptococcal glomerulonephritis, which instruction should the nurse plan to discuss?
- [ ] 1. Restricting dietary protein.
- [ ] 2. Monitoring pulse rate and rhythm.
- [ ] 3. Preventing respiratory infections.
- [ ] 4. Restricting foods high in potassium.

32. An older adolescent with a history of losing weight and feeling tired and irritable has been admitted to the hospital with a diagnosis of chronic glomerulonephritis. Which of the following laboratory results would the nurse most likely see?
- [ ] 1. Serum sodium of 133 mEq/L.
- [ ] 2. Blood urea nitrogen (BUN) of 7 mg/dl.
- [ ] 3. Serum potassium of 3.8 mEq/L.
- [ ] 4. Blood pH of 7.43.

The Client with Nephrotic Syndrome

33. A child with nephrosis is taking prednisone. The nurse should teach the caregivers to report which of the following adverse effects? Select all that apply.
- [ ] 1. Increased urinary output.
- [ ] 2. Hematemesis.
- [ ] 3. Respiratory infection.
- [ ] 4. Bleeding gums.
- [ ] 5. Vision problems.

34. The urinalysis of a toddler diagnosed with nephrotic syndrome reveals +4 for protein. The nurse interprets this result as indicating which of the following?
- [ ] 1. Decreased secretion of aldosterone.
- [ ] 2. Increased glomerular permeability to albumin.
- [ ] 3. Inhibited tubular reabsorption of sodium and water.
- [ ] 4. Loss of red blood cells in the urine.

35. Which of the following statements by the mother of a toddler diagnosed with nephrotic syndrome indicates that the mother has understood the nurse's teaching about this disease?
- [ ] 1. "My child really likes chips and bologna. I guess we'll have to find something else."
- [ ] 2. "We'll have to encourage lots of liquids. Did you say about 4 liters every day?"
- [ ] 3. "We worry about the surgery. Do you think we should do direct donation of blood?"
- [ ] 4. "We understand the need for antibiotics. I just wish the antibiotics could be given by mouth."

36. A toddler diagnosed with nephrotic syndrome has a nursing diagnosis of *Excess fluid volume* related to fluid accumulation in the tissues. Which measure should the nurse anticipate including in the child's plan of care?
- [ ] 1. Limiting visitors to 2 to 3 hours a day.
- [ ] 2. Maintaining strict bed rest.
- [ ] 3. Testing urine specific gravity every shift.
- [ ] 4. Weighing the child before breakfast.

37. The mother of a toddler with nephrotic syndrome asks the nurse what can be done about the child's swollen eyes. Which measure should the nurse suggest?
- [ ] 1. Applying cool compresses to the child's eyes.
- [ ] 2. Elevating the head of the child's bed.
- [ ] 3. Applying eye drops every 8 hours.
- [ ] 4. Limiting the child's television watching.

38. The nurse determines that interventions for decreasing fluid retention have been effective when the child with nephrotic syndrome demonstrates evidence of which of the following?
- [ ] 1. Decreased abdominal girth.
- [ ] 2. Increased caloric intake.
- [ ] 3. Increased respiratory rate.
- [ ] 4. Decreased heart rate.

39. The toddler with nephrotic syndrome exhibits generalized edema. Which of the following measures should the nurse institute for this child with a nursing diagnosis of *Impaired skin integrity* related to edema?
- [ ] **1.** Ambulate every shift while awake.
- [ ] **2.** Apply lotion on opposing skin surfaces.
- [ ] **3.** Apply powder to skinfolds.
- [ ] **4.** Separate opposing skin surfaces with soft cloth.

40. A child with nephrosis is placed on prednisone. The dose is 2 mg/kg/day to be administered twice a day. The child weighs 25 lb. How many milligrams will the child receive at each dose?

_____ mg

41. The toddler with nephrotic syndrome responds to treatment and is ready to go home. When helping the family plan for home care, which of the following instructions should the nurse include in the teaching?
- [ ] **1.** Administer pain medication as needed.
- [ ] **2.** Keep the child away from others with an infection.
- [ ] **3.** Notify the physician if there is an increase in the child's urine output.
- [ ] **4.** Administer acetaminophen (Tylenol) daily.

The Client with Acute or Chronic Renal Failure

42. When explaining the advantages of peritoneal dialysis versus hemodialysis to an adolescent with chronic renal failure, the nurse states that continuous peritoneal dialysis involves which of the following?
- [ ] **1.** Fewer dietary restrictions.
- [ ] **2.** Less chance of infection.
- [ ] **3.** More protein loss.
- [ ] **4.** More rapid fluid removal.

43. While performing daily peritoneal dialysis and catheter exit site care with the mother of a child with chronic renal failure, which of the following would be an important step to stress to the mother?
- [ ] **1.** Applying an occlusive dressing after cleaning the site.
- [ ] **2.** Changing the dressing when the peritoneal space is dry.
- [ ] **3.** Examining the site for signs of infection while cleaning the area.
- [ ] **4.** Pulling on the catheter to hold taut while cleaning the skin.

44. When developing the discharge teaching plan for a child with chronic renal failure and the family, the nurse should emphasize restriction of which of the following nutrients?
- [ ] **1.** Ascorbic acid.
- [ ] **2.** Calcium.
- [ ] **3.** Magnesium.
- [ ] **4.** Phosphorus.

45. After emphasizing to an adolescent with renal failure the importance of maintaining a positive self-concept, which of the following behaviors by the adolescent should the nurse identify as an indicator that the plan is working?
- [ ] **1.** Complaints about headaches, abdominal pain, and nausea.
- [ ] **2.** Insistence on making diet choices even if the foods chosen are restricted.
- [ ] **3.** Verbalization of plans to quit all after-school activities when returning home.
- [ ] **4.** Demonstration of desire to do the dressing changes and take care of the medications.

46. Which of the following diet plans would be appropriate for the nurse to discuss with the family of a child with acute renal failure?
- [ ] **1.** High carbohydrate and protein.
- [ ] **2.** High fat and carbohydrate.
- [ ] **3.** Low fat and protein.
- [ ] **4.** Low in carbohydrate and fat.

47. An adolescent with chronic renal failure is scheduled to go home with a peritoneal dialysis catheter in place. When developing the discharge teaching plan for the client and family focusing on psychosocial needs, which of the following areas should be a top priority to include?
- [ ] **1.** Advantages of limiting social activities and contacts for the first few months.
- [ ] **2.** Not disclosing information about the peritoneal dialysis to people outside the family.
- [ ] **3.** Possible effect on body image of the presence of an abdominal catheter.
- [ ] **4.** Importance of relying on parents to do the dialysis and dressing changes.

48. During a home visit, the public health nurse assesses the peritoneal catheter exit site of a child with chronic renal failure. Which of the following findings should lead the nurse to formulate the nursing diagnosis *Risk for infection*?
- [ ] **1.** Dialysate leakage.
- [ ] **2.** Granulation tissue.
- [ ] **3.** Increased time for drainage.
- [ ] **4.** Tissue swelling.

49. After teaching the mother of a young child with a peritoneal catheter about the signs and symptoms of peritonitis, the nurse determines that the mother has understood the teaching when she identifies which of the following as an important sign?
- [ ] **1.** Cloudy dialysate drainage return.
- [ ] **2.** Distended abdomen.
- [ ] **3.** Shortness of breath.
- [ ] **4.** Weight gain of 3 lb in 2 days.

50. The nurse assesses the child with chronic renal failure who is receiving peritoneal dialysis for edema. Which sign should the nurse expect to find?
☐ **1.** Absence of pulmonary crackles.
☐ **2.** Increased dialysate outflow.
☐ **3.** Normal blood pressure.
☐ **4.** Pallor.

51. The mother of a child with chronic renal failure who is receiving peritoneal dialysis at home asks the public health nurse what she can do if both inflow and drain times are increased. Which of the following instructions would be *most* appropriate for the nurse to include when responding to the mother?
☐ **1.** Assess the child for constipation.
☐ **2.** Decrease the amount of dialysate infused for each dwell.
☐ **3.** Incorporate the increased inflow and drain times into the dialysis schedule.
☐ **4.** Monitor the child for shoulder pain during inflow and drain times.

52. The nurse judges that the mother understands the diet restrictions for her child with chronic renal failure who is receiving peritoneal dialysis when she reports providing a diet involving which of the following?
☐ **1.** Sodium and water restrictions.
☐ **2.** High protein and carbohydrates.
☐ **3.** High potassium and iron.
☐ **4.** Protein and phosphorus restrictions.

The Client with Wilms' Tumor

53. When assessing a child admitted to the pediatric unit with the diagnosis of Wilms' tumor, which of the following findings should the nurse expect?
☐ **1.** Hypotension.
☐ **2.** Proteinemia.
☐ **3.** Pallor.
☐ **4.** Petechiae.

54. When assessing a 2-year-old child with Wilms' tumor, the nurse should keep in mind that it is *most* important to avoid which of the following actions?
☐ **1.** Measuring the child's chest circumference.
☐ **2.** Palpating the child's abdomen.
☐ **3.** Placing the child in an upright position.
☐ **4.** Measuring the child's occipitofrontal circumference.

55. Which statement by the mother of a child with Wilms' tumor tells the nurse that the mother understands what *stage II tumor* means?
☐ **1.** "The tumor has extended beyond the kidney but was completely removed."
☐ **2.** "Although the tumor was in the kidney, it has spread to the lung, liver, and bone."
☐ **3.** "The tumor has extended outside the kidney to the lungs and the liver."
☐ **4.** "The tumor was solely located in the kidney but it was totally removed."

56. A child diagnosed with Wilms' tumor undergoes successful surgery for removal of the diseased kidney. When the child returns to the room, the nurse should place the child in which position?
☐ **1.** Modified Trendelenburg.
☐ **2.** Sims'.
☐ **3.** Semi-Fowler's.
☐ **4.** Supine.

57. After a child undergoes nephrectomy for a Wilms' tumor, the nurse should assess the child postoperatively for which early sign of a complication?
☐ **1.** Increased abdominal distention.
☐ **2.** Elevated blood pressure.
☐ **3.** Increased respiratory rate.
☐ **4.** Increased urine output.

58. When developing the discharge plan for a child who had a nephrectomy for a Wilms' tumor, the nurse identifies outcomes to prevent damage to the child's remaining kidney and accomplish which of the following?
☐ **1.** Minimize pain.
☐ **2.** Prevent dependent edema.
☐ **3.** Prevent urinary tract infection.
☐ **4.** Minimize sodium intake.

Correct Answers and Rationales

The letter in parentheses after each rationale identifies the client need addressed in the item, including management of care (M), safety and infection control (S), health promotion and maintenance (H), psychosocial adaptation (P), basic care and comfort (C), pharmacological and parenteral therapies (D), reduction of risk potential (R), and physiological adaptation (A).

The Client with Cryptorchidism

1. 4. Normally the testes descend by 1 year of age; failure to do so may indicate a problem with patency or a hormonal imbalance. By age 4 weeks, descent may not have occurred. However, telling the father that lack of descent is not a cause for worry is inappropriate and uncaring. Additionally, a statement such as this may be false reassurance. By acknowledging the father's concern, the nurse indicates acceptance of his feelings. If the testes have not descended, then they will not be palpable in the scrotal sac. Surgery is not discussed until after a full assessment is completed. (H)

2. 3. A cold environment can cause the testes to retract. Cold and touch stimulate the cremasteric reflex, which causes a normal retraction of the testes toward the body. Therefore, the nurse should warm the hands and make sure that the environment also is warm. Checking the diaper for urination provides information about the infant's voiding and urinary function, not information about the testes. Giving the infant a pacifier may help to calm the infant and possibly make the examination easier, but the concern here is with the temperature of the environment. Tapping on the inguinal ring would not be helpful in assessing the infant. (H)

3. 2. The nurse needs more information about the father's perceptions and feelings before providing any information or taking action. Determining the exact nature of the father's concern rather than making an assumption about it is essential. Therefore, the nurse should identify what is observed and ask the father how he is feeling. Telling the father that everything will be fine or not to worry is inappropriate and provides false reassurance. It also devalues the father's concern. Later on it may be appropriate for the father to talk to a parent of a child with the same problem for support. (P)

4. 3. When an anomaly is found in one system, such as the genitourinary system, that system requires a more focused assessment to reveal other conditions that also may be occurring. A bulging in the inguinal area may suggest an inguinal hernia. Also, hydrocele or an upper urinary tract anomaly may occur on the same side as the undescended testis. A neuromuscular problem, not a genitourinary problem such as undescended testes, would most likely be the cause of abnormal lower extremity reflexes. A history of frequent emesis may be caused by pyloric stenosis or viral gastroenteritis. Poor weight gain might suggest a metabolic or feeding problem. (H)

5. 1. A trial of human chorionic gonadotrophin may be given to stimulate descent of the affected testis. A trial of adrenocorticotropic hormone will not cause the testis to descend. The cremasteric reflex results in the testis being drawn up, the opposite of the intended effect. Application of warmth, such as warm baths, although soothing and relaxing for the infant, would have little or no effect on stimulating the testis to descend. (D)

6. 2. Preoperative teaching would be directed at the parents, because the child is too young to understand the teaching. Telling the child that his penis and scrotum will be "fixed," telling the child he will not see incisions after surgery, and using a doll to illustrate the surgery are appropriate interventions for a preschool-age child. (P)

7. 3. Because the incidence of testicular cancer is increased in adulthood among children who have had undescended testes, it is extremely important to teach the adolescent how to perform the testicular self-examination monthly. The undescended testicle is removed to reduce the risk of cancer in that testicle. Removal of a testis would not necessarily make the adolescent sterile because the other testicle remains. Although discussing the adolescent's future plans is important, it is not the priority at this time. Because the adolescent has been dealing with the situation for a long time, the need for a sports physical at this time should not be a cause of emotional distress requiring a lot of psychological support. (H)

The Client with Hydrocele

8. 3. A hydrocele is a collection of fluid in the tunica vaginalis of the testicle or along the spermatic cord that results from a patent processus vaginalis. Failure of the upper part of the processus vaginalis to atrophy allows the accumulation of fluid in the testicle and peritoneal cavity, causing an inguinal hernia. (A)

9. 3. A hydrocele is a collection of fluid in the tunica vaginalis of the testicle or along the spermatic cord that results from a patent processus vaginalis. Because scrotal size is decreasing, the fluid is being absorbed. Elevation of the infant's bottom, massage, or keeping the infant quiet or in an infant seat would have no effect in promoting fluid reabsorption in hydrocele. (A)

10. 4. Some swelling and bruising are normal postoperatively. By assessing the area with the mother, the nurse is conveying acceptance of the mother's concern. In addition, the nurse needs to inspect the area to determine if what the mother is describing is accurate. Doing so also provides an opportunity for teaching. Aspirin is not usually prescribed for children because of the link between aspirin and Reye's syndrome. Acetaminophen is commonly administered for fever or pain relief. Asking the mother to wait in the child's room ignores the mother's concerns. There is no need to notify the doctor at this time. (P)

The Client with Hypospadias

11. 2. The condition in which the urethral opening is on the ventral side of the penis or below the glans penis is referred to as *hypospadias*. *Chordee* refers to a ventral curvature of the penis that results from a fibrous band of tissue that has replaced normal tissue. Circumcision is delayed because the foreskin, which is removed with a circumcision, often is used to reconstruct the urethra. The chordee is corrected when the hypospadias is repaired. Circumcision is performed at the same time. Urethral meatal stenosis, which can occur in circumcised infants, results from meatal ulceration, possibly leading to urinary obstruction. It is not associated with hypospadias or circumcision. The infant is not too small to have a circumcision, which is commonly performed on the first or second day of life. (R)

12. In hypospadias, the urethral opening is on the ventral side of the penis. (A)

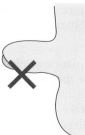

13. 2. The preferred time for surgery is between the ages of 6 and 18 months, before the child develops castration and body image anxiety. Children learn early on about society's emphasis on the importance of genitals. Pain is different for each child and is not related to the preferred time for repair of the hypospadias or chordee. Although the child will probably not remember the experience, this is not the basis for having the surgery at this age. If the condition is not repaired, the child will have difficulty with toilet training because urine is not eliminated through the tip of the penis. (A)

14. 2. Surgical repair of a hypospadias involves use of the skin from the prepuce to extend the urethra to the tip of the penis. An alternative urinary elimination route is needed because the surgical site needs to be kept dry, clean, and free from the pressure of a full bladder. Pressure from a full bladder might cause fluid to leak around the urethral catheter or possibly disrupt the delicate plastic surgery. Although the suprapubic catheter does aid in providing an accurate measurement of urine output, its primary purpose is to provide an alternative route for urinary elimination. After surgical repair of a hypospadias, the bladder does not need to be irrigated. Following surgery, there may be blood clots, but they will drain primarily from the urethral catheter. (R)

15. 2. The main purpose of the urethral catheter is to maintain patency of the reconstructed urethra. The catheter prevents the new tissue inside the urethra from healing on itself. However, the urethral catheter can cause bladder spasms. Recently, stents have been used instead of catheters. The urethral catheter will have no effect on the child's pain level. In fact, because bladder spasms are associated with its use, the child's complaints of pain may actually increase. Urine output can be measured through the suprapubic catheter because it provides an alternative route for urinary elimination, thus keeping the bladder empty and pressure-free. (R)

16. 2. A dusky blue color at the tip of the penis may indicate a problem with circulation, and the nurse should notify the surgeon. Following surgery, it is normal for the penis to be swollen and pink. The penis may be misshapen and is unlikely to look normal even after reconstruction. (A)

17. 4. The most important consideration for a successful outcome of this surgery is maintenance of the catheters or stents. A 12-month-old infant likes to explore his environment but must be prevented from manipulating his dressings or catheters through the use of soft restraints. Allowing the infant to become familiar with the dressings will not prevent him from pulling at them. After surgery the child is allowed limited activity, possibly with sitting in the parent's lap. A 12-month-old infant may or may not be walking. If he is, most likely he will be clumsy and possibly injure himself. Although increasing fluids is important, 2,500 ml/day is an excessive amount for a 12-month-old. Fluid requirements would be 115 ml/kg. (A)

18. 3. A normal white blood cell count in a urinalysis is 1 to 2 cells/ml. A white blood cell count of 25 per high-powered field indicates a urinary tract infection. A urine specific gravity of 1.017 is within the normal range of 1.002 to 1.030. After urologic surgery, it is not unusual for a small number of red blood cells to appear in the urine. The child's urine pH is within the normal range of 4.6 to 8. (R)

The Client with Urinary Tract Infection

19. 1. Abdominal pain frequently accompanies urinary tract infection in children 2 years of age and older. Other associated signs and symptoms include decreased appetite, vomiting, fever, and irritability. The presence of swollen lymph glands (lymphadenopathy) is unrelated to urinary tract infections. Lymphadenopathy is associated with a systemic infection or possibly cancer. Skin rash is associated with exposure to allergens or irritants (for example, poison ivy or harsh soaps); prolonged contact with urine (for example, diaper dermatitis); or illnesses such as measles, rheumatic fever, or juvenile rheumatoid arthritis. Flank or back pain is associated with urinary tract infection in children older than 2 years of age and in adults. (A)

20. 2. To ensure appropriate psychosocial development, a child needs to have normal patterns maintained as much as possible during illness. It is tempting to give ill children special treatment and to relax discipline. However, family routines and discipline should be kept as normal as possible. The child needs to know the limits to ensure feelings of security. When they are ill, children commonly attempt to stretch the rules and limits. If this occurs, returning to the previous well-behavior patterns will take time. (H)

21. 1. The reason that urinary tract infections are a problem in children with vesicoureteral reflux is that urine flows back up the ureter, past the incompetent valve, and back into the bladder after the child has finished voiding. This incomplete emptying of the bladder results in stasis of urine, providing a good medium for bacterial growth and subsequent infection. Vesicoureteral reflux does not cause bladder spasms or painful urination. However, the child may experience painful urination with a urinary tract infection. (A)

The Client with Glomerulonephritis

22. **2.** An adolescent with acute glomerulonephritis has a high urine specific gravity related to oliguria caused by inflammation of the glomeruli. The client will have periorbital edema, but not the generalized edema that occurs in nephrotic syndrome. In glomerulonephritis, there is some albumin in the urine, but there are large amounts of red blood cells, giving the urine a brown color. The urine in glomerulonephritis is scanty, averaging about 400 ml in 24 hours, which leads to fluid volume excess and hypertension. (A)

23. **3.** The best selection of food would include no added salt or salty food. Because sodium cannot be excreted due to the oliguria and to avoid increasing the hypertension, a low-salt diet is recommended. Most canned foods have sodium added as a preservative. Hamburger, ham, hot dogs, canned peas, canned carrots, corn chips, pickles, and milk are high in sodium. (H)

24. **2.** Hypertension occurs with acute glomerulonephritis. The symptoms of headache and blurred vision may indicate an elevated blood pressure. Hypertension in acute glomerulonephritis occurs due to the inability of the kidneys to remove fluid and sodium; the fluid is reabsorbed, causing fluid volume excess. The nurse must verify that these symptoms are due to hypertension. Calling the physician before confirming the cause of the symptoms would not assist the physician in his treatment. Putting the client to bed may help treat an elevated blood pressure, but first the nurse must establish that high blood pressure is the cause of the symptoms. Administering Tylenol for high blood pressure is not recommended. (A)

25. **3.** Most likely, the nurse suspects that the child is exhibiting signs and symptoms of glomerulonephritis, such as periorbital edema and fever. Other signs and symptoms include loss of appetite, dark-colored urine, pallor, headaches, and abdominal pain. To confirm this suspicion, the nurse would ask about the child's urinary elimination patterns. Typically the child with glomerulonephritis experiences a decrease in urine output. Asking about any recent sore throat would provide additional information to confirm the suspicion of glomerulonephritis, because the most common type is acute poststreptococcal glomerulonephritis, which follows a strep throat by 10 to 14 days. Frequently, the children have only mild cold symptoms and do not realize they have a streptococcal infection. Asking whether the child plays with friends as usual is important and gives the nurse information about how the child feels in general. However, this is a general question that would be appropriate to ask later on in the history. Although asking the mother about the color of the child's urine is important, the nurse needs to determine whether there is any change in the child's urinary output first. (A)

26. **3.** The child with acute poststreptococcal glomerulonephritis experiences a problem with renal function that ultimately affects fluid balance. Because weight is the best indicator of fluid balance, obtaining daily weights would be the highest priority. (A)

27. **2.** The most appropriate and effective choice would be ice chips, because they help moisten the mouth and lips while keeping fluid intake low. However, ice chips must still be counted as intake with the fluid restriction. Sweet beverages, such as diet cola or lemonade, commonly increase thirst. Tap water effectively relieves thirst but does not help keep fluid intake low. (A)

28. **4.** The best choice would be fruits such as strawberries and kiwi because they are low in sodium and potassium. Typically, diet is related to the stage and severity of the disease. In children with uncomplicated disease, a regular diet is offered but sodium is usually restricted. In children with hypertension and edema, moderate restriction of sodium is instituted. Pizza and cola, hamburgers and fries, and ice cream are high in sodium and should be avoided. Children with oliguria usually also have potassium restricted. Therefore, foods such as bananas and oranges would be avoided. (A)

29. **1.** Generally, school-age children enjoy activities with their peers first, then family members, and lastly younger children. School-age children like to be busy but also to accomplish something. This helps to meet their task of industry versus inferiority, feeling good about what they are able to accomplish. (H)

30. **1.** The nurse should assess the child's neurologic status, because hypertensive encephalopathy is a major potential complication of the acute phase of glomerulonephritis. Seizure precautions also should be instituted. Hypertensive encephalopathy can result in transient loss of vision, hemiparesis, disorientation, and grand mal seizures. Encouraging the child to drink more water is inappropriate because the child has had a low urine output for 14 hours. Typically, in this situation, fluids would be restricted. Although a low-sodium diet is encouraged, it is not the priority action at this time. Initially, bed rest, not ambulation, is advocated during the acute phase of glomerulonephritis. (R)

31. **3.** Children recovering from glomerulonephritis need to avoid exposure to all types of infections. Glomerulonephritis is caused by group A beta-hemolytic streptococcus, a common cause of sore throat. As the child recovers, he or she may be susceptible to a recurrence if exposed to the organism again. During convalescence from glomerulonephritis, fluid and dietary restrictions are no longer indicated because the kidneys are now functioning normally. There is no need for the parents to assess the child's vital signs. (A)

32. **1.** Because the client with chronic glomerulo-nephritis is in a permanent salt-losing state, the sodium level would be on the low end of normal range of 138 to 145 mEq/L. The blood urea nitrogen level is usually increased above the normal range of 5 to 18 mg/dl. The serum potassium level is usually increased above the normal range of 3.5 to 5.0 mEq/L. Acidosis is usually present. A blood pH of 7.43 is within the normal range of 7.35 to 7.45. (A)

The Client with Nephrotic Syndrome

33. **2, 3.** Adverse effects of steroid therapy include edema of the face and trunk, increased susceptibility to infection, gastric and intestinal mucosal bleeding, sodium and water retention, and hypertension. Urinary output is decreased due to the retention of sodium. Bleeding gums do not result from steroids. Steroid therapy does not cause vision problems. (D)

34. **2.** Nephrotic syndrome involves altered glomerular permeability, which results in increased permeability to albumin, leading to the excretion of large amounts of protein in the urine. Aldosterone secretion is increased, resulting in sodium and water reabsorption. Red blood cells are not lost in the urine in nephrotic syndrome. (R)

35. **1.** Children with nephrotic syndrome usually require sodium restriction. Because potato chips and bologna are high in sodium, the mother's statement about finding something else reflects understanding of this need. Although fluid intake is not restricted in children with nephrotic syndrome, 4 L is an excessive amount for a toddler. The typical fluid requirement for a toddler is 115 ml/kg. Surgical intervention and antibiotic therapy are not parts of the treatment plan for nephrotic syndrome. (A)

36. **4.** The best indicator of fluid balance is weight. Therefore, daily weight measurements help determine fluid losses and gains. Although limiting visitors to 2 to 3 hours per day or maintaining strict bed rest would help to ensure that the child gets adequate rest, this is unrelated to the child's fluid balance. In nephrotic syndrome, urine is tested for protein, not specific gravity. (A)

37. **2.** The child's swollen eyes are caused by fluid accumulation. Elevating the head of the bed allows gravity to increase the downward flow of fluids in the body, away from the face. Applying cool compresses or eye drops, or limiting television, may be comforting but will not relieve the swelling. (A)

38. **1.** Fluid accumulates in the abdomen and interstitial spaces owing to hydrostatic pressure changes. Increased abdominal fluid is evidenced by an increase in abdominal girth. Therefore, decreased abdominal girth is a sign of reduced fluid in the third spaces and tissues. When fluid accumulates in the abdomen and interstitial spaces, the child does not feel hungry and does not eat well. Although increased caloric intake may indicate decreased

intestinal edema, it is not the best and most accurate indicator of fluid retention. Increased respiratory rate may be an indication of increasing fluid in the abdomen (ascites) causing pressure on the diaphragm. Heart rate usually stays in the normal range even with excessive fluid volume. (A)

39. **4.** Placing soft cloth between opposing skin surfaces absorbs moisture and keeps the area dry, thus preventing any further breakdown. The child with nephrotic syndrome and severe edema is usually maintained on bed rest. Therefore, ambulation is not appropriate. Applying lotion or powder to edematous surfaces that touch increases moisture and can lead to maceration, causing further breakdown. (C)

40. **11.3**

$$25 \text{ lb} \times 2.2 = 11.3 \text{ kg}$$

$$11.3 \text{ kg} \times 2 \text{ mg} = 22.7 \text{ mg/day}$$

$$22.7 \text{ mg} \times 2 = 11.3 \text{ mg per dose}$$

(D)

41. **2.** A child recovering from nephrotic syndrome should be protected from infection. Therefore, the nurse would teach the parents to keep the child away from others with an infection. Because pain is not associated with this disorder, pain medication typically is not needed. The physician should be notified if urine output decreases, not increases. In children recovering from nephrotic syndrome, there is no reason to administer acetaminophen daily. (R)

The Client with Acute or Chronic Renal Failure

42. **1.** A client receiving continuous peritoneal dialysis usually requires few dietary restrictions, whereas a client receiving hemodialysis usually has fluid and food restrictions. With continuous peritoneal dialysis, fluid excesses and increased body wastes are removed continuously. With hemodialysis, which is performed two or three times per week, fluid and wastes accumulate between treatments. Although infection is associated with both hemodialysis and peritoneal dialysis, the risk of peritonitis is the major disadvantage of peritoneal dialysis. During peritoneal dialysis, plasma proteins, amino acids, and polypeptides diffuse into the dialysate because of the permeability of the peritoneal membrane. Peritoneal dialysis removes fluid less rapidly than does hemodialysis because peritoneal dialysis uses the peritoneal membrane for diffusion and there is no direct vascular access. (R)

43. **3.** Until it heals, the catheter exit site is particularly vulnerable to invasion by pathogenic organisms. Therefore, the site must be monitored for signs of infection. An occlusive dressing is not needed because there is no danger of air being sucked in or out of the peritoneal space. Furthermore, the catheter used is designed with a cuff, so that the skin grows around the catheter, sealing off the area. Site care may be done at any time, but the child may experience abdominal discomfort if the peritoneal space is dry during site care. Holding the catheter taut or pulling on it may cause irritation of the skin at the exit site, which could lead to infection. (S)

44. **4.** With minimal or absent kidney function, the serum phosphate level rises, and the ionized calcium level falls in response. This causes increased secretion of parathyroid hormone, which releases calcium from the bones. Therefore, the intake of foods high in phosphorus is restricted. Because renal failure results in decreased erythropoietin production, an increase in ascorbic acid intake is needed. Because magnesium is minimally affected by renal failure, its intake need not be restricted. (A)

45. **4.** Demonstration of desire to do the dressing changes and manage medications implies compliance with the medical regimen and acceptance of the condition, thereby indicating a positive self-image. Diffuse somatic complaints could indicate anxiety or problems with coping, with a negative effect on self-concept. Insistence on choosing restricted foods implies that the adolescent has not accepted the diagnosis and is noncompliant, possibly indicating a negative self-concept. Social withdrawal from activities may indicate depression, possibly negatively affecting the self-concept. (A)

46. **2.** The child with acute renal failure needs extra calories to reduce tissue catabolism, metabolic acidosis, and uremia. Using a high-fat and carbohydrate diet helps to supply the necessary extra calories. If the child is able to tolerate oral foods, concentrated food sources that are high in carbohydrate and fat but low in protein, potassium, and sodium may be provided. (A)

47. **3.** For an adolescent, body image is a major concern. The presence of an abdominal catheter can greatly affect the client's body image. The adolescent needs opportunities to discuss feelings about altered body image due to the catheter. Adolescents need to be with their peers and to maintain social activities and contacts in order to meet the developmental tasks for this age group. The adolescent client may choose to confide in friends for both psychological health and physical safety. Because peers are most important to adolescents, they will confide in their peers before confiding in family members. Another major developmental need of the adolescent is achieving independence. Relying on the parents would interfere with the adolescent's ability to do so. (P)

48. **4.** Tissue swelling, pain, redness, and exudate indicate infection. Dialysate leakage is associated with improper catheter function, incomplete healing at the insertion site, or excessive instillation of dialysate. Granulation tissue indicates healing around the exit site, not infection. Increased time for drainage may indicate that the tube is kinked, suggesting an obstruction. (R)

49. **1.** Normally, dialysate drainage return should be clear. With peritonitis, large numbers of bacteria, white blood cells, and fibrin cause the dialysate to appear cloudy. Abdominal distention is unrelated to peritonitis. However, it might suggest an obstruction. Weight gain and shortness of breath are associated with fluid excess, not infection. (A)

50. **4.** With edema, pallor can occur owing to hemodilution as intestinal fluid moves to the vascular space. The child would exhibit pulmonary crackles secondary to pulmonary congestion and edema. Dialysate outflow would decrease, not increase, as the body attempts to conserve fluid. The child's blood pressure would be increased because of excessive fluid volume. (A)

51. **1.** Accumulation of hard stool in the bowel can cause the distended intestine to block the holes of the catheter. Consequently, the dialysate cannot flow freely through the catheter. Decreasing the dialysate infusion may make the dialysis less effective. Altering fluid, electrolyte, and waste product removal can cause fluid and electrolyte imbalance and increased levels of blood urea nitrogen and creatinine. Incorporating the increased times into the dialysis may make the dialysis less effective because fewer cycles can be scheduled. Shoulder pain, which may occur occasionally, can be caused by air in the peritoneal space and diaphragmatic irritation. However, it is unrelated to inflow and drain times. (A)

52. **4.** Regulation of the diet is the most effective means, besides dialysis, for reducing renal excretion. Dietary phosphorus is restricted, which reduces the protein load on the kidneys. Clients are also given substances to bind phosphorus in the intestines to prevent absorption. Limited protein in the diet should include foods high in essential amino acids. Foods high in fat and carbohydrate are used to increase caloric intake. Sodium and water may not be restricted because of the continual loss of sodium and water through the dialysate. Iron-rich foods are commonly high in protein. (A)

The Client with Wilms' Tumor

53. **3.** Wilms' tumor, or *nephroblastoma*, is the most common intra-abdominal tumor of childhood and the most common type of renal cancer. It is highly malignant. Anemia, which is secondary to hemorrhage within the tumor, causes pallor, anorexia, and lethargy. The most common presenting sign is an abdominal mass. Other signs and symptoms are the result of compression from the tumor mass, metabolic alterations secondary to the tumor, or metastasis. Hypertension occurs occasionally, probably owing to excessive excretion of renin by the tumor. Proteinemia and petechiae are not associated with Wilms' tumor. Generally, proteinemia is associated with renal disorders such as nephrotic syndrome and glomerulonephritis. Petechiae are seen with hematologic problems such as idiopathic thrombocytopenia and leukemias. (A)

54. **2.** The abdomen of the child with Wilms' tumor should not be palpated because of the danger of disseminating tumor cells. Techniques such as measuring the occipitofrontal circumference (which is done in children younger than 18 months of age because the anterior fontanel closes between 12 to 18 months of age), upright positioning, and measuring chest circumference are not necessarily contraindicated; however, the child with Wilms' tumor should always be handled gently and carefully. (A)

55. **1.** A stage II tumor is one that extends beyond the kidney but is completely resected. The tumor staging is verified during surgery to maximize treatment protocols. The following criteria for staging are commonly used: *stage I*, tumor is limited to the kidney and completely resected; *stage II*, tumor extends beyond the kidney but is completely resected; *stage III*, residual nonhematogenous tumor is confined to the abdomen; *stage IV*, hematogenous metastasis occurs, with deposits beyond stage III (lung, bone and brain, liver); *stage V*, bilateral renal involvement is present at diagnosis. (A)

56. **3.** The child who has undergone abdominal surgery is usually placed in a semi-Fowler's position to facilitate draining of abdominal contents and promote pulmonary expansion. The modified Trendelenburg position is used for clients in shock. The Sims' position is likely to be uncomfortable for this child because of the large transabdominal incision. The supine position, without the head elevated, puts the child at increased risk for aspiration. (R)

57. **1.** Children who have undergone abdominal surgery are at risk for intestinal obstruction from adynamic ileus. Indications of intestinal obstruction include abdominal distention, decreased or absent bowel sounds, and vomiting. Later signs of intestinal obstruction include tachycardia, fever, hypotension, increased respirations, shock, and decreased urinary output. (R)

58. **3.** Because the child has only one kidney, measures should be recommended to prevent urinary tract infection and injury to the remaining kidney. Severe pain and dependent edema are not associated with surgery for Wilms' tumor. Dietary sodium is not restricted because function in the remaining kidney is not impaired. (R)

The Child with Neurologic Health Problems

The Client with Myelomeningocele

1. Parents bring a 10-month-old boy born with myelomeningocele and hydrocephalus with a ventriculoperitoneal shunt to the emergency department. His symptoms include vomiting, poor feeding, lethargy, and irritability. What interventions by the nurse are appropriate? Select all that apply.
- [ ] **1.** Weigh the child.
- [ ] **2.** Listen to bowel sounds.
- [ ] **3.** Palpate the anterior fontanel.
- [ ] **4.** Obtain vital signs.
- [ ] **5.** Assess pitch and quality of the child's cry.

2. When positioning a neonate with an unrepaired myelomeningocele, which of the following positions is *most* appropriate?
- [ ] **1.** Supine with the hips at 90-degree flexion.
- [ ] **2.** Right side-lying position with the knees flexed.
- [ ] **3.** Prone with hips in abduction.
- [ ] **4.** Supine in semi-Fowler's position with chest and abdomen elevated.

3. Prevention of urinary tract infections in a child with myelomeningocele is an important long-term goal. What should the care plan include for this child? Select all that apply.
- [ ] **1.** Provide meticulous skin care.
- [ ] **2.** Use the Credé maneuver to empty the bladder.
- [ ] **3.** Encourage frequent emptying of the bladder.
- [ ] **4.** Assure adequate fluid intake.
- [ ] **5.** Use tight-fitting diapers around the meatus.

4. When assessing an infant admitted to the pediatric unit with upper lumbar myelomeningocele, which characteristic should the nurse anticipate finding?
- [ ] **1.** Minimal movement of the lower extremities.
- [ ] **2.** Upper extremity paralysis.
- [ ] **3.** Urinary bladder prolapse.
- [ ] **4.** Respiratory problems.

5. When developing the plan of care for an infant diagnosed with myelomeningocele and the parents who have just been informed of the infant's diagnosis, which action should the nurse include as the *priority* when the parents visit the infant for the first time?
- [ ] **1.** Emphasizing the infant's normal and positive features.
- [ ] **2.** Encouraging the parents to discuss their fears and concerns.
- [ ] **3.** Reinforcing the doctor's explanation of the defect.
- [ ] **4.** Having the parents feed their infant.

6. The mother of an infant with myelomeningocele asks if her baby is likely to have any other defects. The nurse responds based on the understanding that myelomeningocele is commonly associated with which disorder?
- [ ] **1.** Excessive cerebrospinal fluid within the cranial cavity.
- [ ] **2.** Abnormally small head.
- [ ] **3.** Congenital absence of the cranial vault.
- [ ] **4.** Overriding of the cranial sutures.

7. The parents of an infant with myelomeningocele ask the nurse about their child's future mental ability. What is the nurse's *best* response?
- [ ] **1.** "About one-third are mentally retarded, but it's too early to tell about your child."
- [ ] **2.** "About two-thirds are significantly retarded, and you'll know soon if this will occur."
- [ ] **3.** "Your child will probably be of normal intelligence since he demonstrates signs of it now."
- [ ] **4.** "You'll need to talk with the doctor about that, but you can ask later."

8. After placing an infant with myelomeningocele in an isolette shortly after birth, which indicator should the nurse use as the *best* way to determine the effectiveness of this intervention?
- [ ] **1.** The partial pressure of arterial oxygen remains between 94 and 100 mm Hg.
- [ ] **2.** The axillary temperature remains between 97° and 98° F (36.1° and 36.7° C).
- [ ] **3.** The bilirubin level remains stable.
- [ ] **4.** Weight increases by about 1 oz (28.35 g) per day.

9. Prior to surgery, a nurse is positioning a neonate with a myelomeningocele. Which action is appropriate for this infant? Select all that apply.
- [ ] **1.** Place the neonate in a prone position.
- [ ] **2.** Keep a diaper over the sac.
- [ ] **3.** Allow the neonate's feet to hang over the mattress edge.
- [ ] **4.** Use a foam pad to maintain hip adduction.
- [ ] **5.** Use a soft pad over the mattress.

10. After surgical repair of a myelomeningocele, which measure should the nurse use to prevent musculoskeletal deformity in the infant?
- [ ] **1.** Placing the feet in flexion.
- [ ] **2.** Allowing the hips to be abducted.
- [ ] **3.** Maintaining knees in the neutral position.
- [ ] **4.** Placing the legs in adduction.

11. Which sign or symptom should alert the nurse initially to suspect hydrocephalus in an infant who has undergone surgical repair of a myelomeningocele?
- [ ] **1.** Seizures and vomiting.
- [ ] **2.** Frontal bossing and sunset eyes.
- [ ] **3.** Increased head circumference and bulging fontanel.
- [ ] **4.** Irritability and shrill cry.

12. When developing the discharge plan for the parents of an infant who has undergone a myelomeningocele repair, what information is *most* important for the nurse to include?
- [ ] **1.** A list of available hospital services.
- [ ] **2.** Schedule for daily home health care.
- [ ] **3.** Chaplain referral for psychological support.
- [ ] **4.** Daily care required by the infant.

13. Which of the following statements by the mother of an infant with a repaired upper lumbar myelomeningocele indicates that she understands the nurse's teaching at the time of discharge?
- [ ] **1.** "I can apply a heating pad to his lower back."
- [ ] **2.** "I'll be sure to keep him away from other infants."
- [ ] **3.** "I will call the doctor if his urine has a funny smell."
- [ ] **4.** "I will prop him with pillows to prevent him from rolling over."

14. A preschooler with a history of repaired lumbar myelomeningocele is in the emergency department with wheezing and skin rash. Which of the following questions should the nurse ask the mother *first*?
- [ ] **1.** "Is your child taking any medications?"
- [ ] **2.** "Who brought your child to the emergency department?"
- [ ] **3.** "Is your child allergic to bananas or milk products?"
- [ ] **4.** "What are you doing to treat your child's skin rash?"

The Client with Hydrocephalus

15. Before placement of a ventriculoperitoneal shunt for hydrocephalus, an infant is irritable, lethargic, and difficult to feed. To maintain the infant's nutritional status, which of the following actions would be *most* appropriate?
- [ ] **1.** Feeding the infant just before doing any procedures.
- [ ] **2.** Giving the infant small, frequent feedings.
- [ ] **3.** Feeding the infant in a horizontal position.
- [ ] **4.** Scheduling the feedings for every 6 hours.

16. A 4-year-old child with hydrocephalus is scheduled to have a ventroperitoneal shunt in the right side of the head. When developing the child's postoperative plan of care, the nurse should expect to place the preschooler in which of the following positions immediately after surgery?

☐ **1.** On the right side, with the foot of the bed elevated.
☐ **2.** On the left side, with the head of the bed elevated.
☐ **3.** Prone, with the head of the bed elevated.
☐ **4.** Supine, with the head of the bed flat.

17. Which action should the nurse take when providing postoperative nursing care to a child after insertion of a ventriculoperitoneal shunt?

☐ **1.** Administer narcotics for pain control.
☐ **2.** Check the urine for glucose and protein.
☐ **3.** Monitoring for increased temperature.
☐ **4.** Test cerebrospinal fluid leakage for protein.

18. A nurse evaluates discharge teaching as successful when the parents of a school-age child with a ventriculoperitoneal shunt insertion identify which sign as signaling a blocked shunt?

☐ **1.** Decreased urine output with stable intake.
☐ **2.** Tense fontanel and increased head circumference.
☐ **3.** Elevated temperature and reddened incisional site.
☐ **4.** Irritability and increasing difficulty with eating.

The Client with Down Syndrome

19. A 7-year-old has been diagnosed as mentally retarded. Which of the parents' expectations for their child is realistic? Select all that apply.

☐ **1.** Difficulty learning.
☐ **2.** An IQ below 70.
☐ **3.** Deficits in adaptive behavior.
☐ **4.** Normal intellectual capacity.
☐ **5.** Behavioral problems.

20. A nurse is assessing a child who is mildly mentally retarded. The best indication of how a mentally retarded child is progressing can be obtained by observing him:

☐ **1.** At school with his teacher.
☐ **2.** At home with his family.
☐ **3.** In the clinic with his mother.
☐ **4.** Playing soccer with his friends.

21. After talking with the parents of a child with Down syndrome, which action should the nurse identify as appropriate?

☐ **1.** Encouraging self-care skills in the child.
☐ **2.** Teaching the child something new each day.
☐ **3.** Encouraging more lenient behavior limits for the child.
☐ **4.** Achieving age-appropriate social skills.

22. The nurse discusses with the parents how best to raise the IQ of their child with Down syndrome. Which of the following would be *most* appropriate?

☐ **1.** Serving hearty, nutritious meals.
☐ **2.** Giving vasodilator medications as prescribed.
☐ **3.** Letting the child play with more able children.
☐ **4.** Providing stimulating, nonthreatening life experiences.

23. Which sign should alert the nurse to suspect a physical problem most commonly associated with Down syndrome?

☐ **1.** Weight loss.
☐ **2.** Irregular heart rate.
☐ **3.** Rapid respirations.
☐ **4.** Increased blood pressure.

24. When developing a teaching plan for the parents of a child with Down syndrome, the nurse focuses on activities to increase which of the following for the parents?

☐ **1.** Affection for their child.
☐ **2.** Responsibility for their child's welfare.
☐ **3.** Understanding of their child's disability.
☐ **4.** Confidence in their ability to care for their child.

25. The nurse mentions that a group meeting for mothers of mentally retarded children is to be held soon. "Not retarded!" the child's mother angrily blazes, "Exceptional." When responding to this outburst, which of the following replies by the nurse would be *most* appropriate?

☐ **1.** "'Retarded' is the commonly used and accepted term."
☐ **2.** "I'm sorry if I offended you by my thoughtless remark."
☐ **3.** "No matter what it's called, the condition is still the same, isn't it?"
☐ **4.** "I'd like to hear more of your thoughts and feelings on that."

The Client with a Seizure Disorder

26. A child with a seizure disorder is hospitalized for an appendectomy. If the child has a seizure, what should the nurse do?
- ☐ **1.** Record the time and pattern of the seizure.
- ☐ **2.** Restrain the extremities.
- ☐ **3.** Insert a padded tongue blade between the teeth.
- ☐ **4.** Keep the child in a prone position.

27. What should be part of the nurse's teaching plan for a child with epilepsy being discharged on a regimen of diphenylhydantoin (Dilantin)?
- ☐ **1.** Drinking plenty of fluids.
- ☐ **2.** Brushing teeth after each meal.
- ☐ **3.** Having someone be with the child during waking hours.
- ☐ **4.** Reporting signs of infection.

28. After teaching a group of school teachers about seizures, the teachers role-play a scenario involving a child experiencing a generalized tonic-clonic seizure. Which of the following actions, when performed *first*, indicates that the nurse's teaching has been successful?
- ☐ **1.** Asking the other children what happened before the seizure.
- ☐ **2.** Moving the child to the nurse's office for privacy.
- ☐ **3.** Removing any nearby objects that could harm the child.
- ☐ **4.** Placing a padded tongue blade between the child's teeth.

29. A nurse is developing a plan of care with the parents of a 6-year-old girl diagnosed with a seizure disorder. The plan focuses on promoting growth and development. Which instruction should the nurse expect to include?
- ☐ **1.** The child will need activity limitation and will be unable to perform as well as her peers.
- ☐ **2.** There is potential for a learning disability and the child may need tutoring to reach her grade level.
- ☐ **3.** The child will likely have normal intelligence and be able to attend regular school.
- ☐ **4.** There will be problems associated with social stigma and parents should consider home schooling.

30. The parents of a child with occasional generalized seizures want to send the child to summer camp. The parents contact the nurse for advice on planning for the camping experience. Which of the following activities should the nurse and family decide is *most* important for the child to avoid?
- ☐ **1.** Rock climbing.
- ☐ **2.** Hiking.
- ☐ **3.** Swimming.
- ☐ **4.** Tennis.

31. Which of the following statements obtained from the nursing history of a toddler should alert the nurse to suspect that the child has had a febrile seizure?
- ☐ **1.** The child has had a low-grade fever for several weeks.
- ☐ **2.** The family history is negative for convulsions.
- ☐ **3.** The seizure resulted in respiratory arrest.
- ☐ **4.** The seizure occurred when the child had a respiratory infection.

32. After teaching the parents of a child with febrile seizures about methods to lower temperature other than medication, which of the following statements indicates successful teaching?
- ☐ **1.** "We'll add extra blankets when he complains of being cold."
- ☐ **2.** "We'll wrap him in a blanket if he starts shivering."
- ☐ **3.** "We'll make the bath water cold enough to make him shiver."
- ☐ **4.** "We'll use a solution of half alcohol and half water when sponging him."

33. An adolescent girl with a seizure disorder controlled with phenytoin (Dilantin) and carbamazepine (Tegretol) asks the nurse about getting married and having children. Which of the following responses by the nurse would be *most* appropriate?
- ☐ **1.** "You probably shouldn't consider having children until your seizures are cured."
- ☐ **2.** "Your children won't necessarily have an increased risk of seizure disorder."
- ☐ **3.** "When you decide to have children, talk to the doctor about changing your medication."
- ☐ **4.** "Women who have seizure disorders commonly have a difficult time conceiving."

34. When teaching an adolescent with a seizure disorder who is receiving valproic acid (Depakene), which sign or symptom should the nurse instruct the client to report to the health care provider?
- ☐ **1.** Three episodes of diarrhea.
- ☐ **2.** Loss of appetite.
- ☐ **3.** Jaundice.
- ☐ **4.** Sore throat.

The Client with Meningitis

35. During the acute stage of meningitis, a 3-year-old child is restless and irritable. Which of the following would be *most* appropriate to institute?
- ☐ **1.** Limiting conversation with the child.
- ☐ **2.** Keeping extraneous noise to a minimum.
- ☐ **3.** Allowing the child to play in the bathtub.
- ☐ **4.** Performing treatments quickly.

36. Which sign should lead the nurse to suspect that a child with meningitis has developed disseminated intravascular coagulation?
- ☐ **1.** Hemorrhagic skin rash.
- ☐ **2.** Edema.
- ☐ **3.** Cyanosis.
- ☐ **4.** Dyspnea on exertion.

37. When interviewing the parents of a 2-year-old child, a history of which of the following illnesses should lead the nurse to suspect pneumococcal meningitis?
- ☐ **1.** Bladder infection.
- ☐ **2.** Middle ear infection.
- ☐ **3.** Fractured clavicle.
- ☐ **4.** Septic arthritis.

38. A preschooler with pneumonococci meningitis is receiving intravenous antibiotic therapy. When discontinuing the intravenous therapy, the nurse allows the child to apply a dressing to the area where the needle is removed. The nurse's rationale for doing so is based on the interpretation that a child in this age-group has a need to accomplish which of the following?
- ☐ **1.** Trust those caring for her.
- ☐ **2.** Find diversional activities.
- ☐ **3.** Protect the image of an intact body.
- ☐ **4.** Relieve the anxiety of separation from home.

39. A child with meningitis is to receive 1,000 ml of dextrose 5% in normal saline over 12 hours. At what rate in milliliters per hour should the nurse set the pump? Round your answer to the nearest whole number.

_____ ml/hour

40. A hospitalized preschooler with meningitis who is to be discharged becomes angry when the discharge is delayed. Which of the following play activities would be most appropriate at this time?
- ☐ **1.** Reading the child a story.
- ☐ **2.** Painting with watercolors.
- ☐ **3.** Pounding on a pegboard.
- ☐ **4.** Stacking a tower of blocks.

The Client with Near-Drowning

41. The nurse caring for a toddler just admitted with the diagnosis of near-drowning in a neighbor's heated swimming pool is most concerned about which of the following?
- ☐ **1.** Hypothermia.
- ☐ **2.** Hypoxia.
- ☐ **3.** Fluid aspiration.
- ☐ **4.** Cutaneous capillary paralysis.

42. When assessing a toddler with near-drowning, which of the following acid-base imbalances should the nurse expect to find?
- ☐ **1.** Respiratory acidosis and metabolic acidosis.
- ☐ **2.** Respiratory acidosis and metabolic alkalosis.
- ☐ **3.** Respiratory alkalosis and metabolic acidosis.
- ☐ **4.** Respiratory alkalosis and metabolic alkalosis.

43. The parents of a child tell the nurse that they feel guilty because their child almost drowned. Which of the following remarks by the nurse would be *most* appropriate?
- ☐ **1.** "I can understand why you feel guilty, but these things happen."
- ☐ **2.** "Tell me a little bit more about your feelings of guilt."
- ☐ **3.** "You should not have taken your eyes off of your child."
- ☐ **4.** "You really shouldn't feel guilty; you're lucky because your child will be all right."

The Client with Guillain-Barré Syndrome (Infectious Polyneuritis)

44. Which of the following assessments would be most important for the nurse to make initially in a school-age child being seen in the clinic for complaints of a sore throat, muscle tenderness, arms feeling weak, and generally not feeling well?
- ☐ 1. Difficulty swallowing.
- ☐ 2. Diet intake for the last 24 hours.
- ☐ 3. Exposure to illnesses.
- ☐ 4. Difficulty urinating.

45. Which of the following actions should be the priority when caring for a school-age child admitted to the pediatric unit with the diagnosis of Guillain-Barré syndrome?
- ☐ 1. Assessing the child's ability to follow simple commands.
- ☐ 2. Evaluating the child's bilateral muscle strength.
- ☐ 3. Making a game of the range-of-motion exercises.
- ☐ 4. Providing the child with a diversional activity.

46. The nurse asks a school-age child with Guillain-Barré syndrome to cough and also assesses the child's speech for decreased volume and clarity. The underlying rationale for these assessments is to determine which of the following?
- ☐ 1. Inflammation of the larynx and epiglottis.
- ☐ 2. Increased intracranial pressure.
- ☐ 3. Involvement of facial and cranial nerves.
- ☐ 4. Regression to an earlier developmental phase.

47. Assessment of a school-age child with Guillain-Barré syndrome reveals absent gag and cough reflexes. Which of the following nursing diagnoses should receive the highest priority during the acute phase?
- ☐ 1. *Risk for infection* due to altered immune system.
- ☐ 2. *Ineffective breathing pattern* related to neuromuscular impairment.
- ☐ 3. *Impaired swallowing* related to neuromuscular impairment.
- ☐ 4. *Total urinary incontinence* related to fluid losses.

48. A 9-year-old child with Guillain-Barré syndrome requires mechanical ventilation. Which action should the nurse take?
- ☐ 1. Maintain the child in a supine position to prevent unnecessary nerve stimulation.
- ☐ 2. Transfer the child to a bedside chair three times a day to prevent postural hypotension.
- ☐ 3. Engage the child in vigorous passive range-of-motion exercises to prevent loss of muscle function.
- ☐ 4. Turn the child slowly and gently from side to side to prevent respiratory complications.

49. The mother brings her child to the clinic after discharge from the hospital for Guillain-Barré syndrome. Which of the following statements by the mother indicates that she is following the discharge plan?
- ☐ 1. "She and her sister argue all day."
- ☐ 2. "I have to bribe her to get her to do her exercises."
- ☐ 3. "I take her to the pool where she can exercise with other children."
- ☐ 4. "She's missed a few of her therapy sessions because she often sleeps."

The Client with a Head Injury

50. The nurse is inserting a nasogastric (NG) tube in a child admitted with head trauma. The nurse should explain to the parents that the NG tube will be used for what purpose?
- ☐ 1. Administer medications.
- ☐ 2. Decompress the stomach.
- ☐ 3. Obtain gastric specimens for analysis.
- ☐ 4. Provide adequate nutrition.

51. A nasogastric tube is ordered to be inserted for a child with severe head trauma. Diagnostic testing reveals that the child has a basilar skull fracture. What should the nurse do next?
- ☐ 1. Ask for the order to be changed to oral gastric tube.
- ☐ 2. Attempt to place the tube into the duodenum.
- ☐ 3. Test the gastric aspirate for blood.
- ☐ 4. Use extra lubrication when inserting the nasogastric tube.

52. The parents of a child with a serious head injury ask the nurse if the child is going to be all right. Which of the following responses by the nurse would be most appropriate?
- ☐ 1. "Children usually don't do very well after head injuries like this."
- ☐ 2. "Children usually recover rapidly from head injuries."
- ☐ 3. "It's hard to tell this early, but we'll keep you informed of the progress."
- ☐ 4. "That's something you'll have to talk to the doctor about."

53. The nurse is caring for a child with a head injury. Place the following assessments in order of priority, starting with the nursing assessment the nurse should perform first.

1. Vital signs.

2. Decreased urine output.

3. Level of consciousness.

4. Motor strength.

5. Vomiting episodes.

54. When developing the plan of care for a child who is unconscious after a serious head injury, in which of the following positions should the nurse expect to place the child?
- ☐ 1. Prone with hips and knees slightly elevated.
- ☐ 2. Lying on the side, with the head of the bed elevated.
- ☐ 3. Lying on the back, in the Trendelenburg position.
- ☐ 4. In the semi-Fowler's position, with arms at the side.

55. The parents ask the nurse why the physician ordered mannitol to be given to their child with a serious head injury. The nurse's response is based on the understanding that mannitol acts in which of the following ways?
- ☐ 1. It helps hold fluid in the vascular bed, to prevent shock.
- ☐ 2. It aids in decreasing fluid, to decrease swelling in the brain.
- ☐ 3. It increases caloric intake, to aid wound healing.
- ☐ 4. It fights off bacteria, to prevent infections.

The Client with a Brain Tumor

56. A child with a brain tumor is less responsive to verbal commands than he was when the nurse assessed the client the previous hour. Which intervention should receive priority now?
- ☐ 1. Raising the head of the bed.
- ☐ 2. Notifying the physician.
- ☐ 3. Administering an ordered analgesic.
- ☐ 4. Obtaining an oximeter reading.

57. A 12-year-old child has had a traumatic head injury from playing in a football game. He is admitted to the emergency department and transferred to the pediatric intensive care unit. He has an I.V. of dextrose 5% in water at a "keep-open" rate and nasal oxygen at 2 L/minute. The nurse is assessing the child at the beginning of the shift (11:00 p.m.) and reviews the Glasgow Coma Scale flow sheet below. The nurse notes that the child responds to pain, is making incomprehensible sounds, and has abnormal flexion of the limbs. What should the nurse do first?
- ☐ 1. Notify the physician.
- ☐ 2. Lower the head of the bed.
- ☐ 3. Increase the rate of nasal oxygen.
- ☐ 4. Increase the rate of the I.V. infusion.

FLOW SHEET

Glasgow Coma Scale

Test	Score	Patient's response
EYE OPENING		
Spontaneously	4	Opens eyes spontaneously
To Speech	3	Opens eyes to verbal command
To Pain	2	Opens eyes to painful stimulus
None	1	Doesn't open eyes in response to stimulus
MOTOR RESPONSE		
Obeys	6	Reacts to verbal command
Localizes	5	Identifies localized pain
Withdraws	4	Flexes and withdraws from painful stimulus
Abnormal Flexion	3	Assumes a decorticate position
Abnormal Extension	2	Assumes a decerebrate position
None	1	No response; lies flaccid
VERBAL RESPONSE		
Oriented	5	Is oriented and converses
Confused	4	Is disoriented and confused
Inappropriate Words	3	Replies randomly with incorrect words
Incomprehensible	2	Moans or screams
None	1	No response

Date	Time	Progress Notes
11/13/07	05:00 pm	GCS = 13
11/13/07	06:00 pm	GCS = 12
11/13/07	07:00 pm	GCS = 13
11/13/07	08:00 pm	GCS = 11
11/13/07	09:00 pm	GCS = 10
11/13/07	10:00 pm	GCS = 9

58. A 13-year-old child has seen the school nurse several times with complaints of headache, vomiting, and difficulty walking. When calling the adolescent's mother about the complaints, what should the nurse suggest the mother do first?
- ☐ 1. Schedule an appointment with the eye doctor.
- ☐ 2. Begin psychological counseling for her adolescent.
- ☐ 3. Make an appointment with the adolescent's physician.
- ☐ 4. Meet with the adolescent's teachers to determine academic progress.

59. A school-age child is admitted to the hospital with the diagnosis of probable infratentorial brain tumor. During the child's admission to the pediatric unit, which action should the nurse anticipate taking?
- ☐ 1. Eliminating the child's anxiety.
- ☐ 2. Implementing seizure precautions.
- ☐ 3. Introducing the child to other clients of the same age.
- ☐ 4. Preparing the child and parents for diagnostic procedures.

60. The nurse is assessing a child diagnosed with a brain tumor. Which of the following signs and symptoms should the nurse expect the child to demonstrate? Select all that apply.
- ☐ 1. Head tilt.
- ☐ 2. Vomiting.
- ☐ 3. Polydipsia.
- ☐ 4. Lethargy.
- ☐ 5. Increased appetite.
- ☐ 6. Increased pulse.

61. After a child undergoes a craniotomy for an infratentorial brain tumor, the nurse places the child in which of the following positions to prevent undue strain on the sutures?
- ☐ 1. Prone.
- ☐ 2. Semi-Fowler's.
- ☐ 3. Side-lying.
- ☐ 4. Trendelenburg.

62. A child who was intubated after a craniotomy now shows signs of decreased level of consciousness. The physician orders manual hyperventilation to keep the $Paco_2$ between 25 and 29 mm Hg and the Pao_2 between 80 and 100 mm Hg. The nurse interprets this order based on the understanding that this action will accomplish which of the following?
- ☐ 1. Decrease intracranial pressure.
- ☐ 2. Ensure a patent airway.
- ☐ 3. Lower the arousal level.
- ☐ 4. Produce hypoxia.

63. Which action should the nurse do first when noting clear drainage on the child's dressing and bed linen after a craniotomy for a brain tumor?
- ☐ 1. Change the dressing.
- ☐ 2. Elevate the head of the bed.
- ☐ 3. Test the fluid for glucose.
- ☐ 4. Notify the physician.

64. An 8-year-old child does well after infratentorial tumor removal and is transferred back to the pediatric unit. Although she had been told about having her head shaved for surgery, she is very upset. After exploring the child's feelings, which action should the nurse take?
- ☐ 1. Ask the child if she'd like to wear a hat.
- ☐ 2. Reassure the child that her hair will grow back.
- ☐ 3. Explain to the child's parents that her reaction is normal.
- ☐ 4. Suggest that the parents buy the child a wig as a surprise.

65. Which of the following statements made by the mother of a school-age child who has had a craniotomy for a brain tumor would warrant further exploration by the nurse?
- ☐ 1. "After this, I'll never let her out of my sight again."
- ☐ 2. "I hope that she'll be able to go back to school soon."
- ☐ 3. "I wonder how long it will be before she can ride her bike."
- ☐ 4. "Her best friend is eager to see her; I hope she won't be upset."

The Client with a Spinal Cord Injury

66. A nurse who witnesses an accident involving an adolescent riding a motorcycle, hitting a tree, and being thrown 30 feet into a field stops to help. The adolescent reports that he is now unable to move his legs. While waiting for the emergency medical service to arrive, what should the nurse do?
- ☐ 1. Flex the adolescent's knees to relieve stress on his back.
- ☐ 2. Leave the adolescent as he is, staying close by.
- ☐ 3. Remove the adolescent's helmet as soon as possible.
- ☐ 4. Assess the adolescent for abdominal trauma.

67. An adolescent sustains a T3 spinal cord injury. After insertion of an intravenous line, a nasogastric tube, and an indwelling urinary (Foley) catheter, the adolescent is admitted to the intensive care unit. What should the nurse do next when assessment reveals that the adolescent's feet and legs are cool to the touch?
☐ **1.** Cover the adolescent's legs with blankets.
☐ **2.** Report this finding to the physician immediately.
☐ **3.** Reposition the adolescent's legs.
☐ **4.** Lay the adolescent flat to aid circulation.

68. During assessment of an adolescent who has sustained a recent thoracic spinal injury, the nurse auscultates the adolescent's abdomen. The nurse explains to the parents that this is necessary because clients with spinal cord injury often develop which of the following?
☐ **1.** Abdominal cramping.
☐ **2.** Hyperactive bowel sounds.
☐ **3.** Paralytic ileus.
☐ **4.** Profuse diarrhea.

69. Which of the following findings should lead the nurse to decide that spinal shock was resolving in the adolescent with a spinal cord injury?
☐ **1.** Atonic urinary bladder.
☐ **2.** Flaccid paralysis.
☐ **3.** Hyperactive reflexes.
☐ **4.** Widened pulse pressure.

70. A school-age boy with a spinal cord injury is moved to the rehabilitation unit. The nurse notes that the child tends to refuse to cooperate in care and to be hostile. The nurse interprets this behavior as indicative of which of the following?
☐ **1.** A stage of grief reaction.
☐ **2.** A phase of rebellion.
☐ **3.** A reaction to sensory overload.
☐ **4.** A response to too much attention.

71. Two months after an adolescent's thoracic spinal cord injury, he complains of a pounding headache. The nurse notes that the client's arms and face are flushed and he is diaphoretic. What should the nurse do next?
☐ **1.** Check the patency of the urinary catheter.
☐ **2.** Lower the adolescent's head below his knees.
☐ **3.** Place the adolescent flat on his back.
☐ **4.** Prepare to administer epinephrine subcutaneously.

Correct Answers and Rationales

The letter in parentheses after each rationale identifies the client need addressed in the item, including management of care (M), safety and infection control (S), health promotion and maintenance (H), psychosocial adaptation (P), basic care and comfort (C), pharmacological and parenteral therapies (D), reduction of risk potential (R), and physiological adaptation (A).

The Client with Myelomeningocele

1. 2, 3, 4, 5. Common shunt complications are obstruction, infection, and disconnection of the tubing. The signs presented by the child indicate increased intracranial pressure from a shunt malformation, which could be caused by an infection, such as peritonitis or meningitis. By listening to bowel sounds, the nurse will note if peritonitis might be a possibility. Palpating the fontanel would indicate increased intracranial pressure if it were bulging and taut. Obtaining vital signs would assess for signs of infection, such as elevated temperature or, possibly, Cushing's triad (elevated blood pressure, slow pulse, and depressed respirations). A high-pitched cry is a sign of increased intracranial pressure. Weighing the child at this time would not be a priority, nor would it add to identifying the cause of the signs and symptoms. (A)

2. 3. Before surgery, the infant is kept flat in the prone position to decrease tension on the sac. This allows for optimal positioning of the hips, knees, and feet because orthopedic problems are common. The supine position is unacceptable because it causes pressure on the defect. Flexing the knees when side lying will increase tension on the sac, as will placing the infant in semi-Fowler's position, even though the chest and abdomen are elevated. (A)

3. 2, 4, 5. Prevention of urinary tract infections includes adequate fluid intake, urine acidification, frequent emptying of the bladder and, if needed, using the Credé maneuver to empty the bladder. Keeping urine close to the urinary meatus by wearing tight-fitting diapers would increase the chance of a urinary tract infection. While the nurse should keep the skin clean and dry, doing so will not prevent urinary tract infections. Urine that stands forms compounds that are suitable for bacteria to grow and multiply. (H)

4. 1. Clinical manifestations of myelomeningocele are related to the anatomic level of the defect and the nerves involved. An upper lumbar (L1 to L2) myelomeningocele is associated with minimal movement of the lower extremities and dribbling of urine and feces. The upper lumbar area of the spinal cord controls leg flexion at the hip and adduction of the thigh. The sacral area of the spinal cord controls foot and toe movement as well as sphincter and perineal muscle contraction. Upper extremity paralysis would be seen with a cervical spine injury. Rectal prolapse, not urinary bladder prolapse, may occur with myelomeningocele due to lack of innervation to the rectum. Respiratory problems are not associated with an upper level myelomeningocele. (A)

5. 1. The parents should see the neonate as soon as possible, because the longer they must wait to see the neonate, the more anxiety they will feel. Because the parents are acutely aware of the deficit, the nurse should emphasize the neonate's normal and positive features during the visit. All parents, but especially those with a child who has a disability or defect, need to hear positive comments and comments that reflect how the infant is normal. Although the parents need to discuss their fears and concerns, the priority on the first visit is to emphasize the neonate's normal and positive features. Reinforcing the doctor's explanation of the defect may be necessary later. Reinforcing the explanation at this initial visit emphasizes the defect, not the child. The parents should spend time with or care for the neonate after birth because parent-infant contact is necessary for attachment. The parents cannot feed the neonate before the defect is repaired because the repair typically occurs within 24 hours. The infant will be prone in an isolette or warmed and watched closely. However, the parents can fondle and stroke the neonate. (P)

6. 1. Excessive cerebrospinal fluid in the cranial cavity, called *hydrocephalus,* is the most common anomaly associated with myelomeningocele. Microencephaly, an abnormally small head, is associated with maternal exposure to rubella or cytomegalovirus. Anencephaly, a congenital absence of the cranial vault, is a different type of neural tube defect. Overriding of the sutures, possibly a normal finding after a vaginal delivery, is not associated with myelomeningocele. (A)

7. 1. Approximately one-third of infants diagnosed with myelomeningocele are mentally retarded, but the degree of retardation is variable and it is difficult to predict intellectual functioning in neonates. The parents are asking for an answer now and should not be told to talk with the physician later. (A)

8. 2. The nurse places the neonate with myelomeningocele in an isolette shortly after birth to help to maintain the infant's temperature. Because of the defect, the neonate cannot be bundled in blankets. Therefore, it may be difficult to prevent cold stress. The isolette can be maintained at higher than room temperature, helping to maintain the temperature of a neonate who cannot be dressed or bundled. Body temperature readings, not arterial oxygen levels, are the best indicator. Typically, an infant loses 5% to 10% of body weight before beginning to regain the weight. (R)

9. 1, 3, 5. Prior to surgery, the neonate with a myelomeningocele should be placed in a prone position. The feet can hang over the edge of the mattress to prevent foot deformities. The neonate should rest on a soft surface to reduce pressure on the skin; the nurse can use a fleece pad or foam over the mattress. The meningeal sac should not be covered. The hips should be maintained in abduction using a diaper roll or small pillow. (C)

10. 2. Because of the potential for hip dislocation, the neonate's legs should be slightly abducted, hips maintained in slight to moderate abduction, and feet maintained in a neutral position. The infant's knees are flexed to help maintain the hips in abduction. (R)

11. 3. In a neonate with open cranial sutures, increasing head circumference is the predominant and earliest sign of increased intracranial pressure. Bulging fontanels also are seen. However, some neonates may exhibit bulging fontanels without head enlargement. Seizures and vomiting are associated with hydrocephalus, but most often these are seen in an older child with closed cranial sutures. Shortly after increasing head circumference and bulging fontanels occur, other signs and symptoms, such as frontal bossing or enlargement with depressed eyes and the sunset sign (sclera visible above the iris), may develop. Although irritability is an early sign, a brief, shrill cry is a later sign of increasing intracranial pressure associated with the development of hydrocephalus. (A)

12. 4. The most important aspect of the discharge plan is to ensure that the parents understand what the daily care of their infant involves and to provide teaching related to carrying out this daily care. In addition to the routine care required by the infant, care also may include physical therapy to the lower extremities. Providing a list of available hospital services may be helpful to the parents, but it is not the most important aspect to include in the discharge plan. Usually, home health care is not needed because the parents are able to care for their child. A referral for counseling is initiated whenever the need arises, not just at discharge. (R)

13. **3.** All children with myelomeningocele are prone to urinary tract infections. Because of the level of the defect, sensory impairment is present and the child is unaware of bladder discomfort. Similarly, the child is insensitive to pressure and other sources of tissue damage, such as heat. Using a heating pad could lead to thermal injury. The immune system is not affected with a myelomeningocele. Keeping the infant away from other infants would be unnecessary. Additionally, the infant needs the stimulation of others for adequate growth and development. Activities that encourage body consciousness, such as rolling over, are encouraged. Because the defect has been repaired, there is no need to keep the infant off his back. (R)

14. **3.** Children with myelomeningocele are at high risk for development of latex allergy because of repeated exposure to latex products during surgery and bladder catheterizations. Cross-reactions to food items such as bananas, kiwi, milk products, chestnuts, and avocados also occur. These allergic reactions vary in severity ranging from mild (such as sneezing) to severe anaphylaxis. While the child could have allergies to medications that caused the wheezing, the latex and food allergies are more common. Asking about the skin rash is not a priority when a child is wheezing. Who brought the child to the emergency department is irrelevant at this time. (R)

The Client with Hydrocephalus

15. **2.** An infant with hydrocephalus is difficult to feed because of poor sucking, lethargy, and vomiting, which are associated with increased intracranial pressure. Small, frequent feedings given at times when the infant is relaxed and calm are tolerated best. Feeding an infant before any procedure is inappropriate because the stress of the procedure may lead to vomiting. Ideally, the infant should be held in a slightly vertical position when feeding to prevent backflow of formula into the eustachian tubes and subsequent development of ear infections. Most infants are fed on demand every 3 to 4 hours. (C)

16. **4.** For at least the first 24 hours after insertion of a ventriculoperitoneal shunt, the child is positioned supine with the head of the bed flat to prevent too rapid a decrease in cerebrospinal fluid pressure. Although elevating the head increases cerebrospinal fluid drainage and reduces intracranial pressure, a rapid reduction in the size of the ventricles can cause subdural hematoma. Positioning on the operative or right side is avoided because it places pressure on the shunt valve, possibly blocking desired drainage of the cerebrospinal fluid. Elevating the foot of the bed could increase intracranial pressure. With continued increased intracranial pressure, the child would be positioned with the head of the bed elevated to allow gravity to aid drainage. The child should be kept off the nonoperative side (side opposite the shunt), or the left side, to help prevent rapid decompression leading to a cerebral hematoma. (R)

17. **3.** Monitoring the temperature allows the nurse to assess for infection, the most common and most hazardous postoperative complication after ventroperitoneal shunt placement. Typically, pain after insertion of a ventriculoperitoneal shunt is mild, requiring the use of mild analgesics. Usually narcotics are not administered because they alter the level of consciousness, making assessment of cerebral function difficult. Neither proteinuria nor glycosuria is associated with shunt placement. Cerebrospinal fluid leakage commonly occurs with head injury. It is not usually associated with shunt placement. (R)

18. **4.** In a school-age child, irritability, lethargy, vomiting, difficulty with eating, and decreased level of consciousness are signs of increased intracranial pressure caused by a blocked shunt. Decreased urine output with stable fluid intake indicates fluid loss from a source other than the kidneys. A tense fontanel and increased head circumference would be signs of a blocked shunt in an infant. Elevated temperature and redness around incisions might suggest an infection. (R)

The Client with Down Syndrome

19. **1, 2, 3.** The definition of mental retardation includes deficits in intellectual functioning and behavior. The child's IQ will be 70 or less and he will have difficult learning. The client cannot adapt to situations in a manner consistent with children with higher IQs. The client does not have a normal intellectual capacity to learn and develop from his experiences. The client may have behavioral problems but these are not considered a result of mental retardation. (H)

20. **1.** Watching the child relate to his teacher and school work is the best indication of how he is progressing. School involves interacting with a person who is not a relative and in a situation that is not totally familiar. Observing the client in situations with family and friends shows social relationships but does not indicate how the child is learning new intellectual skills. (H)

21. **1.** The goal in working with mentally retarded children is to train them to be as independent as possible, focusing on developmental skills. The child may not be capable of learning something new every day but needs to repeat what has been taught previously. Rather than encouraging more lenient behavior limits, the parents need to be strict and consistent when setting limits for the child. Most children with Down syndrome are unable to achieve age-appropriate social skills due to their mental retardation. Rather, they are taught socially appropriate behaviors. (H)

22. **4.** Nonthreatening experiences that are stimulating and interesting to the child have been observed to help raise IQ. Practices such as serving nutritious meals or letting the child play with more able children have not been supported by research as beneficial in increasing intelligence. Vasodilator medications act to increase oxygenation to the tissues, including the brain. However, these medications do not increase the child's IQ. (H)

23. **3.** It is especially important to observe the nature of the child's respirations because children with Down syndrome are prone to develop respiratory infections. Weight loss usually is not a problem for children with Down syndrome. An irregular heart rate and increased blood pressure may be associated with children with Down syndrome and cardiac problems. (A)

24. **4.** When teaching the parents of a child with Down syndrome, activities should focus on increasing the parents' confidence in their ability to care for the child. The parents must continue to work daily with their child. Most parents feel affection and a sense of responsibility for their child regardless of the child's limitations. Parents usually understand the child's disability on the cognitive level but have difficulty accepting it on the emotional level. As the parents' confidence in their caring abilities increases, their understanding of the child's disability also increases on all levels. (P)

25. **4.** When responding to a mother who becomes angry when someone calls her child mentally retarded instead of exceptional, the nurse should give the mother a chance to explore her feelings on the subject. Because the mother obviously has difficulty with the term "retarded," stressing the use of this term would cause further angry feelings. Apologizing, trying to use logic, and defending the comment are not effective ways to handle the situation because the mother's feelings need to be addressed. (P)

The Client with a Seizure Disorder

26. **1.** The nurse should time the seizures and note what area of the body the seizure starts in and where it spreads. This information can help pinpoint the area of the brain involved. If the nurse tries to restrain the child during the tonic-clonic phase of the seizure, the child's bones or tissues may be damaged. When the child has entered the tonic phase of a seizure, trying to insert a tongue blade would damage the teeth and gums as the blade could not be easily inserted past clenched teeth. Until the tonic-clonic seizure has abated, the child is kept supine and objects in the environment that could cause harm during the jerking movements should be removed from the area. After this phase of the seizure when the child's body relaxes, the child is turned on his side to ensure that secretions collected in the mouth can drain and the tongue has not fallen back in the throat and blocked the airway. (A)

27. **2.** Diphenylhydantoin (Dilantin) can cause gingival hyperplasia. Children taking Dilantin should brush their teeth after every meal and at bedtime, and visit their dentist on a regular basis. Drinking plenty of fluids is not required while taking Dilantin. A child on Dilantin does not need to be observed during waking hours because the seizures should be under control. Infections do not occur with an increased incidence in clients receiving Dilantin. (D)

28. **3.** During a generalized tonic-clonic seizure, the first priority is to keep the child safe and protect the child by removing any nearby objects that could cause injury. Although obtaining information about events surrounding the seizure is important, this information can be obtained later, once the child's safety is ensured. During a seizure, the child should not be moved. Although providing privacy is important, the child's safety is the priority. During a seizure, nothing should be forced into the client's mouth because this can cause severe damage to the teeth and mouth. (A)

29. **3.** Most children who develop seizures after infancy are intellectually normal. A child with a seizure disorder needs the same experiences and opportunities to develop intellectual, emotional, and social abilities as any other child. Activity limitation is not needed. Learning disabilities are not associated with seizures. The child is able to attend public school, and social stigma is a rarity. (H)

30. **1.** A child who has generalized seizures should not participate in activities that are potentially hazardous. Even if accompanied by a responsible adult, the child could be seriously injured if a seizure were to occur during rock climbing. Someone also should accompany the child during activities in the water. At summer camp, hiking and swimming would occur most commonly as group activities, so someone should be with the child. Tennis would be considered an appropriate, nonhazardous activity for a child with generalized seizures. (S)

31. **4.** Most febrile seizures occur in the presence of an upper respiratory infection, otitis media, or tonsillitis. Febrile seizures typically occur during a temperature rise rather than after prolonged fever. There appears to be increased susceptibility to febrile seizures within families. Infrequently, febrile seizures may lead to respiratory arrest. (A)

32. **2.** Shivering, the body's defense against rapid temperature decrease, results in an increase in body temperature. Therefore the parents need to take measures to stop the shivering (and the resulting increase in body temperature) by increasing the room temperature or the temperature of the child's immediate environment (such as with blankets) until the shivering stops. Then, attempts are made to lower the temperature more slowly. Shivering does not necessarily correlate with being cold. Alcohol, a toxic substance, can be absorbed through the skin. Its use is to be avoided. (A)

33. **3.** Phenytoin sodium (Dilantin) is a known terato-genic agent, causing numerous fetal problems. Therefore the adolescent should be advised to talk to the doctor about changing the medication. Additionally, anticonvulsant requirements usually increase during pregnancy. Seizures can be controlled but cannot be cured. There is a familial tendency for seizure disorders. Seizure disorders and infertility are not related. (D)

34. **3.** A toxic effect of valproic acid (Depakene) is liver toxicity, which may manifest with jaundice and abdominal pain. If jaundice occurs, the client needs to notify the health care provider as soon as possible. Diarrhea and sore throat are not common side effects of this drug. Increased appetite is common with this drug. (D)

The Client with Meningitis

35. **2.** A child in the acute stage of meningitis is irritable and hypersensitive to loud noise and light. Therefore, extraneous noise should be minimized and bright lights avoided as much as possible. There is no need to limit conversations with the child. However, the nurse should speak in a calm, gentle, reassuring voice. The child needs gentle and calm bathing. Because of the acuteness of the infection, sponge baths would be more appropriate than tub baths. Although treatments need to be completed as quickly as possible to prevent overstressing the child, they should be performed carefully and at a pace that avoids sudden movements to prevent startling the child and subsequently increasing intracranial pressure. (C)

36. **1.** Disseminated intravascular coagulation is characterized by skin petechiae and a purpuric skin rash caused by spontaneous bleeding into the tissues. An abnormal coagulation phenomenon causes the condition. Heparin therapy is often used to interrupt the clotting process. Edema would suggest a fluid volume excess. Cyanosis would indicate decreased tissue oxygenation. Dyspnea on exertion would suggest respiratory problems, such as pulmonary edema. (A)

37. **2.** Organisms that cause bacterial meningitis, such as pneumococci or meningococci, are commonly spread in the body by vascular dissemination from a middle ear infection. The meningitis may also be a direct extension from the paranasal and mastoid sinuses. The causative organism is a pneumococcus. A chronically draining ear is also frequently found. Bladder infections commonly are caused by *Escherichia coli*, unrelated to the development of pneumococcal meningitis. Pneumococcal meningitis is unrelated to a fractured clavicle or to septic arthritis, which is commonly caused by Staphylococcus aureus, group A streptococci, or Haemophilus influenzae. (A)

38. **3.** Preschool-age children worry about having an intact body and become fearful of any threat to body integrity. Allowing the child to participate in required care helps protect her image of an intact body. Development of trust is the task typically associated with infancy. Additionally, allowing the child to apply a dressing over the intravenous insertion site is unrelated to the development of trust. Finding diversional activities is not a priority need for a child in this age group. Separation anxiety is more common in toddlers than in preschoolers. (H)

39. **83**

$$1,000 \text{ ml} \div 12 \text{ hours} = 83 \text{ ml/hour}$$

(D)

40. **3.** The child is angry and needs a positive outlet for expression of feelings. An emotionally tense child with pent-up hostilities needs a physical activity that will release energy and frustration. Pounding on a pegboard offers this opportunity. Listening to a story does not allow the child to express emotions. It also places the child in a passive role and does not allow the child to deal with feelings in a healthy and positive way. Activities such as painting and stacking a tower of blocks require concentration and fine movements, which could add to frustration. However, if the child then knocks the tower over, doing so may help to dispel some of the anger. (H)

The Client with Near-Drowning

41. **2.** Hypoxia is the primary problem because it results in brain cell damage. Irreversible brain damage occurs after 4 to 6 minutes of submersion. Hypothermia occurs rapidly in infants and children because of their large body surface area. Hypothermia is more of a problem when the child is in cold water. Although fluid aspiration occurs in most drownings and results in atelectasis and pulmonary edema, further aggravating hypoxia, hypoxia is the primary problem. Cutaneous capillary paralysis is not a problem. (A)

42. **1.** When a child experiences near-drowning, respiratory acidosis occurs secondary to the retention of carbon dioxide from inadequate pulmonary ventilation, and metabolic acidosis occurs secondary to the buildup of acid metabolites from anaerobic metabolism resulting from tissue hypoxia. (R)

43. **2.** Guilt is a common parental response. The parents need to be allowed to express their feelings openly in a nonthreatening, nonjudgmental atmosphere. Telling the parents that these things happen does not allow them to verbalize their feelings. Telling the parents that they should not have taken their eyes off the child blames them, possibly further contributing to their guilt. Telling the parents that they shouldn't feel guilty denies the parents' feelings of guilt and is inappropriate. Telling the parents that they are lucky that the child will be okay does not remove the feelings of guilt. (P)

The Client with Guillain-Barré Syndrome (Infectious Polyneuritis)

44. **1.** Most children with sore throat have some difficulty swallowing, so it is important for the nurse to determine the extent of difficulty to aid in determining what action is necessary. Typically a sore throat precedes the paralysis of this disorder. Muscle tenderness is an initial symptom. Distal muscle weakness follows proximal muscle weakness, ultimately progressing to paralysis. Diet history and difficulty urinating will not contribute to assessment of the cause of a sore throat or difficulty swallowing. After determining the extent of difficulty swallowing, the nurse can obtain information about exposure to illness. (H)

45. **2.** With Guillain-Barré syndrome, progressive ascending paralysis occurs. Therefore, the nurse should assess the child's muscle strength bilaterally to determine the extent of involvement and progression of the illness. Assessing the child's ability to follow simple commands evaluates brain function. Range-of-motion exercises are an important part of treatment, but they are not a priority initially. Although the child may need diversional activities later, they also are not an initial priority. (A)

46. **3.** In a child with Guillain-Barré syndrome, decreased volume and clarity of speech and decreased ability to cough voluntarily indicate ascending progression of neural inflammation, specifically affecting the cranial nerves. Inflammation of the larynx and epiglottis is manifested by hoarseness, stridor, and dyspnea. A child with laryngeal inflammation still retains the ability to cough. Irritability, behavior changes, headache, and vomiting are common signs of increased intracranial pressure in a school-age child. Regression would be manifested by being more dependent and less able to care for self. (A)

47. **2.** *Ineffective breathing pattern* caused by the ascending paralysis of the disorder interferes with the child's ability to maintain an adequate oxygen supply. Therefore, this nursing diagnosis takes precedence. Additionally, as the neurologic impairment progresses, it will probably have an effect on the child's ability to maintain respirations. *Risk for infection* related to an altered immune system is not involved with Guillain-Barré syndrome. Although impaired swallowing and incontinence may occur with the ascending paralysis of this disorder, oxygenation is the priority. (A)

48. **4.** Even in the absence of respiratory problems or distress, the child must be turned frequently to help prevent the cardiopulmonary complications associated with immobility, such as atelectasis and pneumonia. Maintaining the child in a supine position is unnecessary. Doing so does not prevent unnecessary nerve stimulation. In addition, maintaining a supine position may lead to stasis of secretions, placing the child at risk for pneumonia. Transferring the child to a chair will not prevent postural hypotension. However, doing so will increase vascular tone and help prevent respiratory and skin complications. During the acute disease phase, vigorous physiotherapy is contraindicated because the child may experience muscle pain and be hypersensitive to touch. Careful and gentle handling is essential. (A)

49. **3.** Developmentally appropriate activities and therapeutic play should be used as rehabilitation modalities. Taking the child to the pool to exercise with other children indicates that the child is participating in exercise as well as engaging with other children, thus fostering development. Arguing with the sister does not address the discharge plan. Inappropriate rewards or threats should not be used to coerce a child into compliance. Although the mother is attempting to comply with the discharge plan, bribery is an inappropriate technique to foster compliance. Missing therapy sessions delays recovery. The parents need to help set the child's schedule to ensure that she gets adequate rest to be able to follow her treatment plan. (A)

The Client with a Head Injury

50. **2.** For the child with serious head trauma, a nasogastric tube is inserted initially to decompress the stomach and to prevent vomiting and aspiration. Medications would be administered intravenously in the initial period. The tube will not be used to obtain gastric specimens. Nutrition is not a priority initially. Later on, the tube may be used to administer feedings. (R)

51. **1.** Because a basilar skull fracture can involve the frontal and ethmoid bones, inserting a nasogastric tube carries the risk of introducing the tube into the cranial cavity through the fracture. An oral gastric tube is preferred for a client with a basilar skull fracture. The tube would not be placed into the duodenum. Gastric aspirate is not routinely tested for blood unless there is an indication to suggest bleeding, such as a falling hemoglobin or visible blood in the drainage. (R)

52. **3.** As a rule, children demonstrate more rapid and more complete recovery from coma than do adults. However, it is extremely difficult to predict a specific outcome. Reassuring the parents that they will be kept informed helps open lines of communication and establish trust. Telling the parents that children do not do well would be extremely negative, destroying any hope that the parents might have. Telling the parents that children recover rapidly may give the parents false hopes. Telling the parents to talk to the doctor ignores the parents' concerns and interferes with trust-building. (A)

53.

| **3.** Level of consciousness. |
| **4.** Motor strength. |
| **1.** Vital signs. |
| **5.** Vomiting episodes. |
| **2.** Decreased urine output. |

In order of priority, the nurse would assess level of consciousness, motor strength, vital signs, vomiting episodes, and then decreased urine output. Level of consciousness is the best indication of brain function. If the child's condition deteriorates, the nurse would observe changes in level of consciousness before any other changes. Motor strength is primarily assessed as a voluntary action. With change in level of consciousness there may be changes in motor function. Vomiting episodes would be important to note and include in output record but are not as critical as level of consciousness or vital signs. If the client's fluids are restricted, then the urine output would decrease. In children, the usual urine output is 1 ml/kg/hour. (R)

54. **2.** The unconscious child is positioned to prevent aspiration of saliva and minimize intracranial pressure. The head of the bed should be elevated, and the child should be in either the semiprone or the side-lying position. Lying prone with hips and knees slightly elevated increases intracranial pressure, as does lying on the back in the Trendelenburg position. The semi-Fowler's position with arms at the side is not the best choice. (A)

55. **2.** Mannitol is an osmotic diuretic used to help decrease intracranial pressure by decreasing cerebral edema. Fluid would be eliminated, not held in the vascular bed. Although mannitol does contribute to the calorie intake of the child, it is used for its diuretic effect. Mannitol has no effect on bacteria. (D)

The Client with a Brain Tumor

56. **2.** A decreasing level of consciousness, decerebrate positioning, or Cushing's triad (elevated systolic blood pressure, decreased pulse, and decreased respiratory rate) indicates that there is pressure on the brain stem and the client could require intubation and cardiac resuscitation unless the physician can order a medication or surgical procedure to reduce the intracranial pressure. Raising the head of the bed could offer some reduction in the intracranial pressure by increasing venous blood return from the head, but it is not the priority at this time. An analgesic administered at this time would mask the sign of decreasing level of consciousness and hinder assessment. An oximeter would measure the oxygen level in the blood, but not necessarily in the brain. (A)

57. **1.** This client is experiencing neurological changes consistent with increasing intracranial pressure (ICP). The nurse should first notify the physician. The physician may intubate the child to ensure a patent airway. The nurse should not lower the head of the bed as this will cause increased ICP. The nurse should ensure an adequate fluid balance. The physician will likely order hypertonic saline to draw fluid from the brain. (M)

58. **3.** A child who has symptoms of vomiting, headaches, and problems walking needs to be evaluated by a health care provider to determine the cause. Unexplained headaches and vomiting along with complaints of difficulty walking (for example ataxia) may suggest a brain tumor. Evaluation by an eye doctor would be appropriate once a complete medical evaluation has been accomplished. Psychological counseling may be indicated for this adolescent, but only after medical evaluation to determine that she is physically healthy. Meeting with the child's teachers would be appropriate after medical evaluation. (A)

59. **4.** When a brain tumor is suspected, the child and parents are likely to be very apprehensive and anxious. It is unrealistic to expect to eliminate their fears; rather, the nurse's goal is to decrease them. Preparing both the child and family during hospitalization can help them cope with some of their fears. Although the nurse may be able to decrease some of the child's anxiety, it would be impossible to eliminate it. Children with infratentorial tumors seldom have seizures, so seizure precautions are not indicated. Although introducing the child to other children is a positive action, this action would be more appropriate once the nurse has decreased some of the child's and parents' anxiety by preparing them. (P)

60. 1, 2, 4. Head tilt, vomiting, and lethargy are classic signs assessed in a child with a brain tumor. Clinical manifestations are the result of location and size of the tumor. Polydipsia is rare with a brain tumor. It is more often a sign of diabetes insipidus following a closed head injury. Increased appetite occurs during a growth spurt and is not necessarily a sign of a brain tumor. Increased pulse is a nonspecific sign and can occur with many illnesses, cardiac anomalies, fever, or exercise. (A)

61. 3. After surgery for an infratentorial tumor, the child is usually positioned flat on either side, with the head and neck in midline and the body slightly extended. Pillows against the back, not the head, help maintain position. Such a position helps avoid pressure on the operative site. Placing the child in a prone or semi-Fowler's position will cause pressure on the operative site. The Trendelenburg position is usually contraindicated because keeping the head below the level of the heart increases intracranial pressure as well as the risk of hemorrhage. (A)

62. 1. Hypercapnia, hypoxia, and acidosis are potent cerebral vasodilating mechanisms that can cause increased intracranial pressure. Lowering the carbon dioxide level and increasing the oxygen level through hyperventilation is the most effective short-term method of reducing intracranial pressure. Although ensuring a patent airway is important, this is not accomplished by manual hyperventilation. Manual hyperventilation does not lower the arousal level; in fact, the arousal level may increase. Manual hyperventilation is used to reduce hypoxia, not produce it. (R)

63. 3. Glucose in this clear, colorless fluid indicates the presence of cerebrospinal fluid. Excessive fluid leakage should be reported to the physician. The nurse should not change the dressing of a postoperative craniotomy client unless instructed to do so by the surgeon. Ordinarily, the head of the bed would not be elevated because this would put pressure on the sutures. The nurse should notify the physician after testing the fluid for glucose. (R)

64. 1. It is not uncommon for a child to be concerned about a change in appearance when the entire head or only part of the head has been shaved. The child should be encouraged to participate in decisions about her care when possible. Asking her if she would like to wear a hat is one way to encourage this participation. Reassuring the child that her hair will grow back does not address the immediate change in appearance, and it ignores the child's current feelings. Explaining that this type of reaction is normal does not address the child's feelings. The child

needs to be able to express feelings and be involved in care as much as possible. Buying the child a wig as a surprise does not address the child's feelings and does not allow her to participate in decision making. Rather, the parents should ask the child if she would like a wig and then work with the child to determine what kind of wig she would like. (P)

65. 1. Parents of a child who has undergone neurosurgery can easily become overprotective. Yet the parents must foster independence in the convalescing child. It is important for the child to resume age-appropriate activities, and parents play an important role in encouraging this. Statements about going back to school would be expected. Parents want the child to return to normal activities after a serious illness or injury as a sign that the child is doing well. (P)

The Client with a Spinal Cord Injury

66. 2. The adolescent's signs and symptoms suggest a spinal cord injury. A client with suspected spinal cord injury should not be moved until the spine has been immobilized. Removing the helmet could further aggravate a spinal cord injury. The nurse could assess for abdominal trauma, but only if it can be done without moving the adolescent. (R)

67. 1. In spinal cord injury, temperature regulation is lost below T3. Body temperature must be maintained by adjusting room temperature or bed linens, such as covering the client's legs with blankets. Coolness of the extremities is an expected finding. Therefore, it is not necessary to notify the physician immediately. Repositioning the client's legs does not alleviate the temperature regulation problem and could be harmful, considering the client's diagnosis. Moving the legs before the spine is stabilized could lead to further cord damage. Laying the client flat will not increase the warmth to the legs and feet. (A)

68. 3. A thoracic spinal cord injury involves the muscles of the lower extremities, bladder, and rectum. Paralytic ileus often occurs as a result of decreased gastrointestinal muscle innervation. The nurse evaluates this by auscultating the abdomen. Because the client has a thoracic spinal cord injury, the client may not feel abdominal cramping. Additionally, auscultation would provide no evidence of cramping. Hyperactive bowel sounds would be evidenced with increased peristalsis; peristalsis would probably be diminished with this injury. Profuse diarrhea, resulting from increased peristalsis, would not be an expected finding. Diarrhea would be more commonly associated with a gastrointestinal infection. (A)

69. **3.** Spinal shock causes a loss of reflex activity below the level of the injury, resulting in bladder atony and flaccid paralysis. When the reflex arc returns, it tends to be overactive, resulting in spasticity. The reflexes and bladder becomes hypertonic during this phase of spinal shock resolution; sensation does not return. A widened pulse pressure is not associated with resolution of spinal shock. (A)

70. **1.** After a catastrophic injury, individuals commonly experience grief. Initially, the person experiences denial, the most common response. With gradual awareness of the situation, anger commonly occurs. The child is demonstrating anger, not rebellion, as he gradually becomes aware of his situation. Rebellion is the child's way to maintain autonomy and individuality. It is a reaction to rigid rules. Examples include refusing to follow a treatment protocol when the child had no input and running away. Sensory overload would cause the child to be irritable and tired and to have difficulty sleeping. Too much attention usually would lead to irritability, difficulty sleeping, and mood swings. (P)

71. **1.** The adolescent is exhibiting signs of autonomic dysreflexia, a generalized sympathetic response usually caused by bladder or bowel distention. Immediate treatment involves eliminating the cause. Because bladder distention is a common cause of this problem, the nurse should immediately determine the patency of the indwelling (Foley) catheter. Lowering the head below the knees would increase the blood pressure and is contraindicated because of the spinal cord injury. Lying flat will not decrease blood pressure. Epinephrine is contraindicated because it elevates blood pressure and therefore can exacerbate the problem. (A)

The Child with Musculoskeletal Health Problems

The Client with Musculoskeletal Dysfunction

1. A child who limps and complains of pain has been found to have Legg-Calvé-Perthes disease. What should the nurse expect to include in the child's plan of care?
- [ ] **1.** Initiation of pain control measures, especially at night when acute.
- [ ] **2.** Promotion of ambulation despite child's discomfort in the affected hip.
- [ ] **3.** Prevention of flexion in the affected hip and knee.
- [ ] **4.** Avoidance of weight bearing on the head of the affected femur.

2. When planning home care for the child with Legg-Calvé-Perthes disease, what should be the primary focus for family teaching?
- [ ] **1.** Need for intake of protein-rich foods.
- [ ] **2.** Gentle stretching exercises for both legs.
- [ ] **3.** Management of the corrective appliance.
- [ ] **4.** Relaxation techniques for pain control.

3. A characteristic abnormality in which area should lead the nurse to suspect that an infant has torticollis (wry neck)?
- [ ] **1.** Quadriceps.
- [ ] **2.** Cervical vertebrae.
- [ ] **3.** Trapezius muscle.
- [ ] **4.** Sternocleidomastoid muscle.

4. When assessing a female adolescent for scoliosis, what should the nurse ask the client to do?
- [ ] **1.** Bend forward at the waist with arms hanging freely.
- [ ] **2.** Lie flat on the floor and extend her legs straight from the trunk.
- [ ] **3.** Sit in a chair while lifting her feet and legs to a right angle with the trunk.
- [ ] **4.** Stand against a wall while pressing the length of her back against the wall.

5. After teaching the family of a child with scoliosis who needs to wear a Boston brace, which of the following activities, if stated by the child and family as occasions appropriate for removal of the brace, indicates successful teaching?
- [ ] **1.** When bathing, for about 1 hour per day.
- [ ] **2.** While eating, for a total of 3 hours a day.
- [ ] **3.** During school, for about 8 hours a day.
- [ ] **4.** When sleeping, for a total of 10 hours a day.

6. When teaching the child with scoliosis being treated with a Boston brace about exercises, the nurse explains that the exercises are performed primarily for which of the following purposes?
- [ ] **1.** To decrease back muscle spasms.
- [ ] **2.** To improve the brace's traction effect.
- [ ] **3.** To prevent spinal contractures.
- [ ] **4.** To strengthen the back and abdominal muscles.

7. An adolescent tells the school nurse that the area below his knee has been hurting for several weeks. The nurse should obtain history information about participation in which of the following?
- [ ] **1.** Soccer.
- [ ] **2.** Golf.
- [ ] **3.** Diving.
- [ ] **4.** Swimming.

8. An adolescent is on the football team and practices in the morning and afternoon before school starts for the year. The temperature on the field has been high. The school nurse has been called to the practice field because the adolescent is now complaining of muscle cramps, nausea, and dizziness. Which of the following actions should the school nurse do next?
- [ ] **1.** Administer cold water with ice cubes.
- [ ] **2.** Take the adolescent's temperature.
- [ ] **3.** Have the adolescent go to the swimming pool.
- [ ] **4.** Move the adolescent to a cool environment.

The Client with Cerebral Palsy

9. The mother of a toddler with cerebral palsy comes to the clinic for developmental screening. The nurse explains that the major reason that these tests are done is to recognize primary delays early so as to accomplish which of the following?
- [ ] **1.** Encourage health maintenance.
- [ ] **2.** Facilitate communication.
- [ ] **3.** Prevent secondary developmental delays.
- [ ] **4.** Maintain current development.

10. The nurse judges that the mother understands the term cerebral palsy when she describes it as a term applied to impaired movement resulting from which of the following?
- [ ] **1.** Injury to the cerebrum caused by viral infection.
- [ ] **2.** Malformed blood vessels in the ventricles caused by inheritance.
- [ ] **3.** Nonprogressive brain damage caused by injury.
- [ ] **4.** Inflammatory brain disease caused by metabolic imbalances.

11. When assessing the development of a 15-month-old child with cerebral palsy, which of the following milestones should the nurse expect a toddler of this age to have achieved?
- [ ] **1.** Walking up steps.
- [ ] **2.** Using a spoon.
- [ ] **3.** Copying a circle.
- [ ] **4.** Putting a block in cup.

12. The mother asks the nurse whether her child with hemiparesis due to spastic cerebral palsy will be able to walk normally because he can pull himself to a standing position. Which of the following responses by the nurse would be most appropriate?
- [ ] **1.** "Ask the doctor what he thinks at your next appointment."
- [ ] **2.** "Maybe, maybe not. How old were you when you first walked?"
- [ ] **3.** "It's difficult to predict, but his ability to bear weight is a positive factor."
- [ ] **4.** "If he really wants to walk, and works hard, he probably will eventually."

13. The nurse assesses the family's ability to cope with the child's cerebral palsy. Which action should alert the nurse to the possibility of their inability to cope with the disease?
- [ ] **1.** Limiting interaction with extended family and friends.
- [ ] **2.** Learning measures to meet the child's physical needs.
- [ ] **3.** Requesting teaching about cerebral palsy in general.
- [ ] **4.** Not seeking financial help to pay for medical bills.

The Client with Duchenne's Muscular Dystrophy

14. The mother of a child with Duchenne's muscular dystrophy asks about the chance that her next child will have the disease. The nurse responds based on the understanding of which of the following?
- [ ] **1.** Sons have a 50% chance of being affected.
- [ ] **2.** Daughters have a 1 in 4 chance of being carriers.
- [ ] **3.** Each child has a 1 in 4 chance of developing the disease.
- [ ] **4.** Each child has a 50% chance of being a carrier.

15. A home health nurse is making an initial visit to a family with a 3-year-old child with early Duchenne's muscular dystrophy. What assessment should the nurse expect as most likely with this child?
- [ ] **1.** Contractures of the large joints.
- [ ] **2.** Enlarged calf muscles.
- [ ] **3.** Difficulty riding a tricycle.
- [ ] **4.** Small, weak muscles.

16. The nurse observes as a child with Duchenne's muscular dystrophy attempts to rise from a sitting position on the floor. After attaining a kneeling position, the child "walks" his hands up his legs to stand. The nurse documents this as which of the following?
- [ ] **1.** Galeazzi's sign.
- [ ] **2.** Goodell's sign.
- [ ] **3.** Goodenough's sign.
- [ ] **4.** Gower's sign.

17. When developing the plan of care for a child with early Duchenne's muscular dystrophy, which nursing goal should the nurse identify as the primary nursing goal for the child?
- [ ] **1.** Encouraging early wheelchair use.
- [ ] **2.** Fostering social interactions.
- [ ] **3.** Maintaining function of unaffected muscles.
- [ ] **4.** Prevent circulatory impairment.

18. When interacting with the mother of a child who has Duchenne's muscular dystrophy, the nurse observes behavior indicating that the mother may feel guilty about her child's condition. The nurse interprets this behavior as guilt stemming from which of the following?
- ☐ **1.** The terminal nature of the disease.
- ☐ **2.** The dependent behavior of the child.
- ☐ **3.** The genetic mode of transmission.
- ☐ **4.** The sudden onset of the disease.

19. The nurse teaches the mother of a young child with Duchenne's muscular dystrophy about the disease and its management. Which of the following statements by the mother indicates successful teaching?
- ☐ **1.** "My son will probably be unable to walk independently by the time he is 9 to 11 years old."
- ☐ **2.** "Muscle relaxants are effective for some children; I hope they can help my son."
- ☐ **3.** "When my son is a little older, he can have surgery to improve his ability to walk."
- ☐ **4.** "I need to help my son be as active as possible to prevent progression of the disease."

The Client with Developmental Dysplasia of the Hip

20. The nurse is examining an infant for hip placement and has abducted her flexed legs. The nurse should next:
- ☐ **1.** Rotate the hips.
- ☐ **2.** Extend the legs.
- ☐ **3.** Listen for a "click."
- ☐ **4.** Palpate the hips for a mass.

21. A 16-month-old child is seen in the clinic for a checkup for the first time. The nurse notices that the toddler limps when walking. Which of the following would be appropriate to use when assessing this toddler for developmental dysplasia of the hip?
- ☐ **1.** Ortolani's maneuver.
- ☐ **2.** Barlow's maneuver.
- ☐ **3.** Adam's position.
- ☐ **4.** Trendelenburg's sign.

22. The nurse is assessing the infant shown below. On observing the client from this angle, the nurse should document that this infant has which of the following?
- ☐ **1.** Ortolani's "click."
- ☐ **2.** Limited abduction.
- ☐ **3.** Galeazzi's sign.
- ☐ **4.** Asymmetric gluteal folds.

23. The nurse teaches the parents of an infant with developmental dysplasia of the hip how to handle their child in a Pavlik harness. Which of the following interventions would be most appropriate?
- ☐ **1.** Fitting the diaper under the straps.
- ☐ **2.** Leaving the harness off while the infant sleeps.
- ☐ **3.** Checking for skin redness under straps every other day.
- ☐ **4.** Putting powder on the skin under the straps every day.

24. When developing the teaching plan for parents using the Pavlik harness with their child, what should be the nurse's initial step?
- ☐ **1.** Assessing the parents' current coping strategies.
- ☐ **2.** Determining the parents' knowledge about the device.
- ☐ **3.** Providing the parents with written instructions.
- ☐ **4.** Giving the parents a list of community resources.

25. When teaching the family of an older infant who has had a hip spica cast applied for developmental dysplasia of the hip, which information should the nurse include when describing the abduction stabilizer bar?
- ☐ **1.** It can be adjusted to a position of comfort.
- ☐ **2.** It is used to lift the child.
- ☐ **3.** It adds strength to the cast.
- ☐ **4.** It is necessary to turn the child.

26. The mother asks the nurse about using a car seat for her toddler who is in a hip spica cast. What is the nurse's best reply?
- ☐ **1.** "You can use a seat belt because of the spica cast."
- ☐ **2.** "You will need a specially designed car seat for your toddler."
- ☐ **3.** "You can still use the car seat you already have."
- ☐ **4.** "You'll need to get a special release from the police so that a car seat won't be needed."

The Client with Congenital Clubfoot

27. The parents of a neonate born with congenital clubfoot express feelings of helplessness and guilt, exhibiting anxiety about how the neonate will be treated. Which of the following actions by the nurse would be most appropriate initially?
- ☐ **1.** Ask them to share these concerns with the physician.
- ☐ **2.** Arrange a meeting with other parents whose infants have had successful clubfoot treatment.
- ☐ **3.** Discuss the problem with the parents and the current feelings that they are experiencing.
- ☐ **4.** Suggest that they make an appointment to talk things over with a counselor.

28. After teaching the parents of an infant with club-foot requiring application of a plaster cast how to care for the cast, which of the following statements would indicate that the parents have understood the teaching?

- ☐ 1. "If the cast becomes soiled, we'll clean it with soap and water."
- ☐ 2. "We'll elevate the leg with the cast on pillows, so the leg is above heart level."
- ☐ 3. "We will check the color and temperature of the toes of the casted leg frequently."
- ☐ 4. "The petals on the edge of the cast can be removed after the first 24 hours."

The Client with Juvenile Idiopathic Arthritis

29. The father of a preschool-age child with a tentative diagnosis of juvenile idiopathic arthritis (JIA), formerly known as *juvenile rheumatoid arthritis,* asks about a test to definitively diagnose JIA. The nurse's response is based on knowledge of which of the following?

- ☐ 1. The latex fixation test is diagnostic.
- ☐ 2. An increased erythrocyte sedimentation rate is diagnostic.
- ☐ 3. A positive synovial fluid culture is diagnostic.
- ☐ 4. No specific laboratory test is diagnostic.

30. The parents of a child just diagnosed with juvenile idiopathic arthritis (JIA) tell the nurse that the diagnosis frightens them because they know nothing about the prognosis. What should the nurse include when teaching the parents about the disease?

- ☐ 1. Half of affected children recover without joint deformity.
- ☐ 2. Many affected children go into long remissions but have severe deformities.
- ☐ 3. The disease usually progresses to crippling rheumatoid arthritis.
- ☐ 4. Most affected children recover completely within a few years.

31. The mother of a 4-year-old child with juvenile idiopathic arthritis (JIA) is worried that her child will have to stop attending preschool because of the illness. Which of the following responses by the nurse would be most appropriate?

- ☐ 1. "It may be difficult for your child to attend school because of the side effects of the medications he will be prescribed."
- ☐ 2. "Your child should be encouraged to attend school, but he'll need extra time to work out early morning stiffness."
- ☐ 3. "You should keep your child at home from school whenever he experiences discomfort or pain in his joints."
- ☐ 4. "Your child will probably need to wear splints and braces so that his joints will be supported properly."

32. A preschool-age child with juvenile idiopathic arthritis (JIA) has become withdrawn, and the mother asks the nurse what she should do. Which of the following suggestions by the nurse would be most appropriate?

- ☐ 1. Introduce the child to other children her age who also have JIA.
- ☐ 2. Tell the mother to spend extra time with the child and less time with her other children.
- ☐ 3. Recommend that the mother send the child to see a counselor for therapy.
- ☐ 4. Encourage the mother to be supportive and understanding of the child.

33. Nonsteroidal anti-inflammatory drugs are the first choice in treating a child with juvenile idiopathic arthritis. Which adverse effects should the nurse include in the teaching plan for the parents? Select all that apply.

- ☐ 1. Weight gain.
- ☐ 2. Abdominal pain.
- ☐ 3. Blood in the stool.
- ☐ 4. Folic acid deficiency.
- ☐ 5. Reduced blood clotting ability.

34. What should the nurse include when developing the teaching plan for the parents of a child with juvenile idiopathic arthritis who is being treated with naproxen (Naprosyn)?

- ☐ 1. Anti-inflammatory effect will occur in approximately 8 weeks.
- ☐ 2. Within 24 hours, the child will have anti-inflammatory relief.
- ☐ 3. The nurse should be called before giving the child any over-the-counter medications.
- ☐ 4. If a dose is forgotten or missed, that dose is not made up.

The Client with a Fracture

35. A 10-year-old has 5 lb of Buck's extension traction on his left leg. What should nurse should assess for? Select all that apply.

- ☐ 1. Dryness of the skin, by removing the foam wraps and boot.
- ☐ 2. Alignment of the shoulder, hips, and knees.
- ☐ 3. Frayed rope near pulleys.
- ☐ 4. Correct amount of traction weight on fracture.
- ☐ 5. Pressure on the coccyx.

36. A 14-year-old has just had a plaster cast placed on his lower left leg. What should the nurse do?

- ☐ 1. Petal the cast as soon as it is put on.
- ☐ 2. Keep the child in the same position for 24 hours until the cast is dry.
- ☐ 3. Use only the palms of the hand when handling the cast.
- ☐ 4. Notify the physician if the client complains of heat.

37. A 9-year-old is given morphine for postoperative pain. As the nurse is assessing the client for pain 4 hours later, his mother leaves the room, and the child begins to cry. The nurse's initial assessment of the child's pain is that he is:
☐ **1.** Not in pain because the crying began after the mother leaves.
☐ **2.** Less tolerant of pain because he is upset.
☐ **3.** In pain because he is crying.
☐ **4.** Not in pain because he was medicated 4 hours ago.

38. A 12-year-old is having surgery to repair a fractured left femur. As a part of the preoperative safety procedures, the nurse should ask the client to:
☐ **1.** Point to the area of the fracture.
☐ **2.** Mark the location of the fracture with an "x" and sign his name.
☐ **3.** Confirm with his parents that they have signed the operative permit.
☐ **4.** State the surgery risks as understood from the surgeon.

39. A child is admitted with a fracture of the femur and placed in skeletal traction. What should the nurse assess first?
☐ **1.** The pull of traction on the pin.
☐ **2.** The Ace bandage.
☐ **3.** The pin sites for signs of infection.
☐ **4.** The dressings for tightness.

40. A preschooler with a fractured femur of the left leg in traction is complaining that his leg hurts. It is too early for pain medication. The nurse should do which of the following?
☐ **1.** Place a pillow under the child's buttocks to provide support.
☐ **2.** Remove the weight from the left leg.
☐ **3.** Assess the feet for signs of neurovascular impairment.
☐ **4.** Reposition the pulleys so the traction is looser.

41. The nurse in the emergency department is caring for a 3-year-old child with a fractured humerus. The child is crying and screaming, "I hate you." Which of the following would be most appropriate?
☐ **1.** Tell the parents they will need to wait out in the lobby.
☐ **2.** Ask the charge nurse to assign this client to another nurse.
☐ **3.** Reassure the parents that this a normal behavior under the circumstances.
☐ **4.** Ask the parents to discipline the child so that the physician can treat her.

42. After a plaster cast has been applied to the arm of a child with a fractured right humerus, the nurse completes discharge teaching. The nurse should evaluate the teaching as successful when the mother agrees to seek medical advice if the child experiences which of the following?
☐ **1.** Inability to extend the fingers on the right hand.
☐ **2.** Vomiting after the cast is applied.
☐ **3.** Coolness and dampness of the cast after 5 hours.
☐ **4.** Fussiness with complaints that the cast is heavy.

43. The nurse should teach the mother of a child who has a new cast for a fractured radius to do which of the following for the first few days at home?
☐ **1.** Use a hair dryer to dry the cast more quickly.
☐ **2.** Have the child refrain from strenuous activities.
☐ **3.** Check movement and sensation of the child's fingers once a day.
☐ **4.** Administer acetaminophen every 8 to 12 hours for discomfort.

44. While assessing a 3-year-old child who has had an injury to the leg, complains of pain, and refuses to walk, the nurse notes that the child's left thigh is swollen. What should the nurse do next?
☐ **1.** Assess the neurologic status of the toes.
☐ **2.** Determine the circulatory status of the upper thigh.
☐ **3.** Obtain the child's vital signs.
☐ **4.** Notify the physician immediately.

45. Anticipating that a 3-year-old child in traction will have need for diversion, what should the nurse offer the child?
☐ **1.** A video game.
☐ **2.** Blocks.
☐ **3.** Hand puppets.
☐ **4.** Marbles.

46. The parents of a child who requires skeletal traction are unable to visit their child for more than 1 hour a day because there are five other children at home and both parents work outside of the home. The nurse recognizes expressions of guilt in both parents. To help alleviate this guilt, the nurse should make which of the following remarks?
☐ **1.** "I'm sure you feel guilty about not being able to visit often."
☐ **2.** "It's important that you visit even for 1 hour."
☐ **3.** "Not all parents can stay all the time."
☐ **4.** "Perhaps you could take turns visiting for a bit longer."

47. The child in a new hip spica cast seems to be adjusting to the cast, except that after each meal the child complains that the cast is too tight. Which of the following should the nurse plan to do?
☐ **1.** Give the enema that was ordered as needed.
☐ **2.** Offer smaller, more frequent meals.
☐ **3.** Give the child a mechanical soft diet.
☐ **4.** Offer the child more fruits and grains.

48. The nurse is helping a family plan for the discharge of their child, who will be going home in a spica cast. Which of the following points of information should be most important for the nurse to consider?
- ☐ **1.** The bathrooms are all on the second floor.
- ☐ **2.** The child's bedroom is on the second floor.
- ☐ **3.** A 16-year-old sister will care for the child during the day.
- ☐ **4.** There are three steps up to the front door.

49. The nurse is measuring a child for crutches. What should the nurse consider? Select all that apply.
- ☐ **1.** Type of gait child will be using.
- ☐ **2.** Degree of child's elbow flexion.
- ☐ **3.** Space above the crutch to child's axilla.
- ☐ **4.** Weight of the child.
- ☐ **5.** Whether child has to use the stairs.

The Client with Osteomyelitis

50. During the initial assessment of a child admitted to the pediatric unit with osteomyelitis of the left tibia, what should the nurse expect the area over the tibia to exhibit?
- ☐ **1.** Diffuse tenderness.
- ☐ **2.** Decreased pain.
- ☐ **3.** Increased warmth.
- ☐ **4.** Localized edema.

51. After receiving orders for laboratory tests and antibiotics for a child with osteomyelitis, the nurse should expect to start the antibiotic after blood is drawn for which laboratory test?
- ☐ **1.** Creatinine.
- ☐ **2.** Culture.
- ☐ **3.** Hemoglobin.
- ☐ **4.** White blood cell count.

52. On reviewing preliminary laboratory results for a newly admitted child, which of the following findings should lead the nurse to suspect osteomyelitis?
- ☐ **1.** Hematocrit, 30%.
- ☐ **2.** Erythrocyte sedimentation rate, 35 mm/hour.
- ☐ **3.** Serum potassium concentration, 5.7 mEq/L.
- ☐ **4.** White blood cell count, 12,000/mm^3.

53. The home health nurse is caring for a child with osteomyelitis who will be receiving high-dose intravenous antibiotic therapy for 3 to 4 weeks. What should the nurse plan to monitor?
- ☐ **1.** Blood glucose level.
- ☐ **2.** Thrombin times.
- ☐ **3.** Urine glucose level.
- ☐ **4.** Urine specific gravity.

54. To meet the developmental needs of an 8-year-old child who is confined to home with osteomyelitis, what should the home health nurse expect to include in the care plan?
- ☐ **1.** Encouraging the child to communicate with schoolmates.
- ☐ **2.** Encouraging the parents to stay with the child.
- ☐ **3.** Allowing siblings to visit freely throughout the day.
- ☐ **4.** Talking to the child about his interests twice daily.

55. Which of the following meals would be appropriate for the child with osteomyelitis to choose?
- ☐ **1.** Beef and bean burrito with cheese, carrot and celery sticks, and an orange.
- ☐ **2.** Buttered wheat bread, cream of broccoli soup, tossed salad with dressing, and an apple.
- ☐ **3.** Potato soup; bacon, lettuce, and tomato sandwich; and an orange.
- ☐ **4.** Tomato soup, grilled cheese sandwich, and banana.

The Client with Scoliosis

56. A 14-year-old is being screened for scoliosis. Which of the following statements about routine scoliosis screening is true?
- ☐ **1.** Teenagers ages 14 to 16 should be screened yearly.
- ☐ **2.** A shirt and shorts are worn for screening.
- ☐ **3.** The girl is assessed standing and bending forward.
- ☐ **4.** The girl should refrain from eating 8 hours before the examination.

57. A 10-year-old with scoliosis has to wear a brace. The nurse's teaching plan should include which of the following instructions?
- ☐ **1.** Wear the brace during waking hours.
- ☐ **2.** Use lotions to relieve skin irritations.
- ☐ **3.** Wear a form-fitting, sleeveless T-shirt under the brace.
- ☐ **4.** Bathe the skin under the brace once per week.

The Client Who Is Abused

58. Which parental characteristic is *least* likely to be a risk factor for child abuse?
- ☐ **1.** Low self-esteem.
- ☐ **2.** History of substance abuse.
- ☐ **3.** Inadequate knowledge of normal growth and development patterns.
- ☐ **4.** Being a member of a large family.

59. When obtaining a nursing history from parents who are suspected of abusing their child, which of the following characteristics about the parents should the nurse typically find?
- ☐ **1.** Attentiveness to the child's needs.
- ☐ **2.** Self-blame for the injury to the child.
- ☐ **3.** Ability to relate the child's developmental achievements.
- ☐ **4.** Difficulty with controlling aggression.

60. A 3-year-old child with a history of being abused has blood drawn. The child lies very still and makes no sound during the procedure. Which of the following comments by the nurse would be *most* appropriate?
- ☐ 1. "It's okay to cry when something hurts."
- ☐ 2. "That really didn't hurt, did it?"
- ☐ 3. "We're mean to hurt you that way, aren't we?"
- ☐ 4. "You were very good not to cry with the needle."

61. Which of the following nursing diagnoses should the nurse include as the priority in the plan of care for a preschooler who has been physically abused?
- ☐ 1. *Risk for trauma* related to the characteristics of the child and caregiver.
- ☐ 2. *Impaired physical mobility* related to physical maltreatment.
- ☐ 3. *Self-care deficit* related to the child's developmental level.
- ☐ 4. *Anticipatory grieving* related to the cycle of abuse.

62. While interviewing a 3-year-old girl who has been sexually abused about the event, which approach would be most effective?
- ☐ 1. Describe what happened during the abusive act.
- ☐ 2. Draw a picture and explain what it means.
- ☐ 3. "Play out" the event using anatomically correct dolls.
- ☐ 4. Name the perpetrator.

63. Which of the following observations by the nurse should strongly suggest that a 15-month-old toddler has been abused?
- ☐ 1. The child appears happy when personnel work with him.
- ☐ 2. The child plays alongside others contentedly.
- ☐ 3. The child is underdeveloped for his age.
- ☐ 4. The child sucks his thumb.

64. When planning interventions for parents who are abusive, the nurse should incorporate knowledge of which factor as a common parental indicator?
- ☐ 1. Lower socioeconomic group.
- ☐ 2. Unemployment.
- ☐ 3. Low self-esteem.
- ☐ 4. Loss of emotional family attachments.

Correct Answers and Rationales

The letter in parentheses after each rationale identifies the client need addressed in the item, including management of care (M), safety and infection control (S), health promotion and maintenance (H), psychosocial adaptation (P), basic care and comfort (C), pharmacological and parenteral therapies (D), reduction of risk potential (R), and physiological adaptation (A).

The Client with Musculoskeletal Dysfunction

1. 4. Legg-Calvé-Perthes disease, also known as *coxa plana* or *osteochondrosis,* is characterized by aseptic necrosis at the head of the femur when the blood supply to the area is interrupted. Avoidance of weight bearing is especially important to prevent the head of the femur from leaving the acetabulum, thus preventing hip dislocation. Devices such as an abduction brace, a leg cast, or a harness sling are used to protect the affected joint while revascularization and bone healing occur. Surgical procedures are used in some cases. Although pain control measures may be appropriate, pain is not necessarily more acute at night. Initial therapy involves rest and non–weight bearing to help restore motion. Preventing flexion is not necessary. (A)

2. 3. Because most of the child's care takes place at home, the primary focus of family teaching would be on the care and management of the corrective device. Devices such as an abduction brace, a leg cast, or a harness sling are used to protect the affected joint while revascularization and bone healing occur. As long as the child is eating a well-balanced diet, there is no need for an intake of protein-rich foods. The parents can encourage range of motion in the unaffected leg, but motion in the affected leg is limited until it heals. Once therapy has been initiated, pain is usually not a problem. The key is management of the corrective device. (R)

3. 4. In torticollis, the sternocleidomastoid muscle appears contracted or shortened, and range of motion in the neck is limited. This causes the neck to turn laterally to one side, with the chin directed to the opposite side. Torticollis does not occur in the vertebrae, trapezius muscle, or quadriceps. (A)

4. 1. Scoliosis, a lateral deviation of the spine, is assessed by having the client bend forward at the waist with arms hanging freely, then looking for lateral curvature of the spine and a rib hump. The other positions will not reveal the deviation of the spine. (H)

5. 1. One of the most effective spinal braces for correcting scoliosis, the Boston brace should be worn for at least 16 to 23 hours a day, except when carrying out personal hygiene measures. (R)

6. 4. Exercises are prescribed for the child with scoliosis wearing a Boston brace to help strengthen spinal and abdominal muscles and provide support. Typically, children wearing a Boston brace do not complain of muscle spasms. Performing exercises provides no effect on the brace's traction ability. Spinal contractures do not occur when a Boston brace is worn. (A)

7. 1. The adolescent's complaint should alert the nurse to the possibility of Osgood-Schlatter disease. This disease, found primarily in boys 10 to 15 years of age and in girls 8 to 13 years of age, occurs when the infrapatellar ligament of the quadriceps muscle is not well anchored to the tibial tubercle. Excessive activity of the quadriceps muscle results in microtrauma, which causes swelling and pain. Track, soccer, and football commonly produce this condition. Osgood-Schlatter disease is self-limited and usually responds to rest and application of ice. (A)

8. **4.** The adolescent is most likely experiencing heat exhaustion or heat collapse, which are common after vigorous exercise in a hot environment. Symptoms result from loss of fluids and include nausea, vomiting, dizziness, headache, and thirst. Treatment consists of moving the adolescent to a cool environment and giving cool liquids. Cool liquids are easier to drink than cold liquids. Taking the adolescent's temperature would be appropriate once these actions have been completed. However, the adolescent's temperature is likely to be normal or only mildly elevated. The water in a swimming pool would be too cool, possibly causing the adolescent to shiver and thus raising his temperature. (C)

The Client with Cerebral Palsy

9. **3.** The major goal of early recognition of primary developmental delays in children with cerebral palsy is to prevent secondary and tertiary delays. For example, a young infant who is unable to reach or focus on objects would be unable to attain various levels of sensory-perceptual development described by Piaget. While the nurse can also encourage health maintenance, the focus of this clinic visit is developmental screening. There is no evidence that there is a communication problem. The goal of health promotion is for the child to seek optimal development, not just to maintain current development. (H)

10. **3.** The term *cerebral palsy* (CP) refers to a group of nonprogressive disorders of upper motor neuron impairment that result in motor dysfunction due to injury. In addition, a child may have speech or ocular difficulties, seizures, hyperactivity, or cognitive impairment. The condition of congenital malformed blood vessels in the ventricles is known as arteriovenous malformations. Viral infection and metabolic imbalances do not cause CP. (A)

11. **4.** Delay in achieving developmental milestones is a characteristic of children with cerebral palsy. Ninety percent of 15-month-old children can put a block in a cup. Walking up steps typically is accomplished at 18 to 24 months. A child usually is able to use a spoon at 18 months. The ability to copy a circle is achieved at approximately 3 to 4 years of age. (H)

12. **3.** The nurse needs to respond honestly to the mother. Most children with hemiparesis due to spastic cerebral palsy are able to walk because the motor deficit is usually greater in the upper extremity. There is no need to refer the mother to the physician. The age at which the mother walked may be important to elicit, but this does not influence when the child will walk. The will to walk is important, but without neurologic stability the child may be unable to do so. (A)

13. **1.** Limited interaction or lack of interaction with friends and family may lead the nurse to suspect a possible problem with the family's ability to cope with others' reactions and responses to a child with cerebral palsy. Learning measures to meet the child's physical needs demonstrates some understanding and acceptance of the disease. Requesting teaching about the disease suggests curiosity or a desire for understanding, thus demonstrating the family dealing with the situation. Although not seeking financial help to pay for medical bills may be problem, it does not indicate the type of response the family is having to the child's problems. (P)

The Client with Duchenne's Muscular Dystrophy

14. **1.** Duchenne's muscular dystrophy is an X-linked recessive disorder. The gene is transmitted through female carriers to affected sons 50% of the time. Daughters have a 50% chance of being carriers. (A)

15. **3.** Usually the first clinical manifestations of Duchenne's muscular dystrophy include difficulty with typical age-appropriate physical activities such as running, riding a bicycle, and climbing stairs. Contractures of the large joints typically occur much later in the disease process. Occasionally enlarged calves may be noted, but they are not typical findings in a child with Duchenne's muscular dystrophy. Muscular atrophy and development of small, weak muscles are later signs. (A)

16. **4.** With Gower's sign, the child walks the hands up the legs in an attempt to stand, a common approach used by children with Duchenne's muscular dystrophy when rising from a sitting to a standing position. Galeazzi's sign refers to the shortening of the affected limb in congenital hip dislocation. Goodell's sign refers to the softening of the cervix, considered a sign of probable pregnancy. Goodenough's sign refers to a test of mental age. (A)

17. **3.** The primary nursing goal is to maintain function in unaffected muscles for as long as possible. There is no effective treatment for childhood muscular dystrophy. Children who remain active are able to forestall being confined in wheelchair. Remaining active also minimizes the risk for social isolation. Preventing rather than encouraging wheelchair use by maintaining function for as long as possible is an appropriate nursing goal. Children with muscular dystrophy become socially isolated as their condition deteriorates and they can no longer keep up with friends. Maintaining function helps prevent social isolation. Circulatory impairment is not associated with muscular dystrophy. (A)

18. **3.** The guilt that mothers of children with muscular dystrophy commonly experience usually results from the fact that the disease is genetic and the mother transmitted the defective gene. Although many children die from the disease, the disease is considered chronic and progressive. As the disease progresses, the child becomes more dependent. However, guilt typically stems from the knowledge that the mother transmitted the disease to her son rather than the dependency of the child. The disease onset is usually gradual, not sudden. (P)

19. **1.** Muscular dystrophy is a progressive disease. Children who are affected by this disease usually are unable to walk independently by age 9 to 11 years. There is no effective treatment for childhood muscular dystrophy. Although children who remain active are able to avoid wheelchair confinement for a longer period, activity does not prevent disease progression. (A)

The Client with Developmental Dysplasia of the Hip

20. **3.** Ortolani's manipulation is used to detect congenital hip dysplasia. The infant is supine and a "click" is heard when flexed legs are abducted. This results from pressure causing the femoral head to slip out of the acetabulum. The other maneuvers will not determine the position of the femoral head in the acetabulum. (A)

21. **4.** In a toddler, weight bearing causes the pelvis to tilt downward on the unaffected side instead of upward as it would normally. This is Trendelenburg's sign, and it indicates developmental dysplasia of the hip. Ortolani's maneuver is used during the neonatal period to assess developmental dysplasia of the hip in infants. With the infant quiet, relaxed, and lying on the back, the hips and knees are flexed at right angles. The knees are moved to abduction and pressure is exerted. If the femoral head moves forward, then it is dislocated. Barlow's maneuver is used to assess developmental dysplasia of the hip in infants. As the femur is moved into or out of the acetabulum, a "clunk" is heard, indicating dislocation. Adam's position is used to evaluate for structural scoliosis. The child bends forward with feet together and arms hanging freely or with palms together. (R)

22. **4.** This infant with congenital hip dysplasia has asymmetric gluteal folds. The Ortolani "click" occurs when the nurse feels the femur sliding into the acetabulum with a "click." Limited abduction may be observed during an attempt to abduct the infant's thighs. Galeazzi's sign reveals femoral foreshortening and is observed by flexing the thighs. (H)

23. **1.** The Pavlik harness is worn over a diaper. Knee socks are also worn to prevent the straps and foot and leg pieces from rubbing directly on the skin. For maximum results, the infant needs to wear the harness continuously. The skin should be inspected several times a day, not every other day, for signs of redness or irritation. Lotions and powders are to be avoided because they can cake and irritate the skin. (R)

24. **2.** Assessing the learner's knowledge level is the initial step in any teaching plan to promote the maximum amount of learning. This assessment also provides the nurse with a starting point for teaching. Assessing coping strategies can provide important information to the development of the teaching plan but is not the initial step. Giving parents written instructions or a list of community resources is appropriate once the parents' knowledge level has been determined and teaching has begun. (R)

25. **3.** The abduction bar is incorporated into the cast to increase the cast's strength and maintain the legs in alignment. The bar cannot be removed or adjusted, unless the cast is removed and a new cast is applied. The bar should never be used to lift or turn the client, because doing so may weaken the cast. (R)

26. **2.** The toddler in a hip spica cast needs a specially designed car seat. The one that the mother already has will not be appropriate because of the need for the car seat to accommodate the cast and abductor bar. Legally, all children younger than 4 years of age are required to be restrained in a car seat. (S)

The Client with Congenital Clubfoot

27. **3.** When an infant is born with an unexpected anomaly, parents are faced with questions, uncertainties, and possible disappointments. They may feel inadequate, helpless, and anxious. The nurse can help the parents initially by assessing their concerns and providing appropriate information to help them clarify or resolve the immediate problems. Referring the parents to the physician is not necessary at this time. The nurse can assist the parents by listening to their concerns. Having them talk with other parents would be helpful a little bit later, once the nurse assesses their concerns and discusses the problem and the parents' current feelings. If the parents continue to have difficulties expressing and working through their feelings, referral to a counselor would be appropriate. (P)

28. **3.** A cast that is too tight can cause a tourniquet effect, compromising the neurovascular integrity of the extremity. Manifestations of neurovascular impairment include pain, edema, pulselessness, coolness, altered sensation, and inability to move the distal exposed extremity. The toes of the casted extremity should be assessed frequently to evaluate for changes in neurovascular integrity. Wetting a plaster cast with water and soap softens the plaster, which may alter the cast's effectiveness. There is no reason to elevate the casted extremities when a child with clubfoot is being treated with nonsurgical measures. The legs would be elevated if swelling were present. Petals, which are applied to cover the rough edges of the cast, are to be left in place to minimize the risk for skin irritation from the cast edges. (R)

The Client with Juvenile Idiopathic Arthritis

29. **4.** The nurse's response to the father is based on the knowledge that there is no definitive test for JIA. The latex fixation test, which is commonly used to diagnose arthritis in adults, is negative in 90% of children. The erythrocyte sedimentation rate may or may not be increased during active disease. This test identifies the presence of inflammation only. Synovial fluid cultures are done to rule out septic arthritis, not to diagnose JIA. (R)

30. **1.** In half of the children diagnosed with JIA, recovery occurs without joint deformity. Approximately one third of the children will continue to have the disease into adulthood, and approximately one sixth will experience severe, crippling deformities. (A)

31. **2.** Socialization is important for this preschool-age child, and activity is important to maintain function. Because children with JIA commonly experience the most problems in the early morning after arising, they need more time to "warm up." Adverse effects may or may not occur. The child's normal routine needs to be maintained as much as possible. Although splints and braces may be needed, they are worn during periods of rest, not activity, to maintain function. (A)

32. **4.** Because the child is dealing with grief and loss associated with a chronic illness, parents need to be supportive and understanding. The child needs to feel valued and worthwhile. Introducing the child to others of the same age who also have JIA most probably would be ineffective because preschoolers are developmentally egocentric. Although the child needs to feel valued, the mother's spending more time with the child and less time with her other children is inappropriate because the child with JIA may experience secondary gain from the illness if the family interaction patterns are altered. Also, this action reinforces the child's withdrawal behavior. Psychological counseling is not needed at this time because the child's reaction is normal. (P)

33. **2, 3, 5.** Adverse effects from nonsteroidal anti-inflammatory drugs include abdominal pain, blood in stool, and reduced clotting ability. Weight gain is common with corticosteroids. Folic acid deficiency is associated with methotrexate therapy. (D)

34. **3.** The first group of drugs typically prescribed is the nonsteroidal anti-inflammatory drugs, which include naproxen. Naproxen is included in only a few over-the-counter medications but aspirin is in several. The family should check with the nurse before giving any over-the-counter medications. Once therapy is started, it takes hours or days for relief from pain to occur. However, it takes 3 to 4 weeks for the anti-inflammatory effects to occur, including reduction in swelling and less pain with movement. The missed dose will need to be made up to maintain the serum level and to maintain therapeutic effectiveness of the drug. (D)

The Client with a Fracture

35. **2, 3, 4, 5.** Buck's traction provides a skin traction that keeps the extremity in straight alignment and can be observed by noting a straight line formed between the shoulder, hips, and knees. The rope must be intact to maintain the ordered traction from the weights. The correct amount of traction must be maintained to keep the fractured femur in correct alignment. Because the client is in a recumbent position, the nurse should also inspect the skin on the back and buttocks for integrity. The nurse should not remove the client's wraps and boot unless she has a physician's order to do so. (A)

36. **3.** The wet plaster cast should be handled using only the palms of the hands to prevent indentations of the cast surface. Petaling a cast should be done only when the edges of the cast are rough and are causing irritation to the client's skin. The nurse should not keep the child in the same position until the cast is dry. Doing so would prohibit proper toileting and elimination and would produce undue pressure on the coccyx. The cast typically emits heat as it dries, so notifying a physician is not necessary in this instance. If needed, a fan can be used to circulate the room air. (H)

37. **2.** Emotional or physical stress lowers a person's tolerance of pain. The mother's presence may have distracted him and when she left it caused him to focus on the pain he was having. Crying does not automatically indicate pain. The nurse must further assess the client for pain. Although an analgesic was given 4 hours before, pain may be present. (A)

38. **2.** According to national client safety standards, when possible, the client should mark the surgery site and sign his name on the site. This step should be done prior to receiving preoperative medication. Pointing to the area is not sufficient identification. Because the client is a minor, the parents are responsible for signing the operative permit and accepting the surgery risks. The nurse should determine that the parents understand the surgery risks. (S)

39. **1.** Skeletal traction applies the pull directly to the skeletal structure by tongs, pin, or wire. The nurse should assess the pull of the traction on the pin first. This is critical to the success of the traction. Once this is assessed, then the pin sites are assessed for signs of infection. The dressings would be examined after the pull of the traction, neurovascular status, and pin sites were assessed. The Ace wrap is used to anchor skin traction nonadherent straps, not skeletal traction. (R)

40. **3.** The nurse should assess the client frequently for signs of neurovascular impairment of the feet, such as pallor, coldness, numbness, or tingling. Pillows are not placed under the buttocks because the pillows would alter the alignment of the traction. Weights provide traction and should not be removed. Pulleys help to maintain optimal alignment of the traction and therefore should be left alone. (C)

41. **3.** Explaining to the parents that this is a normal reaction under the circumstances is most appropriate. The child's outburst is related to the child's fears of the unknown. The child is scared and anxious and needs the parents for support. Asking the parents to wait outside would only add to the child's fear and anxiety. The reaction is normal for a child her age and does not usually call for a change in staff assignments. Asking the parents to discipline their child for her behavior is inappropriate. The nurse needs to handle the situation. (H)

42. 1. Inability to extend the fingers of the involved arm may indicate neurologic impairment caused by pressure on soft tissue. It is not unusual for a child to vomit after experiencing a traumatic injury. It may take up to 72 hours for a plaster cast to dry. Until the cast dries, the dampness causes the sensation of coolness. The cast will seem heavy until the child adjusts to the extra weight. The child may exhibit fussiness (such as whining, crying or clinging) as a result of numerous causes, such as placement of the cast, the hospital experience, or pain. These reactions are normal and do not warrant medical advice. (R)

43. 2. For the first few days after application of a plaster or fiberglass cast, the child should not engage in strenuous activities, to minimize swelling that would cause the cast to become too tight. Use of a hair dryer to complete the drying of the cast is not encouraged because the hair dryer only dries the outside of the cast. Movement and sensation of the fingers need to be checked several times a day for the first few days. Typically, the mother would be instructed to administer acetaminophen every 4 to 6 hours, not every 8 to 12 hours, for discomfort. (R)

44. 1. Because the nurse suspects a possible fracture based on the child's presentation, assessing the neurologic and circulatory status of the toes, the tissues distal to the fracture, is important. Soft tissue contusions, which accompany femur fractures, can result in severe hemorrhage into the tissue and subsequent circulatory and neurologic impairment. Once this information has been obtained, vital signs can be assessed and the nurse can notify the physician and report the findings. In fractures, circulation impairment will occur distal to the injury. (A)

45. 3. Hand puppets would enable a 3-year-old child in traction to act out feelings within the constraints imposed by the traction. A 3-year-old needs creative play. The video game would make the child too active in bed and does not meet the child's developmental need for creative play. Blocks would be more appropriate for a younger child. Marbles are unsafe at this age because they can be swallowed. (H)

46. 2. Stressing the importance of the parents' visiting when they can helps to alleviate the guilt they feel. It allows the parents to feel that they are doing what they can. Acknowledging the guilt gives the parents an opportunity to talk about it but does not help alleviate it. Comparing the parents with other parents does not alleviate guilt feelings. The parents need reinforcement that what they are doing is appropriate. Suggesting that the parents take turns visiting implies that they should feel guilty because they may not be doing all they could. (P)

47. 2. A hip spica cast encircles the abdomen. When the child eats a large meal, abdominal pressure increases, causing the cast to feel tight. Therefore, the nurse would plan to offer smaller, more frequent meals to minimize abdominal distention. If the child's appetite were decreased in conjunction with a feeling of fullness, the nurse might suspect that the child was becoming constipated and plan to use laxatives or a higher-fiber diet. A mechanical soft diet is indicated when the child has difficulty chewing food adequately. Giving the child more fruits and grains would contribute to abdominal distention and complaints of the cast tightness after eating. (R)

48. 2. The child with a hip spica cast who is going home and has a bedroom on the second floor of the home needs to have the bed moved to an area that is more central to family life. Negotiating a flight of steps at least twice a day (on awakening in the morning and before going to bed at night) with a child in a hip spica cast would be difficult and most likely dangerous. Because the child in a hip spica cast will need to use a bedpan or urinal, the bathrooms can be on any floor. Because the family is involved in the discharge, the 16-year-old sister should be taught appropriate care along with the rest of the family. The child can be carried up and down the three steps to the house the few times necessary after discharge. (S)

49. 2, 3. To ensure proper fit of crutches, the child's elbow flexion should be 20 degrees, and the area above the top of the crutch to the child's axilla should be 1 to $1\frac{1}{2}$ inches. The type of gait, weight of the child, and use of stairs are not factors in the measurement. (R)

The Client with Osteomyelitis

50. 3. Findings associated with osteomyelitis commonly include pain over the area, increased warmth, localized tenderness, and diffuse swelling over the involved bone. The area over the affected bone is red. (A)

51. 2. Antibiotic therapy starts after blood for culture is drawn. The blood cultures determine the causative organism. Creatine tests kidney function. Hemoglobin tests for oxygen carrying capacity. While blood count reveals the presence of infection, it does not identify the causative organism. (R)

52. 2. In osteomyelitis, the erythrocyte sedimentation rate is increased (for a child, the normal range is 0 to 13 mm/hour). The erythrocyte sedimentation rate rises in the presence of severe localized or systemic inflammation. The hematocrit level would be normal in a child with osteomyelitis. This child's hematocrit is lower than the normal level, which typically is greater than 33%. The serum potassium concentration would be normal in a child with osteomyelitis; in this child it is higher than the normal range of 3.5 to 5.5 mEq/L. The leukocyte count in osteomyelitis is increased, usually 15,000 to 25,000/mm³. This child's leukocyte level is low in light of the diagnosis of osteomyelitis. Normally, the white blood cell count ranges from 5,000 to 10,000/mm³. (A)

53. **4.** Long-term, high-dose antibiotic therapy can adversely affect renal, hepatic, and hematopoietic function. Urine specific gravity would provide valuable information about the kidneys' ability to concentrate or dilute urine, thereby suggesting renal impairment. Blood glucose levels reveal how well the client's body is using glucose. Thrombin times reveal information about the clotting mechanism. Urine glucose levels reveal information about the body's use and excretion of glucose. (D)

54. **1.** Encouraging contact with schoolmates allows the school-age child to maintain and develop socialization with peers, an important developmental task of this age-group. Although having family visits and interacting with the child are important, they do not meet the child's developmental needs. Talking to the child about his interests is important, but encouraging contact with schoolmates is crucial to maintain and develop socialization with peers. (H)

55. **1.** Children with osteomyelitis need a diet that is high in protein and calories. Milk, eggs, cheese, meat, fish, and beans are the best sources of these nutrients. (A)

The Client with Scoliosis

56. **3.** Screening is done with the child wearing minimal clothing, standing and bending forward. The examination should be done on girls ages 10 to 12 years old so a diagnosis can be made early and the scoliosis can be treated with exercises or bracing. Only underwear should be worn for the examination so that symmetry of the shoulders and hips can be observed. If the deviation on the scoliometer is less than 20 degrees, no treatment is indicated. The child does not need to refrain from eating prior to this test. (A)

57. **3.** A form-fitting, sleeveless T-shirt can be worn under the brace to prevent skin irritation and collect perspiration. Braces are worn 23 hours each day. Lotions may cause irritation and should not be used. The skin under the brace should be bathed daily to help prevent irritation from the brace. The brace can be removed for bathing so all the skin can be bathed. (A)

The Client Who Is Abused

58. **4.** From documented cases of child abuse, a profile has emerged of a high-risk parent as a person who is isolated, impulsive, impatient, and single with low self-esteem, a history of substance abuse, a lack of knowledge about a child's normal growth and development, and multiple life stressors. Just because a parent comes from a large family, there is no increase in the incidence of the parent abusing their own children unless they possess the other risk factors. (P)

59. **4.** Parents of an abused child have difficulty controlling their aggressive behaviors. They may blame the child or others for the injury, may not ask questions about treatment, and may not know developmental information. (P)

60. **1.** It is not normal for a preschooler to be totally passive during a painful procedure. Typically a preschooler reacts to a painful procedure by crying or pulling away because of the fear of pain. However, an abused child may become "immune" to pain and may find that crying can bring on more pain. The child needs to learn that appropriate emotional expression is acceptable. Telling the child that it really didn't hurt is inappropriate because it is untrue. Telling the child that nurses are mean does not build a trusting relationship. Praising the child will reinforce the child's response not to cry, even though it is acceptable to do so. (P)

61. **1.** A child who is abused would have as a priority nursing diagnosis *Risk for trauma* because the child is at risk for continued abuse or a recurrence of the abuse. Although *Impaired physical mobility* related to physical maltreatment or *Self-care deficit* related to developmental level may be appropriate after serious abuse has occurred, the priority nursing diagnosis is *Risk for trauma*. A 3-year-old child would not experience anticipatory grieving because of the child's cognitive level of development at this age. (P)

62. **3.** A 3-year-old child has limited verbal skills and should not be asked to describe an event, explain a picture, or respond verbally or nonverbally to questions. More appropriately, the child can act out an event using dolls. The child is likely to be too fearful to name the perpetrator or will not be able to do so. (P)

63. **3.** An almost universal finding in descriptions of abused children is underdevelopment for age. This may be reflected in small physical size or in poor psychosocial development. The child should be evaluated further until a plausible diagnosis can be established. A child who appears happy when personnel work with him is exhibiting normal behavior. Children who are abused often are suspicious of others, especially adults. A child who plays alongside others is exhibiting normal behavior, that of parallel play. A child who sucks his thumb contentedly is also exhibiting normal behavior. (P)

64. **3.** Parents who are abusive often suffer from low self-esteem, commonly because of the way they were parented, including not being able to develop trust in caretakers and not being encouraged or offered emotional support by parents. Therefore, the nurse works to bolster the parents' self-esteem. This can be achieved by praising the parents for appropriate parenting. Employment and socioeconomic status are not indicators of abusive parents. Abusive parents usually are attached to their children and do not want to give them up to foster care. Parents who are abusive love their children and feel close to them emotionally. (P)

The Child with Dermatologic and Endocrine Health Problems

- The Client with Skin Disorders
- The Client with Burns
- The Client with Hyperthyroidism
- The Client with Insulin-Dependent Diabetes Mellitus
- Correct Answers and Rationales

The Client with Skin Disorders

1. When teaching an adolescent with facial acne about skin care, the nurse should instruct the adolescent to:
- ☐ 1. Wash the face twice a day with mild soap and water.
- ☐ 2. Remove whiteheads and comedones after washing his face with antibacterial soap.
- ☐ 3. Apply vitamin E ointment twice daily to the affected skin.
- ☐ 4. Apply tretinoin (Retin-A) daily in the morning and expose the face to the sun.

2. A 10-year old child is admitted to the hospital with complications related to chickenpox. The nurse caring for the child should perform which of the following interventions to prevent the transmission of the infection to other children on the unit? Select all that apply.
- ☐ 1. Place the child on contact isolation.
- ☐ 2. Wear a gown, mask, and gloves before entering the room.
- ☐ 3. Place the child in a room with a 10-year-old who has had chickenpox.
- ☐ 4. Place the child in a negative air-flow room.
- ☐ 5. Maintain isolation until lesions have disappeared.

3. A 9-month-old infant with eczema has lesions that are secondarily infected. Which of the following interventions would be *most* appropriate to help the parents best meet the needs of the child?
- ☐ 1. Preventing siblings from being in close contact.
- ☐ 2. Sending the child to day care as usual.
- ☐ 3. Playing video games for several hours each evening.
- ☐ 4. Playing with the child every day.

4. After the nurse teaches the mother of a child with atopic dermatitis how to bathe her child, which of the following statements by the mother indicates effective teaching?
- ☐ 1. "I let my child play in the tub for 30 minutes every night."
- ☐ 2. "My child loves the bubble bath I put in the tub."
- ☐ 3. "When my child gets out of the tub I just pat the skin dry."
- ☐ 4. "I make sure my child has a bath every night."

5. A 5-year-old child brought to the clinic with several superficial sores on the front of the left leg is diagnosed with impetigo. Which of the following instructions should the nurse give the parent?
- ☐ 1. Wash the child's legs gently three times per day with a mild soap.
- ☐ 2. Cover the sores with loose gauze.
- ☐ 3. Allow the child to go back to school after 24 hours of treatment.
- ☐ 4. Have the child return to the clinic the next week for a follow-up examination.

6. When developing the teaching plan for the mother of a 2-year-old child diagnosed with scabies, which of the following points should the nurse expect to include?
- ☐ 1. The floors of the house should be cleaned with a damp mop.
- ☐ 2. The child should be held frequently.
- ☐ 3. Itching should cease in a few days.
- ☐ 4. The entire family should be treated.

The Client with Burns

7. A 10-year-old has just spilled hot liquid on his arm, and a 4-inch area on his forearm is severely burned. His mother calls the emergency department. What should the nurse advise the mother to do?
- ☐ 1. Keep the child warm.
- ☐ 2. Cover the burned area with an antibiotic cream.
- ☐ 3. Apply cool water to the burned area.
- ☐ 4. Call 911 to transport the child to the hospital.

8. The nurse is assessing a 9-year-old child who has third-degree burns as shown below. Using the "Rule of Nines" adapted for children, the nurse estimates that the extent of burns for this child is:
- ☐ **1.** 9%.
- ☐ **2.** 14%.
- ☐ **3.** 18%.
- ☐ **4.** 24%.

9. A school-age child who has received burns over 60% of his body is to receive 2,000 ml of I.V. fluid over the next 8 hours. At what rate (in milliliters per hour) should the nurse set the infusion pump?

_____ ml/hour

10. Which of the following would be *most* appropriate to institute when a school-age child with burns becomes angry and combative when it is time to change the dressings and apply mafenide acetate (Sulfamylon)?
- ☐ **1.** Ensure parental support during the dressing changes.
- ☐ **2.** Allow the child to assist in removing the dressings and applying the cream.
- ☐ **3.** Give the child permission to cry during the procedure.
- ☐ **4.** Allow the child to schedule the time for dressing changes.

11. A 5-year-old child with burns on the trunk and arms has no appetite. The nurse and mother develop a plan of care to stimulate the child's appetite. Which of the following suggestions made by the mother would indicate that she needs additional teaching?
- ☐ **1.** Deciding that she will feed the child herself.
- ☐ **2.** Withholding dessert and treats unless meals are eaten.
- ☐ **3.** Offering the child finger foods that the child likes.
- ☐ **4.** Serving smaller and more frequent meals.

12. After teaching the mother of a child with severe burns about the importance of specific nutritional support in burn management, which of the following, if chosen by the mother from the child's diet menu, indicates the need for further instruction?
- ☐ **1.** Bacon, lettuce, and tomato sandwich; milk; and celery and carrot sticks.
- ☐ **2.** Cheeseburger, cottage cheese and pineapple salad, chocolate milk, and a brownie.
- ☐ **3.** Chicken nuggets, orange and grapefruit sections, and a vanilla milkshake.
- ☐ **4.** Beef, bean, and cheese burrito; a banana; fruit-flavored yogurt; and skim milk.

13. When caring for a child with moderate burns from the waist down, which of the following should the nurse do when positioning the child?
- ☐ **1.** Place the child in a position of comfort.
- ☐ **2.** Allow the child to lie on the abdomen.
- ☐ **3.** Ensure the application of leg splints.
- ☐ **4.** Have the child flex the hips and knees.

The Client with Hyperthyroidism

14. An 11-year-old child has been diagnosed with Grave's disease and is to start drug therapy. Which of the following instructions should the school nurse include in the teaching plan for the child's mother and teacher?
- ☐ **1.** Continue with the same amount of schoolwork and homework.
- ☐ **2.** Understand that mood swings are rare with this disorder.
- ☐ **3.** Limit the amount of food that is offered to the child.
- ☐ **4.** Provide the child with a calm, nonstimulating environment.

The Client with Insulin-Dependent Diabetes Mellitus

15. An 8-year-old with newly diagnosed diabetes is in the hospital for regulation of diet and medications. The child is using an exchange method for the diet. The nurse should instruct the client that the American Diabetes Association's (ADA's) exchange method for dietary regulation includes:
- ☐ **1.** Choosing food from each exchange list.
- ☐ **2.** Using a scale to weigh all food.
- ☐ **3.** Selecting from lists that group food according to protein, fat, and carbohydrate content.
- ☐ **4.** Carbohydrate counting for each meal and snack.

16. A 10 year-old child has the following blood glucose readings during a 24-hour period. Which reading requires the most immediate intervention?
- ☐ **1.** 50 mg/dl.
- ☐ **2.** 100 mg/dl.
- ☐ **3.** 150 mg/dl.
- ☐ **4.** 200 mg/dl.

17. An 8-year-old with diabetes is placed on neutral protamine Hagedorn (NPH) and regular insulin before breakfast and before dinner. She will receive a snack of milk and cereal at bedtime. The snack will:
- ☐ **1.** Help her regain lost weight.
- ☐ **2.** Provide carbohydrates for immediate use.
- ☐ **3.** Prevent late night hypoglycemia.
- ☐ **4.** Help her stay on her diet.

18. A nurse is teaching an 8-year-old with diabetes and her parents about managing diabetes during illness. The nurse determines the parents understand the instruction when they indicate that, when the child is ill, they will provide:
- ☐ **1.** More calories.
- ☐ **2.** More insulin.
- ☐ **3.** Less insulin.
- ☐ **4.** Less protein and fat.

19. A nurse is assessing an 8-year-old with diabetes who is experiencing hyperglycemia. Which symptom indicates that the hyperglycemia requires immediate intervention? Select all that apply.
- ☐ **1.** Weakness.
- ☐ **2.** Thirst.
- ☐ **3.** Shakiness.
- ☐ **4.** Hunger.
- ☐ **5.** Headache.
- ☐ **6.** Irritability.
- ☐ **7.** Dizziness.

20. The mother of an 8-year-old with diabetes tells the nurse that she does not want the school to know about her daughter's condition. The nurse should reply:
- ☐ **1.** "I think that would be a good idea."
- ☐ **2.** "What is it that concerns you about having the school know about your daughter's condition?"
- ☐ **3.** "It would be fine not to tell your daughter's friends, but the teacher must know."
- ☐ **4.** "In order to keep your daughter safe, it is necessary for all adults in the school to know her condition."

21. After a school-age child with insulin-dependent diabetes mellitus attends a nutritional teaching class, the nurse determines that the teaching has been effective when the child states which of the following?
- ☐ **1.** "If I don't eat all my meal, I can make up the carbohydrates at the next meal."
- ☐ **2.** "If I'm not hungry for a meal, I can eat the carbohydrates for a snack later."
- ☐ **3.** "When I don't finish a meal, I must make up the carbohydrates right then."
- ☐ **4.** "When I don't finish a meal, I just need to take more insulin."

22. The nurse talks to an adolescent about how she can tell her friends about her new diagnosis of diabetes. Which of the following behaviors by the adolescent indicates that the adolescent has responded positively to the discussion?
- ☐ **1.** She asks the nurse for material on diabetes for a school paper.
- ☐ **2.** She introduces the nurse to her friends as "the one who taught me all about my diabetes."
- ☐ **3.** She says, "I'll try to tell my friends, but they'll probably quit hanging out with me."
- ☐ **4.** She asks her friends what they think about someone who has a lifelong illness.

23. When developing the teaching plan for the mother and a child with insulin-dependent diabetes about sick-day management, which of the following instructions should the nurse expect to include?
- ☐ **1.** Adhere to the same schedule and type and amount of insulin.
- ☐ **2.** Immediately call the physician for information about what to do.
- ☐ **3.** Adjust insulin based on more frequent testing of blood glucose levels.
- ☐ **4.** Take the child to the emergency department for immediate care.

24. An adolescent with insulin-dependent diabetes is being taught the importance of rotating the sites of insulin injections. The nurse should judge that the teaching was successful when the adolescent identifies which of the following as a result of using the same site?
- ☐ **1.** Destruction of the fat tissue and poor absorption.
- ☐ **2.** Destruction of nerves and painful neuritis.
- ☐ **3.** Destruction of the tissue and too-rapid insulin uptake.
- ☐ **4.** Development of resistance to insulin and need for increased amounts.

25. Which of the following tests should the nurse expect to be performed as a follow-up measure to periodically assess the effectiveness of treatment for a child with insulin-dependent diabetes?
- ☐ **1.** Hemoglobin electrophoresis.
- ☐ **2.** Glycosylated hemoglobin.
- ☐ **3.** Glucose tolerance test.
- ☐ **4.** Post-postprandial blood test.

Correct Answers and Rationales

The letter in parentheses after each rationale identifies the client need addressed in the item, including management of care (M), safety and infection control (S), health promotion and maintenance (H), psychosocial adaptation (P), basic care and comfort (C), pharmacological and parenteral therapies (D), reduction of risk potential (R), and physiological adaptation (A).

The Client with Skin Disorders

1. 1. Washing the face once or twice a day with a mild soap removes fatty acids from the skin. Acne is an inflammation of the sebaceous glands that produce sebum. Washing the face with mild soap and water keeps the sebaceous glands from becoming plugged. Excessive washing or squeezing the eruptions can cause rupture of these glands, spreading the sebum and causing further inflammation. Applying vitamin E to the lesions does not reduce the inflammation and, due to the greasiness of the preparation, may plug the ducts. Retin-A should be applied at night. Exposure to the sun can result in sunburn and an increased risk of skin cancer and should be avoided. Sunscreen with a sun protection factor of at least 15 must be applied before the client can be exposed to the sun. (A)

2. 2, 4. Gowns, mask, and gloves are needed before the nurse or anyone can enter the room of a client who has chickenpox because the varicella virus is spread by air, droplets, and contact. It is very contagious so a negative-air flow room is recommended. Contact isolation only includes a gown and gloves. Because varicella is spread by air and contact, a private room is needed. The child should remain in isolation until all lesions have crusted. (A)

3. 4. The parents can best meet the needs of their 9-month-old infant by playing with the child every day. All infants need time with their parents to develop trust and thus attain optimal development. The parents of a child with a chronic problem may need more guidance to meet the child's needs because of the focus on medical problems. The child's lesions are secondarily infected and therefore should not be contagious. Siblings do not need to stay away. Even with lesions that are infected, the child can still attend day care, but the child needs attention from the parents as well. Playing video games for several hours is not appropriate for a 9-month-old infant. (H)

4. 3. Atopic dermatitis is a chronic pruritic dermatitis that usually begins in infancy. Many of the children diagnosed with it have a family history of eczema, allergies, or asthma. Atopic dermatitis is best treated with hydrating the skin, controlling the pruritus, and preventing secondary infection. Patting the skin dry removes less natural skin moisturizer and thus maintains skin hydration. Water has a drying effect on the skin. Playing in the tub for 30 minutes each night would deplete the skin of its natural moisturizers, thereby leading to increased pruritus and dry skin. Bubble baths are to be avoided in children with atopic dermatitis because they may act as an irritant, possibly exacerbating the condition. Also, bubble baths deplete the skin of its natural moisturizers. The issue is not whether the child bathes every night. Rather, the goal is to decrease dryness and itching. (A)

5. 3. Impetigo involving several superficial lesions is usually treated topically, including washing the affected areas, removing crusts, and applying antibiotic ointment several times a day. The child can return to day care or school after being treated for 24 hours. The lesions do not need to be covered, they can remain open to the air. There is no need for follow-up unless the lesions have not resolved or have become more severe. (A)

6. 4. Scabies is caused by the scabies mite, *Sarcoptes scabiei*. The mite burrows into the stratum corneum of the epidermis, where the female deposits eggs and fecal material. These burrows are linear. Scabies is highly contagious. The length of time from infestation to physical symptoms is 30 to 60 days, so everyone in close contact with the child will need to be treated. The bed linens and the child's clothing should be washed in hot water and dried on the hot setting. It is not necessary to damp mop the floors to prevent the spread of scabies. The child should be held minimally until treatment is completed. Family members should wash their hands after contact with the child. Itching lasts for 2 to 3 weeks until the stratum corneum is replaced. (S)

The Client with Burns

7. 3. To prevent further injury to the skin, the mother should apply cool water to the burn site. Doing so causes vasoconstriction, retards further damage to tissues, and decreases fluid loss. Keeping the child warm promotes vasodilation, increases fluid loss, and decreases blood pressure and, thus, circulation to the area. Applying ointment to the burn is contraindicated because it does not allow healing to occur and may need to be removed in the hospital. Only a clean cloth should be used to cover the wound to prevent contamination or decrease pain or chilling. If only the arm is burned, a call to 911 for emergency care is not necessary, but the mother should seek health care services immediately. (H)

8. 2. The child has burns of the entire leg. Because of the smaller size of children's legs, the estimate of 14% is used instead of 18%, which is used with adults. The arms of children are estimated at 9%, and the anterior and posterior trunk at 18% each. The head of the child is estimated at 18%, rather than the 9% used for adults. (A)

9. 250

$$2,000 \text{ ml} \div 8 \text{ hours} = 250 \text{ ml/hour}$$

(D)

10. **2.** Expressions of anger and combativeness are often the result of loss of control and a feeling of powerlessness. Some control over the situation is regained by allowing the child to participate in care. Although having parental support during the dressing changes may be helpful, this action does nothing to allow the child control. Giving the child permission to cry may help with verbalizing feelings, but doing so does nothing to provide the child with control over the situation. Although allowing the child to determine the time for dressing changes may provide a sense of control over the situation, doing so is inappropriate because the dressing changes need to be performed as ordered to ensure effectiveness and healing. (A)

11. **2.** Withholding certain foods until the child complies is punitive and rarely successful. Allowing the mother to feed the child, serving smaller and more frequent meals, and offering finger foods are all acceptable interventions for a 5-year-old child. This is true whether the child is well or ill. (C)

12. **1.** Hypoproteinemia is common after severe burns. The child's diet should be high in protein to compensate for protein loss and to promote tissue healing. The child will also require a diet that is high in calories and rich in iron. The menu of bacon, lettuce, and tomato sandwich; milk; and celery sticks is lacking in sufficient protein and calories. (A)

13. **3.** A child with moderate burns is at high risk for contractures. A position of comfort would encourage contracture formation. Therefore, splints need to be applied to maintain proper positioning and joint function, thereby preventing contractures and loss of function. Allowing the child to lie on the abdomen or with hips and knees flexed often encourages contracture formation. (R)

The Client with Hyperthyroidism

14. **4.** Because it takes approximately 2 weeks before the response to drug treatment occurs, much of the child's care focuses on managing the child's physical symptoms. Signs and symptoms of the disorder include inability to sit still or concentrate, increased appetite with weight loss, emotional lability, and fatigue. Nursing care is directed toward ensuring that the mother and teacher know how to handle the child, suggesting a shortened school day, a nonstimulating environment, and decreased stress and workload. The child should be encouraged to eat a well-balanced diet. (A)

The Client with Insulin–Dependent Diabetes Mellitus

15. **4.** Carbohydrate counting identifies the number of grams of carbohydrate to be eaten at each meal and snack. The ADA's exchange diet allows the substitution of one food for another on the same diet list. The exchange list does not require that all food is weighed. Choices are made from lists referred to as *carbohydrate, meat or meat substitute,* and *fat.* The client's prescription identifies how many items from each food group are to be consumed at each meal and snack. The exchange assumes that foods with similar nutrient content affect blood glucose levels in a similar manner. (A)

16. **1.** A normal blood sugar is 70 to 110 mg/dl. Hypoglycemia causes the most immediate concern. When the brain does not have enough glucose, the client will become rapidly unconscious and, if uncorrected, seizures and death can result. A reading of 100 mg/dl is normal and no intervention is necessary. Readings of 150 and 200 mg/dl are elevated and could cause complications, but complications from the elevation would not occur as rapidly. (R)

17. **3.** NPH insulin peaks in 6 to 8 hours, which would occur during sleep. A bedtime snack is needed to prevent late night hypoglycemia. The snack is not given to help regain weight. Milk contains fat and protein which cause delayed absorption into the blood stream and maintains the blood glucose level at night when the NPH insulin will peak. The snack is not used to provide carbohydrates for immediate use because NPH insulin, unlike regular insulin, does not peak immediately. The snack has nothing to do with a diet. (P)

18. **2.** The child needs more insulin during an illness, because the cells becomes more insulin resistant during illness and need more insulin to achieve a normal blood glucose level. During an acute illness, simple carbohydrates and fluids are usually tolerated best. (A)

19. **1, 2, 7.** Weakness, thirst, and dizziness are symptoms related to dehydration caused by excretion of large amounts of glucose and water in the urine. The nurse should notify the physician. Shakiness, hunger, headache, and irritability are related to hypoglycemia and result from the brain and other cells being starved for nutrients. (A)

20. **2.** The nurse's first response should be to obtain more information about the mother's concerns. It is true that the child may have a diabetic reaction anywhere at school, and it is advisable that her teacher, classmates, and other adults know about her diabetes in order to help her; however, it is ultimately the client and her parents who will make the decision about informing the school. The nurse can facilitate a dialogue that will help the mother reach this decision. Dictating to the mother does not explain any rationale for the necessity of the information. (S)

21. **3.** The diabetic diet usually is based on an exchange system that takes into account the fact that some foods have similar fat, carbohydrate, and protein components and therefore can be exchanged one for another. The meal or snack must be eaten in its entirety because it is calculated together with the dose of insulin. If a child does not eat all the meal or snack, then a make-up meal should be given. (A)

22. **2.** The ability to talk about her diabetes indicates that the adolescent feels good enough about herself to share her problem with her peers. Asking for reference material does not specifically indicate that the client's self-esteem has improved or that she has accepted her diagnosis. Saying that her friends will probably desert her if she tells them about the illness indicates that the adolescent still needs to work on her self-esteem and her feelings about the disease. Asking her friends what they think of someone with a lifelong illness would not indicate that the nurse's interventions targeted toward improving self-esteem have been successful. Rather, this statement demonstrates the adolescent's uncertainty about herself. (P)

23. **3.** Sick-day management requires more frequent monitoring of the child's blood glucose to evaluate for changes associated with a decreased intake and absorption of food, commonly associated with illness. Based on the child's glucose levels, insulin adjustments may be needed. In this case, regular insulin is used. Adhering to the same schedule, type, and amount of insulin is inappropriate because the child's ability to take in food and absorb nutrients can change rapidly. Typically, the child and parents are provided with specific instructions about sick-day management rules. Commonly the physician will pre-scribe adjustments to insulin (e.g., on a sliding scale) based on the child's blood glucose levels. Therefore, calling the physician to report that the child is ill and ask what to do is inappropriate. However, the parents do need to notify the physician should any problems arise with management of the child's blood glucose levels. The child who can tolerate oral feedings of simple sugars can be kept at home as long as the parents monitor the child's blood glucose levels frequently for changes. (A)

24. **1.** Repeated use of the same injection site can result in atrophy of the fat in the subcutaneous tissue and lead to poor insulin absorption. The neuritis that develops from diabetes is related to microvascular changes that occur. Subcutaneous tissue is not destroyed and insulin is not rapidly absorbed. Resistance to insulin is caused by an immune response to the insulin protein. (D)

25. **2.** Glycosylated hemoglobin, which reflects the average blood glucose level for the past 2 to 3 months, provides a good indication of how well the blood glucose level has been controlled. Hemoglobin electrophoresis is indicated for differentiation among types of thalassemias, evaluation of hemolytic anemia, and differentiation of sickle cell trait from sickle cell disease; it provides no information about the effectiveness of diabetic treatment. A glucose tolerance test is used to evaluate the client's response to the ingestion of a specific amount of glucose. This test may be used to diagnose diabetes. A post-postprandial blood test reflects the body's metabolic response to the ingestion of a specific amount of glucose. It may be used to help make the medical diagnosis of diabetes. (R)

The Nursing Care of Adults with Medical and Surgical Health Problems

TEST 1

The Client with Cardiac Health Problems

- The Client with Acute Coronary Syndromes
- The Client with Heart Failure
- The Client with Valvular Heart Disease
- The Client with Hypertension
- The Client with a Permanent Pacemaker
- The Client Requiring Cardiopulmonary Resuscitation
- Correct Answers and Rationales

The Client with Acute Coronary Syndromes

1. The nurse is caring for a client admitted 2 days ago for a myocardial infarction (MI). Upon assessment, the nurse notes a new systolic murmur at the cardiac apex. The nurse should assess the client for which of the following conditions?
- [ ] 1. Ventricular aneurysm.
- [ ] 2. Acute pericarditis.
- [ ] 3. Papillary muscle dysfunction.
- [ ] 4. Pulmonary embolism.

2. A client with acute chest pain is receiving I.V. morphine sulfate. Which of the following results are intended effects of morphine in this client? Select all that apply.
- [ ] 1. Reduces myocardial oxygen consumption.
- [ ] 2. Promotes reduction in respiratory rate.
- [ ] 3. Prevents ventricular remodeling.
- [ ] 4. Reduces blood pressure and heart rate.
- [ ] 5. Reduces anxiety and fear.

3. A client receives fibrinolytic therapy upon admission following a myocardial infarction. He is now receiving an I.V. infusion of heparin sodium at 1,200 units/hour. The dilution is 25,000 units/500 ml. How many milliliters per hour will this client receive?

_____ ml/hour

4. A 65-year-old client is admitted to the emergency department with a fractured hip. The client has chest pain and shortness of breath. The health care provider orders nitroglycerin tablets. Which should the nurse instruct the client to do?
- [ ] 1. Put the tablet under the tongue until it is absorbed.
- [ ] 2. Swallow the tablet with 120 ml of water.
- [ ] 3. Chew the tablet until it is dissolved.
- [ ] 4. Place the tablet between his cheek and gums.

5. A 60-year-old male client comes into the emergency department with a complaint of crushing substernal chest pain that radiates to his shoulder and left arm. The admitting diagnosis is acute myocardial infarction (MI). Immediate admission orders include oxygen by nasal cannula at 4 L/minute, blood work, a chest radiograph, a 12-lead electrocardiogram (ECG), and 2 mg of morphine sulfate given I.V. The nurse should first:
☐ **1.** Administer the morphine.
☐ **2.** Obtain a 12-lead ECG.
☐ **3.** Obtain the blood work.
☐ **4.** Order the chest radiograph.

6. When administering a thrombolytic drug to the client experiencing a myocardial infarction (MI), the nurse explains to him that the purpose of the drug is to:
☐ **1.** Help keep him well hydrated.
☐ **2.** Dissolve clots that he may have.
☐ **3.** Prevent kidney failure.
☐ **4.** Treat potential cardiac arrhythmias.

7. The nurse is assessing a client who has had a myocardial infarction (MI). The nurse notes the cardiac rhythm shown on the electrocardiogram strip below. The nurse identifies this rhythm as which of the following?
☐ **1.** Atrial fibrillation.
☐ **2.** Ventricular tachycardia.
☐ **3.** Premature ventricular contractions (PVCs).
☐ **4.** Third-degree heart block.

8. Aspirin is administered to the client experiencing a myocardial infarction (MI) because of its:
☐ **1.** Antipyretic action.
☐ **2.** Antithrombotic action.
☐ **3.** Antiplatelet action.
☐ **4.** Analgesic action.

9. When interpreting the electrocardiogram (ECG), the nurse would keep in mind which of the following about the P wave? Select all that apply.
☐ **1.** Reflects electrical impulse beginning at the sino-atrial (SA) node.
☐ **2.** Indicates electrical impulse beginning at the atrio-ventricular (AV) node.
☐ **3.** Reflects atrial muscle depolarization.
☐ **4.** Identifies ventricular muscle depolarization.
☐ **5.** Has a duration normally of 0.11 second or less.

10. If the client who was admitted for myocardial infarction (MI) develops cardiogenic shock, which characteristic sign should the nurse expect to observe?
☐ **1.** Oliguria.
☐ **2.** Bradycardia.
☐ **3.** Elevated blood pressure.
☐ **4.** Fever.

11. The physician orders continuous I.V. nitroglycerin infusion for the client with myocardial infarction. Essential nursing actions include which of the following?
☐ **1.** Obtaining an infusion pump for the medication.
☐ **2.** Monitoring blood pressure every 4 hours.
☐ **3.** Monitoring urine output hourly.
☐ **4.** Obtaining serum potassium levels daily.

12. When teaching the client with myocardial infarction (MI), the nurse explains that the pain associated with MI is caused by:
☐ **1.** Left ventricular overload.
☐ **2.** Impending circulatory collapse.
☐ **3.** Extracellular electrolyte imbalances.
☐ **4.** Insufficient oxygen reaching the heart muscle.

13. The nurse is assessing a client who has had a myocardial infarction. The nurse notes the cardiac rhythm shown on the electrocardiogram strip below. The nurse identifies this rhythm as which of the following?
☐ **1.** Atrial fibrillation.
☐ **2.** Ventricular tachycardia.
☐ **3.** Premature ventricular contractions.
☐ **4.** Sinus tachycardia.

14. While caring for a client who has sustained a myocardial infarction (MI), the nurse notes eight premature ventricular contractions (PVCs) in 1 minute on the cardiac monitor. The client is receiving an I.V. infusion of 5% dextrose in water (D_5W) and oxygen at 2 L/minute. The nurse's first course of action should be to:
- ☐ **1.** Increase the I.V. infusion rate.
- ☐ **2.** Notify the physician promptly.
- ☐ **3.** Increase the oxygen concentration.
- ☐ **4.** Administer a prescribed analgesic.

15. Which of the following is an expected outcome for a client on the second day of hospitalization after a myocardial infarction (MI)? The client:
- ☐ **1.** Has severe chest pain.
- ☐ **2.** Can identify risk factors for MI.
- ☐ **3.** Agrees to participate in a cardiac rehabilitation walking program.
- ☐ **4.** Can perform personal self-care activities without pain.

16. When teaching a client about the expected outcomes after I.V. administration of furosemide, the nurse would include which outcome?
- ☐ **1.** Increased blood pressure.
- ☐ **2.** Increased urine output.
- ☐ **3.** Decreased pain.
- ☐ **4.** Decreased premature ventricular contractions.

17. After a myocardial infarction, the hospitalized client is taught to move the legs while resting in bed. This type of exercise is recommended primarily to help:
- ☐ **1.** Prepare the client for ambulation.
- ☐ **2.** Promote urinary and intestinal elimination.
- ☐ **3.** Prevent thrombophlebitis and blood clot formation.
- ☐ **4.** Decrease the likelihood of pressure ulcer formation.

18. Which of the following reflects the principle on which a client's diet will most likely be based during the acute phase of myocardial infarction?
- ☐ **1.** Liquids as desired.
- ☐ **2.** Small, easily digested meals.
- ☐ **3.** Three regular meals per day.
- ☐ **4.** Nothing by mouth.

19. Which of the following controllable risk factors for coronary artery disease (CAD) appears most closely linked to the development of the disease?
- ☐ **1.** Age.
- ☐ **2.** Medication usage.
- ☐ **3.** High cholesterol levels.
- ☐ **4.** Gender.

20. Which of the following is an uncontrollable risk factor that has been linked to the development of coronary artery disease (CAD)?
- ☐ **1.** Exercise.
- ☐ **2.** Obesity.
- ☐ **3.** Stress.
- ☐ **4.** Heredity.

21. If a client displays risk factors for coronary artery disease, such as smoking cigarettes, eating a diet high in saturated fat, or leading a sedentary lifestyle, techniques of behavior modification may be used to help the client change the behavior. The nurse can best reinforce new adaptive behaviors by:
- ☐ **1.** Explaining how the old behavior leads to poor health.
- ☐ **2.** Withholding praise until the new behavior is well established.
- ☐ **3.** Rewarding the client whenever the acceptable behavior is performed.
- ☐ **4.** Instilling mild fear into the client to extinguish the behavior.

22. Alteplase recombinant, or tissue plasminogen activator (t-PA), a thrombolytic enzyme, is administered during the first 6 hours after onset of myocardial infarction (MI) to:
- ☐ **1.** Control chest pain.
- ☐ **2.** Reduce coronary artery vasospasm.
- ☐ **3.** Control the arrhythmias associated with MI.
- ☐ **4.** Revascularize the blocked coronary artery.

23. After the administration of t-PA, the nurse understands that a nursing assessment priority is to:
- ☐ **1.** Observe the client for chest pain.
- ☐ **2.** Monitor for fever.
- ☐ **3.** Monitor the 12-lead electrocardiogram (ECG) every 4 hours.
- ☐ **4.** Monitor breath sounds.

24. When monitoring a client who is receiving tissue plasminogen activator (t-PA), the nurse understands it is important to monitor vital signs and have resuscitation equipment available because reperfusion of the cardiac tissue can result in which of the following?
- ☐ **1.** Cardiac arrhythmias.
- ☐ **2.** Hypertension.
- ☐ **3.** Seizure.
- ☐ **4.** Hypothermia.

25. Contraindications to the administration of tissue plasminogen activator (t-PA) include which of the following?
☐ **1.** Age greater than 60 years.
☐ **2.** History of cerebral hemorrhage.
☐ **3.** History of heart failure.
☐ **4.** Cigarette smoking.

26. A client has driven himself to the emergency department. He is 50 years old, has a history of hypertension, and informs the nurse that his father died from a heart attack at age 60. The client is presently complaining of indigestion. The nurse connects him to an electrocardiogram monitor and begins administering oxygen at 2 L/minute per nasal cannula. The nurse's next action would be to:
☐ **1.** Call for the physician.
☐ **2.** Start an I.V. line.
☐ **3.** Obtain a portable chest radiograph.
☐ **4.** Draw blood for laboratory studies.

27. Crackles heard on lung auscultation indicate which of the following?
☐ **1.** Cyanosis.
☐ **2.** Bronchospasm.
☐ **3.** Airway narrowing.
☐ **4.** Fluid-filled alveoli.

28. A 68-year-old female client on day 2 after hip surgery has no cardiac history but starts to complain of chest heaviness. The first nursing action should be to:
☐ **1.** Inquire about the onset, duration, severity, and precipitating factors of the heaviness.
☐ **2.** Administer oxygen via nasal cannula.
☐ **3.** Offer pain medication for the chest heaviness.
☐ **4.** Inform the physician of the chest heaviness.

29. The nurse receives emergency laboratory results for a client with chest pain and immediately informs the physician. An increased myoglobin level suggests which of the following?
☐ **1.** Cancer.
☐ **2.** Hypertension.
☐ **3.** Liver disease.
☐ **4.** Myocardial damage.

30. An older, sedentary adult may not respond to emotional or physical stress as well as a younger individual because of:
☐ **1.** Left ventricular atrophy.
☐ **2.** Irregular heartbeats.
☐ **3.** Peripheral vascular occlusion.
☐ **4.** Pacemaker placement.

31. During the previous few months, a 56-year-old woman felt brief twinges of chest pain while working in her garden and has had frequent episodes of indigestion. She comes to the hospital after experiencing severe anterior chest pain while raking leaves. Her evaluation confirms a diagnosis of stable angina pectoris. After stabilization and treatment, the client is discharged from the hospital. At her follow-up appointment, she is discouraged because she is experiencing pain with increasing frequency. She states that she visits an invalid friend twice a week and now cannot walk up the second flight of steps to the friend's apartment without pain. Which of the following measures that the nurse could suggest would most likely help the client prevent this problem?
☐ **1.** Visit her friend early in the day.
☐ **2.** Rest for at least an hour before climbing the stairs.
☐ **3.** Take a nitroglycerin tablet before climbing the stairs.
☐ **4.** Lie down once she reaches the friend's apartment.

32. The client who experiences angina has been told to follow a low-cholesterol diet. Which of the following meals should the nurse tell the client would be best on her low-cholesterol diet?
☐ **1.** Hamburger, salad, and milkshake.
☐ **2.** Baked liver, green beans, and coffee.
☐ **3.** Spaghetti with tomato sauce, salad, and coffee.
☐ **4.** Fried chicken, green beans, and skim milk.

33. Which of the following symptoms should the nurse teach the client with unstable angina to report immediately to her physician?
☐ **1.** A change in the pattern of her pain.
☐ **2.** Pain during sexual activity.
☐ **3.** Pain during an argument with her husband.
☐ **4.** Pain during or after an activity such as lawn-mowing.

34. The physician refers the client with unstable angina for a cardiac catheterization. The nurse explains to the client that this procedure is being used in this specific case to:
☐ **1.** Open and dilate blocked coronary arteries.
☐ **2.** Assess the extent of arterial blockage.
☐ **3.** Bypass obstructed vessels.
☐ **4.** Assess the functional adequacy of the valves and heart muscle.

35. The client is scheduled for a percutaneous transluminal coronary angioplasty (PTCA) to treat angina. Priority goals for the client immediately after PTCA should include:
☐ **1.** Minimizing dyspnea.
☐ **2.** Maintaining adequate blood pressure control.
☐ **3.** Decreasing myocardial contractility.
☐ **4.** Preventing fluid volume deficit.

36. Which of the following is not generally considered to be a risk factor for the development of atherosclerosis?
☐ **1.** Family history of early heart attack.
☐ **2.** Late onset of puberty.
☐ **3.** Total blood cholesterol level greater than 220 mg/dl.
☐ **4.** Elevated fasting blood glucose concentration.

37. Many more men than women younger than age 50 have coronary artery disease (CAD) as a result of atherosclerosis. The leading cause of death in women is:
☐ **1.** Acquired immunodeficiency syndrome (AIDS).
☐ **2.** Breast cancer.
☐ **3.** CAD.
☐ **4.** Chronic obstructive pulmonary disease (COPD).

38. A client with angina asks the nurse, "What information does an electrocardiogram (ECG) provide?" The nurse would respond that an ECG primarily gives information about the:
☐ **1.** Electrical conduction of the myocardium.
☐ **2.** Oxygenation and perfusion of the heart.
☐ **3.** Contractile status of the ventricles.
☐ **4.** Physical integrity of the heart muscle.

39. As an initial step in treating a client with angina, the physician prescribes nitroglycerin tablets, 0.3 mg given sublingually. This drug's principal effects are produced by:
☐ **1.** Antispasmodic effects on the pericardium.
☐ **2.** Causing an increased myocardial oxygen demand.
☐ **3.** Vasodilation of peripheral vasculature.
☐ **4.** Improved conductivity in the myocardium.

40. The nurse teaches the client with angina about the common expected adverse effects of nitroglycerin, including:
☐ **1.** Headache.
☐ **2.** High blood pressure.
☐ **3.** Shortness of breath.
☐ **4.** Stomach cramps.

41. Sublingual nitroglycerin tablets begin to work within 1 to 2 minutes. How should the nurse instruct the client to use the drug when chest pain occurs?
☐ **1.** Take one tablet every 2 to 5 minutes until the pain stops.
☐ **2.** Take one tablet and rest for 10 minutes. Call the physician if pain persists after 10 minutes.
☐ **3.** Take one tablet, then an additional tablet every 5 minutes for a total of three tablets. Call the physician if pain persists after three tablets.
☐ **4.** Take one tablet. If pain persists after 5 minutes, take two tablets. If pain still persists 5 minutes later, call the physician.

42. A client with angina has been taking nifedipine. The client should be taught to:
☐ **1.** Monitor blood pressure monthly.
☐ **2.** Perform daily weights.
☐ **3.** Inspect gums daily.
☐ **4.** Limit intake of green leafy vegetables.

The Client with Heart Failure

43. A client with chronic heart failure has atrial fibrillation and a left ventricular ejection fraction of 15%. The client is taking warfarin (Coumadin). The expected outcome of this drug is to:
☐ **1.** Decrease circulatory overload.
☐ **2.** Improve the myocardial workload.
☐ **3.** Prevent thrombus formation.
☐ **4.** Regulate cardiac rhythm.

44. A client has a history of heart failure and has been taking several medications, including furosemide (Lasix), digoxin (Lanoxin) and potassium chloride. The client complains of nausea, blurred vision, headache, and weakness. The nurse notes that the client is confused. The telemetry strip shows first-degree atrioventricular block. The nurse should assess the client for signs of which condition?
☐ **1.** Hyperkalemia.
☐ **2.** Digoxin toxicity.
☐ **3.** Fluid deficit.
☐ **4.** Pulmonary edema.

45. A nurse is assessing a client with heart failure. The nurse should assess the client based on which compensatory mechanisms that are activated in the presence of heart failure? Select all that apply.
☐ **1.** Ventricular hypertrophy.
☐ **2.** Parasympathetic nervous stimulation.
☐ **3.** Renin-angiotensin-aldosterone system.
☐ **4.** Jugular venous distention.
☐ **5.** Sympathetic nervous stimulation.

46. Which of the following sets of conditions is an indication that a client with a history of left-sided heart failure is developing pulmonary edema?
☐ **1.** Distended jugular veins and wheezing.
☐ **2.** Dependent edema and anorexia.
☐ **3.** Coarse crackles and tachycardia.
☐ **4.** Hypotension and tachycardia.

47. A 69-year-old female has a history of heart failure. She is admitted to the emergency department with heart failure complicated by pulmonary edema. On admission of this client, which of the following should the nurse assess first?
☐ **1.** Blood pressure.
☐ **2.** Skin breakdown.
☐ **3.** Serum potassium level.
☐ **4.** Urine output.

48. Which of the following nursing diagnoses would be appropriate for a client with heart failure? Select all that apply.
- ☐ **1.** *Ineffective tissue perfusion* related to decreased peripheral blood flow secondary to decreased cardiac output.
- ☐ **2.** *Activity intolerance* related to increased cardiac output.
- ☐ **3.** *Decreased cardiac output* related to structural and functional changes.
- ☐ **4.** *Impaired gas exchange* related to decreased sympathetic nervous system activity.

49. In which of the following positions should the nurse place a client with suspected heart failure?
- ☐ **1.** Semi-sitting (low Fowler's position).
- ☐ **2.** Lying on the right side (Sims' position).
- ☐ **3.** Sitting almost upright (high Fowler's position).
- ☐ **4.** Lying on the back with the head lowered (Trendelenburg's position).

50. Which of the following would be a priority nursing diagnosis for the client with heart failure and pulmonary edema?
- ☐ **1.** *Risk for infection* related to stasis of alveolar secretions.
- ☐ **2.** *Impaired skin integrity* related to pressure.
- ☐ **3.** *Activity intolerance* related to pump failure.
- ☐ **4.** *Constipation* related to immobility.

51. The major goal of therapy for a client with heart failure and pulmonary edema should be to:
- ☐ **1.** Increase cardiac output.
- ☐ **2.** Improve respiratory status.
- ☐ **3.** Decrease peripheral edema.
- ☐ **4.** Enhance comfort.

52. Digoxin is administered intravenously to a client with heart failure, primarily because the drug acts to:
- ☐ **1.** Dilate coronary arteries.
- ☐ **2.** Increase myocardial contractility.
- ☐ **3.** Decrease cardiac arrhythmias.
- ☐ **4.** Decrease electrical conductivity in the heart.

53. Captopril (Capoten), an angiotensin-converting enzyme (ACE) inhibitor, may be administered to a client with heart failure because it acts as a:
- ☐ **1.** Vasopressor.
- ☐ **2.** Volume expander.
- ☐ **3.** Vasodilator.
- ☐ **4.** Potassium-sparing diuretic.

54. Furosemide is administered intravenously to a client with heart failure. How soon after administration should the nurse begin to see evidence of the drug's desired effect?
- ☐ **1.** 5 to 10 minutes.
- ☐ **2.** 30 to 60 minutes.
- ☐ **3.** 2 to 4 hours.
- ☐ **4.** 6 to 8 hours.

55. The nurse teaches a client with heart failure to take oral furosemide in the morning. The primary reason for this is to help:
- ☐ **1.** Prevent electrolyte imbalances.
- ☐ **2.** Retard rapid drug absorption.
- ☐ **3.** Excrete excessive fluids accumulated during the night.
- ☐ **4.** Prevent sleep disturbances during the night.

56. Clients with heart failure are prone to atrial fibrillation. During physical assessment, the nurse should suspect atrial fibrillation when palpation of the radial pulse reveals:
- ☐ **1.** Two regular beats followed by one irregular beat.
- ☐ **2.** An irregular pulse rhythm.
- ☐ **3.** Pulse rate below 60 bpm.
- ☐ **4.** A weak, thready pulse.

57. When teaching the client about complications of atrial fibrillation, the nurse understands that the complications can be caused by:
- ☐ **1.** Stasis of blood in the atria.
- ☐ **2.** Increased cardiac output.
- ☐ **3.** Decreased pulse rate.
- ☐ **4.** Elevated blood pressure.

58. The nurse should teach the client that signs of digoxin toxicity include which of the following?
- ☐ **1.** Rash over the chest and back.
- ☐ **2.** Increased appetite.
- ☐ **3.** Visual disturbances such as seeing yellow spots.
- ☐ **4.** Elevated blood pressure.

59. The nurse should be especially alert for signs and symptoms of digoxin toxicity if serum levels indicate that the client has a:
- ☐ **1.** Low sodium level.
- ☐ **2.** High glucose level.
- ☐ **3.** High calcium level.
- ☐ **4.** Low potassium level.

60. Which of the following foods should the nurse teach a client with heart failure to avoid or limit when following a 2-g sodium diet?
- ☐ **1.** Apples.
- ☐ **2.** Tomato juice.
- ☐ **3.** Whole wheat bread.
- ☐ **4.** Beef tenderloin.

61. To help maintain a normal blood serum level of potassium, the client receiving a loop diuretic should be encouraged to eat foods, such as bananas, orange juice, and:
- ☐ **1.** Spinach.
- ☐ **2.** Skimmed milk.
- ☐ **3.** Baked chicken.
- ☐ **4.** Brown rice.

62. The nurse finds the apical impulse below the fifth intercostal space. The nurse suspects:
- ☐ **1.** Left atrial enlargement.
- ☐ **2.** Left ventricular enlargement.
- ☐ **3.** Right atrial enlargement.
- ☐ **4.** Right ventricular enlargement.

63. The nurse is admitting a 69-year-old male to the clinical unit. The client has a history of left ventricular enlargement. During the assessment, the nurse notes +3 pitting edema of the ankles bilaterally. The client does not have chest pain. The nurse observes that the client does have dyspnea at rest. The nurse infers that the client may have:
- ☐ **1.** Arteriosclerosis.
- ☐ **2.** Heart failure.
- ☐ **3.** Chronic bronchitis.
- ☐ **4.** Acute myocardial infarction.

64. The nurse's discharge teaching plan for the client with heart failure should stress the significance of which of the following?
- ☐ **1.** Maintaining a high-fiber diet.
- ☐ **2.** Walking 2 miles every day.
- ☐ **3.** Obtaining daily weights at the same time each day.
- ☐ **4.** Remaining sedentary for most of the day.

65. When teaching a client with heart failure about preventing complications and future hospitalizations, which problems stated by the client as reasons to call the physician would indicate to the nurse that the client has understood the teaching? Select all that apply.
- ☐ **1.** Becoming increasingly short of breath at rest.
- ☐ **2.** Weight gain of 2 lb or more in 1 day.
- ☐ **3.** High intake of sodium for breakfast.
- ☐ **4.** Having to sleep sitting up in a reclining chair.
- ☐ **5.** Weight loss of 2 lb in 1 day.

The Client with Valvular Heart Disease

66. A client is scheduled for a cardiac catheterization. The nurse should do which of the following preprocedure tasks? Select all that apply.
- ☐ **1.** Administer all ordered oral medications.
- ☐ **2.** Check for iodine sensitivity.
- ☐ **3.** Verify that written consent has been obtained.
- ☐ **4.** Withhold food and oral fluids before the procedure.
- ☐ **5.** Insert a urinary drainage catheter.

67. A client has returned to the medical-surgical unit after a cardiac catheterization. Which is the most important initial postprocedure nursing assessment for this client?
- ☐ **1.** Monitor the laboratory values.
- ☐ **2.** Observe neurologic function every 15 minutes.
- ☐ **3.** Observe the puncture site for swelling and bleeding.
- ☐ **4.** Monitor skin warmth and turgor.

68. A 70-year-old female is scheduled to undergo mitral valve replacement for severe mitral stenosis and mitral regurgitation. Although the diagnosis was made during childhood, she did not have symptoms until 4 years ago. Recently, she noticed increased symptoms, despite daily doses of digoxin and furosemide. During the initial interview with the client, the nurse would most likely learn that the client's childhood health history included:
- ☐ **1.** Chickenpox.
- ☐ **2.** Poliomyelitis.
- ☐ **3.** Rheumatic fever.
- ☐ **4.** Meningitis.

69. A client experiences some initial signs and symptoms of excitation after having an I.V. infusion of lidocaine hydrochloride started. The nurse should assess that the client is demonstrating a typical adverse reaction to lidocaine when the client complains of:
- ☐ **1.** Palpitations.
- ☐ **2.** Tinnitus.
- ☐ **3.** Urinary frequency.
- ☐ **4.** Lethargy.

70. A female with severe mitral stenosis and mitral regurgitation has a pulmonary artery catheter inserted. The physician orders pulmonary artery pressure monitoring, including pulmonary capillary wedge pressures. The purpose of pulmonary artery pressure monitoring is to help assess the:
- ☐ **1.** Degree of coronary artery stenosis.
- ☐ **2.** Peripheral arterial pressure.
- ☐ **3.** Pressure from fluid within the left ventricle.
- ☐ **4.** Oxygen and carbon dioxide concentrations in the blood.

71. Which of the following signs and symptoms would most likely be found in a client with mitral regurgitation?
☐ **1.** Exertional dyspnea.
☐ **2.** Confusion.
☐ **3.** Elevated creatine kinase concentration.
☐ **4.** Chest pain.

72. The nurse expects that a client with mitral stenosis would demonstrate symptoms associated with congestion in the:
☐ **1.** Aorta.
☐ **2.** Right atrium.
☐ **3.** Superior vena cava.
☐ **4.** Pulmonary circulation.

73. Because a client has mitral stenosis and is a prospective valve recipient, the nurse preoperatively assesses the client's past compliance with medical regimens. Lack of compliance with which of the following regimens would pose the greatest health hazard to this client?
☐ **1.** Medication therapy.
☐ **2.** Diet modification.
☐ **3.** Activity restrictions.
☐ **4.** Dental care.

74. In preparing the client and the family for a postoperative stay in the intensive care unit (ICU) after open heart surgery, the nurse should explain that:
☐ **1.** The client will remain in the ICU for 5 days.
☐ **2.** The client will sleep most of the time while in the ICU.
☐ **3.** Noise and activity within the ICU are minimal.
☐ **4.** The client will receive medication to relieve pain.

75. A client who has undergone a mitral valve replacement experiences persistent bleeding from the surgical incision during the early postoperative period. Which of the following pharmaceutical agents should the nurse be prepared to administer to this client?
☐ **1.** Vitamin C.
☐ **2.** Protamine sulfate.
☐ **3.** Quinidine sulfate.
☐ **4.** Warfarin sodium (Coumadin).

76. The most effective measure the nurse can use to prevent wound infection when changing a client's dressing after coronary artery bypass surgery is to:
☐ **1.** Observe careful hand-washing procedures.
☐ **2.** Clean the incisional area with an antiseptic.
☐ **3.** Use prepackaged sterile dressings to cover the incision.
☐ **4.** Place soiled dressings in a waterproof bag before disposing of them.

77. For a client who excretes excessive amounts of calcium during the postoperative period after open heart surgery, which of the following measures should the nurse institute to help prevent complications associated with excessive calcium excretion?
☐ **1.** Ensure a liberal fluid intake.
☐ **2.** Provide an alkaline-ash diet.
☐ **3.** Prevent constipation.
☐ **4.** Enrich the client's diet with dairy products.

78. The nurse teaches the client who is receiving warfarin sodium that:
☐ **1.** Partial thromboplastin time values determine the dosage of warfarin sodium.
☐ **2.** Protamine sulfate is used to reverse the effects of warfarin sodium.
☐ **3.** International Normalized Ratio (INR) is used to assess effectiveness.
☐ **4.** Warfarin sodium will facilitate clotting of the blood.

79. Good dental care is an important measure in reducing the risk of endocarditis. A teaching plan to promote good dental care in a client with mitral stenosis should include demonstration of the proper use of:
☐ **1.** A manual toothbrush.
☐ **2.** An electric toothbrush.
☐ **3.** An irrigation device.
☐ **4.** Dental floss.

80. Before a client's discharge after mitral valve replacement surgery, the nurse should evaluate the client's understanding of postsurgery activity restrictions. Which of the following should the client not engage in until after the 1-month postdischarge appointment with the surgeon?
☐ **1.** Showering.
☐ **2.** Lifting anything heavier than 10 lb.
☐ **3.** A program of gradually progressive walking.
☐ **4.** Light housework.

81. Three days after mitral valve surgery, a 45-year-old female comments that she hears a "clicking" noise coming from her chest and her "rather large" chest incision. The nurse's response should reflect the understanding that the client may be experiencing which of the following?
☐ **1.** Anxiety related to altered body image.
☐ **2.** Anxiety related to altered health status.
☐ **3.** Altered tissue perfusion.
☐ **4.** Lack of knowledge regarding the postoperative course.

The Client with Hypertension

82. A client is taking clonidine (Catapres) for treatment of hypertension. The nurse should teach him about which of the following common adverse effects of this drug? Select all that apply.
☐ **1.** Dry mouth.
☐ **2.** Hyperkalemia.
☐ **3.** Impotence.
☐ **4.** Pancreatitis.
☐ **5.** Sleep disturbance.

83. A client with hypertensive emergency is being treated with sodium nitroprusside (Nipride). In a dilution of 50 mg/250 ml, how many micrograms of Nipride are in each milliliter?

_____ mcg

84. In teaching the hypertensive client to avoid orthostatic hypotension, the nurse should emphasize which of the following instructions? Select all that apply.
☐ **1.** Plan regular times for taking medications.
☐ **2.** Arise slowly from bed.
☐ **3.** Avoid standing still for long periods.
☐ **4.** Avoid excessive alcohol intake.
☐ **5.** Avoid hot baths.

85. An industrial health nurse at a large printing plant finds a male employee's blood pressure to be elevated on two occasions 1 month apart and refers him to his private physician. The employee is about 25 lb overweight and has smoked a pack of cigarettes daily for more than 20 years. The client's physician prescribes atenolol (Tenormin) for the hypertension. The nurse should instruct the client to:
☐ **1.** Avoid sudden discontinuation of the drug.
☐ **2.** Monitor the blood pressure annually.
☐ **3.** Follow a 2-g sodium diet.
☐ **4.** Discontinue the medication if severe headaches develop.

86. The nurse teaches her client, who has recently been diagnosed with hypertension, about his dietary restrictions: a low-calorie, low-fat, low-sodium diet. Which of the following menu selections would best meet the client's needs?
☐ **1.** Mixed green salad with blue cheese dressing, crackers, and cold cuts.
☐ **2.** Ham sandwich on rye bread and an orange.
☐ **3.** Baked chicken, an apple, and a slice of white bread.
☐ **4.** Hot dogs, baked beans, and celery and carrot sticks.

87. A client's job involves working in a warm, dry room, frequently bending and crouching to check the underside of a high-speed press, and wearing eye guards. Given this information, the nurse should assess the client for which of the following?
☐ **1.** Muscle aches.
☐ **2.** Thirst.
☐ **3.** Lethargy.
☐ **4.** Orthostatic hypotension.

88. An exercise program is prescribed for the client with hypertension. Which intervention would be most likely to assist the client in maintaining an exercise program?
☐ **1.** Giving the client a written exercise program.
☐ **2.** Explaining the exercise program to the client's spouse.
☐ **3.** Reassuring the client that he or she can do the exercise program.
☐ **4.** Tailoring a program to the client's needs and abilities.

89. The client realizes the importance of quitting smoking, and the nurse develops a plan to help the client achieve this goal. Which of the following nursing interventions should be the initial step in this plan?
☐ **1.** Review the negative effects of smoking on the body.
☐ **2.** Discuss the effects of passive smoking on environmental pollution.
☐ **3.** Establish the client's daily smoking pattern.
☐ **4.** Explain how smoking worsens high blood pressure.

90. Essential hypertension would be diagnosed in a 40-year-old male whose blood pressure readings were consistently at or above which of the following?
☐ **1.** 120/90 mm Hg.
☐ **2.** 130/85 mm Hg.
☐ **3.** 140/90 mm Hg.
☐ **4.** 160/80 mm Hg.

91. When teaching a client about propranolol hydrochloride, the nurse should base the information on the knowledge that propranolol:
☐ **1.** Blocks beta-adrenergic stimulation and thus causes decreased heart rate, myocardial contractility, and conduction.
☐ **2.** Increases norepinephrine secretion and thus decreases blood pressure and heart rate.
☐ **3.** Is a potent arterial and venous vasodilator that reduces peripheral vascular resistance and lowers blood pressure.
☐ **4.** Is an angiotensin-converting enzyme inhibitor that reduces blood pressure by blocking the conversion of angiotensin I to angiotensin II.

92. The nurse understands that a priority nursing diagnosis for the client with hypertension would be:
☐ 1. *Pain.*
☐ 2. *Deficient fluid volume.*
☐ 3. *Impaired skin integrity.*
☐ 4. *Ineffective health maintenance.*

93. The most important long-term goal for a client with hypertension would be to:
☐ 1. Learn how to avoid stress.
☐ 2. Explore a job change or early retirement.
☐ 3. Make a commitment to long-term therapy.
☐ 4. Lose weight.

94. The client with hypertension is prone to long-term complications of the disease. Which of the following is a long-term complication of hypertension?
☐ 1. Renal insufficiency and failure.
☐ 2. Valvular heart disease.
☐ 3. Endocarditis.
☐ 4. Peptic ulcer disease.

95. Hypertension is known as the silent killer. This phrase is associated with the fact that hypertension often goes undetected until signs and symptoms of other system failures occur. Such signs and symptoms may occur in the form of:
☐ 1. Cerebrovascular accidents (CVAs).
☐ 2. Liver disease.
☐ 3. Myocardial infarction.
☐ 4. Pulmonary disease.

The Client with a Permanent Pacemaker

96. When teaching a client about self-care following placement of a new permanent pacemaker to his left upper chest, the nurse should include which information? Select all that apply.
☐ 1. Take and record daily pulse rate.
☐ 2. Avoid air travel because of airport security alarms.
☐ 3. Immobilize the affected arm for 4 to 6 weeks.
☐ 4. Avoid using a microwave oven.
☐ 5. Avoid lifting anything heavier than 3 lb.

97. A client has been admitted to the coronary care unit. The nurse observes third-degree heart block at a rate of 35 bpm on the client's cardiac monitor. The client is hypotensive. The nurse should take which of the following actions first?
☐ 1. Prepare for transcutaneous pacing.
☐ 2. Prepare to defibrillate the client at 200 joules.
☐ 3. Administer an I.V. lidocaine infusion.
☐ 4. Schedule the operating room for insertion of a permanent pacemaker.

98. A 74-year-old female is admitted to the telemetry unit for placement of a permanent pacemaker because of sinus bradycardia. A priority goal for the client within 24 hours after insertion of a permanent pacemaker would be to:
☐ 1. Maintain skin integrity.
☐ 2. Maintain cardiac conduction stability.
☐ 3. Decrease cardiac output.
☐ 4. Increase activity level.

99. The client who had a permanent pacemaker implanted 2 days earlier is being discharged from the hospital. Outcomes include that the client:
☐ 1. Selects a low-cholesterol diet to control coronary artery disease.
☐ 2. States a need for bed rest for 1 week after discharge.
☐ 3. Verbalizes safety precautions needed to prevent pacemaker malfunction.
☐ 4. Explains signs and symptoms of myocardial infarction (MI).

The Client Requiring Cardiopulmonary Resuscitation

100. Ventricular tachycardia is displayed on the cardiac monitor of a client admitted to the telemetry unit. Which should the nurse do first?
☐ 1. Prepare for immediate cardioversion.
☐ 2. Begin cardiopulmonary resuscitation (CPR).
☐ 3. Check for a pulse.
☐ 4. Prepare for immediate defibrillation.

101. The nurse is preparing the client for cardioversion. Which key points must the nurse remember to do? Select all that apply.
☐ 1. Use a conducting agent between the skin and the paddles.
☐ 2. Place the paddles over the client's clothing.
☐ 3. Call "clear" before discharging the electrical current.
☐ 4. Record the delivered energy and the resulting rhythm.
☐ 5. Exert 5 to 10 lb of pressure on each paddle to ensure good skin contact.

102. A client who has been given cardiopulmonary resuscitation (CPR) is transported by ambulance to the hospital's emergency department, where the admitting nurse quickly assesses the client's condition. Of the following observations, the one most often recommended for determining the effectiveness of CPR is noting whether the:
☐ 1. Pulse rate is normal.
☐ 2. Pupils are reacting to light.
☐ 3. Mucous membranes are pink.
☐ 4. Systolic blood pressure is at least 80 mm Hg.

103. The client receives epinephrine during resuscitation in the emergency department. This drug is administered primarily because of its ability to:
☐ **1.** Dilate bronchioles.
☐ **2.** Constrict arterioles.
☐ **3.** Free glycogen from the liver.
☐ **4.** Enhance myocardial contractility.

104. A nurse is administering cardiopulmonary resuscitation (CPR). The compression-to-ventilation ratio for one-rescuer adult CPR is:
☐ **1.** 5:1.
☐ **2.** 15:1.
☐ **3.** 5:2.
☐ **4.** 15:2.

105. During cardiopulmonary resuscitation (CPR), the xiphoid process at the lower end of the sternum should not be compressed when performing cardiac compressions. Which of the following organs would be most likely at risk for laceration by forceful compressions over the xiphoid process?
☐ **1.** Lung.
☐ **2.** Liver.
☐ **3.** Stomach.
☐ **4.** Diaphragm.

106. When performing external chest compressions on an adult during cardiopulmonary resuscitation (CPR), the rescuer should depress the sternum:
☐ **1.** 0.5 to 1 inch.
☐ **2.** 1 to 1.5 inches.
☐ **3.** 1.5 to 2 inches.
☐ **4.** 2 to 2.5 inches.

107. The American Heart Association guidelines for Basic Cardiac Life Support recommend that the rescuer, after first establishing unresponsiveness, should:
☐ **1.** Perform cardiopulmonary resuscitation (CPR) for 2 minutes on the adult victim.
☐ **2.** Place a call for emergency assistance immediately.
☐ **3.** Begin rescue breathing for the victim.
☐ **4.** Begin CPR on the adult victim and wait until help arrives.

108. If the victim's chest wall fails to rise with each inflation when rescue breathing is administered during cardiopulmonary resuscitation (CPR), the most likely reason is that the:
☐ **1.** Airway is not clear.
☐ **2.** Victim is beyond resuscitation.
☐ **3.** Inflations are being given at too rapid a rate.
☐ **4.** Rescuer is using inadequate force for cardiac compressions.

109. During rescue breathing in cardiopulmonary resuscitation (CPR), the victim will exhale by:
☐ **1.** Normal relaxation of the chest.
☐ **2.** Gentle pressure of the rescuer's hand on the upper chest.
☐ **3.** The pressure of cardiac compressions.
☐ **4.** Turning the head to the side.

110. The nurse understands that the estimated maximum time a person can be without cardiopulmonary function and still not experience permanent brain damage is:
☐ **1.** 1 to 2 minutes.
☐ **2.** 4 to 6 minutes.
☐ **3.** 8 to 10 minutes.
☐ **4.** 12 to 15 minutes.

111. A nurse is helping a suspected choking victim. The nurse should perform the Heimlich maneuver when the victim:
☐ **1.** Starts to become cyanotic.
☐ **2.** Cannot speak due to airway obstruction.
☐ **3.** Can make only minimal vocal noises.
☐ **4.** Is coughing vigorously.

112. When performing the Heimlich maneuver on a conscious adult victim, the rescuer delivers inward and upward thrusts specifically:
☐ **1.** Above the umbilicus.
☐ **2.** At the level of the xiphoid process.
☐ **3.** Over the victim's midabdominal area.
☐ **4.** Below the xiphoid process and above the umbilicus.

113. The monitor technician informs the nurse that the client has started having premature ventricular contractions every other beat. Which is the priority nursing action?
☐ **1.** Call a "code blue" emergency.
☐ **2.** Assess the client's orientation and vital signs.
☐ **3.** Call the physician.
☐ **4.** Give the client a bolus of lidocaine.

Correct Answers and Rationales

The letter in parentheses after each rationale identifies the client need addressed in the item, including management of care (M), safety and infection control (S), health promotion and maintenance (H), psychosocial adaptation (P), basic care and comfort (C), pharmacological and parenteral therapies (D), reduction of risk potential (R), and physiological adaptation (A).

The Client with Acute Coronary Syndromes

1. 3. Infarction of the papillary muscles is a potential complication of MI. This condition results in ineffective mitral valve closure, and blood is forced back into the low-pressure left atrium during ventricular systole. Assessment reveals a systolic murmur that occurs acutely. Ventricular aneurysm, pericarditis, and pulmonary embolism are also potential complications after an MI; however, these are not indicated by a new-onset murmur. (R)

2. 1, 4, 5. Morphine sulfate acts as an analgesic and sedative. It also reduces myocardial oxygen consumption, blood pressure, and heart rate. Morphine also reduces anxiety and fear due to its sedative effects and by slowing the heart rate. It can depress respirations; however, such an effect may lead to hypoxia, which should be avoided in the treatment of chest pain. Angiotensin-converting enzyme–inhibitor drugs, not morphine, may help to prevent ventricular remodeling. (D)

3. 24

First, calculate how many units are in each milliliter of the medication:

$$\frac{25,000 \text{ units}}{500 \text{ ml}} = \frac{50 \text{ units}}{1 \text{ ml}}$$

Next, calculate how many milliliters the client receives per hour:

$$\frac{1,200 \text{ units}}{1 \text{ hour}} \div \frac{50 \text{ units}}{1 \text{ ml}} = \frac{\overset{24}{\cancel{1,200}} \text{ units}}{1 \text{ hour}} \times \frac{1 \text{ ml}}{\underset{1}{\cancel{50}} \text{ units}} = 24 \text{ ml/hr.}$$

(D)

4. 3. The client is having symptoms of a myocardial infarction. The first action is to prevent platelet formation and block prostaglandin synthesis. The nitroglycerin tablet will be absorbed fastest if the client chews the tablet. (A)

5. 1. Although obtaining the ECG, chest radiograph, and blood work are all important, the nurse's priority action should be to relieve the crushing chest pain. Therefore, administering morphine sulfate is the priority action. (A)

6. 2. Thrombolytic drugs are administered within the first 6 hours after onset of an MI to lyse clots and reduce the extent of myocardial damage. (D)

7. 3. PVCs are characterized by a QRS of longer than 0.10 second and by a wide, notched, or slurred QRS complex. There is no P wave related to the QRS complex, and the T wave is usually inverted. (R)

8. 2. Aspirin does have antipyretic, antiplatelet, and analgesic actions, but the primary reason aspirin is administered to the client experiencing an MI is its antithrombotic action. In clinical trials, the antithrombotic action of aspirin has been thought to account for improved outcomes in clients with MI. (D)

9. 1, 3, 5. In a client who has had an ECG, the P wave represents the activation of the electrical impulse in the SA node, which is then transmitted to the AV node. In addition, the P wave represents atrial muscle depolarization, not ventricular depolarization. The normal duration of the P wave is 0.11 second or less in duration and 2.5 mm or more in height. (R)

10. 1. Oliguria occurs during cardiogenic shock because there is reduced blood flow to the kidneys. Typical signs of cardiogenic shock include low blood pressure, rapid and weak pulse, decreased urine output, and signs of diminished blood flow to the brain, such as confusion and restlessness. Cardiogenic shock is a serious complication of MI, with a mortality rate approaching 90%. Fever is not a typical sign of cardiogenic shock. (R)

11. 1. I.V. nitroglycerin infusion requires an infusion pump for precise control of the medication. Blood pressure monitoring would be done with a continuous system, and more frequently than every 4 hours. Hourly urine outputs are not always required. Obtaining serum potassium levels is not associated with nitroglycerin infusion. (D)

12. 4. An MI interferes with or blocks blood circulation to the heart muscle. Decreased blood supply to the heart muscle causes ischemia, or poor myocardial oxygenation. Diminished oxygenation or lack of oxygen to the cardiac muscle results in ischemic pain or angina. The pain is not due to ventricular overload, circulatory collapse, or electrolyte imbalances. (A)

13. 4. Sinus tachycardia is characterized by normal conduction and a regular rhythm, but with a rate exceeding 100 bpm. A P wave precedes each QRS, and the QRS is usually normal. (R)

14. **2.** PVCs are often a precursor of life-threatening arrhythmias, including ventricular tachycardia and ventricular fibrillation. An occasional PVC is not considered dangerous, but if PVCs occur at a rate greater than five or six per minute in the post-MI client, the physician should be notified immediately. More than six PVCs per minute is considered serious and usually calls for decreasing ventricular irritability by administering medications such as lidocaine hydrochloride. Increasing the I.V. infusion rate would not decrease the number of PVCs. Increasing the oxygen concentration should not be the nurse's first course of action; rather, the nurse should notify the physician promptly. Administering a prescribed analgesic would not decrease ventricular irritability. (A)

15. **4.** By day 2 of hospitalization after an MI, clients are expected to be able to perform personal care without chest pain. Severe chest pain should not be present on day 2 after and MI. Day 2 of hospitalization may be too soon for clients to be able to identify risk factors for MI or to begin a walking program; however, the client may be sitting up in a chair as part of the cardiac rehabilitation program. (A)

16. **2.** Furosemide is a loop diuretic that acts to increase urine output. Furosemide does not increase blood pressure, decrease pain, or decrease arrhythmias. (D)

17. **3.** This type of exercise is a preventive strategy taught to all clients who are hospitalized and on bed rest. This activity is taught to the client to promote venous return. The muscular action aids in venous return and prevents venous stasis in the lower extremities. It is venous stasis that increases one's risk for thrombophlebitis and blood clot formation. These exercises are not intended to prepare the client for ambulation. These exercises are not associated with promoting urinary and intestinal elimination. These exercises are not performed to decrease the risk of pressure ulcer formation. (A)

18. **2.** Recommended dietary principles in the acute phase of MI include avoiding large meals because small, easily digested foods are better tolerated. Fluids are given according to the client's needs, and sodium restrictions may be prescribed, especially for clients with manifestations of heart failure. Cholesterol restrictions may be ordered as well. Clients are not prescribed diets of liquids only or restricted to nothing by mouth unless their condition is very unstable. (A)

19. **3.** High cholesterol levels are considered a controllable risk factor for CAD and appear most closely linked to the development of the disease. High cholesterol levels can be modified through diet, exercise, and medication. Age and gender are uncontrollable risk factors for CAD.

Medication usage is not considered a risk factor for CAD. (A)

20. **4.** Heredity has been linked to CAD and is an uncontrollable risk factor. Exercise, obesity, and stress are controllable risk factors for CAD. (A)

21. **3.** A basic principle of behavior modification is that behavior that is learned and continued is behavior that has been rewarded. Other reinforcement techniques have not been found to be as effective as reward. (P)

22. **4.** The thrombolytic agent t-PA, administered intravenously, lyses the clot blocking the coronary artery. The drug is most effective when administered within the first 6 hours after onset of MI. The drug does not reduce coronary artery vasospasm; nitrates are used to promote vasodilation. Arrhythmias are managed by antiarrhythmic drugs. Surgical approaches are used to open the coronary artery and reestablish a blood supply to the area. (D)

23. **1.** Although monitoring the 12-lead ECG and monitoring breath sounds are important, observing the client for chest pain is the nursing assessment priority because closure of the previously obstructed coronary artery may recur. Clients who receive t-PA frequently receive heparin to prevent closure of the artery after administration of t-PA. Careful assessment for signs of bleeding and monitoring of partial thromboplastin time are essential to detect complications. Administration of t-PA should not cause fever. (R)

24. **1.** Cardiac arrhythmias are commonly observed with administration of t-PA. Cardiac arrhythmias are associated with reperfusion of the cardiac tissue. Hypotension is commonly observed with administration of t-PA. Seizures and hypothermia are not generally associated with reperfusion of the cardiac tissue. (R)

25. **2.** A history of cerebral hemorrhage is a contraindication to administration of t-PA because the risk of hemorrhage may be further increased. Age greater than 60 years, history of heart failure, and cigarette smoking are not contraindications. (D)

26. **2.** Advanced cardiac life support recommends that at least one or two I.V. lines be inserted in one or both of the antecubital spaces. Calling the physician, obtaining a portable chest radiograph, and drawing blood for the laboratory are important but secondary to starting the I.V. line. (A)

27. **4.** Crackles are auscultated over fluid-filled alveoli. Crackles heard on lung auscultation do not have to be associated with cyanosis. Bronchospasm and airway narrowing generally are associated with wheezing sounds. (A)

28. **1.** Further assessment is needed in this situation. It is premature to initiate other actions until further data have been gathered. Inquiring about the onset, duration, location, severity, and precipitating factors of the chest heaviness will provide pertinent information to convey to the physician. (R)

29. **4.** Detection of myoglobin is one diagnostic tool to determine whether myocardial damage has occurred. Myoglobin is generally detected about 1 hour after a heart attack is experienced and peaks within 4 to 6 hours after infarction. Myoglobin does not help diagnose cancer, hypertension, or liver disease. (R)

30. **1.** In older adults who are less active and do not exercise the heart muscle, atrophy can result. Disuse or deconditioning can lead to abnormal changes in the myocardium of the older adult. As a result, under sudden emotional or physical stress, the left ventricle is less able to respond to the increased demands on the myocardial muscle. Decreased cardiac output, cardiac hypertrophy, and heart failure are examples of the chronic conditions that may develop in response to inactivity, rather than in response to the aging process. Irregular heartbeats are generally not associated with an older sedentary adult's lifestyle. Peripheral vascular occlusion or pacemaker placement should not affect response to stress. (A)

31. **3.** Nitroglycerin may be used prophylactically before stressful physical activities such as stair-climbing to help the client remain pain free. Visiting her friend early in the day would have no impact on decreasing pain episodes. Resting before or after an activity is not as likely to help prevent an activity-related pain episode. (R)

32. **3.** Pasta, tomato sauce, salad, and coffee would be the best selection for the client following a low-cholesterol diet. Hamburgers, milkshakes, liver, and fried foods tend to be high in cholesterol. (C)

33. **1.** The client should report a change in the pattern of chest pain. It may indicate increasing severity of coronary artery disease. Pain occurring during stress or sexual activity would not be unexpected, and the client may be instructed to take nitroglycerin to prevent this pain. Pain during or after an activity such as lawn-mowing also would not be unexpected; the client may be instructed to take nitroglycerin to prevent this pain or may be restricted from doing such activities. (R)

34. **2.** Cardiac catheterization is done in clients with angina primarily to assess the extent and severity of the coronary artery blockage. A decision about medical management, angioplasty, or coronary artery bypass surgery will be based on the catheterization results. Coronary bypass surgery would be used to bypass obstructed vessels. Although cardiac catheterization can be used to assess the functional adequacy of the valves and heart muscle, in this case the client has unstable angina and therefore would need the procedure to assess the extent of arterial blockage. (R)

35. **4.** Because the contrast medium used in PTCA acts as an osmotic diuretic, the client may experience diuresis with resultant fluid volume deficit after the procedure. Additionally, potassium levels must be closely monitored because the client may develop hypokalemia due to the diuresis. Dyspnea would not be anticipated after this procedure. Maintaining adequate blood pressure control should not be a problem after the procedure. Increased myocardial contractility would be a goal, not decreased contractility. (R)

36. **2.** Late onset of puberty is not generally considered to be a risk factor for the development of atherosclerosis. Risk factors for atherosclerosis include family history of atherosclerosis, cigarette smoking, hypertension, high blood cholesterol level, male gender, diabetes mellitus, obesity, and physical inactivity. (A)

37. **3.** CAD is the leading cause of death in women as well as men. Although it is generally agreed that estrogen helps protect women from atherosclerotic changes before menopause, women are still at risk for CAD. Much attention has been focused on the lack of research studies dealing with cardiac disease in women and minorities, and work is under way to gain a better understanding of cardiac disease in these populations. Homosexual men are at high risk for AIDS. Breast cancer is the second leading cause of death in women. More men than women have COPD. (A)

38. **1.** An ECG directly reflects the transmission of electrical cardiac impulses through the heart. This information makes it possible to evaluate indirectly the functional status of the heart muscle and the contractile response of the ventricles. However, these elements are not measured directly. The ECG does not give information about the oxygenation and perfusion of the heart unless an individual is experiencing an acute episode of angina or infarction. (R)

39. **3.** Nitroglycerin produces peripheral vasodilation, which reduces myocardial oxygen consumption and demand. Vasodilation in coronary arteries and collateral vessels may also increase blood flow to the ischemic areas of the heart. Nitroglycerin decreases myocardial oxygen demand. Nitroglycerin does not have an effect on pericardial spasticity or conductivity in the myocardium. (D)

40. 1. Because of its widespread vasodilating effects, nitroglycerin often produces such adverse effects as headache, hypotension, and dizziness. The client should sit or lie down to avoid fainting. Nitroglycerin does not cause shortness of breath or stomach cramps. (D)

41. 3. The correct protocol for nitroglycerin use involves immediate administration, with subsequent doses taken at 5-minute intervals as needed, for a total dose of three tablets. Sublingual nitroglycerin appears in the bloodstream within 2 to 3 minutes and is metabolized within about 10 minutes. (D)

42. 3. The client taking nifedipine should inspect the gums daily to monitor for gingival hyperplasia. This is an uncommon adverse effect but one that requires monitoring and intervention if it occurs. The client taking nifedipine might be taught to monitor blood pressure, but more often than monthly. These clients would not generally need to perform daily weights or limit intake of green leafy vegetables. (D)

The Client with Heart Failure

43. 3. Coumadin is an anticoagulant, which is used in the treatment of atrial fibrillation and decreased left ventricular ejection fraction (less than 20%) to prevent thrombus formation and release of emboli into the circulation. The client may also take other medication as needed to manage the heart failure. Coumadin does not reduce circulatory load or improve myocardial workload. Coumadin does not affect cardiac rhythm. (R)

44. 2. Early symptoms of digoxin toxicity include anorexia, nausea, and vomiting. Visual disturbances can also occur, including double or blurred vision and visual halos. Hypokalemia is a common cause of digoxin toxicity associated with arrhythmias because low serum potassium can enhance ectopic pacemaker activity. Although vomiting can lead to fluid deficit, given the client's history, the vomiting is likely due to the adverse effects of digoxin toxicity. Pulmonary edema is manifested by dyspnea and coughing. (D)

45. 1, 3, 5. When the heart begins to fail, the body activates three major compensatory systems: ventricular hypertrophy, the renin-angiotensin-aldosterone system, and sympathetic nervous stimulation. Parasympathetic stimulation and jugular venous distention are not compensatory mechanisms associated with heart failure. (A)

46. 3. Signs of pulmonary edema are identical to those of acute heart failure. Signs and symptoms are generally apparent in the respiratory system and include coarse crackles, severe dyspnea, and tachypnea. Severe tachycardia may occur due to sympathetic stimulation in the presence of hypoxemia. Blood pressure may be decreased or elevated depending on the severity of the edema. Jugular vein distention, dependent edema, and anorexia are symptoms of right-sided heart failure. (A)

47. 1. It is a priority to assess blood pressure first because people with pulmonary edema typically experience severe hypertension that requires early intervention. The client probably does not have skin breakdown on admission; however, when the client is stable, the nurse should inspect the skin. Potassium levels are not the first priority. The nurse should monitor urine output after the client is stable. (R)

48. 1, 3. Heart failure is a result of structural and functional abnormalities of the heart tissue muscle. The heart muscle becomes weak and does not adequately pump the blood out of the chambers. As a result, blood pools in the left ventricle and backs up into the left atrium, and eventually into the lungs. Therefore, greater amounts of blood remain in the ventricle after contraction thereby decreasing cardiac output. In addition, this pooling leads to thrombus formation and ineffective tissue perfusion because of the decrease in blood flow to the other organs and tissues of the body. Typically, these clients have an ejection fraction of less than 50% and poorly tolerate activity. Activity intolerance is related to the decrease, not increase, in cardiac output. Gas exchange is impaired. However, the decrease in cardiac output triggers compensatory mechanisms, such as an increase in sympathetic nervous system activity. (A)

49. 3. Sitting almost upright in bed with the feet and legs resting on the mattress decreases venous return to the heart, thus reducing myocardial workload. Also, the sitting position allows maximum space for lung expansion. Low Fowler's position would be used if the client could not tolerate high Fowler's position for some reason. Lying on the right side would not be a good position for the client in heart failure. The client in heart failure would not tolerate the Trendelenburg's position. (R)

50. 3. Activity intolerance is a primary problem for clients with heart failure and pulmonary edema. The decreased cardiac output associated with heart failure leads to reduced oxygen and fatigue. Clients frequently complain of dyspnea and fatigue. The client could be at risk for infection related to stasis of secretions or impaired skin integrity related to pressure. However, these are not the priority nursing diagnoses for the client with heart failure and pulmonary edema, nor is constipation related to immobility (A)

51. **1.** Increasing cardiac output is the main goal of therapy for the client with heart failure or pulmonary edema. Pulmonary edema is an acute medical emergency requiring immediate intervention. Respiratory status and comfort will be improved when cardiac output increases to an acceptable level. Peripheral edema is not typically associated with pulmonary edema. (R)

52. **2.** Digoxin is a cardiac glycoside with positive inotropic activity. This inotropic activity causes increased strength of myocardial contractions and thereby increases output of blood from the left ventricle. Digoxin does not dilate coronary arteries. Although digoxin can be used to treat arrhythmias and does decrease the electrical conductivity of the myocardium, these are not primary reasons for its use in clients with heart failure and pulmonary edema. (D)

53. **3.** Angiotensin-converting enzyme (ACE) inhibitors have become the vasodilators of choice in the client with mild to severe heart failure. Vasodilator drugs are the only class of drugs clearly shown to improve survival in overt heart failure. ACE inhibitors do not act as vasopressors, volume expanders, or diuretics. (D)

54. **1.** After intravenous injection of furosemide, diuresis normally begins in about 5 minutes and reaches its peak within about 30 minutes. Medication effects last 2 to 4 hours. When furosemide is given intramuscularly or orally, drug action begins more slowly and lasts longer than when it is given intravenously. (D)

55. **4.** When diuretics are given early in the day, the client will void frequently during the daytime hours and will not need to void frequently during the night. Therefore, the client's sleep will not be disturbed. Taking furosemide in the morning has no effect on preventing electrolyte imbalances or retarding rapid drug absorption. The client should not accumulate excessive fluids throughout the night. (D)

56. **2.** Characteristics of atrial fibrillation include pulse rate greater than 100 bpm, totally irregular rhythm, and no definite P waves on the ECG. During assessment, the nurse is likely to note the irregular rate and should report it to the physician. A weak, thready pulse is characteristic of a client in shock. Two regular beats followed by an irregular beat may indicate a premature ventricular contraction. (R)

57. **1.** Atrial fibrillation occurs when the sinoatrial node no longer functions as the heart's pacemaker and impulses are initiated at sites within the atria. Because conduction through the atria is disturbed, atrial contractions are reduced and stasis of blood in the atria occurs, predisposing to emboli. Some estimates predict that 30% of

clients with atrial fibrillation develop emboli. Atrial fibrillation is not associated with increased cardiac output, elevated blood pressure, or decreased pulse rate; rather, it is associated with an increased pulse rate. (R)

58. **3.** Colored vision and seeing yellow spots are symptoms of digoxin toxicity. Abdominal pain, anorexia, nausea, and vomiting are other common symptoms of digoxin toxicity. Additional signs of toxicity include arrhythmias, such as atrial fibrillation or bradycardia. Rash, increased appetite, and elevated blood pressure are not associated with digoxin toxicity. (D)

59. **4.** A low serum potassium level (hypokalemia) predisposes the client to digoxin toxicity. Because potassium inhibits cardiac excitability, a low serum potassium level would mean that the client would be prone to increased cardiac excitability. Sodium, glucose, and calcium levels do not affect digoxin or contribute to digoxin toxicity. (D)

60. **2.** Canned foods and juices such as tomato juice are typically high in sodium and should be avoided in a sodium-restricted diet. Canned foods and juices in which sodium has been removed or limited are available. The client should be taught to read labels carefully. Apples and whole wheat breads are not high in sodium. Beef tenderloin would have less sodium than canned foods or tomato juice. (R)

61. **1.** Foods rich in potassium include bananas, orange juice, and green leafy vegetables such as spinach. Honeydew melon, cantaloupe, and watermelons are also rich in potassium. Other good sources of potassium are grapefruit juice, nectarines, potatoes, dried prunes, raisins, and figs. Skimmed milk, baked chicken, and brown rice are not considered high in potassium. (D)

62. **2.** A normal apical impulse is found over the apex of the heart and is typically located and auscultated in the left fifth intercostal space in the midclavicular line. An apical impulse located or auscultated below the fifth intercostal space or lateral to the midclavicular line may indicate left ventricular enlargement. (A)

63. **2.** Peripheral edema is a symptom of heart failure. Heart failure results when the heart chronically pumps against increased resistance or is unable to contract forcefully to pump the blood out into the systemic circulation. As a result, the ventricles become overfilled and there is an accumulation of volume within the closed system. The client's symptoms do not indicate arteriosclerosis, chronic bronchitis, or acute myocardial infarction. (A)

64. **3.** Heart failure is a complex and chronic condition. Education should focus on health promotion and preventive care in the home environment. Signs and symptoms can be monitored by the client. Instructing the client to obtain daily weights at the same time each day is very important. The client should be told to call the physician if there has been a weight gain of 2 lb or more. This may indicate fluid overload, and treatment can be prescribed early and on an outpatient basis, rather than waiting until the symptoms become life-threatening. Following a high-fiber diet is beneficial, but it is not relevant to the teaching needs of the client with heart failure. Prescribing an exercise program for the client, such as walking 2 miles every day, would not be appropriate at discharge. The client's exercise program would need to be planned in consultation with the physician and based on the history and the physical condition of the client. The client may require exercise tolerance testing before an exercise plan is laid out. Although the nurse does not prescribe an exercise program for the client, a sedentary lifestyle should not be recommended. (R)

65. **1, 2, 4.** The client stating that he would call the physician with increasing shortness of breath, weight gain over 2 lb in 1 day, and having to sleep sitting up, indicates that he has understood the teaching because these signs and symptoms suggest worsening of the client's heart failure. Although the client will most likely be placed on a sodium-restricted diet, the client would not need to notify the physician if he or she had consumed a high-sodium breakfast. Instead the client would need to be alert for possible signs and symptoms of worsening heart failure and work to reduce sodium intake for the rest of that day and in the future. (R)

The Client with Valvular Heart Disease

66. **2, 3, 4.** For clients scheduled for a cardiac catheterization it is important to assess for iodine sensitivity, verify written consent, and instruct the client to take nothing by mouth for 6 to 18 hours before the procedure. Oral medications are withheld unless specifically ordered. A urinary drainage catheter is rarely required for this procedure. (R)

67. **3.** Assessment of circulatory status, including observation of the puncture site, is of primary importance after a cardiac catheterization. Laboratory values and skin warmth and turgor are important to monitor but are not the most important initial nursing assessment. Neurologic assessment every 15 minutes is not required. (R)

68. **3.** Most clients with mitral stenosis have a history of rheumatic fever or bacterial endocarditis. Chickenpox, poliomyelitis, and meningitis are not associated with mitral stenosis. (A)

69. **2.** Common adverse effects of lidocaine hydrochloride include dizziness, tinnitus, blurred vision, tremors, numbness and tingling of extremities, excessive perspiration, hypotension, seizures, and finally coma. Cardiac effects include slowed conduction and cardiac arrest. Palpitations, urinary frequency, and lethargy are not considered typical adverse reactions to lidocaine. (D)

70. **3.** The pulmonary artery pressures are used to assess the heart's ability to receive and pump blood. The pulmonary capillary wedge pressure reflects the left ventricular end-diastolic pressure and guides the physician in determining fluid management for the client. The degree of coronary artery stenosis is assessed during a cardiac catheterization. The peripheral arterial pressure is assessed with an arterial line. The oxygen and carbon dioxide concentrations in the arterial blood can be measured by an arterial blood gas determination. (R)

71. **1.** Weight gain, due to fluid retention and worsening heart failure, causes exertional dyspnea in clients with mitral regurgitation. The rise in left atrial pressure that accompanies mitral valve disease is transmitted backward to the pulmonary veins, capillaries, and arterioles and eventually to the right ventricle. Signs and symptoms of pulmonary and systemic venous congestion follow. Confusion, elevated creatine kinase concentration, and chest pain are not typically associated with mitral regurgitation. (A)

72. **4.** When mitral stenosis is present, the left atrium has difficulty emptying its contents into the left ventricle. Hence, because there is no valve to prevent backward flow into the pulmonary vein, the pulmonary circulation is under pressure. Functioning of the aorta, right atrium, and superior vena cava is not immediately influenced by mitral stenosis. (A)

73. **1.** Preoperatively, anticoagulants may be prescribed for the client with advanced valvular heart disease to prevent emboli. Postoperatively, all clients with mechanical valves and some clients with bioprostheses are maintained indefinitely on anticoagulant therapy. Adhering strictly to a dosage schedule and observing specific precautions are necessary to prevent hemorrhage or thromboembolism. Some clients are maintained on lifelong antibiotic prophylaxis to prevent recurrence of rheumatic fever. Episodic prophylaxis is required to prevent infective endocarditis after dental procedures or upper respiratory, gastrointestinal, or genitourinary tract surgery. Diet modification, activity restrictions, and dental care are important; however, they do not have as much significance postoperatively as medication therapy does. (R)

74. **4.** Management of postoperative pain is a priority for the client after surgery, including valve replacement surgery, according to the Agency for Health Care Policy and Research. The client and family should be informed that pain will be assessed by the nurse and medications will be given to relieve the pain. The client will stay in the ICU as long as monitoring and intensive care are needed. Sensory deprivation and overload, high noise levels, and disrupted sleep and rest patterns are some environmental factors that affect recovery from valve replaceent surgery. (R)

75. **2.** Protamine sulfate is used to help combat persistent bleeding in a client who has had open heart surgery. Vitamin C and quinidine sulfate do not influence blood clotting. Warfarin sodium is an anticoagulant, as is heparin, and these two agents would tend to cause the client to bleed even more. (D)

76. **1.** Many factors help prevent wound infections, including washing hands carefully, using sterile prepackaged supplies and equipment, cleaning the incisional area well, and disposing of soiled dressings properly. However, most authorities say that the single most effective measure in preventing wound infections is to wash the hands carefully before and after changing dressings. Careful hand washing is also important in reducing other infections often acquired in hospitals, such as urinary tract and respiratory tract infections. (R)

77. **1.** In an immobilized client, calcium leaves the bone and concentrates in the extracellular fluid. When a large amount of calcium passes through the kidneys, calcium can precipitate and form calculi. Nursing interventions that help prevent calculi include ensuring a liberal fluid intake (unless contraindicated). A diet rich in acid should be provided to keep the urine acidic, which increases the solubility of calcium. Preventing constipation is not associated with excessive calcium excretion. Limiting foods rich in calcium, such as dairy products, will help in preventing renal calculi. (A)

78. **3.** INR is the value used to assess effectiveness of the warfarin sodium therapy. INR is the prothrombin time ratio that would be obtained if the thromboplastin reagent from the World Health Organization was used for the plasma test. It is now the recommended method to monitor effectiveness of warfarin sodium. Generally, the INR for clients administered warfarin sodium should range from 2 to 3. In the past, prothrombin time was used to assess effectiveness of warfarin sodium and was maintained at 1.5 to 2.5 times the control value. Partial thromboplastin time is used to assess the effectiveness of heparin therapy. Fresh frozen plasma or vitamin K is used to reverse warfarin

sodium's anticoagulant effect, whereas protamine sulfate reverses the effects of heparin. Warfarin sodium will help to prevent blood clots. (D)

79. **1.** Daily dental care and frequent checkups by a dentist who is informed about the client's condition are required to maintain good oral health. Use of an electric toothbrush, an irrigation device, or dental floss may cause gums to bleed and allow bacteria to enter mucous membranes and the bloodstream, increasing the risk of endocarditis. (R)

80. **2.** Most cardiac surgical clients have median sternotomy incisions, which take about 3 months to heal. Measures that promote healing include avoiding heavy lifting, performing muscle reconditioning exercises, and using caution when driving. Showering or bathing is allowed as long as the incision is well approximated with no open areas or drainage. Activities should be gradually resumed on discharge. (S)

81. **1.** Verbalized concerns from this client may stem from her anxiety over the changes her body has gone through after open heart surgery. Although the client may experience anxiety related to her altered health status or may have a lack of knowledge regarding her postoperative course, she is pointing out the changes in her body image. The client is not concerned about altered tissue perfusion. (P)

The Client with Hypertension

82. **1, 3, 5.** Clonidine (Catapres) is a central-acting adrenergic antagonist. It reduces sympathetic outflow from the central nervous system. Dry mouth, impotence, and sleep disturbances are possible adverse effects. Hyperkalemia and pancreatitis are not anticipated with use of this drug. (D)

83. **200**

First, calculate the number of milligrams per milliliter:

$$\frac{50 \text{ mg}}{250 \text{ ml}} = \frac{1 \text{ mg}}{5 \text{ ml}} = \frac{0.2 \text{ mg}}{1 \text{ ml}}$$

Next, calculate the number of micrograms in each milligram:

$$0.2 \text{ mg} \times 1{,}000 \text{ mcg} = 200 \text{ mcg}.$$

(D)

84. **2, 3.** Changing positions slowly and avoiding long periods of standing may limit the occurrence of orthostatic hypotension. Scheduling regular medication times is important for blood pressure management but this aspect is not related to the development of orthostatic hypotension.

Excessive alcohol intake and hot baths are associated with vasodilation. (R)

85. **1.** Atenolol is a beta-adrenergic antagonist indicated for management of hypertension. Sudden discontinuation of this drug is dangerous because it may exacerbate symptoms. The medication should not be discontinued without a physician's order. Blood pressure needs to be monitored more frequently than annually in a client who is newly diagnosed and treated for hypertension. Clients are not usually placed on a 2-g sodium diet for hypertension. (D)

86. **3.** Processed and cured meat products, such as cold cuts, ham, and hot dogs, are all high in both fat and sodium and should be avoided on a low-calorie, low-fat, low-salt diet. Dietary restrictions of all types are complex and difficult to implement with clients who are basically asymptomatic. (C)

87. **4.** Possible dizziness from orthostatic hypotension when rising from a crouched or bent position increases the client's risk of being injured by the equipment. The nurse should assess the client's blood pressure in all three positions (lying, sitting, and standing) at all routine visits. The client may experience muscle aches, or thirst from working in a warm, dry room, but these are not as potentially dangerous as orthostatic hypotension. The client should not be experiencing lethargy. (R)

88. **4.** Tailoring or individualizing a program to the client's lifestyle has been shown to be an effective strategy for changing health behaviors. Providing a written program, explaining the program to the client's spouse, and reassuring the client that he or she can do the program may be helpful but are not as likely to promote adherence as individualizing the program. (P)

89. **3.** A plan to reduce or stop smoking begins with establishing the client's personal daily smoking pattern and activities associated with smoking. It is important that the client understands the associated health and environmental risks, but this knowledge has not been shown to help clients change their smoking behavior. (P)

90. **3.** American Heart Association standards define hypertension as a consistent systolic blood pressure level greater than 140 mm Hg and a consistent diastolic blood pressure level greater than 90 mm Hg. (R)

91. **1.** Propranolol is a beta-adrenergic blocking agent. Actions of propranolol include reducing heart rate, decreasing myocardial contractility, and slowing conduction. Propranolol does not increase norepinephrine secretion, cause vasodilation, or block conversion of angiotensin I to angiotensin II. (D)

92. **4.** Managing hypertension is a priority for the client with hypertension. Clients with hypertension frequently do not experience other signs and symptoms, such as pain, deficient fluid volume, or impaired skin integrity. It is the asymptomatic nature of hypertension that makes it so difficult to treat, because clients may not recognize they are hypertensive or may not perceive the need for aggressive management of the disease. (A)

93. **3.** Compliance is the most critical element of hypertension therapy. In most cases, hypertensive clients require lifelong treatment and their hypertension cannot be managed successfully without drug therapy. Stress management is an important component of hypertension therapy, but the priority goal is related to compliance. It is not necessary for the client to change jobs or retire, but rather to learn to manage stress if the job is stressful. Losing weight may be necessary and will contribute to lower blood pressure, but the client must first accept the need for a lifelong management plan to control the hypertension. (P)

94. **1.** Renal disease, including renal insufficiency and failure, is a complication of hypertension. Effective treatment of hypertension assists in preventing this complication. Valvular heart disease, endocarditis, and peptic ulcer disease are not complications of hypertension. (R)

95. **1.** Hypertension is referred to as the silent killer for adults, because until the adult has significant damage to other systems, the hypertension may go undetected. CVAs can be related to long-term hypertension. Liver or pulmonary disease is not generally associated with hypertension. Myocardial infarction is generally related to coronary artery disease. (R)

The Client with a Permanent Pacemaker

96. **1, 5.** The nurse must teach the client how to take and record his pulse daily. The client should be instructed to avoid lifting the operative-side arm above shoulder level for 1 week postinsertion. It takes up to 2 months for the incision site to heal and full range of motion to return. The client should avoid heavy lifting until approved by the physician. The pacemaker metal casing does not set off airport security alarms, so there are no travel restrictions. Prolonged immobilization is not required. Microwave ovens are safe to use and do not alter pacemaker function. (R)

97. **1.** Transcutaneous pacemaker therapy provides an adequate heart rate to a client in an emergency situation. Defibrillation and a lidocaine infusion are not indicated for the treatment of third-degree heart block. Transcutaneous pacing is used temporarily until a transvenous or permanent pacemaker can be inserted. (A)

98. **2.** Maintaining cardiac conduction stability to prevent arrhythmias is a priority immediately after artificial pacemaker implantation. The client should have continuous electrocardiographic monitoring until proper pacemaker functioning is verified. Skin integrity, while important, is not an immediate concern. The pacemaker is used to increase heart rate and cardiac output, not decrease it. The client should limit activity for the first 24 to 48 hours after pacemaker insertion. The client should also restrict movement of the affected extremity for 24 hours. (R)

99. **3.** Education is a major component of the discharge plan for a client with an artificial pacemaker. The client with a permanent pacemaker needs to be able to state specific information about safety precautions, such as to refrain from lifting more than 3 lb or stretching and bending and to count the pulse once per week, that are necessary to maintain proper pacemaker function. The client will not necessarily be placed on a low cholesterol diet. The client should resume activities as he is able, and does not need to remain on bed rest. The client should know signs and symptoms of MI, but is not at risk because of the pacemaker. (C)

The Client Requiring Cardiopulmonary Resuscitation

100. **3.** The presence of a pulse determines the treatment for ventricular tachycardia. It is also important to assess the client's heart rate and level of consciousness. Cardioversion may be used to treat hemodynamically unstable tachycardias. Assessment of instability is required before cardioversion. It is not appropriate to begin CPR unless the pulse is absent. Defibrillation is used to treat ventricular fibrillation or pulseless ventricular tachycardia. (A)

101. **1, 3, 4.** A conducting agent is placed between the skin and the paddles to conduct the electrical current when discharged. The nurse must make sure to call "clear" before discharging the electrical current to prevent injury to others who may be helping with the client. Each paddle is placed directly on the conductive pads that are on the client's skin. Applying approximately 20 to 25 lb of pressure on each paddle is recommended to ensure good skin contact. The nurse must record the amount of electrical current delivered and the resulting rhythm. (R)

102. **2.** Pupillary reaction is the best indication of whether oxygenated blood has been reaching the client's brain. Pupils that remain widely dilated and do not react to light probably indicate that serious brain damage has occurred. The pulse rate may be normal, mucous membranes may still be pink, and systolic blood pressure may be 80 mm Hg or higher, and serious brain damage may still have occurred. (R)

103. **4.** Epinephrine is administered during resuscitation efforts primarily for its ability to improve cardiac activity. Epinephrine has great affinity for adrenergic receptors in cardiac tissue and acts to strengthen and speed the heart rate as well as to increase impulse conduction from atria to ventricles. Epinephrine dilates bronchioles and constricts arterioles, but these are not the primary reasons for administering it during resuscitation. Epinephrine is not associated with freeing glycogen from the liver. (D)

104. **4.** With one-rescuer CPR, the compression-to-ventilation ratio is 15:2. (R)

105. **2.** Because of its location near the xiphoid process, the liver is the organ most easily damaged from pressure exerted over the xiphoid process during CPR. The pressure on the victim's chest wall should be sufficient to compress the heart but not so great as to damage internal organs. Injury may result, however, even when CPR is performed properly. (R)

106. **3.** An adult's sternum must be depressed 1.5 to 2 inches with each compression to ensure adequate heart compression. (R)

107. **2.** The American Heart Association guidelines for Basic Cardiac Life Support now recommends that the rescuer call for emergency assistance immediately after establishing unresponsiveness in the adult victim. A call for emergency assistance takes precedence over initiating CPR in the adult victim, in an effort to get emergency personnel and an automatic external defibrillator to the scene. Early defibrillation and prompt bystander CPR have increased sudden cardiac arrest survival rates. (R)

108. **1.** If the airway is not opened properly, it is impossible to inflate the lungs during CPR. A common sign of airway obstruction is failure of the victim's chest wall to rise with each breath given by the rescuer. The victim should not be considered beyond resuscitation; rather, the airway should be opened properly. Inflations may be being given too rapidly. However, this is not the usual cause of not being able to adequately ventilate the victim. If the rescuer is using inadequate force for cardiac compression, it should not interfere with how ventilations are delivered. (R)

109. **1.** The exhalation phase of ventilation is a passive activity that occurs during CPR as part of the normal relaxation of the victim's chest. No action by the rescuer is necessary. (R)

110. **2.** After a person is without cardiopulmonary function for 4 to 6 minutes, permanent brain damage is almost certain. To prevent permanent brain damage, it is important to begin CPR promptly after a cardiopulmonary arrest. (R)

111. **2.** The Heimlich maneuver should be administered only to a victim who cannot make *any* sounds due to airway obstruction. If the victim can whisper words or cough, some air exchange is occurring and the emergency medical system should be called instead of attempting the Heimlich maneuver. Cyanosis may accompany or follow choking; however, the Heimlich maneuver should only be initiated when the victim cannot speak. (R)

112. **4.** The thrusts should be delivered below the xiphoid process, but above the umbilicus, to minimize the risk of internal injuries. (R)

113. **2.** The priority action is to assess the client and determine whether the rhythm is life-threatening. More information, including vital signs, should be obtained and the physician should be quickly notified. A bolus of lidocaine may be ordered to treat this arrhythmia. This is not a code-type situation unless the client has been determined to be in a life-threatening situation. (A)

The Client with Vascular Disease

The Client with Peripheral Vascular Disease

1. The nurse is assigned to a client with peripheral vascular disease (PVD). Which of the following nursing diagnoses should be addressed as the priority in the plan of care?
- [ ] **1.** *Disturbed body image.*
- [ ] **2.** *Disturbed sensory perception.*
- [ ] **3.** *Risk for fluid overload.*
- [ ] **4.** *Risk for fluid deficit.*

2. An overweight client taking warfarin (Coumadin) has a nursing diagnosis of *Ineffective tissue perfusion* related to decreased arterial blood flow. What should the nurse instruct the client to do? Select all that apply.
- [ ] **1.** Apply lanolin or petroleum jelly to intact skin.
- [ ] **2.** Encourage a reduced-calorie, reduced-fat diet.
- [ ] **3.** Inspect the involved areas daily for new ulcerations.
- [ ] **4.** Instruct the client to limit activities of daily living (ADLs).
- [ ] **5.** Use an electric razor to shave.

3. Peripheral blood flow is dependent on which of the following variables?
- [ ] **1.** Blood viscosity and diameter of vessels.
- [ ] **2.** Diameter and resistance of vessels.
- [ ] **3.** Force of contraction of the heart and resistance of vessels.
- [ ] **4.** Pressure differences in the arterial and venous systems and resistance.

4. Blood pressure in the systemic circulation is highest in the:
- [ ] **1.** Arterioles.
- [ ] **2.** Capillaries.
- [ ] **3.** Aorta.
- [ ] **4.** Venules.

5. Which of the following factors is the most important in determining the resistance of a vessel?
- [ ] **1.** Length of the vessel.
- [ ] **2.** Diameter of the vessel.
- [ ] **3.** Blood being too thin.
- [ ] **4.** Blood being too thick.

6. A common abnormal laboratory result associated with the development of peripheral vascular disease (PVD) is:
- [ ] **1.** High serum calcium level.
- [ ] **2.** High serum lipid levels.
- [ ] **3.** Low serum potassium level.
- [ ] **4.** Low serum lipid levels.

7. Which of the following is an important regulator of blood flow in the peripheral circulation of the human body?
- [ ] **1.** Autonomic nervous system.
- [ ] **2.** Central nervous system.
- [ ] **3.** Parasympathetic nervous system.
- [ ] **4.** Sympathetic nervous system.

8. The nurse has been assigned to a client with a history of peripheral vascular disease who has symptoms of claudication. These symptoms result when:
☐ 1. Oxygen demand by the muscle exceeds the supply.
☐ 2. Oxygen demand and supply of the working muscle are in balance.
☐ 3. Oxygen supply exceeds the demand of the working muscle.
☐ 4. Oxygen is absent.

9. To assess the client's pedal pulses, the nurse should palpate the:
☐ 1. Medial aspect of the foot and the ventral aspect of the ankle.
☐ 2. Top of the foot and inner side of each foot.
☐ 3. Popliteal space and the medial aspect of the ankle.
☐ 4. Posterior aspect of the foot and anterior aspect of the ankle.

10. Which of the following explains the influence of aging on the development of peripheral vascular disease?
☐ 1. Decreased resistance.
☐ 2. Increased resistance.
☐ 3. Decreased viscosity.
☐ 4. Increased viscosity.

11. The client admitted with peripheral vascular disease (PVD) asks the nurse why her legs hurt when she walks. The nurse bases a response on the knowledge that the main characteristic of PVD is:
☐ 1. Decreased blood flow.
☐ 2. Increased blood flow.
☐ 3. Slow blood flow.
☐ 4. Thrombus formation.

12. The nurse notes on the client's chart that he has peripheral vascular disease (PVD) and a history of heart failure. The nurse must plan care and anticipate that the client may have a low tolerance for exercise related to:
☐ 1. Decreased blood flow.
☐ 2. Increased blood flow.
☐ 3. Decreased pain.
☐ 4. Increased blood viscosity.

13. When assessing the lower extremities of a client with peripheral vascular disease (PVD), the nurse notes bilateral ankle edema. The edema is related to:
☐ 1. Competent venous valves.
☐ 2. Decreased blood volume.
☐ 3. Increase in muscular activity.
☐ 4. Increased venous pressure.

14. When assessing lower-extremity pulses in older adults with peripheral vascular disease (PVD), the nurse first notes whether or not the pulses are palpable. The nurse then assesses for which of the following characteristics?
☐ 1. Rhythm.
☐ 2. Quality.
☐ 3. Rate.
☐ 4. Pattern.

15. Atherosclerosis results in stenosis of the arteries. Which of the following vascular problems is also a result of atherosclerosis?
☐ 1. Thickened endothelial lining of the vessels walls.
☐ 2. Formation of an aneurysm.
☐ 3. Hardening of the arteries.
☐ 4. Formation of varicose veins.

16. The nurse realizes that the underlying etiology for the nursing diagnosis of *Pain* related to peripheral vascular disease is atherosclerotic lesions resulting from:
☐ 1. Atheromas.
☐ 2. Calcium plaques and hardening.
☐ 3. Thickened intima and calcium plaques.
☐ 4. Fibrous plaque and fatty streaks.

17. The nurse reviews with the client the risk factors associated with atherosclerosis. Nonmodifiable risk factors that the nurse instructs the client about include:
☐ 1. Diabetes.
☐ 2. Age.
☐ 3. Exercise level.
☐ 4. Dietary preferences.

18. The nurse is assessing the lower extremities of the client with peripheral vascular disease (PVD). During the assessment, the nurse should expect to find which of the following clinical manifestations of PVD?
☐ 1. Hairy legs.
☐ 2. Mottled skin.
☐ 3. Pink, cool skin.
☐ 4. Warm, moist skin.

19. The client complains of experiencing midcalf pain when walking a block or more. The client states that the discomfort is relieved with rest. The nurse suspects that this client may be experiencing intermittent claudication. Intermittent claudication occurs when arterial occlusion reaches which of the following percentages?
☐ 1. 20%.
☐ 2. 40%.
☐ 3. 50%.
☐ 4. 100%.

20. The nurse is unable to palpate the client's left pedal pulses. Which of the following actions should the nurse take next?

☐ **1.** Auscultate the pulses with a stethoscope.
☐ **2.** Call the physician.
☐ **3.** Use a Doppler ultrasound device.
☐ **4.** Inspect the lower left extremity.

21. When using a Doppler instrument to assess peripheral pulses, the nurse understands that correct placement of the transducer is important because it is difficult to differentiate between:

☐ **1.** Arterial and capillary blood flow.
☐ **2.** Arterial and venous blood flow.
☐ **3.** Arterial and arteriole blood flow.
☐ **4.** Capillary and venous blood flow.

22. Which of the following lipid abnormalities is a risk factor for the development of atherosclerosis and peripheral vascular disease?

☐ **1.** Low concentration of triglycerides.
☐ **2.** High levels of high-density lipid (HDL) cholesterol.
☐ **3.** High levels of low-density lipid (LDL) cholesterol.
☐ **4.** Low levels of LDL cholesterol.

23. When assessing an individual with peripheral vascular disease, which clinical manifestation would indicate complete arterial obstruction in the lower left leg?

☐ **1.** Aching pain in the left calf.
☐ **2.** Burning pain in the left calf.
☐ **3.** Numbness and tingling in the left leg.
☐ **4.** Coldness of the left foot and ankle.

24. One goal of care for a client with PVD is to decrease anxiety, so as to decrease or prevent vasoconstriction of the:

☐ **1.** Arteries.
☐ **2.** Capillaries.
☐ **3.** Lymphatics.
☐ **4.** Veins.

25. A 70-year-old male with the diagnosis of claudication has been hospitalized for an evaluation of his increasingly impaired mobility and complaints of pain. The client tells the nurse that he can no longer walk a block without having severe pain in his left calf and foot. Based on these data, which nursing diagnosis would be most appropriate for this client?

☐ **1.** *Activity intolerance* related to decreased blood supply and pain.
☐ **2.** *Self-care deficit* related to increased leg pain.
☐ **3.** *Ineffective coping* related to chronic pain.
☐ **4.** *Impaired skin integrity* related to poor circulation.

26. A client with peripheral vascular disease returns to the surgical care unit after having femoral-popliteal bypass grafting. Indicate in which order the nurse should conduct assessment of this client.

| 1. Postoperative pain. |
| 2. Peripheral pulses. |
| 3. Urine output. |
| 4. Incision site. |

| |
| |
| |
| |

27. A client with a history of heart failure has bilateral +4 edema of her right ankle that extends up to midcalf. She is sitting out of bed and has her legs in a dependent position. The nurse will choose interventions to obtain which of the following outcomes?

☐ **1.** Decrease venous congestion.
☐ **2.** Maintain normal respirations.
☐ **3.** Maintain body temperature.
☐ **4.** Prevent injury to lower extremities.

28. The nurse is assessing an older Caucasian male who has a history of peripheral vascular disease. The nurse observes that the man's left great toe is black. The discoloration is probably a result of:

☐ **1.** Atrophy.
☐ **2.** Contraction.
☐ **3.** Gangrene.
☐ **4.** Rubor.

29. The nurse uses a Doppler ultrasound device to assess the client's lower extremities. In addition, the nurse calculates the ankle-brachial index to estimate stenosis of the:

☐ **1.** Arteries.
☐ **2.** Aorta.
☐ **3.** Carotid.
☐ **4.** Veins.

30. A client is scheduled for an arteriogram. The nurse should explain to the client that the arteriogram will confirm the diagnosis of occlusive arterial disease by:

☐ **1.** Showing the location of the obstruction and the collateral circulation.

☐ **2.** Scanning the affected extremity and identifying the areas of volume changes.

☐ **3.** Using ultrasound to estimate the velocity changes in the blood vessels.

☐ **4.** Determining how long the client can walk.

31. A client is scheduled to have an arteriogram. During the arteriogram, the client complains of nausea, tingling, and dyspnea. The nurse's immediate action should be to:

☐ **1.** Administer epinephrine.

☐ **2.** Inform the physician.

☐ **3.** Administer oxygen.

☐ **4.** Inform the client that the procedure is almost over.

32. A client with peripheral vascular disease has chronic, severe pretibial and ankle edema bilaterally. Because the client is on complete bed rest and circulation is compromised, one goal is to maintain tissue integrity. Which of the following interventions will help achieve this outcome?

☐ **1.** Administering pain medication.

☐ **2.** Encouraging fluids.

☐ **3.** Turning the client every 1 to 2 hours.

☐ **4.** Maintaining hygiene.

33. A client who has been diagnosed with peripheral vascular disease (PVD) is being discharged. The client needs further instruction if she says she will:

☐ **1.** Avoid heating pads.

☐ **2.** Not cross her legs.

☐ **3.** Wear leather shoes.

☐ **4.** Use iodine on an injured site.

34. A client with peripheral vascular disease has bypass surgery. The primary goal of the plan of care after surgery is to:

☐ **1.** Maintain circulation.

☐ **2.** Prevent infection.

☐ **3.** Relieve pain.

☐ **4.** Provide education.

35. A client has been admitted with the diagnosis of occlusion of the left subclavian artery. The nurse anticipates that which of the following procedures will be done?

☐ **1.** Amputation.

☐ **2.** Bypass grafting.

☐ **3.** Coronary artery bypass grafting.

☐ **4.** Percutaneous transluminal angioplasty (PTA).

36. A client is scheduled to undergo right axillary-to-axillary artery bypass surgery. Which of the following interventions is most important for the nurse to implement in the preoperative period?

☐ **1.** Assess the temperature in the affected arm.

☐ **2.** Monitor the radial pulse in the affected arm.

☐ **3.** Protect the extremity from cold.

☐ **4.** Avoid using the arm for a venipuncture.

The Client with Peripheral Vascular Disease Having an Amputation

37. A client is admitted to the hospital with peripheral vascular disease (PVD) of the lower extremities. He is scheduled for an amputation of the left leg. The client says, "I've really tried to manage my condition well." Which of the following routines should the nurse evaluate as having been appropriate for him?

☐ **1.** Resting with his legs elevated above the level of his heart.

☐ **2.** Walking slowly but steadily for 30 minutes twice a day.

☐ **3.** Minimizing activity.

☐ **4.** Wearing antiembolism stockings at all times when out of bed.

38. While the nurse is providing preoperative teaching, the client says, "I hate the idea of being an invalid after they cut off my leg." The nurse's most therapeutic response should be:

☐ **1.** "You'll still have one good leg to use."

☐ **2.** "Tell me more about how you're feeling."

☐ **3.** "Let's finish the preoperative teaching."

☐ **4.** "You're fortunate to have a wife who can take care of you."

39. The client asks the nurse, "Why can't the doctor tell me exactly how much of my leg they're going to take off? Don't you think I should know that?" The nurse responds, knowing that the final decision on the level of the amputation will depend primarily on:

☐ **1.** The need to remove as much of the leg as possible.

☐ **2.** The adequacy of the blood supply to the tissues.

☐ **3.** The ease with which a prosthesis can be fitted.

☐ **4.** The client's ability to walk with a prosthesis.

40. A client has undergone an amputation of several toes and a femoral-popliteal bypass. The nurse should teach the client that after surgery which of the following leg positions is contraindicated for her while sitting in a chair?

☐ **1.** Crossing her legs.

☐ **2.** Elevating her legs.

☐ **3.** Flexing her ankles.

☐ **4.** Extending her knees.

41. The room for the client who has had an amputation should contain which emergency equipment when the client returns from surgery?
☐ **1.** Suction equipment.
☐ **2.** Emergency cart.
☐ **3.** Airway.
☐ **4.** Tourniquet.

42. The client has had a below-the-knee amputation secondary to arterial occlusive disease. The nurse is instructing the client in stump care. Which of the following statements by the client indicates that she understands how to implement her plan of care?
☐ **1.** "I should inspect the incision carefully when I change the dressing every other day."
☐ **2.** "I should wash the incision, dry it, and apply moisturizing lotion daily."
☐ **3.** "I should rewrap the stump as often as needed."
☐ **4.** "I should elevate the stump on pillows to decrease swelling."

43. One goal in caring for a client with arterial occlusive disease is to promote vasodilation in the affected extremity. To achieve this goal, the nurse encourages the client to:
☐ **1.** Avoid eating low-fat foods.
☐ **2.** Elevate the legs above the heart.
☐ **3.** Stop smoking.
☐ **4.** Begin a jogging program.

44. The client complains of aching, weakness, and a cramping sensation in both of his lower extremities while walking. The nurse knows that exercise enhances blood circulation and utilization of oxygen by the tissues. To promote health and maintain the client's level of activity, the nurse suggests that the client try:
☐ **1.** Cross-country skiing.
☐ **2.** Jogging.
☐ **3.** Golfing.
☐ **4.** Riding a stationary bike.

45. The client with peripheral vascular disease has been prescribed diltiazem (Cardizem). The purpose of using diltiazem for this client would be to promote:
☐ **1.** Relief of anxiety.
☐ **2.** Sedation.
☐ **3.** Vasoconstriction.
☐ **4.** Vasodilation.

46. Pentoxifylline (Trental) is a drug used to decrease platelet aggregation and blood viscosity. The nurse should anticipate that pentoxifylline would be useful in the treatment of clients with which of the following conditions?
☐ **1.** Angina.
☐ **2.** Gastric reflux.
☐ **3.** Intermittent claudication.
☐ **4.** Transient ischemic attacks.

47. A client with peripheral vascular disease and chronic obstructive pulmonary disease takes theophylline (Theo-Dur) 200 mg twice daily every day. The doctor now prescribes pentoxifylline (Trental). To prevent problematic adverse effects, the nurse should monitor the client's:
☐ **1.** Digoxin level.
☐ **2.** Partial thromboplastin time (PTT).
☐ **3.** Serum cholesterol level.
☐ **4.** Theophylline level.

48. A client with a history of coronary artery disease (CAD) has been diagnosed with peripheral vascular disease. The physician started the client on pentoxifylline (Trental) once daily. Approximately 1 hour after receiving the initial dose of pentoxifylline, the client complained of chest pain, which he stated he had not experienced before. Which of the following interventions represents the most appropriate nursing action?
☐ **1.** Advise the client to rest.
☐ **2.** Inform the physician.
☐ **3.** Encourage the client to relax.
☐ **4.** Document the episode in the chart.

49. A client with peripheral vascular disease is recovering from an aortofemoral-popliteal bypass graft. When developing a postoperative education plan, which question by the nurse will provide the most helpful information?
☐ **1.** "How did you manage your health before admission?"
☐ **2.** "How far could you walk without pain before surgery?"
☐ **3.** "What is your home environment like?"
☐ **4.** "Do you have problems with urine retention?"

50. The client with peripheral vascular disease and a history of hypertension is to be discharged on a low-fat, low-cholesterol, low-sodium diet. Which should be the nurse's first step in planning the dietary instructions?
☐ **1.** Determine the client's knowledge level about cholesterol.
☐ **2.** Ask the client to name foods high in fat, cholesterol, and salt.
☐ **3.** Explain the importance of complying with the diet.
☐ **4.** Assess the family's food preferences.

The Client with Buerger's Disease

51. The nurse has been assigned to a client with Buerger's disease (thromboangiitis obliterans). Which of the following anatomic areas are most often affected by this vascular condition?
☐ **1.** Hands and fingers.
☐ **2.** Lower legs and feet.
☐ **3.** Head and neck.
☐ **4.** Lower back.

52. A 30-year-old male client is admitted with Buerger's disease. Which of the following factors has increased the client's risk of developing Buerger's disease?
☐ **1.** History of cigarette smoking.
☐ **2.** Occupational exposure to radiation.
☐ **3.** Age and gender.
☐ **4.** History of hypertension.

53. The primary goal for the client with Buerger's disease is to prevent:
☐ **1.** Embolus formation.
☐ **2.** Fat embolus formation.
☐ **3.** Thrombus formation.
☐ **4.** Thrombophlebitis.

54. A client with Buerger's disease smokes two packs of cigarettes a day. Smoking cessation is critical or the client may lose the affected extremity. When helping a client change behavior, it is important to know the client's:
☐ **1.** Ability to attend support groups.
☐ **2.** Goals of the treatment.
☐ **3.** Perception of the negative behavior.
☐ **4.** Motivation.

55. Because smoking cessation is a critical strategy for the client diagnosed with Buerger's disease, the nurse anticipates that the client will go home with a prescription for which of the following medications?
☐ **1.** nicotine (Nicotrol).
☐ **2.** nitroglycerin.
☐ **3.** furosemide (Lasix).
☐ **4.** ibuprofen.

56. The client with Buerger's disease experiences which of the following signs or symptoms?
☐ **1.** Thickening of the intima and media of the artery.
☐ **2.** Inflammation and fibrosis of arteries, veins, and nerves.
☐ **3.** Vasospasm lasting several minutes.
☐ **4.** Pain, pallor, and pulselessness.

The Client with Vasospastic Disorder

57. A client has been diagnosed with vasospastic disorder (Raynaud's disease) on the tip of the nose and fingertips. The physician has prescribed reserpine (Serpasil) to determine if the client will obtain relief. The client's history reveals that he lives in Vermont and works outside in the logging industry. He smokes two packs of cigarettes per day. Which of the following components are an important part of the discharge plan for this client? Select all that apply.
☐ **1.** Stopping smoking.
☐ **2.** Wearing a face covering and gloves in the winter.
☐ **3.** Placing fingertips in cool water to rewarm them.
☐ **4.** Finding employment that can be done in a warm environment.
☐ **5.** Reporting signs of orthostatic hypotension.

58. A nurse assesses a 40-year-old female client with vasospastic disorder (Raynaud's disease) involving her right hand. The nurse notes the information in the progress notes, as shown below. From these findings, the nurse should formulate which priority nursing diagnosis?

PROGRESS NOTES

Date	Time	Progress Notes
06/10/07	03:00 pm	The client has a palpable but faint right radial pulse. Capillary refill on all five digits less than 8 seconds. No observable swelling. The client is reporting numbness in the tips of all five digits. The skin is warm, dry, and red. ——— *G. Fuentes, RN*

☐ **1.** *Acute pain* related to hyperemic stage.
☐ **2.** *Disturbed sensory perception (tactile)* related to vasospastic process.
☐ **3.** *Ineffective tissue perfusion (peripheral)* related to vasospastic process.
☐ **4.** *Risk for impaired skin integrity* related to vasospastic process.

59. A nurse is assessing a group of clients. Which clients are at risk for vasospastic disorder (Raynaud's disease)?
- ☐ 1. Young women.
- ☐ 2. Old women.
- ☐ 3. Old men.
- ☐ 4. Young men.

60. The nurse has been assigned to a client with vasospastic disorder (Raynaud's disease). The nurse realizes that the underlying etiology of Raynaud's disease is unknown but that it is characterized by:
- ☐ 1. Episodic vasospastic disorder of the small arteries.
- ☐ 2. Episodic vasospastic disorder of the small veins.
- ☐ 3. Episodic vasospastic disorder of the capillaries.
- ☐ 4. Episodic vasospastic disorder of the aorta.

61. The client with vasospastic disorder (Raynaud's disease) complains of cold and numbness in her fingers. The nurse assesses the client for effects of vasoconstriction. Which of the following is an early sign of vasoconstriction?
- ☐ 1. Cyanosis.
- ☐ 2. Gangrene.
- ☐ 3. Pallor.
- ☐ 4. Rubor.

62. A female client has vasospastic disorder (Raynaud's disease). During the initial assessment, the nurse notes that the client is experiencing a vasospastic episode. The nurse should immediately assess the:
- ☐ 1. Brachial artery.
- ☐ 2. Carotid artery.
- ☐ 3. Femoral artery.
- ☐ 4. Radial artery.

63. The nurse should instruct a client who has been diagnosed with vasospastic disorder (Raynaud's disease) to:
- ☐ 1. Immerse her hands in cold water during an episode.
- ☐ 2. Wear light garments when the temperature gets below 50° F (10° C).
- ☐ 3. Wear gloves when handling ice or frozen foods.
- ☐ 4. Live in a cold climate.

64. Stress can produce vasospasm in clients with vasospastic disorder (Raynaud's disease). The client states she is worried about making the necessary behavioral changes to control the vasospastic episodes. Which of the following nursing diagnoses is appropriate?
- ☐ 1. *Activity intolerance* related to Raynaud's disease.
- ☐ 2. *Anxiety* related to change in health status.
- ☐ 3. *Disturbed body image* related to illness treatment.
- ☐ 4. *Impaired social interaction* related to self-concept disturbance.

65. The physician has prescribed a beta-adrenergic blocking medication for the client with vasospastic disorder (Raynaud's disease). An example of a beta-adrenergic blocker is:
- ☐ 1. Tamsulosin hydrochloride (Flomax).
- ☐ 2. Terazosin hydrochloride (Hytrin).
- ☐ 3. Propranolol (Inderal).
- ☐ 4. Labetalol hydrochloride (Trandate).

66. When giving discharge instructions to the client with vasospastic disorder (Raynaud's disease), the nurse should explain that the expected outcome of taking a beta-adrenergic blocking medication is to control the symptoms by:
- ☐ 1. Decreasing the influence of the sympathetic nervous system on the tissues in the hands and feet.
- ☐ 2. Decreasing the pain by producing analgesia.
- ☐ 3. Increasing the blood supply to the affected area.
- ☐ 4. Increasing monoamine oxidase.

67. A client with vasospastic disorder (Raynaud's disease) is scheduled for sympathectomy. This surgery is performed:
- ☐ 1. In the early stages of the disease to prevent further circulatory disturbances.
- ☐ 2. When the disease is controlled by medication.
- ☐ 3. When the client is unable to control stress-related vasospasm.
- ☐ 4. When all other treatment alternatives have failed.

The Client with Thrombophlebitis and Embolus Formation

68. A client is being treated for deep vein thrombosis (DVT) in the left femoral artery. The physician has ordered 60 mg of enoxaparin (Lovenox) subcutaneously. Before administering the drug, the nurse checks the client's laboratory results, noted below.

LABORATORY RESULTS	
Test	**Result**
Prothrombin time	12.5 seconds
INR	2.0 seconds
Platelet count	50,000/µl

Based on these results, the nurse should:
- ☐ 1. Assess the client for bleeding.
- ☐ 2. Administer the medication.
- ☐ 3. Inform the physician.
- ☐ 4. Withhold the dose of Lovenox.

69. The nurse is caring for a client with acute arterial occlusion of the left lower extremity. To prevent further tissue damage, it is important for the nurse to observe for which of the following?
- ☐ 1. Blood pressure and heart rate changes.
- ☐ 2. Gradual or acute loss of sensory and motor function.
- ☐ 3. Metabolic acidosis.
- ☐ 4. Swelling in the left lower extremity.

70. A nurse is assigned to a client with venous thrombus. The nurse identifies a nursing diagnosis of *Impaired physical mobility* related to pain. Which should the nurse do first?
- ☐ 1. Elevate the legs.
- ☐ 2. Elevate the legs by using a pillow under the knees.
- ☐ 3. Encourage adequate fluid intake.
- ☐ 4. Massage the lower legs.

71. A 45-year-old client had a complete abdominal hysterectomy with bilateral salpingo-oophorectomy 2 days ago. The client's abdominal dressing is dry and intact. In addition, the client is taking liquids and voiding a sufficient quantity of straw-colored urine. While sitting up in the chair after her bath, the client complains of severe pain and numbness in her left leg. The nurse should respond immediately by:
- ☐ 1. Administering pain medication.
- ☐ 2. Assessing for edema in the left leg.
- ☐ 3. Assessing color and temperature of the left leg.
- ☐ 4. Encouraging the client to change her position.

72. A client is discharged after being hospitalized for thrombophlebitis. She will be driving home with her daughter, who lives 2 hours away. During the 2-hour ride, the client should:
- ☐ 1. Perform arm circles while riding in the car.
- ☐ 2. Perform ankle pumps and foot range-of-motion exercises.
- ☐ 3. Elevate her legs while riding in the car.
- ☐ 4. Take an ambulance home.

73. A client is admitted from a nursing home with an acute onset of shortness of breath. A diagnosis of pulmonary embolism is made. One common cause of pulmonary embolism is:
- ☐ 1. Arteriosclerosis.
- ☐ 2. Aneurysm formation.
- ☐ 3. Deep vein thrombosis (DVT).
- ☐ 4. Varicose veins.

74. A client receives a thrombolytic agent. The expected outcome of this drug therapy includes:
- ☐ 1. Improved cerebral perfusion.
- ☐ 2. Decreased vascular permeability.
- ☐ 3. Dissolved emboli.
- ☐ 4. Prevention of further cerebral hemorrhage.

75. A client who weighs 187 lb has an order to receive enoxaparin (Lovenox) 1 mg/kg. This drug is available in a concentration of 30 mg/0.3 ml. What dose would the nurse administer in milliliters?

_____ ml

76. The nurse understands that a client on complete bed rest is at risk for developing which of the following complications involving the venous system?
- ☐ 1. Air embolus.
- ☐ 2. Fat embolus.
- ☐ 3. Stress fractures.
- ☐ 4. Thrombophlebitis.

77. The client has an I.V. catheter in the left antecubital space. The nurse notes that the area is swollen and red, and the client complains of discomfort at the site. The nurse realizes that 65% of the clients receiving I.V. therapy will develop:
- ☐ 1. Deep vein thrombosis (DVT).
- ☐ 2. Deep vein thrombophlebitis.
- ☐ 3. Superficial vein thrombus.
- ☐ 4. Superficial vein thrombophlebitis.

78. A client is receiving an I.V. infusion of 5% dextrose in water (D_5W). The skin around the I.V. insertion site is red, warm to touch, and painful. The nurse should first:
- ☐ 1. Administer acetaminophen (Tylenol).
- ☐ 2. Change the D_5W to normal saline.
- ☐ 3. Discontinue the I.V.
- ☐ 4. Place a warm compress on the area.

79. Bed rest is related to an increased incidence of thrombophlebitis. The plan of care for a client on bed rest should not include:
- ☐ 1. Turning every 2 hours.
- ☐ 2. Passive and active range-of-motion exercises.
- ☐ 3. Use of thromboembolic disease support (TED) hose.
- ☐ 4. Maintaining the client in the supine position.

80. The client is admitted with left lower leg pain, a positive Homans' sign, and a temperature of 100.4° F (38° C). The nurse should assess the client further for signs of:
- [ ] **1.** Aortic aneurysm.
- [ ] **2.** Deep vein thrombosis (DVT) in the left leg.
- [ ] **3.** I.V. drug abuse.
- [ ] **4.** Intermittent claudication.

81. The nurse understands that certain risk factors are related to deep vein thrombosis (DVT). Which of the following is one such risk factor?
- [ ] **1.** The client exercises on a regular basis.
- [ ] **2.** The client lives alone at home.
- [ ] **3.** The client recently had abdominal surgery.
- [ ] **4.** The client wears antithrombotic hose on a regular basis.

82. A client is admitted to the unit with a diagnosis of thrombophlebitis and deep vein thrombosis of the right leg. A loading dose of heparin has been given in the emergency room, and I.V. heparin will be continued for the next several days. Care of this client will involve:
- [ ] **1.** Administering aspirin as ordered.
- [ ] **2.** Encouraging green leafy vegetables in the diet.
- [ ] **3.** Monitoring the client's prothrombin time (PT).
- [ ] **4.** Monitoring the client's activated partial thromboplastin time (aPTT) and International Normalized Ratio (INR).

83. With a client who has undergone abdominal or pelvic surgery, the nurse implements strategies to prevent deep vein thrombosis (DVT). Interventions for promoting the circulation in the lower extremities include:
- [ ] **1.** Avoiding fluids.
- [ ] **2.** Practicing deep breathing.
- [ ] **3.** Remaining sedentary.
- [ ] **4.** Using pneumatic compression stockings.

84. A client with deep vein thrombosis (DVT) has an edematous right lower extremity. The client lies on her right side frequently. Rubor is noted on the lateral aspect of the right ankle. From the data collected, the appropriate nursing diagnosis for this client would be:
- [ ] **1.** *Activity intolerance* related to complaints of pain in lower right extremity.
- [ ] **2.** *Ineffective health maintenance* related to lack of knowledge about DVT.
- [ ] **3.** *Pain* related to edema.
- [ ] **4.** *Risk for impaired skin integrity.*

85. The nurse interviews a 22-year-old female client who is scheduled for abdominal surgery the following week. The client is obese and uses estrogen-based oral contraceptives. This client is at high risk for development of:
- [ ] **1.** Atherosclerosis.
- [ ] **2.** Diabetes.
- [ ] **3.** Vasospastic disorder (Raynaud's disease).
- [ ] **4.** Thrombophlebitis.

86. The nurse observes that an older female has small to moderate, distended and tortuous veins running along the inner aspect of her lower legs. These are commonly called:
- [ ] **1.** Aneurysms.
- [ ] **2.** Lipomas.
- [ ] **3.** Ulcers.
- [ ] **4.** Varicose veins.

87. Which of the following clients is at risk for varicose veins?
- [ ] **1.** A client who has had a cerebrovascular accident.
- [ ] **2.** A client who has had anemia.
- [ ] **3.** A client who has had thrombophlebitis.
- [ ] **4.** A client who has had transient ischemic attacks.

88. A client weighs 300 lb (136 kg) and has a history of deep vein thrombosis and thrombophlebitis. When reviewing a teaching plan with this client, the nurse knows that the client has understood the nurse's instructions when he states he will:
- [ ] **1.** Avoid exercise.
- [ ] **2.** Lose weight.
- [ ] **3.** Perform leg lifts every 4 hours.
- [ ] **4.** Wear support hose, using rubber bands to hold the stockings up.

89. Which instructions should the nurse include when developing a teaching plan for a client being discharged from the hospital on anticoagulant therapy after having deep vein thrombosis (DVT)? Select all that apply.
- [ ] **1.** Checking urine for bright blood and a dark smoky color.
- [ ] **2.** Daily walking as a good exercise.
- [ ] **3.** Using garlic and ginger, which may decrease bleeding time.
- [ ] **4.** Performing foot/leg exercises and walking around the airplane cabin on long flights.
- [ ] **5.** Prevention as the best treatment for DVT.
- [ ] **6.** Avoiding surface bumps because the skin is prone to injury.

90. A client has an emergency embolectomy for an embolus in the femoral artery. After the client returns from the recovery room, in what order should the nurse provide care?

| 1. Administer pain medication. |
| 2. Draw blood for laboratory studies. |
| 3. Regulate the I.V. infusion. |
| 4. Monitor the pulses. |

| |
| |
| |
| |

The Client with an Aneurysm

91. The nurse is developing a discharge teaching plan for a client who underwent a repair of abdominal aortic aneurysm 4 days ago. The nurse reviews the client's chart for information about the client's history. Key findings are noted in the chart below.

HISTORY AND PHYSICAL

1) Smokes four cigars a month.

2) Vital signs: blood pressure, ranges from 150/76 mm Hg to 170/98 mm Hg; heart rate, 90 to 100 beats per minute; respirations, 12-18 per minute; temperature, 99.9° F (37.8° C).

3) +1 bilateral ankle edema.

Based on the data and expected outcomes, which should the nurse emphasize in the teaching plan?
- ☐ 1. Food intake.
- ☐ 2. Fluid volume.
- ☐ 3. Skin integrity.
- ☐ 4. Tissue perfusion.

92. A client is admitted with a 6.5-cm thoracic aneurysm. The nurse records findings from the initial assessment in the client's chart, as shown below.

VITAL SIGNS

Date Time	05/07/07 10:00 am	
Blood pressure	160/90 mm Hg	
Heart rate	74 bpm	
Respirations	20 per minute	
	G. Fuentes, RN	

At 10:30 a.m., the client complains of sharp midchest pain after having a bowel movement. What should the nurse do first?
- ☐ 1. Assess the client's vital signs.
- ☐ 2. Administer a bolus of lactated Ringer's solution.
- ☐ 3. Assess the client's neurologic status.
- ☐ 4. Contact the physician.

93. Nursing assessment of a 55-year-old client seen in the emergency department reveals complaints of severe abdominal pain, distention, and nausea; blood pressure of 100/40 mm Hg; heart rate of 118 bpm; respirations of 24 per minute. Based on the data, the nurse should anticipate the potential for which condition?
- ☐ 1. Anaphylactic shock.
- ☐ 2. Cardiogenic shock.
- ☐ 3. Hypovolemic shock.
- ☐ 4. Neurogenic shock.

94. A client had a repair of a thoracoabdominal aneurysm 2 days ago. Which of the following findings should the nurse consider unexpected and report to the physician immediately?
- ☐ 1. Complains of abdominal pain at 5 on a scale of 0 to 10 for the last 2 days.
- ☐ 2. Heart rate of 100 beats per minute after ambulating 200 feet.
- ☐ 3. Urine output of 2,000 ml in 24 hours.
- ☐ 4. Complains of weakness and numbness in the lower extremities.

95. A client is admitted to the emergency department complaining of severe abdominal pain. A radiograph reveals a large abdominal aortic aneurysm. The primary goal at this time is to:
☐ **1.** Maintain circulation.
☐ **2.** Manage pain.
☐ **3.** Prepare the client for emergency surgery.
☐ **4.** Teach postoperative breathing exercises.

96. Before surgery for a known aortic aneurysm, the client's pulse pressure begins to widen, suggesting increased aortic valvular insufficiency. If the branches of the aortic arch are involved, the client will have:
☐ **1.** Loss of consciousness.
☐ **2.** Anxiety.
☐ **3.** Headache.
☐ **4.** Disorientation.

97. A client complains of sudden, severe pain in his back and chest, accompanied by shortness of breath. The individual describes the pain as a "tearing" sensation. The physician suspects the client is experiencing a dissecting aortic aneurysm. The code cart is brought into the room because one complication of a dissecting aneurysm is:
☐ **1.** Cardiac tamponade.
☐ **2.** Stroke.
☐ **3.** Pulmonary edema.
☐ **4.** Myocardial infarction.

98. Which of the following increases the risk of having a large abdominal aortic aneurysm rupture?
☐ **1.** Anemia.
☐ **2.** Dehydration.
☐ **3.** High blood pressure.
☐ **4.** Hyperglycemia.

99. Which of the following represents a significant risk immediately after surgery for repair of an aortic aneurysm?
☐ **1.** Potential alteration in renal perfusion.
☐ **2.** Potential electrolyte imbalance.
☐ **3.** Potential ineffective coping.
☐ **4.** Potential wound infection.

100. A client underwent surgery to repair an abdominal aortic aneurysm. The surgeon made an incision that extends from the xiphoid process to the pubis. At 12 noon 2 days after surgery, the client complains of abdominal distention. The nurse checks the progress notes in the medical record, as shown below.

NURSES PROGRESS NOTES

Date	Time	Progress Notes
07/07/07	10:00 am	The client is receiving D$_5$W, 1,000 ml q 8 h. The NG tube is attached to low suction and draining well. The client has been NPO except ice chips. The client has had 10 mg morphine for pain at 6 a.m. ———— *E. Levine, RN*

What is most likely contributing to the client's abdominal distention?
☐ **1.** Nasogastric (NG) tube.
☐ **2.** Ice chips.
☐ **3.** I.V. fluid intake.
☐ **4.** Morphine.

101. A client is discharged after an aortic aneurysm repair with a synthetic graft to replace part of the aorta. The nurse should instruct the client to notify the physician before having:
☐ **1.** Blood drawn.
☐ **2.** An I.V. line inserted.
☐ **3.** Major dental work.
☐ **4.** An X-ray examination.

102. A client with deep vein thrombosis has been receiving warfarin (Coumadin) for 2 months. The client reports bleeding gums, increased bruising, and dark stools. These symptoms indicate that the medication:
☐ **1.** Does not need to be changed.
☐ **2.** Needs to be decreased.
☐ **3.** Needs to be increased.
☐ **4.** Is not being taken as prescribed.

The Client with Stasis Ulcers

103. A well-nourished client is admitted with a stasis ulcer. The nurse assesses the ulcer and finds excavation of the skin surface as a result of sloughing of inflammatory necrotic tissue. The physician has ordered the ulcer to be flushed with a fibrinolytic agent. Which of the following goals are appropriate for this client? Select all that apply.
☐ 1. Increase oxygen to the tissues.
☐ 2. Prevent direct trauma to the ulcer.
☐ 3. Improve nutrition.
☐ 4. Prevent infection.
☐ 5. Reduce pain.

104. A client has had a stasis ulcer of the left ankle with 2+ pitting edema for 2 years. The client is taking chlorothiazide (Diuril). The expected outcome of this drug is:
☐ 1. Improved capillary circulation.
☐ 2. Decreased blood pressure.
☐ 3. Wound healing.
☐ 4. Absence of infection.

105. The nurse assesses a client with a 5 × 2 stasis ulcer just above the left malleolus. The wound is open with irregular, reddened, swollen edges and there is a moderate amount of yellowish tan drainage coming from the wound. The client verbalizes pressure-type pain and rates the discomfort at 7 on a scale of 0 to 10. To maintain tissue integrity, the primary nursing goal should focus on:
☐ 1. Administering prescribed analgesics.
☐ 2. Applying lanolin lotions to the left ankle stasis ulcer.
☐ 3. Encouraging the client to sit up in a chair four times per day.
☐ 4. Providing an over-the-bed cradle to protect the left ankle from the pressure of bed linens.

106. The nurse is discharging a male Chinese client with a chronic right ankle stasis ulcer. Before discharge, the nurse realizes that the client needs further teaching about wound care when he indicates that he:
☐ 1. Has made an appointment with a physical therapist.
☐ 2. Will apply a home herb mixture to his wound to promote healing.
☐ 3. Will need to be patient with the healing process.
☐ 4. Will eat a balanced diet.

The Client with Peripheral Arterial Occlusive Disease

107. The nurse is caring for a client who has just had an ankle-brachial index (ABI) test. The left arm blood pressure was 160/80 mm Hg and a palpable systolic blood pressure of the left lower extremity was 130/60 mm Hg. These findings suggest that the client has:
☐ 1. Mild peripheral artery disease.
☐ 2. Moderate peripheral artery disease.
☐ 3. No apparent occlusion in the left lower extremity.
☐ 4. Severe peripheral artery disease.

108. A client is admitted for a revascularization procedure for arteriosclerosis in his left iliac artery. To promote circulation in the extremities, the nurse should:
☐ 1. Position the client on a firm mattress.
☐ 2. Keep the involved extremity warm with blankets.
☐ 3. Position the left leg at or below the body's horizontal plane.
☐ 4. Encourage the client to raise and lower his leg four times every hour.

109. A client has acute arterial occlusion. The physician has ordered I.V. heparin. Before starting the medication the nurse should:
☐ 1. Review the blood coagulation laboratory values.
☐ 2. Test the client's stools for occult blood.
☐ 3. Count the client's apical pulse for 1 minute.
☐ 4. Check the 24-hour urine output record.

110. A sedentary, obese, middle-aged client is recovering from a right iliac blood clot. The nurse should develop a discharge plan with the client that will focus on participating in which of the following activities? Select all that apply.
☐ 1. Aerobic activity.
☐ 2. Strength training.
☐ 3. Weight control.
☐ 4. Stress management.

111. The nurse is assessing the pulse in a client with aortic iliac disease. On the illustration below, indicate the pulse site that will give the nurse the most useful data.

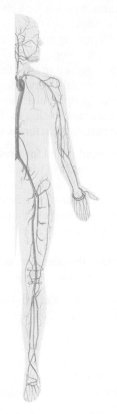

Correct Answers and Rationales

The letter in parentheses after each rationale identifies the client need addressed in the item, including management of care (M), safety and infection control (S), health promotion and maintenance (H), psychosocial adaptation (P), basic care and comfort (C), pharmacological and parenteral therapies (D), reduction of risk potential (R), and physiological adaptation (A).

The Client with Peripheral Vascular Disease

1. **2.** Ineffective tissue perfusion leads to damage to the nerves of the area. Therefore, this client will probably have disturbed sensory perception and will need to focus on health-promoting strategies that prevent injury to the involved extremity. Although skin color changes are associated with PVD, most people can wear clothing to cover up the discoloration. Thus, *Disturbed body image* would not be a priority nursing diagnosis. Edema may be associated with PVD; however, *Risk for fluid overload* is usually associated with heart problems rather than vascular problems. There is no indication that the client is at risk for fluid deficit. (A)

2. **1, 2, 3, 5.** Maintaining skin integrity is important in preventing chronic ulcers and infections. The client should be taught to routinely inspect the skin on a daily basis. The client should reduce weight to promote circulation; a diet lower in calories and fat is appropriate. Because the client is receiving Coumadin, the client is at risk for bleeding from cuts. To decrease the risk of cuts, the nurse should suggest that the client use an electric razor. The client with decreased arterial blood flow should be encouraged to participate in ADLs. In fact, the client should be encouraged to consult an exercise physiologist for an exercise program that enhances the aerobic capacity of the body. (H)

3. **4.** Blood flows in a unidirectional manner, and the blood flow involves the differences in pressure between the arterial and venous systems. The two variables influencing blood flow within this closed system are the pressure differences and the resistance to blood flow throughout the system. The greater the resistance, the greater the driving force needed, which results in an increase in the force of the contraction of the heart. Blood viscosity is important, and diameter influences resistance, but flow is dependent on pressure differences and resistance. The force of the contraction of the heart and resistance of vessels influence flow, but it is the pressure differences that control blood flow. (H)

4. **3.** Blood pressure is the highest in the aorta as the blood is being ejected out of the left ventricle into the aorta. The pressure declines as the blood flows through the arteries, capillaries, arterioles, veins, capillaries, and venules. The force of the contraction of the heart and resistance of vessels influence flow; however, it is the pressure differences that control blood flow. (H)

5. **2.** The diameter of the vessel is the most important component in determining resistance in the systemic circulation. The length of the vessel is also a factor in determining resistance. Viscosity, whether the blood is "thin" or "thick," is less important when discussing blood flow. (H)

6. **2.** High serum lipid levels are associated with an increased incidence of PVD. High serum calcium level, low serum potassium level, and low serum lipid levels have no relation to PVD. (R)

7. **4.** It is the sympathetic nervous system (adrenergic) that is involved in regulating the blood flow in the peripheral blood vessels. The autonomic nervous system is divided into two branches, the sympathetic branch and the parasympathetic branch. The parasympathetic nervous system does not control peripheral blood flow. The central nervous system is composed of the brain and the spinal cord and does not have an influential effect on peripheral blood flow. (H)

8. **1.** *Claudication* is the term used to describe the discomfort a person experiences when oxygen demand in the leg muscles is greater than the supply. The pain is a result of tissue hypoxia in the working muscle. Symptoms include aching, cramping, and weakness. (A)

9. **2.** Assessing pedal pulses involves palpating both the dorsalis pedis and the posterior tibial arteries. These pulses are located on the top of the foot (ventral aspect) and the inner aspect of the ankle (medial surface of the ankle). (H)

10. **2.** As people age, the accumulation of collagen in the intima of the blood vessels results in the vessels' becoming stiff and less flexible. Consequently, there is an increased resistance within the aging adult's circulatory system. (H)

11. **1.** Decreased blood flow is a common characteristic of all PVD. When the demand for oxygen to the working muscles becomes greater than the supply, pain is the outcome. Slow blood flow throughout the circulatory system may suggest pump failure. Thrombus formation can result from stasis or damage to the intima of the vessels. (R)

12. **1.** A client with PVD and pump failure will experience decreased blood flow. In this situation, low exercise tolerance (oxygen demand becomes greater than the oxygen supply) may be related to less blood being ejected from the left ventricle into the systemic circulation. Decreased blood supply to the tissues results in pain. Increased blood viscosity may be a component, but it is of much less importance than the disease processes. (R)

13. **4.** In PVD, decreased blood flow can result in increased venous pressure. The increase in venous pressure results in an increase in capillary hydrostatic pressure, which causes a net filtration of fluid out of the capillaries into the interstitial space, resulting in edema. Valves often become incompetent with PVD. Blood volume is not decreased in this condition. Decreased muscular action would contribute to the formation of edema in the lower extremities. (R)

14. **2.** Presence or absence of a peripheral pulse is essential data when assessing peripheral pulses in clients with PVD. The quality of the pulse is the next important piece of information needed. The client's cardiac rhythm, or pattern, is not assessed by evaluating pulses in the lower extremities. The heart rate is not assessed during evaluation of the peripheral pulses. (A)

15. **2.** A common result of atherosclerosis is the formation of an aneurysm. Arteriosclerosis, or "hardening" of the arteries, involves the endothelial lining and results in thickened arterial walls. Varicose veins are the outcome of incompetent valves in the venous system. (A)

16. **4.** Yellowish, smooth, fatty streaks are associated with atherosclerosis of the arteries. Atheromas, calcium plaques, and thickening of the intima are associated with arteriosclerosis. (R)

17. **2.** Age is a nonmodifiable risk factor for atherosclerosis. The nurse instructs the client to manage modifiable risk factors such as comorbid diseases (e.g., diabetes), activity level, and diet. Controlling serum blood glucose levels, engaging in regular aerobic activity, and choosing a diet low in saturated fats can reduce the risk of developing atherosclerosis. (H)

18. **2.** Reduction of blood flow to a specific area results in decreased oxygen and nutrients. As a result, the skin may appear mottled. Loss of hair and cool, dry skin are other signs that the nurse may observe in a client with PVD of the lower extremities. (H)

19. **3.** Generally, a 50% to 75% occlusion in the arterial lumen causes symptoms associated with intermittent claudication. When the demand for oxygen becomes greater than the supply in the working muscle, the client experience pain (aching, cramping). When the individual sits down and rests, the demand and supply of oxygen become balanced and the discomfort dissipates. Occlusion of 100% would result in ischemia and necrosis of tissue distal to the artery and would require immediate surgical intervention. (R)

20. **3.** When pedal pulses are not palpable, the nurse should obtain a Doppler ultrasound device. Auscultation is not likely to be helpful if the pulse isn't palpable. Inspection of the lower extremity can be done simultaneously when palpating, but the nurse should first try to locate a pulse by Doppler. Calling the physician may be necessary if there is a change in the client's condition. (A)

21. **2.** The sound produced by the Doppler instrument reflects all of the vascular structures in the path of the sound beam; therefore, it may be hard to differentiate between arterial and venous blood flow. Capillary and arteriole blood flow cannot be auscultated with a Doppler instrument. (A)

22. **3.** An increased LDL cholesterol concentration has been documented as a risk factor for the development of atherosclerosis. LDL cholesterol is not broken down in the liver but is deposited into the intima of the blood vessels. Low triglyceride levels are desirable. High HDL and low LDL levels are beneficial and are known to be protective for the cardiovascular system. (R)

23. **4.** Coldness in the left foot and ankle is consistent with complete arterial obstruction. Other expected findings would include paralysis and pallor. Aching pain, a burning sensation, or numbness and tingling are earlier signs of tissue hypoxia and ischemia and are commonly associated within incomplete obstruction. (A)

24. **1.** Anxiety stimulates the sympathetic nervous system, which results in the secretion of epinephrine, angiotensin, and serum proteins that cause vasoconstriction in the arteries of the peripheral circulatory system. As a result, peripheral vascular resistance is increased. This vasoconstriction may increase pain in the areas where PVD is the greatest. The lymphatic system does not affect the blood supply of tissues. (A)

25. **1.** Activity intolerance related to decreased blood supply and pain is a common problem with clients experiencing claudication. The goal should be to educate the client to maintain his level of activity and incorporate frequent rest periods to prevent episodes of decreased blood supply. The data do not suggest that the client cannot perform self-care activities, is not coping with his chronic pain, or that his skin integrity is impaired. It should be appropriate to incorporate the nursing diagnosis of *Risk for impaired skin integrity* into the client's plan of care. (H)

26.

| 2. Peripheral pulses. |
| 4. Incision site. |
| 3. Urine output. |
| 1. Postoperative pain. |

Because assessment of the presence and quality of the pedal pulses in the affected extremity is essential after surgery to make sure that the bypass graft is functioning, this step should be done first. The nurse should next ensure that the dressing is intact, and then that the client has adequate urine output. Lastly, the nurse should determine the client's level of pain. (A)

27. **1.** Decreasing venous congestion in the extremities is a desired outcome for clients with heart failure. The nurse should elevate the client's legs above the level of the heart to achieve this goal. The client is not demonstrating difficulty breathing or being cold. The nurse should prevent injury to the swollen extremity; however, this is not the priority. (H)

28. **3.** The term *gangrene* refers to blackened, decomposing tissue that is devoid of circulation. Chronic ischemia and death of the tissue can lead to gangrene in the affected extremity. Injury, edema, and decreased circulation lead to infection, gangrene, and tissue death. Atrophy is the shrinking of tissue, and contraction is joint stiffening secondary to disuse. The term *rubor* denotes a reddish color of the skin. (A)

29. **1.** The ankle-brachial index is based on the ratio of the ankle systolic blood pressure to arm systolic blood pressure. It allows one to quantify the degree of arterial stenosis. (R)

30. **1.** An arteriogram involves injecting a radiopaque contrast agent directly into the vascular system to visualize the vessels. It usually involves computed tomographic scanning. The velocity of the blood flow can be estimated by duplex ultrasound. The client's ankle-brachial index is determined, and then the client is requested to walk. The normal response is little or no drop in ankle systolic pressure after exercise. (R)

31. **2.** Clients may have an immediate or a delayed reaction to the radiopaque dye. The physician should be notified immediately because the symptoms suggest an allergic reaction. Treatment may involve administering oxygen and epinephrine. Explaining that the procedure is over does not address the current symptoms. (A)

32. **3.** The client is at greater risk for skin breakdown in the lower extremities related to the edema and to remaining in one position, which increases capillary pressure. Turning the client every 1 to 2 hours promotes vasodilation and prevents vascular compression. Administering pain medication will not have an effect on skin integrity. Encouraging fluids is not a direct intervention for maintaining skin integrity, although being well hydrated is a goal for most clients. Maintaining hygiene does influence skin integrity but is secondary in this situation. (A)

33. **4.** The client should avoid using iodine or over-the-counter medications. Iodine is a highly toxic solution. An individual who has known PVD should be seen by a physician for treatment to avoid infection. The client with PVD should avoid heating pads and crossing the legs, and should wear leather shoes. A heating pad can cause injury, which, because of the decreased blood supply, can be difficult to heal. Crossing the legs can further impede blood flow. Leather shoes provide better protection. (H)

34. **1.** Maintaining circulation in the affected extremity after surgery is the focus of care. The graft can become occluded, and the client must be assessed frequently to determine whether the graft is patent. Preventing infection and relieving pain are important but are secondary to maintaining graft patency. Education should have taken place in the preoperative phase and then continued during the recovery phase. (A)

35. **4.** PTA should be attempted first. If the blood flow is being diverted from the cranial circulation, other surgical procedures involving bypass grafts may be indicated. Amputation is necessary only if gangrene from complete loss of blood supply develops. Coronary artery bypass grafting is a specific procedure involving the arteries in the heart. (A)

36. **4.** If surgery is scheduled, the nurse should avoid venipunctures in the affected extremity. The goal should be to prevent unnecessary trauma and possible infection in the affected arm. Disruptions in skin integrity and even minor skin irritations can cause the surgery to be canceled. The nurse can continue to monitor the temperature and radial pulse in the affected arm; however, doing so is not the priority. Keeping the client warm is important but is not the priority at this time. (R)

The Client with Peripheral Vascular Disease Having an Amputation

37. **2.** Slow, steady walking is a recommended activity for clients with peripheral vascular disease because it stimulates the development of collateral circulation. The client with PVD should not remain inactive. Elevating the legs above the heart or wearing antiembolism stockings is a strategy for alleviating venous congestion and may worsen peripheral arterial disease. (C)

38. **2.** Encouraging the client who is undergoing amputation to verbalize feelings is the most therapeutic nursing intervention. By eliciting concerns, the nurse may be able to provide information to help the client cope. The nurse should avoid value-laden responses, such as "You'll still have one good leg," that may make the client feel guilty or hostile and block further communication. The nurse should not ignore the client's expressed concerns, nor should the nurse reinforce the client's concern about invalidism and dependency or assume that his wife is willing to care for him. (P)

39. **2.** The level of amputation commonly cannot be accurately determined until surgery, when the surgeon can directly assess the adequacy of the circulation of the residual limb. A longer residual limb facilitates prosthesis fitting and will make it easier for the client to walk. However, although these aspects will be considered in the final decision, they are not the primary factors influencing the decision. (A)

40. **1.** Leg crossing is contraindicated because it causes adduction of the hips and decreases the flow of blood into the lower extremities. This may result in increased pressure in the graft in the affected leg. Elevating the legs, flexing the ankles, and extending the knees are not necessarily contraindicated. (R)

41. **4.** Because amputation requires severing and tying off major arteries and veins, hemorrhage, although unexpected, is a possible complication. A tourniquet should be available at the bedside during the early postoperative period to manage such a complication. Suction equipment, as an emergency precaution, should be available for the client who has undergone head and neck surgery; however, it is not likely that the client will require suctioning after an amputation. There is no reason to have an emergency cart or an airway in the room of a client who has undergone an amputation. (A)

42. **3.** The purpose of wrapping the stump is to shape the residual limb to accept a prosthesis and bear weight. The compression bandaging should be worn at all times for many weeks after surgery and should be reapplied as needed to keep it free of wrinkles and snug. The dressing should be changed daily to allow for inspection of the stump incision. No lotions should be applied to the stump unless specifically ordered by the physician. The stump should not be elevated on pillows because this will contribute to the formation of flexion contractures. Contractures will prevent the client from wearing a prosthesis and ambulating. (A)

43. **3.** Nicotine causes vasospasm and impedes blood flow. Stopping smoking is the most significant lifestyle change the client can make. The client should eat low-fat foods as part of a balanced diet. The legs should not be elevated above the heart because this will impede arterial flow. The legs should be in a slightly dependent position. Jogging is not necessary and probably is not possible for many clients with arterial occlusive disease. A rehabilitation program that includes daily walking is suggested. (H)

44. **4.** In this case, the exercise prescription needs to be individualized because walking causes discomfort. To maintain the level of activity and decrease venous congestion, riding a stationary bike is another appropriate exercise behavior. Use of a stationary bike provides a non-weight-bearing exercise modality, which allows a longer duration of activity. Jogging and cross-country skiing are weight-bearing activities. In addition, cross-country skiing involves a cold environment, and maintaining warmth is essential in promoting arterial blood flow and preventing vasoconstriction. Golfing is a good activity, but it is not typically considered an exercise that causes aerobic changes in the body. (H)

45. **4.** Diltiazem is a calcium channel blocker that blocks the influx of calcium into the cell. In this situation, the primary use of diltiazem is to promote vasodilation and prevent spasms of the arteries. As a result of the vasodilation, blood, oxygen, and nutrients can reach the muscle and tissues. Diltiazem is not an antianxiety agent and does not promote sedation. It also does not cause vasoconstriction, which would be contraindicated for the client with PVD. (D)

46. **3.** Although pentoxifylline's precise mechanism of action is unknown, its therapeutic effect is to increase blood flow. It is commonly prescribed for clients experiencing intermittent claudication. Pentoxifylline should not be used for clients with coronary artery disease; an adverse effect of pentoxifylline is angina. It does not have a therapeutic effect on gastric reflux, and it is not a treatment for transient ischemic attacks. (D)

47. **4.** Pentoxifylline can potentiate the effects of theophylline and increase the risk of theophylline toxicity. Therefore, the nurse should monitor the client's theophylline level. Pentoxifylline does not interact with digoxin. Pentoxifylline can interact with heparin, and the client's PTT would need to be monitored closely if the client were taking heparin. It does not affect cholesterol levels. (D)

48. **2.** Angina is an adverse reaction to pentoxifylline, which should be used cautiously in clients with CAD. The nurse should report the client's symptoms to the physician, who may order nitroglycerin and possibly discontinue the pentoxifylline. The client should rest until the chest pain subsides, and documentation is essential when a client experiences an adverse reaction with medications that have been prescribed; however, the nurse's top priority is to call the physician, report the problem, and obtain an order for nitroglycerin. The client's complaints should never be dismissed. (A)

49. **1.** Assessing the individual's health behavior before surgery will help the nurse and client develop strategies to manage the postoperative course. Asking open-ended questions will illicit the most helpful information. The client's ability to walk after surgery will be improved after surgery. The nurse can ask direct questions after obtaining general information. (H)

50. **4.** Before beginning dietary interventions, the nurse must assess the client's pattern of food intake, life style, food preferences, and ethnic, cultural, and financial influences. (C)

The Client with Buerger's Disease

51. **1.** Buerger's disease is an inflammation of the intermediate and small arteries and veins. The tibial artery and vessels of the feet are affected in about 70% of clients with this disease. The forearms and hands are affected in approximately 30% of cases. The head, neck, and lower back are not affected. (A)

52. **1.** Daily use of nicotine, either by smoking or by use of smokeless tobacco products, is associated with Buerger's disease. Occupational exposure to radiation and hypertension are not associated with the condition. Although this disorder is commonly observed in males ages 20 to 40, smoking is the most strongly associated risk factor; the disease does not occur in nonsmokers. (H)

53. **3.** Because of the inflammation, a common complication of Buerger's disease is thrombus formation and potential occlusion of the vessel. Inflammation of the immediate and small arteries and veins is involved in the disease process. Embolus is a potential risk if a thrombus has developed. Fat embolus is associated with fractures of the bones. Thrombophlebitis occurs after thrombus formation. (H)

54. **3.** When helping a client change detrimental health behavior, it is critical to learn how the client perceives the situation or problem. The client is more likely to change detrimental health behaviors if he realizes that there is a problem and that these behaviors lead to the problem. While understanding the client's ability to attend group meetings, his goals for treatment, and his motivation may help facilitate change, the nurse should first understand the client's perception of the problem and then determine what strategies might work from his perspective. (H)

55. **1.** Pharmacologic nicotine (e.g., Nicotrol) is given in controlled and decreasing doses for the management of nicotine withdrawal symptoms as an adjunct to a smoking cessation program. Pharmacologic nicotine can be administered by various routes: transdermal, topical, oral, or nasal sprays. The nicotine dosage is titrated in declining dosage over 4 to 6 weeks. Nitroglycerin is used for anginal symptoms, furosemide is a diuretic, and ibuprofen is an anti-inflammatory medication; these agents have no role in a smoking cessation program. (D)

56. **2.** Buerger's disease is characterized by inflammation and fibrosis of arteries, veins, and nerves. White blood cells infiltrate the area and become fibrotic, which results in occlusion of the vessels. Signs and symptoms include slowly developing claudication, cyanosis, coldness, and pain at rest. Thickening of the intima and media of the artery is characteristic of atherosclerosis. Vasospasm lasting several minutes is characteristic of Raynaud's disease. Pain, pallor, and pulselessness are symptoms of acute occlusion of an artery by an embolus or other cause (e.g., compartment syndrome). (H)

The Client with Vasospastic Disorder

57. **1, 2.** Vasospastic disorder (Raynaud's disease) is a form of intermittent arteriolar vasoconstriction that results in coldness, pain, and pallor of the fingertips, toes, or tip of the nose, and a rebound circulation with redness and pain. The nurse should instruct the client to stop smoking because nicotine is a vasoconstrictor. An adverse effect of reserpine is orthostatic hypotension. The client should report dizziness and low blood pressure as it may be necessary to consider stopping the drug. The client should prevent vasoconstriction by covering affected parts when in cold environments. The nurse can teach the client to rewarm exposed extremities by using warm water or placing them next to the body, such as under the axilla. It is not realistic to ask this client to change jobs at this time. (H)

58. **2.** The client complains of numbness in her fingertips, thus *Disturbed sensory perception (tactile)* is the priority nursing diagnosis. The client does not complain of acute pain. The other data suggest that the circulation is adequate at this time, so neither *Ineffective tissue perfusion* nor *Risk for impaired skin integrity* is the priority nursing diagnosis. (A)

59. **1.** Vasospastic disorder (Raynaud's disease) is more common in young women and is associated with collagen diseases such as rheumatoid arthritis and lupus. (A)

60. **1.** Vasospastic disorder (Raynaud's disease) is characterized by vasospasms of the small cutaneous arteries involving the fingers and toes. (A)

61. **3.** Initially the vasoconstriction effect produces pallor or a whitish coloring, followed by cyanosis (bluish) and finally rubor (red). Gangrene is the end result of complete arterial occlusion; the skin is blackened and without a blood supply. (R)

62. **4.** Vasospastic disorder (Raynaud's disease) involves the small cutaneous arteries of the fingers and toes. The nurse should palpate the radial artery to detect circulation. If the disease process affects the lower extremities, the nurse should palpate the femoral and dorsalis pedis arteries during a vasospastic episode. Vasospastic disease primarily affects the extremities. The pulses in the brachial and carotid arteries should be present and strong. (A)

63. **3.** Extreme changes in temperature can precipitate a vasospastic episode and should be avoided by clients with vasospastic disorder (Raynaud's disease). The client should be encouraged to wear gloves when handling frozen foods or ice. The client should immerse the involved extremity in warm water during an episode to promote vasodilation and relaxation of the small arteries that are in spasm. The client can help prevent vasospasm brought on by temperature changes by wearing warm clothes. Living in a cold climate will exacerbate the symptoms. (H)

64. **2.** The data suggest a nursing diagnosis of *Anxiety* related to change in health status. The client's statements support this diagnosis. The goal for the client is to learn strategies for effective coping with anxiety-producing situations because stress can cause vasospasm. There are no data to support the diagnoses of *Activity intolerance, Disturbed body image,* or *Impaired social interaction.* (P)

65. **3.** Propranolol (Inderal) is the only beta-adrenergic medication listed. Tamsulosin hydrochloride (Flomax) blocks the smooth muscle alpha-adrenergic receptors in the prostate, leading to relaxation of the prostate and bladder. Terazosin hydrochloride (Hytrin) is classified as an alpha-adrenergic blocker and selectively blocks postsynaptic alpha-adrenergic receptors. This blocking action decreases sympathetic tone on the vasculature, dilating arterioles and veins. Labetalol hydrochloride (Trandate) competitively blocks alpha and beta receptors. (D)

66. **1.** Beta-adrenergic medications block the beta-adrenergic receptors. Therefore, the expected outcome of the medication is to decrease the influence of the sympathetic nervous system on the blood vessels in the hands. Beta-adrenergic blockers have no analgesic effects. Increasing blood supply to the affected area is an indirect effect of beta-adrenergic blockers. They do not increase monoamine oxidase, which does not play a role in Raynaud's disease. (D)

67. **4.** Sympathectomy is scheduled only after other treatment alternatives have been explored and have failed. Medication and stress management are beneficial strategies to prevent advancement of the disease process. If the disease is controlled by medication, there is no reason for surgery. (A)

The Client with Thrombophlebitis and Embolus Formation

68. **4.** Based on the laboratory findings, prothrombin time and INR are at acceptable anticoagulation levels for the treatment of DVT. However, the platelets are below the acceptable level. Clients taking enoxaparin are at risk for thrombocytopenia. Because of the low platelet level, the nurse should withhold the enoxaparin, assess the client for bleeding, and then contact the physician. (D)

69. **2.** Acute arterial occlusion is a sudden interruption of blood flow. The interruption can be the result of complete or partial obstruction. Acute pain, loss of sensory and motor function, and a pale, mottled, numb extremity are the most dramatic and observable changes that indicate a life-threatening interruption of tissue perfusion. Blood pressure and heart rate changes may be associated with the acute pain episode. Metabolic acidosis is a complication of irreversible ischemia. Swelling may result but may also indicate venous stasis or arterial insufficiency. (A)

70. **1.** Venous stasis can increase pain. Therefore, proper positioning in bed or when sitting up in a chair can help promote venous drainage, reduce swelling, and reduce the amount of pain the client might experience. Placing a pillow under the knees causes flexion of the joint, resulting in a dependent position of the lower leg an causing a decrease in blood flow. Fluids are encouraged to maintain normal fluid and electrolyte balance but do little to relieve pain. Therapeutic massage to the legs is discouraged because of the danger of breaking up the clot. (C)

71. **3.** The client is likely suffering from an embolus as a result of abdominal surgery. The nurse should inspect the left leg for color and temperature changes associated with tissue perfusion. Administering pain medication without gathering more information about the pain can mask important signs and symptoms. Although assessing for edema is important, it is not critical to this situation. Encouraging the client to change her position does not adequately address the need for gathering more data. (R)

72. **2.** Performing active ankle and foot range-of-motion exercises periodically during the ride home will promote muscular contraction and provide support to the venous system. It is the muscular action that facilitates return of the blood from the lower extremities, especially when in the dependent position. Arm circle exercises will not promote circulation in the leg. It is not necessary for the client to elevate her legs as long as she does not occlude blood flow to her legs and does her leg exercises. It is not necessary to take an ambulance because the client is able to sit in the car safely. (R)

73. **3.** DVT is commonly associated with venous stasis in the legs when there is a lack of the skeletal muscle pump that enhances venous return to the heart. When a client is confined to bed rest, venous compression occurs because of the position of the lower extremities. This increased pressure causes damage to the intima lining of the veins and causes platelets to adhere to the damaged site. DVT increases the risk that a displaced plaque will become a pulmonary embolus. Arteriosclerosis is hardening of the arteries; aneurysm is the abnormal dilation of a vessel; and varicose veins are swollen, tortuous veins. These are not generally considered causes of pulmonary embolism. (A)

74. 3. Thrombolytic agents are used for clients with a history of thrombus formation, cerebrovascular accidents, and chronic atrial fibrillation. The thrombolytic agents act by dissolving emboli. Thrombolytic agents do not directly improve perfusion or increase vascular permeability, nor do they prevent cerebral hemorrhage. (D)

75. 0.85

First convert pounds (lb) to kilograms (kg) by using the formula:

$$1 \text{ kg} = 2.2 \text{ lb } [187 \text{ lb} \div 2.2 = 85 \text{ kg}].$$

The physician's order is for the client to receive enoxaparin (Lovenox) 1 mg/kg. Therefore, the client is to receive 85 mg. The desired dose in milliliters then can be calculated by using the formula of desired dose (D) divided by dose or strength of dose on hand (H) times volume (V).

$$85 \text{ (mg)} \times 0.3 \text{ ml} = 25.5 \text{ mg/ml}$$

$$25.5 \text{ mg} \div 30 = 0.85 \text{ ml}.$$

(D)

76. 4. Thrombophlebitis is an inflammation of a vein. The underlying etiology involves stasis of blood, increased blood coagulability, and vessel wall injury. The symptoms of thrombophlebitis are pain, swelling, and deep muscle tenderness. Air embolus is a result of air entering the vascular system. Fat embolus is associated with the presence of intracellular fat globules in the lung parenchyma and peripheral circulation after long-bone fractures. Stress fractures are associated with the musculoskeletal system. (H)

77. 4. Current literature suggests that approximately 65% of the clients receiving I.V. therapy will develop superficial vein thrombophlebitis. (R)

78. 3. The first action should be to discontinue the I.V. The nurse should restart the I.V. elsewhere and then apply a warm compress to the affected area. The nurse should administer acetaminophen or an anti-inflammatory agent only if ordered by the physician. The type of infusion cannot be changed without a physician's order, and such a change would not help in this case. (R)

79. 4. Three factors contribute to the formation of venous thrombus and thrombophlebitis: damage to the inner lining of the vein (prolonged pressure), hypercoagulability of the blood, and venous stasis. Bed rest and immobilization are associated with decreased blood flow and venous pooling in the lower extremities. Keeping the client in the supine position would not be appropriate. Turning the client every 1 to 2 hours, passive and active range-of-motion exercises, and use of TED hose help prevent venous stasis in the lower extremities. (R)

80. 2. The client demonstrates classic symptoms of DVT, and the nurse should continue to assess the client. Signs and symptoms of an aortic aneurysm include abdominal pain and a pulsating abdominal mass. Clients with drug abuse demonstrate confusion and decreased levels of consciousness. Claudication is an intermittent pain in the leg. (P)

81. 3. A history of recent abdominal surgery is a risk factor for developing DVT, thrombophlebitis, or thromboembolism. Exercising on a regular basis helps prevent venous stasis and DVT. Living alone has no link to development of DVT. Wearing antithrombotic hose is a measure to help prevent venous stasis. (A)

82. 4. Heparin dosage is usually determined by the physician based on the client's aPTT and INR laboratory values. Therefore, the nurse monitors these values to prevent complications. Administering aspirin when the client is on heparin is contraindicated. Green leafy vegetables are high in vitamin K and therefore are not recommended for clients receiving heparin. Monitoring of the client's PT is done when the client is receiving warfarin sodium (Coumadin). (D)

83. 4. The use of pneumatic compression stockings is an intervention used to prevent DVT. Other strategies include early ambulation, leg exercises if the client is confined to bed, adequate fluid intake, and administering anticoagulant medication as ordered. Deep breathing would be encouraged postoperatively, but it does not prevent DVT. (H)

84. 4. *Risk for impaired skin integrity* is the primary nursing diagnosis. With rubor or hyperemia, there is increased blood flow to the area, raising filtration pressure. As a result, capillary permeability is altered, causing damage to capillary walls. The increased permeability, obstruction of lymphatic drainage, elevation of venous pressure, and decrease in plasma protein osmotic force result in edema. The data do not support the nursing diagnoses of *Activity intolerance, Ineffective health maintenance,* or *Pain.* (A)

85. 4. The data suggest an increased risk of thrombophlebitis. The risk factors in this situation include abdominal surgery, obesity, and use of estrogen-based oral contraceptives. Risk factors for atherosclerosis include genetics, older age, and a high-cholesterol diet. Risk factors for diabetes include genetics and obesity. Risk factors for vasospastic disorders include cold climate, age (16 to 40), and immunologic disorders. (R)

86. **4.** Varicose veins are tortuous, distended veins where blood has pooled. Varicose veins are commonly observed in the lower extremities. An aneurysm is a localized, abnormal dilation of a blood vessel. A lipoma is a fatty tumor. An ulcer is an open sore or lesion of the skin or mucous membrane, accompanied by sloughing of inflamed necrotic tissue. (H)

87. **3.** Secondary varicosities can result from previous thrombophlebitis of the deep femoral veins, with subsequent valvular incompetence. Cerebrovascular accident, anemia, and transient ischemic attacks are not associated with an increased risk of varicose veins. (H)

88. **2.** The client is at risk for development of varicose veins. Therefore, prevention is key in the treatment plan. Maintaining ideal body weight is the goal. In order to achieve this, the client should consume a balanced diet and participate in a regular exercise program. Depending on the individual, leg lifts may or may not be an appropriate activity. Performing leg lifts provides muscular activity and should be done more often than every 4 hours. Wearing support hose is helpful. However, the client should not use rubber bands to hold the stockings up. (R)

89. **1, 2, 4, 5, 6.** Clients with resolving DVT being sent home on anticoagulant therapy need instructions about assessing and preventing bleeding episodes and preventing a recurrence of DVT. Blood in the urine (hematuria) is often one of the first symptoms of anticoagulant overdose. Fresh blood in the urine is red; however, blood in the urine may also be a dark smoky color. Daily ambulation is an excellent activity to keep the venous blood circulating and thus to prevent blood clots from forming in the lower extremities. Garlic and ginger increase the bleeding time and should not be used when a client is on anticoagulant therapy. Clients who have had previous DVTs should avoid activities that cause stagnation and pooling of venous blood. Prolonged sitting coupled with change of air pressure without foot or leg exercises or ambulation in the cabin are activities that prevent venous return. Instructing the client about prevention measures is important because clients with DVT are at high risk for pulmonary emboli (PE), which can be fatal. The client can be taught risk factors for DVT and PE. In addition, recommendations for prevention of these events also are standard protocol in practice and should be shared with the client for home care purposes. Older adults should be monitored closely for bleeding because the skin becomes thinner and the capillaries become more fragile with the aging process. (H)

90.

4. Monitor the pulses.
3. Regulate the I.V. infusion.
1. Administer pain medication.
2. Draw blood for laboratory studies.

The nurse should first monitor the popliteal and pedal pulses in the affected extremity after arterial embolectomy. Monitoring peripheral pulses below the site of occlusion checks the arterial circulation in the involved extremity. The nurse should next regulate the I.V. infusion to prevent fluid overload. Then the nurse should assess pain and administer pain medications as ordered. Last, the nurse can obtain blood for laboratory studies. (A)

The Client with an Aneurysm

91. **4.** The underlying pathophysiology in this client is atherosclerosis. The findings from the assessment indicate the risk factors of smoking and high blood pressure. Therefore, tissue perfusion is a priority for health promoting education. The data do not support education that focuses on food or fluid intake. Although edema is a potential problem and could contribute to poor skin integrity, the edema will likely be resolved by the aneurysm repair. (A)

92. **1.** The size of the thoracic aneurysm is rather large, so the nurse should anticipate rupture. A sudden incidence of pain may indicate leakage or rupture. The blood pressure and heart rate will provide useful information in assessing for hypovolemic shock. The nurse needs more data before initiating other interventions. After assessment of vital signs, neurologic status, and pain, the nurse can then contact the physician. Administering lactated Ringer's solution would require a physician's order. (A)

93. **3.** Onset of sudden abdominal pain with changes in vital signs strongly suggests a potential bleeding problem. Therefore, based on the data given, the nurse should consider the possibility of an abdominal aneurysm and the potential that the aneurysm is leaking or has ruptured. (A)

94. **4.** One of the complications of a thoracoabdominal aneurysm repair is spinal cord injury. Therefore, it is important for the nurse to assess for signs and symptoms of neurologic changes at and below the site where the aneurysm was repaired. The client is expected to have moderate pain following surgery. An elevated heart rate is expected after physical exertion. It is important to monitor urine output following aneurysm surgery, but a urine output of 2,000 ml in 24 hours is adequate following surgery. (S)

95. **3.** The primary goal is to prepare the client for emergency surgery. The goal would be to prevent rupture of the aneurysm and potential death. Circulation is maintained, unless the aneurysm ruptures. When the client is prepared for surgery, the nurse should place the client in a recumbent position to promote circulation, teach the client about postoperative breathing exercises, and administer pain medication if ordered. (A)

96. **1.** If the aortic arch is involved, there will be a decrease in the blood flow to the cerebrum. Therefore, loss of consciousness will be observed. A sudden loss of consciousness is a primary symptom of rupture and no blood flow to the brain. Anxiety is not a sign of aortic valvular insufficiency. The end result of decreased cerebral blood flow is loss of consciousness, not headache or disorientation. (R)

97. **1.** Cardiac tamponade is a life-threatening complication of a dissecting thoracic aneurysm. The sudden, painful "tearing" sensation is typically associated with the sudden release of blood, and the client may experience cardiac arrest. Stroke, pulmonary edema, and myocardial infarction are not common complications of a dissecting aneurysm. (A)

98. **3.** In the preoperative phase, the goal is to prevent rupture. The client is placed in a semi-Fowler's position and in a quiet environment. The systolic blood pressure is maintained at the lowest level the client can tolerate. Anemia, dehydration, and hyperglycemia do not put the client at risk for rupture. (H)

99. **1.** There is a potential for an alteration in renal perfusion, manifested by decreased urine output. The altered renal perfusion may be related to renal artery embolism, prolonged hypotension, or prolonged aortic cross-clamping during surgery. Electrolyte imbalance, ineffective coping, and wound infection may occur after any surgery. (A)

100. **4.** The client is experiencing paralytic ileus. One of the adverse effects of morphine used to manage pain is decreased GI motility. Bowel manipulation and immobility also contribute to a postoperative ileus. Insertion of an NG tube generally prevents a postoperative ileus. The ice chips and I.V. fluids will not affect the ileus. (C)

101. **3.** The client with a synthetic graft may need to be treated with prophylactic antibiotics before undergoing major dental work. This reduces the danger of systemic infection caused by bacteria from the oral cavity. Venous access for drawing blood, I.V. line insertion, and X-rays do not contribute to the risk of infection. (D)

102. **2.** These symptoms suggest that the client is receiving too much Coumadin. Coumadin hinders the hepatic synthesis of vitamin K–dependent clotting factors and prolongs the clotting time. Because many factors influence the effectiveness of Coumadin, the dosage is monitored closely. Signs and symptoms of blood loss include bleeding gums, petechiae, bruises, dark stools, and dark urine. (D)

The Client with Stasis Ulcers

103. **1, 2, 4, 5.** The underlying pathophysiology in stasis ulcers of the skin surface is a result of inadequate oxygen and other nutrients to the tissues because of edema and decreased circulation. The nurse should first initiate care that will increase oxygen and improve tissue integrity. It is also important to prevent trauma to the tissues and prevent infections, which result from decreased microcirculation that limits the body's response to infection. Stasis ulcers are painful. The nurse can administer prescribed analgesics 30 minutes before changing the dressing. There is no indication that the client's overall nutrition needs to be improved. (A)

104. **1.** The result of chronic venous stasis is swelling and edema and superficial varicose veins. Diuretics will help reduce the swelling, thus improving capillary circulation. Although diuretics may decrease blood pressure, that is not the intended outcome of this drug. The nurse should teach the client to prevent infection and monitor wound healing, but these are not the primary outcomes of chlorothiazide. (D)

105. **4.** Providing an over-the-bed cradle will decrease the amount of pressure that the linens exert upon the lower extremity and prevent further tissue breakdown. Administering prescribed analgesics would be an intervention for reducing the pain. Applying lanolin lotions to the left ankle ulcer will not promote healing. Encouraging the client to sit up in a chair four times per day is an intervention to promote activity. The nurse would elevate the involved extremity while the client is sitting up to reduce venous stasis and capillary pressure. (H)

106. **2.** The nurse should first determine what the client means when he says he will apply an herb mixture to his ulcer. The nurse should then encourage the client to consult the physician because home remedies may be beneficial or may interfere with the medical treatment plan. In many cultures, home remedies are commonly used and may be helpful. The nurse must be sensitive to these traditions and cultural beliefs. The other statements demonstrate that the client understands the plan of care for his ulcer. (H)

The Client with Peripheral Arterial Occlusive Disease

107. **1.** The ABI test is a noninvasive test that compares the systolic blood pressure in the arm with that of the ankle. It may be done before or after exercise. The client's highest brachial systolic pressure is divided by the left ankle systolic blood pressure to get 0.81. This score is between 0.71 and 0.90, which suggests mild peripheral artery disease. Moderate peripheral artery disease would yield a score of 0.41 to 0.70. Severe peripheral artery disease would result in a score of 0.00 to 0.40. (A)

108. **3.** Keeping the involved extremity at or below the body's horizontal plane will facilitate tissue perfusion and prevent tissue damage. The nurse should avoid placing the affected extremity on a hard surface, such as a firm mattress, to avoid pressure ulcers. In addition, the involved extremity should be free from heavy overlying bed linens. The nurse should handle the involved extremity in a gentle fashion to prevent friction or pressure. Raising the leg would cause occlusion to the iliac artery, which is contrary to the goal to promote arterial circulation. (A)

109. **1.** Before starting a heparin infusion, it is essential for the nurse to know the client's baseline blood coagulation values (hematocrit, hemoglobin, and red blood cell and platelet counts). In addition, the partial thromboplastin time should be monitored closely during the process. The client's stools would be tested only if internal bleeding is suspected. Although monitoring vital signs such as apical pulse is important in assessing potential signs and symptoms of hemorrhage or potential adverse reactions to the medication, vital signs are not the most important data to collect before administering the heparin. Intake and output are not important assessments for heparin administration unless the client has fluid and volume problems or kidney disease. (D)

110. **1, 3.** Discharge teaching begins when the client enters the hospital. One of the risk factors for clot formation is a sedentary lifestyle, and the client should engage in daily aerobic activity, such as biking or swimming (non-weight-bearing). The client is also overweight and should plan to control his weight through dietary counseling or attending weight management programs in the community. Strength training is beneficial by increasing strength and lean body mass, but not helpful in preventing vascular disease. Stress management is not a focus based on the client's needs at this time. (H)

111. The nurse should assess the femoral artery. Weak or absent femoral pulses are symptomatic of aortoiliac disease. (A)

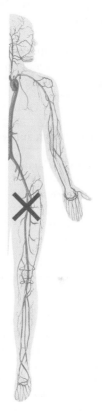

The Client with Hematologic Health Problems

- The Client with Red Blood Cell Disorders
- The Client with Platelet Disorders
- The Client with White Blood Cell Disorders
- The Client with Lymphoma
- The Client Who Is in Shock
- Correct Answers and Rationales

The Client with Red Blood Cell Disorders

1. The nurse is assisting with a bone marrow aspiration and biopsy. In which order of priority should the nurse complete the following tasks?

| 1. Position the client in a side-lying position. |
| 2. Clean the skin with an antiseptic solution. |
| 3. Verify the client has signed an informed consent. |
| 4. Apply ice to the biopsy site. |

| |
| |
| |
| |

2. A client with iron deficiency anemia is refusing to take the prescribed oral iron medication because the medication is causing nausea. The nurse should do which of the following? Select all that apply.
- [ ] 1. Suggest that the client use ginger when taking the medication.
- [ ] 2. Ask the client what she thinks is causing the nausea.
- [ ] 3. Tell the client to use stool softeners to minimize constipation.
- [ ] 4. Offer to administer the medication by an intramuscular injection.
- [ ] 5. Suggest that the client take the iron with orange juice.

3. A client had a mastectomy followed by chemotherapy 6 months ago. She reports that she is now "unable to concentrate at her card game" and "it seems harder and harder to finish her errands because of exhaustion." Based on this information, the nurse should suggest that the client do which of the following?
- [ ] 1. Take frequent naps.
- [ ] 2. Limit activities.
- [ ] 3. Increase fluid intake.
- [ ] 4. Avoid contact with others.

4. A client is to have a transfusion of packed red blood cells from a designated donor. The client asks if any diseases can be transmitted by this donor. The nurse should inform the client that which of the following diseases can be transmitted by a designated donor? Select all that apply.
- [ ] 1. Epstein-Barr virus.
- [ ] 2. Human immunodeficiency virus (HIV).
- [ ] 3. Cytomegalovirus (CMV).
- [ ] 4. Hepatitis A.
- [ ] 5. Malaria.

5. A client has been admitted with active rectal bleeding. He has been typed and cross-matched for 2 units of packed red blood cells (RBCs). Within 10 minutes of admission the client faints when getting up to go to the bedside commode. The nurse notifies the health care provider, who orders a unit of blood immediately. The nurse should expect which type of packed RBCs will be used for immediate transfusion?
- [ ] 1. A negative.
- [ ] 2. B negative.
- [ ] 3. AB negative.
- [ ] 4. O negative.

6. A nurse has two clients that have an order to receive a blood transfusion of packed red blood cells at the same time. The first client's blood pressure dropped from the preoperative value of 120/80 mm Hg to a postoperative value of 100/50. The second client is 58 years old, and is hospitalized because he developed dehydration and anemia following pneumonia. After checking the patency of their I.V. lines and vital signs, which should the nurse do next?

☐ **1.** Call for both clients' blood transfusions at the same time.
☐ **2.** Ask another nurse to verify the compatibility of both units at the same time.
☐ **3.** Call for and hang the first client's blood transfusion.
☐ **4.** Ask another nurse to call for and hang the blood for the second client.

7. The nurse is preparing to teach a client with microcytic hypochromic anemia about the diet to follow after discharge. Which of the following foods should be included in the diet?

☐ **1.** Eggs.
☐ **2.** Lettuce.
☐ **3.** Citrus fruits.
☐ **4.** Cheese.

8. The nurse should instruct the client to eat which of the following foods to obtain the best supply of vitamin B_{12}?

☐ **1.** Whole grains.
☐ **2.** Green leafy vegetables.
☐ **3.** Meats and dairy products.
☐ **4.** Broccoli and brussels sprouts.

9. The nurse has just admitted a 35-year-old female client who has a serum vitamin B_{12} concentration of 800 pg/ml. Which of the following laboratory findings should cue the nurse to focus the client history assessment on specific drug or alcohol use?

☐ **1.** Total bilirubin, 0.3 mg/dl.
☐ **2.** Serum creatinine, 0.5 mg/dl.
☐ **3.** Hemoglobin, 16 g/dl.
☐ **4.** Folate, 1.5 ng/ml.

10. The nurse understands that the client with pernicious anemia will have which distinguishing laboratory findings?

☐ **1.** Schilling's test, elevated.
☐ **2.** Intrinsic factor, absent.
☐ **3.** Sedimentation rate, 16 mm/hour.
☐ **4.** Red blood cells (RBCs), 5.0 million/µl.

11. The nurse devises a teaching plan for the client with aplastic anemia. Which of the following is the most important concept to teach for health promotion and maintenance?

☐ **1.** Eat animal protein and dark green, leafy vegetables every day.
☐ **2.** Avoid exposure to others with acute infections.
☐ **3.** Practice yoga and meditation to decrease stress and anxiety.
☐ **4.** Get 8 hours of sleep at night and take naps during the day.

12. A client comes to the health clinic 3 years after undergoing a resection of the terminal ileum complaining of weakness, shortness of breath, and a sore tongue. Which client statement indicates a need for intervention and client teaching?

☐ **1.** "I have been drinking plenty of fluids."
☐ **2.** "I have been gargling with warm salt water for my sore tongue."
☐ **3.** "I have three to four loose stools per day."
☐ **4.** "I take a vitamin B_{12} tablet every day."

13. A vegetarian client was referred to a dietitian for nutritional counseling for anemia. Which client outcome indicates that the client does not understand nutritional counseling? The client:

☐ **1.** Adds dried fruit to cereal and baked goods.
☐ **2.** Cooks tomato-based foods in iron pots.
☐ **3.** Drinks coffee or tea with meals.
☐ **4.** Adds vitamin C to all meals.

14. A client was admitted with iron deficiency anemia and blood-streaked emesis. Which question is most appropriate for the nurse to ask in determining the extent of the client's activity intolerance?

☐ **1.** "What daily activities were you able to do 6 months ago compared with the present?"
☐ **2.** "How long have you had this problem?"
☐ **3.** "Have you been able to keep up with all your usual activities?"
☐ **4.** "Are you more tired now than you used to be?"

15. A physician orders vitamin B_{12} for a client with pernicious anemia. Which site is appropriate for the nurse to administer vitamin B_{12}? Select all that apply.

☐ **1.** Median cutaneous.
☐ **2.** Greater femur trochanter.
☐ **3.** Acromion muscle.
☐ **4.** Ventrogluteal.
☐ **5.** Upper back.
☐ **6.** Dorsogluteal.

16. Which position would most help to decrease a client's discomfort when the client's spouse injects vitamin B$_{12}$ using the ventrogluteal site?
- ☐ **1.** Lying on the side with legs extended.
- ☐ **2.** Lying on the abdomen with toes pointed inward.
- ☐ **3.** Leaning over the edge of a low table with hips flexed.
- ☐ **4.** Standing upright with the feet one shoulder-width apart.

17. A client is admitted from the emergency department after falling down a flight of stairs at home. Her vital signs are stable and her history states that she had a gastric stapling 2 years ago and takes neomycin for acne. The client jokes about how she is clumsy lately and trips over things. The nurse should ask the client which of the following questions? Select all that apply.
- ☐ **1.** "Are you experiencing numbness in your extremities?"
- ☐ **2.** "How much vitamin B$_{12}$ are you getting?"
- ☐ **3.** "Are you feeling depressed?"
- ☐ **4.** "Do you feel safe at home?"
- ☐ **5.** "Are you getting sufficient iron in your diet?"

18. A client returned home from an overseas tour of duty complaining of fatigue. He has a temperature of 99.5° F (37.5° C). His skin is dark bronze, and his urine has a dark color. His hemoglobin level is 9 g/dl; his hematocrit is 49, and red blood cells are 2.75 million/µl. What should the nurse do?
- ☐ **1.** Initiate an intake and output record.
- ☐ **2.** Place the client on bed rest.
- ☐ **3.** Place the client on contact isolation.
- ☐ **4.** Keep the client out of sunlight.

19. The primary purpose of the Schilling test is to measure the client's ability to:
- ☐ **1.** Store vitamin B$_{12}$.
- ☐ **2.** Digest vitamin B$_{12}$.
- ☐ **3.** Absorb vitamin B$_{12}$.
- ☐ **4.** Produce vitamin B$_{12}$.

20. The nurse implements which of the following for the client who is starting a Schilling test?
- ☐ **1.** Administering methylcellulose (Citrucel).
- ☐ **2.** Starting a 24- to 48-hour urine specimen collection.
- ☐ **3.** Maintaining nothing-by-mouth (NPO) status.
- ☐ **4.** Starting a 72-hour stool specimen collection.

21. A 16-year-old client from a Mediterranean country is admitted with thalassemia, jaundice, splenomegaly, and hepatomegaly. Which of the following should be the primary focus of nursing care for this client?
- ☐ **1.** Providing activities of daily living on the time schedule of his homeland.
- ☐ **2.** Offering foods of his preference to increase his intake of calories.
- ☐ **3.** Decreasing his cardiac demands by promoting a 1:3 ratio of rest to activity as tolerated.
- ☐ **4.** Listening to his concerns about his hospitalization.

22. A client with pernicious anemia asks why she must take vitamin B$_{12}$ injections for the rest of her life. Which is the nurse's *best* response?
- ☐ **1.** "The reason for your vitamin deficiency is an inability to absorb the vitamin because the stomach is not producing sufficient acid."
- ☐ **2.** "The reason for your vitamin deficiency is an inability to absorb the vitamin because the stomach is not producing sufficient intrinsic factor."
- ☐ **3.** "The reason for your vitamin deficiency is an excessive excretion of the vitamin because of kidney dysfunction."
- ☐ **4.** "The reason for your vitamin deficiency is an increased requirement for the vitamin because of rapid red blood cell production."

23. An African-American woman had experienced severe palpitations, weakness, and shortness of breath after taking bacitracin (Bactrim). As a part of the discharge planning, the nurse evaluates the client's knowledge about her:
- ☐ **1.** Increased folic acid needs.
- ☐ **2.** Congenital enzyme deficiency.
- ☐ **3.** Restricted activity in hot weather.
- ☐ **4.** Need for blood transfusions.

24. The nurse is assessing a client's activity tolerance by having the client walk on a treadmill for 5 minutes. Which of the following indicates an abnormal response?
- ☐ **1.** Pulse rate increased by 20 beats per minute (bpm) immediately after the activity.
- ☐ **2.** Respiratory rate decreased by 5 breaths/minute.
- ☐ **3.** Diastolic blood pressure increased by 7 mm Hg.
- ☐ **4.** Pulse rate within 6 bpm of resting pulse after 3 minutes of rest.

25. When comparing the hematocrit levels of a postoperative client, the nurse notes that the hematocrit decreased from 36% to 34% on the third day even though the RBC count and hemoglobin value remained stable at 4.5 million/µl and 11.9 g/dl, respectively. Which nursing intervention is most appropriate?
☐ **1.** Check the dressing and drains for frank bleeding.
☐ **2.** Call the physician.
☐ **3.** Continue to monitor vital signs.
☐ **4.** Start oxygen at 2 L/minute per nasal cannula.

26. The nurse administers packed red blood cells (PRBCs) to a client. Which of the following nursing actions is appropriate?
☐ **1.** Discontinue the I.V. catheter if a blood transfusion reaction occurs.
☐ **2.** Administer the PRBCs through a percutaneously inserted central catheter line with a 20-gauge needle.
☐ **3.** Flush PRBCs with 5% dextrose and 0.45% normal saline solution.
☐ **4.** Stay with the client during the first 15 minutes of infusion.

27. A young adult female has sickle cell anemia. The nurse should remind this client to do which of the following? Select all that apply.
☐ **1.** Drink plenty of fluids when outside in hot weather.
☐ **2.** Avoid high altitudes where oxygen levels are lower.
☐ **3.** Be aware that since she is homozygous for HbS, she carries the sickle cell trait.
☐ **4.** Understand that pregnancy with sickle cell disease increases the risk of a crisis.

28. The nurse is teaching a client and his family about the client's new diagnosis of hemochromatosis. Which of the following details should the nurse include?
☐ **1.** Hemochromatosis is an autoimmune disorder that affects the HFE gene.
☐ **2.** Individuals who are heterozygous for hemochromatosis rarely develop the disease.
☐ **3.** Individuals who are homozygous for hemochromatosis are carriers of hemochromatosis.
☐ **4.** Men are at greater risk for hemochromatosis.

29. Which safety measures would be most important to implement when caring for a client who is receiving 2 units of packed red blood cells (PRBCs)? Select all that apply.
☐ **1.** Verify that the ABO and Rh of the 2 units are the same.
☐ **2.** Infuse a unit of PRBCs in less than 4 hours.
☐ **3.** Stop the transfusion if a reaction occurs, but keep the line open.
☐ **4.** Take vital signs every 15 minutes while the unit is transfusing.
☐ **5.** Inspect the blood bag for leaks, abnormal color, and clots.
☐ **6.** Use a 22-gauge catheter for optimal flow of a blood transfusion.

30. A client had received 25 ml of packed red blood cells (PRBCs) when she began to experience low back pain and mild itching. After stopping the infusion, the nurse should:
☐ **1.** Administer prescribed aspirin and antihistamines.
☐ **2.** Collect blood and urine samples to be sent to the laboratory.
☐ **3.** Administer prescribed diuretics, oxygen, and morphine.
☐ **4.** Administer prescribed vasopressors.

31. A client is to receive epoetin (Epogen) injections. What laboratory value should the nurse assess before giving the injection?
☐ **1.** Hematocrit.
☐ **2.** Partial thromboplastin time.
☐ **3.** Hemoglobin concentration.
☐ **4.** Prothrombin time.

32. When beginning I.V. erythropoietin (Epogen, Procrit) therapy, which of the following nursing interventions would be appropriate? Select all that apply.
☐ **1.** Checking the hemoglobin levels before administering subsequent doses.
☐ **2.** Shaking the vial thoroughly to mix the concentrated white, milky solution.
☐ **3.** Keeping the multidose vial refrigerated between scheduled twice-a-day doses.
☐ **4.** Administering the medication through the I.V. line without other medications.
☐ **5.** Adjusting the initial doses according to the client's changes in blood pressure.
☐ **6.** Educating the client to avoid driving and performing hazardous activity during the initial treatment.

33. A client states that she is afraid of receiving vitamin B$_{12}$ injections because of potential toxic reactions. Which is the nurse's best response to relieve these fears?
- ☐ 1. "Vitamin B$_{12}$ will cause ringing in the ears before a toxic level is reached."
- ☐ 2. "Vitamin B$_{12}$ may cause a very mild rash initially."
- ☐ 3. "Vitamin B$_{12}$ cause mild nausea but nothing toxic."
- ☐ 4. "Vitamin B$_{12}$ is generally free of toxicity because it is water-soluble."

34. A client with microcytic anemia is having trouble selecting food from the hospital menu. Which food is best for the nurse to suggest for satisfying the client's nutritional needs?
- ☐ 1. Egg yolks.
- ☐ 2. Brown rice.
- ☐ 3. Vegetables.
- ☐ 4. Tea.

35. A client with macrocytic anemia has a burn on her foot and states that she had been watching television while lying on a heating pad. Which action should be the nurse's first response?
- ☐ 1. Assess for potential abuse.
- ☐ 2. Check for diminished sensations.
- ☐ 3. Document the findings.
- ☐ 4. Clean and dress the area.

36. Which of the following nursing assessment findings is a late symptom of polycythemia vera?
- ☐ 1. Headache.
- ☐ 2. Dizziness.
- ☐ 3. Pruritus.
- ☐ 4. Shortness of breath.

37. The nurse is teaching a client with polycythemia vera about potential complications from this disease. Which manifestations should the nurse include in the client's teaching plan? Select all that apply.
- ☐ 1. Hearing loss.
- ☐ 2. Visual disturbance.
- ☐ 3. Headache.
- ☐ 4. Orthopnea.
- ☐ 5. Gout.
- ☐ 6. Weight loss.

38. When a client is diagnosed with aplastic anemia, the nurse monitors for changes in which of the following physiologic functions?
- ☐ 1. Bleeding tendencies.
- ☐ 2. Intake and output.
- ☐ 3. Peripheral sensation.
- ☐ 4. Bowel function.

The Client with Platelet Disorders

39. A health care provider orders 0.5 mg of protamine sulfate for a client who is showing signs of bleeding after receiving a 100-unit dose of heparin. The nurse should expect the effects of the protamine sulfate to be noted in which of the following time frames?
- ☐ 1. 5 minutes.
- ☐ 2. 10 minutes.
- ☐ 3. 20 minutes.
- ☐ 4. 30 minutes.

40. The nurse is to administer subcutaneous heparin to an older adult. What facts should the nurse keep in mind when administering this dose? Select all that apply.
- ☐ 1. It should be administered in the anterior area of the iliac crest.
- ☐ 2. The onset is immediate.
- ☐ 3. Use a 27G, ⅝″ needle.
- ☐ 4. Cephalosporin potentiates the effects of heparin.
- ☐ 5. Double check the dose with another nurse.

41. Which of the following nursing interventions is appropriate for a client with a platelet count of 31,000/μl?
- ☐ 1. Pad sharp surfaces to avoid minor trauma when walking.
- ☐ 2. Assess for spontaneous petechiae in the extremities.
- ☐ 3. Keep the room darkened.
- ☐ 4. Check for blood in the urine.

42. A client with a history of systemic lupus erythematosus was admitted with a severe viral respiratory tract infection and diffuse petechiae. Based on these data, it is most important that the nurse further evaluate the client's recent:
- ☐ 1. Quality and quantity of food intake.
- ☐ 2. Type and amount of fluid intake.
- ☐ 3. Weakness, fatigue, and ability to get around.
- ☐ 4. Length and amount of menstrual flow.

43. When a client with thrombocytopenia complains of a severe headache, the nurse interprets that this may indicate which of the following?
- ☐ 1. Stress of the disease.
- ☐ 2. Cerebral bleeding.
- ☐ 3. Migraine headache.
- ☐ 4. Sinus congestion.

44. The nurse evaluates that the client correctly understands how to report signs and symptoms of bleeding when the client makes which of the following statements?
- ☐ 1. "Petechiae are large, red skin bruises."
- ☐ 2. "Ecchymoses are large, purple skin bruises."
- ☐ 3. "Purpura is an open cut on the skin."
- ☐ 4. "Abrasions are small pinpoint red dots on the skin."

45. The client states she does not understand what causes idiopathic thrombocytopenic purpura (ITP). The nurse provides which of the following explanations?
- ☐ **1.** It is believed that the platelets are coated with antibodies and the spleen sees them as foreign bodies.
- ☐ **2.** It is believed that the liver identifies the platelets as foreign bodies.
- ☐ **3.** It is now believed that the syndrome is related to an underactive immune system.
- ☐ **4.** The cause is unknown.

46. The nurse should instruct the client with a platelet count of less than 150,000/µl to avoid which of the following activities?
- ☐ **1.** Ambulation.
- ☐ **2.** Valsalva's maneuver.
- ☐ **3.** Visiting with children.
- ☐ **4.** Semi-Fowler's position.

47. If a client who is taking Bufferin Arthritis Strength caplets develops prolonged bleeding from a superficial injury, the nurse recognizes that this clinical manifestation most likely reflects:
- ☐ **1.** A prothrombin time (PT) of 10 seconds.
- ☐ **2.** An activated partial thromboplastin time (aPTT) of 40 seconds.
- ☐ **3.** A bleeding time of 8 minutes.
- ☐ **4.** A coagulation time (CT) of 8 minutes.

48. A client's bone marrow report reveals normal stem cells and precursors of platelets (megakaryocytes) in the presence of decreased circulating platelets. The nurse recognizes a knowledge deficit when the client makes which of the following statements?
- ☐ **1.** "I need to stop flossing and throw away my hard toothbrush."
- ☐ **2.** "I am glad that my report turned out normal."
- ☐ **3.** "Now I know why I have all these bruises."
- ☐ **4.** "I shouldn't jump off that last step anymore."

49. Which early symptom does the nurse observe in a client with thrombocytopenia who has developed a hemorrhage?
- ☐ **1.** Tachycardia.
- ☐ **2.** Bradycardia.
- ☐ **3.** Decreased Pa_{CO_2}.
- ☐ **4.** Narrowed pulse pressure.

50. The client with idiopathic thrombocytopenic purpura (ITP) asks the nurse why she has to take steroids. Which is the nurse's best response?
- ☐ **1.** Steroids destroy the antibodies and prolong the life of platelets.
- ☐ **2.** Steroids neutralize the antigens and prolong the life of platelets.
- ☐ **3.** Steroids increase phagocytosis and increase the life of platelets.
- ☐ **4.** Steroids alter the spleen's recognition of platelets and increase the life of platelets.

51. A client is to be discharged on prednisone. Which of the following statements indicates that the client understands important concepts about the medication therapy?
- ☐ **1.** "I need to take the medicine in divided doses at morning and bedtime."
- ☐ **2.** "I am to take 40 mg of prednisone for 2 months and then stop."
- ☐ **3.** "I need to wear or carry identification that I am taking prednisone."
- ☐ **4.** "Prednisone will give me extra protection from colds and flu."

52. When teaching the client older than age 50 who is receiving long-term prednisone therapy, which of the following actions does the nurse recommend?
- ☐ **1.** Take the prednisone with food.
- ☐ **2.** Take over-the-counter drugs as needed.
- ☐ **3.** Exercise three to four times a week.
- ☐ **4.** Eat foods that are low in potassium.

53. The nurse is preparing a teaching plan about increased exercise for a female client who is receiving long-term corticosteroid therapy. What type of exercise is most appropriate for this client?
- ☐ **1.** Floor exercises.
- ☐ **2.** Stretching.
- ☐ **3.** Running.
- ☐ **4.** Walking.

54. A client with a history of acquired thrombocytopenia has been instructed on how to prevent and control hemorrhage. Which statement indicates that the client needs further intervention?
- ☐ **1.** "I can apply direct pressure over small cuts for at least 5 to 10 minutes to stop a venous bleed."
- ☐ **2.** "I can count the number of tissues saturated to detect blood loss during a nosebleed."
- ☐ **3.** "I can take hormones to decrease blood loss during menses."
- ☐ **4.** "I can count the number of sanitary napkins to detect excess blood loss during menses."

55. Which of the following clinical manifestations does the nurse find in the client who has systemic adverse effects from long-term corticosteroid therapy?
- ☐ **1.** Weight gain.
- ☐ **2.** High serum albumin.
- ☐ **3.** Low sodium.
- ☐ **4.** Hyperkalemia.

56. Platelets should not be administered under which of the following conditions?
- [ ] **1.** The platelet bag is cold.
- [ ] **2.** The platelets are 2 days old.
- [ ] **3.** The platelet bag is at room temperature.
- [ ] **4.** The platelets are 12 hours old.

57. The nurse is preparing to administer platelets. The nurse should:
- [ ] **1.** Check the ABO compatibility.
- [ ] **2.** Administer the platelets slowly.
- [ ] **3.** Gently rotate the bag.
- [ ] **4.** Use a whole blood tubing set.

58. Which of the following indicates that a client has achieved the goal of correctly demonstrating deep breathing for an upcoming splenectomy? The client:
- [ ] **1.** Breathes in through the nose and out through the mouth.
- [ ] **2.** Breathes in through the mouth and out through the nose.
- [ ] **3.** Uses diaphragmatic breathing in the lying, sitting, and standing positions.
- [ ] **4.** Takes a deep breath in through the nose, holds it for 5 seconds, and blows out through pursed lips.

59. A client is scheduled for an elective splenectomy. Before the client goes to surgery, the nurse's final assessment is the client's:
- [ ] **1.** Empty bladder.
- [ ] **2.** Signed consent.
- [ ] **3.** Vital signs.
- [ ] **4.** Name band.

60. When receiving a client from the postanesthesia care unit after a splenectomy, which should the nurse assess after obtaining vital signs?
- [ ] **1.** Nasogastric drainage.
- [ ] **2.** Urinary catheter.
- [ ] **3.** Dressing.
- [ ] **4.** Need for pain medication.

61. The client's family asks why the client who had a splenectomy has a nasogastric (NG) tube. An NG tube is used to:
- [ ] **1.** Move the stomach away from where the spleen was removed.
- [ ] **2.** Irrigate the operative site.
- [ ] **3.** Decrease abdominal distention.
- [ ] **4.** Assess for the gastric pH as peristalsis returns.

62. A client who had a splenectomy is being discharged. Of the following discharge instructions, which is most specific to the client's surgical procedure?
- [ ] **1.** Do not drive.
- [ ] **2.** Alternate rest and activity.
- [ ] **3.** Make an appointment for the staples to be removed.
- [ ] **4.** Report early signs of infection.

63. What is the earliest and most obvious clinical manifestation in a client with acute disseminated intravascular coagulation (DIC)?
- [ ] **1.** Severe shortness of breath.
- [ ] **2.** Bleeding without history or cause.
- [ ] **3.** Orthopnea.
- [ ] **4.** Hematuria.

64. Which of the following is contraindicated for a client diagnosed with disseminated intravascular coagulation (DIC)?
- [ ] **1.** Treating the underlying cause.
- [ ] **2.** Administering heparin.
- [ ] **3.** Administering warfarin sodium (Coumadin).
- [ ] **4.** Replacing depleted blood products.

65. A client with disseminated intravascular coagulation develops clinical manifestations of microvascular thrombosis. The nurse should assess the client for:
- [ ] **1.** Hemoptysis.
- [ ] **2.** Focal ischemia.
- [ ] **3.** Petechiae.
- [ ] **4.** Hematuria.

66. Which of the following is an assessment finding associated with internal bleeding with disseminated intravascular coagulation?
- [ ] **1.** Bradycardia.
- [ ] **2.** Hypertension.
- [ ] **3.** Increasing abdominal girth.
- [ ] **4.** Petechiae.

The Client with White Blood Cell Disorders

67. A 10-year-old client is diagnosed with infectious mononucleosis. Her white blood cell (WBC) count is 19,000/µl. She has a streptococcal throat infection and her spleen is enlarged. She is complaining of aching muscles. Which of the following instructions should the nurse include in discharge planning with the client and her parents? Select all that apply.
- [ ] **1.** Stay on bed rest until the temperature is normal.
- [ ] **2.** Gargle with warm saline while the throat is irritated.
- [ ] **3.** Increase intake of fluids until the infection subsides.
- [ ] **4.** Take aspirin as long as the fever and myalgia persist.
- [ ] **5.** Avoid contact sports while the spleen is enlarged.

68. The nurse notes that the daily white blood cell (WBC) count in a client with aplastic anemia has dropped overnight from 3,900 to 2,900/μl. Which is the appropriate nursing intervention?
☐ **1.** Continue monitoring the client.
☐ **2.** Call the laboratory to verify the report.
☐ **3.** Document the finding.
☐ **4.** Call the physician and place the client in reverse isolation.

69. A client who had an exploratory laparotomy 3 days ago has a white blood cell (WBC) differential with a shift to the left. The nurse instructs unlicensed personnel to report which clinical manifestation?
☐ **1.** Swelling around the incision.
☐ **2.** Redness around the incision.
☐ **3.** Elevated temperature.
☐ **4.** Purulent wound drainage.

70. What does the nurse calculate as the absolute neutrophil count (ANC) for a client with a white blood cell count of 1,200/μl with bands, 1%; neutrophils, 34%; eosinophils, 3%; and basophils, 4%?
☐ **1.** 440.
☐ **2.** 420.
☐ **3.** 468.
☐ **4.** 456.

71. A client with neutropenia has an absolute neutrophil count of 900. What is the client's risk of infection?
☐ **1.** Normal risk.
☐ **2.** Moderate risk.
☐ **3.** High risk.
☐ **4.** Extremely high risk.

72. Which factor besides the degree of neutropenia does the nurse assess in determining the client's risk of infection?
☐ **1.** Length of time neutropenia has existed.
☐ **2.** Health status before neutropenia.
☐ **3.** Body build and weight.
☐ **4.** Resistance to infection in childhood.

73. Which nursing action is important in preventing cross-contamination?
☐ **1.** Change gloves immediately after use.
☐ **2.** Stand 2 feet from the client.
☐ **3.** Speak minimally when in the room.
☐ **4.** Wear long-sleeved shirts.

74. The nurse should teach the neutropenic client and the family to avoid which of the following?
☐ **1.** Using suppositories or enemas.
☐ **2.** Using a high-efficiency particulate air (HEPA) filter mask.
☐ **3.** Performing perianal care after every bowel movement.
☐ **4.** Performing oral care after every meal.

75. The nurse should remind family members who are visiting a client with granulocytopenia to:
☐ **1.** Visit only if they do not have a cold.
☐ **2.** Wash their hands.
☐ **3.** Leave the children at home.
☐ **4.** Avoid kissing the client on the lips.

76. The nurse should remind the unlicensed personnel that which of the following is the most important goal in the care of the neutropenic client in isolation?
☐ **1.** Listening to the client's feelings of concern.
☐ **2.** Completing the client's care in a nonhurried manner.
☐ **3.** Completing all of the client's care at one time.
☐ **4.** Instructing the client to dispose of tissue after blowing the nose.

77. A nurse is obtaining consent for a bone marrow aspiration. What should the nurse do? Select all that apply.
☐ **1.** Witness the client signing the consent form.
☐ **2.** Evaluate that the client understands the procedure.
☐ **3.** Explain the risks of the procedure to the client.
☐ **4.** Verify that the client is signing the consent form of his own free will.
☐ **5.** Determine that the client understands postprocedure care.

78. A client is about to undergo bone marrow aspiration of the sternum. Which of the following statements should the nurse include to provide sensory information to the client?
☐ **1.** "You may feel a warm solution being wiped over your entire front from your neck down to your navel and out to your shoulders."
☐ **2.** "You will not feel the local anesthetic being applied because it will be sprayed on."
☐ **3.** "You will feel a pulling type of discomfort for a few seconds."
☐ **4.** "After the needle is removed, a bandage will be applied around your chest for the first 24 hours."

79. Twenty-four hours after a bone marrow aspiration, the nurse evaluates which of the following as an appropriate client outcome?
☐ **1.** The client maintains bed rest.
☐ **2.** There is redness and swelling at the aspiration site.
☐ **3.** The client requests morphine sulfate for pain.
☐ **4.** There is no bleeding at the aspiration site.

80. A client states, "I don't want any more tests. Who cares what kind of leukemia I have? I just want to be treated now." Which is the nurse's *best* response?
☐ **1.** "I'm sure you are frustrated and want to be well now."
☐ **2.** "Your treatment can be more effective if it is based on more specific information about your disease."
☐ **3.** "Now, you know the tests are necessary and that you are just upset right now."
☐ **4.** "I understand how you feel."

81. During the induction stage for treatment of leukemia, the nurse should remove which items that the family has brought into the room?
- ☐ **1.** A Bible.
- ☐ **2.** A picture.
- ☐ **3.** A sachet of lavender.
- ☐ **4.** A hairbrush.

82. The nurse identifies deficient knowledge when the client undergoing induction therapy for leukemia makes which of the following statements?
- ☐ **1.** "I will have to pace my activities with rest periods."
- ☐ **2.** "I can't wait to get home to my cat!"
- ☐ **3.** "I will use warm saline gargle instead of brushing my teeth."
- ☐ **4.** "I must report a temperature of 100° F."

83. A 60-year-old client with acute myeloid leukemia (AML) states that he overheard one of the other clients say that AML had a very poor prognosis. The client explains to the nurse that he had understood his doctor to say that he had a relatively good prognosis. Which is the nurse's *best* response?
- ☐ **1.** "You must have misunderstood. Whom did you hear that from?"
- ☐ **2.** "AML does have a very poor prognosis for poorly differentiated cells."
- ☐ **3.** "AML is the most common nonlymphocytic leukemia."
- ☐ **4.** "Your doctor stated your prognosis based on the differentiation of your cells."

84. The goal of nursing care for a client with acute myeloid leukemia (AML) is to prevent:
- ☐ **1.** Cardiac arrhythmias.
- ☐ **2.** Liver failure.
- ☐ **3.** Renal failure.
- ☐ **4.** Hemorrhage.

85. Which of the following does the nurse observe in the client with chronic myeloid leukemia (CML)?
- ☐ **1.** Lymphadenopathy.
- ☐ **2.** Hyperplasia of the gum.
- ☐ **3.** Bone pain from expansion of marrow.
- ☐ **4.** Shortness of breath or slight confusion.

86. Which is the peak age range for acquiring acute lymphocytic leukemia (ALL)?
- ☐ **1.** 4 to 12 years.
- ☐ **2.** 20 to 30 years.
- ☐ **3.** 40 to 50 years.
- ☐ **4.** 60 to 70 years.

87. The client with acute lymphocytic leukemia (ALL) is at risk for infection. What should the nurse do?
- ☐ **1.** Place the client in a private room.
- ☐ **2.** Have the client wear a mask.
- ☐ **3.** Have staff wear gowns and gloves.
- ☐ **4.** Restrict visitors.

88. In assessing a client in the early stage of chronic lymphocytic leukemia (CLL), the nurse is aware that the client is prone to experiencing which of the following?
- ☐ **1.** Enlarged, painless lymph nodes.
- ☐ **2.** Headache.
- ☐ **3.** Hyperplasia of the gums.
- ☐ **4.** Unintentional weight loss.

89. Which does the nurse suggest as the most appropriate intervention to manage mucositis for a client with acute leukemia?
- ☐ **1.** "After each meal or every 4 hours while awake, use lemon-glycerin swabs."
- ☐ **2.** "After each meal or every 4 hours while awake, use a commercial mouthwash."
- ☐ **3.** "After each meal or every 4 hours while awake, use a saline or baking soda solution."
- ☐ **4.** "After each meal or every 4 hours while awake, use your own toothpaste and brush."

90. The client with acute leukemia and the health care team establish mutual client outcomes of improved tidal volume and activity tolerance. Which measure would be least likely to promote outcome achievement?
- ☐ **1.** Ambulating in the hallway.
- ☐ **2.** Sitting up in a chair.
- ☐ **3.** Lying in bed and taking deep breaths.
- ☐ **4.** Using a stationary bicycle in the room.

91. The nurse is evaluating the client's learning about combination chemotherapy. Which of the following statements by the client about reasons for using combination chemotherapy indicates the need for *further* explanation?
- ☐ **1.** "Combination chemotherapy is used to interrupt cell growth cycle at different points."
- ☐ **2.** "Combination chemotherapy is used to destroy cancer cells and treat side effects simultaneously."
- ☐ **3.** "Combination chemotherapy is used to decrease resistance."
- ☐ **4.** "Combination chemotherapy is used to minimize the toxicity from using high doses of a single agent."

92. In providing care to the client with leukemia who has developed thrombocytopenia, the nurse assesses the most common sites for bleeding. Which of the following is not a common site?
☐ **1.** Biliary system.
☐ **2.** Gastrointestinal tract.
☐ **3.** Brain and meninges.
☐ **4.** Pulmonary system.

93. The nurse's best explanation for why the severely neutropenic client is placed in reverse isolation is that reverse isolation helps prevent the spread of organisms:
☐ **1.** To the client from sources outside the client's environment.
☐ **2.** From the client to health care personnel, visitors, and other clients.
☐ **3.** By using special techniques to dispose of contaminated materials.
☐ **4.** By using special techniques to handle the client's linens and personal items.

The Client with Lymphoma

94. Which of the following clinical manifestations does the nurse most likely observe in a client with Hodgkin's disease?
☐ **1.** Difficulty swallowing.
☐ **2.** Painless, enlarged cervical lymph nodes.
☐ **3.** Difficulty breathing.
☐ **4.** A feeling of fullness over the liver.

95. A client with a suspected diagnosis of Hodgkin's disease is to have a lymph node biopsy. Which action is correct for handling the lymph node biopsy specimen for histologic examination for this client?
☐ **1.** Maintain sterile technique.
☐ **2.** Use a mask, gloves, and a gown when assisting with the procedure.
☐ **3.** Place the specimen in a container and send it to the laboratory when someone is available to take it.
☐ **4.** Call for a laboratory technician to assist the physician.

96. The client with Hodgkin's disease undergoes an excisional cervical lymph node biopsy under local anesthesia. After the procedure, which does the nurse assess first?
☐ **1.** Vital signs.
☐ **2.** The incision.
☐ **3.** The airway.
☐ **4.** Neurologic signs.

97. The nurse explains to the client that a biopsy of the enlarged lymph node is important because, if Hodgkin's disease is present, the histologic examination will reveal which of the following?
☐ **1.** Tay-Sachs cells.
☐ **2.** Sarcoidosis cells.
☐ **3.** Reed-Sternberg cells.
☐ **4.** Duchenne's cells.

98. When assessing the client with Hodgkin's disease, the nurse is alert for which of the following findings?
☐ **1.** Herpes zoster infections.
☐ **2.** Discolored teeth.
☐ **3.** Hemorrhage.
☐ **4.** Hypercellular immunity.

99. The client with Hodgkin's disease develops B symptoms. These manifestations indicate which of the following?
☐ **1.** The client has a low-grade fever (temperature lower than 100° F [37.8° C]).
☐ **2.** The client has a weight loss of 5% or less of body weight.
☐ **3.** The client has night sweats.
☐ **4.** The client probably has not progressed to an advanced stage.

100. The client tells the nurse that he wants to be sure that he is receiving the latest staging technique for his lymphoma. The nurse tells the client that which of the following is being used *less* frequently in the staging of lymphomas?
☐ **1.** Body scans.
☐ **2.** Radiography.
☐ **3.** Blood studies.
☐ **4.** Exploratory laparotomy with lymph node biopsy.

101. The client asks the nurse to explain what it means that his Hodgkin's disease is diagnosed at stage 1A. Which of the following describes the involvement of the disease?
☐ **1.** Involvement of a single lymph node.
☐ **2.** Involvement of two or more lymph nodes on the same side of the diaphragm.
☐ **3.** Involvement of lymph node regions on both sides of the diaphragm.
☐ **4.** Diffuse disease of one or more extralymphatic organs.

102. A client is undergoing a bone marrow aspiration and biopsy. What is the best way for the nurse to help the client handle her stress?
- ☐ 1. Allow the client's family to stay with her as long as possible.
- ☐ 2. Stay with the client and hold her hand without speaking.
- ☐ 3. Encourage the client to take slow, deep breaths to relax.
- ☐ 4. Allow the client time to express her feelings.

103. The nurse explains to the client with Hodgkin's disease that a bone marrow biopsy will be taken after the aspiration. What should the nurse explain about the biopsy?
- ☐ 1. "Your biopsy will be performed before the aspiration because enough tissue may be obtained so that you won't have to go through the aspiration."
- ☐ 2. "You will feel a pressure sensation when the biopsy is taken but should not feel actual pain; if you do, tell the doctor so that you can be given extra numbing medicine."
- ☐ 3. "You may hear a crunch as the needle passes through the bone, but when the biopsy is taken, you will feel a suction-type pain that will last for just a moment."
- ☐ 4. "You will be shaved and cleaned with an antiseptic agent, after which the doctor will inject a needle without making an incision to aspirate out the bone marrow."

104. A client with advanced Hodgkin's disease is readmitted because death is imminent. The goal of nursing care is to help relieve the client's:
- ☐ 1. Fear of pain.
- ☐ 2. Fear of further therapy.
- ☐ 3. Feelings of isolation.
- ☐ 4. Feelings of social inadequacy.

105. The client is a survivor of non-Hodgkin's lymphoma. Which of the following statements indicates the client needs additional information?
- ☐ 1. "Regular screening is very important for me."
- ☐ 2. "The survivor rate is directly proportional to the incidence of second malignancy."
- ☐ 3. "The survivor rate is indirectly proportional to the incidence of second malignancy."
- ☐ 4. "It is important for survivors to know the stage of the disease and their current treatment plan."

The Client Who Is in Shock

106. Which of the following is the most important goal of nursing care for a client who is in shock?
- ☐ 1. Manage fluid overload.
- ☐ 2. Manage increased cardiac output.
- ☐ 3. Manage inadequate tissue perfusion.
- ☐ 4. Manage vasoconstriction of vascular beds.

107. Which of the following nursing assessment findings indicates hypovolemic shock in a client who has had a 15% blood loss?
- ☐ 1. Pulse rate less than 60 bpm.
- ☐ 2. Respiratory rate of 4 breaths/minute.
- ☐ 3. Pupils unequally dilated.
- ☐ 4. Systolic blood pressure less than 90 mm Hg.

108. Which of the following findings is the best indication that fluid replacement for the client in hypovolemic shock is adequate?
- ☐ 1. Urine output greater than 30 ml/hour.
- ☐ 2. Systolic blood pressure greater than 110 mm Hg.
- ☐ 3. Diastolic blood pressure greater than 90 mm Hg.
- ☐ 4. Respiratory rate of 20 breaths/minute.

109. Which of the following is a risk factor for hypovolemic shock?
- ☐ 1. Hemorrhage.
- ☐ 2. Antigen-antibody reaction.
- ☐ 3. Gram-negative bacteria.
- ☐ 4. Vasodilation.

110. Which is a priority assessment for the client in shock who is receiving an I.V. infusion of packed red blood cells and normal saline solution?
- ☐ 1. Fluid balance.
- ☐ 2. Anaphylactic reaction.
- ☐ 3. Pain.
- ☐ 4. Altered level of consciousness.

111. The client who does not respond adequately to fluid replacement has an order for an I.V. infusion of dopamine hydrochloride at 5 μg/kg/minute. The desired effect of this drug is:
- ☐ 1. Increased renal and mesenteric blood flow.
- ☐ 2. Increased cardiac output.
- ☐ 3. Vasoconstriction.
- ☐ 4. Reduced preload and afterload.

112. Which of the following should be an essential nursing action for the client who is receiving dopamine hydrochloride for treatment of shock?
- ☐ 1. Administer pain medication concurrently.
- ☐ 2. Monitor blood pressure continuously.
- ☐ 3. Evaluate arterial blood gases at least every 2 hours.
- ☐ 4. Monitor for signs of infection.

113. A male client who has been taking warfarin (Coumadin) has been admitted with severe acute rectal bleeding and the following laboratory results: International Normalized Ratio (INR), 8; hemoglobin, 11 g/dl; and hematocrit, 33%. Which of the following physician orders should the nurse expect to implement initially? Select all that apply.
- ☐ 1. Administer I.V. dextrose 5% in 0.45% normal saline solution.
- ☐ 2. Schedule client for a sigmoidoscopy in the morning.
- ☐ 3. Give 1 unit fresh frozen plasma (FFP).
- ☐ 4. Administer vitamin K (AquaMEPHYTON) 2.5 mg P.O.
- ☐ 5. Begin giving polyethylene glycol-electrolyte solution (GoLYTELY) in preparation for sigmoidoscopy.
- ☐ 6. Administer Fleet enema.

114. The nurse in the preoperative holding area keeps a client with gastric bleeding in a dimly lit environment with one family member present. What is the primary rationale for these nursing interventions?
- ☐ 1. To stabilize fluid and electrolyte balance.
- ☐ 2. To minimize oxygen consumption.
- ☐ 3. To increase client and family comfort.
- ☐ 4. To prevent infection.

115. When assessing a client for early septic shock, the nurse observes for which of the following?
- ☐ 1. Cool, clammy skin.
- ☐ 2. Warm, flushed skin.
- ☐ 3. Decreased systolic blood pressure.
- ☐ 4. Hemorrhage.

116. A client with toxic shock has been receiving ceftriaxone sodium (Rocephin), 1 g every 12 hours. In addition to culture and sensitivity studies, which other laboratory findings does the nurse monitor?
- ☐ 1. Serum creatinine.
- ☐ 2. Spinal fluid analysis.
- ☐ 3. Arterial blood gases.
- ☐ 4. Serum osmolality.

117. Which nursing intervention is *most* important in preventing septic shock?
- ☐ 1. Administering I.V. fluid replacement therapy as ordered.
- ☐ 2. Obtaining vital signs every 4 hours for all clients.
- ☐ 3. Monitoring red blood cell counts for elevation.
- ☐ 4. Maintaining asepsis of indwelling urinary catheters.

118. Which of the following is an indication of a complication of septic shock?
- ☐ 1. Anaphylaxis.
- ☐ 2. Acute respiratory distress syndrome (ARDS).
- ☐ 3. Chronic obstructive pulmonary disease (COPD).
- ☐ 4. Mitral valve prolapse.

Correct Answers and Rationales

The letter in parentheses after each rationale identifies the client need addressed in the item, including management of care (M), safety and infection control (S), health promotion and maintenance (H), psychosocial adaptation (P), basic care and comfort (C), pharmacological and parenteral therapies (D), reduction of risk potential (R), and physiological adaptation (A).

The Client with Red Blood Cell Disorders

1.

3.	Verify the client has signed an informed consent.
1.	Position the client in a side-lying position.
2.	Clean the skin with an antiseptic solution.
4.	Apply ice to the biopsy site.

First, the nurse must verify that the client has voluntarily signed a consent form before the procedure begins, and check that the client understands the procedure. The nurse then positions the client in a side-lying, or *lateral decubitus*, position with the affected side up. Then she must clean the skin site and surrounding area with an antiseptic solution such as Betadine before the health care provider numbs the site and collects the specimen. When the procedure is finished, the nurse must apply ice to the biopsy site to reduce pain. (M)

2. 1, 2, 5. Nausea and vomiting are common adverse effects of oral iron preparations. The nurse should first ask the client why she does not want to take the oral medication, and then suggest ways to decrease the nausea and vomiting. Ginger may help minimize the nausea and the client can try this remedy and evaluate its effectiveness. Iron should be taken on an empty stomach but can be taken with orange juice. The client can evaluate if this helps the nausea. Stool softeners should not be used in clients with iron deficiency anemia. Instead, constipation can be prevented by following a high-fiber diet. Administering iron intramuscularly is done only if other approaches are not effective. (H)

3. 1. This client is likely experiencing fatigue and should increase her periods of rest. The fatigue may be caused by anemia from depletion of red blood cells due to the chemotherapy. Asking the client to limit her activities may cause the client to become withdrawn. The information given does not support limiting activity. Increasing fluid intake will not reduce the fatigue. The information does not indicate that the client is immunosuppressed and should avoid contact with others. (A)

4. 1, 2, 3. Using designated donors does not decrease the risk of contracting infectious diseases, such as the Epstein-Barr virus, HIV, or CMV. Hepatitis A is transmitted by the oral-fecal route, not the blood route; however, hepatitis B and C can be contracted from a designated donor. Malaria is transmitted by mosquitoes. (S)

5. 4. A routine serology study to confirm compatibility between a blood donor and recipient takes about 1 hour. In an emergency, O negative RBCs can be safely administered to most clients, which is why a person with O-negative blood is called a *universal donor.* The other types of RBCs may cause an adverse reaction. (S)

6. 3. When two clients are to receive blood at the same time, the nurse should call and hang the clients' transfusions separately to avoid error. The nurse should call for and hang the first client's blood first because this client has experienced a change in blood pressure over a short period of time. The nurse should next call and hang the second client's blood transfusion as there is no indication that this client is unstable at this time. The nurse should not call for both units of transfusions at the same time due to the increased risk of misidentification. The nurse should not verify compatibility of both units at the same time due to the increased risk of misidentification. It is not necessary to involve two nurses because the second client can wait until the nurse has time to hang the blood. (A)

7. 1. One of the microcytic, hypochromic anemias is iron deficiency anemia. A rich source of iron is needed in the diet, and eggs are high in iron. Other foods high in iron include organ and muscle (dark) meats; shellfish, shrimp, and tuna; enriched, whole-grain, and fortified cereals and breads; legumes, nuts, dried fruits, and beans; oatmeal; and sweet potatoes. Dark green, leafy vegetables and citrus fruits are good sources of vitamin C. Cheese is a good source of calcium. (R)

8. 3. Good sources of vitamin B_{12} include meats and dairy products. Whole grains are a good source of thiamine. Green, leafy vegetables are good sources of niacin, folate, and carotenoids (precursors of vitamin A). Broccoli and brussels sprouts are good sources of ascorbic acid (vitamin C). (R)

9. 4. The normal range of folic acid is 1.8 to 9 ng/ml, and the normal range of vitamin B_{12} (cyanocobalamin) is 200 to 900 pg/ml. A low folic acid level in the presence of a normal vitamin B_{12} level is indicative of a primary folic acid deficiency anemia. Factors that affect the absorption

of folic acid are drugs such as methotrexate, oral contraceptives, antiseizure drugs, and alcohol. The total bilirubin, serum creatinine, and hemoglobin values are within normal limits. (A)

10. 2. The defining characteristic of pernicious anemia, a megaloblastic anemia, is lack of the intrinsic factor, which results from atrophy of the stomach wall. Without the intrinsic factor, vitamin B_{12} cannot be absorbed in the small intestines, and folic acid needs vitamin B_{12} for deoxyribonucleic acid synthesis of RBCs. The gastric analysis was done to determine the primary cause of the anemia. An elevated excretion of the injected radioactive vitamin B_{12}, which is protocol for the first and second stage of the Schilling test, indicates that the client has the intrinsic factor and can absorb vitamin B_{12} into the intestinal tract. A sedimentation rate of 16 mm/hour is normal for both men and women and is a nonspecific test to detect the presence of inflammation. It is not specific to anemias. An RBC value of 5.0 million/µl is a normal value for both men and women and does not indicate an anemia. (A)

11. 2. Clients with aplastic anemia are severely immunocompromised and at risk for infection and possible death related to bone marrow suppression and pancytopenia. Strict aseptic technique and reverse isolation are important measures to prevent infection. Although diet, reduced stress, and rest are valued in supporting health, the potentially fatal consequence of an acute infection places it as a priority for teaching the client about health maintenance. Animal meat and dark green leafy vegetables, good sources of vitamin B_{12} and folic acid, should be included in the daily diet. Yoga and meditation are good complementary therapies to reduce stress. Eight hours of rest and naps are good for spacing and pacing activity and rest. (R)

12. 4. Vitamin B_{12} combines with intrinsic factor in the stomach and is then carried to the ileum, where it is absorbed into the bloodstream. In this situation, vitamin B_{12} cannot be absorbed regardless of the amount of oral intake of sources of vitamin B_{12}, such as animal protein or vitamin B_{12} tablets. Vitamin B_{12} needs to be injected every month because the ileum has been surgically removed. Replacement of fluids and electrolytes is important when the client has continuous multiple loose stools on a daily basis. Warm salt water is used to soothe sore mucous membranes. Crohn's disease and a small-bowel resection may cause several loose stools a day. (A)

13. 3. Coffee and tea increase gastrointestinal motility and inhibit the absorption of nonheme iron. Clients are instructed to add dried fruits to dishes at every meal because dried fruits are a nonheme or nonanimal iron source. Cooking in iron cookware, especially acid-based foods such as tomatoes, adds iron to the diet. Clients are instructed to add a rich supply of vitamin C to every meal because the absorption of iron is increased when food with vitamin C or ascorbic acid is consumed. (R)

14. 1. It is difficult to determine activity intolerance without objectively comparing activities from one time frame to another. Because iron deficiency anemia can occur gradually and individual endurance varies, the nurse can best assess the client's activity tolerance by asking the client to compare activities 6 months ago and at present. Asking a client how long a problem has existed is a very open-ended question that allows for too much subjectivity for any definition of the client's activity tolerance. Also, the client may not even identify that a "problem" exists. Asking the client whether he is staying abreast of usual activities addresses whether the tasks were completed, not the tolerance of the client while the tasks were being completed or the resulting condition of the client after the tasks were completed. Asking the client if he is more tired now than usual does not address his activity tolerance. Tiredness is a subjective evaluation and again can be distorted by factors such as the gradual onset of the anemia or the endurance of the individual. (R)

15. 4, 6. A client with pernicious anemia has lost the ability to absorb vitamin B_{12} either because of the lack of an acidic gastric environment or the lack of the intrinsic factor. Vitamin B_{12} must be administered by a deep intramuscular route. The ventrogluteal and dorsogluteal locations are the most acceptable sites for a deep intramuscular injection. The other sites are not acceptable. (D)

16. 2. To promote comfort when injecting at the ventrogluteal site, the position of choice is with the client lying on the abdomen with toes pointed inward. This positioning promotes muscle relaxation, which decreases the discomfort of making an injection into a tense muscle. Lying on the side with legs extended will not provide the greatest muscle relaxation. Leaning over the edge of a table with the hips flexed and standing upright with the feet apart will increase muscular tension. (A)

17. 1, 2, 3, 4. The nurse should ask the client about symptoms related to pernicious anemia because she had her stomach stapled 2 years ago and shows no history of supplemental vitamin B_{12}. Numbness and tingling relate to a loss of intrinsic factor from the gastric stapling. Intrinsic factor is necessary for absorption of vitamin B_{12}. The nurse should suspect pernicious anemia if the client is not taking supplemental vitamin B_{12}. Other signs and symptoms of pernicious anemia include cognitive problems and depression. The nurse also should ask about the client's support at home in case the fall was not an acci-

dent. Pernicious anemia is not related to dietary intake of iron. (R)

18. 1. The nurse should prepare to start an intake and output record because the client is exhibiting clinical manifestations of anemia with jaundice and is demonstrating a fluid imbalance. The client does not need to be on bed rest at this point. The client is not contagious and does not need to be placed in contact isolation. The changes in the color of the skin and urine are related to the jaundice and will not be affected by sunlight. (A)

19. 3. Pernicious anemia is caused by the body's inability to absorb vitamin B_{12}. This results from a lack of intrinsic factor in the gastric juices. Schilling's test helps diagnose pernicious anemia by determining the client's ability to absorb vitamin B_{12}. (A)

20. 2. Urinary vitamin B_{12} levels are measured after the ingestion of radioactive vitamin B_{12}. A 24- to 48-hour urine specimen is collected after administration of an oral dose of radioactively tagged vitamin B_{12} and an injection of nonradioactive vitamin B_{12}. In a healthy state of absorption, excess vitamin B_{12} is excreted in the urine; in a malabsorptive state or when the intrinsic factor is missing, vitamin B_{12} is excreted in the feces. Citrucel is a bulk-forming agent. Laxatives interfere with the absorption of vitamin B_{12}. The client is NPO 8 to 12 hours before the test but is not NPO during the test. A stool collection is not a part of the Schilling test. If stool contaminates the urine collection, the results will be altered. (D)

21. 3. This client has clinical manifestations of thalassemia major, a disease found in descendants from the Mediterranean Sea area whose mother and father both possess the gene for thalassemia (i.e., the client is homozygous for the gene). The severe hemolytic anemia causes sequestration of red blood cells in the spleen and liver, which leads to engorgement of the organs, and chronic bone marrow hyperplasia, which leads to widening of the bones. Mental and physical growth is retarded, and the only treatment is blood transfusion, and chelation therapy if numerous transfusions have been administered. Death may result from cardiac enlargement and failure. (A)

22. 2. Most clients with pernicious anemia have deficient production of intrinsic factor in the stomach. Intrinsic factor attaches to the vitamin in the stomach and forms a complex that allows the vitamin to be absorbed in the small intestine. The stomach is producing enough acid, there is not an excessive excretion of the vitamin, and there is not a rapid production of red blood cells in this condition. (A)

23. **2.** This client presented with the typical signs of glucose-6-phosphate dehydrogenase (G6PD)–deficiency anemia. Ten percent of African Americans inherit an X-linked recessive disorder of the G6PD enzyme in the red blood cell (RBC). When cells with decreased levels of G6PD are exposed to certain drugs, such as sulfonamides, acetylsalicylic acid, thiazide diuretics, and vitamin K, the RBC may hemolyze and anemia and jaundice may occur. The reaction is self-limited as soon as the causative agent is withheld. No further treatment is necessary except counseling to prevent acute incidence by avoiding exposure to specific drugs. There is no need for increased folic acid, restricted activity in hot weather, or blood transfusions. (A)

24. **2.** The normal physiologic response to activity is an increased metabolic rate over the resting basal rate. The decrease in respiratory rate indicates that the client is not strong enough to complete the mechanical cycle of respiration needed for gas exchange. The postactivity pulse is expected to increase immediately after activity but by no more than 50 bpm if it is strenuous activity. The diastolic blood pressure is expected to rise but by no more than 15 mm Hg. The pulse returns to within 6 bpm of the resting pulse after 3 minutes of rest. (A)

25. **3.** The nurse should continue to monitor the client because this value reflects a normal physiologic response. The physician does not need to be called, and oxygen does not need to be started based on these laboratory findings. Immediately after surgery, the client's hematocrit reflects a falsely high value related to the body's compensatory response to the stress of sudden loss of fluids and blood. Activation of the intrinsic pathway and the renin-angiotensin cycle via antidiuretic hormone produces vasoconstriction and retention of fluid for the first 1 to 2 days postoperatively. By the second to third day, this response decreases and the client's hematocrit level is more reflective of the amount of RBCs in the plasma. Fresh bleeding is a less likely occurrence on the third postoperative day but is not impossible; however, the nurse should have expected to see a decrease in the RBC count and hemoglobin value accompanying the hematocrit. (A)

26. **4.** The most likely time for a blood transfusion reaction to occur is during the first 15 minutes or first 50 ml of the infusion. If a blood transfusion reaction does occur, it is imperative to keep an established I.V. line so that medication can be administered to prevent or treat cardiovascular collapse in case of anaphylaxis. PRBCs should be administered through a 19-gauge or larger needle; a peripherally inserted central catheter line is not recommended, in order to avoid a slow flow. RBCs will hemolyze in dextrose or lactated Ringer's solution and should be infused with only normal saline solution. (D)

27. **1, 2, 4.** The nurse should teach the client to drink plenty of fluids when outside in hot weather to avoid becoming dehydrated. The client should avoid high altitudes such as mountains where the oxygen levels are low and may precipitate a sickle cell crisis. The nurse should alert young women with sickle cell anemia that pregnancy increases the risk of a crisis. People who are homozygous for HbS have sickle cell anemia; the heterozygous form is the sickle cell carrier trait. (H)

28. **2.** The nurse should teach the client and family that individuals who are heterozygous for hemochromatosis rarely develop the disease. The nurse should teach that men and women are equally at risk for hemochromatosis, but men are diagnosed earlier because women do not usually have manifestations until menopause. Hemochromatosis is the most common genetic disorder in the United States. Individuals who are homozygous for hemochromatosis received a defective gene from each parent. Those with homozygous genes may develop the disease. (H)

29. **2, 3, 5.** The American Association of Blood Banks recommends that two qualified people, such as two registered nurses or a physician and a registered nurse, compare the name and number on the identification bracelet with the tag on the blood bag. Verifying that the two units are the same is not a recommendation. Rather, the verification is always with the client, not with bags of blood. A unit of blood should infuse in 4 hours or less to avoid the risk of septicemia since no preservatives are used. When a blood transfusion reaction occurs, the blood transfusion should be stopped immediately, but the I.V. line should be kept open so that emergency medications and fluids can be administered. The unit of PRBCs should be inspected for contamination by looking for leaks, abnormal color, clots, and excessive air bubbles. When a unit of PRBCs is being transfused, vital signs are assessed before the transfusion begins, after the first 15 minutes, and then every hour until 1 hour after the transfusion has been completed. When PRBCs are being administered, a 20-gauge or larger needle is needed to avoid destroying the RBCs passing through the lumen and to allow for maximal flow rate. (D)

30. **1.** Low back pain occurs when the RBCs of the recipient's serum antibodies react with the donor RBC antigens. The renal tubules become obstructed with the hemoglobin freed from the hemolysis of RBCs. Hemoglobinuria can lead to acute renal failure. Freed hemoglobin in the urine and blood samples taken at the time of the reaction provide evidence of a hemolytic blood transfusion reaction. Antipyretics are administered with febrile, nonhemolytic transfusion reactions. Diuretics, oxygen, and morphine are administered with circulatory overload. Vasopressors are administered with septic transfusion reactions. (D)

31. 1. Epoetin (Epogen) is a recombinant DNA form of erythropoietin, which stimulates the production of RBCs and therefore causes the hematocrit to rise. The elevation in hematocrit causes an elevation in the blood pressure; therefore, the blood pressure is a vital sign that should be checked. The partial thromboplastin time, hemoglobin level, and prothrombin time are not monitored for this drug. (D)

32. 4, 5, 6. Erythropoietin is administered to decrease the need for blood transfusions by stimulating RBC production. The medication should be administered through the I.V. line without other medications to avoid a reaction. The hematocrit, a simple measurement of the percent of RBCs in the total blood volume, is used to monitor this therapy. When initiating I.V. erythropoietin therapy, the nurse should monitor the hematocrit level so that it rises no more than four points in any 2-week period. In addition, the initial doses of erythropoietin are adjusted according to the client's changes in blood pressure. The nurse should tell the client to avoid driving and performing hazardous activity during the initial treatment due to possible dizziness and headaches secondary to the adverse effect of hypertension. The hematocrit, not the hemoglobin level, is used for monitoring the effectiveness of therapy. The vial of erythropoietin should not be shaken because it may be biologically inactive. The solution should not be used if it is discolored. The nurse should not reenter the vial once it has been entered; it is a one-time use vial. All remaining erythropoietin should be discarded since it does not contain preservatives. (D)

33. 4. Vitamin B_{12} is a water-soluble vitamin. When water-soluble vitamins are taken in excess of the body's needs, they are filtered through the kidneys and excreted. Vitamin B_{12} is considered to be nontoxic. Adverse reactions that have occurred are believed to be related to impurities or to the preservative in B_{12} preparations. Ringing in the ears, rash, and nausea are not considered to be related to vitamin B_{12} administration. (D)

34. 2. Brown rice is a source of iron from plant sources (nonheme iron). Other sources of nonheme iron are whole-grain cereals and breads, dark green vegetables, legumes, nuts, dried fruits (apricots, raisins, dates), oatmeal, and sweet potatoes. Egg yolks have iron but it is not as well absorbed as iron from other sources. Vegetables are a good source of vitamins that may facilitate iron absorption. Tea contains tannin, which combines with nonheme iron, preventing its absorption. (A)

35. 2. Macrocytic anemias can result from deficiencies in vitamin B_{12} or ascorbic acid. Only vitamin B_{12} deficiency causes diminished sensations of peripheral nerve endings. The nurse should assess for peripheral neuropathy and instruct the client in self-care activities for her diminished sensation to heat and pain (e.g., using a heating pad at a lower heat setting, making frequent checks to protect against skin trauma). The burn could be related to abuse, but this conclusion would require more supporting data. The findings should be documented, but the nurse would want to address the client's sensations first. The decision of how to treat the burn should be determined by the physician. (R)

36. 3. Pruritus is a late symptom that results from abnormal histamine metabolism. Headache and dizziness are early symptoms from engorged veins. Shortness of breath is an early symptom from congested mucous membranes and ineffective gas exchange. (A)

37. 2, 3, 4, 5. Polycythemia vera, a condition in which too many RBCs are produced in the blood serum, can lead to an increase in the hematocrit and hypervolemia, hyperviscosity, and hypertension. Subsequently, the client can experience dizziness, tinnitus, visual disturbances, headaches, or a feeling of fullness in the head. The client may also experience cardiovascular symptoms such as heart failure (shortness of breath and orthopnea) and increased clotting time or symptoms of an increased uric acid level such as painful, swollen joints (usually the big toe). Hearing loss and weight loss are not manifestations associated with polycythemia vera. (R)

38. 1. Aplastic anemia decreases the bone marrow production of RBCs, white blood cells, and platelets. The client is at risk for bruising and bleeding tendencies. A change in the client's intake and output is important, but assessment for the potential for bleeding takes priority. Change in the peripheral nervous system is a priority problem specific to clients with vitamin B_{12} deficiency. Change in bowel function is not associated with aplastic anemia. (A)

The Client with Platelet Disorders

39. 3. A dose of 0.5 mg of protamine sulfate reverses a 100-unit dose of heparin within 20 minutes. The nurse should administer protamine sulfate by I.V. push slowly to avoid adverse effects, such as hypotension, dyspnea, bradycardia, and anaphylaxis. (D)

40. 1, 3, 4, 5. Older adults may have little subcutaneous tissue, so the area around the anterior iliac crest is a suitable site for these clients. The nurse should use a 27G,

⅝″ needle. Cephalosporin and penicillin potentiate the effects of heparin. Two nurses should check the dose because a dose error could cause hemorrhage. The onset of heparin is not immediate when given subcutaneously. (D)

41. **1.** A client with a platelet count of 30,000 to 50,000/µl is susceptible to bruising with minor trauma. Padding areas that the client might bump, scratch, or hit may help prevent minor trauma. A platelet count of 15,000 to 30,000/µl may result in spontaneous petechiae and bruising, especially on the extremities. Safety measures to pad surfaces would still be used, but the focus would be on assessing for new spontaneous petechiae. Keeping the room dark does not help the client with a low platelet count. When the count is lower than 20,000/µl, the client is at risk for spontaneous bleeding from the mucous membranes (oral, nasal, urinary, and rectal) and intracranial bleeding. (R)

42. **4.** A recent viral infection in a female client between the ages of 20 and 30 with a history of systemic lupus erythematosus and an insidious onset of diffuse petechiae are hallmarks of idiopathic thrombocytopenic purpura. It is important to ask whether the client's recent menses have been lengthened or are heavier. Determining her ability to clot can help determine her risk of increased bleeding tendency until a platelet count is drawn. Petechiae are not caused by poor nutrition. Because of poor food and fluid intake or weakness and fatigue, the client may have gotten bruises from falling or bumping into things, but not petechiae. (R)

43. **2.** When the platelet count is very low, RBCs leak out of the blood vessels and into the tissue. If the blood pressure is elevated and the platelet count falls to less than 15,000/µl, internal bleeding in the brain can occur. A severe headache occurs from meningeal irritation when blood leaks out of the cerebral vasculature. When a client has thrombocytopenia, the nurse should always assess for cerebral bleeding by checking vital signs and performing neurologic checks. Headaches can be caused by stress, migraines, and sinus congestion. However, the concern here is the risk of internal bleeding into the brain. (H)

44. **2.** Large, purplish skin lesions caused by hemorrhage are called ecchymoses. Small, flat, red pinpoint lesions are petechiae. Numerous petechiae result in a reddish, bruised appearance called purpura. An abrasion is a wound caused by scraping. (H)

45. **1.** Previously the cause was unknown, but recent research suggests that idiopathic thrombocytopenic purpura occurs when antibody-coated platelets are identified as foreign bodies and destroyed by macrophages in the spleen. It is not an idiosyncratic response and is not related to a depressed immune system. (H)

46. **2.** When the platelet count is less than 150,000/µl, prolonged bleeding can occur from trauma, injury, or straining such as with Valsalva's maneuver. Clients should avoid any activity that causes straining to evacuate the bowel. Clients can ambulate, but pointed or sharp surfaces should be padded. Clients can visit with their families but should avoid any scratches, bumps, or scrapes. Clients can sit in a semi-Fowler's position but should change positions to promote circulation and check for petechiae. (H)

47. **3.** Bufferin contains aspirin, which is an antiplatelet agent that prevents platelet aggregation. After a 300-mg dose of aspirin, the bleeding time can be prolonged as long as 5 days. One of the best methods to check for platelet deficiency is the bleeding time test. A number of other drugs, such as alcohol, sulfonamides, and thiazide diuretics, can prolong the bleeding time. The PT evaluates the extrinsic pathway (coagulation factor VIII) and represents the time it takes to form a firm clot. The PT value is normal in severe thrombocytopenia. The aPTT evaluates the intrinsic and common coagulation pathway and represents the time it takes to form a firm clot. It is basically the same as the partial thromboplastin time but is considered to be more reliably reproducible and faster. The aPTT value is normal in severe thrombocytopenia. The CT, or Lee-White coagulation time, is normal, but it is an old and insensitive test that does not rule out a coagulation defect. (D)

48. **2.** The client who states that the test results are normal has only heard that the bone marrow is functioning. The etiology is in the destruction of circulating platelets. Further tests must be completed to determine the cause (e.g., a coating of the platelets with antibodies that are seen as foreign bodies). The bone marrow result does rule out other potential diagnoses such as anemia, leukemia, or myeloproliferative disorders that involve bone marrow depression. The client needs to stop flossing and throw away his hard toothbrush, which can lead to bleeding of the gums. The destruction of the circulating platelets accounts for the easy bruising and the need to protect oneself from further bruising. The client should not jump or increase exertion of joints, which may lead to bleeding in the joints and joint pain. (R)

49. **1.** The nurse observes tachycardia in the hemorrhaging client because the heart beats faster to compensate for decreased circulating volume and decreased numbers of oxygen-carrying RBCs. The degree of cardiopulmonary distress and anemia will be related to the amount of hemorrhage that occurred and the period of time over which it occurred. Bradycardia is a late symptom of hemorrhage; it occurs after the client is no longer able to compromise and is debilitating further into shock. If bradycardia is left untreated, the client will die from cardiovascular collapse. Decreased Paco$_2$ is a late symptom of hemorrhage, after transport of oxygen to the tissue has been affected. A narrowed pulse pressure is not an early sign of hemorrhage. (A)

50. 4. ITP is treated with steroids to suppress the splenic macrophages from phagocytizing the antibody-coated platelets, which are recognized as foreign bodies, so that the platelets live longer. The steroids also suppress the binding of the autoimmune antibody to the platelet surface. Steroids do not destroy the antibodies on the platelets, neutralize antigens, or increase phagocytosis. (D)

51. 3. The client needs to wear or carry information containing the name of the drug, dosage, physician and contact information, and emergency instructions because additional corticosteroid drug therapy would be needed during emergency situations. Prednisone should be taken in the morning because it can cause insomnia and because exogenous corticosteroid suppression of the adrenal cortex is less when it is administered in the morning. Prednisone must never be stopped suddenly. It must be tapered off to allow for the adrenal cortex to recover from drug-induced atrophy so that it can resume its function. Prednisone suppresses the immune response and masks infections. It does not provide extra protection against infection. (D)

52. 1. Nausea, vomiting, and peptic ulcers are gastrointestinal adverse effects of prednisone, so it is recommended that clients take the prednisone with food. In some instances, the client may be advised to take a prescribed antacid prophylactically. The client should never take over-the-counter drugs without notifying the physician who prescribed the prednisone. The client should ask the physician about the amount and kind of exercise because of the need to establish baseline physical values before starting an exercise program and because of the increased potential for comorbidity with increasing age. The client should eat foods that are high in potassium to prevent hypokalemia. (D)

53. 4. The best exercise for females who are on long-term corticosteroid therapy is a low-impact, weight-bearing exercise such as walking or weight lifting. Floor exercises do not provide for the weight bearing. Stretching is appropriate but does not offer sufficient weight bearing. Running provides for weight bearing but is hard on the joints and may cause bleeding. (D)

54. 2. The client needs further teaching if she thinks that the number of tissues saturated represents all of the blood lost during a nosebleed. During a nosebleed, a significant amount of blood can be swallowed and go undetected. It is important that clients with severe thrombocytopenia do not take a nosebleed lightly. Clients with thrombocytopenia can apply pressure for 5 to 10 minutes over a small, superficial cut. Clients with thrombocytopenia can take hormones to suppress menses and control menstrual blood loss. Clients can also count the number of saturated sanitary napkins to approximate blood loss during menses. Some authorities estimate that a completely soaked sanitary napkin holds 50 ml. (R)

55. 1. Adverse effects of prednisone are weight gain, retention of sodium and fluids with hypertension and cushingoid features, a low serum albumin level, suppressed inflammatory processes with masked symptoms, and osteoporosis. A diet high in protein, potassium, calcium, vitamin D, and vitamin C is recommended. (D)

56. 1. Platelets cannot survive cold temperatures. The platelets should be stored at room temperature and last for no more than 5 days. (D)

57. 3. The bag containing platelets needs to be gently rotated to prevent clumping. ABO compatibility is not a necessary requirement, but human leukocyte antigen (HLA) matching of lymphocytes may be completed to avoid development of anti-HLA antibodies when multiple platelet transfusions are necessary. Platelets should be administered as fast as can be tolerated by the client to avoid aggregation. Most institutions use tubing especially for platelets instead of tubing for blood and blood products. (D)

58. 4. The correct technique for deep breathing postoperatively to avoid atelectasis and pneumonia is to take in a deep breath through the nose, hold it for 5 seconds, then blow it out through pursed lips. The goal is to fully expand and empty the lungs for pulmonary hygiene. (R)

59. 3. An elective surgical procedure is scheduled in advance so that all preparations can be completed ahead of time. The vital signs are the final check that must be completed before the client leaves the room so that continuity of care and assessment is provided for. The first assessment that will be completed in the preoperative holding area or operating room will be the client's vital signs. The client should have emptied the bladder before receiving preoperative medications so that the bladder is empty when it is time for transport into the operating room. The client should have signed the consent before the transport time so that if there were any questions or concerns there was time to meet with the surgeon. Also, the consent form must be signed before any sedative medications are given. The client's name band should be placed as soon as the client arrives in the perioperative setting, and it remains in place through discharge. (A)

60. 3. After a splenectomy, the client is at high risk for hypovolemia and hemorrhage. The dressing should be checked often; if drainage is present, a circle should be drawn around the drainage and the time noted to help determine how fast bleeding is occurring. The nasogastric tube should be connected, but this can wait until the dressing has been checked. A urinary catheter is not needed. The last pain medication administration and the client's current pain level should be communicated in the exchange report. Checking for hemorrhage is a greater priority than assessing pain level. (A)

61. 3. A splenectomy may involve manipulation of the upper abdominal organs, such as diaphragm, stomach, liver, spleen, and small intestines. Manipulation of these organs and resulting inflammation lead to a slowed peristalsis. An NG tube is placed to decrease abdominal distention in the immediate postoperative phase. The stomach does not need to be manipulated away from the spleen postoperatively, nor would an NG tube accomplish this. The NG tube drains gastric contents and air in the stomach; it is not in the operative site, and therefore cannot be used to irrigate it. The gastric juices are not checked as an indicator that peristalsis has returned; instead, bowel sounds are auscultated in all four quadrants to indicate the return of peristalsis. (A)

62. 4. Clients who have had a splenectomy are especially prone to infection. The reduction of immunoglobulin M leaves the client especially at risk for immunologic deficiency infections. All clients who have had major abdominal surgery usually receive discharge instructions not to drive because the stomach muscles are not strong enough to brake hard or quickly after the abdominal muscles have been separated. All clients need to pace activity and rest when going home after major surgery. Rest and sleep allow the growth hormone to repair the tissue, and activity allows the energy and strength to build endurance and muscle strength. An appointment is usually made to see the surgeon in the office 1 week after discharge for follow-up and to remove sutures or staples if this has not already been done. (R)

63. 2. There is no well-defined sequence for acute DIC other than that the client starts bleeding without a history or cause and does not stop bleeding. Later signs may include severe shortness of breath, hypotension, pallor, petechiae, hematoma, orthopnea, hematuria, vision changes, and joint pain. (A)

64. 3. DIC has not been found to respond to oral anticoagulants such as warfarin sodium (Coumadin). Treatments for DIC are controversial but include treating the underlying cause, administering heparin, and replacing depleted blood products. (D)

65. 2. Clinical manifestations of microvascular thrombosis are those that represent a blockage of blood flow and oxygenation to the tissue that results in eventual death of the organ. Examples of microvascular thrombosis include acute respiratory distress syndrome, focal ischemia, superficial gangrene, oliguria, azotemia, cortical necrosis, acute ulceration, delirium, and coma. Hemoptysis, petechiae, and hematuria are signs of hemorrhage. (A)

66. 3. As blood collects in the peritoneal cavity, it causes dilation and distention, which is reflected in increased abdominal girth. The client would be tachycardic and hypotensive. Petechiae reflect bleeding in the skin. (A)

The Client with White Blood Cell Disorders

67. 1, 2, 3, 5. The nurse should teach this client to stay on bed rest if she has a fever, gargle with warm saline, and increase her oral fluids to prevent dehydration from the elevated temperature. The client with an enlarged spleen should avoid contact sports due to the increased risk of injury due to the enlargement. The nurse should tell the client to avoid aspirin if she has a fever because of the risk of Reye's syndrome. Instead, nonsteroidal anti-inflammatory drugs should be used to treat fever and myalgia. (C)

68. 4. The client will need an order to be placed in reverse (protective) isolation because his normal defenses are ineffective and place him at risk for infection (leukopenia, less than 5,000 cells/µl). The faster the decrease in WBCs, the greater the bone marrow suppression, and the more susceptible the client is to infection from not only pathogenic but nonpathogenic organisms. The client will continue to be monitored, the laboratory may be called, and the report will be placed on the chart, but protection of the client must be instituted immediately. (A)

69. 3. A shift to the left means that more immature than mature WBCs are at the site of inflammation or infection. Immature WBCs are less effective at phagocytosis and do not produce classic signs of inflammation, such as pus, redness, swelling, or heat. Fever is the only sign; therefore, it is a significant sign of infection in a client with immature or depressed WBCs. (A)

70. **2.** The ANC is calculated by multiplying the total WBC count by the sum of percentage of neutrophils and the percentage of bands and dividing by 100. In this case,

$$1,200 (1 + 34) = 420.100.$$

(A)

71. **2.** A client is at moderate risk when the ANC is less than 1,000. The ANC decreases proportionately to the increased risk for infection. The client is at normal risk for infection if the ANC is 1,500 or greater. The client is at high risk for infection if the ANC is less than 500. An ANC of 100 or less is life-threatening. (A)

72. **1.** The one factor that may be more important than the degree of neutropenia in determining the risk for infection is the duration of the neutropenia. (A)

73. **1.** Bedside rails, call bells, drug-administration controls operated by the client, and other surface areas are frequently touched by caregivers with used gloves. Changing gloves immediately after use protects the client from contamination by organisms. Cross-contamination is a break in technique of serious consequence to the severely compromised client. Standing 2 feet from the client, speaking minimally, and wearing long-sleeved shirts are not required in standard interventions for risk of infection. (S)

74. **1.** The neutropenic client is at risk for infection, especially bacterial infection of the respiratory and gastrointestinal tracts. Breaks in the mucous membranes, such as those that could be caused by the insertion of a suppository or enema tube, would be a break in the first line of the body's defense and a direct port of entry for infection. The client with neutropenia is encouraged to wear a HEPA filter mask and to use an incentive spirometer for pulmonary hygiene. The client needs to know the importance of completing meticulous total body hygiene daily, including perianal care after every bowel movement, to decrease the flora at normal body orifices. The client also needs to know the importance of performing oral care after every meal and every 4 hours while the client is awake to decrease the bacterial buildup in the oropharynx. (H)

75. **2.** The Centers for Disease Control and Prevention advises that washing hands before, during, and after care has a significant effect in reducing infections. It is advisable to avoid introducing a cold or children's germs and to avoid kissing on the lips, but the primary prevention technique is hand washing. (H)

76. **4.** The most common source of infection and microbial colonization in neutropenic clients is their own nonpathogenic normal flora. Attention to personal hygiene, such as oral, pulmonary, urinary, and rectal care, is essential. It is important to acknowledge the client's concerns and fears and to provide organized, nonhurried, caring care, but it is more important to teach the client how to prevent an infection that could be life-threatening. (H)

77. **1, 2, 4, 5.** The nurse can serve as a witness for consent for procedures. The nurse also ascertains whether the client has an understanding that is consistent with the procedure listed on the form, determines that the client is signing the consent of his own free will, and determines that the client understands postprocedure care. The nurse's role does not include explaining the risks of the procedure. That responsibility belongs to the person who is to perform the procedure, such as the physician. (M)

78. **3.** As the bone marrow is being aspirated, the client will feel a suction or pulling type of sensation or discomfort that lasts a few seconds. A systemic premedication may be given to decrease this discomfort. A small area over the sternum is cleaned with an antiseptic. It is unnecessary to paint the entire anterior chest. The local anesthetic is injected through the subcutaneous tissue to numb the tissue for the larger-bore needle that is used for aspiration and biopsy. After the needle is removed, pressure is held over the aspiration site for 5 to 10 minutes to achieve hemostasis. A small dressing is applied; a large pressure dressing, such as an Ace bandage, would restrict the expansion of the lungs and is not used. (P)

79. **4.** After a bone marrow aspiration, the puncture site should be checked every 10 to 15 minutes for bleeding. For a short period after the procedure, bed rest may be ordered. Signs of infection, such as redness and swelling, are not anticipated at the aspiration site. A mild analgesic may be ordered. If the client continues to need the morphine for longer than 24 hours, the nurse should suspect that internal bleeding or increased pressure at the puncture site may be the cause of the pain and should consult the physician. (A)

80. **2.** The nurse is an advocate for the client with leukemia who can be empowered with knowledge of the treatment. Immunologic, cytogenic, morphologic, histochemical, and other means are used to identify cell subtypes and stages of leukemia cell development for very specific and optimal treatment. The nurse should not label the client's feeling, such as frustration or emotional; only the client can identify her own feelings. Chastising the client is not helpful. It disavows the client's emotional state and responses to her diagnosis and involved treatment. Unless nurses have had leukemia, they cannot possibly know how the client feels even though they may be trying to offer her empathy. (P)

81. 3. The induction phase of chemotherapy is an aggressive treatment to kill leukemia cells. The client is severely immunocompromised and severely at risk for infection. Flowers, herbs, and plants should be avoided during this time. The client's Bible, pictures, and other personal belongings can be cleaned before being brought into the room to prevent client contact with pathogenic and non-pathogenic organisms. (S)

82. 2. The nurse identifies that the client does not understand that contact with animals must be avoided because they carry infection and the induction therapy will destroy the client's WBCs. The induction therapy will cause anemia, and the client will experience fatigue and will have to pace activities with rest periods. Platelet production will be decreased, and the client will be at risk for bleeding tendencies; oral hygiene will have to be provided by using a warm saline gargle instead of brushing the teeth and gums. The client will be at risk for infection owing to the decrease in WBC production and should report a temperature of 100° F (37.8° C) or higher. (S)

83. 4. The statement, "Your doctor stated your prognosis based on the differentiation of your cells" addresses the client's situation on an individual basis. The nurse is clarifying that clients have different prognoses—even though they may have the same type of leukemia—because of the cell differentiation. Stating that the client misunderstood is inappropriate for an advocate of the client and serves no useful purpose. The other statements are true but do not address this client's individual concern. (P)

84. 4. Bleeding and infection are the major complications and causes of death for clients with AML. Bleeding is related to the degree of thrombocytopenia, and infection is related to the degree of neutropenia. Cardiac arrhythmias rarely occur as a result of AML. Liver or renal failure may occur, but neither is a major cause of death in AML. (R)

85. 4. Although the clinical manifestations of CML vary, clients usually have confusion and shortness of breath related to decreased capillary perfusion to the brain and lungs. Lymphadenopathy is rare in CML. Hyperplasia of the gum and bone pain are clinical manifestations of AML. (R)

86. 1. The peak incidence of ALL is at 4 years of age. ALL is uncommon after 15 years of age. The median age at incidence of CML is 40 to 50 years. The peak incidence of AML occurs at 60 years of age. Two-thirds of cases of chronic lymphocytic leukemia occur in clients older than 60 years of age. (A)

87. 1. Clients with ALL are at risk for infection due to granulocytopenia. The nurse should place the client in a private room. Strict hand-washing procedures should be enforced and will be the most effective way to prevent infection. It is not necessary to have the client wear a mask. The client is not contagious and the staff does not need to wear gloves. The client can have visitors; however, they should be screened for infection and use hand-washing procedures. (A)

88. 4. Clients with CLL develop unintentional weight loss; fever and drenching night sweats; enlarged, painful lymph nodes, spleen, and liver; decreased reaction to skin sensitivity tests (anergy); and susceptibility to viral infections. Enlarged, painless lymph nodes are a clinical manifestation of Hodgkin's lymphoma. A headache would not be one of the early signs and symptoms expected in CLL because CLL does not cross the blood-brain barrier and would not irritate the meninges. Hyperplasia of the gums is a clinical manifestation of AML. (A)

89. 3. Simple rinses with saline or baking soda solution are effective and moisten the oral mucosa. Commercial mouthwashes and lemon-glycerin swabs contain glycerin and alcohol, which are drying to the mucosa and should be avoided. Brushing after each meal is recommended, but every 4 hours may be too traumatic. During acute leukemia, the neutrophil and platelet counts are often low and a soft-bristle toothbrush, instead of the client's usual brush, should be used to prevent bleeding gums. (R)

90. 3. The client with acute leukemia experiences fatigue and deconditioning. Lying in bed and taking deep breaths will not help achieve the goals. The client must get out of bed to increase activity tolerance and improve tidal volume. Ambulating in the hall (using a HEPA filter mask if neutropenic) is a sensible activity and helps improve conditioning. Sitting up in a chair facilitates lung expansion. Using a stationary bicycle in the room allows the client to increase activity as tolerated. (R)

91. 2. Combination chemotherapy does not mean two groups of drugs, one to kill the cancer cells and one to treat the adverse effects of the chemotherapy. Combination chemotherapy means that multiple drugs are given to interrupt the cell growth cycle at different points, to decrease resistance to a chemotherapy agent, and to minimize the toxicity associated with use of a high dose of a single agent (i.e., by using multiple agents with different toxicities). (D)

92. 1. The biliary system is not especially prone to hemorrhage. Thrombocytopenia (a low platelet count) leaves the client at risk for a potentially life-threatening spontaneous hemorrhage in the gastrointestinal, respiratory, and intracranial cavities. (A)

93. **1.** The primary purpose of reverse isolation is to reduce transmission of organisms to the client from sources outside the client's environment. (S)

The Client with Lymphoma

94. **2.** Painless and enlarged cervical lymph nodes, tachycardia, weight loss, weakness and fatigue, and night sweats are signs of Hodgkin's disease. Difficulty swallowing and breathing may occur, but only with mediastinal node involvement. Hepatomegaly is a late-stage manifestation. (A)

95. **1.** The nurse must ensure that sterile technique is used when a biopsy is obtained. In most cases, a lymph node biopsy is sent immediately to the laboratory once it is placed in a specific solution in a closed container. It is not necessary to wear a gown and mask when obtaining the specimen. The nurse can assist with the procedure because the client may be at increased risk for infection. (M)

96. **3.** Assessing for an open airway is always first. The procedure involves the neck; the anesthesia may have affected the swallowing reflex, or the inflammation may have closed in on the airway, leading to ineffective air exchange. Once a patent airway is confirmed and an effective breathing pattern established, the circulation is checked. Vital signs and the incision are assessed as soon as possible, but only after it is established that the airway is patent and the client is breathing normally. A neurologic assessment is completed as soon as possible after other important assessments. (A)

97. **3.** A definitive diagnosis of Hodgkin's disease is made if Reed-Sternberg cells are found in the histologic examination of the excisional lymph node biopsy. Tay-Sachs disease is an inherited disease carried by an autosomal recessive gene. Sarcoidosis is an inflammatory granulomatous disease. Duchenne's disease is a type of muscular disorder. (A)

98. **1.** Herpes zoster infections are common in clients with Hodgkin's disease. Discoloring of the teeth is not related to Hodgkin's disease but rather to the ingestion of iron supplements or some antibiotics such as tetracycline. Mild anemia is common in Hodgkin's disease, but the platelet count is not affected until the tumor has invaded the bone marrow. A cellular immunity defect occurs in Hodgkin's disease in which there is little or no reaction to skin sensitivity tests. This is called anergy. (A)

99. **3.** A temperature higher than 100.4° F (38° C), profuse night sweats, and an unintentional weight loss of 10% of body weight represent the cluster of clinical manifestations known as the B symptoms. Forty percent of clients

with Hodgkin's disease have B symptoms, and B symptoms are more common in advanced stages of the disease. (A)

100. **4.** Invasive procedures such as exploratory laparotomy and lymphangiography are being used less often because noninvasive technologies, such as radiography, body scans, and blood tests, provide reliable indications of lymph node and surrounding tissue or organ involvement. (A)

101. **1.** In the staging process, the designations A and B signify, respectively, that symptoms were or were not present when Hodgkin's disease was found. The Roman numerals I through IV indicate the extent and location of involvement of the disease. Stage I indicates involvement of a single lymph node; stage II, two or more lymph nodes on the same side of the diaphragm; stage III, lymph node regions on both sides of the diaphragm; and stage IV, diffuse disease of one or more extralymphatic organs. (A)

102. **3.** Encouraging the client to take slow, deep breaths during uncomfortable parts of procedures is the best method of decreasing the stress response of tightening and tensing the muscles. Slow, deep breathing affects the level of carbon dioxide in the brain to increase the client's sense of well-being. Allowing the client's family to stay with her may be appropriate if the family has a calming effect on the client. Silence can be therapeutic, but when the client is faced with a potentially life-threatening diagnosis and a new, invasive procedure, she really needs words in addition to touch unless another health care provider is talking to her. Expressing feelings is important, but the client will have to hold still for the procedure. (P)

103. **2.** A biopsy needle is inserted through a separate incision in the anesthetized area. The client will feel a pressure sensation when the biopsy is taken but should not feel actual pain. The client should be instructed to inform the physician if pain is felt so that more anesthetic agent can be administered to keep the client comfortable. The biopsy is performed after the aspiration and from a slightly different site so that the tissue is not disturbed by either test. The client will feel a suction-type pain for a moment when the aspiration is being performed, not the biopsy. A small incision is made for the biopsy to accommodate the larger-bore needle. This may require a stitch. (P)

104. **3.** Terminally ill clients most often describe feelings of isolation because they tend to be ignored; they are often left out of conversations (especially those dealing with the future); and they sense the attitudes of discomfort that many people feel in their presence. Helpful nursing measures include taking the time to be with the client; offering opportunities to talk about feelings; and answering questions honestly. (P)

105. **2.** It is incorrect that the survivor rate is directly proportional to the incidence of second malignancy. The survivor rate is indirectly proportional to the incidence of second malignancy, and regular screening is very important to detect a second malignancy, especially acute myeloid leukemia or myelodysplastic syndrome. Survivors should know the stage of the disease and their current treatment plan so that they can remain active participants in their health care. (A)

The Client Who Is in Shock

106. **3.** Nursing interventions and collaborative management are focused on correcting and maintaining adequate tissue perfusion. Inadequate tissue perfusion may be caused by hemorrhage, as in hypovolemic shock; by decreased cardiac output, as in cardiogenic shock; or by massive vasodilation of the vascular bed, as in neurogenic, anaphylactic, and septic shock. Fluid deficit, not fluid overload, occurs in shock. (A)

107. **4.** Typical signs and symptoms of hypovolemic shock include systolic blood pressure less than 90 mm Hg, narrowing pulse pressure, tachycardia, tachypnea, cool and clammy skin, decreased urine output, and mental status changes, such as irritability or anxiety. Unequal dilation of the pupils is related to central nervous system injury or possibly to a previous history of eye injury. (A)

108. **1.** Urine output provides the most sensitive indication of the client's response to therapy for hypovolemic shock. Urine output should be consistently greater than 35 ml/hour. Blood pressure is a more accurate reflection of the adequacy of vasoconstriction than of tissue perfusion. Respiratory rate is not a sensitive indicator of fluid balance in the client recovering from hypovolemic shock. (D)

109. **1.** Causes of hypovolemic shock include external fluid loss, such as hemorrhage; internal fluid shifting, such as ascites and severe edema; and dehydration. Massive vasodilation is the initial phase of vasogenic or distributive shock, which can be further subdivided into three types of shock: septic, neurogenic, and anaphylactic. A severe antigen-antibody reaction occurs in anaphylactic shock. Gram-negative bacterial infection is the most common cause of septic shock. Loss of sympathetic tone (vasodilation) occurs in neurogenic shock. (A)

110. **2.** The client who is receiving a blood product requires astute assessment for signs and symptoms of allergic reaction and anaphylaxis, including pruritus (itching), urticaria (hives), facial or glottal edema, and shortness of breath. If such a reaction occurs, the nurse should stop the transfusion immediately, but leave the I.V. line intact, and notify the physician. Usually, an antihistamine such as diphenhydramine hydrochloride (Benadryl) is administered. Epinephrine and corticosteroids may be administered in severe reactions. Fluid balance is not an immediate concern during the blood administration. The administration should not cause pain unless it is extravasating out of the vein, in which case the I.V. administration should be stopped. Administration of a unit of blood should not affect the level of consciousness. (D)

111. **2.** At medium doses (4 to 8 µg/kg/minute), dopamine hydrochloride slightly increases the heart rate and improves contractility to increase cardiac output and improve tissue perfusion. When given at low doses (0.5 to 3.0 µg/kg/minute), dopamine increases renal and mesenteric blood flow. At high doses (8 to 10 µg/kg/minute), dopamine produces vasoconstriction, which is an undesirable effect. Dopamine is not given to affect preload and afterload. (D)

112. **3.** The client who is receiving dopamine hydrochloride requires continuous blood pressure monitoring with an invasive or noninvasive device. The nurse may titrate the I.V. infusion to maintain a systolic blood pressure of 90 mm Hg. Administration of a pain medication concurrently with dopamine hydrochloride, which is a potent sympathomimetic with dose-related alpha-adrenergic agonist, beta$_1$-selective adrenergic agonist, and dopaminergic blocking effects, is not an essential nursing action for a client who is in shock with already low hemodynamic values. Arterial blood gas concentrations should be monitored according to the client's respiratory status and acid-base balance status and are not directly related to the dopamine hydrochloride dosage. Monitoring for signs of infection is not related to the nursing action for the client receiving dopamine hydrochloride. (D)

113. **1, 3, 4.** Analysis of the client's laboratory results would indicate that an INR of 8 is increased beyond therapeutic ranges. The client is also experiencing severe acute rectal bleeding and has a hemoglobin level in the low range of normal and a hematocrit reflecting fluid volume loss. Getting the I.V. line started is crucial so that this client can receive FFP immediately. FFP contains concentrated clotting factors and provides an immediate reversal of the prolonged INR. Vitamin K 2.5 mg P.O. should be given next because it reverses the warfarin by returning the PT to normal values. However, the reversal process occurs over 1 to 2 hours. The other orders should be completed after these initial orders are in progress. (D)

114. 2. Nursing interventions to provide warmth and rest and minimize anxiety decrease the body's need for oxygen and nutrients. This is important for a client who has lost 500 ml or a unit of blood in a short period from a gastric hemorrhage. If the client has been stabilized, the fluid and electrolyte balance has already been established for the present. The comfort of the client and family is always important and is actually accomplished while the client's oxygen consumption is being minimized, which is a priority and the primary rationale. These nursing interventions are not specific to the prevention of infection. (A)

115. 2. Warm, flushed skin from a high cardiac output with vasodilation occurs in warm shock or the hyperdynamic phase (first phase) of septic shock. Other signs and symptoms of early septic shock include fever with restlessness and confusion; decreased blood pressure with tachypnea and tachycardia; increased or normal urine output; and nausea and vomiting or diarrhea. Cool, clammy skin occurs in the hypodynamic or cold phase (later phase). Hemorrhage is not a factor in septic shock. (A)

116. 1. The nurse monitors the blood levels of antibiotics, white blood cells, serum creatinine, and blood urea nitrogen because of the decreased perfusion to the kidneys, which are responsible for filtering out the Rocephin. It is possible that the clearance of the antibiotic has been decreased enough to cause toxicity. Increased levels of these laboratory values should be reported to the physician immediately. A spinal fluid analysis is done to examine cerebral spinal fluid, but there is no indication of central nervous system involvement in this case. Arterial blood gases are used to determine actual blood gas levels and assess acid-base balance. Serum osmolality is used to monitor fluid and electrolyte balance. (D)

117. 4. Maintaining asepsis of indwelling urinary catheters is essential to prevent infection. Preventing septic shock is a major focus of nursing care because the mortality rate for septic shock is as high as 90% in some populations. Very young and elderly clients (those younger than age 2 or older than age 65) are at increased risk for septic shock. Administering I.V. fluid replacement therapy, obtaining vital signs every 4 hours on all clients, and monitoring red blood cell counts for elevation do not pertain to septic shock prevention. (S)

118. 2. ARDS is a complication associated with septic shock. ARDS causes respiratory failure and may lead to death, even after the client has recovered from shock. Anaphylaxis is a type of distributive or vasogenic shock. COPD is a functional category of pulmonary disease that consists of persistent obstruction of bronchial airflow and involves chronic bronchitis and chronic emphysema. Mitral valve prolapse is a condition in which the mitral valve is pushed back too far during ventricular contraction. (A)

The Client with Respiratory Health Problems

The Client with an Upper Respiratory Tract Infection

1. A nurse is completing the health history for a client who has been taking echinacea for a head cold. The client asks, "Why isn't this helping me feel better?" Which of the following responses by the nurse would be the most accurate?

☐ 1. "There is limited information as to the effectiveness of herbal products."

☐ 2. "Antibiotics are the agents needed to treat a head cold."

☐ 3. "The head cold should be gone within the month."

☐ 4. "Combining herbal products with prescription antiviral medications is sure to help you."

2. A client has developed a hospital-acquired pneumonia. When preparing to administer cephalexin (Keflex) 500 mg, the nurse notices that the pharmacy sent cefazolin (Kefzol). What should the nurse do? Select all that apply.

☐ 1. Administer the cefazolin (Kefzol).

☐ 2. Verify the medication order as written by the physician.

☐ 3. Contact the pharmacy and speak to a pharmacist.

☐ 4. Request that cephalexin (Keflex) be sent promptly.

☐ 5. Return the cefazolin (Kefzol) to the pharmacy.

3. A nurse is teaching a client about taking antihistamines. Which of the following instructions should the nurse include in the teaching plan? Select all that apply.

☐ 1. Operating machinery and driving may be dangerous while taking antihistamines.

☐ 2. Continue taking antihistamines even if nasal infection develops.

☐ 3. The effect of antihistamines is not felt until a day later.

☐ 4. Do not use alcohol with antihistamines.

☐ 5. Increase fluid intake to 2,000 ml/day.

4. A client with allergic rhinitis is instructed on the correct technique for using an intranasal inhaler. Which of the following statements would demonstrate to the nurse that the client understands the instructions?

☐ 1. "I should limit the use of the inhaler to early morning and bedtime use."

☐ 2. "It is important to not shake the canister because that can damage the spray device."

☐ 3. "I should hold one nostril closed while I insert the spray into the other nostril."

☐ 4. "The inhaler tip is inserted into the nostril and pointed toward the inside nostril wall."

5. Which of the following would be an expected outcome for a client recovering from an upper respiratory tract infection? The client will:

☐ 1. Maintain a fluid intake of 800 ml every 24 hours.

☐ 2. Experience chills only once a day.

☐ 3. Cough productively without chest discomfort.

☐ 4. Experience less nasal obstruction and discharge.

6. The nurse teaches the client how to instill nose drops. Which of the following techniques is correct?

☐ **1.** The client uses sterile technique when handling the dropper.

☐ **2.** The client blows the nose gently before instilling drops.

☐ **3.** The client uses a new dropper for each instillation.

☐ **4.** The client sits in a semi-Fowler's position with the head tilted forward after administration of the drops.

7. A client with acute sinusitis is examined in an ambulatory clinic. The nurse can anticipate the use of which of the following medications in the client's treatment plan?

☐ **1.** Antibiotics.

☐ **2.** Antihistamines.

☐ **3.** Bronchodilators.

☐ **4.** Oral corticosteroids.

8. The nurse should include which of the following instructions in the teaching plan for a client with chronic sinusitis?

☐ **1.** Avoid the use of caffeinated beverages.

☐ **2.** Perform postural drainage every day.

☐ **3.** Take hot showers twice daily.

☐ **4.** Report a temperature of 102° F (38.9° C) or higher.

9. Which of the following individuals should the nurse consider to have the highest priority for receiving an influenza vaccination?

☐ **1.** A 60-year-old man with a hiatal hernia.

☐ **2.** A 36-year-old woman with three children.

☐ **3.** A 50-year-old woman caring for a spouse with cancer.

☐ **4.** A 60-year-old woman with osteoarthritis.

10. A client with allergic rhinitis asks the nurse what he should do to decrease his symptoms. Which of the following instructions would be appropriate for the nurse to give the client?

☐ **1.** "Use your nasal decongestant spray regularly to help clear your nasal passages."

☐ **2.** "Ask the doctor for antibiotics. Antibiotics will help decrease the secretion."

☐ **3.** "It is important to increase your activity. A daily brisk walk will help promote drainage."

☐ **4.** "Keep a diary of when your symptoms occur. This can help you identify what precipitates your attacks."

11. An elderly client has been ill with the flu, experiencing headache, fever, and chills. After 3 days, she develops a cough producing yellow sputum. The nurse auscultates her lungs and hears diffuse crackles. How would the nurse best interpret these assessment findings?

☐ **1.** It is likely that the client is developing a secondary bacterial pneumonia.

☐ **2.** The assessment findings are consistent with influenza and are to be expected.

☐ **3.** The client is getting dehydrated and needs to increase her fluid intake to decrease secretions.

☐ **4.** The client has not been taking her decongestants and bronchodilators as prescribed.

12. Guaifenesin (Robitussin) 300 mg four times a day has been ordered as an expectorant. The dosage strength of the liquid is 200 mg/5 ml. How many milliliters should the nurse administer for each dose?

_____ ml

13. Pseudoephedrine (Sudafed) has been ordered as a nasal decongestant. Which of the following is a possible adverse effect of this drug?

☐ **1.** Constipation.

☐ **2.** Bradycardia.

☐ **3.** Diplopia.

☐ **4.** Restlessness.

The Client Undergoing Nasal Surgery

14. A health care provider has just inserted nasal packing for a client with epistaxis. The client is taking ramipril (Altace) for hypertension. What should the nurse instruct the client to do?

☐ **1.** Use 81 mg of aspirin daily for relief of discomfort.

☐ **2.** Omit the next dose of ramipril (Altace).

☐ **3.** Remove the packing if there is difficulty swallowing.

☐ **4.** Avoid rigorous aerobic exercise.

15. A 27-year-old female has had elective nasal surgery for a deviated septum. Which of the following would be an important initial clue that bleeding was occurring even if the nasal drip pad remained dry and intact?

☐ **1.** Complaints of nausea.

☐ **2.** Repeated swallowing.

☐ **3.** Increased respiratory rate.

☐ **4.** Increased pain.

16. A client who has undergone outpatient nasal surgery is ready for discharge and has nasal packing in place. Which of the following discharge instructions would be appropriate for the client?
☐ **1.** Avoid activities that elicit the Valsalva maneuver.
☐ **2.** Take aspirin to control nasal discomfort.
☐ **3.** Avoid brushing the teeth until the nasal packing is removed.
☐ **4.** Apply heat to the nasal area to control swelling.

17. Which of the following statements should indicate to the nurse that a client has understood the discharge instructions provided after her nasal surgery?
☐ **1.** "I should not shower until my packing is removed."
☐ **2.** "I will take stool softeners and modify my diet to prevent constipation."
☐ **3.** "Coughing every 2 hours is important to prevent respiratory complications."
☐ **4.** "It is important to blow my nose each day to remove the dried secretions."

18. The nurse is planning to give preoperative instructions to a client who will be undergoing rhinoplasty. Which of the following instructions should be included?
☐ **1.** After surgery, nasal packing will be in place for 7 to 10 days.
☐ **2.** Normal saline nose drops will need to be administered preoperatively.
☐ **3.** The results of the surgery will be immediately obvious postoperatively.
☐ **4.** Aspirin-containing medications should not be taken for 2 weeks before surgery.

19. Which of the following assessments should be a priority immediately after nasal surgery?
☐ **1.** Assessing the client's pain.
☐ **2.** Inspecting for periorbital ecchymosis.
☐ **3.** Assessing respiratory status.
☐ **4.** Measuring intake and output.

20. After nasal surgery, the client expresses concern about how to decrease facial pain and swelling while recovering at home. Which of the following discharge instructions would be most effective for decreasing pain and edema?
☐ **1.** Take analgesics every 4 hours around the clock.
☐ **2.** Use corticosteroid nasal spray as needed to control symptoms.
☐ **3.** Use a bedside humidifier while sleeping.
☐ **4.** Apply cold compresses to the area.

21. A client is being discharged with nasal packing in place. He should be told to implement which of the following activities into his home care?
☐ **1.** Perform frequent mouth care.
☐ **2.** Use normal saline nose drops daily.
☐ **3.** Sneeze and cough with mouth closed.
☐ **4.** Gargle every 4 hours with salt water.

22. Which of the following activities should the nurse teach the client to implement after the removal of nasal packing on the second postoperative day?
☐ **1.** Avoid cleaning the nares until swelling has subsided.
☐ **2.** Apply water-soluble jelly to lubricate the nares.
☐ **3.** Keep a nasal drip pad in place to absorb secretions.
☐ **4.** Use a bulb syringe to gently irrigate nares.

23. The nurse is teaching a client how to manage a nosebleed. Which of the following instructions would be appropriate to give the client?
☐ **1.** "Tilt your head backward and pinch your nose."
☐ **2.** "Lie down flat and place an ice compress over the bridge of the nose."
☐ **3.** "Blow your nose gently with your neck flexed."
☐ **4.** "Sit down, lean forward, and pinch the soft portion of your nose."

24. An elderly client had posterior packing inserted to control a severe nosebleed. After insertion of the packing, the client should be closely monitored for which of the following complications?
☐ **1.** Vertigo.
☐ **2.** Bell's palsy.
☐ **3.** Hypoventilation.
☐ **4.** Loss of gag reflex.

The Client with Cancer of the Larynx

25. Which of the following is a priority nursing diagnosis for the client with a total laryngectomy due to cancer?
☐ **1.** *Deficient fluid volume* related to difficulty swallowing.
☐ **2.** *Impaired verbal communication* related to inability to speak.
☐ **3.** *Feeding self-care deficit* related to inability to swallow.
☐ **4.** *Powerlessness* related to diagnosis of cancer.

26. A client who has had a total laryngectomy appears withdrawn and depressed. He keeps the curtain drawn, refuses visitors, and indicates a desire to be left alone. Which nursing intervention would most likely be therapeutic for the client?
☐ **1.** Discussing his behavior with his wife to determine the cause.
☐ **2.** Exploring his future plans.
☐ **3.** Respecting his need for privacy.
☐ **4.** Encouraging him to express his feelings nonverbally and in writing.

27. The nurse is suctioning a client who had a laryngectomy. What is the maximum amount of time the nurse should suction the client?
☐ **1.** 10 seconds.
☐ **2.** 15 seconds.
☐ **3.** 25 seconds.
☐ **4.** 30 seconds.

28. When suctioning a tracheostomy or laryngectomy tube, the nurse should follow which of the following procedures?
☐ **1.** Use a sterile catheter each time the client is suctioned.
☐ **2.** Clean the catheter in sterile water after each use and reuse for no longer than 8 hours.
☐ **3.** Protect the catheter in sterile packaging between suctioning episodes.
☐ **4.** Use a clean catheter with each suctioning, and disinfect it in hydrogen peroxide between uses.

29. The client with a laryngectomy communicates to the nurse that he does not want his family to see him. He indicates that he thinks the opening in his throat is disgusting. Which of the following nursing diagnoses would be most appropriate?
☐ **1.** *Deficient knowledge* about the care of a stoma.
☐ **2.** *Disturbed personal identity* related to change in appearance.
☐ **3.** *Disturbed body image* related to neck surgery.
☐ **4.** *Hopelessness* related to irreversible changes in body functioning.

30. The nurse is preparing a community presentation on the prevention of cancer. Which of the following should be included as a primary risk factor for developing laryngeal cancer?
☐ **1.** Chronic allergy.
☐ **2.** Chewing tobacco.
☐ **3.** Exposure to airborne environmental toxins.
☐ **4.** Smoking.

31. Which of the following signs and symptoms should the nurse include in a teaching plan as an early warning sign of laryngeal cancer?
☐ **1.** Dysphagia.
☐ **2.** Hoarseness.
☐ **3.** Airway obstruction.
☐ **4.** Stomatitis.

32. A client has just returned from the postanesthesia care unit after undergoing a laryngectomy. Which of the following interventions should the nurse include in the plan of care?
☐ **1.** Maintain the head of the bed at 30 to 40 degrees.
☐ **2.** Teach the client how to use esophageal speech.
☐ **3.** Initiate small feedings of soft foods.
☐ **4.** Irrigate drainage tubes as needed.

33. Which of the following is an appropriate expected outcome for a client recovering from a total laryngectomy? The client will:
☐ **1.** Regain the ability to taste and smell food.
☐ **2.** Demonstrate appropriate care of the gastrostomy tube.
☐ **3.** Communicate feelings about body image changes.
☐ **4.** Demonstrate sterile suctioning technique for stoma care.

34. Which of the following home care instructions would be appropriate for a client with a laryngectomy?
☐ **1.** Perform mouth care every morning and evening.
☐ **2.** Provide adequate humidity in the home.
☐ **3.** Maintain a soft, bland diet.
☐ **4.** Limit physical activity to shoulder and neck exercises.

35. The nurse has reported to the hospital to work the evening shift on a respiratory unit. The nurse's assignment consists of four clients. Prioritize in order from highest to lowest priority how the nurse would assess the clients after receiving report.

---

1. An 85-year-old client with bacterial pneumonia, temperature of 102.2° F (42° C), and shortness of breath.

---

2. A 60-year-old client with chest tubes who is 2 days postoperative following a thoracotomy for lung cancer and is requesting something for pain.

---

3. A 35-year-old client with suspected tuberculosis who is complaining of a cough.

---

4. A 56-year-old client with emphysema who has a scheduled dose of a bronchodilator due to be administered, with no report of acute respiratory distress.

The Client with Pneumonia

36. A nurse notes that a client has kyphosis and generalized muscle atrophy. Which of the following problems is a priority when the nurse develops a nursing plan of care?
☐ **1.** Infection.
☐ **2.** Confusion.
☐ **3.** Ineffective coughing and deep breathing.
☐ **4.** Difficulty chewing solid foods.

37. A client with deep vein thrombosis suddenly develops dyspnea, tachypnea, and chest discomfort. What should the nurse do first?
☐ **1.** Elevate the head of the bed 30 to 45 degrees.
☐ **2.** Encourage the client to cough and deep breathe.s
☐ **3.** Auscultate the lungs to detect abnormal breath sounds.
☐ **4.** Contact the physician.

38. A 79-year-old female client is admitted to the hospital with a diagnosis of bacterial pneumonia. While obtaining the client's health history, the nurse learns that the client has osteoarthritis, follows a vegetarian diet, and is very concerned with cleanliness. Which of the following would most likely be a predisposing factor for the diagnosis of pneumonia?
☐ **1.** Age.
☐ **2.** Osteoarthritis.
☐ **3.** Vegetarian diet.
☐ **4.** Daily bathing.

39. Which of the following would be priority assessment data to gather from a client who has been diagnosed with pneumonia? Select all that apply.
☐ **1.** Auscultation of breath sounds.
☐ **2.** Auscultation of bowel sounds.
☐ **3.** Presence of chest pain.
☐ **4.** Presence of peripheral edema.
☐ **5.** Color of nail beds.

40. A client with bacterial pneumonia is to be started on I.V. antibiotics. Which of the following diagnostic tests must be completed before antibiotic therapy begins?
☐ **1.** Urinalysis.
☐ **2.** Sputum culture.
☐ **3.** Chest radiograph.
☐ **4.** Red blood cell count.

41. When caring for the client who is receiving an aminoglycoside antibiotic, the nurse monitors which of the following laboratory values?
☐ **1.** Serum sodium.
☐ **2.** Serum potassium.
☐ **3.** Serum creatinine.
☐ **4.** Serum calcium.

42. A client with pneumonia has a temperature of 102.6° F (39.2° C), is diaphoretic, and has a productive cough. The nurse should include which of the following measures in the plan of care?
☐ **1.** Position changes every 4 hours.
☐ **2.** Nasotracheal suctioning to clear secretions.
☐ **3.** Frequent linen changes.
☐ **4.** Frequent offering of a bedpan.

43. Bed rest is prescribed for a client with pneumonia during the acute phase of the illness. Bed rest serves which of the following purposes?
☐ **1.** It reduces the cellular demand for oxygen.
☐ **2.** It decreases the episodes of coughing.
☐ **3.** It promotes safety.
☐ **4.** It promotes clearance of secretions.

44. The cyanosis that accompanies bacterial pneumonia is primarily caused by which of the following?
- [ ] **1.** Decreased cardiac output.
- [ ] **2.** Pleural effusion.
- [ ] **3.** Inadequate peripheral circulation.
- [ ] **4.** Decreased oxygenation of the blood.

45. A client with pneumonia is experiencing pleuritic chest pain. Which of the following describes pleuritic chest pain?
- [ ] **1.** A mild but constant aching in the chest.
- [ ] **2.** Severe midsternal pain.
- [ ] **3.** Moderate pain that worsens on inspiration.
- [ ] **4.** Muscle spasm pain that accompanies coughing.

46. Which of the following measures would most likely be successful in reducing pleuritic chest pain in a client with pneumonia?
- [ ] **1.** Encourage the client to breathe shallowly.
- [ ] **2.** Have the client practice abdominal breathing.
- [ ] **3.** Offer the client incentive spirometry.
- [ ] **4.** Teach the client to splint the rib cage when coughing.

47. Aspirin is administered to clients with pneumonia because of its antipyretic and:
- [ ] **1.** Analgesic effects.
- [ ] **2.** Anticoagulant effects.
- [ ] **3.** Adrenergic effects.
- [ ] **4.** Antihistamine effects.

48. Which of the following mental status changes may occur when a client with pneumonia is first experiencing hypoxia?
- [ ] **1.** Coma.
- [ ] **2.** Apathy.
- [ ] **3.** Irritability.
- [ ] **4.** Depression.

49. The client with pneumonia develops mild constipation, and the nurse administers docusate sodium (Colace) as ordered. This drug works by:
- [ ] **1.** Softening the stool.
- [ ] **2.** Lubricating the stool.
- [ ] **3.** Increasing stool bulk.
- [ ] **4.** Stimulating peristalsis.

50. A client with pneumonia has a temperature ranging between 101° and 102° F (38.3° and 38.8° C) and periods of diaphoresis. Based on this information, which of the following nursing interventions would be a priority?
- [ ] **1.** Maintain complete bed rest.
- [ ] **2.** Administer oxygen therapy.
- [ ] **3.** Provide frequent linen changes.
- [ ] **4.** Provide fluid intake of 3 L/day.

51. Which of the following would be an appropriate expected outcome for an elderly client recovering from bacterial pneumonia?
- [ ] **1.** A respiratory rate of 25 to 30 breaths/minute.
- [ ] **2.** The ability to perform activities of daily living without dyspnea.
- [ ] **3.** A maximum loss of 5 to 10 lb of body weight.
- [ ] **4.** Chest pain that is minimized by splinting the rib cage.

The Client with Tuberculosis

52. Which of the following symptoms is common in clients with active tuberculosis?
- [ ] **1.** Weight loss.
- [ ] **2.** Increased appetite.
- [ ] **3.** Dyspnea on exertion.
- [ ] **4.** Mental status changes.

53. The nurse obtains a sputum specimen from a client with suspected tuberculosis for laboratory study. Which of the following laboratory techniques is most commonly used to identify tubercle bacilli in sputum?
- [ ] **1.** Acid-fast staining.
- [ ] **2.** Sensitivity testing.
- [ ] **3.** Agglutination testing.
- [ ] **4.** Dark-field illumination.

54. Which of the following antituberculosis drugs can cause damage to the eighth cranial nerve?
- [ ] **1.** Streptomycin.
- [ ] **2.** Isoniazid (INH).
- [ ] **3.** Para-aminosalicylic acid (PAS).
- [ ] **4.** Ethambutol hydrochloride (Myambutol).

55. The client who experiences eighth cranial nerve damage will most likely report which of the following symptoms?
- [ ] **1.** Vertigo.
- [ ] **2.** Facial paralysis.
- [ ] **3.** Impaired vision.
- [ ] **4.** Difficulty swallowing.

56. The nurse should teach clients that the most common route of transmitting tubercle bacilli from person to person is through contaminated:
- [ ] **1.** Dust particles.
- [ ] **2.** Droplet nuclei.
- [ ] **3.** Water.
- [ ] **4.** Eating utensils.

57. What is the rationale that supports multidrug treatment for clients with tuberculosis?
☐ **1.** Multiple drugs potentiate the drugs' actions.
☐ **2.** Multiple drugs reduce undesirable drug adverse effects.
☐ **3.** Multiple drugs allow reduced drug dosages to be given.
☐ **4.** Multiple drugs reduce development of resistant strains of the bacteria.

58. The client with tuberculosis is to be discharged home with community health nursing follow-up. Of the following interventions, which should have the highest priority?
☐ **1.** Offering the client emotional support.
☐ **2.** Teaching the client about the disease and its treatment.
☐ **3.** Coordinating various agency services.
☐ **4.** Assessing the client's environment for sanitation.

59. Which of the following techniques for administering the Mantoux test is correct?
☐ **1.** Hold the needle and syringe almost parallel to the client's skin.
☐ **2.** Pinch the skin when inserting the needle.
☐ **3.** Aspirate before injecting the medication.
☐ **4.** Massage the site after injecting the medication.

60. Which of the following family members exposed to tuberculosis would be at highest risk for contracting the disease?
☐ **1.** 45-year-old mother.
☐ **2.** 17-year-old daughter.
☐ **3.** 8-year-old son.
☐ **4.** 76-year-old grandmother.

61. The nurse is teaching a client who has been diagnosed with tuberculosis how to avoid spreading the disease to family members. Which statement(s) by the client indicate(s) that he has understood the nurse's instructions? Select all that apply.
☐ **1.** "I will need to dispose of my old clothing when I return home."
☐ **2.** "I should always cover my mouth and nose when sneezing."
☐ **3.** "It is important that I isolate myself from family when possible."
☐ **4.** "I should use paper tissues to cough in and dispose of them promptly."
☐ **5.** "I can use regular plates and utensils whenever I eat."

62. A client has a positive reaction to the Mantoux test. The nurse correctly interprets this reaction to mean that the client has:
☐ **1.** Active tuberculosis.
☐ **2.** Had contact with *Mycobacterium tuberculosis*.
☐ **3.** Developed a resistance to tubercle bacilli.
☐ **4.** Developed passive immunity to tuberculosis.

63. Isoniazid (INH) treatment is associated with the development of peripheral neuropathies. Which of the following interventions should the nurse teach the client to help prevent this complication?
☐ **1.** Adhere to a low-cholesterol diet.
☐ **2.** Supplement the diet with pyridoxine (vitamin B_6).
☐ **3.** Get extra rest.
☐ **4.** Avoid excessive sun exposure.

64. The nurse should caution sexually active female clients taking isoniazid (INH) that the drug has which of the following effects?
☐ **1.** Increases the risk of vaginal infection.
☐ **2.** Has mutagenic effects on ova.
☐ **3.** Decreases the effectiveness of hormonal contraceptives.
☐ **4.** Inhibits ovulation.

65. Clients who have had active tuberculosis are at risk for recurrence. Which of the following conditions increases that risk?
☐ **1.** Cool and damp weather.
☐ **2.** Active exercise and exertion.
☐ **3.** Physical and emotional stress.
☐ **4.** Rest and inactivity.

66. In which areas of the United States is the incidence of tuberculosis highest?
☐ **1.** Rural farming areas.
☐ **2.** Inner-city areas.
☐ **3.** Areas where clean water standards are low.
☐ **4.** Suburban areas with significant industrial pollution.

67. The nurse should include which of the following instructions when developing a teaching plan for a client who is receiving isoniazid and rifampin (Rifamate) for treatment of tuberculosis?
☐ **1.** Take the medication with antacids.
☐ **2.** Double the dosage if a drug dose is missed.
☐ **3.** Increase intake of dairy products.
☐ **4.** Limit alcohol intake.

68. A client who has been diagnosed with tuberculosis has been placed on drug therapy. The medication regimen includes rifampin (Rifadin). Which of the following instructions should the nurse include in the client's teaching plan related to the potential adverse effects of rifampin? Select all that apply.
- ☐ 1. Having eye examinations every 6 months.
- ☐ 2. Maintaining follow-up monitoring of liver enzymes.
- ☐ 3. Decreasing protein intake in the diet.
- ☐ 4. Avoiding alcohol intake.
- ☐ 5. The urine may have an orange color.

69. The public health nurse is providing follow-up care to a client with tuberculosis who does not regularly take his medication. Which nursing action would be most appropriate for this client?
- ☐ 1. Ask the client's spouse to supervise the daily administration of the medications.
- ☐ 2. Visit the client weekly to ask him whether he is taking his medications regularly.
- ☐ 3. Notify the physician of the client's noncompliance and request a different prescription.
- ☐ 4. Remind the client that tuberculosis can be fatal if it is not treated promptly.

The Client with Chronic Obstructive Pulmonary Disease

70. A client with chronic obstructive pulmonary disease (COPD) reports steady weight loss and being "too tired from just breathing to eat." Which of the following nursing diagnoses would be most appropriate when planning nutritional interventions for this client?
- ☐ 1. *Imbalanced nutrition: Less than body requirements* related to fatigue.
- ☐ 2. *Activity intolerance* related to dyspnea.
- ☐ 3. *Weight loss* related to COPD.
- ☐ 4. *Ineffective breathing pattern* related to alveolar hypoventilation.

71. When developing a discharge plan to manage the care of a client with chronic obstructive pulmonary disease (COPD), the nurse should anticipate that the client will do which of the following?
- ☐ 1. Develop respiratory infections easily.
- ☐ 2. Maintain current status.
- ☐ 3. Require less supplemental oxygen.
- ☐ 4. Show permanent improvement.

72. Which of the following outcomes would be appropriate for a client with chronic obstructive pulmonary disease (COPD) who has been discharged to home?
- ☐ 1. The client promises to do pursed-lip breathing at home.
- ☐ 2. The client states actions to reduce pain.
- ☐ 3. The client states that he will use oxygen via a nasal cannula at 5 L/minute.
- ☐ 4. The client agrees to call the physician if dyspnea on exertion increases.

73. Which of the following physical assessment findings would the nurse expect to find in a client with advanced chronic obstructive pulmonary disease (COPD)?
- ☐ 1. Increased anteroposterior chest diameter.
- ☐ 2. Underdeveloped neck muscles.
- ☐ 3. Collapsed neck veins.
- ☐ 4. Increased chest excursions with respiration.

74. When instructing clients on how to decrease the risk of chronic obstructive pulmonary disease (COPD), the nurse should emphasize which of the following behaviors?
- ☐ 1. Participate regularly in aerobic exercises.
- ☐ 2. Maintain a high-protein diet.
- ☐ 3. Avoid exposure to people with known respiratory infections.
- ☐ 4. Abstain from cigarette smoking.

75. Which of the following is the primary reason to teach pursed-lip breathing to clients with emphysema?
- ☐ 1. To promote oxygen intake.
- ☐ 2. To strengthen the diaphragm.
- ☐ 3. To strengthen the intercostal muscles.
- ☐ 4. To promote carbon dioxide elimination.

76. Which of the following is a priority goal for the client with chronic obstructive pulmonary disease (COPD)?
- ☐ 1. Maintaining functional ability.
- ☐ 2. Minimizing chest pain.
- ☐ 3. Increasing carbon dioxide levels in the blood.
- ☐ 4. Treating infectious agents.

77. A client's arterial blood gas values are as follows: pH, 7.31; Pao_2, 80 mm Hg; $Paco_2$, 65 mm Hg; HCO_3^-, 36 mEq/L. Which of the following signs or symptoms should the nurse expect?
- ☐ 1. Cyanosis.
- ☐ 2. Flushed skin.
- ☐ 3. Irritability.
- ☐ 4. Anxiety.

78. When performing postural drainage, which of the following factors promotes the movement of secretions from the lower to the upper respiratory tract?
☐ **1.** Friction between the cilia.
☐ **2.** Force of gravity.
☐ **3.** Sweeping motion of cilia.
☐ **4.** Involuntary muscle contractions.

79. When teaching a client with chronic obstructive pulmonary disease to conserve energy, the nurse should teach the client to lift objects:
☐ **1.** While inhaling through an open mouth.
☐ **2.** While exhaling through pursed lips.
☐ **3.** After exhaling but before inhaling.
☐ **4.** While taking a deep breath and holding it.

80. The nurse teaches a client with chronic obstructive pulmonary disease (COPD) to assess for signs and symptoms of right-sided heart failure. Which of the following signs and symptoms should be included in the teaching plan?
☐ **1.** Clubbing of nail beds.
☐ **2.** Hypertension.
☐ **3.** Peripheral edema.
☐ **4.** Increased appetite.

81. The nurse assesses the respiratory status of a client who is experiencing an exacerbation of chronic obstructive pulmonary disease (COPD) secondary to an upper respiratory tract infection. Which of the following findings would be expected?
☐ **1.** Normal breath sounds.
☐ **2.** Prolonged inspiration.
☐ **3.** Normal chest movement.
☐ **4.** Coarse crackles and rhonchi.

82. Which of the following blood gas abnormalities should the nurse anticipate in a client with advanced chronic obstructive pulmonary disease (COPD)?
☐ **1.** Increased $Paco_2$.
☐ **2.** Increased Pao_2.
☐ **3.** Increased pH.
☐ **4.** Increased oxygen saturation.

83. A client with chronic obstructive pulmonary disease (COPD) is experiencing dyspnea and has a low Pao_2 level. The nurse plans to administer oxygen as ordered. Which of the following statements is true concerning oxygen administration to a client with COPD?
☐ **1.** High oxygen concentrations will cause coughing and dyspnea.
☐ **2.** High oxygen concentrations may inhibit the hypoxic stimulus to breathe.
☐ **3.** Increased oxygen use will cause the client to become dependent on the oxygen.
☐ **4.** Administration of oxygen is contraindicated in clients who are using bronchodilators.

84. Which of the following diets would be most appropriate for a client with chronic obstructive pulmonary disease (COPD)?
☐ **1.** Low-fat, low-cholesterol diet.
☐ **2.** Bland, soft diet.
☐ **3.** Low-sodium diet.
☐ **4.** High-calorie, high-protein diet.

85. The nurse administers theophylline (Theo-Dur) to a client. To evaluate the effectiveness of this medication, which of the following drug actions should the nurse anticipate?
☐ **1.** Suppression of the client's respiratory infection.
☐ **2.** Decrease in bronchial secretions.
☐ **3.** Relaxation of bronchial smooth muscle.
☐ **4.** Thinning of tenacious, purulent sputum.

86. The nurse is planning to teach a client with chronic obstructive pulmonary disease how to cough effectively. Which of the following instructions should be included?
☐ **1.** Take a deep abdominal breath, bend forward, and cough three or four times on exhalation.
☐ **2.** Lie flat on the back, splint the thorax, take two deep breaths, and cough.
☐ **3.** Take several rapid, shallow breaths and then cough forcefully.
☐ **4.** Assume a side-lying position, extend the arm over the head, and alternate deep breathing with coughing.

The Client with Asthma

87. A client uses a metered-dose inhaler (MDI) to aid in management of his asthma. Which action by the client indicates to the nurse that he needs further instruction regarding its use? Select all that apply.
☐ **1.** Activation of the MDI is not coordinated with inspiration.
☐ **2.** The client inspires rapidly when using the MDI.
☐ **3.** The client holds his breath for 3 seconds after inhaling with the MDI.
☐ **4.** The client shakes the MDI after use.
☐ **5.** The client performs puffs in rapid succession.

88. A 34-year-old female with a history of asthma is admitted to the emergency department. The nurse notes that the client is dyspneic, with a respiratory rate of 35 breaths/minute, nasal flaring, and use of accessory muscles. Auscultation of the lung fields reveals greatly diminished breath sounds. Based on these findings, which action should the nurse take to initiate care of the client?
☐ **1.** Initiate oxygen therapy and reassess the client in 10 minutes.
☐ **2.** Draw blood for an arterial blood gas analysis and send the client for a chest X-ray.
☐ **3.** Encourage the client to relax and breathe slowly through the mouth.
☐ **4.** Administer bronchodilators.

89. The nurse should anticipate which of the following arterial blood gas results in a client experiencing a prolonged, severe asthma attack?
- ☐ **1.** Decreased $Paco_2$, increased Pao_2, and decreased pH.
- ☐ **2.** Increased $Paco_2$, decreased Pao_2, and decreased pH.
- ☐ **3.** Increased $Paco_2$, increased Pao_2, and increased pH.
- ☐ **4.** Decreased $Paco_2$, decreased Pao_2, and increased pH.

90. A client with acute asthma is prescribed short-term corticosteroid therapy. Which is the rationale for the use of steroids in clients with asthma?
- ☐ **1.** Corticosteroids promote bronchodilation.
- ☐ **2.** Corticosteroids act as an expectorant.
- ☐ **3.** Corticosteroids have an anti-inflammatory effect.
- ☐ **4.** Corticosteroids prevent development of respiratory infections.

91. The nurse is teaching the client how to use a metered-dose inhaler (MDI) to administer a corticosteroid. Which of the following client actions indicates that he is using the MDI correctly? Select all that apply.
- ☐ **1.** The inhaler is held upright.
- ☐ **2.** The head is tilted down while inhaling the medicine.
- ☐ **3.** The client waits 5 minutes between puffs.
- ☐ **4.** The mouth is rinsed with water following administration.
- ☐ **5.** The client lies supine for 15 minutes following administration.

92. A client is prescribed metaproterenol (Alupent) via a metered-dose inhaler, two puffs every 4 hours. The nurse instructs the client to report adverse effects. Which of the following are potential adverse effects of metaproterenol?
- ☐ **1.** Irregular heartbeat.
- ☐ **2.** Constipation.
- ☐ **3.** Pedal edema.
- ☐ **4.** Decreased pulse rate.

93. A client has been taking flunisolide (AeroBid), two inhalations a day, for treatment of asthma. He tells the nurse that he has painful, white patches in his mouth. Which response by the nurse would be most appropriate?
- ☐ **1.** "This is an anticipated adverse effect of your medication. It should go away in a couple of weeks."
- ☐ **2.** "You are using your inhaler too much and it has irritated your mouth."
- ☐ **3.** "You have developed a fungal infection from your medication. It will need to be treated with an antifungal agent."
- ☐ **4.** "Be sure to brush your teeth and floss daily. Good oral hygiene will treat this problem."

94. A nurse is teaching a client to use a metered-dose inhaler (MDI) to administer his bronchodilator medication. Indicate the correct order of the steps the client should take to use the MDI appropriately.

1. Shake the inhaler immediately before use.
2. Hold breath for 5 to 10 seconds and then exhale.
3. Activate the MDI on inhalation.
4. Breathe out through the mouth.

95. Which of the following would be an appropriate expected outcome for an adult client with well-controlled asthma?
- ☐ **1.** Chest X-ray demonstrates minimal hyperinflation.
- ☐ **2.** Temperature remains lower than 100° F (37.8° C).
- ☐ **3.** Arterial blood gas analysis demonstrates a decrease in Pao_2.
- ☐ **4.** Breath sounds are clear.

96. Which of the following health promotion activities should the nurse include in the discharge teaching plan for a client with asthma?
- ☐ **1.** Incorporate physical exercise as tolerated into the daily routine.
- ☐ **2.** Monitor peak flow numbers after meals and at bedtime.
- ☐ **3.** Eliminate stressors in the work and home environment.
- ☐ **4.** Use sedatives to ensure uninterrupted sleep at night.

97. The client with asthma should be taught that which of the following is one of the most common precipitating factors of an acute asthma attack?
- ☐ **1.** Occupational exposure to toxins.
- ☐ **2.** Viral respiratory infections.
- ☐ **3.** Exposure to cigarette smoke.
- ☐ **4.** Exercising in cold temperatures.

98. Which of the following findings would most likely indicate the presence of a respiratory infection in a client with asthma?
- ☐ 1. Cough productive of yellow sputum.
- ☐ 2. Bilateral expiratory wheezing.
- ☐ 3. Chest tightness.
- ☐ 4. Respiratory rate of 30 breaths/minute.

The Client with Lung Cancer

99. A female client diagnosed with lung cancer is to have a left lower lobectomy. Which of the following assessment findings obtained during the nurse's admission interview would increase the client's risk of developing postoperative pulmonary complications?
- ☐ 1. Height is 5 feet, 7 inches and weight is 110 lb.
- ☐ 2. The client tends to keep her real feelings to herself.
- ☐ 3. She ambulates and can climb one flight of stairs without dyspnea.
- ☐ 4. The client is 58 years of age.

100. The nurse in the perioperative area is preparing a client for surgery and notices that the client looks sad. The client says, "I'm scared of having cancer. It's so horrible and I brought it on myself. I should have quit smoking years ago." What would be the nurse's best response to the client?
- ☐ 1. "It's okay to be scared. What is it about cancer that you're afraid of?"
- ☐ 2. "It's normal to be scared. I would be, too. We'll help you through it."
- ☐ 3. "Don't be so hard on yourself. You don't know if your smoking caused the cancer."
- ☐ 4. "Do you feel guilty because you smoked?"

101. A client who underwent a left lower lobectomy has been out of surgery for 48 hours. She is receiving morphine sulfate via a patient-controlled analgesia (PCA) system. She complains of moderately severe pain in her left thorax that worsens when she coughs. The nurse should:
- ☐ 1. Let the client rest, so that she is not stimulated to cough.
- ☐ 2. Encourage the client to take deep breaths to help control the pain.
- ☐ 3. Check that the PCA device is functioning properly, and then reassure the client that the machine is working and will relieve her pain.
- ☐ 4. Assess the pain systematically with the hospital-approved scale.

102. Which of the following areas is a priority to evaluate when completing discharge planning for a client who has had a lobectomy for treatment of lung cancer?
- ☐ 1. The support available to assist the client at home.
- ☐ 2. The distance the client lives from the hospital.
- ☐ 3. The client's ability to do home blood pressure monitoring.
- ☐ 4. The client's knowledge of the causes of lung cancer.

103. Which of the following would be a major intervention to help prevent lung cancer?
- ☐ 1. Encourage cigarette smokers to have yearly chest radiographs.
- ☐ 2. Instruct people about techniques for smoking cessation.
- ☐ 3. Recommend that people have their houses and apartments checked for asbestos leakage.
- ☐ 4. Encourage people to install central air cleaners in their homes.

104. After a thoracotomy, clients should be instructed to perform deep-breathing exercises for which of the following reasons?
- ☐ 1. Deep breathing elevates the diaphragm, which enlarges the thorax and increases the lung surface available for gas exchange.
- ☐ 2. Deep breathing increases blood flow to the lungs to allow them to recover from the trauma of surgery.
- ☐ 3. Deep breathing controls the rate of air flow to the remaining lobe so that it will not become hyperinflated.
- ☐ 4. Deep breathing expands the alveoli and increases the lung surface available for ventilation.

105. Which of the following is the most important aspect of pain management for the client after a thoracotomy?
- ☐ 1. Repositioning the client immediately after administering pain medication.
- ☐ 2. Reassessing the client 30 minutes after administering pain medication.
- ☐ 3. Verbally reassuring the client after administering pain medication.
- ☐ 4. Readjusting the pain medication dosage as needed according to the client's condition.

106. While assessing a thoracotomy incisional area from which a chest tube exits, the nurse feels a crackling sensation under the fingertips along the entire incision. Which of the following should be the nurse's first action?
- ☐ 1. Lower the head of the bed and call the physician.
- ☐ 2. Prepare an aspiration tray.
- ☐ 3. Mark the area with a skin pencil at the outer periphery of the crackling.
- ☐ 4. Turn off the suction of the chest drainage system.

107. When teaching a client to deep breathe effectively after a lobectomy, the nurse should instruct the client to do which of the following?

☐ **1.** Contract the abdominal muscles, take a slow deep breath through the nose and hold it for 3 to 5 seconds, then exhale.

☐ **2.** Contract the abdominal muscles, take a deep breath through the mouth, and exhale slowly as if trying to blow out a candle.

☐ **3.** Relax the abdominal muscles, take a slow deep breath through the nose, and hold it for 3 to 5 seconds.

☐ **4.** Relax the abdominal muscles, take a deep breath through the mouth, and exhale slowly over 10 seconds.

108. Which of the following rehabilitative measures should the nurse teach the client who has undergone chest surgery to prevent shoulder ankylosis?

☐ **1.** Turn from side to side.

☐ **2.** Raise and lower the head.

☐ **3.** Raise the arm on the affected side over the head.

☐ **4.** Flex and extend the elbow on the affected side.

109. When caring for a client with a chest tube and water-seal drainage system, the nurse should implement which of the following interventions?

☐ **1.** Verify that the air vent on the water-seal drainage system is capped when the suction is off.

☐ **2.** Strip the chest drainage tubes at least every 4 hours if excessive bleeding occurs.

☐ **3.** Ensure that the chest tube is clamped when moving the client out of the bed.

☐ **4.** Make sure that the drainage apparatus is always below the client's chest level.

110. A client has a chest tube attached to a water-seal drainage system and the nurse notes that the fluid in the chest tube and in the water-seal column has stopped fluctuating. Which of the following is the explanation?

☐ **1.** The lung has fully expanded.

☐ **2.** The lung has collapsed.

☐ **3.** The chest tube is in the pleural space.

☐ **4.** The mediastinal space has decreased.

111. The nurse observes a constant gentle bubbling in the water-seal column of a water-seal chest drainage system. This observation should prompt the nurse to do which of the following?

☐ **1.** Continue monitoring as usual; this is expected.

☐ **2.** Check the connectors between the chest and drainage tubes and where the drainage tube enters the collection bottle.

☐ **3.** Decrease the suction to –15 cm H_2O and continue observing the system for changes in bubbling during the next several hours.

☐ **4.** Drain half of the water from the water-seal chamber.

112. A client who underwent a lobectomy and has a water-seal chest drainage system is breathing with a little more effort and at a faster rate than 1 hour ago. The client's pulse rate is also increased. Which of the following actions should the nurse implement?

☐ **1.** Check the tubing to ensure that the client is not lying on it or kinking it.

☐ **2.** Increase the suction.

☐ **3.** Lower the drainage bottles 2 to 3 feet below the level of the client's chest.

☐ **4.** Ensure that the chest tube has two clamps on it to prevent air leaks.

113. The nurse is assessing a client who has a chest tube connected to a water-seal chest tube drainage system. According to the illustration below, which should the nurse do?

☐ **1.** Clamp the chest tube near the insertion site to prevent air from entering the pleural cavity.

☐ **2.** Chart the amount of chest tube drainage.

☐ **3.** Add water to maintain the water seal.

☐ **4.** Change the chest tube drainage system.

114. Which of the following should be readily available at the bedside of a client with a chest tube in place?
☐ **1.** A tracheostomy tray.
☐ **2.** Another sterile chest tube.
☐ **3.** A bottle of sterile water.
☐ **4.** A spirometer.

The Client with Chest Trauma

115. A nurse is to administer 10 mg of morphine sulfate to a client with three fractured ribs. The available concentration for this drug is 15 mg/ml. How many milliliters should the nurse administer? Round to one decimal point.

_____ ml

116. A 21-year-old male client is transported by ambulance to the emergency department after a serious automobile accident. He complains of severe pain in his right chest where he struck the steering wheel. Which is the primary client goal at this time?
☐ **1.** Reduce the client's anxiety.
☐ **2.** Maintain adequate oxygenation.
☐ **3.** Decrease chest pain.
☐ **4.** Maintain adequate circulating volume.

117. A client with rib fractures and a pneumothorax has a chest tube inserted that is connected to a water-seal chest tube drainage system. The nurse notes that the fluid in the water-seal column is fluctuating with each breath that the client takes. What is the significance of this fluctuation?
☐ **1.** An obstruction is present in the chest tube.
☐ **2.** The client is developing subcutaneous emphysema.
☐ **3.** The chest tube system is functioning properly.
☐ **4.** There is a leak in the chest tube system.

118. A client who is recovering from chest trauma is to be discharged home with a chest tube drainage system intact. The nurse should instruct the client to call the physician for which of the following?
☐ **1.** Respiratory rate greater than 16 breaths/minute.
☐ **2.** Continuous bubbling in the water-seal chamber.
☐ **3.** Fluid in the chest tube.
☐ **4.** Fluctuation of fluid in the water-seal chamber.

119. Which of the following findings would suggest pneumothorax in a trauma victim?
☐ **1.** Pronounced crackles.
☐ **2.** Inspiratory wheezing.
☐ **3.** Dullness on percussion.
☐ **4.** Absent breath sounds.

120. For a client with rib fractures and a pneumothorax, the physician prescribes morphine sulfate, 1 to 2 mg/hour, given I.V. as needed for pain. The primary objective of this order is to provide adequate pain control so that the client can breathe effectively. Which of the following outcomes would indicate successful achievement of this objective?
☐ **1.** Pain rating of 0 on a scale of 0 to 10 by the client.
☐ **2.** Decreased client anxiety.
☐ **3.** Respiratory rate of 26 breaths/minute.
☐ **4.** Pao_2 of 70 mm Hg.

121. A client undergoes surgery to repair lung injuries. Postoperative orders include the transfusion of one unit of packed red blood cells at a rate of 60 ml/hour. How long would this transfusion take to infuse?
☐ **1.** 2 hours.
☐ **2.** 4 hours.
☐ **3.** 6 hours.
☐ **4.** 8 hours.

122. The primary reason for infusing blood at a rate of 60 ml/hour is to help prevent which of the following complications?
☐ **1.** Emboli formation.
☐ **2.** Fluid volume overload.
☐ **3.** Red blood cell hemolysis.
☐ **4.** Allergic reaction.

123. A client's chest tube is to be removed by the physician. Which of the following items should the nurse have ready to be placed directly over the wound when the chest tube is removed?
☐ **1.** Butterfly dressing.
☐ **2.** Montgomery strap.
☐ **3.** Fine-mesh gauze dressing.
☐ **4.** Petroleum gauze dressing.

124. Which of the following is a sign or symptom of a moderate pneumothorax?
☐ **1.** Sudden, sharp chest pain.
☐ **2.** Wheezing breath sounds over affected side.
☐ **3.** Hemoptysis.
☐ **4.** Cyanosis.

125. A chest tube is inserted in a client with a pneumothorax for which of the following reasons?
☐ **1.** For administration of oxygen.
☐ **2.** To promote formation of lung scar tissue.
☐ **3.** To insert antibiotics into the pleural space.
☐ **4.** To remove air and fluid.

The Client with Acute Respiratory Distress Syndrome

126. A client with acute respiratory distress syndrome (ARDS) has fine crackles at lung bases and the respirations are shallow at a rate of 28 breaths per minute. The client is restless and anxious. In addition to monitoring the arterial blood gas results, the nurse should do which of the following? Select all that apply.
- ☐ 1. Monitor serum creatinine and blood urea nitrogen levels.
- ☐ 2. Administer a sedative.
- ☐ 3. Keep the head of the bed flat.
- ☐ 4. Administer humidified oxygen.
- ☐ 5. Auscultate the lungs.

127. Which of the following interventions would be most likely to prevent the development of acute respiratory distress syndrome (ARDS)?
- ☐ 1. Teaching cigarette smoking cessation.
- ☐ 2. Maintaining adequate serum potassium levels.
- ☐ 3. Monitoring clients for signs of hypercapnia.
- ☐ 4. Replacing fluids adequately during hypovolemic states.

128. Which of the following nursing diagnoses would be a priority for a client with acute respiratory distress syndrome (ARDS)?
- ☐ 1. *Ineffective breathing pattern.*
- ☐ 2. *Pain.*
- ☐ 3. *Ineffective health maintenance.*
- ☐ 4. *Risk for infection.*

129. The nurse interprets which of the following as an early sign of acute respiratory distress syndrome (ARDS) in a client at risk?
- ☐ 1. Elevated carbon dioxide level.
- ☐ 2. Hypoxia not responsive to oxygen therapy.
- ☐ 3. Metabolic acidosis.
- ☐ 4. Severe, unexplained electrolyte imbalance.

130. A client has metabolic acidosis with compensatory respiratory alkalosis. Which of the following is a priority nursing diagnosis?
- ☐ 1. *Impaired gas exchange* related to intermittent hypoventilation.
- ☐ 2. *Impaired tissue integrity* related to hypertension.
- ☐ 3. *Fluid volume deficit* related to insufficient peristalsis.
- ☐ 4. *Ineffective breathing pattern* related to hyperventilation.

131. A client with acute respiratory distress syndrome (ARDS) is showing signs of increased dyspnea. The nurse reviews a report of blood gas values that recently arrived, shown below.

LABORATORY RESULTS	
Blood chemistry	**Result**
pH	7.35
$Paco_2$	25 mm Hg
HCO_3^-	22 mEq/L
Pao_2	95 mm Hg

Which finding should the nurse report to the physician?
- ☐ 1. pH.
- ☐ 2. $Paco_2$.
- ☐ 3. HCO_3^-.
- ☐ 4. Pao_2.

132. A client has the following arterial blood gas values: pH, 7.52; Pao_2, 50 mm Hg; $Paco_2$, 28 mm Hg; HCO_3^-, 24 mEq/L. From the client's $Paco_2$ level, the nurse determines that the client is experiencing which of the following conditions?
- ☐ 1. Hypoxemia.
- ☐ 2. Hypoventilation.
- ☐ 3. Hyperventilation.
- ☐ 4. Oxygen toxicity.

133. A client has the following arterial blood gas values: pH, 7.52; Pao_2, 50 mm Hg; $Paco_2$, 28 mm Hg; HCO_3^-, 24 mEq/L. Based upon the client's Pao_2, which of the following conclusions would be accurate?
- ☐ 1. The client is severely hypoxic.
- ☐ 2. The oxygen level is low but poses no risk for the client.
- ☐ 3. The client's Pao_2 level is within normal range.
- ☐ 4. The client requires oxygen therapy with very low oxygen concentrations.

134. A client has the following arterial blood gas values: pH, 7.52; Pao_2, 50 mm Hg; $Paco_2$, 28 mm Hg; HCO_3^-, 24 mEq/L. The nurse determines that which of the following is a possible cause for these findings?
- ☐ 1. Chronic obstructive pulmonary disease (COPD).
- ☐ 2. Diabetic ketoacidosis with Kussmaul's respirations.
- ☐ 3. Myocardial infarction.
- ☐ 4. Pulmonary embolus.

135. Which of the following interventions should the nurse anticipate in a client who has been diagnosed with acute respiratory distress syndrome (ARDS)?
- ☐ **1.** Tracheostomy.
- ☐ **2.** Use of a nasal cannula.
- ☐ **3.** Mechanical ventilation.
- ☐ **4.** Insertion of a chest tube.

136. The nurse should anticipate that which of the following conditions can place a client at risk for acute respiratory distress syndrome (ARDS)?
- ☐ **1.** Septic shock.
- ☐ **2.** Chronic obstructive pulmonary disease.
- ☐ **3.** Asthma.
- ☐ **4.** Heart failure.

137. Which one of the following assessments would be most appropriate for determining the correct placement of an endotracheal tube in a mechanically ventilated client?
- ☐ **1.** Assessing the client's skin color.
- ☐ **2.** Monitoring the respiratory rate.
- ☐ **3.** Verifying the amount of cuff inflation.
- ☐ **4.** Auscultating breath sounds bilaterally.

138. Which of the following nursing interventions would promote effective airway clearance in a client with acute respiratory distress?
- ☐ **1.** Administering oxygen every 2 hours.
- ☐ **2.** Turning the client every 4 hours.
- ☐ **3.** Administering sedatives to promote rest.
- ☐ **4.** Suctioning if cough is ineffective.

139. Which of the following complications is associated with mechanical ventilation?
- ☐ **1.** Gastrointestinal hemorrhage.
- ☐ **2.** Immunosuppression.
- ☐ **3.** Increased cardiac output.
- ☐ **4.** Pulmonary emboli.

140. A client experiences a headache, weakness, and slight confusion. A neighbor brings the client to the emergency department, where the physician diagnoses carbon monoxide poisoning. What should the nurse do?
- ☐ **1.** Initiate gastric lavage.
- ☐ **2.** Maintain body temperature.
- ☐ **3.** Administer 100% oxygen by mask.
- ☐ **4.** Obtain a psychiatric referral.

141. A confused client with carbon monoxide poisoning experiences dizziness when ambulating to the bathroom. Which action should the nurse perform?
- ☐ **1.** Put all four side rails up on the bed.
- ☐ **2.** Ask the unlicensed personnel to place restraints on the client's upper extremities.
- ☐ **3.** Request that the client's roommate put the call light on when the client is attempting to get out of bed.
- ☐ **4.** Check on the client at regular intervals to ascertain the need to use the bathroom.

142. A nurse receives the taped change-of-shift report for her assigned clients and prioritizes client rounds. In what order should the nurse assess these clients?

> **1.** A client with an endotracheal tube transferred out of the intensive care unit that day.

> **2.** A client with type 2 diabetes who had a cerebrovascular accident 4 days ago.

> **3.** A client with cellulitis of the left lower extremity with a fever of 100.8° F (38.2° C).

> **4.** A client receiving D_5W I.V. at 125 ml/hour with 75 ml remaining.

>

>

>

>

143. Interventions by a nurse for a client with pulmonary disease are aimed at attaining which of the following outcomes?
- ☐ **1.** A relatively matched ventilation-to-perfusion ratio.
- ☐ **2.** A low ventilation-to-perfusion ratio.
- ☐ **3.** A high ventilation-to-perfusion ratio.
- ☐ **4.** An equal Pao_2 and $Paco_2$ ratio.

Correct Answers and Rationales

The letter in parentheses after each rationale identifies the client need addressed in the item, including management of care (M), safety and infection control (S), health promotion and maintenance (H), psychosocial adaptation (P), basic care and comfort (C), pharmacological and parenteral therapies (D), reduction of risk potential (R), and physiological adaptation (A).

The Client with an Upper Respiratory Tract Infection

1. 1. At this time, there is no strong research evidence to warrant recommendations of herbal products for management of colds; further study is needed to show evidence of therapeutic effects and indications. Antibiotics are effective against bacteria; the head cold may have a viral cause. An uncomplicated upper respiratory tract infection subsides within 2 to 3 weeks. There may be a drug-drug interaction with herbal products and prescriptions. (C)

2. 2, 3, 4, 5. One of the "five rights" of drug administration is "right medication." Kefzol was not the medication ordered. The pharmacist is the professional resource and serves as a check to ensure that clients receive the right medication. Returning unwanted medications to the pharmacy will decrease the opportunity for a medication error by the nurse who follows the current nurse. (S)

3. 1, 4, 5. Antihistamines have an anticholinergic action and a drying effect and reduce nasal, salivary, and lacrimal gland hypersecretion (runny nose, tearing, and itching eyes). An adverse effect is drowsiness, so operating machinery and driving are not recommended. There is also an additive depressant effect when alcohol is combined with antihistamines, so alcohol should be avoided during antihistamine use. The client should ensure adequate fluid intake of at least 8 glasses per day due to the drying effect of the drug. Antihistamines have no antibacterial action. The effect of antihistamines is prompt, not delayed. (D)

4. 3. When using an intranasal inhaler, it is important to close off one nostril while inhaling the spray into the other nostril to ensure the best inhalation of the spray. Use of the inhaler is not limited to mornings and bedtime. The canister should be shaken immediately before use. The inhaler tip should be inserted into the nostril and pointed toward the outside nostril wall to maximize inhalation of the medication. (D)

5. 4. A client recovering from an upper respiratory tract infection should report decreasing or no nasal discharge and obstruction. Daily fluid intake should be increased to more than 1 L every 24 hours to liquefy secretions. The temperature should be below 100° F (37.8° C) with no chills or diaphoresis. A productive cough with chest pain indicates a pulmonary infection, not an upper respiratory tract infection. (A)

6. 2. The client should blow the nose before instilling nose drops. Instilling nose drops is a clean technique. The dropper should be cleaned after each administration, but it does not need to be changed. The client should assume a position that will allow the medication to reach the desired area; this is usually a supine position. (D)

7. 1. The plan of care for a client who has acute sinusitis includes antibiotics to treat the bacterial infection. In addition, nasal corticosteroids and decongestants are frequently ordered to decrease mucosal inflammation and edema. Nasal corticosteroids are preferred to oral corticosteroids because they do not produce systematic adverse effects when used as prescribed. Bronchodilators are ineffective in sinusitis. Antihistamines can promote an increase in secretion viscosity and continued symptoms; they should be avoided. (D)

8. 3. The client with chronic sinusitis should be instructed to take hot showers in the morning and evening to promote drainage of secretions. There is no need to limit caffeine intake. Performing postural drainage will inhibit removal of secretions, not promote it. Clients should elevate the head of the bed to promote drainage. Clients should report all temperatures higher than 100.4° F (38° C), because a temperature that high can indicate infection. (R)

9. 3. Individuals who are household members or home care providers for high-risk individuals are high-priority targeted groups for immunization against influenza to prevent transmission to those who have a decreased capacity to deal with the disease. The wife who is caring for a husband with cancer has the highest priority of the clients described because her husband is likely to be immunocompromised and particularly susceptible to the flu. A healthy 60-year-old man or a healthy 36-year-old woman is not in a high-priority category for influenza vaccination. A 60-year-old woman with osteoarthritis does not have a higher priority for influenza vaccination than a home care provider. (R)

10. 4. It is important for clients with allergic rhinitis to determine the precipitating factors so that they can be avoided. Keeping a diary can help identify these triggers. Nasal decongestant sprays should not be used regularly because they can cause a rebound effect. Antibiotics are not appropriate for allergic rhinitis because an infection is not present. Increasing activity will not control the client's symptoms; in fact, walking outdoors may increase them if the client is allergic to pollen. (H)

11. 1. Pneumonia is the most common complication of influenza, especially in the elderly. The development of a purulent cough and crackles may be indicative of a bacterial infection and is not consistent with a diagnosis of influenza. These findings are not indicative of dehydration. Decongestants and bronchodilators are not typically prescribed for the flu. (A)

12. 7.5

$$300 \text{ mg}/X = 200 \text{ mg}/5 \text{ ml}$$

$$X = 7.5 \text{ ml}.$$

(D)

13. 4. Adverse effects of pseudoephedrine (Sudafed) are experienced primarily in the cardiovascular system and through sympathetic effects on the central nervous system (CNS). The most common CNS adverse effects include restlessness, dizziness, tension, anxiety, insomnia, and weakness. Common cardiovascular adverse effects include tachycardia, hypertension, palpitations, and arrhythmias. Constipation and diplopia are not adverse effects of pseudoephedrine. Tachycardia, not bradycardia, is a adverse effect of pseudoephedrine. (D)

The Client Undergoing Nasal Surgery

14. **4.** Epistaxis, or *nosebleed*, is a common, sudden emergency. Commonly, no apparent explanation for the bleeding is known. With significant blood loss, systemic symptoms, such as vertigo, increased pulse, shortness of breath, decreased blood pressure, and pallor, will occur. Because aerobic exercise may increase blood pressure and increased blood pressure can cause epistaxis, the client with hypertension should avoid it. Aspirin inhibits platelet aggregation, reducing the ability of the blood to clot. The client should continue to take his antihypertension medication, ramipril (Altace). Posterior nasal packing should be left in place for 1 to 3 days. (H)

15. **2.** Because of the dense nasal packing, bleeding may not be apparent through the nasal drip pad. Instead, the blood may run down the throat, causing the client to swallow frequently. The back of the throat, where the blood will be apparent, can be assessed with a flashlight. An accumulation of blood in the stomach can cause nausea and vomiting, but nausea would not be the initial indicator of bleeding. An increased respiratory rate occurs in shock but is not an early sign of bleeding in a client who has undergone nasal surgery. Increased pain warrants further assessment but is not an indicator of bleeding. (R)

16. **1.** The client should be instructed to avoid any activities that cause Valsalva's maneuver (e.g., constipation, vigorous coughing, exercise) in order to reduce bleeding and stress on suture lines. The client should not take aspirin because of its antiplatelet properties, which may cause bleeding. Oral hygiene is important to rid the mouth of old dried blood and to enhance the client's appetite. Cool compresses, not heat, should be applied to decrease swelling and control discoloration of the area. (A)

17. **2.** Constipation can cause straining during defecation, which can induce bleeding. Showering is not contraindicated. The client should take measures to prevent coughing, which can cause bleeding. The client should avoid blowing her nose for 48 hours after the packing is removed. Thereafter, she should blow her nose gently, using the open-mouth technique to minimize bleeding in the surgical area. (A)

18. **4.** Aspirin-containing medications should be discontinued for 2 weeks before surgery to decrease the risk of bleeding. Nasal packing is usually removed the day after surgery. Normal saline nose drops are not routinely administered preoperatively. The results of the surgery will not be obvious immediately after surgery because of edema and ecchymosis. (R)

19. **3.** Immediately after nasal surgery, ineffective breathing patterns may develop as a result of the nasal packing and nasal edema. Nasal packing may dislodge, leading to obstruction. Assessing for airway obstruction is a priority. Assessing for pain is important, but it is not as high a priority as assessment of the airways. It is too early to detect ecchymosis. Measuring intake and output is not typically a priority nursing assessment after nasal surgery. (A)

20. **4.** Applying cold compresses helps to decrease facial swelling and pain from edema. Analgesics may decrease pain, but they do not decrease edema. A corticosteroid nasal spray would not be administered postoperatively because it can impair healing. Use of a bedside humidifier promotes comfort by providing moisture for nasal mucosa, but it does not decrease edema. (C)

21. **1.** Frequent mouth care is important to provide comfort and encourage eating. Mouth care promotes moist mucous membranes. Nose drops cannot be used with nasal packing in place. When sneezing and coughing, the client should do so with the mouth open to decrease the chance of dislodging the packing. Gargling should not be attempted with packing in place. (C)

22. **2.** After removal of nasal packing, the client should be instructed to apply water-soluble jelly to the nares to lubricate the nares and promote comfort. Swelling gradually subsides over several weeks; the client can gently clean the nares as soon as packing is removed. A nasal drip pad is not needed after removal of packing. Irrigation with a bulb syringe may interfere with healing and introduce infection. (C)

23. **4.** The client should assume a sitting position and lean forward. Firm pressure should be applied to the soft portion of the nose for approximately 10 minutes. Tilting the head backward can cause the client to swallow blood, which can obscure the amount of bleeding and also can lead to nausea. Ice compresses may be applied, but the client should not lie flat. Blowing the nose is to be avoided because it can increase bleeding. (R)

24. **3.** Posterior packing may alter the respiratory status of the client, especially in elderly clients, causing hypoventilation. Clients should be observed carefully for changes in level of consciousness, respiratory rate, and heart rate and rhythm after the insertion of the packing. Vertigo does not occur as a result of the insertion of posterior packing. Bell's palsy, a disorder of the seventh cranial nerve, is not associated with epistaxis or nasal packing. Loss of gag reflex does not occur as a result of the insertion of posterior packing. (R)

The Client with Cancer of the Larynx

25. 2. The client will be unable to speak after the laryngectomy, and an alternative method of communication must be used. The method (writing or using a communication board with letters, words, or pictures as desired) should be determined and practiced preoperatively. The client with a laryngectomy is able to swallow but may have difficulty swallowing initially. Intravenous fluids will be administered to maintain an adequate fluid volume. Although *Powerlessness* may be an important diagnosis for clients with cancer, there are no data to support that it is indicated for this client. (A)

26. 4. The client has undergone body changes and permanent loss of verbal communication. He may feel isolated and insecure. The nurse can encourage him to express his feelings and use this information to develop an appropriate plan of care. Discussing the client's behavior with his wife may not reveal his feelings. Exploring future plans is not appropriate at this time because more information about the client's behavior is needed before proceeding to this level. The nurse can respect the client's need for privacy while also encouraging him to express his feelings. (P)

27. 1. A client should be suctioned for no longer than 10 seconds at a time. Suctioning for longer than 10 seconds may reduce the client's oxygen level so much that he becomes hypoxic. (R)

28. 1. The recommended technique is to use a sterile catheter each time the client is suctioned. There is a danger of introducing organisms into the respiratory tract when strict aseptic technique is not used. Reusing a suction catheter is not consistent with aseptic technique. The nurse does not use a clean catheter when suctioning a tracheostomy or a laryngectomy; it is a sterile procedure. (R)

29. 3. *Disturbed body image* is the most appropriate nursing diagnosis based on the client's statements at this time. Most clients are concerned about how their family members will respond to the physical changes that have occurred as a result of radical neck surgery. The nurse should allow the client to communicate any negative feelings or concerns that exist because of the surgery. Referral

to a support group for laryngectomy clients may be helpful to the client and family members in coping with the changes in their lives. The client's feelings are not related to a knowledge deficit, but rather to a permanent change in physical appearance and functioning. The diagnosis of *Disturbed personal identity* refers to a client's inability to distinguish self from nonself. *Hopelessness* may be an issue for the client experiencing a body image disturbance; however, there are no data to support this diagnosis at this time. (P)

30. 4. The primary risk factor for laryngeal cancer is cigarette smoking. The use of alcohol, in combination with smoking, appears to increase the risk. Approximately 90% of head and neck cancers, including laryngeal cancer, develop after prolonged use of tobacco and alcohol. Chronic allergy conditions are not implicated in cancer of the larynx. The use of chewing tobacco and snuff can lead to the development of oral cancer. Exposure to noxious fumes or polluted air and voice abuse are also factors in the development of laryngeal cancer, but they are not primary factors. (H)

31. 2. Early warning signs of laryngeal cancer can vary depending on tumor location. Hoarseness lasting longer than 2 weeks should be evaluated because it is one of the most common warning signs. Other early warning signs include a lump in the neck, persistent sore throat, cough, earache, or the feeling of a lump in the throat. Later signs and symptoms include dysphagia, hemoptysis, pain, and airway obstruction. Stomatitis is not a sign of laryngeal cancer. (H)

32. 1. Immediately after surgery, the client should be maintained in a position with the head of the bed elevated 30 to 40 degrees (semi-Fowler's position) to decrease tissue edema, facilitate breathing, and decrease pain related to edema formation. Immediately postoperatively, the client should be provided alternative means of communicating, such as a communication board. As healing progresses and edema subsides, a speech therapist should work with the client to explore various voice restoration options, such as the use of a voice prosthesis, electrolarynx, artificial larynx, or esophageal speech. Food is not initiated in the immediate postoperative phase; enteral feedings are usually used to meet nutritional needs until edema subsides. Irrigation of the drainage tubes is an inappropriate action. (C)

33. 3. It is important that the client be able to communicate his or her feelings about the body image changes that have occurred as a result of surgery. Open communication helps promote adjustment. The client may not regain the ability to taste and smell food because of no longer breathing through the nose or because of radiation therapy treatments, or both. A gastrostomy tube would not typically be placed after a total laryngectomy, nor would it be necessary for the client to demonstrate sterile suctioning technique for stoma care. The client would use clean technique. (A)

34. **2.** Adequate humidity should be provided in the home to help keep secretions moist. A bedside humidifier is recommended. A high fluid intake is also important to liquefy secretions. Mouth care is important to prevent drying of mucous membranes and should be performed frequently throughout the day, especially before and after meals, to help stimulate appetite. The client may eat any food that can be chewed and swallowed comfortably. The client may resume physical activity as tolerated. (R)

35.

> **1.** An 85-year-old client with bacterial pneumonia, temperature of 102.2° F (42° C), and shortness of breath.

> **2.** A 60-year-old client with chest tubes who is 2 days postoperative following a thoracotomy for lung cancer and is requesting something for pain.

> **4.** A 56-year-old client with emphysema who has a scheduled dose of a bronchodilator due to be administered, with no report of acute respiratory distress.

> **3.** A 35-year-old client with suspected tuberculosis who is complaining of a cough.

The elderly client with pneumonia, an elevated temperature, and shortness of breath is the most acutely ill client described and should be the client with the highest priority. The elevated temperature and shortness of breath can lead to a decrease in the client's oxygen levels, and can predispose the client to dehydration and confusion. Then the nurse should assess the client with the thoracotomy who is requesting pain medication and administer any needed medication. The client with emphysema should be the next priority so that the bronchodilator can be administered on schedule as close as possible. The nurse would then assess the client with suspected tuberculosis and a cough. (M)

The Client with Pneumonia

36. **3.** In kyphosis, the thoracic spine bends forward with convexity of the curve in a posterior direction, making effective coughing and deep breathing difficult. Al-

though the client may develop other problems because respiratory status deteriorates when pulmonary secretions are not adequately cleared from airways, ineffective coughing and deep breathing should receive priority attention. (A)

37. **1.** Elevating the head of the bed facilitates breathing because the lungs are able to expand as the diaphragm descends. Coughing and deep breathing do not alleviate the symptoms of a pulmonary embolus, nor does lung auscultation. The physician must be kept informed of changes in a client's status, but the priority in this case is alleviating the symptoms. (R)

38. **1.** The client's age is a predisposing factor for pneumonia; pneumonia is more common in elderly or debilitated clients. Other predisposing factors include smoking, upper respiratory tract infections, malnutrition, immunosuppression, and the presence of a chronic illness. Osteoarthritis, a nutritionally sound vegetarian diet, and frequent bathing are not predisposing factors for pneumonia. (R)

39. **1, 3, 5.** A respiratory assessment, which includes auscultating breath sounds and assessing the color of the nail beds, is a priority for clients with pneumonia. Assessing for the presence of chest pain is also an important respiratory assessment as chest pain can interfere with the client's ability to breathe deeply. Auscultating bowel sounds and assessing for peripheral edema may be appropriate assessments, but these are not priority assessments for the client with pneumonia. (A)

40. **2.** A sputum specimen is obtained for culture to determine the causative organism. After the organism is identified, an appropriate antibiotic can be prescribed. Beginning antibiotic therapy before obtaining the sputum specimen may alter the results of the test. Neither a urinalysis, a chest radiograph, nor a red blood cell count needs to be obtained before initiation of antibiotic therapy for pneumonia. (R)

41. **3.** It is essential to monitor serum creatinine in the client receiving an aminoglycoside antibiotic because of the potential of this type of drug to cause acute tubular necrosis. Aminoglycoside antibiotics do not affect serum sodium, potassium, or calcium levels. (D)

42. **3.** Frequent linen changes are appropriate for this client because of the diaphoresis. Diaphoresis produces general discomfort. The client should be kept dry to promote comfort. Position changes need to be done every 2 hours. Nasotracheal suctioning is not indicated with the client's productive cough. Frequent offering of a bedpan is not indicated by the data provided in this scenario. (C)

43. 1. Exudate in the alveoli interferes with ventilation and the diffusion of gases in clients with pneumonia. During the acute phase of the illness, it is essential to reduce the body's need for oxygen at the cellular level; bed rest is the most effective method for doing so. Bed rest does not decrease coughing or promote clearance of secretions, and it does not necessarily provide a safe environment. (A)

44. 4. A client with pneumonia has less lung surface available for the diffusion of gases because of the inflammatory pulmonary response that creates lung exudate and results in reduced oxygenation of the blood. The client becomes cyanotic because blood is not adequately oxygenated in the lungs before it enters the peripheral circulation. Decreased cardiac output may be a comorbid condition in some clients with pneumonia; however, it is not the cause of cyanosis. Pleural effusions are a potential complication of pneumonia but are not the primary cause of decreased oxygenation. Inadequate peripheral circulation is also not the cause of the cyanosis that develops with bacterial pneumonia. (A)

45. 3. Chest pain in pneumonia is generally caused by friction between the pleural layers. It is more severe on inspiration than on expiration, secondary to chest wall movement. Pleuritic chest pain is usually described as sharp, not mild or aching. Pleuritic chest pain is not localized to the sternum, and it is not the result of a muscle spasm. (A)

46. 4. The pleuritic pain is triggered by chest movement and is particularly severe during coughing. Splinting the chest wall will help reduce the discomfort of coughing. Deep breathing is essential to prevent further atelectasis. Abdominal breathing is not as effective in decreasing pleuritic chest pain as is splinting of the rib cage. Incentive spirometry facilitates effective deep breathing but does not decrease pleuritic chest pain. (A)

47. 1. Aspirin is administered to clients with pneumonia because it is an analgesic that helps control chest discomfort and an antipyretic that helps reduce fever. It is also an anti-inflammatory agent that reduces inflammation. Aspirin has an anticoagulant effect, but that is not the reason for prescribing it for a client with pneumonia. Aspirin does not have adrenergic or antihistamine effects, and drugs with adrenergic or antihistamine effects are not used for the treatment of pneumonia. (D)

48. 3. Clients who are experiencing hypoxia characteristically exhibit irritability, restlessness, or anxiety as initial mental status changes. As the hypoxia becomes more pronounced, the client may become confused and combative. Coma is a late clinical manifestation of hypoxia. Apathy and depression are not symptoms of hypoxia. (A)

49. 1. Docusate sodium (Colace) is a stool softener that allows fluid and fatty substances to enter the stool and soften it. Docusate sodium does not lubricate the stool, increase stool bulk, or stimulate peristalsis. (D)

50. 4. A fluid intake of at least 3 L/day should be provided to replace any fluid loss occurring as a result of the fever and diaphoresis; this is a high-priority intervention. Although clients with pneumonia may be prescribed bed rest, complete bed rest is not necessary solely because of the elevated temperature. Administration of oxygen therapy also is not indicated for the purposes of treating the fever. Frequent linen changes is an appropriate intervention, but it is not of the highest priority among the options given. (R)

51. 2. An expected outcome for a client recovering from pneumonia would be the ability to perform activities of daily living without experiencing dyspnea. A respiratory rate of 25 to 30 breaths/minute indicates the client is experiencing tachypnea, which would not be expected on recovery. A weight loss of 5 to 10 lb is undesirable; the expected outcome would be to maintain normal weight. A client who is recovering from pneumonia should experience decreased or no chest pain. (M)

The Client with Tuberculosis

52. 1. Tuberculosis typically produces anorexia and weight loss. Other signs and symptoms may include fatigue, low-grade fever, and night sweats. Increased appetite is not a symptom of tuberculosis; dyspnea on exertion and change in mental status are not common symptoms of tuberculosis. (A)

53. 1. The most commonly used technique to identify tubercle bacilli is acid-fast staining. The bacilli have a waxy surface, which makes them difficult to stain in the laboratory. However, once they are stained, the stain is resistant to removal, even with acids. Therefore, tubercle bacilli are often called acid-fast bacilli. Sensitivity testing, agglutination testing, and dark-field illumination are not used to identify tubercle bacilli. (R)

54. 1. Streptomycin is an aminoglycoside, and eighth cranial nerve damage (ototoxicity) is a common adverse effect of aminoglycosides. A common adverse effect of isoniazid (INH) is peripheral neuritis. A common adverse effect of para-aminosalicylic acid (PAS) is gastrointestinal disturbance. A common adverse effect of ethambutol hydrochloride (Myambutol) is optic neuritis. (D)

55. 1. The eighth cranial nerve is the vestibulocochlear nerve, which is responsible for hearing and equilibrium. Streptomycin can damage this nerve (ototoxicity). Symptoms of ototoxicity include vertigo, tinnitus, hearing loss, and ataxia. Facial paralysis would result from damage to the facial nerve (VII). Impaired vision would result from damage to the optic (II), oculomotor (III), or the trochlear (IV) nerves. Difficulty swallowing would result from damage to the glossopharyngeal (IX) or the vagus (X) nerve. (D)

56. 2. Tubercle bacilli are spread by airborne droplet nuclei. Droplet nuclei are the residue of evaporated droplets containing the bacilli, which remain suspended and are circulated in the air. Dust particles and water do not spread tubercle bacilli. Tuberculosis is not spread by eating utensils, dishes, or other fomites. (S)

57. 4. Use of a combination of antituberculosis drugs slows the rate at which organisms develop drug resistance. Combination therapy also appears to be more effective than single-drug therapy. Many drugs potentiate (or inhibit) the actions of other drugs; however, this is not the rationale for using multiple drugs to treat tuberculosis. Treatment with multiple drugs does not reduce adverse effects and may expose the client to more adverse effects. Combination therapy may allow some medications (e.g., antihypertensives) to be given in reduced dosages; however, reduced dosages are not prescribed for antibiotics and antituberculosis drugs. (D)

58. 2. Ensuring that the client is well educated about tuberculosis is the highest priority. Education of the client and family is essential to help the client understand the need for completing the prescribed drug therapy to cure the disease. Offering the client emotional support, coordinating various agency services, and assessing the environment may be part of the care for the client with tuberculosis; however, these interventions are of less importance than education about the disease process and its treatment. (C)

59. 1. The Mantoux test is administered via intradermal injection. The appropriate technique for an intradermal injection includes holding the needle and syringe almost parallel to the client's skin, keeping the skin slightly taut when the needle is inserted, and inserting the needle with the bevel side up. There is no need to aspirate, a technique that assesses for incorrect placement in a blood vessel, when giving an intradermal injection. The injection site is not massaged. (D)

60. 4. Elderly persons are believed to be at higher risk for contracting tuberculosis because of decreased immunocompetence. Other high-risk populations in the United States include the urban poor, clients with acquired immunodeficiency syndrome, and minority groups. (S)

61. 2, 4, 5. When teaching the client how to avoid the transmission of tubercle bacilli, it is important for the client to understand that the organism is transmitted by droplet infection. Therefore, covering the mouth and nose when sneezing, using paper tissues to cough in with prompt disposal, and using regular plates and utensils indicate that the client has understood the nurse's instructions about preventing the spread of airborne droplets. It is not essential to discard clothing, nor does the client need to isolate himself from family members. (H)

62. 2. A positive Mantoux skin test indicates that the client has been exposed to tubercle bacilli. Exposure does not necessarily mean that active disease exists. A positive Mantoux test does not mean that the client has developed resistance. Unless involved in treatment, the client may still develop active disease at any time. Immunity to tuberculosis is not possible. (R)

63. 2. INH competes for the available vitamin B_6 in the body and leaves the client at risk for development of neuropathies related to vitamin deficiency. Supplemental vitamin B_6 is routinely prescribed. Following a low-cholesterol diet, getting extra rest, and avoiding excessive sun exposure will not prevent the development of peripheral neuropathies. (D)

64. 3. INH interferes with the effectiveness of hormonal contraceptives, and female clients of childbearing age should be counseled to use an alternative form of birth control while taking the drug. INH does not increase the risk of vaginal infection, nor does it affect the ova or ovulation. (D)

65. 3. Tuberculosis can be controlled but never completely eradicated from the body. Periods of intense physical or emotional stress increase the likelihood of recurrence. Clients should be taught to recognize the signs and symptoms of a potential recurrence. Weather and activity levels are not related to recurrences of tuberculosis. (A)

66. 2. Statistics show that of the four geographic areas described, most cases of tuberculosis are found in inner-core residential areas of large cities, where health and sanitation standards tend to be low. Substandard housing, poverty, and crowded living conditions also generally characterize these city areas and contribute to the spread of the disease. Farming areas have a low incidence of tuberculosis. Variations in water standards and industrial pollution are not correlated to tuberculosis incidence. (S)

67. 4. Isoniazid and rifampin (Rifamate) is a hepatotoxic drug. The client should be warned to limit intake of alcohol during drug therapy. The drug should be taken on an empty stomach. If antacids are needed for gastrointestinal distress, they should be taken 1 hour before or 2 hours after the drug is administered. The client should not double the dose of the drug because of potential toxicity. The client taking the drug should avoid foods that are rich in tyramine, such as cheese and dairy products, or he may develop hypertension. (D)

68. **2, 4, 5.** A potential adverse effect of rifampin (Rifadin) is hepatotoxicity. Clients should be instructed to avoid alcohol intake while taking rifampin and keep follow-up appointments for periodic monitoring of liver enzyme levels to detect liver toxicity. Rifampin causes the urine to turn an orange color and the client should understand that this is normal. It is not necessary to restrict protein intake in the diet or have the eyes examined due to rifampin therapy. (D)

69. **1.** Directly observed therapy (DOT) can be implemented with clients who are not compliant with drug therapy. In DOT, a responsible person, who may be a family member or a health care provider, observes the client taking the medication. Visiting the client, changing the prescription, or threatening the client will not ensure compliance if the client will not or cannot follow the prescribed treatment. (S)

The Client with Chronic Obstructive Pulmonary Disease

70. **1.** The client's problem is imbalanced nutrition—specifically, less than required. The cause, as stated by the client, is the fatigue associated with the disease process. *Activity intolerance* is a likely diagnosis but is not related to the client's nutritional problems. *Weight loss* is not a nursing diagnosis. *Ineffective breathing pattern* may be a problem, but this diagnosis does not specifically address the problem of weight loss described by the client. (C)

71. **1.** A client with COPD is at high risk for development of respiratory infections. COPD is slowly progressive; therefore, maintaining current status and establishing a goal that the client will require less supplemental oxygen are unrealistic expectations. Treatment may slow progression of the disease, but permanent improvement is highly unlikely. (M)

72. **4.** Increasing dyspnea on exertion indicates that the client may be experiencing complications of COPD. Therefore, the nurse should notify the physician. Extracting promises from clients is not an outcome criterion. Pain is not a common symptom of COPD. Clients with COPD use low-flow oxygen supplementation (1 to 2 L/minute) to avoid suppressing the respiratory drive, which, for these clients, is stimulated by hypoxia. (C)

73. **1.** Increased anteroposterior chest diameter is characteristic of advanced COPD. Air is trapped in the overextended alveoli, and the ribs are fixed in an inspiratory position. The result is the typical barrel-chested appearance. Overly developed, not underdeveloped, neck muscles are associated with COPD because of their increased use in the work of breathing. Distended, not collapsed, neck veins are associated with COPD as a symptom of the heart failure that the client may experience secondary to the increased workload on the heart to pump blood into the pulmonary vasculature. Diminished, not increased, chest excursion is associated with COPD. (A)

74. **4.** Cigarette smoking is the primary cause of COPD. Other risk factors include exposure to environmental pollutants and chronic asthma. Participating in an aerobic exercise program, although beneficial, will not decrease the risk of COPD. Insufficient protein intake and exposure to people with respiratory infections do not increase the risk of COPD. (H)

75. **4.** Pursed-lip breathing prolongs exhalation and prevents air trapping in the alveoli, thereby promoting carbon dioxide elimination. By prolonging exhalation and helping the client relax, pursed-lip breathing helps the client learn to control the rate and depth of respiration. Pursed-lip breathing does not promote the intake of oxygen, strengthen the diaphragm, or strengthen intercostal muscles. (A)

76. **1.** A priority goal for the client with COPD is to manage the signs and symptoms of the disease process so as to maintain the client's functional ability. Chest pain is not a typical symptom of COPD. The carbon dioxide concentration in the blood is increased to an abnormal level in clients with COPD; it would not be a goal to increase the level further. Preventing infection would be a goal of care for the client with COPD. (C)

77. **2.** The high $Paco_2$ level causes flushing due to vasodilation. The client also becomes drowsy and lethargic because carbon dioxide has a depressant effect on the central nervous system. Cyanosis is a sign of hypoxia. Irritability and anxiety are not common with a $Paco_2$ level of 65 mm Hg but are associated with hypoxia. (R)

78. **2.** The principle behind using postural drainage is that gravity will help move secretions from smaller to larger airways. Postural drainage is best used after percussion has loosened secretions. Coughing or suctioning is then used to remove secretions. Movement of cilia is not sufficient to move secretions. Muscle contractions do not move secretions within the lungs. (A)

79. 2. Exhaling requires less energy than inhaling. Therefore, lifting while exhaling saves energy and reduces perceived dyspnea. Pursing the lips prolongs exhalation and provides the client with more control over breathing. Lifting after exhaling but before inhaling is similar to lifting with the breath held. This should not be recommended because it is similar to the Valsalva maneuver, which can stimulate cardiac arrhythmias. (C)

80. 3. Right-sided heart failure is a complication of COPD that occurs because of pulmonary hypertension. Signs and symptoms of right-sided heart failure include peripheral edema, jugular venous distention, hepatomegaly, and weight gain due to increased fluid volume. Clubbing of nail beds is associated with conditions of chronic hypoxemia. Hypertension is associated with left-sided heart failure. Clients with heart failure have decreased appetites. (A)

81. 4. Exacerbations of COPD are commonly caused by respiratory infections. Coarse crackles and rhonchi would be auscultated as air moves through airways obstructed with secretions. In COPD, breath sounds are diminished because of an enlarged anteroposterior diameter of the chest. Expiration, not inspiration, becomes prolonged. Chest movement is decreased as lungs become overdistended. (A)

82. 1. As COPD progresses, the client typically develops increased Pa_{CO_2} levels and decreased Pa_{O_2} levels. This results in decreased pH and decreased oxygen saturation. These changes are the result of air trapping and hypoventilation. (R)

83. 2. Clients who have a long history of COPD may retain carbon dioxide (CO_2). Gradually the body adjusts to the higher CO_2 concentration, and the high levels of CO_2 no longer stimulate the respiratory center. The major respiratory stimulant then becomes hypoxemia. Administration of high concentrations of oxygen eliminates this respiratory stimulus and leads to hypoventilation. Oxygen can be drying if it is not humidified, but it does not cause coughing and dyspnea. Increased oxygen use will not create an oxygen dependency; clients should receive oxygen as needed. Oxygen is not contraindicated with the use of bronchodilators. (A)

84. 4. The client should eat high-calorie, high-protein meals to maintain nutritional status and prevent weight loss that results from the increased work of breathing. The client should be encouraged to eat small, frequent meals. A low-fat, low-cholesterol diet is indicated for clients with coronary artery disease. The client with COPD does not necessarily need to follow a sodium-restricted diet, unless otherwise medically indicated. There is no need for the client to eat bland, soft foods. (C)

85. 3. Theophylline (Theo-Dur) is a bronchodilator that is administered to relax airways and decrease dyspnea. Theophylline is not used to treat infections and does not decrease or thin secretions. (D)

86. 1. The goal of effective coughing is to conserve energy, facilitate removal of secretions, and minimize airway collapse. The client should assume a sitting position with feet on the floor if possible. The client should bend forward slightly and, using pursed-lip breathing, exhale. After resuming an upright position, the client should use abdominal breathing to slowly and deeply inhale. After repeating this process three or four times, the client should take a deep abdominal breath, bend forward, and cough three or four times upon exhalation ("huff" cough). Lying flat does not enhance lung expansion; sitting upright promotes full expansion of the thorax. Shallow breathing does not facilitate removal of secretions, and forceful coughing promotes collapse of airways. A side-lying position does not allow for adequate chest expansion to promote deep breathing. (C)

The Client with Asthma

87. 1, 2, 3, 4, 5. Utilization of an MDI requires coordination between activation and inspiration; deep breaths to ensure that medication is distributed into the lungs, holding the breath for 10 seconds or as long as possible to disperse the medication into the lungs, shaking up the medication in the MDI before use, and a sufficient amount of time between puffs to provide an adequate amount of inhalation medication. (D)

88. 4. In an acute asthma attack, diminished or absent breath sounds can be an ominous sign indicating lack of air movement in the lungs and impending respiratory failure. The client requires immediate intervention with inhaled bronchodilators, I.V. corticosteroids and, possibly, I.V. theophylline (Theo-Dur). Administering oxygen and reassessing the client 10 minutes later would delay needed medical intervention, as would drawing blood for an arterial blood gas analysis and obtaining a chest X-ray. It would be futile to encourage the client to relax and breathe slowly without providing the necessary pharmacologic intervention. (M)

89. 2. As the severe asthma attack worsens, the client becomes fatigued and alveolar hypoventilation develops. This leads to carbon dioxide retention and hypoxemia. The client develops respiratory acidosis. Therefore, the Pa_{CO_2}

level increases, the Pa_{O_2} level decreases, and the pH decreases, indicating acidosis. (A)

90. 3. Corticosteroids have an anti-inflammatory effect and act to decrease edema in the bronchial airways and decrease mucus secretion. Corticosteroids do not have a bronchodilator effect, act as expectorants, or prevent respiratory infections. (D)

91. 1, 4. The client should shake the inhaler and hold it upright when administering the drug. The head should be tilted back slightly. The client should wait about 1 to 2 minutes between puffs. The mouth should be rinsed following the use of a corticosteroid MDI to decrease the likelihood of developing an oral infection. The client does not need to lie supine; instead, the client will likely to be able to breathe more freely if sitting upright. (D)

92. 1. Irregular heartbeats should be reported promptly to the care provider. Metaproterenol (Alupent) may cause irregular heartbeat, tachycardia, or anginal pain because of its adrenergic effect on beta-adrenergic receptors in the heart. It is not recommended for use in clients with known cardiac disorders. Metaproterenol does not cause constipation, pedal edema, or bradycardia. (D)

93. 3. Use of oral inhalant corticosteroids such as flunisolide (AeroBid) can lead to the development of oral thrush, a fungal infection. Once developed, thrush must be treated by antifungal therapy; it will not resolve on its own. Fungal infections can develop even without overuse of the corticosteroid inhaler. Although good oral hygiene can help prevent development of a fungal infection, it cannot be used alone to treat the problem. (D)

94.

| 1. Shake the inhaler immediately before use. |
| 4. Breathe out through the mouth. |
| 3. Activate the MDI on inhalation. |
| 2. Hold breath for 5 to 10 seconds and then exhale. |

When using inhalers, clients should first shake the inhaler to activate the MDI, and then breathe out through the mouth. Next, the client should activate the MDI while inhaling, hold the breath for 5 to 10 seconds, and then exhale normally. (D)

95. 4. Between attacks, breath sounds should be clear on auscultation with good air flow present throughout lung fields. Chest X-rays should be normal. The client should remain afebrile. Arterial blood gases should be normal. (A)

96. 1. Physical exercise is beneficial and should be incorporated as tolerated into the client's schedule. Peak flow numbers should be monitored daily, usually in the morning (before taking medication). Peak flow does not need to be monitored after each meal. Stressors in the client's life should be modified but cannot be totally eliminated. Although adequate sleep is important, it is not recommended that sedatives be routinely taken to induce sleep. (R)

97. 2. The most common precipitator of asthma attacks is viral respiratory infection. Clients with asthma should avoid people who have the flu or a cold and should get yearly flu vaccinations. Environmental exposure to toxins or heavy particulate matter can trigger asthma attacks; however, far fewer asthmatics are exposed to such toxins than are exposed to viruses. Cigarette smoke can also trigger asthma attacks, but to a lesser extent than viral respiratory infections. Some asthmatic attacks are triggered by exercising in cold weather. (R)

98. 1. A cough productive of yellow sputum is the most likely indicator of a respiratory infection. The other signs and symptoms—wheezing, chest tightness, and increased respiratory rate—are all findings associated with an asthma attack and do not necessarily mean an infection is present. (A)

The Client with Lung Cancer

99. 1. Risk factors for postoperative pulmonary complications include malnourishment, which is indicated by this client's height and weight. It is thought that emotional responses can affect overall health; however, not verbalizing one's feelings is not a contributing factor in postoperative pulmonary complications. The client's current activity level and age do not place her at increased risk for complications. (A)

100. 1. Acknowledging the basic feeling the client expresses—fear—and asking an open-ended question allows the client to explain any fears. The other options dismiss the client's feelings and may give false reassurance or label the client's feelings. The client should be encouraged to explore feelings about a cancer diagnosis. (P)

101. 4. Systematic pain assessment is necessary for adequate pain management in the postoperative client. Guidelines from a variety of health care agencies and nursing groups recommend that institutions adopt a pain assessment scale to assist in facilitating pain management. Even though the client is receiving morphine sulfate by PCA, assessment is needed if she is experiencing pain. The concern is not to eliminate coughing but to control pain adequately. Coughing is necessary to prevent postoperative atelectasis and pneumonia. Breathing exercises may help control pain in some circumstances; however, most clients with thoracic surgery require parenteral opioid analgesics in the early postoperative period. Although it is necessary that the PCA device be checked periodically to ensure that it is functioning properly, if the machine is functional and the client's pain is not relieved, further intervention, beginning with a pain assessment, is indicated. (C)

102. **1.** Because clients are discharged as soon as possible from the hospital, it is essential to evaluate the support they have to assist them with self-care at home. The distance the client lives from the hospital is not a critical factor in discharge planning. There are no data indicating that home blood pressure monitoring is needed. Knowledge of the causes of lung cancer, although important, is not the most essential area to evaluate given the client's postoperative status. (P)

103. **2.** Epidermoid cancer involving the larger bronchi is almost entirely associated with heavy cigarette smoking. The American Cancer Society reports that smoking is responsible for more than 80% of lung cancers in men and women. The prevalence of lung cancer is related to the duration and intensity of the smoking, so nurses can best prevent lung cancer by persuading clients to stop smoking. Chest radiographs aid in detection of lung cancer; they do not prevent it. Exposure to asbestos has been implicated as a risk factor for lung cancer, but cigarette smoking is the major risk factor. There are no data to support the use of home air cleaners in the prevention of lung cancer. (H)

104. **4.** Deep breathing helps prevent microatelectasis and pneumonitis and also helps force air and fluid out of the pleural space into the chest tubes. More than half of the ventilatory process is accomplished by the rise and fall of the diaphragm. The diaphragm is the major muscle of respiration; deep breathing causes it to descend, not elevate, thereby increasing the ventilating surface. Deep breathing increases blood flow to the lungs; however, the primary reason for deep breathing is to expand alveoli and prevent atelectasis. The remaining lobe naturally hyperinflates to fill the space created by the resected lobe. This is an expected phenomenon. (A)

105. **2.** It is essential that the nurse evaluate the effects of pain medication after the medication has had time to act; reassessment is necessary to determine the effectiveness of the pain management plan. Although it is prudent to check for discomfort related to positioning when assessing the client's pain, repositioning the client immediately after administering pain medication is not necessary. Verbally reassuring the client after administering pain medication may be useful to help instill confidence in the treatment plan; however, it is not as important as evaluating the effectiveness of the medication. Readjusting the pain medication dosage as needed according to the client's condition is essential, but the effectiveness of the medication must be evaluated first. (A)

106. **3.** This crackling sensation is subcutaneous emphysema. Subcutaneous emphysema is not an unusual finding, and it is not dangerous if confined. But progression can be serious, especially if the neck is involved; a tracheotomy may be needed. If emphysema progresses noticeably in 1 hour, the physician should be notified. Lowering the head of the bed will not arrest the progress or provide any further information. A tracheotomy tray would be useful if subcutaneous emphysema progresses to the neck. Subcutaneous emphysema may progress if the chest drainage system does not adequately remove air and fluid; therefore, the system should not be turned off. (A)

107. **1.** The recommended procedure for teaching clients postoperatively to deep breathe includes contracting (pulling in) the abdominal muscles and taking a slow, deep breath through the nose. This breath is held 3 to 5 seconds, which facilitates alveolar ventilation by improving the inspiratory phase of ventilation. Exhaling slowly as if trying to blow out a candle is a technique used in pursed-lip breathing to facilitate exhalation in clients with chronic obstructive pulmonary disease. It is recommended that the abdominal muscles be contracted, not relaxed, to promote deep breathing. The client should breathe through the nose. (A)

108. **3.** A client who has undergone chest surgery should be taught to raise the arm on the affected side over the head to help prevent shoulder ankylosis. This exercise helps restore normal shoulder movement, prevents stiffening of the shoulder joint, and improves muscle tone and power. Turning from side to side, raising and lowering the head, and flexing and extending the elbow on the affected side do not exercise the shoulder joint. (C)

109. **4.** The drainage apparatus is always kept *below* the client's chest level to prevent back flow of fluid into the pleural space. The air vent must always be open in the closed chest drainage system to allow air from the client to escape. Stripping a chest tube causes excessive negative intrapleural pressure and is not recommended. Clamping a chest tube when moving a client is not recommended. (A)

110. **1.** Cessation of fluid fluctuation in the tubing can mean one of several things: the lung has fully expanded and negative intrapleural pressure has been re-established; the chest tube is occluded; or the chest tube is not in the pleural space. Fluid fluctuation occurs because, during inspiration, intrapleural pressure exceeds the negative pressure generated in the water-seal system. Therefore, drainage moves toward the client. During expiration, the pleural pressure exceeds that generated in the water-seal system, and fluid moves away from the client. When the lung is collapsed or the chest tube is in the pleural space, fluid fluctuation is likely to be noted. The chest tube is not inserted in the mediastinal space. (A)

111. **2.** There should never be constant bubbling in the water-seal bottle; normally the bubbling is intermittent. Constant bubbling in the water-seal bottle indicates an air leak, which means that less negative pressure is being exerted on the pleural space. Decreasing the suction or draining part of the water in the water-seal chamber will not reduce the leak. (A)

112. **1.** In this case, there may be some obstruction to the flow of air and fluid out of the pleural space, causing air and fluid to collect and build up pressure. This prevents the remaining lung from re-expanding and can cause a mediastinal shift to the opposite side. The nurse's first response is to assess the tubing for kinks or obstruction. Increasing the suction is not done without a physician's order. The normal position of the drainage bottles is 2 to 3 feet below chest level. Clamping the tubes obstructs the flow of air and fluid out of the pleural space and should not be done. (A)

113. **2.** The chest drainage system is set up properly. The chest tube is attached to the drainage system and does not need to be clamped; there is sufficient water to maintain the water seal; the drainage from the client has not exceeded the capacity of the drainage system. The nurse should chart the amount and color of the drainage every 4 to 8 hours. (A)

114. **3.** A bottle of sterile water should be readily available and in view when a client has a chest tube so that the tube can be immediately submersed in the water if the chest tube system becomes disconnected. The chest tube should be reconnected to the water-seal system as soon as a sterile functioning system can be re-established. There is no need for a tracheostomy tray, another chest tube, or a spirometer to be placed at the bedside for emergency use. (A)

The Client with Chest Trauma

115. **0.7**

$$10 \, \text{mg} : X \, \text{ml} = 15 \, \text{mg} : 1 \, \text{ml}$$
$$15 \, \text{mg} \times X \, \text{ml} = 10 \, \text{mg} \times 1 \, \text{ml}$$
$$15X = 10$$
$$X = 0.6667$$
$$X = 0.67 \, \text{ml}.$$

(D)

116. **2.** Blunt chest trauma may lead to respiratory failure, and maintenance of adequate oxygenation is the priority for the client. Decreasing the client's anxiety is related to maintaining effective respirations and oxygenation. Although pain is distressing to the client and can increase anxiety and decrease respiratory effectiveness, pain control is secondary to maintaining oxygenation. Maintaining adequate circulatory volume is also secondary to maintaining adequate oxygenation. (A)

117. **3.** Fluctuation of fluid in the water-seal column with respirations indicates that the system is functioning properly. If an obstruction were present in the chest tube, fluid fluctuation would be absent. Subcutaneous emphysema occurs when air pockets can be palpated beneath the client's skin around the chest tube insertion site. A leak in the system is indicated when continuous bubbling occurs in the water-seal column. (A)

118. **2.** Continuous bubbling in the water-seal chamber indicates a leak in the system, and the client needs to be instructed to notify the physician if continuous bubbling occurs. A respiratory rate of more than 16 breaths/minute may not be unusual and does not necessarily mean that the client should notify the physician. Fluid in the chest tube is expected, as is fluctuation of the fluid in the water-seal chamber. (A)

119. **4.** Pneumothorax means that the lung has collapsed and is not functioning. The nurse will hear no sounds of air movement on auscultation. Movement of air through mucus produces crackles. Wheezing occurs when airways become obstructed. Dullness on percussion indicates increased density of lung tissue, usually caused by accumulation of fluid. (A)

120.   1. If the client reports no pain, then the objective of adequate pain relief has been met. Decreased anxiety is not related only to pain control; it could also be related to other factors. A respiratory rate of 26 breaths/minute is not within normal limits. A PaO_2 of 70 mm Hg is not within normal limits. (A)

121.   2. One unit of packed red blood cells is about 250 ml. If the blood is delivered at a rate of 60 ml/hour, it will take about 4 hours to infuse the entire unit. The transfusion of a single unit of packed red blood cells should not exceed 4 hours to prevent the growth of bacteria and minimize the risk of septicemia. (D)

122.   2. Too-rapid infusion of blood, or any intravenous fluid, can cause fluid volume overload and related problems such as pulmonary edema. Emboli formation, red blood cell hemolysis, and allergic reaction are not related to rapid infusion. (D)

123.   4. Immediately after chest tube removal, a petroleum gauze is placed over the wound and covered with a dry sterile dressing. This serves as an airtight seal to prevent air leakage or air movement in either direction. Bandages are not applied directly over wounds. Montgomery straps are used in place of adhesive tape when a dressing requires very frequent changes and the constant removal of adhesive tape would damage the skin. Montgomery straps are not placed over open wounds. Mesh gauze would allow air movement. (A)

124.   1. Pneumothorax signs and symptoms include sudden, sharp chest pain; tachypnea; and tachycardia. Other signs and symptoms include diminished or absent breath sounds over the affected lung, anxiety, and restlessness. Breath sounds are diminished or absent over the affected side. Hemoptysis and cyanosis are not typically present with a moderate pneumothorax. (A)

125.   4. A chest tube is inserted to re-expand the lung and remove air and fluid. Oxygen is not administered through a chest tube. Chest tubes are not inserted to promote scar tissue formation. Antibiotics are not used to treat a pneumothorax. (C)

The Client with Acute Respiratory Distress Syndrome

126.   1, 4, 5. Acute respiratory distress syndrome (ARDS) may cause renal failure and superinfection, so the nurse should monitor urine output and urine chemistries. Treatment of hypoxemia can be complicated because changes in lung tissue leave less pulmonary tissue available for gas exchange, thereby causing inadequate perfusion. Humidi-fied oxygen may be one means of promoting oxygenation. The client has crackles in the lung bases, so the nurse should continue to assess breath sounds. Sedatives should be used with caution in clients with ARDS. The nurse should try other measures to relieve the client's restlessness and anxiety. The head of the bed should be elevated to 30 degrees to promote chest expansion and prevent atelectasis. (M)

127.   4. One of the major risk factors for development of ARDS is hypovolemic shock. Adequate fluid replacement is essential to minimize the risk of ARDS in these clients. Teaching smoking cessation does not prevent ARDS. An abnormal serum potassium level and hypercapnia are not risk factors for ARDS. (A)

128.   1. *Ineffective breathing pattern* is a priority nursing diagnosis for the client with ARDS. The massive shift of fluid from the capillaries to the alveoli, as well as the reduced surfactant, greatly increases the work of breathing. The lungs become stiff and noncompliant, and the client becomes severely hypoxic. The client with ARDS usually requires endotracheal intubation and mechanical ventilation. *Pain* and *Ineffective health maintenance* are not priority nursing diagnoses for a client with ARDS. Although the client may be at risk for development of an infection, a higher nursing priority is maintaining an airway. (A)

129.   2. A hallmark of early ARDS is refractory hypoxemia. The client's PaO_2 level continues to fall, despite higher concentrations of administered oxygen. Elevated carbon dioxide and metabolic acidosis occur late in the disorder. Severe electrolyte imbalances are not indicators of ARDS. (A)

130.   4. Kussmaul's respirations in metabolic acidosis are deep and rapid, thus hyperventilation is a concern, not hypoventilation. Fluid volume deficit is related to nausea, vomiting, and decreased fluid intake, not hypoperistalsis. There are no data to indicate that the client has hypertension or is at risk for impaired skin integrity. (A)

131.   2. The normal range for partial pressure of arterial carbon dioxide ($PaCO_2$) is 35 to 45 mm Hg. Thus, this client's $PaCO_2$ level is low. The client is experiencing respiratory alkalosis (carbonic acid deficit) due to hyperventilation. The nurse should report this finding to the physician because it requires intervention. The increase in ventilation decreases the $PaCO_2$ level, which leads to decreased carbonic acid and alkalosis. The bicarbonate level is normal in uncompensated respiratory alkalosis along with the normal PaO_2 level. Normal serum pH is 7.35 to 7.45; in uncompensated respiratory alkalosis, the serum pH is greater than 7.45. (R)

132. **3.** The Pa_{CO_2} level of 28 mm Hg indicates that the client is hyperventilating. Normal Pa_{CO_2} levels are between 35 and 45 mm Hg. In hyperventilation, carbon dioxide is excreted at an increased rate, and the Pa_{CO_2} falls below 35 mm Hg. The client develops respiratory alkalosis. Pa_{CO_2} levels do not measure arterial blood oxygen. Hypoventilation causes increased Pa_{CO_2} levels. Oxygen toxicity does not cause decreased Pa_{CO_2} levels. (A)

133. **1.** Normal Pa_{O_2} level ranges from 80 to 100 mm Hg. When the Pa_{O_2} value falls to 50 mm Hg, the nurse should be alert for signs of hypoxia and impending respiratory failure. An oxygen level this low poses a severe risk for respiratory failure. The Pa_{O_2} is not within normal range. The client will require oxygenation at a concentration that maintains the Pa_{O_2} at 55 to 60 mm Hg or more. (A)

134. **4.** A Pa_{CO_2} of 28 mm Hg and Pa_{O_2} of 50 mm Hg are both abnormal; the Pa_{O_2} of 50 mm Hg signifies acute respiratory failure. In evaluating possible causes for this disorder, the nurse should consider conditions that lead to hypoxia and hyperventilation, such as pulmonary embolus. COPD is typically associated with respiratory acidosis and elevated Pa_{CO_2}. The client with diabetic ketoacidosis most often has metabolic acidosis. A myocardial infarction does not often cause an acid-base imbalance because the primary problem is cardiac in origin. (A)

135. **3.** Endotracheal intubation and mechanical ventilation are required in ARDS to maintain adequate respiratory support. Endotracheal intubation, not a tracheostomy, is usually the initial method of maintaining an airway. The client requires mechanical ventilation; nasal oxygen will not provide adequate oxygenation. Chest tubes are used to remove air or fluid from intrapleural spaces. (A)

136. **1.** The two risk factors most commonly associated with the development of ARDS are gram-negative septic shock and gastric content aspiration. Nurses should be particularly vigilant in assessing a client for onset of ARDS if the client has experienced direct lung trauma or a systemic inflammatory response syndrome (which can be caused by any physiologic insult that leads to widespread inflammation). Chronic obstructive pulmonary disease, asthma, and heart failure are not direct causes of ARDS. (R)

137. **4.** Auscultation for bilateral breath sounds is the most appropriate method for determining cuff placement. The nurse should also look for the symmetrical rise and fall of the chest and should note the location of the exit mark on the tube. Assessments of skin color, respiratory rate, and the amount of cuff inflation cannot validate the placement of the endotracheal tube. (C)

138. **4.** The nurse should suction the client if the client is not able to cough up secretions and clear the airway. Administering oxygen will not promote airway clearance. The client should be turned every 2 hours to help move secretions; every 4 hours is not often enough. Administering sedatives is contraindicated in acute respiratory distress because sedatives can depress respirations. (A)

139. **1.** Gastrointestinal hemorrhage occurs in about 25% of clients receiving prolonged mechanical ventilation because of the development of stress ulcers. Clients who are receiving steroid therapy and those with a previous history of ulcers are most likely to be at risk. Other possible complications include incorrect ventilation, oxygen toxicity, fluid imbalance, decreased cardiac output, pneumothorax, infection, and atelectasis. (A)

140. **3.** Carbon monoxide poisoning develops when carbon monoxide combines with hemoglobin. Because carbon monoxide combines more readily with hemoglobin than oxygen does, tissue anoxia results. The nurse should administer 100% oxygen by mask to reduce the half-life of carboxyhemoglobin. Gastric lavage is used for ingested poisons. With tissue anoxia, metabolism is diminished, with a subsequent lowering of the body's temperature, thus steps to increase body temperature would be required. Unless the carbon monoxide poisoning is intentional, a psychiatric referral would be inappropriate. (A)

141. **4.** Confusion and vertigo are risk factors for falls. Measures must be taken to minimize the risk of injury. The nurse or unlicensed personnel should check on the client regularly to determine needs regarding elimination. Restraints, including bed rails and extremity restraints, should be used only to ensure the person's safety or the safety of others, and there must be a written order from a physician before using them. The nurse should never ask the roommate of a client to be responsible for the client's safety. (S)

142.

1. An 85-year-old client with bacterial pneumonia, temperature of 102.2° F (42° C), and shortness of breath.

3. A 35-year-old client with suspected tuberculosis who is complaining of a cough.

4. A 56-year-old client with emphysema who has a scheduled dose of a bronchodilator due to be administered, with no report of acute respiratory distress.

2. A 60-year-old client with chest tubes who is 2 days postoperative following a thoracotomy for lung cancer and is requesting something for pain.

Because two major complications of endotracheal tube intubation, inadvertent extubation and aspiration, can be catastrophic events, assessment of this client is the first priority. Cellulitis is a serious infection as there is inflammation of subcutaneous tissues; third spacing of fluid may promote the formation of a fluid volume deficit, which can be exacerbated by the fever due to insensible fluid loss. The nurse should assess this client next to determine current vital signs and fluid status. The nurse should assess the client with the I.V. fluids next because the new bag of fluids will need to be hung in 30 to 40 minutes. I.V. therapy necessitates that the client be assessed for signs and symptoms of adequate hydration (moist mucous membranes, elastic skin turgor, vital signs within normal limits, adequate urine output, and level of consciousness within normal limits), and the I.V. access site needs to be assessed. From the information provided, there is no indication that the client who had the cerebrovascular accident is unstable. Thus, this client is the last priority for assessment. (M)

143. **1.** In the normal lung, the volume of blood perfusing the lungs each minute is approximately equal to the amount of fresh gas that reaches the alveoli each minute. Blood gas analysis evaluates respiratory function; the level of dissolved oxygen (Pa_{O_2}) should be greater than the level of dissolved carbon dioxide (Pa_{CO_2}). (A)

The Client with Upper Gastrointestinal Tract Health Problems

- The Client with Disorders of the Oral Cavity
- The Client with Peptic Ulcer Disease
- The Client with Cancer of the Stomach
- The Client with Gastroesophageal Reflux Disease
- Correct Answers and Rationales

The Client with Disorders of the Oral Cavity

1. The nurse is teaching a group of teenage boys who are on a baseball team about the risks of chewing tobacco. Which of the following signs or symptoms should the nurse instruct the teenagers to report to their parents and physicians? Select all that apply.

☐ **1.** Dysphagia.
☐ **2.** Sensitive teeth.
☐ **3.** Unexplained mouth pain.
☐ **4.** Lump in the neck.
☐ **5.** Decreased saliva.
☐ **6.** White patch on the mucosa.

2. Which of the following hospitalized clients would be most likely to develop parotitis?

☐ **1.** A 50-year-old client with nausea and vomiting who is on nothing-by-mouth status.
☐ **2.** A 75-year-old client with diabetes who has ill-fitting dentures.
☐ **3.** An 80-year-old client who has poor oral hygiene and is dehydrated.
☐ **4.** A 65-year-old client with lung cancer who has a feeding tube in place.

3. A nurse is caring for a client who has just returned from surgery to treat a fractured mandible. Which of the following items should always be available at this client's bedside? Select all that apply.

☐ **1.** Nasogastric tube.
☐ **2.** Wire cutters.
☐ **3.** Oxygen cannula.
☐ **4.** Suction equipment.
☐ **5.** Code cart.

4. Which of the following interventions is most appropriate for a client who has stomatitis?

☐ **1.** Drinking hot tea at frequent intervals.
☐ **2.** Gargling with antiseptic mouthwash.
☐ **3.** Using an electric toothbrush.
☐ **4.** Eating a soft, bland diet.

5. A client who has a history of a mitral valve prolapse tells the nurse during a clinic visit that she is scheduled to get her teeth cleaned. Which of the following replies by the nurse is *most* appropriate?

☐ **1.** "The physician will need to reevaluate the status of your heart condition before your dental appointment."
☐ **2.** "Be sure to remind your dentist that you have a heart condition."
☐ **3.** "It is important for you to care for your teeth because your heart condition makes you more susceptible to developing oral infections."
☐ **4.** "We will prescribe a prophylactic antibiotic for you to take before getting your teeth cleaned."

6. The nurse instructs the nursing assistant on how to provide oral hygiene for a client who cannot perform this task for himself. Which of the following techniques should the nurse tell the assistant to incorporate into the client's daily care?

☐ **1.** Assess the oral cavity each time mouth care is given and record observations.
☐ **2.** Use a soft toothbrush to brush the client's teeth after each meal.
☐ **3.** Swab the client's tongue, gums, and lips with a soft foam applicator every 2 hours.
☐ **4.** Rinse the client's mouth with mouthwash several times a day.

7. Amoxicillin trihydrate (Amoxil) 300 mg P.O. has been prescribed for a client with an oral infection. The medication is available in a liquid suspension that is available as 250 mg/5 ml. How many milliliters would the nurse administer?

_____ ml

8. During the assessment of a client's mouth, the nurse notes the absence of saliva. The client is also complaining of pain in the area of the ear. The client has been nothing-by-mouth (NPO) for several days because of the insertion of a nasogastric tube. Based on these findings, the nurse suspects that the client may be developing which of the following mouth conditions?
- ☐ **1.** Stomatitis.
- ☐ **2.** Oral candidiasis.
- ☐ **3.** Parotitis.
- ☐ **4.** Gingivitis.

9. The nurse is preparing a community presentation on oral cancer. Which of the following is a primary risk factor for oral cancer that the nurse should include in the presentation?
- ☐ **1.** Use of alcohol.
- ☐ **2.** Frequent use of mouthwash.
- ☐ **3.** Lack of vitamin B_{12}.
- ☐ **4.** Lack of regular teeth cleaning by a dentist.

10. A client has entered a smoking cessation program to quit a two-pack-a-day cigarette habit. He tells the occupational health nurse at his place of employment that he has not smoked a cigarette for 3 weeks, but is afraid he is going to "slip up" and smoke because of current job pressures. What would be the most appropriate reply for the nurse to make in response to the client's comments?
- ☐ **1.** "Don't worry about it. Everybody has difficulty quitting smoking, and you should expect to as well."
- ☐ **2.** "If you increase your self-control, I am sure you will be able to avoid smoking."
- ☐ **3.** "Try taking a couple of days of vacation to relieve the stress of your job."
- ☐ **4.** "It is good that you can talk about your concerns. Try calling a friend when you want to smoke."

11. A client who was in a motor vehicle accident has a fractured mandible. Surgery has been performed to immobilize the injury by wiring the jaw. Which is the nurse's priority in regard to care in the immediate postoperative phase?
- ☐ **1.** Prevent nausea and vomiting.
- ☐ **2.** Maintain a patent airway.
- ☐ **3.** Provide frequent oral hygiene.
- ☐ **4.** Establish a way for the client to communicate.

12. A client has returned from surgery during which her jaws were wired as treatment for a fractured mandible. The client is in stable condition. The nurse is instructing the assistant on how to properly position the client. Which instructions about positioning would be appropriate for the nurse to give the assistant?
- ☐ **1.** Keep the client in a side-lying position with the head slightly elevated.
- ☐ **2.** Do not reposition the client without the assistance of a registered nurse.
- ☐ **3.** The client can assume any position that is comfortable.
- ☐ **4.** Keep the client's head elevated on two pillows at all times.

13. A client who has had her jaws wired begins to vomit. What should be the nurse's *first* action?
- ☐ **1.** Insert a nasogastric (NG) tube and connect it to suction.
- ☐ **2.** Use wire cutters to cut the wire.
- ☐ **3.** Suction the client's airway as needed.
- ☐ **4.** Administer an antiemetic intravenously.

The Client with Peptic Ulcer Disease

14. A nurse teaches a client experiencing heartburn to take 1½ oz of Maalox when symptoms appear. How many milliliters should the client take?

_____ ml

15. The nurse has been assigned to provide care for four clients at the beginning of the day shift. In what order should the nurse assess these clients?

1. A client awaiting surgery for a hiatal hernia repair at 11 a.m.

2. A client with suspected gastric cancer who is on nothing-by-mouth (NPO) status for tests.

3. A client with peptic ulcer disease experiencing a sudden onset of acute stomach pain.

4. A client who is requesting pain medication 2 days after surgery to repair a fractured jaw.

16. The nurse is caring for a client who has just had an upper GI endoscopy. The client's vital signs must be taken every 30 minutes for 2 hours after the procedure. The nurse assigns an unlicensed assistant to take the vital signs. One hour later, the assistant reports the client, who was previously afebrile, has developed a temperature of 101.8° F (38.8° C). What should the nurse do in response to this reported assessment data?
☐ **1.** Promptly assess the client for potential perforation.
☐ **2.** Tell the assistant to change thermometers and retake the temperature.
☐ **3.** Plan to give the client acetaminophen (Tylenol) to lower the temperature.
☐ **4.** Ask the assistant to bathe the client with tepid water.

17. A client is admitted to the hospital after vomiting bright red blood and is diagnosed with a bleeding duodenal ulcer. The client develops a sudden, sharp pain in the midepigastric region along with a rigid, boardlike abdomen. These clinical manifestations most likely indicate which of the following?
☐ **1.** An intestinal obstruction has developed.
☐ **2.** Additional ulcers have developed.
☐ **3.** The esophagus has become inflamed.
☐ **4.** The ulcer has perforated.

18. When obtaining a nursing history on a client with a suspected gastric ulcer, which signs and symptoms should the nurse expect to assess? Select all that apply.
☐ **1.** Epigastric pain at night.
☐ **2.** Relief of epigastric pain after eating.
☐ **3.** Vomiting.
☐ **4.** Weight loss.
☐ **5.** Melena.

19. The nurse is caring for a client who has had a gastroscopy. Which of the following signs and symptoms may indicate that the client is developing a complication related to the procedure? Select all that apply.
☐ **1.** The client complains of a sore throat.
☐ **2.** The client has a temperature of 100° F (37.8° C).
☐ **3.** The client appears drowsy following the procedure.
☐ **4.** The client complains of epigastric pain.
☐ **5.** The client experiences hematemesis.

20. A client with peptic ulcer disease tells the nurse that he has black stools, which he has not reported to his physician. Based on this information, which nursing diagnosis would be appropriate for this client?
☐ **1.** *Ineffective coping* related to fear of diagnosis of chronic illness.
☐ **2.** *Deficient knowledge* related to unfamiliarity with significant signs and symptoms.
☐ **3.** *Constipation* related to decreased gastric motility.
☐ **4.** *Imbalanced nutrition: Less than body requirements* related to gastric bleeding.

21. The client asks the nurse what causes a peptic ulcer to develop. The nurse responds that recent research indicates that many peptic ulcers are the result of which of the following?
☐ **1.** Work-related stress.
☐ **2.** *Helicobacter pylori* infection.
☐ **3.** Diets high in fat.
☐ **4.** A genetic defect in the gastric mucosa.

22. A client with a peptic ulcer reports epigastric pain that frequently awakens her during the night, a feeling of fullness in the abdomen, and a feeling of anxiety about her health. Based on this information, which nursing diagnosis would be *most* appropriate?
☐ **1.** *Imbalanced nutrition: Less than body requirements* related to anorexia.
☐ **2.** *Insomnia* related to epigastric pain.
☐ **3.** *Ineffective coping* related to exacerbation of duodenal ulcer.
☐ **4.** *Activity intolerance* related to abdominal pain.

23. A client with peptic ulcer disease reports that he has been nauseated most of the day and is now feeling light-headed and dizzy. Based upon these findings, which nursing actions would be most appropriate for the nurse to take? Select all that apply.
☐ 1. Administering an antacid hourly until nausea subsides.
☐ 2. Monitoring the client's vital signs.
☐ 3. Notifying the physician of the client's symptoms.
☐ 4. Initiating oxygen therapy.
☐ 5. Reassessing the client in an hour.

24. The nurse is preparing to teach a client with a peptic ulcer about the diet that should be followed after discharge. The nurse should explain that the diet will most likely consist of which of the following?
☐ 1. Bland foods.
☐ 2. High-protein foods.
☐ 3. Any foods that are tolerated.
☐ 4. Large amounts of milk.

25. The nurse finds a client who has been diagnosed with a peptic ulcer surrounded by papers from his briefcase and arguing on the telephone with a coworker. The nurse's response to observing these actions should be based on knowledge that:
☐ 1. Involvement with his job will keep the client from becoming bored.
☐ 2. A relaxed environment will promote ulcer healing.
☐ 3. Not keeping up with his job will increase the client's stress level.
☐ 4. Setting limits on the client's behavior is an important nursing responsibility.

26. A client with a peptic ulcer has been instructed to avoid intense physical activity and stress. Which strategy should the client incorporate into the home care plan?
☐ 1. Conduct physical activity in the morning so that he can rest in the afternoon.
☐ 2. Have the family agree to perform the necessary yard work at home.
☐ 3. Give up jogging and substitute a less demanding hobby.
☐ 4. Incorporate periods of physical and mental rest in his daily schedule.

27. A client is to take one daily dose of ranitidine (Zantac) at home to treat her peptic ulcer. The nurse knows that the client understands proper drug administration of ranitidine when she says that she will take the drug at which of the following times?
☐ 1. Before meals.
☐ 2. With meals.
☐ 3. At bedtime.
☐ 4. When pain occurs.

28. A client has been taking aluminum hydroxide (Amphojel) 30 ml six times per day at home to treat his peptic ulcer. He tells the nurse that he has been unable to have a bowel movement for 3 days. Based on this information, the nurse would determine that which of the following is the most likely cause of the client's constipation?
☐ 1. The client has not been including enough fiber in his diet.
☐ 2. The client needs to increase his daily exercise.
☐ 3. The client is experiencing an adverse effect of the aluminum hydroxide.
☐ 4. The client has developed a gastrointestinal obstruction.

29. A client is taking an antacid for treatment of a peptic ulcer. Which of the following statements best indicates that the client understands how to correctly take the antacid?
☐ 1. "I should take my antacid before I take my other medications."
☐ 2. "I need to decrease my intake of fluids so that I don't dilute the effects of my antacid."
☐ 3. "My antacid will be most effective if I take it whenever I experience stomach pains."
☐ 4. "It is best for me to take my antacid 1 to 3 hours after meals."

30. Which of the following would be an expected outcome for a client with peptic ulcer disease? The client will:
☐ 1. Demonstrate appropriate use of analgesics to control pain.
☐ 2. Explain the rationale for eliminating alcohol from the diet.
☐ 3. Verbalize the importance of monitoring hemoglobin and hematocrit every 3 months.
☐ 4. Eliminate contact sports from his or her lifestyle.

The Client with Cancer of the Stomach

31. A nurse is assessing a client who has been admitted with a diagnosis of upper GI bleeding. Which of the following signs and symptoms should the nurse expect to find? Select all that apply.
☐ 1. Dry, flushed skin.
☐ 2. Decreased urine output.
☐ 3. Tachycardia.
☐ 4. Widening pulse pressure.
☐ 5. Rapid respirations.
☐ 6. Thirst.

32. A client with suspected gastric cancer undergoes an endoscopy of the stomach. Which of the following assessments made after the procedure would indicate the development of a potential complication?
- [ ] **1.** The client complains of a sore throat.
- [ ] **2.** The client displays signs of sedation.
- [ ] **3.** The client experiences a sudden increase in temperature.
- [ ] **4.** The client demonstrates a lack of appetite.

33. A client has been diagnosed with adenocarcinoma of the stomach and is scheduled to undergo a subtotal gastrectomy (Billroth II procedure). During preoperative teaching, the nurse is reinforcing information about the surgical procedure. Which of the following explanations is most accurate?
- [ ] **1.** The procedure will result in enlargement of the pyloric sphincter.
- [ ] **2.** The procedure will result in anastomosis of the gastric stump to the jejunum.
- [ ] **3.** The procedure will result in removal of the duodenum.
- [ ] **4.** The procedure will result in repositioning of the vagus nerve.

34. The client tells the nurse that since his diagnosis of stomach cancer, he has been having trouble sleeping and is frequently preoccupied with thoughts about how his life will change. He says, "I wish my life could stay the same." Based on this information, which one of the following nursing diagnoses would be appropriate at this time?
- [ ] **1.** *Ineffective coping* related to the diagnosis of cancer.
- [ ] **2.** *Insomnia* related to fear of the unknown.
- [ ] **3.** *Grieving* related to the diagnosis of cancer.
- [ ] **4.** *Anxiety* related to the need for gastric surgery.

35. After a subtotal gastrectomy, the nurse should anticipate that nasogastric tube drainage will be what color for about 12 to 24 hours after surgery?
- [ ] **1.** Dark brown.
- [ ] **2.** Bile green.
- [ ] **3.** Bright red.
- [ ] **4.** Cloudy white.

36. After a subtotal gastrectomy, care of the client's nasogastric (NG) tube and drainage system should include which of the following nursing interventions?
- [ ] **1.** Irrigate the tube with 30 ml of sterile water every hour, if needed.
- [ ] **2.** Reposition the tube if it is not draining well.
- [ ] **3.** Monitor the client for nausea, vomiting, and abdominal distention.
- [ ] **4.** Turn the machine to high suction if the drainage is sluggish on low suction.

37. A client who is recovering from gastric surgery is receiving I.V. fluids to be infused at 100 ml/hour. The I.V. tubing delivers 15 gtt/ml. The nurse should infuse the solution at a flow rate of how many drops per minute to ensure that the client receives 100 ml/hour?

_____ gtt/minute

38. The nurse understands that the best position for the client who has undergone a gastrectomy is:
- [ ] **1.** Prone.
- [ ] **2.** Supine.
- [ ] **3.** Low Fowler's.
- [ ] **4.** Right or left Sims.

39. As part of the client's discharge planning after a subtotal gastrectomy, the nurse has identified *Imbalanced nutrition: Less than body requirements* as a major nursing diagnosis. To help the client meet nutritional goals at home, the nurse should develop a plan of care that includes which of the following interventions?
- [ ] **1.** Instruct the client to increase the amount eaten at each meal.
- [ ] **2.** Encourage the client to eat smaller amounts more frequently.
- [ ] **3.** Explain that if vomiting occurs after a meal, nothing more should be eaten that day.
- [ ] **4.** Inform the client that bland foods are typically less nutritional and should be used minimally.

40. As a result of a gastric resection, the client is at risk for development of dumping syndrome. The nurse should prepare a plan of care for this client based on knowledge that this problem stems primarily from which of the following gastrointestinal changes?
- [ ] **1.** Excess secretion of digestive enzymes in the intestines.
- [ ] **2.** Rapid emptying of stomach contents into the small intestine.
- [ ] **3.** Excess glycogen production by the liver.
- [ ] **4.** Loss of gastric enzymes.

41. To reduce the risk of dumping syndrome, the nurse should teach the client which of the following interventions?
- [ ] **1.** Sit upright for 30 minutes after meals.
- [ ] **2.** Drink liquids with meals, avoiding caffeine.
- [ ] **3.** Avoid milk and other dairy products.
- [ ] **4.** Decrease the carbohydrate content of meals.

42. A client who is recovering from a subtotal gastrectomy experiences dumping syndrome. The client asks the nurse, "When will I be able to eat three meals a day again like I used to?" Which of the following responses by the nurse is most appropriate?
- ☐ **1.** "Eating six meals a day is time-consuming, isn't it?"
- ☐ **2.** "You will have to eat six small meals a day for the rest of your life."
- ☐ **3.** "You will be able to tolerate three meals a day before you are discharged."
- ☐ **4.** "Most clients can resume their normal meal patterns in about 6 to 12 months."

43. Which of the following signs and symptoms would be indicative of the dumping syndrome?
- ☐ **1.** Hunger.
- ☐ **2.** Vomiting.
- ☐ **3.** Diaphoresis.
- ☐ **4.** Heartburn.

44. After surgery for gastric cancer, a client is scheduled to undergo radiation therapy. It will be most important for the nurse to include information about which of the following in the client's teaching plan?
- ☐ **1.** Nutritional intake.
- ☐ **2.** Management of alopecia.
- ☐ **3.** Exercise and activity levels.
- ☐ **4.** Access to community resources.

45. Which of the following would be an expected nutritional outcome for a client who has undergone a subtotal gastrectomy for cancer? The client will:
- ☐ **1.** Regain weight loss within 1 month after surgery.
- ☐ **2.** Resume normal dietary intake of three meals a day.
- ☐ **3.** Control nausea and vomiting through regular use of antiemetics.
- ☐ **4.** Achieve optimal nutritional status through oral or parenteral feedings.

The Client with Gastroesophageal Reflux Disease

46. Which of the following instructions should the nurse include in the teaching plan for a client who is experiencing gastroesophageal reflux disease (GERD)?
- ☐ **1.** Limit caffeine intake to two cups of coffee per day.
- ☐ **2.** Do not lie down for 2 hours after eating.
- ☐ **3.** Follow a low-protein diet.
- ☐ **4.** Take medications with milk to decrease irritation.

47. The client is scheduled to have an upper gastrointestinal tract series. Which of the following treatments should the nurse anticipate after the examination?
- ☐ **1.** Administering a laxative.
- ☐ **2.** Placing the client on a clear liquid diet.
- ☐ **3.** Giving the client a tap water enema.
- ☐ **4.** Starting an I.V. infusion.

48. A client who has been diagnosed with gastroesophageal reflux disease (GERD) complains of heartburn. To decrease the heartburn, the nurse should instruct the client to eliminate which of the following items from the diet?
- ☐ **1.** Lean beef.
- ☐ **2.** Air-popped popcorn.
- ☐ **3.** Hot chocolate.
- ☐ **4.** Raw vegetables.

49. The client with gastroesophageal reflux disease (GERD) complains of a chronic cough. The nurse understands that in a client with GERD this symptom may be indicative of which of the following conditions?
- ☐ **1.** Development of laryngeal cancer.
- ☐ **2.** Irritation of the esophagus.
- ☐ **3.** Esophageal scar tissue formation.
- ☐ **4.** Aspiration of gastric contents.

50. Bethanechol (Urecholine) has been ordered for a client with gastroesophageal reflux disease (GERD). The nurse should evaluate the client for which of the following adverse effects?
- ☐ **1.** Constipation.
- ☐ **2.** Urinary urgency.
- ☐ **3.** Hypertension.
- ☐ **4.** Dry oral mucosa.

51. The client attends two sessions with the dietitian to learn about diet modifications to minimize gastroesophageal reflux. The teaching would be considered successful if the client says that she will decrease her intake of which of the following foods?
- ☐ **1.** Fats.
- ☐ **2.** High-sodium foods.
- ☐ **3.** Carbohydrates.
- ☐ **4.** High-calcium foods.

52. Which of the following dietary measures would be useful in preventing esophageal reflux?
- ☐ **1.** Eating small, frequent meals.
- ☐ **2.** Increasing fluid intake.
- ☐ **3.** Avoiding air swallowing with meals.
- ☐ **4.** Adding a bedtime snack to the dietary plan.

53. The nurse understands that the primary symptoms of a sliding hiatal hernia are associated with reflux. Therefore, the nurse should assess the client with a hiatal hernia for which of the following symptoms?
- ☐ **1.** Heartburn.
- ☐ **2.** Jaundice.
- ☐ **3.** Anorexia.
- ☐ **4.** Stomatitis.

54. Which of the following factors would most likely contribute to the development of a client's hiatal hernia?
- ☐ **1.** Having a sedentary desk job.
- ☐ **2.** Being 5 feet, 3 inches tall and weighing 190 lb.
- ☐ **3.** Using laxatives frequently.
- ☐ **4.** Being 40 years old.

55. Which of the following nursing interventions would most likely promote self-care behaviors in the client with a hiatal hernia?
- ☐ 1. Introduce the client to other people who are successfully managing their care.
- ☐ 2. Include the client's daughter in the teaching so that she can help implement the plan.
- ☐ 3. Ask the client to identify other situations in which he demonstrated responsibility for himself.
- ☐ 4. Reassure the client that he will be able to implement all aspects of the plan successfully.

56. The client has been taking magnesium hydroxide (milk of magnesia) at home in an attempt to control hiatal hernia symptoms. The nurse should assess the client for which of the following conditions most commonly associated with the ongoing use of magnesium-based antacids?
- ☐ 1. Anorexia.
- ☐ 2. Weight gain.
- ☐ 3. Diarrhea.
- ☐ 4. Constipation.

57. Which of the following lifestyle modifications should the nurse encourage the client with a hiatal hernia to include in activities of daily living?
- ☐ 1. Daily aerobic exercise.
- ☐ 2. Eliminating smoking and alcohol use.
- ☐ 3. Balancing activity and rest.
- ☐ 4. Avoiding high-stress situations.

58. In developing a teaching plan for the client with a hiatal hernia, the nurse's assessment of which work-related factors would be most useful?
- ☐ 1. Number and length of breaks.
- ☐ 2. Body mechanics used in lifting.
- ☐ 3. Temperature in the work area.
- ☐ 4. Cleaning solvents used.

59. The nurse instructs the client on health maintenance activities to help control symptoms from her hiatal hernia. Which of the following statements would indicate that the client has understood the instructions?
- ☐ 1. "I'll avoid lying down after a meal."
- ☐ 2. "I can still enjoy my potato chips and cola at bedtime."
- ☐ 3. "I wish I didn't have to give up swimming."
- ☐ 4. "If I wear a girdle, I'll have more support for my stomach."

60. The physician prescribes metoclopramide hydrochloride (Reglan) for the client with hiatal hernia. The nurse plans to instruct the client that this drug is used in hiatal hernia therapy to accomplish which of the following objectives?
- ☐ 1. Increase tone of the esophageal sphincter.
- ☐ 2. Neutralize gastric secretions.
- ☐ 3. Delay gastric emptying.
- ☐ 4. Reduce secretion of digestive juices.

61. The nurse should instruct the client to avoid which of the following drugs while taking metoclopramide hydrochloride (Reglan)?
- ☐ 1. Antacids.
- ☐ 2. Antihypertensives.
- ☐ 3. Anticoagulants.
- ☐ 4. Alcohol.

62. Cimetidine (Tagamet) may also be used to treat hiatal hernia. The nurse should understand that this drug is used to prevent which of the following?
- ☐ 1. Esophageal reflux.
- ☐ 2. Dysphagia.
- ☐ 3. Esophagitis.
- ☐ 4. Ulcer formation.

63. The client asks the nurse whether he will need surgery to correct his hiatal hernia. Which reply by the nurse would be most accurate?
- ☐ 1. "Surgery is usually required, although medical treatment is attempted first."
- ☐ 2. "Hiatal hernia symptoms can usually be successfully managed with diet modifications, medications, and lifestyle changes."
- ☐ 3. "Surgery is not performed for this type of hernia."
- ☐ 4. "A minor surgical procedure to reduce the size of the diaphragmatic opening will probably be planned."

Correct Answers and Rationales

The letter in parentheses after each rationale identifies the client need addressed in the item, including management of care (M), safety and infection control (S), health promotion and maintenance (H), psychosocial adaptation (P), basic care and comfort (C), pharmacological and parenteral therapies (D), reduction of risk potential (R), and physiological adaptation (A).

The Client with Disorders of the Oral Cavity

1. **1, 3, 4, 6.** Chewing tobacco has become a more common practice among teenagers. It is important that they understand that this increases their risk for oral cancer. They should be instructed to inspect their mouth frequently and report any observed lesions or other changes in the oral mucosa. Signs and symptoms that are potential indicators of oral cancer are dysphagia, unexplained mouth pain, a lump in the neck, and white patches on the mucosa (leukoplakia). Other indications may be a painless mouth ulcer, a reddened patch (erythroplasia), and rough patches on the mucosa. Sensitive teeth and decreased saliva are not associated with oral cancer. (H)

2. 3. Parotitis is inflammation of the parotid gland. Although any of the clients listed could develop parotitis, given the data provided, the one most likely to develop parotitis is the elderly client who is dehydrated with poor oral hygiene. Any client who experiences poor oral hygiene is at risk for developing parotitis. To help prevent parotitis, it is essential for the nurse to ensure the client receives oral hygiene at regular intervals and has an adequate fluid intake. (R)

3. 2, 4. Following surgery for a fractured mandible, the client's jaws will be wired. The nurse should be prepared to intervene quickly in case the client develops respiratory distress or begins to choke or vomit. Wire cutters or scissors should always be available in case the wires need to be cut in a medical emergency. Suction equipment should be available to help clear the client's airway if necessary. It is not necessary to keep a nasogastric tube or oxygen cannula at the client's bedside. Cardiopulmonary arrest is unlikely, so a code cart is not needed at the bedside. (S)

4. 4. Clients with stomatitis (inflammation of the mouth) have significant discomfort, which impacts their ability to eat and drink. They will be most comfortable eating soft, bland foods, and avoiding temperature extremes in their food and liquids. Gargling with an antiseptic mouthwash will be irritating to the mucosa. Mouth care should include gentle brushing with a soft toothbrush and flossing. (C)

5. 4. Clients who are at risk for developing infective endocarditis due to cardiac conditions such as mitral valve prolapse must take prophylactic antibiotics before any dental procedure that may cause bleeding. The client is not more susceptible to developing oral infections. Rather, the client is more susceptible to developing endocarditis that results from oral bacteria that enter the circulation during the dental procedure. The physician does not necessarily need to re-evaluate the heart condition of a client who is stable, but antibiotics must be prescribed. It is not enough to simply remind the dentist about the heart condition. (R)

6. 2. A soft toothbrush should be used to brush the client's teeth after every meal and more often as needed. Mechanical cleaning is necessary to maintain oral health, stimulate gingiva, and remove plaque. Assessing the oral cavity and recording observations is the responsibility of the nurse, not the nursing assistant. Swabbing with a safe foam applicator does not provide enough friction to clean the mouth. Mouthwash can be a drying irritant and is not recommended for frequent use. (C)

7. 6

To administer 300 mg P.O., the nurse will need to administer 6 ml. The following formula is used to calculate the correct dosage:

$$300 \text{ mg}/X \text{ ml} = 250 \text{ mg}/5 \text{ ml.}$$

(D)

8. 3. The lack of saliva, pain near the area of the ear, and the prolonged NPO status of the client should lead the nurse to suspect the development of parotitis, or inflammation of the parotid gland. Parotitis usually develops in cases of dehydration combined with poor oral hygiene or when clients have been NPO for an extended period. Preventive measures include the use of sugarless hard candy or gum to stimulate saliva production, adequate hydration, and frequent mouth care. Stomatitis (inflammation of the mouth) produces excessive salivation and a sore mouth. Oral candidiasis (thrush) causes bluish white mouth lesions. Gingivitis can be recognized by the inflamed gingiva and bleeding that occur during toothbrushing. (C)

9. 1. Chronic and excessive use of alcohol can lead to oral cancer. Smoking and use of smokeless tobacco are other significant risk factors. Additional risk factors include chronic irritation such as a broken tooth or ill-fitting dentures, poor dental hygiene, overexposure to sun (lip cancer), and syphilis. Use of mouthwash, lack of vitamin B_{12}, and lack of regular teeth cleaning appointments have not been implicated as primary risk factors for oral cancer. (H)

10. 4. It is important for individuals who are engaged in smoking cessation efforts to feel comfortable with sharing their fears of failure with others and seeking support. Although fewer than 5% of smokers successfully quit on their first attempt, it is not helpful to tell a client that he should anticipate failure. Telling the client to exercise more self-control does not provide him with support. Taking a vacation to avoid job pressures does not address the issue of fearing he will smoke a cigarette when in a stressful situation. (P)

11. 2. The priority of care in the immediate postoperative phase is to maintain a patent airway. The nurse should observe the client carefully for signs of respiratory distress. If the client becomes nauseated, antiemetics should be administered to decrease the chance of vomiting with obstruction of the airway and aspiration of vomitus. Providing frequent oral hygiene and an alternative means of communication are important aspects of nursing care, but maintaining a patent airway is most important. (A)

12. **1.** Immediately after surgery the client should be placed on the side with the head slightly elevated. This position helps facilitate removal of secretions and decreases the likelihood of aspiration should vomiting occur. A registered nurse does not need to be present to reposition the client, unless the client's condition warrants the presence of the nurse. Although it is important to elevate the head, there is no need to keep the client's head elevated on two pillows unless that position is comfortable for the client. (R)

13. **3.** The nurse's first action is to clear the client's airway as necessary. Inserting an NG tube or administering an antiemetic may prevent future vomiting episodes, but these procedures are not helpful when the client is actually vomiting. Cutting the wires is done only as a last resort or in case of respiratory or cardiac arrest. (A)

The Client with Peptic Ulcer Disease

14. **45**

$$1 \text{ oz} = 30 \text{ ml}$$

$$\frac{1 \text{ oz}}{1.5 \text{ oz}} = \frac{30 \text{ ml}}{X \text{ ml}}$$

$$1X = 1.5 \times 30$$

$$X = 45 \text{ ml}.$$

(D)

15.

3. A client with peptic ulcer disease experiencing a sudden onset of acute stomach pain.

4. A client who is requesting pain medication 2 days after surgery to repair a fractured jaw.

2. A client with suspected gastric cancer who is on nothing-by-mouth (NPO) status for tests.

1. A client awaiting surgery for a hiatal hernia repair at 11 a.m.

The client with peptic ulcer disease who is experiencing a sudden onset of acute stomach pain should be assessed first by the nurse. The sudden onset of stomach pain could be indicative of a perforated ulcer, which would require immediate medical attention. It is also important for the nurse to thoroughly assess the nature of the client's pain. The client with the fractured jaw is experiencing pain and should be assessed next. The nurse should then assess the client who is NPO for tests to ensure NPO status and comfort. Last, the nurse can assess the client before surgery. (M)

16. **1.** A sudden spike in temperature following an endoscopic procedure may indicate perforation of the GI tract. The nurse should promptly conduct a further assessment of the client, looking for further indicators of perforation, such as a sudden onset of acute upper abdominal pain; a rigid, boardlike abdomen; and developing signs of shock. Telling the assistant to change thermometers is not an appropriate action and only further delays the appropriate action of assessing the client. The nurse would not administer acetaminophen without further assessment of the client or without a physician's order; a suspected perforation would require that the client be placed on nothing-by-mouth status. Asking the assistant to bathe the client before any assessment by the nurse is inappropriate. (M)

17. **4.** The body reacts to perforation of an ulcer by immobilizing the area as much as possible. This results in boardlike abdominal rigidity, usually with extreme pain. Perforation is a medical emergency requiring immediate surgical intervention because peritonitis develops quickly after perforation. An intestinal obstruction would not cause midepigastric pain. The development of additional ulcers or esophageal inflammation would not cause a rigid, boardlike abdomen. (A)

18. **3, 4, 5.** Vomiting and weight loss are common with gastric ulcers. The client may also have blood in the stools (melena) from gastric bleeding. Clients with a gastric ulcer are most likely to complain of a burning epigastric pain that occurs about 1 hour after eating. Eating frequently aggravates the pain. Clients with duodenal ulcers are more likely to complain about pain that occurs during the night and is frequently relieved by eating. (A)

19. **2, 4, 5.** Following a gastroscopy, the nurse should monitor the client for complications, which include perforation and the potential for aspiration. An elevated temperature, complaints of epigastric pain, or the vomiting of blood (hematemesis) are all indications of a possible perforation and should be reported promptly. A sore throat is a common occurrence following a gastroscopy. Clients are usually sedated to decrease anxiety and the nurse would anticipate that the client will be drowsy following the procedure. (R)

20. **2.** Black, tarry stools are an important warning sign of bleeding in peptic ulcer disease. Digested blood in the stool causes it to be black. The odor of the stool is very offensive. Clients with peptic ulcer disease should be instructed to report the incidence of black stools promptly to their primary health care provider. The data do not support the other diagnoses. (R)

21. **2.** Most peptic ulcers are caused by *Helicobacter pylori*, which is a gram-negative bacterium. If this organism is detected through diagnostic tests, treatment of the ulcer will include the use of antibiotics and bismuth compounds such as Pepto-Bismol. It has not been proven that work-related stress or a genetic defect causes ulcers. Diets high in fat do not cause peptic ulcer disease. The data do not support the other diagnoses. (A)

22. **2.** Based on the data provided, the most appropriate nursing diagnosis would be *Insomnia*. A client with a duodenal ulcer commonly awakens during the night with pain. The client's feelings of anxiety do not necessarily indicate that she is coping ineffectively. There are no data to indicate that the client has anorexia or is not able to carry out daily activities. (C)

23. **2, 3.** The symptoms of nausea and dizziness in a client with peptic ulcer disease may be indicative of hemorrhage and should not be ignored. The appropriate nursing actions at this time are for the nurse to monitor the client's vital signs and notify the physician of the client's symptoms. To administer an antacid hourly or to wait 1 hour to reassess the client would be inappropriate; prompt intervention is essential in a client who is potentially experiencing a gastrointestinal hemorrhage. The nurse would notify the physician of assessment findings and then initiate oxygen therapy if ordered by the physician. (A)

24. **3.** Diet therapy for ulcer disease is a controversial issue. There is no scientific evidence that diet therapy promotes healing. Most clients are instructed to follow a diet that they can tolerate. There is no need for the client to ingest only a bland or high-protein diet. Milk may be included in the diet, but it is not recommended in excessive amounts. (C)

25. **2.** A relaxed environment is an essential component of ulcer healing. Nurses can help clients understand the importance of relaxation and explore with them ways to balance work and family demands to promote healing. Being involved with his work may prevent boredom; however, this client is upset and argumentative. Not keeping up with his job will probably increase the client's stress level, but the nurse's response is best if it is based on the fact that a relaxed environment is an essential component of ulcer healing. Nurses cannot set limits on a client's behavior; clients must make the decision to make lifestyle changes. (C)

26. **4.** It would be most effective for the client to develop a health maintenance plan that incorporates regular periods of physical and mental rest in the daily schedule. Strategies should be identified to deal with the types of physical and mental stressors that the client needs to cope with in the home and work environments. Scheduling physical activity to occur only in the morning would not be restful or practical. There is no need for the client to

avoid yard work or jogging if these activities are not stressful. (P)

27. **3.** Ranitidine blocks secretion of hydrochloric acid. Clients who take only one daily dose of ranitidine are usually advised to take it at bedtime to inhibit nocturnal secretion of acid. Clients who take the drug twice a day are advised to take it in the morning and at bedtime. It is not necessary to take the drug before meals. The client should take the drug regularly, not just when pain occurs. (D)

28. **3.** It is most likely that the client is experiencing an adverse effect of the antacid. Antacids with aluminum salt products, such as aluminum hydroxide, form insoluble salts in the body. These precipitate and accumulate in the intestines, causing constipation. Increasing dietary fiber intake or daily exercise may be a beneficial lifestyle change for the client but is not likely to relieve the constipation caused by the aluminum hydroxide. Constipation, in isolation from other symptoms, is not a sign of a bowel obstruction. (D)

29. **4.** Antacids are most effective if taken 1 to 3 hours after meals and at bedtime. When an antacid is taken on an empty stomach, the duration of the drug's action is greatly decreased. Taking antacids 1 to 3 hours after a meal lengthens the duration of action, thus increasing the therapeutic action of the drug. Antacids should be administered about 2 hours after other medications to decrease the chance of drug interactions. It is not necessary to decrease fluid intake when taking antacids. If antacids are taken more frequently than recommended, the likelihood of developing adverse effects increases. Therefore, the client should not take antacids as often as desired to control pain. (D)

30. **2.** Alcohol is a gastric irritant that should be eliminated from the intake of the client with peptic ulcer disease. Analgesics are not used to control ulcer pain; many analgesics are gastric irritants. The client's hemoglobin and hematocrit typically do not need to be monitored every 3 months, unless gastrointestinal bleeding is suspected. The client can maintain an active lifestyle and does not need to eliminate contact sports as long as they are not stress-inducing. (R)

The Client with Cancer of the Stomach

31. **2, 3, 5, 6.** The client who is experiencing upper GI bleeding is at risk for developing hypovolemic shock from blood loss. Therefore, the signs and symptoms the nurse should expect to find are those related to hypovolemia, including decreased urine output, tachycardia, rapid respirations, and thirst. The client's skin would be cool and clammy, not dry and flushed. The client would also be likely to develop hypotension, which would lead to a narrowing pulse pressure, not a widening pulse pressure. (A)

32. 3. The most likely complication of an endoscopic procedure is perforation. A sudden temperature spike within 1 to 2 hours after the procedure is indicative of a perforation and should be reported immediately to the physician. A sore throat is to be anticipated after an endoscopy. Clients are given sedatives during the procedure, so it is expected that they will display signs of sedation after the procedure is completed. A lack of appetite could be the result of many factors, including the disease process. (R)

33. 2. A Billroth II procedure bypasses the duodenum and connects the gastric stump directly to the jejunum. The pyloric sphincter is removed, along with some of the stomach fundus. (A)

34. 3. The information presented most clearly supports a nursing diagnosis of *Grieving*. The feelings expressed in this situation are more related to grieving about the changes that will occur in the client's life as a result of the diagnosis of gastric cancer than to fear of the unknown or anxiety about the surgery. There is no evidence of ineffective coping at this time. (P)

35. 1. About 12 to 24 hours after a subtotal gastrectomy, gastric drainage is normally brown, which indicates digested blood. Bile green or cloudy white drainage is not expected during the first 12 to 24 hours after a subtotal gastrectomy. Drainage during the first 6 to 12 hours contains some bright red blood, but large amounts of blood or excessive bloody drainage should be reported to the physician promptly. (R)

36. 3. Nausea, vomiting, or abdominal distention indicates that gas and secretions are accumulating within the gastric pouch due to impaired peristalsis or edema at the operative site and may indicate that the drainage system is not working properly. Saline solution is used to irrigate NG tubes. Hypotonic solutions such as water increase electrolyte loss. In addition, a physician's order is needed to irrigate the NG tube because this procedure could disrupt the suture line. After gastric surgery, only the surgeon repositions the NG tube because of the danger of rupturing or dislodging the suture line. The amount of suction varies with the type of tube used and is ordered by the physician. High suction may create too much tension on the gastric suture line. (R)

37. 25

To administer I.V. fluids at 100 ml/hour using tubing that has a drip factor of 15 gtt/ml, the nurse should use the following formula:

$$100 \text{ ml}/60 \text{ minutes} \times 15 \text{ gtts}/1 \text{ ml} = 25 \text{ gtt}/\text{minute}.$$

(D)

38. 3. A client who has had abdominal surgery is best placed in a low Fowler's position postoperatively. This positioning relaxes abdominal muscles and provides for maximum respiratory and cardiovascular function. The prone, supine, or Sims position would not be tolerated by a client who has had abdominal surgery, nor do those positions support respiratory or cardiovascular functioning. (A)

39. 2. Because of the client's reduced stomach capacity, frequent small feedings are recommended. Early satiety can result, and large quantities of food are not well tolerated. Each client should progress at his or her own pace, gradually increasing the amount of food eaten. The goal is three meals daily if possible, but this can take 6 months or longer to achieve. Nausea can be episodic and can result from eating too fast or eating too much at one time. Eating less and eating more slowly, rather than not eating at all, can be a solution. Bland foods are recommended as starting foods because they are easily digested and are less irritating to the healing mucosa. Bland foods are not less nutritional. (C)

40. 2. After a gastric resection, ingested food moves rapidly from the remaining stomach into the duodenum or jejunum. The food has not undergone adequate preliminary digestion in the stomach. It is concentrated (hypertonic), distends the intestine, and stimulates significant secretion of insulin by the pancreas, as well as a shift of fluid into the bowel. The dumping syndrome results from these factors, which are initiated by the rapid movement of food out of the stomach. After gastric resection, excess digestive enzymes are not secreted and the liver does not produce glycogen. Dumping syndrome is not caused by loss of gastric secretions. (R)

41. 4. Carbohydrates are restricted, but protein, including meat and dairy products, is recommended because it is digested more slowly. Lying down for 30 minutes after a meal is encouraged to slow movement of the food bolus. Fluids are restricted to reduce the bulk of food. There is no need to avoid caffeine. (C)

42. 4. The symptoms related to dumping syndrome that occur after a gastrectomy usually disappear by 6 to 12 months after surgery. Most clients can begin to resume normal meal patterns after signs of the dumping syndrome have stopped. Acknowledging that eating six meals a day is time-consuming does not address the client's question and makes an assumption about the client's concerns. It is not necessarily true that a six-meal-a-day dietary pattern will be required for the rest of the client's life. Clients will not be able to eat three meals a day before hospital discharge. (A)

43. 3. Signs and symptoms of the dumping syndrome usually begin 15 to 30 minutes after eating and include weakness, dizziness, diaphoresis, palpitations, a sense of fullness, abdominal cramps, and diarrhea. These symptoms result when a large bolus of hypertonic fluid enters the small intestine and causes a sudden decrease in plasma volume as fluid is shifted into the bowel. Heartburn is the result of gastric reflex, not the dumping syndrome. (A)

44. **1.** Clients who have had gastric surgery are prone to postoperative complications, such as dumping syndrome and postprandial hypoglycemia, that can affect nutritional intake. Vitamin absorption can also be an issue, depending on the extent of the gastric surgery. Radiation therapy to the upper gastrointestinal area also can affect nutritional intake by causing anorexia, nausea, and esophagitis. The client would not be expected to develop alopecia. Exercise and activity levels as well as access to community resources are important teaching areas, but nutritional intake is a priority need. (R)

45. **4.** An appropriate expected outcome is for the client to achieve optimal nutritional status through the use of oral feedings or total parenteral nutrition (TPN). TPN may be used to supplement oral intake, or it may be used alone if the client cannot tolerate oral feedings. The client would not be expected to regain lost weight within 1 month after surgery or to tolerate a normal dietary intake of three meals a day. Nausea and vomiting would not be considered an expected outcome of gastric surgery, and regular use of antiemetics would not be anticipated. (A)

The Client with Gastroesophageal Reflux Disease

46. **2.** The nurse should instruct the client to not lie down for about 2 hours after eating to prevent reflux. Caffeinated beverages decrease pressure in the lower esophageal sphincter and milk increases gastric acid secretion, so these beverages should be avoided. The client is encouraged to follow a high-protein, low-fat diet, and avoid foods that are irritating. (R)

47. **1.** A laxative is administered after an upper gastrointestinal series to stimulate a bowel movement. This examination involves the administration of barium, which must be promptly eliminated from the body because it may harden and cause an obstruction. A clear liquid diet or an I.V. infusion would have no effect on stimulating removal of the barium. An enema would be ineffective because the barium is too high in the gastrointestinal tract. (R)

48. **3.** With GERD, eating substances that decrease lower esophageal sphincter pressure causes heartburn. A decrease in the lower esophageal sphincter pressure allows gastric contents to reflux into the lower end of the esophagus. Foods that can cause a decrease in esophageal sphincter pressure include fatty foods, chocolate, caf-feinated beverages, peppermint, and alcohol. A diet high in protein and low in fat is recommended for clients with GERD. Lean beef, popcorn, and raw vegetables would be acceptable. (A)

49. **4.** Clients with GERD can develop pulmonary symptoms, such as coughing, wheezing, and dyspnea, that are caused by the aspiration of gastric contents. GERD does not predispose the client to the development of laryngeal cancer. Irritation of the esophagus and esophageal scar tissue formation can develop as a result of GERD. However, GERD is more likely to cause painful and difficult swallowing. (A)

50. **2.** Bethanechol (Urecholine), a cholinergic drug, may be used in GERD to increase lower esophageal sphincter pressure and facilitate gastric emptying. Cholinergic adverse effects may include urinary urgency, diarrhea, abdominal cramping, hypotension, and increased salivation. To avoid these adverse effects, the client should be closely monitored to establish the minimum effective dose. (D)

51. **1.** Fats are associated with decreased esophageal sphincter tone, which increases reflux. Obesity contributes to the development of hiatal hernia, and a low-fat diet might also aid in weight loss. Carbohydrates and foods high in sodium or calcium do not affect gastroesophageal reflux. (C)

52. **1.** Esophageal reflux worsens when the stomach is overdistended with food. Therefore, an important measure is to eat small, frequent meals. Fluid intake should be decreased during meals to reduce abdominal distention. Avoiding air swallowing does not prevent esophageal reflux. Food intake in the evening should be strictly limited to reduce the incidence of nighttime reflux, so bedtime snacks are not recommended. (C)

53. **1.** Heartburn, the most common symptom of a sliding hiatal hernia, results from reflux of gastric secretions into the esophagus. Regurgitation of gastric contents and dysphagia are other common symptoms. Jaundice, which results from a high concentration of bilirubin in the blood, is not associated with hiatal hernia. Anorexia is not a typical symptom of hiatal hernia. Stomatitis is inflammation of the mouth. (A)

54. **2.** Any factor that increases intra-abdominal pressure, such as obesity, can contribute to the development of hiatal hernia. Other factors include abdominal straining, frequent heavy lifting, and pregnancy. Hiatal hernia is also associated with older age and occurs in women more frequently than in men. Having a sedentary desk job, using laxatives frequently, or being 40 years old is not likely to be a contributing factor in development of a hiatal hernia. (R)

55. **3.** Self-responsibility is the key to individual health maintenance. Using examples of situations in which the client has demonstrated self-responsibility can be reinforcing and supporting. The client has ultimate responsibility for his personal health habits. Meeting other people who are managing their care and involving family members can be helpful, but individual motivation is more important. Reassurance can be helpful but is less important than individualization of care. (C)

56. **3.** The magnesium salts in magnesium hydroxide are related to those found in laxatives and may cause diarrhea. Aluminum salt products can cause constipation. Many clients find that a combination product is required to maintain normal bowel elimination. The use of magnesium hydroxide does not cause anorexia or weight gain. (D)

57. **2.** Smoking and alcohol use both reduce esophageal sphincter tone and can result in reflux. They therefore should be avoided by clients with hiatal hernia. Daily aerobic exercise, balancing activity and rest, and avoiding high-stress situations may increase the client's general health and well-being, but they are not directly associated with hiatal hernia. (H)

58. **2.** Bending, especially after eating, can cause gastroesophageal reflux. Lifting heavy objects increases intra-abdominal pressure. Assessing the client's lifting techniques enables the nurse to evaluate the client's knowledge of factors contributing to hiatal hernia and how to prevent complications. Number and length of breaks, temperature in the work area, and cleaning solvents used are not directly related to treatment of hiatal hernia. (C)

59. **1.** A client with a hiatal hernia should avoid the recumbent position immediately after meals to minimize gastric reflux. Bedtime snacks, as well as high-fat foods and carbonated beverages, should be avoided. Excessive vigorous exercise also should be avoided, especially after meals, but there is no reason why the client must give up swimming. Wearing tight, constrictive clothing such as a girdle can increase intra-abdominal pressure and thus lead to reflux of gastric juices. (C)

60. **1.** Metoclopramide hydrochloride (Reglan) increases esophageal sphincter tone and facilitates gastric emptying; both actions reduce the incidence of reflux. Other drugs, such as antacids or histamine receptor antagonists, may also be prescribed to help control reflux and esophagitis and to decrease or neutralize gastric secretions. Reglan is not effective in decreasing or neutralizing gastric secretions. (D)

61. **4.** Metoclopramide hydrochloride (Reglan) can cause sedation. Alcohol and other central nervous system depressants add to this sedation. A client who is taking this drug should be cautioned to avoid driving or performing other hazardous activities for a few hours after taking the drug. Clients may take antacids, antihypertensives, and anticoagulants while on metoclopramide. (D)

62. **3.** Cimetidine (Tagamet) is a histamine receptor antagonist that decreases the quantity of gastric secretions. It may be used in hiatal hernia therapy to prevent or treat the esophagitis and heartburn associated with reflux. Cimetidine is not used to prevent reflux, dysphagia, or ulcer development. (D)

63. **2.** Most clients can be treated successfully with a combination of diet restrictions, medications, weight control, and lifestyle modifications. Surgery to correct a hiatal hernia, which commonly produces complications, is performed only when medical therapy fails to control the symptoms. (R)

The Client with Lower Gastrointestinal Tract Health Problems

- The Client with Cancer of the Colon
- The Client with Hemorrhoids
- The Client with Inflammatory Bowel Disease
- The Client with an Intestinal Obstruction
- The Client with an Ileostomy
- The Client Receiving Total Parenteral Nutrition
- The Client with Diverticular Disease
- The Client with Appendicitis
- The Client with an Inguinal Hernia
- Correct Answers and Rationales

The Client with Cancer of the Colon

1. Which of the following guidelines reflects the current American Cancer Society recommendations for screening for colon cancer in individuals who are not at high risk?
- ☐ **1.** Annual digital rectal examination should begin at age 40.
- ☐ **2.** Annual fecal testing for occult blood should begin at age 50.
- ☐ **3.** Individuals should obtain a baseline barium enema at age 40.
- ☐ **4.** Individuals should obtain a baseline colonoscopy at age 45.

2. A client refuses to look at or care for her colostomy. Which of the following statements by the nurse would be most appropriate?
- ☐ **1.** "It has been 4 days since your surgery and you will soon be discharged. You have to learn to care for your colostomy before you leave the hospital."
- ☐ **2.** "I think we will need to teach your husband to care for your colostomy if you are not going to be able to do it."
- ☐ **3.** "I understand how you are feeling. It is important for you to feel attractive and you think having a colostomy changes your attractiveness."
- ☐ **4.** "I can see that you are upset. Would you like to share your concerns with me?"

3. Which of the following has been identified as a potential risk factor for the development of colon cancer?
- ☐ **1.** Chronic constipation.
- ☐ **2.** Long-term use of laxatives.
- ☐ **3.** History of smoking.
- ☐ **4.** History of inflammatory bowel disease.

4. The nurse is preparing a teaching plan for a community presentation on the prevention and early detection of colon cancer. Which of the following should the nurse identify to the audience as the most common symptom of colon cancer?
- ☐ **1.** Abdominal pain.
- ☐ **2.** Diarrhea.
- ☐ **3.** Rectal bleeding.
- ☐ **4.** Abdominal distention.

5. When teaching a client with signs and symptoms of colon cancer about the diagnostic workup, the nurse instructs the client to take which of the following types of medication after a barium enema?
- ☐ **1.** Laxative.
- ☐ **2.** Anticholinergic.
- ☐ **3.** Antacid.
- ☐ **4.** Demulcent.

6. The client with colon cancer has an abdominal-perineal resection with a colostomy. Which of the following nursing interventions is most appropriate for this client in the postoperative period?
- ☐ **1.** Maintain the client in a semi-Fowler's position.
- ☐ **2.** Assist the client with warm sitz baths.
- ☐ **3.** Administer 30 ml of milk of magnesia to stimulate colostomy activity.
- ☐ **4.** Remove the ostomy pouch as needed so the stoma can be assessed.

7. The nurse evaluates the client's stoma during the initial postoperative period. Which of the following observations should be reported immediately to the physician?
- [ ] **1.** The stoma is slightly edematous.
- [ ] **2.** The stoma is dark red to purple.
- [ ] **3.** The stoma oozes a small amount of blood.
- [ ] **4.** The stoma does not expel stool.

8. While changing the client's colostomy bag and dressing, the nurse assesses that the client is ready to participate in her care by noting which of the following?
- [ ] **1.** The client asks what time the doctor will visit that day.
- [ ] **2.** The client asks about the supplies used during the dressing change.
- [ ] **3.** The client talks about something she read in the morning newspaper.
- [ ] **4.** The client complains about the way the night nurse changed the dressing.

9. Which of the following skin preparations would be best to apply around the client's colostomy?
- [ ] **1.** Karaya.
- [ ] **2.** Petroleum jelly.
- [ ] **3.** Cornstarch.
- [ ] **4.** Antiseptic cream.

10. A client is recovering from an abdominal-perineal resection. Which of the following measures would most effectively promote wound healing after the perineal drains have been removed?
- [ ] **1.** Taking sitz baths.
- [ ] **2.** Taking daily showers.
- [ ] **3.** Applying warm, moist dressings to the area.
- [ ] **4.** Applying a protected heating pad to the area.

11. When planning diet teaching for the client with a colostomy, the nurse should develop a plan that emphasizes which of the following dietary instructions?
- [ ] **1.** Foods containing roughage should not be eaten.
- [ ] **2.** Liquids are best limited to prevent diarrhea.
- [ ] **3.** Clients should experiment to find the diet that is best for them.
- [ ] **4.** A high-fiber diet will produce a regular passage of stool.

12. Which of the following would be an expected outcome for a client who is recovering from an abdominal-perineal resection with a colostomy? The client will:
- [ ] **1.** Maintain a fluid intake of 3,000 ml/day.
- [ ] **2.** Eliminate fiber from the diet.
- [ ] **3.** Limit physical activity to light exercise.
- [ ] **4.** Accept that sexual activity will be diminished.

The Client with Hemorrhoids

13. A 36-year-old female client has been diagnosed with hemorrhoids. Which of the following factors in the client's history would most likely be a primary cause of her hemorrhoids?
- [ ] **1.** Her age.
- [ ] **2.** Three vaginal delivery pregnancies.
- [ ] **3.** Her job as a schoolteacher.
- [ ] **4.** Varicosities in her legs.

14. Which position would be ideal for the client in the early postoperative period after a hemorrhoidectomy?
- [ ] **1.** High Fowler's.
- [ ] **2.** Supine.
- [ ] **3.** Side-lying.
- [ ] **4.** Trendelenburg's.

15. The nurse instructs the client who has had a hemorrhoidectomy not to use sitz baths until at least 12 hours postoperatively to avoid inducing which of the following complications?
- [ ] **1.** Hemorrhage.
- [ ] **2.** Rectal spasm.
- [ ] **3.** Urine retention.
- [ ] **4.** Constipation.

16. The nurse teaches the client who has had rectal surgery the proper timing for sitz baths. The nurse knows that the client has understood the teaching when the client states that it is most important to take a sitz bath:
- [ ] **1.** First thing each morning.
- [ ] **2.** As needed for discomfort.
- [ ] **3.** After a bowel movement.
- [ ] **4.** At bedtime.

The Client with Inflammatory Bowel Disease

17. A client has been placed on long-term sulfasalazine (Azulfidine) therapy for treatment of his ulcerative colitis. The nurse should encourage the client to eat which of the following foods to help avoid the nutrient deficiencies that may develop as a result of this medication?
- [ ] **1.** Citrus fruits.
- [ ] **2.** Green, leafy vegetables.
- [ ] **3.** Eggs.
- [ ] **4.** Milk products.

18. The nurse is assigning clients for the evening shift. Which of the following clients are appropriate for the nurse to assign to a licensed practical nurse to provide client care? Select all that apply.
☐ 1. A client with Crohn's disease who is receiving total parenteral nutrition (TPN).
☐ 2. A client who underwent inguinal hernia repair surgery 3 hours ago.
☐ 3. A client with an intestinal obstruction who needs a Cantor tube inserted.
☐ 4. A client with diverticulitis who needs teaching about his take-home medications.
☐ 5. A client who is experiencing an exacerbation of his ulcerative colitis.

19. A client who has had ulcerative colitis for the past 5 years is admitted to the hospital with an exacerbation of the disease. Which of the following factors was most likely of greatest significance in causing an exacerbation of ulcerative colitis?
☐ 1. A demanding and stressful job.
☐ 2. Changing to a modified vegetarian diet.
☐ 3. Beginning a weight-training program.
☐ 4. Walking 2 miles every day.

20. A client who is experiencing an exacerbation of ulcerative colitis is receiving I.V. fluids that are to be infused at 125 ml/hour. The I.V. tubing delivers 15 gtt/ml. How quickly should the nurse infuse the fluids in drops per minute to infuse the fluids at the prescribed rate?

_____ gtt/minute

21. When planning care for a client with ulcerative colitis who is experiencing an exacerbation of symptoms, which client care activities can the nurse appropriately delegate to an unlicensed assistant? Select all that apply.
☐ 1. Assessing the client's bowel sounds.
☐ 2. Providing skin care following bowel movements.
☐ 3. Evaluating the client's response to antidiarrheal medications.
☐ 4. Maintaining intake and output records.
☐ 5. Obtaining the client's weight.

22. Which goal for the client's care should take priority during the first days of hospitalization for an exacerbation of ulcerative colitis?
☐ 1. Promoting self-care and independence.
☐ 2. Managing diarrhea.
☐ 3. Maintaining adequate nutrition.
☐ 4. Promoting rest and comfort.

23. The client with ulcerative colitis is following orders for bed rest with bathroom privileges. What would be the primary rationale for this activity restriction?
☐ 1. To conserve energy.
☐ 2. To reduce intestinal peristalsis.
☐ 3. To promote rest and comfort.
☐ 4. To prevent injury.

24. A client's ulcerative colitis signs and symptoms have been present for longer than 1 week. The nurse recognizes that the client should be assessed carefully for signs and symptoms of which of the following complications?
☐ 1. Heart failure.
☐ 2. Deep vein thrombosis.
☐ 3. Hypokalemia.
☐ 4. Hypocalcemia.

25. A client who has ulcerative colitis says to the nurse, "I can't take this anymore! I'm constantly in pain, and I can't leave my room because I need to stay by the toilet. I don't know how to deal with this." Based on these comments, an appropriate nursing diagnosis for this client would be:
☐ 1. *Impaired physical mobility* related to fatigue.
☐ 2. *Disturbed thought processes* related to pain.
☐ 3. *Social isolation* related to chronic fatigue.
☐ 4. *Ineffective coping* related to chronic abdominal pain.

26. A client newly diagnosed with ulcerative colitis has been placed on steroids. He states that he has heard that taking steroids can be dangerous and asks the nurse why steroids are prescribed. Which of the following statements by the nurse provides the client with accurate information about the use of steroid therapy in the treatment of ulcerative colitis?
☐ 1. "Ulcerative colitis can be cured by the use of steroids."
☐ 2. "Steroids are used in severe flare-ups because they can decrease the incidence of bleeding."
☐ 3. "Long-term use of steroids will prolong periods of remission."
☐ 4. "The side effects of steroids outweigh their benefits to clients with ulcerative colitis."

27. A client who has ulcerative colitis has persistent diarrhea. He is thin and has lost 12 lb since the exacerbation of his ulcerative colitis. The nurse should anticipate that the physician will order which of the following treatment approaches to help the client meet his nutritional needs?
☐ 1. Initiate continuous enteral feedings.
☐ 2. Encourage a high-calorie, high-protein diet.
☐ 3. Implement total parenteral nutrition (TPN).
☐ 4. Provide six small meals a day.

28. The physician prescribes sulfasalazine (Azulfidine) for the client with ulcerative colitis to continue taking at home. Which instruction should the nurse give the client about taking this medication?
- ☐ **1.** Avoid taking it with food.
- ☐ **2.** Take the total dose at bedtime.
- ☐ **3.** Take it with a full glass (240 ml) of water.
- ☐ **4.** Stop taking it if urine turns orange-yellow.

29. The nurse has an order to administer sulfasalazine (Azulfidine) 2 g. The medication is available in 500-mg tablets. How many tablets should the nurse administer?

_____ tablets

30. A client with ulcerative colitis expresses serious concerns about her career as an attorney because of the effects of stress on ulcerative colitis. Which of the following nursing interventions will be most helpful to the client?
- ☐ **1.** Review her current coping mechanisms and develop alternatives, if needed.
- ☐ **2.** Suggest a less stressful career in which she would still use her education and experience.
- ☐ **3.** Suggest that she ask her colleagues to help decrease her stress by giving her the easier cases.
- ☐ **4.** Prepare family members for the fact that she will have to work part-time.

31. Which of the following diets would be most appropriate for the client with ulcerative colitis?
- ☐ **1.** High-calorie, low-protein.
- ☐ **2.** High-protein, low-residue.
- ☐ **3.** Low-fat, high-fiber.
- ☐ **4.** Low-sodium, high-carbohydrate.

32. A client who has a history of Crohn's disease is admitted to the hospital with fever, diarrhea, cramping, abdominal pain, and weight loss. Which of the following laboratory findings would be anticipated for the client?
- ☐ **1.** Hyperalbuminemia.
- ☐ **2.** Thrombocytopenia.
- ☐ **3.** Hypokalemia.
- ☐ **4.** Hypercalcemia.

33. A client with Crohn's disease experiences rectal bleeding along with 15 to 20 watery stools per day. Which of the following signs and symptoms would be indicative of dehydration?
- ☐ **1.** Sunken eyeballs.
- ☐ **2.** Decreased pulse rate.
- ☐ **3.** Moist skin.
- ☐ **4.** Pitting edema.

34. The nurse is developing a plan of care for a client with Crohn's disease who is receiving total parenteral nutrition (TPN). Which of the following interventions should the nurse include? Select all that apply.
- ☐ **1.** Monitoring vital signs once a shift.
- ☐ **2.** Weighing the client daily.
- ☐ **3.** Changing the central venous line dressing daily.
- ☐ **4.** Monitoring the I.V. infusion rate hourly.
- ☐ **5.** Taping all I.V. tubing connections securely.

35. Which of the following should be a priority focus of care for a client experiencing an exacerbation of Crohn's disease?
- ☐ **1.** Encouraging regular ambulation.
- ☐ **2.** Promoting bowel rest.
- ☐ **3.** Maintaining current weight.
- ☐ **4.** Decreasing episodes of rectal bleeding.

The Client with an Intestinal Obstruction

36. A nurse is assessing a client who has been admitted with a diagnosis of an obstruction in the small intestine. What should the nurse assess the client for? Select all that apply.
- ☐ **1.** Projectile vomiting.
- ☐ **2.** Significant abdominal distention.
- ☐ **3.** Copious diarrhea.
- ☐ **4.** Rapid onset of dehydration.
- ☐ **5.** Increased bowel sounds.

37. A client is admitted to the hospital complaining of nausea, vomiting, and abdominal pain. Bowel obstruction is suspected. During the initial assessment, the nurse hears high-pitched tinkling bowel sounds on auscultation and flat sounds on percussion. The flat sounds are caused by:
- ☐ **1.** Hyperactive peristalsis.
- ☐ **2.** Excessive gas trapped in the intestine.
- ☐ **3.** The presence of a mass or tumor in the bowel.
- ☐ **4.** Fluid trapped in the intestine.

38. The physician orders intestinal decompression with a Cantor tube for the client. The primary purpose of a nasoenteric tube such as a Cantor tube is to accomplish which of the following?
- ☐ **1.** Remove fluid and gas from the intestine.
- ☐ **2.** Prevent fluid accumulation in the stomach.
- ☐ **3.** Break up the obstruction.
- ☐ **4.** Provide an alternative route for drug administration.

39. After insertion of a nasoenteric tube, the nurse should place the client in which position?
☐ **1.** Supine.
☐ **2.** Right side-lying.
☐ **3.** Semi-Fowler's.
☐ **4.** Upright in a bedside chair.

40. Which of the following statements about nasoenteric tubes is correct?
☐ **1.** The tube cannot be attached to suction.
☐ **2.** The tube contains a soft rubber bag filled with mercury.
☐ **3.** The tube is taped securely to the client's cheek after insertion.
☐ **4.** The tube can have its placement determined only by auscultation.

41. Which of the following nursing diagnoses would be most appropriate for a client with an intestinal obstruction?
☐ **1.** *Impaired swallowing* related to nothing-by-mouth (NPO) status.
☐ **2.** *Urinary retention* related to deficient fluid volume.
☐ **3.** *Deficient fluid volume* related to nausea and vomiting.
☐ **4.** *Chronic pain* related to abdominal distention.

42. The client with an intestinal obstruction continues to have acute pain even though the nasoenteric tube is patent and draining. Which action by the nurse would be most appropriate?
☐ **1.** Reassure the client that the nasoenteric tube is functioning.
☐ **2.** Assess the client for a rigid abdomen.
☐ **3.** Administer an opioid as ordered.
☐ **4.** Reposition the client on the left side.

43. Before abdominal surgery for an intestinal obstruction, the nurse monitors the client's urine output and finds that the total output for the past 2 hours was 35 ml. The nurse then assesses the client's total intake and output over the last 24 hours and notes that he had 2,000 ml of I.V. fluid for intake, 500 ml of drainage from the nasogastric tube, and 700 ml of urine for a total output of 1,200 ml. This would indicate which of the following?
☐ **1.** Decreased renal function.
☐ **2.** Inadequate pain relief.
☐ **3.** Extension of the obstruction.
☐ **4.** Inadequate fluid replacement.

The Client with an Ileostomy

44. The nurse is teaching the client how to care for her ileostomy. The client asks the nurse how long she can wear her pouch before changing it. The nurse responds:
☐ **1.** "The pouch is changed only when it leaks."
☐ **2.** "You can wear the pouch for about 4 to 7 days."
☐ **3.** "You should change the pouch every evening before bedtime."
☐ **4.** "It depends on your activity level and your diet."

45. A client is scheduled for an ileostomy. Which of the following interventions would be most helpful in preparing the client psychologically for the surgery?
☐ **1.** Include family members in preoperative teaching sessions.
☐ **2.** Encourage the client to ask questions about managing an ileostomy.
☐ **3.** Provide a brief, thorough explanation of all preoperative and postoperative procedures.
☐ **4.** Invite a member of the ostomy association to visit the client.

46. A client who is scheduled for an ileostomy has an order for oral neomycin (Mycifradin) to be administered before surgery. The nurse understands that the rationale for administering oral neomycin before surgery is to:
☐ **1.** Prevent postoperative bladder infection.
☐ **2.** Reduce the number of intestinal bacteria.
☐ **3.** Decrease the potential for postoperative hypostatic pneumonia.
☐ **4.** Increase the body's immunologic response to the stressors of surgery.

47. Of the following outcomes for client care after an ileostomy, which has the *highest* priority?
☐ **1.** Providing relief from constipation.
☐ **2.** Assisting the client with self-care activities.
☐ **3.** Maintaining fluid and electrolyte balance.
☐ **4.** Minimizing odor formation.

48. The client asks the nurse, "Is it really possible to lead a normal life with an ileostomy?" Which action by the nurse would be the most effective to address this question?
☐ **1.** Have the client talk with a member of the clergy about these concerns.
☐ **2.** Tell the client to worry about those concerns after surgery.
☐ **3.** Arrange for a person with an ostomy to visit the client preoperatively.
☐ **4.** Notify the surgeon of the client's question.

49. The nurse explains to the client that some form of skin barrier must be used around the stoma at all times. The primary function of a skin barrier is to:
- ☐ 1. Help prevent the formation of odor.
- ☐ 2. Help maintain an accurate output record.
- ☐ 3. Protect against irritation from ileostomy effluent.
- ☐ 4. Allow the client to keep the ostomy pouch on longer.

50. The nurse should instruct the client with an ileostomy to report which of the following signs and symptoms immediately?
- ☐ 1. Passage of liquid stool from the stoma.
- ☐ 2. Occasional presence of undigested food in the effluent.
- ☐ 3. Absence of drainage from the ileostomy for 6 or more hours.
- ☐ 4. Temperature of 99.8° F (37.7° C).

51. The nurse finds the client crying. The client explains to the nurse, "I'm upset because I know I won't be able to have children now that I have an ileostomy." Which of the following would be the best response for the nurse?
- ☐ 1. "Many women with ileostomies decide to adopt. Why don't you consider that option?"
- ☐ 2. "Having an ileostomy does not necessarily mean that you can't bear children. Let's talk about your concerns."
- ☐ 3. "I can understand your reasons for being upset. Having children must be important to you."
- ☐ 4. "I'm sure you will adjust to this situation with time. Try not to be too upset."

52. The nurse evaluates the client's understanding of ileostomy care. Which of the following statements indicates that discharge teaching has been effective?
- ☐ 1. "I should be able to resume weight lifting in 2 weeks."
- ☐ 2. "I can return to work in 2 weeks."
- ☐ 3. "I need to drink at least 3,000 ml a day of fluid."
- ☐ 4. "I will need to avoid getting my stoma wet while bathing."

53. A client calls the nurse at a clinic to report the sudden onset of abdominal cramps, vomiting, and watery discharge from his ileostomy. How should the nurse respond to this client?
- ☐ 1. Tell the client to come into the clinic for an examination if the symptoms persist for longer than 24 hours.
- ☐ 2. Encourage the client to increase fluid intake to 3 L/day to replace fluid lost through vomiting.
- ☐ 3. Instruct the client to take 30 ml of milk of magnesia to stimulate a bowel movement.
- ☐ 4. Tell the client that he needs to be examined immediately by the physician.

The Client Receiving Total Parenteral Nutrition

54. The nurse is changing the subclavian dressing of a client who is receiving total parenteral nutrition. When assessing the catheter insertion site, the nurse notes the presence of yellow drainage from around the sutures that are anchoring the catheter. Which action should the nurse take first?
- ☐ 1. Clean the insertion site and redress the area.
- ☐ 2. Document assessment findings in the client's chart.
- ☐ 3. Obtain a culture specimen of the drainage.
- ☐ 4. Notify the physician.

55. Using a sliding-scale schedule, the nurse is preparing to administer an evening dose of regular insulin to a client who is receiving total parenteral nutrition (TPN). Which action is most appropriate for the nurse to take to determine the amount of insulin to give?
- ☐ 1. Base the dosage on the glucometer reading of the client's glucose level obtained immediately before administering the insulin.
- ☐ 2. Base the dosage on the fasting blood glucose level obtained earlier in the day.
- ☐ 3. Calculate the amount of TPN fluid the client has received since the last dose of insulin and adjust the dosage accordingly.
- ☐ 4. Assess the client's dietary intake for the evening meal and snack and adjust the dosage accordingly.

56. A client with inflammatory bowel disease is receiving total parenteral nutrition (TPN). The basic component of the client's TPN solution is most likely to be:
- ☐ 1. An isotonic dextrose solution.
- ☐ 2. A hypertonic dextrose solution.
- ☐ 3. A hypotonic dextrose solution.
- ☐ 4. A colloidal dextrose solution.

57. TPN is ordered for a client with Crohn's disease. While administering the TPN solution, it is important for the nurse to remember that total parental solutions are used to:
- ☐ 1. Increase cell nutrition.
- ☐ 2. Treat metabolic acidosis.
- ☐ 3. Provide hydration.
- ☐ 4. Reverse a positive nitrogen balance.

58. The nurse would regularly assess a client's ability to metabolize the TPN solution adequately by monitoring the client for which of the following signs?
- ☐ 1. Tachycardia.
- ☐ 2. Hypertension.
- ☐ 3. Elevated blood urea nitrogen concentration.
- ☐ 4. Hyperglycemia.

59. Which of the following interventions should the nurse include in the client's plan of care to prevent complications associated with TPN administered through a central line?
- ☐ 1. Use a clean technique for all dressing changes.
- ☐ 2. Tape all connections of the system.
- ☐ 3. Encourage bed rest.
- ☐ 4. Cover the insertion site with a moisture-proof dressing.

60. When developing a plan of care for a client who is receiving TPN, which of the following potential nursing diagnoses would be most appropriate?
- ☐ 1. *Impaired swallowing.*
- ☐ 2. *Impaired gas exchange.*
- ☐ 3. *Risk for fluid volume excess.*
- ☐ 4. *Ineffective tissue perfusion.*

61. A client's TPN fluid is being administered through central I.V. tubing. Which complication can occur if the tubing becomes disconnected?
- ☐ 1. Phlebitis.
- ☐ 2. Pneumothorax.
- ☐ 3. Hemorrhage.
- ☐ 4. Air embolus.

62. The nurse discovers that a client's TPN solution was running at an incorrect rate and is now 2 hours behind schedule. Which action is most appropriate for the nurse to take to correct the problem?
- ☐ 1. Readjust the solution to infuse the desired amount.
- ☐ 2. Continue the infusion at the current rate, but run the next bottle at an increased rate.
- ☐ 3. Double the infusion rate for 2 hours.
- ☐ 4. Notify the physician.

63. The nurse administers fat emulsion solution during TPN as ordered based on the understanding that this type of solution:
- ☐ 1. Provides essential fatty acids.
- ☐ 2. Provides extra carbohydrates.
- ☐ 3. Promotes effective metabolism of glucose.
- ☐ 4. Maintains a normal body weight.

64. Which of the following should the nurse interpret as an indication of a complication after the first few days of TPN therapy?
- ☐ 1. Glycosuria.
- ☐ 2. A 1- to 2-pound weight gain.
- ☐ 3. Decreased appetite.
- ☐ 4. Elevated temperature.

65. Which of the following adverse effects would the nurse expect the client to exhibit in the event of too rapid an infusion of TPN solution?
- ☐ 1. Negative nitrogen balance.
- ☐ 2. Circulatory overload.
- ☐ 3. Hypoglycemia.
- ☐ 4. Hypokalemia.

The Client with Diverticular Disease

66. Which foods should the nurse encourage a client with diverticulosis to incorporate into his diet? Select all that apply.
- ☐ 1. Bran cereal.
- ☐ 2. Broccoli.
- ☐ 3. Tomato juice.
- ☐ 4. Navy beans.
- ☐ 5. Cheese.

67. Which of the following laboratory findings would the nurse expect to find in a client with diverticulitis?
- ☐ 1. Elevated red blood cell count.
- ☐ 2. Decreased platelet count.
- ☐ 3. Elevated white blood cell count.
- ☐ 4. Elevated serum blood urea nitrogen concentration.

68. The nurse is aware that the diagnostic tests typically ordered for acute diverticulitis do not include a barium enema. The reason for this is that a barium enema:
- ☐ 1. Can perforate an intestinal abscess.
- ☐ 2. Would greatly increase the client's pain.
- ☐ 3. Is of minimal diagnostic value in diverticulitis.
- ☐ 4. Is too lengthy a procedure for the client to tolerate.

69. Which of the following measures should the client with diverticulitis be taught to integrate into his daily routine at home?
- ☐ 1. Using enemas to relieve constipation.
- ☐ 2. Decreasing fluid intake to increase the formed consistency of the stool.
- ☐ 3. Eating a high-fiber diet when symptomatic with diverticulitis.
- ☐ 4. Refraining from straining and lifting activities.

70. After instructing a client with diverticulosis about appropriate self-care activities, which of the following client comments indicate effective teaching? Select all that apply.
- ☐ 1. "With careful attention to my diet, my diverticulosis can be cured."
- ☐ 2. "Using a cathartic laxative weekly is okay to control bowel movements."
- ☐ 3. "I should follow a diet that's high in fiber."
- ☐ 4. "It is important for me to drink at least 2,000 ml of fluid every day."
- ☐ 5. "I should exercise regularly."

71. Which of the following medications should the nurse anticipate administering to a client with diverticular disease?
- ☐ 1. Psyllium hydrophilic mucilloid (Metamucil).
- ☐ 2. Diphenoxylate with atropine sulfate (Lomotil).
- ☐ 3. Diazepam (Valium).
- ☐ 4. Aluminum hydroxide (Amphojel).

72. Which of the following signs and symptoms would be indicative of peritonitis in a client with diverticulitis?
- ☐ **1.** Hyperactive bowel sounds.
- ☐ **2.** Rigid abdominal wall.
- ☐ **3.** Explosive diarrhea.
- ☐ **4.** Excessive flatulence.

The Client with Appendicitis

73. A nurse is providing wound care to a client 1 day after the client underwent an appendectomy. A drain was inserted into the incisional site during surgery. Which action should the nurse perform when providing wound care?
- ☐ **1.** Remove the dressing and leave the incision open to air.
- ☐ **2.** Remove the drain if wound drainage is minimal.
- ☐ **3.** Gently irrigate the drain to remove exudate.
- ☐ **4.** Clean the area around the drain moving away from the drain.

74. In a client with acute appendicitis, the nurse should anticipate which of the following treatments?
- ☐ **1.** Administration of enemas to clean the bowel.
- ☐ **2.** Insertion of a nasogastric (NG) tube.
- ☐ **3.** Placement of client on nothing-by-mouth (NPO) status.
- ☐ **4.** Administration of heat to the abdomen.

75. A client with acute appendicitis develops a fever, tachycardia, and hypotension. Based on these assessment findings, the nurse suspects which of the following complications?
- ☐ **1.** Deficient fluid volume.
- ☐ **2.** Intestinal obstruction.
- ☐ **3.** Bowel ischemia.
- ☐ **4.** Peritonitis.

76. Postoperative nursing care for a client after an appendectomy should include which of the following interventions?
- ☐ **1.** Administering sitz baths four times a day.
- ☐ **2.** Noting the first bowel movement after surgery.
- ☐ **3.** Limiting the client's activity to bathroom privileges.
- ☐ **4.** Measuring abdominal girth every 2 hours.

77. A client who had an appendectomy for a perforated appendix returns from surgery with a drain inserted in the incisional site. The nurse understands that the purpose of the drain is to accomplish which of the following?
- ☐ **1.** Provide access for wound irrigation.
- ☐ **2.** Promote drainage of wound exudates.
- ☐ **3.** Minimize development of scar tissue.
- ☐ **4.** Decrease postoperative discomfort.

The Client with an Inguinal Hernia

78. A client who has a history of an inguinal hernia is admitted to the hospital with complaints of sudden, severe abdominal pain; vomiting; and abdominal distention. Based on these assessment findings, the nurse suspects that which of the following complications has developed?
- ☐ **1.** Peritonitis.
- ☐ **2.** Incarcerated hernia.
- ☐ **3.** Strangulated hernia.
- ☐ **4.** Intestinal perforation.

79. A client has just had an inguinal herniorrhaphy. Which of the following instructions would be most appropriate to include in his discharge plan?
- ☐ **1.** Turning, coughing, and deep breathing every 2 hours.
- ☐ **2.** Applying an ice bag to the scrotum.
- ☐ **3.** Applying a truss before the client ambulates.
- ☐ **4.** Maintaining a high Fowler's position while resting.

80. After an inguinal herniorrhaphy, the nurse should evaluate the client carefully for which of the following likely complications?
- ☐ **1.** Hypostatic pneumonia.
- ☐ **2.** Deep vein thrombosis.
- ☐ **3.** Paralytic ileus.
- ☐ **4.** Urine retention.

Correct Answers and Rationales

The letter in parentheses after each rationale identifies the client need addressed in the item, including management of care (M), safety and infection control (S), health promotion and maintenance (H), psychosocial adaptation (P), basic care and comfort (C), pharmacological and parenteral therapies (D), reduction of risk potential (R), and physiological adaptation (A).

The Client with Cancer of the Colon

1. 2. Annual fecal testing for occult blood should begin at age 50. Annual digital rectal examinations are recommended in men beginning at age 50 to screen for prostate cancer. Baseline barium enemas or colonoscopies are recommended at age 50. Baseline barium enemas and colonoscopies are not performed on individuals in their 40s unless they experience signs or symptoms that indicate the need for such diagnostic testing, or are considered to be at high risk. (H)

2. **4.** It is important for the nurse to recognize that individuals go through a grieving process when adjusting to a colostomy. The nurse should be accepting and provide the client with opportunities to share her concerns and feelings when she is ready. Lecturing the client about the need to learn how to care for the colostomy is not productive, nor is attempting to shame her into caring for the colostomy by implying her husband will have to provide the care if she does not. It is not possible for the nurse to understand what the client is feeling. (P)

3. **4.** A history of inflammatory bowel disease is a risk factor for colon cancer. Other risk factors include age (older than 40 years), history of familial polyposis, colorectal polyps, and high-fat or low-fiber diet. (R)

4. **3.** Rectal bleeding is the most common symptom of colon cancer. Other commonly seen symptoms include alternating constipation and diarrhea, narrowing of stool caliber, and a sense of incomplete evacuation. Iron deficiency anemia and occult bleeding may also be present. Colon cancer may be asymptomatic in early stages. Abdominal pain and distention are not necessarily present in the early stages of colon cancer. (R)

5. **1.** After a barium enema, a laxative is ordinarily prescribed. This is done to promote elimination of the barium. Retained barium predisposes the client to constipation and fecal impaction. Anticholinergic drugs decrease gastrointestinal motility. Antacids decrease gastric acid secretion. Demulcents soothe mucous membranes of the gastrointestinal tract and are used to treat diarrhea. (R)

6. **2.** Appropriate nursing interventions after an abdominal-perineal resection with a colostomy include assisting the client with warm sitz baths three to four times a day to clean the perineal incision. The client will be more comfortable assuming a side-lying position because of the perineal incision. It would be inappropriate to administer milk of magnesia to stimulate colostomy activity. Stool passage will begin as peristalsis returns. It is not necessary or desirable to change the ostomy pouch daily to assess the stoma. The ostomy pouch should be transparent to allow easy observation of the stoma and drainage. (A)

7. **2.** A dark red to purple stoma indicates inadequate blood supply. Mild edema and slight oozing of blood are normal in the early postoperative period. The colostomy would typically not begin functioning until 2 to 4 days after surgery. (A)

8. **2.** A client who displays interest in the procedure and asks about supplies used for dressings may be ready to participate in self-care. Inquiring about the physician's visit, discussing news events, and complaining about a dressing change are behaviors that avoid the subject of the colostomy. (C)

9. **1.** Karaya and Stomahesive are both effective agents for protecting the skin around a colostomy. They keep the skin healthy and prevent skin irritation from stoma drainage. Petroleum jelly, cornstarch, and antiseptic creams do not protect the skin adequately and may prevent an adequate seal between the skin and the colostomy bag. (C)

10. **1.** Sitz baths are an effective way to clean the operative area after an abdominal-perineal resection. Sitz baths bring warmth to the area, improve circulation, and promote healing and cleanliness. Most clients find them comfortable and relaxing. Between sitz baths, the area should be kept clean and dry. A shower will not adequately clean the perineal area. Moist dressings may promote wound contamination and delay healing. A heating pad applied to the area for longer than 20 minutes may cause excessive vasodilation, leading to congestion and discomfort. (A)

11. **3.** It is best to adjust the diet of a client with a colostomy in a manner that suits the client rather than trying special diets. Severe restriction of roughage is not recommended. The client is encouraged to drink 2 to 3 L of fluid per day. A high-fiber diet may produce loose stools. (C)

12. **1.** An expected outcome is that the client will maintain a fluid intake of 3,000 ml/day unless contraindicated. There is no need to eliminate fiber from the diet; the client can eat whatever foods are desired, avoiding those that are bothersome. Physical activity does not need to be limited to light exercise. The client can resume normal activities as tolerated, usually within 6 to 8 weeks. The client's sexual activity may be affected, but it does not need to be diminished. (A)

The Client with Hemorrhoids

13. **2.** Hemorrhoids are associated with prolonged sitting or standing, portal hypertension, chronic constipation, and prolonged increased intra-abdominal pressure, as associated with pregnancy and the strain of vaginal delivery. Her job as a schoolteacher does not require prolonged sitting or standing. Age and leg varicosities are not related to the development of hemorrhoids. (R)

14. **3.** Positioning in the early postoperative phase should avoid stress and pressure on the operative site. The prone and side-lying positions are ideal from a comfort perspective. A high Fowler's or supine position will place pressure on the operative site and is not recommended. There is no need for Trendelenburg's position. (A)

15. 1. Applying heat during the immediate postoperative period may cause hemorrhage at the surgical site. Moist heat may relieve rectal spasms after bowel movements. Urine retention caused by reflex spasm may also be relieved by moist heat. Increasing fiber and fluid in the diet can help prevent constipation. (A)

16. 3. Adequate cleaning of the anal area is difficult but essential. After rectal surgery, sitz baths assist in this process, so the client should take a sitz bath after a bowel movement. Other times are dictated by client comfort. (R)

The Client with Inflammatory Bowel Disease

17. 2. In long-term sulfasalazine therapy, the client may develop folic acid deficiency. The client can take folic acid supplements, but the nurse should also encourage the client to increase the intake of folic acid in his diet. Green, leafy vegetables are a good source of folic acid. Citrus fruits, eggs, and milk products are not good sources of folic acid. (D)

18. 2, 5. The nurse should consider client needs and scope of practice when assigning staff to provide care. The client who is recovering from inguinal hernia repair surgery and the client who is experiencing an exacerbation of his ulcerative colitis are appropriate clients to assign to a licensed practical nurse as the care they require fall within the scope of practice for a licensed practical nurse. It is not within the scope of practice for the licensed practical nurse to administer TPN, insert nasoenteric tubes, or provide client teaching related to medications. (M)

19. 1. Stressful and emotional events have been clearly linked to exacerbations of ulcerative colitis, although their role in the etiology of the disease has been disproved. A modified vegetarian diet or an exercise program is an unlikely cause of the exacerbation. (A)

20. 31

To administer I.V. fluids at 125 ml/hour using tubing that has a drip factor of 15 gtt/ml, the nurse should use the following formula:

$$125 \text{ ml}/60 \text{ minutes} \times 15 \text{ gtt}/1 \text{ ml} = 31 \text{ gtt/minute.}$$

(D)

21. 2, 4, 5. The nurse can delegate the following basic care activities to the unlicensed assistant: providing skin care following bowel movements, maintaining intake and output records, and obtaining the client's weight. Assessing the client's bowel sounds and evaluating the client's response to medication are registered nurse activities that cannot be delegated. (M)

22. 2. Diarrhea is the primary symptom in an exacerbation of ulcerative colitis, and decreasing the frequency of stools is the first goal of treatment. The other goals are ongoing and will be best achieved by halting the exacerbation. The client may receive antidiarrheal agents, antispasmodic agents, bulk hydrophilic agents, or anti-inflammatory drugs. (A)

23. 2. Although modified bed rest does help conserve energy and promotes comfort, its primary purpose in this case is to help reduce the hypermotility of the colon. Preventing injury is accomplished by other means, such as providing assistance, education, and monitoring of clients at risk for injury. (A)

24. 3. Excessive diarrhea causes significant depletion of the body's stores of sodium and potassium as well as fluid. The client should be closely monitored for hypokalemia and hyponatremia. Ulcerative colitis does not place the client at risk for heart failure, deep vein thrombosis, or hypocalcemia. (R)

25. 4. It is not uncommon for clients with ulcerative colitis to become apprehensive and upset about the frequency of stools and the presence of abdominal cramping. During these acute exacerbations, clients need emotional support and encouragement to verbalize their feelings about their chronic health concerns and assistance in developing effective coping methods. The client has not expressed feelings of fatigue or isolation or demonstrated disturbed thought processes. (P)

26. 2. Steroids are effective in management of the acute symptoms of ulcerative colitis. Steroids do not cure ulcerative colitis, which is a chronic disease. Long-term use is not effective in prolonging the remission and is not advocated. Clients should be assessed carefully for side effects related to steroid therapy, but the benefits of short-term steroid therapy usually outweigh the potential adverse effects. (D)

27. 3. Food will be withheld from the client with severe symptoms of ulcerative colitis to rest the bowel. To maintain the client's nutritional status, the client will be started on TPN. Enteral feedings or dividing the diet into six small meals does not allow the bowel to rest. A high-calorie, high-protein diet will worsen the client's symptoms. (A)

28. 3. Adequate fluid intake of at least 8 glasses a day prevents crystalluria and stone formation during sulfasalazine therapy. Sulfasalazine can cause gastrointestinal distress and is best taken after meals and in equally divided doses. Sulfasalazine gives alkaline urine an orange-yellow color, but it is not necessary to stop the drug when this occurs. (D)

29. 4

To administer 2 g sulfasalazine (Azulfidine), the nurse will need to administer 4 tablets. The following formula is used to calculate the correct dosage:

The first step is to convert grams into milligrams:

$$1 \text{ g}/1{,}000 \text{ mg} = 2 \text{ g}/X \text{ mg}$$

$$X = 2{,}000 \text{ mg}.$$

Then,

$$2{,}000 \text{ mg}/X \text{ tablets} = 500 \text{ mg}/1 \text{ tablet}$$

$$X = 4 \text{ tablets}.$$

(D)

30. **1.** A client with ulcerative colitis need not curtail career goals. Self-care is the cornerstone of long-term management, and learning to cope with and modify stressors will enable the client to live with the disease. Giving up a desired career could discourage and even depress the client. Placing the responsibility for minimizing stressors at work in the hands of others leads to a feeling of loss of control and decreases the sense of responsibility needed for sound self-care. Working part-time rather than full-time is unnecessary. (P)

31. **2.** Clients with ulcerative colitis should follow a well-balanced high-protein, high-calorie, low-residue diet, avoiding such high-residue foods as whole-wheat grains, nuts, and raw fruits and vegetables. Clients with ulcerative colitis need more protein for tissue healing and should avoid excess roughage. There is no need for clients with ulcerative colitis to follow low-sodium diets. (C)

32. **3.** Hypokalemia is the most expected laboratory finding owing to the diarrhea. Hypoalbuminemia can also occur in Crohn's disease; however, the client's potassium level is of greater importance at this time because a low potassium level can cause cardiac arrest. Anemia is an expected development, but thrombocytopenia is not. Calcium levels are not affected. (A)

33. **1.** Signs and symptoms of dehydration include sunken eyeballs, orthostatic hypotension, increased pulse rate, dry skin, weight loss, thirst, dry oral mucosa, and restlessness. Pitting edema is an indication of fluid excess. (A)

34. **2, 4, 5.** When caring for a client who is receiving TPN, the nurse should plan to weigh the client daily, monitor the I.V. fluid infusion rate hourly (even when using an I.V. fluid pump), and securely tape all I.V. tubing connections to prevent disconnections. Vital signs should be monitored at least every 4 hours to facilitate early detection of complications. It is recommended that the I.V.

dressing be changed once or twice per week or when it becomes soiled, loose, or wet. (D)

35. **2.** A priority goal of care during an acute exacerbation of Crohn's disease is to promote bowel rest. This is accomplished through decreasing activity, encouraging rest, and initially placing client on nothing-by-mouth status while maintaining nutritional needs parenterally. Regular ambulation is important, but the priority is bowel rest. The client will probably lose some weight during the acute phase of the illness. Diarrhea is nonbloody in Crohn's disease, and episodes of rectal bleeding are not expected. (A)

The Client with an Intestinal Obstruction

36. **1, 4, 5.** Signs and symptoms of intestinal obstructions in the small intestine may include projectile vomiting and rapidly developing dehydration and electrolyte imbalances. The client will also have increased bowel sounds, usually high-pitched and tinkling. The client would not normally have diarrhea and would have minimal abdominal distention. Pain is intermittent, being relieved by vomiting. Intestinal obstructions in the large intestine usually evolve slowly, produce persistent pain, and vomiting is less common. Clients with a large-intestine obstruction may develop obstipation and significant abdominal distention. (A)

37. **4.** On percussion, air or gas produces a resonant sound, and fluid produces a flat sound. An intestinal obstruction traps large amounts of fluid in the intestine. Hyperactive peristalsis resulting in the frequent high-pitched tinkling sounds would be apparent on auscultation above the area of obstruction. Masses cause a dull sound when percussed. (A)

38. **1.** Intestinal decompression is accomplished with a Cantor, Harris, or Miller-Abbott tube. These 6- to 10-foot tubes are passed into the small intestine to the obstruction. They remove accumulated fluid and gas, relieving the pressure. A nasogastric tube is used to remove fluid from the stomach. Obstructions are not "broken up" but resolve with decompression or surgical intervention. The length of the nasoenteric tubes prohibits its use as an alternative route for medication administration. (R)

39. **2.** The client is placed in a right side-lying position to facilitate movement of the mercury-weighted tube through the pyloric sphincter. After the tube is in the intestine, the client is turned from side to side or encouraged to ambulate to facilitate tube movement through the intestinal loops. Placing the client in the supine or semi-Fowler's position, or having the client sitting out of bed in a chair will not facilitate tube progression. (R)

40. **2.** A nasoenteric tube has a small balloon at its tip that is weighted with mercury. The weight of the mercury helps advance the tube by gravity through the intestine. Nasoenteric tubes are attached to suction. A nasoenteric tube is not taped in position until it has reached the obstruction. Because the tube has a radiopaque strip, its progress through the intestinal tract can be followed by fluoroscopy. (R)

41. **3.** A client with an intestinal obstruction is particularly susceptible to deficient fluid volume and electrolyte imbalances. NPO status does not impair swallowing. Urine retention is not caused by deficient fluid volume. The client's pain is acute in nature, not chronic. (A)

42. **2.** The client's pain may be indicative of peritonitis, and the nurse should assess for signs and symptoms, such as a rigid abdomen, elevated temperature, and increasing pain. Reassuring the client is important, but accurate assessment of the client is essential. The full assessment should occur before pain relief measures are employed. Repositioning the client to the left side will not resolve the pain. (R)

43. **4.** Considering that there is usually 1 L of insensible fluid loss, this client's output exceeds his intake (intake, 2,000 ml; output, 2,200 ml), indicating deficient fluid volume. The kidneys are concentrating urine in response to low circulating volume, as evidenced by a urine output of less than 30 ml/hour. This indicates that increased fluid replacement is needed. Decreasing urine output can be a sign of decreased renal function, but the data provided suggest that the client is dehydrated. Pain does not affect urine output. There are no data to suggest that the obstruction has worsened. (R)

The Client with an Ileostomy

44. **2.** Unless the pouch leaks, the client can wear her ileostomy pouch for about 4 to 7 days. If leakage occurs, it is important to promptly change the pouch to avoid skin irritation. It is not necessary to change the pouch daily or in the evening. Diet and activity typically do not affect the schedule for changing the pouch. (C)

45. **3.** Providing explanations of preoperative and postoperative procedures helps the client prepare and understand what to expect. It also provides an opportunity for the client to share concerns. Including family members in the teaching sessions is beneficial but does not focus on the client's psychological preparation. Encouraging the client to ask questions about managing the ileostomy may be rushing the client psychologically into accepting the change in body image and function. The client may need time to first handle the stress of surgery and then observe the care of the ileostomy by others before it is appropriate to begin discussing self-management. The nurse should

gently explore whether the client is ready to ask questions about management throughout the hospitalization. The client should have the opportunity to express concerns and to agree to an ostomy association visitor before an invitation is extended. (P)

46. **2.** The rationale for the administration of oral neomycin is to decrease intestinal bacteria and thereby decrease the potential for peritonitis and wound infection postoperatively. Neomycin will not alter the client's potential for developing a urinary or respiratory infection. Neomycin does not affect the body's immune system. (D)

47. **3.** A high-priority outcome after ileostomy surgery is the maintenance of fluid and electrolyte balance. The client will experience continuous liquid to semiliquid stools. The client should be engaged in self-care activities, and minimizing odor formation is important; however, these goals do not take priority over maintaining fluid and electrolyte balance. (A)

48. **3.** If the client agrees, having a visit by a person who has successfully adjusted to living with an ileostomy would be the most helpful measure. This would let the client actually see that typical activities of daily living can be pursued postoperatively. Someone who has felt some of the same concerns can answer the client's questions. A visit from the clergy may be helpful to some clients but would not provide this client with the information sought. Disregarding the client's concerns is not helpful. Although the physician should know about the client's concerns, this in itself will not reassure the client about life after an ileostomy. (P)

49. **3.** Because of high concentrations of digestive enzymes, ileostomy effluent is irritating to skin and can cause excoriation and ulceration. Some form of protection must be used to keep the effluent from contacting the skin. A skin barrier does not decrease odor formation; odor is controlled by diet. The barrier does not affect the accuracy of output records. Pouches are usually worn for 4 to 7 days before being changed. (C)

50. **3.** Any sudden decrease in drainage or onset of severe abdominal pain should be reported to the physician immediately because it could mean that an obstruction has developed. The ileostomy drains liquid stool at frequent intervals throughout the day. Undigested food may be present at times. A temperature of 99.8° F is not necessarily abnormal or a cause for concern. (R)

51. **2.** The fact that the client has an ileostomy does not necessarily mean that she cannot get pregnant and bear children. It may be recommended, however, that the number of pregnancies be limited. Women of childbearing age should be encouraged to discuss their concerns with their physician. Discussing their concerns about sexual functioning and pregnancy will help decrease fears and anxiety. Empathizing or telling the woman that she can adopt does not address her concerns. Her current fears may be based on erroneous understanding. Telling the client that she will adjust to the situation ignores her concerns. (P)

52. 3. To maintain an adequate fluid balance, the client needs to drink at least 3,000 ml/day. Heavy lifting should be avoided; the physician will indicate when the client can participate in sports again. The client will not resume working as soon as 2 weeks after surgery. Water does not harm the stoma, so the client does not have to worry about getting it wet. (A)

53. 4. Sudden onset of abdominal cramps, vomiting, and watery discharge with no stool from an ileostomy are likely indications of an obstruction. It is imperative that the client be examined immediately. If an obstruction is present, ingesting fluids or taking milk of magnesia will increase the severity of symptoms. Oral intake is avoided when a bowel obstruction is suspected. In addition, the client is vomiting and, although he may very well need fluid replacement, he will not be able to tolerate oral fluids. Laxatives are contraindicated in cases of suspected bowel obstruction. (R)

The Client Receiving Total Parenteral Nutrition

54. 3. The nurse should first obtain a culture specimen. The presence of drainage is a potential indication of an infection and the catheter may need to be removed. A culture specimen should be obtained and sent for analysis so that treatment can be promptly initiated. Since removing the catheter will be required in the presence of an infection, the nurse would not clean and redress the area. After the culture report is obtained, the nurse should notify the physician and document all assessments and client care activities in the client's record. (S)

55. 1. When using a sliding-scale insulin schedule, the nurse obtains a glucometer reading of the client's blood glucose level immediately before giving the insulin and bases the dosage on those findings. The fasting blood glucose level obtained earlier in the day is not relevant to an evening sliding-scale insulin dosage. The nurse cannot calculate insulin dosage by assessing the amount of TPN intake or dietary intake. (D)

56. 2. The TPN solution is usually a hypertonic dextrose solution. The greater the concentration of dextrose in solution, the greater the tonicity. Hypertonic dextrose solutions are used to meet the body's calorie demands in a volume of fluid that will not overload the cardiovascular system. An isotonic dextrose solution (e.g., 5% dextrose in water) or a hypotonic dextrose solution will not provide enough calories to meet metabolic needs. Colloids are plasma expanders and blood products and are not used in TPN. (D)

57. 1. The goal of TPN is to meet the client's nutritional needs. TPN is not used to treat metabolic acidosis; ketoacidosis can actually develop as a result of administering TPN. TPN is a hypertonic solution containing carbohydrates, amino acids, electrolytes, trace elements, and vitamins. It is not used to meet the hydration needs of clients. TPN is administered to provide a positive nitrogen balance. (D)

58. 4. During TPN administration, the client should be monitored regularly for hyperglycemia. The client may require small amounts of insulin to improve glucose metabolism. The client should also be observed for signs and symptoms of hypoglycemia, which may occur if the body overproduces insulin in response to a high glucose intake or if too much insulin is administered to help improve glucose metabolism. Tachycardia or hypertension is not indicative of the client's ability to metabolize the solution. An elevated blood urea nitrogen concentration is indicative of renal status and fluid balance. (D)

59. 2. Complications associated with administration of TPN through a central line include infection and air embolism. To prevent these complications, strict aseptic technique is used for all dressing changes, the insertion site is covered with an air-occlusive dressing, and all connections of the system are taped. Ambulation and activities of daily living are encouraged and not limited during the administration of TPN. (D)

60. 3. The most appropriate nursing diagnosis *is Risk for excess fluid volume.* Clients receiving TPN are at high risk for development of fluid overload. To prevent fluid imbalances, the nurse must carefully monitor the rate of the infusion and the client's response to the infusion. The diagnoses of *Impaired swallowing, Impaired gas exchange,* and *Ineffective tissue perfusion* have no application specifically related to administration of TPN. (D)

61. 4. An air embolus can occur if the I.V. tubing becomes disconnected. The tubing connection should be carefully secured to prevent separation of tubing. The client should be instructed to take a deep breath and hold it when the tubing is changed to prevent an air embolus. Phlebitis can occur as a result of irritation from the hypertonic infusion. Pneumothorax and hemorrhage are complications of catheter placement. (R)

62. 4. When TPN fluids are infused too rapidly or too slowly, the physician should be notified. TPN solutions must be carefully and accurately infused. Rate adjustments should not be made without a written order from the physician. Significant alterations in rate (10% increase or decrease) can result in fluctuations of blood glucose levels. Speeding up the solution can result in too much glucose entering the system. (D)

63. **1.** The administration of fat emulsion solution provides additional calories and essential fatty acids to meet the body's energy needs. Fatty acids are lipids, not carbohydrates. Fatty acids do not aid in the metabolism of glucose. Although they are necessary for meeting the complete nutritional needs of the client, fatty acids do not necessarily help a client maintain normal body weight. (D)

64. **4.** An elevated temperature can be an indication of an infection at the insertion site or in the catheter. Vital signs should be taken every 2 to 4 hours after initiation of TPN therapy to detect early signs of complications. Glycosuria is to be expected during the first few days of therapy until the pancreas adjusts by secreting more insulin. A gradual weight gain is to be expected as the client's nutritional status improves. Some clients experience a decreased appetite during TPN therapy. (R)

65. **2.** Too rapid infusion of a TPN solution can lead to circulatory overload. The client should be assessed carefully for indications of excessive fluid volume. A negative nitrogen balance occurs in nutritionally depleted individuals, not when TPN fluids are administered in excess. When TPN is administered too rapidly the client is at risk for receiving an excess of dextrose and electrolytes. Therefore, the client is at risk for hyperglycemia and hyperkalemia. (D)

The Client with Diverticular Disease

66. **1, 2, 4.** Clients with diverticulosis are encouraged to follow a high-fiber diet. Bran, broccoli, and navy beans are foods high in fiber. Tomato juice and cheese are low-residue foods. (R)

67. **3.** Because of the inflammatory nature of diverticulitis, the nurse would anticipate an elevated white blood cell count. The remaining laboratory findings are not associated with diverticulitis. Elevated red blood cell counts occur in clients with polycythemia vera or fluid volume deficit. Decreased platelet counts can occur as a result of aplastic anemias or malignant blood disorders, as an adverse effect of some drugs, and as a result of some heritable conditions. Elevated serum blood urea nitrogen concentration is usually associated with renal conditions. (R)

68. **1.** Barium enemas and colonoscopies are contraindicated in clients with acute diverticulitis because they can lead to perforation of the colon and peritonitis. A barium enema may be ordered after the client has been treated with antibiotic therapy and the inflammation has

subsided. A barium enema is diagnostic in diverticulitis. A barium enema could increase the client's pain; however, that is not a reason for excluding this test. The client may be able to tolerate the procedure but the concern is the potential for perforation of the intestine. (R)

69. **4.** Clients with diverticular disease should refrain from any activities, such as lifting, straining, or coughing, that increase intra-abdominal pressure and may precipitate an attack. Enemas are contraindicated because they increase intestinal pressure. Fluid intake should be increased, rather than decreased, to promote soft, formed stools. A low-fiber diet is used when inflammation is present. (R)

70. **3, 4, 5.** Clients who have diverticulosis should be instructed to maintain a diet high in fiber and, unless contraindicated, should increase their fluid intake to a minimum of 2,000 ml/day. Participating in a regular exercise program is also strongly encouraged. Diverticulosis can be controlled with treatment but cannot be cured. Clients should be instructed to avoid the regular use of cathartic laxatives. Bulk laxatives and stool softeners may be helpful to maintain regularity and decrease straining. (R)

71. **1.** Diverticular disease is treated with a high-fiber diet and bulk laxatives such as psyllium hydrophilic mucilloid (Metamucil). Fiber decreases the intraluminal pressure and makes it easier for stool to pass through the colon. Antidiarrheals such as Lomotil and tranquilizers such as Valium are not used to treat diverticular disease. Antacids such as aluminum hydroxide (Amphojel) are used to decrease gastric acidity and are not useful for treating diverticular disease. (D)

72. **2.** Diverticular rupture causes peritonitis from the release of intestinal contents (chemicals and bacteria) into the peritoneal cavity. The inflammatory response of the peritoneal tissue produces severe abdominal rigidity and pain, diminished intestinal motility, and retention of intestinal contents (air, fluid, and stool). Because of decreased intestinal motility, bowel sounds will be hypoactive or absent and the client will not experience bowel movements or flatulence. (A)

The Client with Appendicitis

73. **4.** The nurse should gently clean the area around the drain by moving in a circular motion away from the drain. Doing so prevents the introduction of microorganisms to the wound and drain site. The incision cannot be left open to air as long as the drain is intact. The nurse should note the amount and character of wound drainage, but the surgeon will determine when the drain should be removed. Surgical wound drains are not irrigated. (S)

74. **3.** A client who is diagnosed with acute appendicitis is placed on NPO status in anticipation of surgery. Enemas are not administered because they can lead to perforation and peritonitis. An NG tube is not usually inserted, unless the client has suffered a perforation. Heat is contraindicated because it may lead to perforation of the appendix. (R)

75. **4.** Complications of acute appendicitis are perforation, peritonitis, and abscess development. Signs of the development of peritonitis include abdominal pain and distention, tachycardia, tachypnea, nausea, vomiting, and fever. Because peritonitis can cause hypovolemic shock, hypotension can develop. Deficient fluid volume would not cause a fever. Intestinal obstruction would cause abdominal distention, diminished or absent bowel sounds, and abdominal pain. Bowel ischemia has signs and symptoms similar to those found with intestinal obstruction. (A)

76. **2.** Noting the client's first bowel movement after surgery is important because this indicates that normal peristalsis has returned. Sitz baths are used after rectal surgery, not appendectomy. Ambulation is started the day of surgery and is not confined to bathroom privileges. The abdomen should be auscultated for bowel sounds and palpated for softness, but there is no need to measure the girth every 2 hours. (A)

77. **2.** Drains are inserted postoperatively in appendectomies when an abscess was present or the appendix was perforated. The purpose is to promote drainage of exudate from the wound and facilitate healing. A drain is not used for irrigation of the wound. The drain will not minimize scar tissue development or decrease postoperative discomfort. (R)

The Client with an Inguinal Hernia

78. **3.** The symptoms are indicative of a strangulated hernia. In a strangulated hernia, the hernia cannot be reduced back into the abdominal cavity. The intestinal lumen and the blood supply to the intestine are obstructed, causing an acute intestinal obstruction. Without immediate intervention, necrosis and gangrene may develop. Surgery is required to release the strangulation. Although many of these signs and symptoms are present with peritonitis or perforated bowel, abdominal rigidity, a cardinal sign of peritonitis and perforated bowel, is not mentioned. Therefore, the nurse would not immediately suspect these conditions. An incarcerated hernia refers to a hernia that is irreducible but has not necessarily resulted in an obstruction. (A)

79. **2.** After inguinal herniorrhaphy, an ice bag to the scrotum will help decrease pain and edema. The client is encouraged to turn and deep-breathe, but coughing is not encouraged, to decrease straining on the surgical area. A truss is not needed for support after surgery. While resting, the client may be most comfortable in a semi-Fowler's position, but there is no need to maintain a high Fowler's position. (A)

80. **4.** The most common complication after an inguinal hernia repair is the inability to void, especially in men. The nurse should evaluate the client carefully for urine retention. Hypostatic pneumonia, deep vein thrombosis, and paralytic ileus are potential postoperative problems with any surgical client but are not as likely to occur after an inguinal hernia repair as is urine retention. (R)

The Client with Biliary Tract Disorders

- **The Client with Cholecystitis**
- **The Client with Pancreatitis**
- **The Client with Viral Hepatitis**
- **The Client with Cirrhosis**
- **Correct Answers and Rationales**

The Client with Cholecystitis

1. A client has undergone a laparoscopic cholecystectomy. Which of the following instructions should the nurse include in the discharge teaching?
- ☐ **1.** Empty the bile bag daily.
- ☐ **2.** If you become nauseated, breathe deeply into a paper bag.
- ☐ **3.** Keep all adhesive dressings on for at least 6 weeks.
- ☐ **4.** Report bile-colored drainage from any incision.

2. A 40-year-old client is admitted to the hospital with a diagnosis of abdominal pain. Following numerous diagnostic tests, it is concluded that the client has acute cholecystitis. The nurse should contact the physician to question which of the following orders?
- ☐ **1.** I.V. fluid therapy of normal saline solution to be infused at 100 ml/hour until further orders.
- ☐ **2.** Administer morphine sulfate 10 mg I.M. every 4 hours as needed for severe abdominal pain.
- ☐ **3.** Nothing by mouth (NPO) until further orders.
- ☐ **4.** Insert a nasogastric tube and connect to low intermittent suction.

3. A client is admitted to the hospital with a diagnosis of cholecystitis from cholelithiasis. The client is complaining of severe abdominal pain and extreme nausea and has vomited several times. Based on these data, which nursing diagnosis would have the *highest* priority for intervention at this time?
- ☐ **1.** *Anxiety* related to severe abdominal discomfort.
- ☐ **2.** *Deficient fluid volume* related to vomiting.
- ☐ **3.** *Pain* related to gallbladder inflammation.
- ☐ **4.** *Imbalanced nutrition: Less than body requirements* related to vomiting.

4. If a gallstone becomes lodged in the common bile duct, the nurse should anticipate that the client's stools would most likely become what color?
- ☐ **1.** Green.
- ☐ **2.** Gray.
- ☐ **3.** Black.
- ☐ **4.** Brown.

5. When the client's common bile duct is obstructed, the nurse should evaluate the client for signs and symptoms of which of the following complications?
- ☐ **1.** Respiratory distress.
- ☐ **2.** Circulatory overload.
- ☐ **3.** Urinary tract infection.
- ☐ **4.** Prolonged bleeding time.

6. A client who has been scheduled to have a choledocholithotomy expresses anxiety about having surgery. Which nursing intervention would be the most appropriate to achieve the outcome of anxiety reduction?
- ☐ **1.** Providing the client with information about what to expect postoperatively.
- ☐ **2.** Telling the client it is normal to be afraid.
- ☐ **3.** Reassuring the client by telling her that surgery is a common procedure.
- ☐ **4.** Stressing the importance of following the physician's instructions after surgery.

7. A client undergoes a traditional cholecystectomy and choledochotomy and returns from surgery with a T-tube. To evaluate the effectiveness of the T-tube, the nurse should understand that the primary reason for the T-tube is to accomplish which of the following?
- ☐ **1.** Promote wound drainage.
- ☐ **2.** Provide a way to irrigate the biliary tract.
- ☐ **3.** Minimize the passage of bile into the duodenum.
- ☐ **4.** Prevent bile from entering the peritoneal cavity.

8. How much bile should the nurse expect the T-tube to drain during the first 24 hours after a choledocholithotomy?

☐ **1.** 50 to 100 ml.
☐ **2.** 150 to 250 ml.
☐ **3.** 300 to 500 ml.
☐ **4.** 550 to 700 ml.

9. The nurse measures the amount of bile drainage from a T-tube and records it by which one of the following methods?

☐ **1.** Adding it to the client's urine output.
☐ **2.** Charting it separately on the output record.
☐ **3.** Adding it to the amount of wound drainage.
☐ **4.** Subtracting it from the total intake for each day.

10. After a cholecystectomy, it is recommended that the client follow a low-fat diet at home. Which of the following foods would be most appropriate to include in a low-fat diet?

☐ **1.** Cheese omelet.
☐ **2.** Peanut butter.
☐ **3.** Ham salad sandwich.
☐ **4.** Roast beef.

11. A client with cholecystitis is complaining of severe right upper quadrant pain. Which of the following medications should the nurse anticipate administering to relieve the client's pain?

☐ **1.** Meperidine (Demerol).
☐ **2.** Acetaminophen (Tylenol) with codeine.
☐ **3.** Promethazine (Phenergan).
☐ **4.** Morphine sulfate.

12. The nurse prepares to administer promethazine (Phenergan) 35 mg I.M. as ordered p.r.n. for a client with cholecystitis complaining of nausea. The ampule label reads that the medication is available in 25 mg/ml. How many milliliters should the nurse administer?

_____ ml

13. A client undergoes a laparoscopic cholecystectomy. Which of the following dietary instructions should the nurse give the client immediately after surgery?

☐ **1.** "You cannot eat or drink anything for 24 hours."
☐ **2.** "You may resume your normal diet the day after your surgery."
☐ **3.** "Drink liquids today and eat lightly for a few days."
☐ **4.** "You can progress from a liquid to a bland diet as tolerated."

14. Which of the following discharge instructions would be appropriate for a client who has had a laparoscopic cholecystectomy?

☐ **1.** Avoid showering for 48 hours after surgery.
☐ **2.** Return to work within 1 week.
☐ **3.** Leave dressings in place until you see the surgeon at the postoperative visit.
☐ **4.** Use acetaminophen (Tylenol) to control any fever.

15. After a client who has had a laparoscopic cholecystectomy receives discharge instructions, which of the following client statements would indicate that the teaching has been successful? Select all that apply.

☐ **1.** "I can resume my normal diet when I want."
☐ **2.** "I need to avoid driving for about 4 weeks."
☐ **3.** "I may experience some pain in my right shoulder."
☐ **4.** "I should spend 2 to 3 days in bed before resuming activity."
☐ **5.** "I can wash the puncture site with mild soap and water."

The Client with Pancreatitis

16. The nurse has reported to the hospital to work the day shift on a medical-surgical unit. The nurse's assignment consists of the following four clients. From highest to lowest priority, in which order should the nurse assess the clients after receiving morning report?

1. The client with cirrhosis who became confused and disoriented during the night.

2. The client who is 1 day postoperative following a cholecystectomy and has a T-tube inserted.

3. The client with acute pancreatitis who is requesting pain medication.

4. The client with hepatitis B who has questions about his discharge instructions.

17. The initial diagnosis of pancreatitis is confirmed if the client's blood work shows a significant elevation in which of the following serum values?
- [ ] **1.** Amylase.
- [ ] **2.** Glucose.
- [ ] **3.** Potassium.
- [ ] **4.** Trypsin.

18. The client who has been hospitalized with pancreatitis does not drink alcohol because of her religious convictions. She becomes upset when the physician persists in asking her about alcohol intake. The nurse should explain that the reason for these questions is that:
- [ ] **1.** There is a strong link between alcohol use and acute pancreatitis.
- [ ] **2.** Alcohol intake can interfere with the tests used to diagnose pancreatitis.
- [ ] **3.** Alcoholism is a major health problem, and all clients are questioned about alcohol intake.
- [ ] **4.** The physician must obtain the pertinent facts, regardless of religious beliefs.

19. The nurse monitors the client with pancreatitis for early signs of shock. Which of the following conditions is primarily responsible for making it difficult to manage shock in pancreatitis?
- [ ] **1.** Severity of intestinal hemorrhage.
- [ ] **2.** Vasodilating effects of kinin peptides.
- [ ] **3.** Tendency toward heart failure.
- [ ] **4.** Frequent incidence of acute tubular necrosis.

20. Which of the following signs and symptoms should the nurse expect to see in a client with acute pancreatitis?
- [ ] **1.** Diarrhea.
- [ ] **2.** Jaundice.
- [ ] **3.** Hypertension.
- [ ] **4.** Ascites.

21. The nurse evaluates the client's most recent laboratory data. Which laboratory finding would be consistent with a diagnosis of acute pancreatitis?
- [ ] **1.** Hyperglycemia.
- [ ] **2.** Leukopenia.
- [ ] **3.** Thrombocytopenia.
- [ ] **4.** Hyperkalemia.

22. The initial treatment plan for a client with pancreatitis most likely would focus on which of the following as a priority?
- [ ] **1.** Resting the gastrointestinal tract.
- [ ] **2.** Ensuring adequate nutrition.
- [ ] **3.** Maintaining fluid and electrolyte balance.
- [ ] **4.** Preventing the development of an infection.

23. When providing care for a client with acute pancreatitis, the nurse should anticipate which of the following orders?
- [ ] **1.** Increase oral intake to 3,000 ml every 24 hours.
- [ ] **2.** Insert a nasogastric tube and connect it to low suction.
- [ ] **3.** Place the client in the reverse Trendelenburg position.
- [ ] **4.** Place the client on enteric precautions.

24. The nurse carefully monitors the client with acute pancreatitis for which of the following complications?
- [ ] **1.** Heart failure.
- [ ] **2.** Duodenal ulcer.
- [ ] **3.** Cirrhosis.
- [ ] **4.** Pneumonia.

25. When providing care for a client hospitalized with acute pancreatitis who is complaining of acute abdominal pain, which of the following nursing interventions would be most appropriate for this client? Select all that apply.
- [ ] **1.** Placing the client in a side-lying position.
- [ ] **2.** Administering morphine sulfate for pain as needed.
- [ ] **3.** Maintaining the client on a high-calorie, high-protein diet.
- [ ] **4.** Monitoring the client's respiratory status.
- [ ] **5.** Obtaining daily weights.

26. The nurse notes that a client with acute pancreatitis occasionally experiences muscle twitching and jerking. How should the nurse interpret the significance of these symptoms?
- [ ] **1.** The client may be developing hypocalcemia.
- [ ] **2.** The client is experiencing a reaction to meperidine (Demerol).
- [ ] **3.** The client has a nutritional imbalance.
- [ ] **4.** The client needs a muscle relaxant to help him rest.

27. Which of the following medications would most likely be given to the client with acute pancreatitis to augment pain control?
- [ ] **1.** Ibuprofen (Motrin).
- [ ] **2.** Magnesium hydroxide (Maalox).
- [ ] **3.** Propantheline bromide (Pro-Banthine).
- [ ] **4.** Propranolol (Inderal).

28. Which of the following would most likely be a major nursing diagnosis for a client with acute pancreatitis?
- [ ] **1.** *Ineffective airway clearance.*
- [ ] **2.** *Excess fluid volume.*
- [ ] **3.** *Impaired swallowing.*
- [ ] **4.** *Imbalanced nutrition: Less than body requirements.*

29. Which of the following dietary instructions would be appropriate for the nurse to give a client who is recovering from acute pancreatitis?
☐ **1.** Avoid crash dieting.
☐ **2.** Restrict carbohydrate intake.
☐ **3.** Eat six small meals a day.
☐ **4.** Decrease sodium in the diet.

30. Pancreatic enzyme replacements are ordered for the client with chronic pancreatitis. When should the nurse instruct the client to take them to obtain the most therapeutic effect?
☐ **1.** Three times daily between meals.
☐ **2.** With each meal and snack.
☐ **3.** In the morning and at bedtime.
☐ **4.** Every 4 hours, at specified times.

31. The nurse should teach the client with chronic pancreatitis to monitor the effectiveness of pancreatic enzyme replacement therapy by doing which of the following?
☐ **1.** Monitoring fluid intake.
☐ **2.** Performing regular glucose fingerstick tests.
☐ **3.** Observing stools for steatorrhea.
☐ **4.** Testing urine for ketones.

32. The client with chronic pancreatitis should be monitored closely for the development of which of the following disorders?
☐ **1.** Cholelithiasis.
☐ **2.** Hepatitis.
☐ **3.** Irritable bowel syndrome.
☐ **4.** Diabetes mellitus.

The Client with Viral Hepatitis

33. The nurse is planning a community education program on how to prevent the transmission of viral hepatitis. Which of the following types of hepatitis is considered to be primarily a sexually transmitted disease?
☐ **1.** Hepatitis A.
☐ **2.** Hepatitis B.
☐ **3.** Hepatitis C.
☐ **4.** Hepatitis D.

34. The nurse should expect the client to exhibit which of the following signs and symptoms during the icteric phase of viral hepatitis?
☐ **1.** Tarry stools.
☐ **2.** Yellowed sclera.
☐ **3.** Shortness of breath.
☐ **4.** Light, frothy urine.

35. The nurse plans care for the client with hepatitis A with the understanding that the causative virus will be excreted from the client's body primarily through the:
☐ **1.** Skin.
☐ **2.** Feces.
☐ **3.** Urine.
☐ **4.** Blood.

36. The nurse is planning a staff development program on how to care for clients with hepatitis A. Which of the following precautions should the nurse indicate as essential when caring for clients with hepatitis A?
☐ **1.** Gowning when entering a client's room.
☐ **2.** Wearing a mask when providing care.
☐ **3.** Assigning the client to a private room.
☐ **4.** Wearing gloves when giving direct care.

37. A client who is recovering from hepatitis A continues to complain of fatigue and malaise. The client asks the nurse, "When will my strength return?" Which of the following responses by the nurse is most appropriate?
☐ **1.** "Your fatigue should be gone by now. We will evaluate you for a secondary infection."
☐ **2.** "Your fatigue is an adverse effect of your drug therapy. It will disappear when your treatment regimen is complete."
☐ **3.** "It is important for you to increase your activity level. That will help decrease your fatigue."
☐ **4.** "It is normal for you to feel fatigued. The fatigue should go away in the next 2 to 4 months."

38. When developing a plan of care for the client with viral hepatitis, the nurse should incorporate nursing orders that reflect the primary treatment. Emphasis will be on ensuring that the client receives which of the following?
☐ **1.** Adequate bed rest.
☐ **2.** Generous fluid intake.
☐ **3.** Regular antibiotic therapy.
☐ **4.** Daily intravenous electrolyte therapy.

39. Which of the following test results should the nurse use to assess the liver function of a client with viral hepatitis?
☐ **1.** Glucose tolerance.
☐ **2.** Creatinine clearance.
☐ **3.** Serum transaminase.
☐ **4.** Serum electrolytes.

40. In a client with viral hepatitis, the nurse should closely assess for indications of which of the following abnormal laboratory values?
☐ **1.** Prolonged prothrombin time.
☐ **2.** Decreased blood glucose level.
☐ **3.** Elevated serum potassium level.
☐ **4.** Decreased serum calcium level.

41. Which of the following diets would most likely be prescribed for a client with viral hepatitis?
☐ **1.** High-fat, low-protein.
☐ **2.** High-protein, low-carbohydrate.
☐ **3.** High-carbohydrate, high-calorie.
☐ **4.** Low-sodium, low-fat.

42. The nurse develops a teaching plan for the client about how to prevent the transmission of hepatitis A. Which of the following discharge instructions is appropriate for the client?
☐ **1.** Spray the house to eliminate infected insects.
☐ **2.** Tell family members to try to stay away from the client.
☐ **3.** Tell family members to wash their hands frequently.
☐ **4.** Disinfect all clothing and eating utensils.

43. The nurse assesses that the client with hepatitis is experiencing fatigue, weakness, and a general feeling of malaise. The client tires rapidly during morning care. Based on this information, which of the following would be an appropriate nursing diagnosis?
☐ **1.** *Impaired physical mobility* related to malaise.
☐ **2.** *Self-care deficit* related to fatigue.
☐ **3.** *Ineffective coping* related to long-term illness.
☐ **4.** *Activity intolerance* related to fatigue.

44. A client has been admitted to the hospital with a diagnosis of hepatitis B. The client tells the nurse, "I feel so isolated from my friends and family. Nobody wants to be around me." What would be the most appropriate nursing diagnosis for this client?
☐ **1.** *Anxiety* related to feelings of isolation.
☐ **2.** *Social isolation* related to significant others' fear of contracting disease.
☐ **3.** *Powerlessness* related to lack of social support.
☐ **4.** *Low self-esteem* related to feelings of rejection.

45. What would be the nurse's *best* response to the client's expressed feelings of isolation as a result of having hepatitis?
☐ **1.** "Don't worry. It's normal to feel that way."
☐ **2.** "Your friends are probably afraid of contracting hepatitis from you."
☐ **3.** "I'm sure you're imagining that!"
☐ **4.** "Tell me more about your feelings of isolation."

46. Which of the following measures would prevent transmission of the hepatitis C virus to health care personnel?
☐ **1.** Administering hepatitis C vaccine to all health care personnel.
☐ **2.** Decreasing contact with blood and blood-contaminated fluids.
☐ **3.** Wearing gloves when emptying the bedpan.
☐ **4.** Wearing a gown and mask when providing direct care.

47. Interferon alfa-2b (Intron A) has been prescribed to treat a client with chronic hepatitis B. What adverse effect is most commonly associated with the administration of interferon alfa-2b?
☐ **1.** Retinopathy.
☐ **2.** Constipation.
☐ **3.** Flulike symptoms.
☐ **4.** Hypoglycemia.

48. The nurse is preparing a community education program about preventing hepatitis B infection. Which of the following would be appropriate to incorporate into the teaching plan?
☐ **1.** Hepatitis B is relatively uncommon among college students.
☐ **2.** Frequent ingestion of alcohol can predispose an individual to development of hepatitis B.
☐ **3.** Good personal hygiene habits are most effective at preventing the spread of hepatitis B.
☐ **4.** The use of a condom is advised for sexual intercourse.

49. Which of the following expected outcomes would be appropriate for a client with viral hepatitis? The client will:
☐ **1.** Demonstrate a decrease in fluid retention related to ascites.
☐ **2.** Verbalize the importance of reporting bleeding gums or bloody stools.
☐ **3.** Limit use of alcohol to two to three drinks per week.
☐ **4.** Restrict activity to within the home to prevent disease transmission.

The Client with Cirrhosis

50. A client has advanced cirrhosis of the liver. The client's spouse asks the nurse why his abdomen is swollen, making it very difficult for him to fasten his pants. How should the nurse respond to provide the most accurate explanation of the disease process?

☐ 1. "He must have been eating too many foods with salt in them. Salt pulls water with it."

☐ 2. "The swelling in his ankles must have moved up closer to his heart so the fluid circulates better."

☐ 3. "He must have forgotten to take his daily water pill."

☐ 4. "Blood is not able to flow readily through the liver now, and the liver cannot make protein to keep fluid inside the blood vessels."

51. A nurse is caring for a client with hepatic encephalopathy. How should the nurse direct care for this client? Select all that apply.

☐ 1. Preventing constipation.

☐ 2. Administering lactulose (Cephulac).

☐ 3. Monitoring coordination while walking.

☐ 4. Checking the pupil reaction.

☐ 5. Providing food and fluids high in carbohydrate.

☐ 6. Encouraging physical activity.

52. The nurse is assessing a client who is in the early stages of cirrhosis of the liver. Which sign should the nurse anticipate finding?

☐ 1. Peripheral edema.

☐ 2. Ascites.

☐ 3. Anorexia.

☐ 4. Jaundice.

53. A client with cirrhosis begins to develop ascites. Spironolactone (Aldactone) is prescribed to treat the ascites. The nurse should monitor the client closely for which of the following drug-related adverse effects?

☐ 1. Constipation.

☐ 2. Hyperkalemia.

☐ 3. Irregular pulse.

☐ 4. Dysuria.

54. What diet should be implemented for a client who is in the early stages of cirrhosis?

☐ 1. High-calorie, high-carbohydrate.

☐ 2. High-protein, low-fat.

☐ 3. Low-fat, low-protein.

☐ 4. High-carbohydrate, low-sodium.

55. A client with cirrhosis complains that his skin always feels itchy and that he "scratches himself raw" while he sleeps. The nurse should recognize that the itching is the result of which abnormality associated with cirrhosis?

☐ 1. Folic acid deficiency.

☐ 2. Prolonged prothrombin time.

☐ 3. Increased bilirubin levels.

☐ 4. Hypokalemia.

56. Which of the following health promotion activities would be appropriate for the nurse to suggest that the client with cirrhosis add to the daily routine at home?

☐ 1. Supplement the diet with daily multivitamins.

☐ 2. Limit daily alcohol intake.

☐ 3. Take a sleeping pill at bedtime.

☐ 4. Limit contact with other people whenever possible.

57. The client with cirrhosis has developed ascites. The nurse should recognize that the pathologic basis for the development of ascites in clients with cirrhosis is portal hypertension and:

☐ 1. An excess serum sodium level.

☐ 2. An increased metabolism of aldosterone.

☐ 3. A decreased flow of hepatic lymph.

☐ 4. A decreased serum albumin level.

58. Which of the following positions would be appropriate for a client with severe ascites?

☐ 1. Fowler's.

☐ 2. Side-lying.

☐ 3. Reverse Trendelenburg.

☐ 4. Sims.

59. The client with cirrhosis receives 100 ml of 25% serum albumin I.V. Which finding would best indicate that the albumin is having its desired effect?

☐ 1. Increased urine output.

☐ 2. Increased serum albumin level.

☐ 3. Decreased anorexia.

☐ 4. Increased ease of breathing.

60. A client with cirrhosis vomits bright red blood and the physician suspects bleeding esophageal varices. The physician decides to insert a Sengstaken-Blakemore tube. The nurse should explain to the client that the tube acts by:

☐ 1. Providing a large diameter for effective gastric lavage.

☐ 2. Applying direct pressure to gastric bleeding sites.

☐ 3. Blocking blood flow to the stomach and esophagus.

☐ 4. Applying direct pressure to the esophagus.

61. About 30 minutes after a Sengstaken-Blakemore tube is inserted, the nurse observes that the client appears to be having difficulty breathing. The nurse's first action should be to:
- ☐ **1.** Remove the tube.
- ☐ **2.** Deflate the esophageal portion of the tube.
- ☐ **3.** Determine whether the tube is obstructing the airway.
- ☐ **4.** Increase the oxygen flow rate.

62. The physician orders oral neomycin (Mycifradin) as well as a neomycin enema for a client with cirrhosis. The nurse understands that the purpose of this therapy is to:
- ☐ **1.** Reduce abdominal pressure.
- ☐ **2.** Prevent straining during defecation.
- ☐ **3.** Block ammonia formation.
- ☐ **4.** Reduce bleeding within the intestine.

63. The nurse monitors a client with cirrhosis for the development of hepatic encephalopathy. Which of the following would be an indication that hepatic encephalopathy is developing?
- ☐ **1.** Decreased mental status.
- ☐ **2.** Elevated blood pressure.
- ☐ **3.** Decreased urine output.
- ☐ **4.** Labored respirations.

64. A client's serum ammonia level is elevated, and the physician orders 30 ml of lactulose (Cephulac). Which of the following adverse effects of this drug should the nurse expect to see?
- ☐ **1.** Increased urine output.
- ☐ **2.** Improved level of consciousness.
- ☐ **3.** Increased bowel movements.
- ☐ **4.** Nausea and vomiting.

65. The nurse has an order to administer 2 oz of lactulose (Cephulac) to a client who has cirrhosis. How many milliliters of lactulose should the nurse administer?

_____ ml

66. A client is to be discharged with a prescription for lactulose (Cephulac). The nurse teaches the client and the client's spouse how to administer this medication. Which of the following statements would indicate that the client has understood the information?
- ☐ **1.** "I'll take it with Maalox."
- ☐ **2.** "I'll mix it with apple juice."
- ☐ **3.** "I'll take it with a laxative."
- ☐ **4.** "I'll mix the crushed tablets in some gelatin."

67. The nurse is providing discharge instructions for a client with cirrhosis. Which of the following statements best indicates that the client has understood the teaching?
- ☐ **1.** "I should eat a high-protein, high-carbohydrate diet to provide energy."
- ☐ **2.** "It is safer for me to take acetaminophen (Tylenol) for pain instead of aspirin."
- ☐ **3.** "I should avoid constipation to decrease chances of bleeding."
- ☐ **4.** "If I get enough rest and follow my diet, it is possible for my cirrhosis to be cured."

68. The nurse is preparing a client for a paracentesis. Which of the following activities would be appropriate before the procedure?
- ☐ **1.** Have the client void immediately before the procedure.
- ☐ **2.** Place the client in a side-lying position.
- ☐ **3.** Initiate an I.V. line to administer sedatives.
- ☐ **4.** Place the client on nothing-by-mouth (NPO) status 6 hours before the procedure.

69. Which of the following interventions should the nurse anticipate incorporating into the client's plan of care when hepatic encephalopathy initially develops?
- ☐ **1.** Inserting a nasogastric (NG) tube.
- ☐ **2.** Restricting fluids to 1,000 ml/day.
- ☐ **3.** Administering I.V. salt-poor albumin.
- ☐ **4.** Implementing a low-protein diet.

70. A client with ascites and peripheral edema is at risk for impaired skin integrity. Which of the following interventions should be implemented to prevent skin breakdown?
- ☐ **1.** Range-of-motion (ROM) exercise every 4 hours.
- ☐ **2.** Massage of the abdomen once a shift.
- ☐ **3.** Use of alternating air pressure mattress.
- ☐ **4.** Elevation of the lower extremities.

Correct Answers and Rationales

The letter in parentheses after each rationale identifies the client need addressed in the item, including management of care (M), safety and infection control (S), health promotion and maintenance (H), psychosocial adaptation (P), basic care and comfort (C), pharmacological and parenteral therapies (D), reduction of risk potential (R), and physiological adaptation (A).

The Client with Cholecystitis

1. 4. There should be no bile-colored drainage coming from any of the incisions postoperatively. A laparoscopic cholecystectomy does not involve a bile bag. Breathing deeply into a paper bag will prevent a person from passing out due to hyperventilation; it does not alleviate nausea. If the adhesive dressings have not already fallen off, they are removed by the surgeon in 7 to 10 days, not 6 weeks. (M)

2. 2. A nurse should question the order for morphine sulfate because it is believed to cause biliary spasm. Thus, the preferred opioid analgesic to treat cholecystitis is meperidine (Demerol). Elderly clients should not be given meperidine because of the risk of acute confusion and seizures in this population. An alternative pain medication will be necessary. I.V. fluid therapy is used to maintain fluid and electrolyte balance that may result from NPO status and gastric suctioning. NPO status and gastric decompression prevent further gallbladder stimulation. (S)

3. 3. The priority for nursing care at this time is to decrease the client's severe abdominal pain. The pain, which is frequently accompanied by nausea and vomiting, is caused by biliary spasm. Opioid analgesics are given to relieve the severe pain and spasm of cholecystitis. Relief of pain may decrease nausea and vomiting and thereby decrease the client's likelihood of developing further complications, such as deficient fluid volume and imbalanced nutrition. There are no data to suggest that the client is anxious. (A)

4. 2. When bile is not reaching the intestine, the feces do not contain bile pigments. The stool then becomes gray, claylike, or putty-like in color. Dark green color in the stool is the result of bile pigment. Black stool can be caused by upper gastrointestinal bleeding and by certain medications, such as iron supplements. Brown stool is normal. (A)

5. 4. A client with an obstructed common bile duct should be monitored for prolonged bleeding time. Such an obstruction prevents bile from entering the intestinal tract, thus decreasing the absorption of fat-soluble vitamins A, D, E, and K. Vitamin K is necessary for prothrombin formation. Prothrombin deficiency causes delayed blood clotting, which results in prolonged bleeding time. An obstructed bile duct does not cause respiratory distress, circulatory overload, or urinary tract infection. (A)

6. 1. Providing information can help to answer the client's questions and decrease anxiety. Fear of the unknown can increase anxiety. Telling the client not to be afraid, that the procedure is common, or to follow her physician's orders will not necessarily decrease anxiety. (P)

7. 4. A T-tube is used after exploration of the common bile duct to help prevent bile from spilling into the peritoneal cavity. The tube also helps maintain patency of the common bile duct and helps ensure bile drainage out of the body, until the edema in the common bile duct subsides. After this occurs, bile can drain into the duodenum. (R)

8. 3. The T-tube usually drains 300 to 500 ml in the first 24 hours after a choledocholithotomy. After 3 to 4 days, as the edema subsides in the common bile duct, the amount decreases to less than 200 ml per 24 hours. (R)

9. 2. T-tube bile drainage is recorded separately on the output record. Adding the T-tube drainage to the urine output or wound drainage makes it difficult to accurately determine the amounts of bile, urine, or drainage. The client's total intake will be incorrect if drainage is subtracted from it. (R)

10. 4. Lean meats, such as beef, lamb, veal, and well-trimmed lean ham and pork, are low in fat. Rice, pasta, and vegetables are low in fat when not served with butter, cream, or sauces. Fruits are low in fat. The amount of fat allowed in a client's diet after a cholecystectomy will depend on the client's ability to tolerate fat. Typically, the client does not require a special diet but is encouraged to avoid excessive fat intake. A cheese omelet and peanut butter have high fat content. Ham salad is high in fat from the fat in salad dressing. (C)

11. 1. Meperidine (Demerol) would be the opioid analgesic of choice for a client with cholecystitis. Acetaminophen (Tylenol) with codeine would not be appropriate to administer because the codeine could cause biliary duct spasm and increase pain, as could opiates such as morphine sulfate. Promethazine (Phenergan) is an antiemetic. (D)

12. 1.4

The following formula is used to calculate the correct dosage:

$$35 \text{ mg}/X \text{ ml} = 25 \text{ mg}/1 \text{ ml}$$

$$X = 1.4.$$

(D)

13. **3.** Immediately after surgery, the client will drink liquids. A light diet can be resumed the day after surgery. There is no need for the client to remain on nothing-by-mouth status after surgery because peristaltic bowel activity should not be affected. The client will probably not be able to tolerate a full meal comfortably the day after surgery. There is no need for the client to stay on a bland diet after a laparoscopic cholecystectomy. The client should, however, avoid excessive fats. (A)

14. **3.** After a laparoscopic cholecystectomy, the client should not remove dressings from the puncture sites but should wait until visiting the surgeon. The client may shower the day after surgery. A client can return to work within 1 week, but only if approved by the surgeon and no strenuous activity is involved. The client should report any fever, which could be an indication of a complication. (R)

15. **1, 3, 5.** Following a laparoscopic cholecystectomy, the client can resume a normal diet as tolerated. The client may experience right shoulder pain from the gas that was used to inflate the abdomen during surgery. The puncture site should be cleansed daily with mild soap and water. Driving can usually be resumed in 3 to 4 days following surgery and there is no need for the client to maintain bed rest in the days following surgery. Light exercise such as walking can be resumed immediately. (A)

The Client with Pancreatitis

16.

> **1.** The client with cirrhosis who became confused and disoriented during the night.

> **3.** The client with acute pancreatitis who is requesting pain medication.

> **2.** The client who is 1 day postoperative following a cholecystectomy and has a T-tube inserted.

> **4.** The client with hepatitis B who has questions about his discharge instructions.

The nurse should first assess the client with cirrhosis to ensure the client's safety and to assess the client for the onset of hepatic encephalopathy. The nurse should then assess the client with acute pancreatitis who is requesting pain medication and administer the needed medication. The nurse should next assess the client who underwent a cholecystectomy and is 1 day postoperative to make sure that the T-tube is draining and that the client is performing postoperative breathing exercises. This client's safety is not at risk and the client is not indicating that he is in pain, so his care is a lower priority. The nurse can speak last with the client with hepatitis B who has questions about his discharge instructions because this client's issues are not urgent. (M)

17. **1.** The primary diagnostic tests for pancreatitis are serum amylase, serum lipase, and urine amylase. All three laboratory results are typically elevated. Serum amylase is the most common test; the result is usually higher than 200 units/dl. Serum glucose level may be elevated in pancreatitis because of beta-cell damage, but this is not used to diagnose pancreatitis. Serum potassium and trypsin levels are not affected in pancreatitis. (R)

18. **1.** Alcoholism is a major cause of acute pancreatitis in the United States. Because some clients are reluctant to discuss alcohol use, staff may inquire about it in several ways. Generally, alcohol intake does not interfere with the tests used to diagnose pancreatitis. Recent ingestion of large amounts of alcohol, however, may cause an increased serum amylase level. Large amounts of ethyl and methyl alcohol may produce an elevated urinary amylase concentration. All clients are asked about alcohol and drug use on hospital admission, but this information is especially pertinent for clients with pancreatitis. Physicians do need to seek facts, but this can be done while respecting the client's religious beliefs. Respecting religious beliefs is important in providing holistic client care. (H)

19. **2.** Life-threatening shock is a potential complication of pancreatitis. Kinin peptides activated by the trapped trypsin cause vasodilation and increased capillary permeability. These effects exacerbate shock and are not easily reversed with pharmacologic agents such as vasopressors. Hemorrhage may occur into the pancreas, but not in the intestines. Systemic complications include pulmonary complications, but not heart failure or acute tubular necrosis. (A)

20. **2.** Jaundice may be present in acute pancreatitis owing to obstruction of the biliary tract. Bowel sounds may be decreased or absent, so diarrhea would not be expected. Hypotension is likely to develop because of pancreatic hemorrhage or toxemia. Ascites develops as a result of portal hypertension and is common in liver disease, but not in pancreatitis. (A)

21. **1.** Pancreatitis interferes with beta-cell functioning, and clients must be monitored carefully for hyperglycemia. The client may also develop hypocalcemia and hyperlipidemia. Pancreatitis does not decrease blood cell counts or affect platelet production or potassium levels. (A)

22. **1.** There is little definitive treatment for pancreatitis. It is crucial to decrease pancreatic enzymes to reduce stimulation of the pancreas. This is done by keeping the client on nothing-by-mouth status to rest the gastrointestinal tract and thereby suppress pancreatic enzyme secretion. Ensuring adequate nutrition, maintaining fluid and electrolyte balance, and preventing the development of an infection are issues for the client with pancreatitis but are not the primary focus of treatment. (A)

23. **2.** Nasogastric suction is frequently used in the treatment of pancreatitis to decrease pancreatic secretions and gastric distention. Foods and fluids are withheld during the acute phase of pancreatitis to rest the pancreas. Intravenous fluids are administered to provide hydration. Placing the client in the reverse Trendelenburg position is not appropriate. Most clients will be more comfortable if they are placed in a side-lying position with the head of the bed elevated to relieve abdominal tension. There is no need to place the client on enteric precautions. (R)

24. **4.** The client with acute pancreatitis is prone to complications associated with the respiratory system. Pneumonia, atelectasis, and pleural effusion are examples of respiratory complications that can develop as a result of pancreatic enzyme exudate. Pancreatitis does not cause heart failure, ulcer formation, or cirrhosis. (R)

25. **1, 4, 5.** The client with acute pancreatitis usually experiences acute abdominal pain. Placing the client in a side-lying position relieves the tension on the abdominal area and promotes comfort. A semi-Fowler's position is also appropriate. The nurse should also monitor the client's respiratory status because clients with pancreatitis are prone to develop respiratory complications. Daily weights are obtained to monitor the client's nutritional and fluid volume status. While the client will likely need opioid analgesics to treat the pain, morphine sulfate is not appropriate as it stimulates spasm of the sphincter of Oddi, thus increasing the client's discomfort. During the acute phase of the illness while the client is experiencing pain, the pancreas is rested by withholding food and drink. When the diet is reintroduced, it is a high-carbohydrate, low-fat, bland diet. (A)

26. **1.** Hypocalcemia develops in severe cases of acute pancreatitis. The exact cause is unknown. Signs and symptoms of hypocalcemia include jerking and muscle twitching, numbness of fingers and lips, and irritability. Meperidine (Demerol) may cause tremors or seizures as an adverse effect, but not muscle twitching. Muscle twitching is not caused by a nutritional deficit, nor does it indicate that the client needs a muscle relaxant. (R)

27. **3.** Antispasmodic drugs such as propantheline bromide (Pro-Banthine) may be administered along with opioids to deal with the intense pain associated with pancreatitis. Antispasmodics relax smooth muscle and decrease gastric motility and pancreatic enzyme secretion, thereby decreasing pain. Ibuprofen (Motrin) does not have an antispasmodic effect and would not be as effective in relieving pain. Propranolol (Inderal) and magnesium hydroxide (Maalox) do not have antispasmodic effects and would not be effective in relieving pain. Antacids may be given to neutralize gastric secretions. (D)

28. **4.** *Imbalanced nutrition: Less than body requirements* is likely to be a priority nursing diagnosis because the abdominal pain, nausea, and vomiting that are typical of pancreatitis can affect the client's food and fluid intake. Treatment of pancreatitis also frequently involves stopping all oral intake until the inflammation is resolved. Clients with pancreatitis are at risk for development of malnutrition. Intravenous therapy is used for fluid replacement, and total parenteral nutrition may be ordered to prevent malnourishment. Clients with pancreatitis do not have airway clearance or swallowing difficulties. Clients with pancreatitis are more likely to develop deficient fluid volume and to require fluid replacement. (A)

29. 1. Crash dieting or bingeing may cause an acute attack of pancreatitis and should be avoided. Carbohydrate intake should be increased because carbohydrates are less stimulating to the pancreas. There is no need to maintain a dietary pattern of six meals a day; the client can eat whenever desired. There is no need to place the client on a sodium-restricted diet because pancreatitis does not promote fluid retention. (A)

30. 2. In chronic pancreatitis, destruction of pancreatic tissue requires pancreatic enzyme replacement. Pancreatic enzymes are prescribed to facilitate the digestion of proteins and fats and should be taken in conjunction with every meal and snack. Specified hours or limited times for administration are ineffective because the enzymes must be taken in conjunction with food ingestion. (D)

31. 3. If the dosage and administration of pancreatic enzymes are adequate, the client's stool will be relatively normal. Any increase in odor or fat content would indicate the need for dosage adjustment. Stable body weight would be another indirect indicator. Fluid intake does not affect enzyme replacement therapy. If diabetes has developed, the client will need to monitor glucose levels. However, glucose and ketone levels are not affected by pancreatic enzyme therapy and would not indicate effectiveness of the therapy. (D)

32. 4. Clients with chronic pancreatitis are likely to develop diabetes as a result of the pancreatic fibrosis that occurs. The pancreas becomes unable to secrete insulin. Cholelithiasis, hepatitis, and irritable bowel syndrome are not caused by chronic pancreatitis. (R)

The Client with Viral Hepatitis

33. 2. Hepatitis B is considered to be a sexually transmitted disease. It can also be transmitted by percutaneous exposure to infected blood. Hepatitis A is transmitted via the fecal-oral route. Hepatitis C is primarily transmitted percutaneously and, less frequently, sexually. Hepatitis D is transmitted percutaneously. (S)

34. 2. Liver inflammation and obstruction block the normal flow of bile. Excess bilirubin turns the skin and sclera yellow and the urine dark and frothy. Profound anorexia is also common. Tarry stools are indicative of gastrointestinal bleeding and would not be expected in hepatitis. Light- or clay-colored stools may occur in hepatitis owing to bile duct obstruction. Shortness of breath would be unexpected. (A)

35. 2. The organism causing hepatitis A is transmitted primarily through feces. Viral hepatitis is not transmitted via the skin or urine. Hepatitis B, C, and D are transmitted through exposure to blood, but hepatitis A is not. (S)

36. 4. Contact precautions are recommended for clients with hepatitis A. This includes wearing gloves for direct care. These recommendations are made by the Centers for Disease Control and Prevention. A gown is not required unless substantial contact with the client is anticipated. It is not necessary to wear a mask. The client does not need a private room unless incontinent of stool. (S)

37. 4. During the convalescent or posticteric stage of hepatitis, fatigue and malaise are the most common complaints. These symptoms usually disappear within 2 to 4 months. Fatigue and malaise are not evidence of a secondary infection. Hepatitis A is not treated by drug therapy. It is important that the client continue to balance activity with periods of rest. (R)

38. 1. Treatment of hepatitis consists primarily of bed rest with bathroom privileges. Bed rest is maintained during the acute phase to reduce metabolic demands on the liver, thus increasing its blood supply and promoting liver cell regeneration. When activity is gradually resumed, the client should be taught to rest before becoming overly tired. Although adequate fluid intake is important, it is not necessary to force fluids to treat hepatitis. Antibiotics are not used to treat hepatitis. Electrolyte imbalances are not typical of hepatitis. (C)

39. 3. Serum levels of bilirubin and liver enzymes, such as alanine aminotransferase and aspartate aminotransferase, are carefully monitored during hepatitis. They provide important data about liver function. Blood glucose levels, the creatinine clearance, and serum electrolyte levels provide no information about liver function. (R)

40. 1. The prothrombin time may be prolonged because of decreased absorption of vitamin K and decreased production of prothrombin by the liver. The client should be assessed carefully for bleeding tendencies. Blood glucose and serum potassium and calcium levels are not affected by hepatitis. (R)

41. 3. Unlike the cirrhosis of alcoholism, viral forms of hepatitis are not usually associated with nutritional depletion. A well-balanced diet is advocated. It is a challenge to ensure that clients with hepatitis ingest a balanced diet with sufficient carbohydrates and calories because these clients are generally anorexic and have little interest in eating. Low-fat, high-protein foods are encouraged with hepatitis clients. There is no need to restrict sodium intake. (C)

42. 3. The hepatitis A virus is transmitted via the fecal-oral route. It spreads through contaminated hands, water, and food, especially shellfish growing in contaminated water. Certain animal handlers are at risk for hepatitis A, particularly those handling primates. Frequent hand washing is probably the single most important preventive action. Insects do not transmit hepatitis A. Family members do not need to stay away from the client with hepatitis. It is not necessary to disinfect food and clothing. (S)

43. 4. The most appropriate diagnosis for this client is *Activity intolerance* related to fatigue. The major goal of care for the client with hepatitis is to increase activity gradually as tolerated. Periods of alternating rest and activity should be included in the plan of care. There is no evidence that the client is physically immobile, unable to provide self-care, or coping ineffectively. (C)

44. 2. The client expresses feelings of isolation. The most appropriate nursing diagnosis for this client is *Social isolation.* Clients with hepatitis frequently feel guilty about possibly exposing others to the disease. Family and friends may experience fear of contracting the disease. The data provided do not indicate that the client is necessarily anxious, feeling powerless, or experiencing low self-esteem. (P)

45. 4. The nurse should encourage the client to further verbalize feelings of isolation. Instead of dismissing these feelings or making assumptions about the cause of isolation, the nurse should allow clients to verbalize their fears and provide education on how to prevent infection transmission. (P)

46. 2. Hepatitis C is usually transmitted through blood exposure or needlesticks. A hepatitis C vaccine is currently under development, but it is not available for use. The first line of defense against hepatitis B is the hepatitis B vaccine. Hepatitis C is not transmitted through feces or urine. Wearing a gown and mask will not prevent transmission of the hepatitis C virus if the caregiver comes in contact with infected blood or needles. (S)

47. 3. Interferon alfa-2b (Intron A) most commonly causes flulike adverse effects, such as myalgia, arthralgia, headache, nausea, fever, and fatigue. Retinopathy is a potential adverse effect, but not a common one. Diarrhea may develop as an adverse effect. Clients are advised to administer the drug at bedtime and get adequate rest. Medications may be prescribed to treat the symptoms. The drug may also cause hematologic changes; therefore, labo-

ratory tests such as a complete blood count and differential should be conducted monthly during drug therapy. Blood glucose laboratory values should be monitored for the development of hyperglycemia. (D)

48. 4. Hepatitis B is spread through exposure to blood or blood products and through high-risk sexual activity. Hepatitis B is considered to be a sexually transmitted disease. High-risk sexual activities include sex with multiple partners, unprotected sex with an infected individual, male homosexual activity, and sexual activity with I.V. drug users. The Centers for Disease Control and Prevention recommends immunization of all newborns and adolescents. College students are at high risk for development of hepatitis B and are encouraged to be immunized. Alcohol intake by itself does not predispose an individual to hepatitis B, but it can lead to high-risk behaviors such as unprotected sex. Good personal hygiene alone will not prevent the transmission of hepatitis B. (S)

49. 2. The client should be able to verbalize the importance of reporting any bleeding tendencies that could be the result of a prolonged prothrombin time. Ascites is not typically a clinical manifestation of hepatitis; it is associated with cirrhosis. Alcohol use should be eliminated for at least 1 year after the diagnosis of hepatitis to allow the liver time to fully recover. There is no need for a client to be restricted to the home because hepatitis is not spread through casual contact between individuals. (A)

The Client with Cirrhosis

50. 4. Portal hypertension and hypoalbuminemia as a result of cirrhosis cause a fluid shift into the peritoneal space causing ascites. In a cardiac or kidney problem, not cirrhosis, sodium can promote edema formation and subsequent decreased urine output. Edema does not migrate upward toward the heart to enhance its circulation. Although diuretics promote the excretion of excess fluid, occasionally forgetting or omitting a dose will not yield the ascites found in cirrhosis of the liver. (A)

51. 1, 2, 3, 4, 5. Constipation leads to increased ammonia production. Lactulose (Cephulac) is a hyperosmotic laxative that reduces blood ammonia by acidifying the colon contents, which retards diffusion of nonionic ammonia from the colon to the blood while promoting its migration from the blood to the colon. Hepatic encephalopathy is considered a toxic or metabolic condition that causes cerebral edema; it affects a person's coordination and pupil reaction to light and accommodation. Food and fluids high in carbohydrates should be given because the liver is not synthesizing and storing glucose. Because exercise produces ammonia as a byproduct of metabolism, physical activity should be limited, not encouraged. (M)

52. 3. Early clinical manifestations of cirrhosis are subtle and usually include gastrointestinal symptoms, such as anorexia, nausea, vomiting, and changes in bowel patterns. These changes are caused by the liver's altered ability to metabolize carbohydrates, proteins, and fats. Peripheral edema, ascites, and jaundice are later signs of liver failure and portal hypertension. (A)

53. 2. Spironolactone (Aldactone) is a potassium-sparing diuretic; therefore, clients should be monitored closely for hyperkalemia. Other common adverse effects include abdominal cramping, diarrhea, dizziness, headache, and rash. Constipation and dysuria are not common adverse effects of spironolactone. An irregular pulse is not an adverse effect of spironolactone but could develop if serum potassium levels are not closely monitored. (D)

54. 1. For clients who have cirrhosis without complications, a high-calorie, high-carbohydrate diet is preferred to provide an adequate supply of nutrients. In the early stages of cirrhosis, there is no need to restrict fat, protein, or sodium. (A)

55. 3. Excess retained bilirubin produces an irritating effect on the peripheral nerves, causing intense itching. Folic acid deficiency causes varied symptoms, but not itching. Itching is not a symptom of a prolonged prothrombin time or of hypokalemia. (R)

56. 1. General health promotion measures include maintaining good nutrition, avoiding infection, and abstaining from alcohol. Rest and sleep are essential, but an impaired liver may not be able to detoxify sedatives and barbiturates. Such drugs must be used cautiously, if at all, by clients with cirrhosis. The client does not need to limit contact with others but should exercise caution to stay away from ill people. (H)

57. 4. Ascites results from increased pressure in the venous system caused by a low level of serum albumin (which contributes to decreased colloid osmotic pressure) and sodium retention. The serum sodium level is not increased. There is a decreased aldosterone clearance and an increased flow of hepatic lymph. (A)

58. 1. Ascites can compromise the action of the diaphragm and increase the client's risk of respiratory problems. Ascites also greatly increases the risk of skin breakdown. Frequent position changes are important, but the preferred position is Fowler's. Placing the client in Fowler's position helps facilitate the client's breathing by relieving pressure on the diaphragm. The other positions do not relieve pressure on the diaphragm. (R)

59. 1. Normal serum albumin is administered to reduce ascites. Hypoalbuminemia, a mechanism underlying ascites formation, results in decreased colloid osmotic pressure. Administering serum albumin increases the plasma colloid osmotic pressure, which causes fluid to flow from the tissue space into the plasma. Increased urine output is the best indication that the albumin is having the desired effect. An increased serum albumin level and increased ease of breathing may indirectly imply that the administration of albumin is effective in relieving the ascites. However, it is not as direct an indicator as increased urine output. Anorexia is not affected by the administration of albumin. (D)

60. 4. The Sengstaken-Blakemore tube has a small gastric balloon that anchors the tube and applies pressure to the area of the cardiac sphincter. The large esophageal balloon applies direct pressure on the bleeding sites in the esophagus. A tube passing through the balloons allows for aspiration and irrigation. The Sengstaken-Blakemore tube is not used for gastric lavage. It would not be desirable to block blood flow to the stomach and esophageal tissue. (R)

61. 3. If the gastric balloon should rupture or deflate, the esophageal balloon can move and partially or totally obstruct the airway, causing respiratory distress. The client must be observed closely. No direct action should be taken until the condition is accurately diagnosed. (R)

62. 3. Neomycin (Mycifradin) is administered to decrease the bacterial action on protein in the intestines, which results in ammonia production. This ammonia, if not detoxified by the liver, can result in hepatic encephalopathy and coma. The antibiotic does not reduce abdominal pressure, prevent straining during defecation, or decrease hemorrhaging within the intestine. (D)

63. 1. The client should be monitored closely for changes in mental status. Ammonia has a toxic effect on central nervous system tissue and produces an altered level of consciousness, marked by drowsiness and irritability. If this process is unchecked, the client may lapse into coma. Increasing ammonia levels are not detected by changes in blood pressure, urine output, or respirations. (A)

64. 3. Lactulose (Cephulac) increases intestinal motility, thereby trapping and expelling ammonia in the feces. An increase in the number of bowel movements is expected as an adverse effect. Lactulose does not affect urine output. Any improvements in mental status would be the result of increased ammonia elimination, not an adverse effect of the drug. Nausea and vomiting are not common adverse effects of lactulose. (D)

65. 60

$$30 \text{ ml} = 1 \text{ oz}$$

The following formula is used to calculate the correct dosage:

$$30 \text{ ml}/1 \text{ oz} = X \text{ ml}/2 \text{ oz}$$

$$X = 60 \text{ ml}.$$

(D)

66. **2.** The taste of lactulose (Cephulac) is a problem for some clients. Mixing it with fruit juice, water, or milk can make it more palatable. Lactulose should not be given with antacids, which may inhibit its action. Lactulose should not be taken with a laxative because diarrhea is an adverse effect of the drug. Lactulose comes in the form of syrup for oral or rectal administration. (D)

67. **3.** Clients with cirrhosis should be instructed to avoid constipation and straining at stool to prevent hemorrhage. The client with cirrhosis has bleeding tendencies because of the liver's inability to produce clotting factors. A low-protein and high-carbohydrate diet is recommended.

Clients with cirrhosis should not take acetaminophen (Tylenol), which is potentially hepatotoxic. Aspirin also should be avoided if esophageal varices are present. Cirrhosis is a chronic disease. (R)

68. **1.** Immediately before a paracentesis, the client should empty the bladder to prevent perforation. The client will be placed in a high Fowler's position or seated on the side of the bed for the procedure. I.V. sedatives are not usually administered. The client does not need to be NPO. (R)

69. **4.** When hepatic encephalopathy develops, measures are taken to reduce ammonia formation. Protein is restricted in the diet. An NG tube is not inserted initially but may be necessary as the disease progresses. Fluid restriction and salt-poor albumin are incorporated into the treatment of ascites, but not hepatic encephalopathy. (A)

70. **3.** Edematous tissue is easily traumatized and must receive meticulous care. An alternating air pressure mattress will help decrease pressure on the edematous tissue. ROM exercises are important to maintain joint function, but they do not necessarily prevent skin breakdown. When abdominal skin is stretched taut due to ascites, it must be cleaned very carefully. The abdomen should not be massaged. Elevation of the lower extremities promotes venous return and decreases swelling. (R)

The Client with Endocrine Health Problems

The Client with Thyrotoxicosis

1. The nurse is completing a health assessment of a 42-year-old female with suspected Graves' disease. The nurse should assess this client for:
- ☐ **1.** Anorexia.
- ☐ **2.** Tachycardia.
- ☐ **3.** Weight gain.
- ☐ **4.** Cold skin.

2. A female client with thyrotoxicosis would probably report which changes related to the menstrual cycle during initial assessment?
- ☐ **1.** Dysmenorrhea.
- ☐ **2.** Metrorrhagia.
- ☐ **3.** Oligomenorrhea.
- ☐ **4.** Menorrhagia.

3. A 34-year-old female is diagnosed with hypothyroidism. Which signs and symptoms would the nurse expect to assess? Select all that apply.
- ☐ **1.** Rapid pulse.
- ☐ **2.** Decreased energy and fatigue.
- ☐ **3.** Weight gain of 10 lb.
- ☐ **4.** Fine, thin hair with hair loss.
- ☐ **5.** Constipation.
- ☐ **6.** Menorrhagia.

4. Propylthiouracil (PTU) is prescribed for a client with Graves' disease to decrease circulating thyroid hormone. The nurse should teach the client to immediately report which of the following signs and symptoms?
- ☐ **1.** Sore throat.
- ☐ **2.** Painful, excessive menstruation.
- ☐ **3.** Constipation.
- ☐ **4.** Increased urine output.

5. A client with thyrotoxicosis says to the nurse, "I am so irritable. I am having problems at work because I lose my temper very easily." Which of the following responses by the nurse would give the client the most accurate explanation of her behavior?
- ☐ **1.** "Your behavior is caused by temporary confusion brought on by your illness."
- ☐ **2.** "Your behavior is caused by the excess thyroid hormone in your system."
- ☐ **3.** "Your behavior is caused by your worrying about the seriousness of your illness."
- ☐ **4.** "Your behavior is caused by the stress of trying to manage a career and cope with illness."

6. Serum concentrations of thyroid hormones and thyroid-stimulating hormone (TSH) are tests ordered for the client with thyrotoxicosis. Which of the following laboratory values are indicative of thyrotoxicosis?
- ☐ **1.** Elevated thyroid hormone concentrations and normal TSH.
- ☐ **2.** Elevated TSH and normal thyroid hormone concentrations.
- ☐ **3.** Decreased thyroid hormone concentrations and elevated TSH.
- ☐ **4.** Elevated thyroid hormone concentrations and decreased TSH.

7. The nurse should teach the client to prevent corneal irritation from mild exophthalmos by:
- ☐ **1.** Massaging the eyes at regular intervals.
- ☐ **2.** Instilling an ophthalmic anesthetic as ordered.
- ☐ **3.** Wearing dark-colored glasses.
- ☐ **4.** Covering both eyes with moistened gauze pads.

8. A client with Graves' disease is treated with radioactive iodine (RAI) in the form of sodium iodide ^{131}I. Which of the following statements by the nurse will explain to the client how the drug works?
- ☐ **1.** "The radioactive iodine stabilizes the thyroid hormone levels before a thyroidectomy."
- ☐ **2.** "The radioactive iodine reduces uptake of thyroxine and thereby improves your condition."
- ☐ **3.** "The radioactive iodine lowers the levels of thyroid hormones by slowing your body's production of them."
- ☐ **4.** "The radioactive iodine destroys thyroid tissue so that thyroid hormones are no longer produced."

9. Which of the following nursing diagnoses would most likely be appropriate for a client with Graves' disease performing self-care after treatment with radioactive iodine (RAI) in the form of sodium iodide ^{131}I?
- ☐ **1.** *Risk for injury* related to altered level of consciousness.
- ☐ **2.** *Ineffective breathing pattern* related to effects of radioactive iodine.
- ☐ **3.** *Total self-care deficit* related to the need for immobilization after RAI therapy.
- ☐ **4.** *Ineffective health maintenance* related to lack of knowledge about disease.

10. After treatment with radioactive iodine (RAI) in the form of sodium iodide ^{131}I, the nurse teaches the client to:
- ☐ **1.** Monitor for signs and symptoms of hyperthyroidism.
- ☐ **2.** Rest for 1 week to prevent complications of the medication.
- ☐ **3.** Take thyroxine replacement for the remainder of the client's life.
- ☐ **4.** Assess for hypertension and tachycardia resulting from altered thyroid activity.

11. A client with a large goiter is scheduled for a subtotal thyroidectomy to treat thyrotoxicosis. Saturated solution of potassium iodide (SSKI) is prescribed preoperatively for the client. The primary reason for using this drug is that it helps:
- ☐ **1.** Slow progression of exophthalmos.
- ☐ **2.** Reduce the vascularity of the thyroid gland.
- ☐ **3.** Decrease the body's ability to store thyroxine.
- ☐ **4.** Increase the body's ability to excrete thyroxine.

12. Which of the following measures is most commonly recommended when preparing a saturated solution of potassium iodide (SSKI) for administration?
- ☐ **1.** Pour the solution over ice chips.
- ☐ **2.** Mix the solution with an antacid.
- ☐ **3.** Dilute the solution with water, milk, or fruit juice and have the client drink it with a straw.
- ☐ **4.** Disguise the solution in a pureed fruit or vegetable.

13. The nurse asks the client to state her name as soon as she regains consciousness postoperatively after a subtotal thyroidectomy and at each assessment. The nurse does this primarily to monitor for signs of which of the following?
- ☐ **1.** Internal hemorrhage.
- ☐ **2.** Decreasing level of consciousness.
- ☐ **3.** Laryngeal nerve damage.
- ☐ **4.** Upper airway obstruction.

14. A client who has undergone a subtotal thyroidectomy is subject to complications in the first 48 hours after surgery. The nurse should obtain and keep at the bedside equipment to:
- ☐ **1.** Begin total parenteral nutrition.
- ☐ **2.** Start a cutdown infusion.
- ☐ **3.** Administer tube feedings.
- ☐ **4.** Perform a tracheotomy.

15. Which of the following symptoms might indicate that a client was developing tetany after a subtotal thyroidectomy?
- ☐ **1.** Pains in the joints of the hands and feet.
- ☐ **2.** Tingling in the fingers.
- ☐ **3.** Bleeding on the back of the dressing.
- ☐ **4.** Tension on the suture line.

16. Which of the following medications should be available to provide emergency treatment if a client develops tetany after a subtotal thyroidectomy?
- ☐ **1.** Sodium phosphate.
- ☐ **2.** Calcium gluconate.
- ☐ **3.** Echothiophate iodide.
- ☐ **4.** Sodium bicarbonate.

17. A 60-year-old female is diagnosed with hypothyroidism. Signs and symptoms of hypothyroidism include:
- ☐ **1.** Tachycardia.
- ☐ **2.** Weight gain.
- ☐ **3.** Diarrhea.
- ☐ **4.** Nausea.

18. Appropriate nursing diagnoses for a client with hypothyroidism would include which of the following?

☐ **1.** *Risk for injury* (corneal abrasion) related to incomplete closure of the eyelid.

☐ **2.** *Imbalanced nutrition: Less than body requirements* related to hypermetabolism.

☐ **3.** *Deficient fluid volume* related to diarrhea.

☐ **4.** *Activity intolerance* related to fatigue associated with the disorder.

19. When discussing recent onset of feelings of sadness and depression in a client with hypothyroidism, the nurse should inform the client that these feelings are:

☐ **1.** The effects of thyroid hormone replacement therapy and will diminish over time.

☐ **2.** Related to thyroid hormone replacement therapy and will not diminish over time.

☐ **3.** A normal part of having a chronic illness.

☐ **4.** Most likely related to low thyroid hormone levels and will improve with treatment.

The Client with Diabetes Mellitus

20. A nurse is participating in a diabetes screening program. Which client is at risk for developing type 2 diabetes? Select all that apply.

☐ **1.** A 32-year-old female who delivered a 9½-lb infant.

☐ **2.** A 44-year-old Native American Indian who has a body mass index (BMI) of 32.

☐ **3.** An 18-year-old Hispanic who jogs four times a week.

☐ **4.** A 55-year-old Asian American who has hypertension and two siblings with type 2 diabetes.

☐ **5.** A 12-year-old who is overweight.

21. A 57-year-old with diabetes insipidus is hospitalized for care. Which finding should the nurse report to the physician?

☐ **1.** Urine output of 350 ml in 8 hours.

☐ **2.** Urine specific gravity of 1.001.

☐ **3.** Potassium of 4.0 mEq.

☐ **4.** Weight gain.

22. The nurse is checking the laboratory results on a 52-year-old client with type 1 diabetes (shown below). What laboratory result indicates a problem that should be managed?

☐ **1.** Blood glucose.

☐ **2.** Total cholesterol.

☐ **3.** Hemoglobin.

☐ **4.** Low-density lipoprotein (LDL) cholesterol.

LABORATORY RESULTS	
Test	**Result**
Blood glucose	192 mg/dl
Total cholesterol	250 mg/dl
Hemoglobin	12.3 mg/dl
Low-density lipoprotein cholesterol	125 mg/dl

23. A client with type 1 diabetes is admitted to the emergency department with dehydration following the flu. The client has a blood glucose level of 325 mg/dl and a serum potassium level of 3.5 mEq. The nurse should question orders for which of the following I.V. fluids for this client?

☐ **1.** Lactated Ringer's solution.

☐ **2.** Normal saline solution.

☐ **3.** 5% dextrose in water.

☐ **4.** Half-normal saline solution.

24. A client with type 1 diabetes mellitus has diabetic ketoacidosis. Which of the following findings has the greatest effect on fluid loss?

☐ **1.** Hypotension.

☐ **2.** Decreased serum potassium level.

☐ **3.** Rapid, deep respirations.

☐ **4.** Warm, dry skin.

25. A client is to receive glargine (Lantus) insulin in addition to a dose of aspart (NovoLog). When the nurse checks his blood glucose level at the bedside, it is greater than 200 mg/dl. How should the nurse administer the insulins?

☐ **1.** Put air into the glargine insulin vial, and then air into the aspart insulin vial, and draw up the correct dose of aspart insulin first.

☐ **2.** Roll the glargine insulin vial, then roll the aspart insulin vial. Draw up the longer-acting glargine insulin first.

☐ **3.** Shake both vials of insulin before drawing up each dose in separate insulin syringes.

☐ **4.** Put air into the glargine insulin vial, and draw up the correct dose in an insulin syringe; then, with a different insulin syringe, put air into the aspart vial and draw up the correct dose.

26. Glulisine (Apidra) insulin is ordered to be administered to a client before each meal. To assist the day-shift nurse who is receiving the report, the night-shift nurse gives the morning dose of glulisine. When the day-shift nurse goes to the room of the client who requires glulisine, the nurse finds that the client is not in the room. The client's roommate tells the nurse that the client "went for a test." What should the nurse do next?

☐ **1.** Bring a small glass of juice, and locate the client.

☐ **2.** Call the client's physician.

☐ **3.** Check the computerized care plan to determine what test was scheduled.

☐ **4.** Send the nurse's assistant to the X-ray department to bring the client back to his room.

27. A young adult client has been diagnosed with type 1 diabetes. He has an insulin drip to aid in lowering the serum blood glucose level of 600 mg/dl. He is also receiving ciprofloxacin (Cipro) I.V. The physician orders discontinuation of the insulin drip. Which of the following steps should the nurse anticipate taking?

☐ **1.** Discontinue the insulin drip, as ordered.

☐ **2.** Hang the next I.V. dose of antibiotic before discontinuing the insulin drip.

☐ **3.** Contact the physician to inform him that the client has not received any subcutaneous insulin yet.

☐ **4.** Add glargine (Lantus) to the insulin drip before discontinuing it.

28. An adult client with type 2 diabetes is taking metformin (Glucophage) 1,000 mg two times every day. A nurse provides instructions regarding the interaction of alcohol and metformin. When the nurse evaluates the client's understanding, she notes that learning is evident because the client makes which of the following statements?

☐ **1.** "If I know I'll be having alcohol, I must not take metformin; I could develop lactic acidosis."

☐ **2.** "If my physician approves, I may drink alcohol with my metformin."

☐ **3.** "Adverse effects I should watch for are feeling excessively energetic, unusual muscle stiffness, low back pain, and a rapid heartbeat."

☐ **4.** "If I feel bloated, I should call my physician."

29. A 55-year-old male client has recently been diagnosed with type 2 diabetes mellitus and is prescribed the sulfonylurea compound tolbutamide (Orinase). He is concerned about the diagnosis and says he knows nothing about diabetes. The nurse determines that the client needs teaching and support. The nurse explains that tolbutamide is believed to lower the blood glucose level by which of the following actions?

☐ **1.** Potentiating the action of insulin.

☐ **2.** Lowering the renal threshold of glucose.

☐ **3.** Stimulating insulin release from functioning beta cells in the pancreas.

☐ **4.** Combining with glucose to render it inert.

30. Which information should the nurse include when developing a teaching plan for a client newly diagnosed with type 2 diabetes mellitus. Select all that apply.

☐ **1.** A major risk factor for complications is obesity and central abdominal obesity.

☐ **2.** Supplemental insulin is mandatory for controlling the disease.

☐ **3.** Exercise increases insulin resistance.

☐ **4.** The primary nutritional source requiring monitoring in the diet is carbohydrates.

☐ **5.** Annual eye and foot examinations are recommended by the American Diabetes Association (ADA).

31. When teaching the diabetic client about foot care, the nurse should instruct the client to do which of the following?

☐ **1.** Avoid going barefoot.

☐ **2.** Buy shoes a half size larger.

☐ **3.** Cut toenails at angles.

☐ **4.** Use heating pads for sore feet.

32. A client with diabetes mellitus asks the nurse to recommend something to remove corns from his toes. The nurse should advise him to:
☐ 1. Apply a high-quality corn plaster to the area.
☐ 2. Consult his physician or podiatrist about removing the corns.
☐ 3. Apply iodine to the corns before peeling them off.
☐ 4. Soak his feet in borax solution to peel off the corns.

33. A client with diabetes mellitus comes to the clinic for a regular 3-month follow-up appointment. The nurse notes several small bandages covering cuts on the client's hands. The client says, "I'm so clumsy. I'm always cutting my finger cooking or burning myself on the iron." Which of the following responses by the nurse would be most appropriate?
☐ 1. "Wash all wounds in isopropyl alcohol."
☐ 2. "Keep all cuts clean and covered."
☐ 3. "Why don't you have your children do the cooking and ironing?"
☐ 4. "You really should be fine as long as you take your daily medication."

34. The client with diabetes mellitus says, "If I could just avoid what you call carbohydrates in my diet, I guess I would be okay." The nurse should base the response to this comment on the knowledge that diabetes affects metabolism of which of the following?
☐ 1. Carbohydrates only.
☐ 2. Fats and carbohydrates only.
☐ 3. Protein and carbohydrates only.
☐ 4. Proteins, fats, and carbohydrates.

35. A client with type 1 diabetes mellitus is admitted to the emergency department. Which of the following respiratory patterns requires immediate action?
☐ 1. Deep, rapid respirations with long expirations.
☐ 2. Shallow respirations alternating with long expirations.
☐ 3. Regular depth of respirations with frequent pauses.
☐ 4. Short expirations and inspirations.

36. Which of the following findings should the nurse report for a client with unstable type 1 diabetes mellitus? Select all that apply.
☐ 1. Systolic blood pressure, 145 mm Hg.
☐ 2. Diastolic blood pressure, 87 mm Hg.
☐ 3. High-density lipoprotein (HDL), 30 mg/dl.
☐ 4. Glycosylated hemoglobin (HbA$_{1c}$), 10.2%.
☐ 5. Triglycerides, 425 mg/dl.
☐ 6. Urine ketones, negative.

37. The nurse should caution the client with diabetes mellitus who is taking a sulfonylurea that alcoholic beverages should be avoided while taking these drugs because they can cause which of the following?
☐ 1. Hypokalemia.
☐ 2. Hyperkalemia.
☐ 3. Hypocalcemia.
☐ 4. Disulfiram (Antabuse)–like symptoms.

38. Which of the following conditions is the most significant risk factor for the development of type 2 diabetes mellitus?
☐ 1. Cigarette smoking.
☐ 2. High-cholesterol diet.
☐ 3. Obesity.
☐ 4. Hypertension.

39. Which of the following indicates a potential complication of diabetes mellitus?
☐ 1. Inflamed, painful joints.
☐ 2. Blood pressure of 160/100 mm Hg.
☐ 3. Stooped appearance.
☐ 4. Hemoglobin of 9 g/dl.

40. The nurse is teaching the client about home blood glucose monitoring. Which of the following blood glucose measurements indicates hypoglycemia?
☐ 1. 59 mg/dl.
☐ 2. 75 mg/dl.
☐ 3. 108 mg/dl.
☐ 4. 119 mg/dl.

41. Assessment of the diabetic client for common complications should always include examination of the:
☐ 1. Abdomen.
☐ 2. Lymph glands.
☐ 3. Pharynx.
☐ 4. Eyes.

42. The client with type 1 diabetes mellitus is taught to take isophane insulin suspension NPH (Humulin N) at 5 p.m. each day. The client should be instructed that the greatest risk of hypoglycemia will occur at about what time?
☐ 1. 11 a.m., shortly before lunch.
☐ 2. 1 p.m., shortly after lunch.
☐ 3. 6 p.m., shortly after dinner.
☐ 4. 1 a.m., while sleeping.

43. A nurse is teaching a client with type 1 diabetes mellitus who jogs daily about the preferred sites for insulin absorption. What is the most appropriate site for a client who jogs?
- [ ] **1.** Arms.
- [ ] **2.** Legs.
- [ ] **3.** Abdomen.
- [ ] **4.** Iliac crest.

44. The diabetic client who is taking insulin lispro (Humalog) injections would be advised to eat:
- [ ] **1.** Within 10 to 15 minutes after the injection.
- [ ] **2.** 1 hour after the injection.
- [ ] **3.** At any time, because timing of meals with lispro injections is unnecessary.
- [ ] **4.** 2 hours before the injection.

45. The best indicator that allows the nurse to judge that the client has learned how to give an insulin self-injection correctly is when the client can do which of the following?
- [ ] **1.** Perform the procedure safely and correctly.
- [ ] **2.** Critique the nurse's performance of the procedure.
- [ ] **3.** Explain all steps of the procedure correctly.
- [ ] **4.** Correctly answer a posttest about the procedure.

46. The nurse is instructing the client on insulin administration. The client is performing a return demonstration for preparing the insulin. The client's morning dose of insulin is 10 units of regular and 22 units of NPH. The nurse checks the dose accuracy with the client. The nurse determines that the client has prepared the correct dose when the syringe reads how many units?

_____ units

47. Angiotensin-converting enzyme (ACE) inhibitors may be prescribed for the client with diabetes mellitus to reduce vascular changes and possibly prevent or delay development of:
- [ ] **1.** Chronic obstructive pulmonary disease.
- [ ] **2.** Pancreatic cancer.
- [ ] **3.** Renal failure.
- [ ] **4.** Cerebrovascular accident.

48. The nurse should teach the diabetic client that which of the following is the most common symptom of hypoglycemia?
- [ ] **1.** Nervousness.
- [ ] **2.** Anorexia.
- [ ] **3.** Kussmaul's respirations.
- [ ] **4.** Bradycardia.

49. The nurse is assessing the client's use of medications. Which of the following medications may cause a complication with the treatment plan of a client with diabetes?
- [ ] **1.** Aspirin.
- [ ] **2.** Steroids.
- [ ] **3.** Sulfonylureas.
- [ ] **4.** Angiotensin-converting enzyme (ACE) inhibitors.

50. A female client with type 1 diabetes mellitus is experiencing minor illness with the flu. The nurse should instruct the client:
- [ ] **1.** To increase the frequency of self-monitoring (blood glucose testing).
- [ ] **2.** That she should try to reduce food intake to diminish nausea.
- [ ] **3.** That she does not need to take the insulin if she cannot eat.
- [ ] **4.** To take half of the normal dose of insulin.

51. Which of the following is a priority nursing diagnosis for the diabetic client who is taking insulin and has nausea and vomiting from a viral illness or influenza?
- [ ] **1.** *Imbalanced nutrition: Less than body requirements.*
- [ ] **2.** *Ineffective health maintenance* related to ineffective coping skills.
- [ ] **3.** *Acute pain.*
- [ ] **4.** *Activity intolerance.*

52. During a home visit, a diabetic client begins to cry and says, "I just cannot stand the thought of having to give myself a shot every day." Which of the following would be the best response by the nurse?
- [ ] **1.** "If you do not give yourself your insulin shots, you will die."
- [ ] **2.** "We can teach your daughter to give the shots so you will not have to do it."
- [ ] **3.** "I can arrange to have a home care nurse give you the shots every day."
- [ ] **4.** "What is it about giving yourself the insulin shots that bothers you?"

53. A client comes to the emergency department with diabetic ketoacidosis. The nurse should identify which of the following nursing diagnoses as a priority problem?
- [ ] **1.** *Insomnia.*
- [ ] **2.** *Ineffective health maintenance.*
- [ ] **3.** *Imbalanced nutrition: Less than body requirements.*
- [ ] **4.** *Deficient fluid volume.*

The Client with Pituitary Adenoma

54. Galactorrhea is caused by overproduction of which hormone?
- [ ] **1.** Prolactin.
- [ ] **2.** Adrenocorticotropic hormone (ACTH).
- [ ] **3.** Growth hormone (GH).
- [ ] **4.** Thyroid-stimulating hormone (TSH).

55. Which of the following signs and symptoms are common in male clients with prolactin-secreting tumors?
- [ ] **1.** Severe lethargy and fatigue.
- [ ] **2.** Decreased libido and impotence.
- [ ] **3.** Bony proliferation of the hands, jaw, and feet.
- [ ] **4.** Deepening or coarsening of the voice.

56. Surgical management for large, invasive pituitary tumors is a transsphenoidal hypophysectomy. The nurse should explain that the surgery will be performed through an incision in the:
- [ ] **1.** Back of the mouth.
- [ ] **2.** Nose.
- [ ] **3.** Sinus channel below the right eye.
- [ ] **4.** Upper gingival mucosa in the space between the upper gums and lip.

57. To help minimize the risk of postoperative respiratory complications after a hypophysectomy, the nurse would focus the client's preoperative teaching on the importance of:
- [ ] **1.** Using blow bottles.
- [ ] **2.** Making frequent position changes.
- [ ] **3.** Deep breathing.
- [ ] **4.** Coughing.

58. Which of the following activities should be a major focus of monitoring when planning nursing care for a client who has undergone transsphenoidal hypophysectomy?
- [ ] **1.** Cerebrospinal fluid (CSF) leak.
- [ ] **2.** Fluctuating blood glucose levels.
- [ ] **3.** Cushing's syndrome.
- [ ] **4.** Cardiac arrest.

59. A client expresses concern about how a hypophysectomy will affect his sexual function. Which of the following statements provides the most accurate information about the physiologic effects of hypophysectomy?
- [ ] **1.** Removing the source of excess hormone should restore the client's libido, erectile function, and fertility.
- [ ] **2.** Potency will be restored, but the client will remain infertile.
- [ ] **3.** Fertility will be restored, but impotence and decreased libido will persist.
- [ ] **4.** Exogenous hormones will be needed to restore erectile function after the adenoma is removed.

60. Before undergoing a transsphenoidal hypophysectomy for pituitary adenoma, the client asks the nurse how the surgeon will close the incision made in the dura. The nurse should respond based on the knowledge that:
- [ ] **1.** Dissolvable sutures are used to close the dura.
- [ ] **2.** Nasal packing provides pressure until normal wound healing occurs.
- [ ] **3.** A patch is made with a piece of fascia.
- [ ] **4.** A synthetic mesh is placed to facilitate healing.

61. Initial treatment for a cerebrospinal fluid (CSF) leak after transsphenoidal hypophysectomy would most likely involve:
- [ ] **1.** Repacking the nose.
- [ ] **2.** Returning the client to surgery.
- [ ] **3.** Enforcing bed rest with the head of the bed elevated.
- [ ] **4.** Administering high-dose corticosteroid therapy.

62. Oral hygiene for a client recovering from transsphenoidal hypophysectomy would include which of the following?
- [ ] **1.** Rinsing the mouth with saline solution.
- [ ] **2.** Performing frequent toothbrushing.
- [ ] **3.** Cleaning the teeth with an electric toothbrush.
- [ ] **4.** Vigorous flossing.

63. The nurse teaches the client to monitor for signs and symptoms of which potential complication after hypophysectomy?
- [ ] **1.** Acromegaly.
- [ ] **2.** Cushing's disease.
- [ ] **3.** Diabetes mellitus.
- [ ] **4.** Hypopituitarism.

64. After pituitary surgery, the nurse should assess the client for which of the following?
☐ **1.** Urine specific gravity less than 1.010.
☐ **2.** Urine output between 1 and 2 L/day.
☐ **3.** Blood glucose level higher than 300 mg/dl.
☐ **4.** Urine negative for glucose and ketones.

65. Vasopressin (Pitressin) is administered to the client with diabetes insipidus because it:
☐ **1.** Decreases blood pressure.
☐ **2.** Increases tubular reabsorption of water.
☐ **3.** Increases release of insulin from the pancreas.
☐ **4.** Decreases glucose production within the liver.

66. Which of the following constitutes a priority outcome for the client with diabetes insipidus?
☐ **1.** The client will maintain normal fluid and electrolyte balance.
☐ **2.** The client will select American Diabetes Association diet correctly.
☐ **3.** The client will state dietary restrictions.
☐ **4.** The client will exhibit serum glucose level within normal range.

The Client with Addison's Disease

67. The nurse is assessing a young adult with Addison's disease. The nurse should recognize that the client may need an increased dosage of glucocorticoids in which of the following situations?
☐ **1.** Completing the spring semester of school.
☐ **2.** Gaining 4 lb.
☐ **3.** Getting engaged.
☐ **4.** Undergoing a root canal.

68. Which of the following is the priority for a client in addisonian crisis?
☐ **1.** Controlling hypertension.
☐ **2.** Preventing irreversible shock.
☐ **3.** Preventing infection.
☐ **4.** Relieving anxiety.

69. Which of the following would be an expected finding in a client with adrenal crisis (addisonian crisis)?
☐ **1.** Fluid retention.
☐ **2.** Pain.
☐ **3.** Peripheral edema.
☐ **4.** Hunger.

70. The client is receiving an I.V. infusion of 5% dextrose in normal saline running at 125 ml/hour. When hanging a new bag of fluid, the nurse notes swelling and hardness at the infusion site. Which immediate action would be indicated?
☐ **1.** Discontinue the infusion.
☐ **2.** Apply a warm soak to the site.
☐ **3.** Stop the flow of solution temporarily.
☐ **4.** Irrigate the needle with normal saline.

71. The client's wife asks the nurse whether the I.V. infusion is meeting her husband's nutritional needs because he has vomited several times. The nurse's response should be based on the knowledge that 1 L of 5% dextrose in normal saline solution delivers:
☐ **1.** 170 calories.
☐ **2.** 250 calories.
☐ **3.** 340 calories.
☐ **4.** 500 calories.

72. A client with Addison's disease is admitted to the medical unit. The nurse diagnoses the client with *Deficient fluid volume* related to inadequate fluid intake and to fluid loss secondary to inadequate adrenal hormone secretion. As the client's oral intake increases, which of the following fluids would be most appropriate?
☐ **1.** Milk and diet soda.
☐ **2.** Water and eggnog.
☐ **3.** Bouillon and juice.
☐ **4.** Coffee and milkshakes.

73. After stabilization of Addison's disease, a client attends a stress management class because stress can precipitate addisonian crisis. Which of the following actions taught by the nurse in the class is based on principles of stress management?
☐ **1.** Remove all sources of stress from your life.
☐ **2.** Use relaxation techniques such as music.
☐ **3.** Take antianxiety drugs daily.
☐ **4.** Avoid discussing stressful experiences.

74. When teaching a client newly diagnosed with primary Addison's disease, the nurse should explain that the disease results from:
☐ **1.** Insufficient secretion of growth hormone (GH).
☐ **2.** Dysfunction of the hypothalamic pituitary.
☐ **3.** Idiopathic atrophy of the adrenal gland.
☐ **4.** Oversecretion of the adrenal medulla.

75. The nurse is conducting discharge education with a client newly diagnosed with Addison's disease. Which information should be included in the client and family teaching plan? Select all that apply.
☐ **1.** Addison's disease will resolve over a few weeks, requiring no further treatment.
☐ **2.** Avoiding stress and maintaining a balanced lifestyle will minimize risk for exacerbations.
☐ **3.** Fatigue, weakness, dizziness, and mood changes need to be reported to the physician.
☐ **4.** A medical identification bracelet should be worn.
☐ **5.** Family members need to be informed about the warning signals of adrenal crisis.
☐ **6.** Dental work or surgery will require adjustment of daily medication.

76. The nurse would expect the client with Addison's disease to exhibit which of the following signs and symptoms?
- [ ] **1.** Weight gain.
- [ ] **2.** Hunger.
- [ ] **3.** Lethargy.
- [ ] **4.** Muscle spasms.

77. A nurse is assessing a client with Addison's disease. The nurse should review laboratory reports for which condition?
- [ ] **1.** Hypokalemia.
- [ ] **2.** Hypernatremia.
- [ ] **3.** Hypoglycemia.
- [ ] **4.** Decreased blood urea nitrogen (BUN) level.

78. The client with Addison's disease is taking glucocorticoids at home. Which of the following statements correctly reflects the principle governing administration and dosage of glucocorticoids?
- [ ] **1.** Various circumstances increase the need for glucocorticoids, so dosage adjustments will be needed.
- [ ] **2.** The need for glucocorticoids stabilizes, and a predetermined dose is taken once a day.
- [ ] **3.** Glucocorticoids are cumulative, so a dose is taken every third day.
- [ ] **4.** A dose is taken every 6 hours to ensure consistent blood levels of glucocorticoids.

79. Cortisone acetate (Cortone) and fludrocortisone acetate (Florinef Acetate) are prescribed as replacement therapy for a client with Addison's disease. What administration schedule should be followed for this therapy?
- [ ] **1.** Take both drugs three times a day.
- [ ] **2.** Take the entire dose of both drugs first thing in the morning.
- [ ] **3.** Take all the fludrocortisone acetate and two-thirds of the cortisone acetate in the morning, and take the remaining cortisone acetate in the afternoon.
- [ ] **4.** Take half of each drug in the morning and the remaining half of each drug at bedtime.

80. Which statement should the nurse make when teaching the client about taking oral glucocorticoids?
- [ ] **1.** "Take your medication with a full glass of water."
- [ ] **2.** "Take your medication on an empty stomach."
- [ ] **3.** "Take your medication at bedtime to increase absorption."
- [ ] **4.** "Take your medication with meals or with an antacid."

81. Which of the following is the best indicator for determining whether a client with Addison's disease is receiving the correct amount of glucocorticoid replacement?
- [ ] **1.** Skin turgor.
- [ ] **2.** Temperature.
- [ ] **3.** Thirst.
- [ ] **4.** Daily weight.

82. Which of the following signs and symptoms would probably indicate that the client with Addison's disease is receiving too much glucocorticoid replacement?
- [ ] **1.** Anorexia.
- [ ] **2.** Dizziness.
- [ ] **3.** Rapid weight gain.
- [ ] **4.** Poor skin turgor.

83. Which of the following is a priority outcome for the client with Addison's disease?
- [ ] **1.** Maintenance of medication compliance.
- [ ] **2.** Avoidance of normal activities with stress.
- [ ] **3.** Adherence to a 2-g sodium diet.
- [ ] **4.** Prevention of hypertensive episodes.

84. The client with Addison's disease should anticipate the need for increased glucocorticoid supplementation in which of the following situations?
- [ ] **1.** Returning to work after a weekend.
- [ ] **2.** Going on vacation.
- [ ] **3.** Having oral surgery.
- [ ] **4.** Having a routine medical checkup.

85. The nurse should teach the client with Addison's disease that the adverse effect of bronze-colored skin is thought to be caused by which of the following?
- [ ] **1.** Hypersensitivity to sun exposure.
- [ ] **2.** Increased serum bilirubin level.
- [ ] **3.** Adverse effects of the glucocorticoid therapy.
- [ ] **4.** Increased secretion of adrenocorticotropic hormone (ACTH).

86. Which of the following would most likely be a priority nursing diagnosis for the client experiencing addisonian crisis?
- [ ] **1.** *Fatigue.*
- [ ] **2.** *Imbalanced nutrition: More than body requirements* related to increased appetite.
- [ ] **3.** *Imbalanced nutrition: More than body requirements* related to decreased exercise.
- [ ] **4.** *Excess fluid volume* related to reduced urinary excretion of fluid.

The Client with Cushing's Disease

87. A 42-year-old female client reports that she has gained weight and that her face and body are "rounder," while her legs and arms have become thinner. A tentative diagnosis of Cushing's disease is made. When examining this client, the nurse would expect to find:
- [ ] **1.** Orthostatic hypotension.
- [ ] **2.** Muscle hypertrophy in the extremities.
- [ ] **3.** Bruised areas on the skin.
- [ ] **4.** Decreased body hair.

88. Signs and symptoms of Cushing's disease include:
- [ ] **1.** Weight loss.
- [ ] **2.** Thin, fragile skin.
- [ ] **3.** Hypotension.
- [ ] **4.** Abdominal pain.

89. Cushing's disease is manifested by the excessive secretion of corticosteroids. The hormones involved are:
- [ ] **1.** Glucocorticoids and aldosterone.
- [ ] **2.** Adrenocorticotropic hormone (ACTH).
- [ ] **3.** Glucocorticoids, aldosterone, and androgens.
- [ ] **4.** Catecholamines.

90. Which of the following test results would be consistent with a diagnosis of Cushing's disease?
- [ ] **1.** Postprandial hypoglycemia.
- [ ] **2.** Hypokalemia.
- [ ] **3.** Hyponatremia.
- [ ] **4.** Decreased urine calcium level.

91. A client with Cushing's disease tells the nurse that the physician said her morning serum cortisol level was within normal limits. She asks, "How can that be? I'm not imagining all these symptoms!" The nurse's response will be based on which of the following concepts?
- [ ] **1.** Some clients are very sensitive to the effects of cortisol and develop symptoms even with normal levels.
- [ ] **2.** A single random blood test cannot provide reliable information about endocrine levels.
- [ ] **3.** The excessive cortisol levels seen in Cushing's disease commonly result from loss of the normal diurnal secretion pattern.
- [ ] **4.** Tumors tend to secrete hormones irregularly, and the hormones are generally not present in the blood.

92. The client with Cushing's disease needs to modify dietary intake to control symptoms. In addition to increasing protein, which strategy would be most appropriate?
- [ ] **1.** Increase calories.
- [ ] **2.** Restrict sodium.
- [ ] **3.** Restrict potassium.
- [ ] **4.** Reduce fat to 10%.

93. Bone resorption is a possible complication of Cushing's disease. Which of the following interventions should the nurse recommend to help the client prevent this complication?
- [ ] **1.** Increase the amount of potassium in the diet.
- [ ] **2.** Maintain a regular program of weight-bearing exercise.
- [ ] **3.** Limit dietary vitamin D intake.
- [ ] **4.** Perform isometric exercises.

94. A client has been found to have an adrenal tumor and is scheduled for a bilateral adrenalectomy. The nurse begins preoperative teaching, which includes the importance of deep breathing. Which of the following would be the most accurate instructions?
- [ ] **1.** "Sit in an upright position and take a deep breath."
- [ ] **2.** "Hold your abdomen firmly with a pillow and take several deep breaths."
- [ ] **3.** "Tighten your stomach muscles as you inhale and breathe normally."
- [ ] **4.** "Raise your shoulders to expand your chest."

95. A priority in the first 24 hours after a bilateral adrenalectomy is:
- [ ] **1.** Beginning oral nutrition.
- [ ] **2.** Promoting self-care activities.
- [ ] **3.** Preventing adrenal crisis.
- [ ] **4.** Ambulating in the hallway.

96. A client undergoing a bilateral adrenalectomy has postoperative orders for hydromorphone hydrochloride (Dilaudid) 2 mg to be given subcutaneously every 4 hours p.r.n. for pain. This drug is administered in relatively small doses primarily because it is:
- [ ] **1.** Less likely to cause dependency in small doses.
- [ ] **2.** Less irritating to subcutaneous tissues in small doses.
- [ ] **3.** As potent as most other analgesics in larger doses.
- [ ] **4.** Excreted before accumulating in toxic amounts in the body.

97. Adrenal function is affected by the drug ketoconazole (Nizoral), an antifungal agent used to treat severe fungal infections. How is this effect manifested?
- [ ] **1.** Ketoconazole suppresses adrenal steroid secretion.
- [ ] **2.** Ketoconazole destroys adrenocortical cells, resulting in a "medical" adrenalectomy.
- [ ] **3.** Ketoconazole increases adrenocorticotropic hormone (ACTH)–induced corticosteroid serum levels.
- [ ] **4.** Ketoconazole decreases duration of adrenal suppression when administered with corticosteroids.

98. In the early postoperative period after a bilateral adrenalectomy, the nurse should recognize that the most probable cause of temperature elevation is:
- ☐ **1.** Dehydration.
- ☐ **2.** Poor lung expansion.
- ☐ **3.** Wound infection.
- ☐ **4.** Urinary tract infection.

99. A client who is recovering from a bilateral adrenalectomy has a patient-controlled analgesia (PCA) system with morphine sulfate. Which of the following actions is a priority nursing intervention for the client?
- ☐ **1.** Observing the client at regular intervals for opioid addiction.
- ☐ **2.** Encouraging the client to reduce analgesic use and tolerate the pain.
- ☐ **3.** Evaluating pain control at least every 2 hours.
- ☐ **4.** Increasing the amount of morphine if the client does not administer the medication.

100. After surgery for bilateral adrenalectomy, the client is kept on bed rest for several days to stabilize the body's need for steroids postoperatively. Which of the following exercises has been found to be especially helpful in preparing a client for ambulation after a period of bed rest?
- ☐ **1.** Alternately flexing and extending the knees.
- ☐ **2.** Alternately abducting and adducting the legs.
- ☐ **3.** Alternately stretching the Achilles tendons.
- ☐ **4.** Alternately flexing and relaxing the quadriceps femoris muscles.

101. As the nurse helps the postoperative client out of bed, the client complains of gas pains in her abdomen. Which of the following is the most effective nursing intervention to relieve this discomfort?
- ☐ **1.** Encourage the client to ambulate.
- ☐ **2.** Insert a rectal tube.
- ☐ **3.** Insert a nasogastric (NG) tube.
- ☐ **4.** Encourage the client to drink carbonated liquids.

102. Because of steroid excess, the client who has undergone a bilateral adrenalectomy is at an increased risk for:
- ☐ **1.** Postoperative confusion.
- ☐ **2.** Delayed wound healing.
- ☐ **3.** Emboli.
- ☐ **4.** Malnutrition.

103. The client who has undergone a bilateral adrenalectomy is ready to return home. She tells the nurse that she is concerned about persistent body changes and the fact that her moods are still so unpredictable. She says, "I thought surgery was supposed to fix all that." The nurse should base teaching about recovery on which of the following concepts?
- ☐ **1.** The body changes are permanent and the client will not be the same as before this condition.
- ☐ **2.** The body and mood will gradually return to normal.
- ☐ **3.** The physical changes are permanent, but the mood swings will disappear.
- ☐ **4.** The physical changes are temporary, but the mood swings are permanent.

104. After bilateral adrenalectomy for Cushing's disease, the client is told by her physician that she needs periodic testosterone injections. She asks the nurse, "What is that for? Did he forget I'm a woman?" What would be the nurse's best response?
- ☐ **1.** "Testosterone is needed to balance the reproductive cycle."
- ☐ **2.** "Testosterone is needed to restore the body's sodium and potassium balance."
- ☐ **3.** "Testosterone is given to stimulate protein anabolism."
- ☐ **4.** "Testosterone is given to stabilize mood swings."

105. Which of the following should the nurse include in the teaching plan of a female client with bilateral adrenalectomy?
- ☐ **1.** Emphasizing that the client will need steroid replacement for the rest of her life.
- ☐ **2.** Instructing the client about the importance of tapering steroid medication carefully to prevent crisis.
- ☐ **3.** Informing the client that steroids will be required only until her body can manufacture sufficient quantities.
- ☐ **4.** Emphasizing that the client will need to take steroids whenever her life involves physical or emotional stress.

The Female Client with Perimenopausal or Menopausal Syndrome

106. The client with perimenopausal or menopausal syndrome is primarily experiencing a deficiency of the hormone:
- ☐ **1.** Progesterone.
- ☐ **2.** Estrogen.
- ☐ **3.** Prolactin.
- ☐ **4.** Oxytocin.

107. A woman with perimenopausal syndrome asks the nurse why she is having irregular periods. The nurse explains that she has a deficiency of estrogen caused by decreased function of the:
- ☐ **1.** Ovarian follicle.
- ☐ **2.** Pituitary gland.
- ☐ **3.** Adrenal cortex.
- ☐ **4.** Thyroid.

108. A menopausal woman with an intact uterus is taking a combined estrogen and progesterone replacement medication, Prempro 0.625 mg/2.5 mg, for severe hot flashes. Combined hormonal therapy is given because estrogen alone:
- ☐ **1.** Would not be effective for hot flashes.
- ☐ **2.** Could be a risk factor for endometrial cancer.
- ☐ **3.** Would not be sufficient to maintain libido.
- ☐ **4.** Could be a risk factor for ovarian cancer.

109. A woman in menopause is a good candidate for hormone replacement therapy (HRT) if she:
- ☐ **1.** Has a family history of breast cancer.
- ☐ **2.** Had breast cancer a year ago.
- ☐ **3.** Has severe hot flashes.
- ☐ **4.** Had an estrogen-dependent dysplasia.

110. The nurse teaches the postmenopausal client prescribed hormone replacement therapy (HRT) to contact her health care provider immediately if she experiences which of the following?
- ☐ **1.** Hot flashes.
- ☐ **2.** Irregular vaginal bleeding.
- ☐ **3.** Vaginal dryness.
- ☐ **4.** Vaginal pH changes.

The Client with Pheochromocytoma

111. A client is admitted with pheochromocytoma. The nurse assesses the client's blood pressure frequently. This is based on the knowledge that pheochromocytoma of the adrenal medulla releases excessive amounts of:
- ☐ **1.** Renin.
- ☐ **2.** Aldosterone.
- ☐ **3.** Catecholamines.
- ☐ **4.** Glucocorticoids.

112. The primary feature of pheochromocytoma's effect on blood pressure is:
- ☐ **1.** Systolic hypertension.
- ☐ **2.** Diastolic hypertension.
- ☐ **3.** Hypertension that is resistant to treatment with drugs.
- ☐ **4.** Widening pulse pressure.

113. The client with pheochromocytoma is scheduled for surgical resection of the tumor in the adrenal medulla. The nurse should monitor the client postoperatively for which of the following potential complications?
- ☐ **1.** Orthostatic hypotension.
- ☐ **2.** Hemorrhage.
- ☐ **3.** Hypoglycemia.
- ☐ **4.** Hypertensive crisis.

114. The client with pheochromocytoma should be instructed to avoid activities that precipitate hypertensive crises or paroxysms, such as:
- ☐ **1.** Jogging.
- ☐ **2.** The Valsalva maneuver.
- ☐ **3.** Anxiety.
- ☐ **4.** Hypoglycemia.

115. Which of the following therapeutic classes of drugs is used to treat tachycardia and angina in a client with pheochromocytoma?
- ☐ **1.** Angiotensin-converting enzyme (ACE) inhibitors.
- ☐ **2.** Calcium channel blockers.
- ☐ **3.** Beta blockers.
- ☐ **4.** Diuretics.

Correct Answers and Rationales

The letter in parentheses after each rationale identifies the client need addressed in the item, including management of care (M), safety and infection control (S), health promotion and maintenance (H), psychosocial adaptation (P), basic care and comfort (C), pharmacological and parenteral therapies (D), reduction of risk potential (R), and physiological adaptation (A).

The Client with Thyrotoxicosis

1. **2.** Graves' disease, the most common type of thyrotoxicosis, is a state of hypermetabolism. The increased metabolic rate generates heat and produces tachycardia and fine muscle tremors. Anorexia is associated with hypothyroidism. Loss of weight, despite a good appetite and adequate caloric intake, is a common feature of hyperthyroidism. Cold skin is associated with hypothyroidism. (A)

2. 3. A change in the menstrual interval, diminished menstrual flow (oligomenorrhea), or even the absence of menstruation (amenorrhea) may result from the hormonal imbalances of thyrotoxicosis. Oligomenorrhea in women and decreased libido and impotence in men are common features of thyrotoxicosis. Dysmenorrhea is painful menstruation. Metrorrhagia, blood loss between menstrual periods, is a symptom of hypothyroidism. Menorrhagia, excessive bleeding during menstrual periods, is a symptom of hypothyroidism. (A)

3. 2, 3, 5, 6. Clients with hypothyroidism exhibit symptoms indicating a lack of thyroid hormone. Bradycardia, decreased energy and lethargy, memory problems, weight gain, coarse hair, constipation, and menorrhagia are common signs and symptoms of hypothyroidism. (A)

4. 1. The most serious adverse effects of PTU are leukopenia and agranulocytosis, which usually occur within the first 3 months of treatment. The client should be taught to promptly report to the health care provider signs and symptoms of infection, such as a sore throat and fever. Clients complaining of a sore throat and fever should have an immediate white blood cell count and differential performed, and the drug must be withheld until the results are obtained. Painful menstruation, constipation, and increased urine output are not associated with PTU therapy. (D)

5. 2. A typical sign of thyrotoxicosis is irritability caused by the high levels of circulating thyroid hormones in the body. This symptom decreases as the client responds to therapy. Thyrotoxicosis does not cause confusion. The client may be worried about her illness, and stress may influence her mood; however, irritability is a common symptom of thyrotoxicosis and the client should be informed of that fact rather than blamed. (P)

6. 4. Elevated serum concentrations of thyroid hormones and suppressed serum TSH are the features of thyrotoxicosis. Decreased or absent serum TSH is a very accurate indicator of thyrotoxicosis. Increased levels of circulating thyroid hormones cause the feedback mechanism to the brain to suppress TSH secretion. (A)

7. 3. Treatment of mild ophthalmopathy that may accompany thyrotoxicosis includes measures such as wearing sunglasses to protect the eyes from corneal irritation. Treatment of ophthalmopathy should be performed in consultation with an ophthalmologist. Massaging the eyes will not help to protect the cornea. An ophthalmic anesthetic is used to examine and possibly treat a painful eye, not protect the cornea. Covering the eyes with moist gauze pads is not a satisfactory nursing measure to protect the eyes of a client with exophthalmos because treatment is not focused on moisture to the eye but rather on protecting the cornea and optic nerve. In exophthalmos, the retrobulbar connective tissues and extraocular muscle volume are expanded because of fluid retention. The pressure is also increased. (R)

8. 4. Sodium iodide ^{131}I destroys the thyroid follicular cells, and thyroid hormones are no longer produced. RAI is commonly recommended for clients with Graves' disease, especially the elderly. The treatment results in a "medical thyroidectomy." RAI is given in lieu of surgery, not before surgery. RAI does not reduce uptake of thyroxine. The outcome of giving RAI is the destruction of the thyroid follicular cells. It is possible to slow the production of thyroid hormones with RAI. (D)

9. 4. Health maintenance is a priority for the client who has undergone RAI therapy with sodium iodide ^{131}I because signs and symptoms of hyperthyroidism usually persist for 1 to 2 months and may still be present for up to 1 year until thyroid hormone production stops. Permanent hypothyroidism is the major complication of radioactive ^{131}I treatment. At that time, the client will need to have sufficient knowledge to be able to recognize signs and symptoms of hypothyroidism. Changes in level of consciousness or breathing pattern are not expected. The client does not need to be immobilized after RAI treatment. (D)

10. 3. The client needs to be educated about the need for lifelong thyroid hormone replacement. Permanent hypothyroidism is the major complication of RAI ^{131}I treatment. Lifelong medical follow-up and thyroid replacement are warranted. The client needs to monitor for signs and symptoms of hypothyroidism, not hyperthyroidism. Resting for 1 week is not necessary. Hypertension and tachycardia are signs of hyperthyroidism, not hypothyroidism. (D)

11. 2. SSKI is frequently administered before a thyroidectomy because it helps decrease the vascularity of the thyroid gland. A highly vascular thyroid gland is very friable, a condition that presents a hazard during surgery. Preparation of the client for surgery includes depleting the gland of thyroid hormone and decreasing vascularity. SSKI does not decrease the progression of exophthalmos, and it does not decrease the body's ability to store thyroxine or increase the body's ability to excrete thyroxine. (D)

12. 3. SSKI should be diluted well in milk, water, juice, or a carbonated beverage before administration to help disguise the strong, bitter taste. Also, this drug is irritating to mucosa if taken undiluted. The client should sip the diluted preparation through a drinking straw to help prevent staining of the teeth. Pouring the solution over ice chips will not sufficiently dilute the SSKI or cover the taste. Antacids are not used to dilute or cover the taste of SSKI. Mixing in a puree would put the SSKI in contact with the teeth. (D)

13. **3.** Laryngeal nerve damage is a potential complication of thyroid surgery because of the proximity of the thyroid gland to the recurrent laryngeal nerve. Asking the client to speak helps assess for signs of laryngeal nerve damage. Persistent or worsening hoarseness and weak voice are signs of laryngeal nerve damage and should be reported to the physician immediately. Internal hemorrhage is detected by changes in vital signs. The client's level of consciousness can be partially assessed by asking her to speak, but that is not the primary reason for doing so in this situation. Upper airway obstruction is detected by color and respiratory rate and pattern. (R)

14. **4.** Equipment for an emergency tracheotomy should be kept in the room, in case tracheal edema and airway occlusion occur. Laryngeal nerve damage can result in vocal cord spasm and respiratory obstruction. A tracheostomy set, oxygen and suction equipment, and a suture removal set (for respiratory distress from hemorrhage) make up the emergency equipment that should be readily available. Total parenteral nutrition is not anticipated for the client undergoing thyroidectomy. Intravenous infusion via a cutdown is not an expected possible treatment after thyroidectomy. Tube feedings are not anticipated emergency care. (R)

15. **2.** Tetany may occur after thyroidectomy if the parathyroid glands are accidentally injured or removed during surgery. This would cause a disturbance in serum calcium levels. An early sign of tetany is numbness and tingling of the fingers or toes and in the circumoral region. Tetany may occur from 1 to 7 days postoperatively. Late signs and symptoms of tetany include seizures, contraction of the glottis, and respiratory obstruction. Pains in the joints of the hands and feet are not early symptoms of tetany. Bleeding on the back of the dressing is related to possible incisional complications. Tension on the suture line may indicate swelling, infection, or internal bleeding, but it is not related to tetany. (A)

16. **2.** The client with tetany is suffering from hypocalcemia, which is treated by administering an I.V. preparation of calcium, such as calcium gluconate or calcium chloride. Oral calcium is then necessary until normal parathyroid function returns. Sodium phosphate is a laxative. Echothiophate iodide is an eye preparation used as a miotic for an antiglaucoma effect. Sodium bicarbonate is a potent systemic antacid. (D)

17. **2.** Typical signs and symptoms of hypothyroidism include weight gain, fatigue, decreased energy, apathy, brittle nails, dry skin, cold intolerance, hair loss, constipation, and numbness and tingling in the fingers. Tachycardia is a sign of hyperthyroidism, not hypothyroidism. Diarrhea and nausea are not symptoms of hypothyroidism. (A)

18. **4.** A major problem for the person with hypothyroidism is fatigue. Other signs and symptoms include lethargy, personality changes, generalized edema, impaired memory, slowed speech, cold intolerance, dry skin, muscle weakness, constipation, weight gain, and hair loss. Incomplete closure of the eyelids, hypermetabolism, and diarrhea are associated with hyperthyroidism. (C)

19. **4.** Hypothyroidism may contribute to sadness and depression. It is good practice for clients with newly diagnosed depression to be monitored for hypothyroidism by checking serum thyroid hormone and thyroid-stimulating hormone levels. This client needs to know that these feelings may be related to her low thyroid hormone levels and may improve with treatment. Replacement therapy does not cause depression. Depression may accompany chronic illness, but it is not "normal." (P)

The Client with Diabetes Mellitus

20. **1, 2, 4, 5.** The risk factors for developing type 2 diabetes include giving birth to an infant weighing more than 9 lb; obesity (BMI over 30); ethnicity of Asian, African American, or Native American Indian; age greater than 45 years; hypertension; and family history in parents or siblings. Childhood obesity is also a risk factor for type 2 diabetes. Maintaining an ideal weight, eating a low-fat diet, and exercising regularly decrease the risk of type 2 diabetes. (R)

21. **2.** Diabetes insipidus is caused by a deficiency of antidiuretic hormone, which results in excretion of a large volume of dilute urine. Therefore, a urine specific gravity of less than 1.005 should be reported. Urine output should be 30 to 50 ml/hour; thus, 350 ml is a normal urinary output over 8 hours. The potassium level is normal. Weight loss, not weight gain, should be monitored as a sign of dehydration. (R)

22. **1.** The elevated blood glucose level indicates hyperglycemia. The hemoglobin is normal. The client's cholesterol and LDL levels are both normal. The nurse should determine if there are standing orders for the hyperglycemia or notify the physician. (R)

23. **3.** The client needs fluid volume replacement due to the dehydration. However, the nurse should question the order for I.V. dextrose due to the risk of hyperglycemia that dextrose would present when administered to a client with diabetes. Lactated Ringer's solution and normal saline solution are isotonic fluids used to restore circulating volume without additional glucose. Half-normal saline solution would also restore fluids, although it has a lower concentration of sodium than that of body fluids. (D)

24. 3. Due to the rapid, deep respirations, the client is losing fluid from vaporization from the lungs and skin (insensible fluid loss). Normally, about 900 ml of fluid is lost per day through vaporization. Decreased serum potassium level has no effect on insensible fluid loss. Hypotension occurs due to polyurea and inadequate fluid intake. It may decrease the flow of blood to the skin, causing skin to be warm and dry. (R)

25. 4. Glargine (Lantus) is a long-acting recombinant human insulin analog. Glargine should not be mixed with any other insulin product. Insulins should not be shaken; instead, if the insulin is cloudy, roll the vial or insulin pen between the palms of the hands. (D)

26. 3. Glulisine (Apidra) is a rapid-acting insulin with an action onset of 15 minutes. The client could experience hypoglycemia with the insulin in the bloodstream and no breakfast. It is not necessary to call the client's physician; the nurse should determine what test was scheduled and then locate the client and provide either breakfast or 4 oz of fruit juice. To bring the client back to the room would be wasting valuable time needed to prevent or correct hypoglycemia. (M)

27. 3. Because subcutaneous administration of insulin has a slower rate of absorption than I.V. insulin, there must be an adequate level of insulin in the bloodstream before discontinuing the insulin drip; otherwise, the glucose level will rise. Adding an I.V. antibiotic has no influence on the insulin drip; it should not be piggy-backed into the insulin drip. Glargine (Lantus) cannot be administered I.V., and should not be mixed with other insulins or solutions. (M)

28. 1. A rare but serious adverse effect of metformin (Glucophage) is lactic acidosis; half the cases are fatal. Ideally, one should stop metformin for 2 days before and 2 days after drinking alcohol. Signs and symptoms of lactic acidosis are weakness, fatigue, unusual muscle pain, dyspnea, unusual stomach discomfort, dizziness or lightheadedness, and bradycardia or cardiac arrhythmias. Bloating is not an adverse effect of metformin. (D)

29. 3. Oral hypoglycemic agents of the sulfonylurea group, such as tolbutamide (Orinase), lower the blood glucose level by stimulating functioning beta cells in the pancreas to release insulin. These agents also increase insulin's ability to bind to the body's cells. They may also act to increase the number of insulin receptors in the body. Tolbu-

tamide does not potentiate the action of insulin. Tolbutamide does not lower the renal threshold of glucose, which would not be a factor in the treatment of diabetes in any case. Tolbutamide does not combine with glucose to render it inert. (D)

30. 1, 5. Being overweight and having a large waist-hip ratio (central abdominal obesity) increase insulin resistance, making control of diabetes more difficult. The ADA recommends a yearly referral to an ophthalmologist and podiatrist. Exercise and weight management decrease insulin resistance. Insulin is not always needed for type 2 diabetes; diet, exercise, and oral medications are the first-line treatment. The client must monitor all nutritional sources for a balanced diet—fats, carbohydrates, and protein. (R)

31. 1. The client with diabetes is prone to serious foot injuries secondary to peripheral neuropathy and decreased circulation. The client should be taught to avoid going barefoot to prevent injury. Shoes that do not fit properly should not be worn because they will cause blisters that can become nonhealing, serious wounds for the diabetic client. Toenails should be cut straight across. A heating pad should not be used because of the risk of burns due to insensitivity to temperature. (R)

32. 2. A client with diabetes should be advised to consult a physician or podiatrist for corn removal because of the danger of traumatizing the foot tissue and potential development of ulcers. The diabetic client should never self-treat foot problems but should consult a physician or podiatrist. (R)

33. 2. Proper and careful first-aid treatment is important when a client with diabetes has a skin cut or laceration. The skin should be kept supple and as free of organisms as possible. Washing and bandaging the cut will accomplish this. Washing wounds with alcohol is too caustic and drying to the skin. Having the children help is an unrealistic suggestion and does not educate the client about proper care of wounds. Tight control of blood glucose levels through adherence to the medication regimen is vitally important; however, it does not mean that careful attention to cuts can be ignored. (R)

34. 4. Diabetes mellitus is a multifactorial, systemic disease associated with problems in the metabolism of all food types. The client's diet should contain appropriate amounts of all three nutrients, plus adequate minerals and vitamins. (C)

35. 1. Deep, rapid respirations with long expirations is indicative of Kussmaul's respirations, which occur in metabolic acidosis. The respirations increase in rate and depth, and the breath has a "fruity" or acetone-like odor.

This breathing pattern is the body's attempt to blow off carbon dioxide and acetone, thus compensating for the acidosis. The other breathing patterns listed are not related to ketoacidosis and would not compensate for the acidosis. (A)

36. 1, 2, 3, 4, 5. The client with unstable diabetes mellitus is at risk for many microvascular and macrovascular complications. Heart disease is the leading cause of mortality in clients with diabetes. The goal blood pressure for diabetics is less than 130/80 mm Hg. Therefore, the nurse would need to report any findings greater than 130/80 mm Hg. The goal of HbA_{1c} is less than 7%; thus, a level of 10.2% must be reported. HDL less than 40 mg/dl and triglycerides greater than 150 mg/dl are risk factors for heart disease. The nurse would need to report the client's HDL and triglyceride levels. The urine ketones are negative, but this is a late sign of complications when there is a profound insulin deficiency. (R)

37. 4. A client with diabetes who takes any first- or second-generation sulfonylurea should be advised to avoid alcohol intake. Sulfonylureas in combination with alcohol can cause serious disulfiram (Antabuse)–like reactions, including flushing, angina, palpitations, and vertigo. Serious reactions, such as seizures and possibly death, may also occur. Hypokalemia, hyperkalemia, and hypocalcemia do not result from taking sulfonylureas in combination with alcohol. (A)

38. 3. The most important factor predisposing to the development of type 2 diabetes mellitus is obesity. Insulin resistance increases with obesity. Cigarette smoking is not a predisposing factor, but it is a risk factor that increases complications of diabetes mellitus. A high-cholesterol diet does not necessarily predispose to diabetes mellitus, but it may contribute to obesity and hyperlipidemia. Hypertension is not a predisposing factor, but it is a risk factor for developing complications of diabetes mellitus. (H)

39. 2. The client with diabetes mellitus is especially prone to hypertension due to atherosclerotic changes, which leads to problems of the microvascular and macrovascular systems. This can result in complications in the heart, brain, and kidneys. Heart disease and stroke are twice as common among people with diabetes mellitus than among people without the disease. Painful, inflamed joints accompany rheumatoid arthritis. A stooped appearance accompanies osteoporosis with narrowing of the vertebral column. A low hemoglobin concentration accompanies anemia, especially iron deficiency anemia and anemia of chronic disease. (R)

40. 1. Although some individual variation exists, when the blood glucose level decreases to less than 70 mg/dl, the client experiences or is at risk for hypoglycemia. Hypoglycemia can occur in both type 1 and type 2 diabetes mellitus, although it is more common when the client is taking insulin. The nurse should instruct the client on the prevention, detection, and treatment of hypoglycemia. (A)

41. 4. Diabetic retinopathy, cataracts, and glaucoma are common complications in diabetics, necessitating eye assessment and examination. The feet should also be examined at each client encounter, monitoring for thickening, fissures, or breaks in the skin; ulcers; and thickened nails. Although assessments of the abdomen, pharynx, and lymph glands are included in a thorough examination, they are not pertinent to common diabetic complications. (R)

42. 4. The client with diabetes mellitus who is taking NPH insulin (Humulin N) in the evening is most likely to become hypoglycemic shortly after midnight because this insulin peaks in 6 to 8 hours. The client should eat a bedtime snack to help prevent hypoglycemia while sleeping. (D)

43. 3. If the client engages in an activity or exercise that focuses on one area of the body, that area may cause inconsistent absorption of insulin. A good regimen for a jogger is to inject the abdomen for 1 week and then rotate to the buttock. A jogger may have inconsistent absorption in the legs or arms with strenuous running. The iliac crest is not an appropriate site due to a lack of loose skin and subcutaneous tissue in that area. (D)

44. 1. Insulin lispro (Humalog) begins to act within 10 to 15 minutes and lasts approximately 4 hours. A major advantage of Humalog is that the client can eat almost immediately after the insulin is administered. The client needs to be instructed regarding the onset, peak, and duration of all insulin, as meals need to be timed with these parameters. Waiting 1 hour to eat may precipitate hypoglycemia. Eating 2 hours before the insulin lispro could cause hyperglycemia if the client does not have circulating insulin to metabolize the carbohydrate. (D)

45. 1. The nurse should judge that learning has occurred from evidence of a change in the client's behavior. A client who performs a procedure safely and correctly demonstrates that he has acquired a skill. Evaluation of this skill acquisition requires performance of that skill by the client with observation by the nurse. The client must also demonstrate cognitive understanding, as shown by the ability to critique the nurse's performance. Explaining the steps demonstrates acquisition of knowledge at the cognitive level only. A posttest does not indicate the degree to which the client has learned a psychomotor skill. (D)

46. 32

Clients commonly need to mix insulin, requiring careful mixing and calculation. The total dosage is 10 units plus 22 units, for a total of 32 units. (D)

47. 3. Renal failure frequently results from the vascular changes associated with diabetes mellitus. ACE inhibitors increase renal blood flow and are effective in decreasing diabetic nephropathy. Chronic obstructive pulmonary disease is not a complication of diabetes, nor is it prevented by ACE inhibitors. Pancreatic cancer is neither prevented by ACE inhibitors nor considered a complication of diabetes. Cerebrovascular accident is not directly prevented by ACE inhibitors, although management of hypertension will decrease vascular disease. (D)

48. 1. The four most commonly reported signs and symptoms of hypoglycemia are nervousness, weakness, perspiration, and confusion. Other signs and symptoms include hunger, incoherent speech, tachycardia, and blurred vision. Anorexia and Kussmaul's respirations are clinical manifestations of hyperglycemia or ketoacidosis. Bradycardia is not associated with hypoglycemia; tachycardia is. (R)

49. 2. Steroids can cause hyperglycemia because of their effects on carbohydrate metabolism, making diabetic control more difficult. Aspirin is not known to affect glucose metabolism. Sulfonylureas are oral hypoglycemic agents used in the treatment of diabetes mellitus. ACE inhibitors are not known to affect glucose metabolism. (D)

50. 1. Colds and influenza present special challenges to the client with diabetes mellitus because the body's need for insulin increases during illness. Therefore, the client must take the prescribed insulin dose, increase the frequency of blood glucose testing, and maintain an adequate fluid intake to counteract the dehydrating effect of hyperglycemia. Clear fluids, juices, and Gatorade are encouraged. Not taking insulin when sick, or taking half the normal dose, may cause the client to develop ketoacidosis. (R)

51. 1. *Imbalanced nutrition: Less than body requirements* is a priority nursing diagnosis for the client with diabetes mellitus who is experiencing vomiting with influenza. The diabetic client should eat small, frequent meals of 50 g of carbohydrate or food equal to 200 calories every 3 to 4 hours. If the client cannot eat the carbohydrates or take fluids, the health care provider should be called or the client should go to the emergency department. The diabetic client is in danger of complications with dehydration, electrolyte imbalance, and ketoacidosis. Increasing the client's coping skills is important to lifestyle behaviors, but it is not a priority during this acute illness of influenza.

Pain relief may be a need for this client, but it is not the priority at this time; neither is intolerance for activity. (C)

52. 4. The best response is to allow the client to verbalize her fears about giving herself a shot each day. Tactics that increase fear are not effective in changing behavior. If possible, the client needs to be responsible for her own care, including giving self-injections. It is unlikely that the client's insurance company will pay for home-care visits if the client is capable of self-administration. (P)

53. 4. Deficient fluid volume, causing dehydration and possible hypovolemic shock, is the main problem in diabetic ketoacidosis because increased osmolarity from the glucose leads to a fluid shift from the intracellular to the extracellular space. The fluid shift leads to increased renal excretion of glucose and fluid. Severe dehydration, electrolyte imbalance, and possible hypovolemic shock is a medical emergency requiring immediate administration of insulin and I.V. fluid and electrolytes. *Insomnia* is not a priority nursing diagnosis for the critically ill client. It is possible that the client's condition has resulted from ineffective health maintenance; however, physiologic problems and diagnoses take priority over psychosocial problems and diagnoses. There are no data to support the diagnosis of *Imbalanced nutrition*. (A)

The Client with Pituitary Adenoma

54. 1. Galactorrhea, or abnormal flow of breast milk, results from overproduction of prolactin. Pituitary tumors are almost always secreting tumors, and they are classified by the specific hormone secreted. Pituitary tumors can cause oversecretion of ACTH, GH, or TSH. Overproduction of ACTH results in Cushing's disease. Overproduction of GH results in gigantism. Overproduction of TSH results in hyperthyroidism. (A)

55. 2. Excessive prolactin secretion in men results in decreased libido and impotence; these are often the only significant signs and symptoms until the tumor becomes large. Signs and symptoms of pituitary tumors result from both the presence of a space-occupying mass in the cranium and the excess secretion of hormones. Lethargy and fatigue are associated with hypothyroidism or Addisonian crisis. Bony proliferation and voice changes are associated with excessive growth hormone. (A)

56. 4. With transsphenoidal hypophysectomy, the sella turcica is entered from below, through the sphenoid sinus. There is no external incision; the incision is made between the upper lip and gums. (R)

57. 3. Deep breathing is the best choice for helping prevent atelectasis. The client should be placed in the semi-Fowler's position (or as ordered) and taught deep breathing, sighing, mouth breathing, and how to avoid coughing. Blow bottles are not effective in preventing atelectasis because they do not promote sustained alveolar inflation to maximal lung capacity. Frequent position changes help loosen lung secretions, but deep breathing is most important in preventing atelectasis. Coughing is contraindicated because it increases intracranial pressure and can cause cerebrospinal fluid to leak from the point at which the sella turcica was entered. (R)

58. **1.** A major focus of nursing care after transsphenoidal hypophysectomy is prevention of and monitoring for a CSF leak. CSF leakage can occur if the patch or incision is disrupted. The nurse should monitor for signs of infection, including elevated temperature, increased white blood cell count, rhinorrhea, nuchal rigidity, and persistent headache. Hypoglycemia and adrenocortical insufficiency may occur. Monitoring for fluctuating blood glucose levels is not related specifically to transsphenoidal hypophysectomy. The client will be given I.V. fluids postoperatively to supply carbohydrates. Cushing's disease results from adrenocortical excess, not insufficiency. Monitoring for postoperative complications contributing to possible cardiac arrest is always important, but it is not related specifically to transsphenoidal hypophysectomy. (R)

59. **1.** The client's sexual problems are directly related to the excessive prolactin level. Removing the source of excessive hormone secretion should allow the client to return gradually to a normal physiologic pattern. Fertility will return, and erectile function and sexual desire will return to baseline as hormone levels return to normal. (A)

60. **3.** The dural opening is typically repaired with a patch of muscle or fascia taken from the abdomen or thigh. The client should be prepared preoperatively for the presence of this additional incision in the abdomen or thigh. The client will need the patch of muscle or fascia to replace the dura. Disposable sutures alone will not provide an intact suture line. Nasal packing will not provide closure for the dural opening. A synthetic mesh is not the tissue of choice for surgical repair of the dura. (R)

61. **3.** If CSF leakage is suspected or confirmed, the client is treated initially with bed rest with the head of the bed elevated to decrease pressure on the graft site. Most leaks heal spontaneously, but occasionally surgical repair of the site in the sella turcica is needed. Repacking the nose will not heal the leak at the graft site in the dura. The client will not be returned to surgery immediately because most leaks heal spontaneously. High-dose corticosteroid therapy is not effective in healing a CSF leak. (A)

62. **1.** After transsphenoidal surgery, the client must be careful not to disturb the suture line while healing occurs. Frequent oral care should be provided with rinses of saline, and the teeth may be gently cleaned with Toothettes. Frequent or vigorous toothbrushing or flossing is contraindicated because it may disturb or cause tension on the suture line. (A)

63. **4.** Most clients who undergo adenoma removal experience a gradual return of normal pituitary secretion and do not experience complications. However, hypopituitarism can cause growth hormone, gonadotropin, thyroid-stimulating hormone, and adrenocorticotropic hormone deficits. The client should be taught to monitor for change in mental status, energy level, muscle strength, and cognitive function. In adults, changes in sexual function, impotence, or decreased libido should be reported. Acromegaly and Cushing's disease are conditions of hypersecretion. Diabetes mellitus is related to the function of the pancreas and is not directly related to the function of the pituitary. (R)

64. **1.** Pituitary diabetes insipidus is a potential complication after pituitary surgery because of possible interference with the production of antidiuretic hormone (ADH). One major manifestation of diabetes insipidus is polyuria because lack of ADH results in insufficient water reabsorption by the kidneys. The polyuria leads to a decreased urine specific gravity (between 1.001 and 1.010). The client may drink and excrete 5 to 40 L of fluid daily. Diabetes insipidus does not affect metabolism. A blood glucose level higher than 300 mg/dl is associated with impaired glucose metabolism or diabetes mellitus. Urine negative for sugar and ketones is normal. (R)

65. **2.** The major characteristic of diabetes insipidus is decreased tubular reabsorption of water due to insufficient amounts of antidiuretic hormone (ADH). Vasopressin (Pitressin) is administered to the client with diabetes insipidus because it has pressor and ADH activities. Vasopressin works to increase the concentration of the urine by increasing tubular reabsorption, thus preserving up to 90% water. Vasopressin is administered to the client with diabetes insipidus because it is a synthetic ADH. The administration of vasopressin results in increased tubular reabsorption of water, and it is effective for emergency treatment or daily maintenance of mild diabetes insipidus. Vasopressin does not decrease blood pressure or affect insulin production or glucose metabolism, nor is insulin production a factor in diabetes insipidus. (D)

66. **1.** Because diabetes insipidus involves excretion of large amounts of fluid, maintaining normal fluid and electrolyte balance is a priority for this client. Special dietary programs or restrictions are not indicated in treatment of diabetes insipidus. Serum glucose levels are priorities in diabetes mellitus but not in diabetes insipidus. (A)

The Client with Addison's Disease

67. 4. Adrenal crisis can occur with physical stress, such as surgery, dental work, infection, flu, trauma, and pregnancy. In these situations, glucocorticoid and mineralocorticoid dosages are increased. Weight loss, not gain, occurs with adrenal insufficiency. Psychological stress has less effect on corticosteroid need than physical stress. (R)

68. 2. Addison's disease is caused by a deficiency of adrenal corticosteroids and can result in severe hypotension and shock because of uncontrolled loss of sodium in the urine and impaired mineralocorticoid function. This results in loss of extracellular fluid and dangerously low blood volume. Glucocorticoids must be administered to reverse hypotension. Preventing infection is not an appropriate goal of care in this life-threatening situation. Relieving anxiety is appropriate when the client's condition is stabilized, but the calm, competent demeanor of the emergency department staff will be initially reassuring. (A)

69. 2. Adrenal hormone deficiency can cause profound physiologic changes. The client may experience severe pain (headache, abdominal pain, back pain, or pain in the extremities). Inhibited gluconeogenesis commonly produces hypoglycemia, and impaired sodium retention causes decreased, not increased, fluid volume. Edema would not be expected. Gastrointestinal disturbances, including nausea and vomiting, are expected findings in Addison's disease, not hunger. (A)

70. 1. Signs of infiltration include slowing of the infusion and swelling, pain, hardness, pallor, and coolness of the skin at the site. If these signs occur, the I.V. line should be discontinued and restarted at another infusion site. The new anatomic site, time, and type of cannula used should be documented. The nurse may apply a warm soak to the site, but only after the I.V. line is discontinued. Parenteral administration of fluids should not be stopped intermittently. Stopping the flow does not treat the problem, nor does it address the client's needs for fluid replacement. Infiltrated I.V. sites should not be irrigated; doing so will only cause more swelling and pain. (D)

71. 1. Each liter of 5% dextrose in normal saline solution contains 170 calories. The nurse should consult with the physician and dietitian when a client is on I.V. therapy or is on nothing-by-mouth status for an extended period because further electrolyte supplementation or alimentation therapy may be needed. (D)

72. 3. Electrolyte imbalances associated with Addison's disease include hypoglycemia, hyponatremia, and hyperkalemia. Salted bouillon and fruit juices provide glucose and sodium to replenish these deficits. Diet soda does not contain sugar. Water could cause further sodium dilution. Coffee's diuretic effect would aggravate the fluid deficit. Milk contains potassium and sodium. (C)

73. 2. Finding alternative methods of dealing with stress, such as relaxation techniques, is a cornerstone of stress management. Removing all sources of stress from one's life is not possible. Antianxiety drugs are prescribed for temporary management during periods of major stress, and they are not an intervention in stress management classes. Avoiding discussion of stressful situations will not necessarily reduce stress. (P)

74. 3. Primary Addison's disease refers to a problem in the gland itself that results from idiopathic atrophy of the glands. The process is believed to be autoimmune in nature. The most common causes of primary adrenocortical insufficiency are autoimmune destruction (70%) and tuberculosis (20%). Insufficient secretion of GH causes dwarfism or growth delay. Hyposecretion of glucocorticoids, aldosterone, and androgens occur with Addison's disease. Pituitary dysfunction can cause Addison's disease, but this is not a primary disease process. Oversecretion of the adrenal medulla causes pheochromocytoma. (A)

75. 2, 3, 4, 5, 6. Addison's disease occurs when the client does not produce enough steroids from the adrenal cortex. Lifetime steroid replacement is needed. The client should be taught lifestyle management techniques to avoid stress and maintain rest periods. A medical identification bracelet should be worn and the family should be taught signs and symptoms that indicate an impending adrenal crisis, such as fatigue, weakness, dizziness, or mood changes. Dental work, infections, and surgery commonly require an adjusted dosage of steroids. (A)

76. 3. Although many of the disease signs and symptoms are vague and nonspecific, most clients experience lethargy and depression as early symptoms. Other early signs and symptoms include mood changes, emotional lability, irritability, weight loss, muscle weakness, fatigue, nausea, and vomiting. Most clients experience a loss of appetite. Muscles become weak, not spastic, because of adrenocortical insufficiency. (A)

77. 3. Decreased hepatic gluconeogenesis and increased tissue glucose uptake cause hypoglycemia in clients with Addison's disease. Hyperkalemia and hyponatremia are characteristic of Addison's disease. There is decreased renal perfusion and excretion of waste products, which causes an elevated BUN level. (R)

78. 1. The need for glucocorticoids changes with circumstances. The basal dose is established when the client is discharged, but this dose covers only normal daily needs and does not provide for additional stressors. As the manager of the medication schedule, the client needs to know signs and symptoms of excessive and insufficient dosages. Glucocorticoid needs fluctuate. Glucocorticoids are not cumulative and must be taken daily. They must never be discontinued suddenly; in the absence of endogenous production, addisonian crisis could result. Two-thirds of the daily dose should be taken at about 8 a.m. and the remainder at about 4 p.m. This schedule approximates the diurnal pattern of normal secretion, with highest levels between 4 a.m. and 6 a.m. and lowest levels in the evening. (D)

79. 3. Fludrocortisone acetate (Florinef Acetate) can be administered once a day, but cortisone acetate (Cortone) administration should follow the body's natural diurnal pattern of secretion. Greater amounts of cortisol are secreted during the day to meet increased demand of the body. Typically, baseline administration of cortisone acetate is 25 mg in the morning and 12.5 mg in the afternoon. Taking it three times a day would result in an excessive dose. Taking the drug only in the morning would not meet the needs of the body later in the day and evening. (D)

80. 4. Oral steroids can cause gastric irritation and ulcers and should be administered with meals, if possible, or otherwise with an antacid. Only instructing the client to take the medication with a full glass of water will not help prevent gastric complications from steroids. Steroids should never be taken on an empty stomach. Glucocorticoids should be taken in the morning, not at bedtime. (D)

81. 4. Measuring daily weight is a reliable, objective way to monitor fluid balance. Rapid variations in weight reflect changes in fluid volume, which suggests insufficient control of the disease and the need for more glucocorticoids in the client with Addison's disease. Nurses should instruct clients taking oral steroids to weigh themselves daily and to report any unusual weight loss or gain. Skin turgor testing does supply information about fluid status, but daily weight monitoring is more reliable. Temperature is not a direct measurement of fluid balance. Thirst is a nonspecific and very late sign of weight loss. (D)

82. 3. Rapid weight gain, because it reflects excess fluids, is a warning sign that the client is receiving too much hormone replacement. It may be difficult to individualize the correct dosage for a client taking glucocorticoids, and the therapeutic range between underdosage and overdosage is narrow. Maintaining the client on the lowest dose that provides satisfactory clinical response is always the goal of pharmacotherapeutics. Fluid balance is an important indicator of the adequacy of hormone replacement. Anorexia is not present with glucocorticoid therapy because these drugs increase the appetite. Dizziness is not specific to the effects of glucocorticoid therapy. Poor skin turgor is a late sign of fluid volume deficit. (D)

83. 1. Medication compliance is an essential part of the self-care required to manage Addison's disease. The client must learn to adjust the glucocorticoid dose in response to the normal and unexpected stresses of daily living. The nurse should instruct the client never to stop taking the drug without consulting the health care provider to avoid an addisonian crisis. Regularity in daily habits makes adjustment easier, but the client should not be encouraged to withdraw from normal activities to avoid stress. The client does not need to restrict sodium. The client is at risk for hyponatremia. Hypotension, not hypertension, is more common with Addison's disease. (R)

84. 3. Illness or surgery places tremendous stress on the body, necessitating increased glucocorticoid dosage. Extreme emotional or psychological stress also necessitates dosage adjustment. Increased dosages are needed in times of stress to prevent drug-induced adrenal insufficiency. Returning to work after the weekend, going on a vacation, or having a routine checkup usually will not alter glucocorticoid dosage needs. (R)

85. 4. Bronzing, or general deepening of skin pigmentation, is a classic sign of Addison's disease and is caused by melanocyte-stimulating hormone produced in response to increased ACTH secretion. The hyperpigmentation is typically found in the distal portion of extremities and in areas exposed to sun. Additionally, areas that may not be exposed to sun, such as the nipples, genitalia, tongue, and knuckles, become bronze-colored. Treatment of Addison's disease usually reverses the hyperpigmentation. Bilirubin level is not related to the pathophysiology of Addison's disease. Hyperpigmentation is not related to the effects of the glucocorticoid therapy. (A)

86. 1. Weakness, fatigue, lethargy, and inability to perform usual activities are major problems for the client experiencing addisonian crisis. A client in crisis requires bed rest until the crisis has been resolved and hormone levels return to normal. A client with addisonian crisis experiences nausea, not increased appetite, and a nursing diagnosis of *Imbalanced nutrition: Less than body requirements. Deficient fluid volume,* not excess, is another priority diagnosis. (A)

The Client with Cushing's Disease

87. 3. Skin bruising from increased skin and blood vessel fragility is a classic sign of Cushing's disease. Hyperpigmentation and bruising are caused by the hypersecretion of glucocorticoids. Fluid retention causes hypertension, not hypotension. Muscle wasting occurs in the extremities. Hair on the head thins, while body hair increases. (A)

88. 2. In Cushing's disease, excessive cortisol secretion causes rapid protein catabolism, depleting the collagen support of the skin. The skin becomes thin and fragile and susceptible to easy bruising. The typical "cushingoid" appearance of the client includes a moon face, buffalo hump, central obesity, and thin musculature. Weight gain, mood swings, and slow wound healing are other signs and symptoms of Cushing's disease. Hypertension, not hypotension, is a sign of Cushing's disease. Abdominal pain is not a symptom of Cushing's disease. (A)

89. 3. Excessive levels of glucocorticoids, aldosterone, and androgens secreted from the adrenal cortex result in the constellation of symptoms known as Cushing's disease. Cushing's disease can be caused by a tumor, overstimulation from the pituitary, or the use of prescription steroid drugs. Androgens are also secreted in excess. ACTH is only one hormone that is abnormal in Cushing's disease. Excessive secretion of catecholamines accompanies pheochromocytoma, a disease of the adrenal medulla. (A)

90. 2. Sodium retention is typically accompanied by potassium depletion. Hypertension, hypokalemia, edema, and heart failure may result from the hypersecretion of aldosterone. The client with Cushing's disease exhibits postprandial or persistent hyperglycemia. Clients with Cushing's disease have hypernatremia, not hyponatremia. Bone resorption of calcium increases the urine calcium level. (R)

91. 3. Cushing's disease is commonly caused by loss of the diurnal cortisol secretion pattern. The client's random morning cortisol level may be within normal limits, but secretion continues at that level throughout the entire day. Cortisol levels should normally decrease after the morning peak. Analysis of a 24-hour urine specimen is often useful in identifying the cumulative excess. Clients will not have symptoms with normal cortisol levels. Hormones are present in the blood. (R)

92. 2. A primary dietary intervention is to restrict sodium, thereby reducing fluid retention. Increased protein catabolism results in loss of muscle mass and necessitates supplemental protein intake. The client may be asked to restrict total calories to reduce weight. The client should be encouraged to eat potassium-rich foods because serum levels are typically depleted. Although reducing fat intake as part of an overall plan to restrict calories is appropriate, fat intake of less than 20% of total calories is not recommended. (C)

93. 2. Osteoporosis is a serious outcome of prolonged cortisol excess because calcium is resorbed out of the bone. Regular daily weight-bearing exercise (e.g., brisk walking) is an effective way to drive calcium back into the bones. The client should also be instructed to have a dietary or supplemental intake of calcium of 1,500 mg daily. Potassium levels are not relevant to prevention of bone resorption. Vitamin D is needed to aid in the absorption of calcium. Isometric exercises condition muscle tone but do not build bones. (R)

94. 2. Effective splinting for a high incision reduces stress on the incision line, decreases pain, and increases the client's ability to deep-breathe effectively. Deep breathing should be done hourly by the client after surgery. Sitting upright ignores the need to splint the incision to prevent pain. Tightening the stomach muscles is not an effective strategy for promoting deep breathing. Raising the shoulders is not a feature of deep-breathing exercises. (A)

95. 3. The priority in the first 24 hours after adrenalectomy is to identify and prevent adrenal crisis. Monitoring of vital signs is the most important evaluation measure. Hypotension, tachycardia, orthostatic hypotension, and arrhythmias can be indicators of pending vascular collapse and hypovolemic shock that can occur with adrenal crisis. Beginning oral nutrition is important, but not necessarily in the first 24 hours after surgery, and it is not more important than preventing adrenal crisis. Promoting self-care activities is not as important as preventing adrenal crisis. Ambulating in the hallway is not a priority in the first 24 hours after adrenalectomy. (A)

96. 3. Hydromorphone hydrochloride (Dilaudid) is about five times more potent than morphine sulfate, from which it is prepared. Therefore, it is administered only in small doses. Hydromorphone hydrochloride can cause dependency in any dose; however, fear of dependency developing in the postoperative period is unwarranted. The dose is determined by the client's need for pain relief. Hydromorphone hydrochloride is not irritating to subcutaneous tissues. As with opioid analgesics, excretion depends on normal liver function. (D)

97. 1. Ketoconazole (Nizoral) suppresses adrenal steroid secretion and may cause acute hypoadrenalism. The adverse effect should reverse when the drug is discontinued. Ketoconazole does not destroy adrenal cells; mitotane (Lysodren) destroys the cells and may be used to obtain a medical adrenalectomy. Ketoconazole decreases, not increases, ACTH-induced serum corticosteroid levels. It increases the duration of adrenal suppression when given with steroids. (D)

98. 2. Poor lung expansion from bed rest, pain, and retained anesthesia is a common cause of slight postoperative temperature elevation. Nursing care includes turning the client and having the client cough and deep-breathe every 1 to 2 hours, or more frequently as ordered. The client will have postoperative I.V. fluid replacement ordered to prevent dehydration. Wound infections typically appear 4 to 7 days after surgery. Urinary tract infections would not be typical with this surgery. (A)

99. 3. Pain control should be evaluated at least every 2 hours for the client with a PCA system. Addiction is not a common problem for the postoperative client. A client should not be encouraged to tolerate pain; in fact, other nursing actions besides PCA should be implemented to enhance the action of opioids. One of the purposes of PCA is for the client to determine frequency of administering the medication; the nurse should not interfere unless the client is not obtaining pain relief. The nurse should ensure that the client is instructed on the use of the PCA control button and that the button is always within reach. (D)

100. 4. Alternately flexing and relaxing the quadriceps femoris muscles helps prepare the client for ambulation. This exercise helps maintain the strength in the quadriceps, which is the major muscle group used when walking. The other exercises listed do not increase a client's readiness for walking. (C)

101. 1. Decreased mobility is one of the most common causes of abdominal distention related to retained gas in the intestines. Peristalsis has been inhibited by the general anesthesia, analgesics, and inactivity during the immediate postoperative period. Ambulation increases peristaltic activity and helps move gas. Walking can prevent the need for a rectal tube, which is a more invasive procedure. An NG tube is also a more invasive procedure and requires a physician's order. It is not a preferred treatment for gas postoperatively. Walking should prevent the need for further interventions. Carbonated liquids can increase gas formation. (R)

102. 2. Persistent cortisol excess undermines the collagen matrix of the skin, impairing wound healing. It also carries an increased risk of infection and of bleeding. The wound should be observed and documentation performed regarding the status of healing. Confusion and emboli are not expected complications after adrenalectomy. Malnutrition also is not an expected complication after adrenalectomy. Nutritional status should be regained postoperatively. (R)

103. 2. As the body readjusts to normal cortisol levels, mood and physical changes will gradually return to a normal state. The body changes are not permanent, and the mood swings should level off. (A)

104. 3. Testosterone is an androgen hormone that is responsible for protein metabolism as well as maintenance of secondary sexual characteristics. Therefore, it is needed by both males and females. Removal of both adrenal glands necessitates replacement of glucocorticoids and androgens. Testosterone does not balance the reproductive cycle, stabilize mood swings, or, in this situation, stimulate protein anabolism. (A)

105. 1. Bilateral adrenalectomy requires lifelong adrenal hormone replacement therapy. If unilateral surgery is performed, most clients gradually reestablish a normal secretion pattern. The client and family will require extensive teaching and support to maintain self-care management at home. Information on dosing, adverse effects, what to do if a dose is missed, and follow-up examinations is needed in the teaching plan. Although steroids are tapered when given for an intermittent or one-time problem, they are not discontinued when given to clients who have undergone bilateral adrenalectomy because the clients will not regain the ability to manufacture steroids. Steroids must be taken on a daily basis, not just during periods of physical or emotional stress. (A)

The Female Client with Perimenopausal or Menopausal Syndrome

106. 2. Deficiency of estrogen causes the major characteristics of perimenopause and menopause. As estrogen decreases, many physiologic changes occur with perimenopause. Although many of the changes occur in the female reproductive system, other organs and systems are affected as well. Progesterone is the hormone responsible for maintaining pregnancy. Prolactin is one of the hormones responsible for lactation. Oxytocin is secreted by the posterior pituitary and is responsible for labor. (A)

107. 1. As the ovarian follicle ceases to produce estrogen, menopause occurs. The endocrine changes that occur in menopause due to cessation of the ovarian follicle include hot flashes, headaches, and mood changes with irritability and anxiety. (A)

108. 2. Unopposed estrogen in a woman with an intact uterus can cause overgrowth of the endometrium, or endometrial hyperplasia. This hyperplasia can be a precursor to endometrial cancer. Estrogen is effective in the control of hot flashes. If libido is a major problem, testosterone is usually deficient. Hormone replacement therapy (HRT) is not known to be related to the incidence of ovarian cancer but it is considered a risk factor for breast cancer. HRT should be used at the lowest dosage for the shortest period of time to control hot flashes. (D)

109. 3. A woman with severe hot flashes is a candidate for HRT for a short time in the lowest dosage possible. A family or personal history of breast cancer or a history of estrogen-dependent dysplasia is an absolute contraindication for HRT. (D)

110. 2. Endometrial or uterine cancer is a potential complication for postmenopausal women on HRT. Unfortunately, no signs or symptoms except irregular vaginal bleeding are evident in endometrial or uterine cancer. A menopausal or postmenopausal woman with irregular bleeding requires a biopsy to rule out endometrial or uterine cancer. Hot flashes may occur but are not a danger sign. Vaginal dryness, a common complaint during menopause, can be treated with vaginal lubricants. However, this condition is not life-threatening. Changes in vaginal pH may occur but need not be reported. (R)

The Client with Pheochromocytoma

111. 3. Pheochromocytomas release catecholamines, both epinephrine and norepinephrine. The excessive hormone secretion can be constant or episodic, producing constant or episodic severe hypertension. The pheochromocytoma does not cause release of renin, aldosterone, or glucocorticoids. (A)

112. 3. The release of catecholamines, epinephrine and norepinephrine, causes hypertension that is resistant to treatment. Although pheochromocytoma accounts for fewer than 1% of the cases of hypertension, it is important to diagnose so the client may be correctly treated. The hypertension occurs with both systolic and diastolic pressures, and the pressures may be very labile. Widening pulse pressure is not related to pheochromocytoma. (R)

113. 4. Postoperative management is directed at maintaining a normal blood pressure because the client may be hypertensive immediately after surgery. The nurse must monitor blood pressure frequently and report abnormalities. Clients in hypertensive crisis should be in an intensive care unit for cardiac, blood pressure, and neurologic monitoring. Orthostatic hypotension may be a concern for clients on prolonged bed rest or with fluid deficits. Although hemorrhage may accompany surgery, it is unlikely with this surgery. Elevated blood glucose concentrations, not hypoglycemia, occur with pheochromocytoma. (R)

114. 2. Bending, lifting, and the Valsalva maneuver can precipitate hypertensive crises or paroxysms. These activities increase transabdominal pressure and may cause cardiac-stimulating effects. The blood pressure is very labile with these activities, and paroxysms may be accompanied by tachycardia, palpitations, angina, or electrocardiographic changes. Jogging, anxiety, and hypoglycemia are not triggers for hypertensive crises or paroxysms. (M)

115. 3. A beta blocker such as propranolol (Inderal) is administered to block the cardiac-stimulating effects of epinephrine. ACE inhibitors and calcium channel blockers do not block sympathetic activity as beta blockers do. Diuretics decrease fluid volume and peripheral resistance, but they do not block sympathetic activity. (D)

The Client with Urinary Tract Health Problems

- The Client with Cancer of the Bladder
- The Client with Renal Calculi
- The Client with Acute Renal Failure
- The Client with Urinary Tract Infection
- The Client with Pyelonephritis
- The Client with Chronic Renal Failure
- The Client with Urinary Incontinence
- Correct Answers and Rationales

The Client with Cancer of the Bladder

1. A client has undergone a cystectomy and an ileal conduit diversion. What should the nurse incorporate into the discharge instructions? Select all that apply.
- [ ] **1.** Drink at least 3,000 ml of fluid each day.
- [ ] **2.** Minimize daily activities.
- [ ] **3.** Keep urine alkaline to prevent urinary tract infections.
- [ ] **4.** Avoid odor-producing foods, such as onions, fish, eggs, and cheese.
- [ ] **5.** Wear snug clothing over the stoma to encourage urine flow into the drainage bag.

2. A nurse is caring for a client with an ileal conduit. Which undesirable outcome can occur if the nurse and client do not take meticulous care of the stoma? Select all that apply.
- [ ] **1.** Dermatitis.
- [ ] **2.** Bleeding.
- [ ] **3.** Fungal infection.
- [ ] **4.** Flow of adhesive solvent into the stoma.
- [ ] **5.** Partial obstruction of the stoma from skin cement.

3. Which of the following symptoms is the most common clinical finding associated with bladder cancer?
- [ ] **1.** Suprapubic pain.
- [ ] **2.** Dysuria.
- [ ] **3.** Painless hematuria.
- [ ] **4.** Urine retention.

4. A client is to have a cystoscopy to rule out cancer of the bladder. Which of the following signs and symptoms would indicate that the client has developed a complication after the cystoscopy?
- [ ] **1.** Dizziness.
- [ ] **2.** Chills.
- [ ] **3.** Pink-tinged urine.
- [ ] **4.** Bladder spasms.

5. If the client develops lower abdominal pain after a cystoscopy, the nurse should instruct the client to do which of the following?
- [ ] **1.** Apply an ice pack to the pubic area.
- [ ] **2.** Massage the abdomen gently.
- [ ] **3.** Ambulate as much as possible.
- [ ] **4.** Sit in a tub of warm water.

6. A client who has been diagnosed with bladder cancer is scheduled for an ileal conduit. Preoperatively, the nurse reinforces the client's understanding of the surgical procedure by explaining that an ileal conduit:
- [ ] **1.** Is a temporary procedure that can be reversed later.
- [ ] **2.** Diverts urine into the sigmoid colon, where it is expelled through the rectum.
- [ ] **3.** Conveys urine from the ureters to a stoma opening on the abdomen.
- [ ] **4.** Creates an opening in the bladder that allows urine to drain into an external pouch.

7. After surgery for an ileal conduit, the nurse should closely evaluate the client for the occurrence of which of the following complications related to pelvic surgery?
- [ ] **1.** Peritonitis.
- [ ] **2.** Thrombophlebitis.
- [ ] **3.** Ascites.
- [ ] **4.** Inguinal hernia.

8. The nurse is assessing the urine of a client who has had an ileal conduit and notes that the urine is yellow with a moderate amount of mucus. Based on the data, which of the following nursing interventions would be most appropriate at this time?
☐ **1.** Change the appliance bag.
☐ **2.** Notify the physician.
☐ **3.** Obtain a urine specimen for culture.
☐ **4.** Encourage a high fluid intake.

9. When teaching the client to care for an ileal conduit, the nurse instructs the client to empty the appliance frequently, primarily to help prevent which of the following problems?
☐ **1.** Rupture of the ileal conduit.
☐ **2.** Interruption of urine production.
☐ **3.** Development of odor.
☐ **4.** Separation of the appliance from the skin.

10. The nurse should teach the client with an ileal conduit to prevent urine leakage when changing the appliance by using which of the following procedures?
☐ **1.** Insert a gauze wick into the stoma.
☐ **2.** Close the opening temporarily with a cellophane seal.
☐ **3.** Suction the stoma before changing the appliance.
☐ **4.** Avoid oral fluids for several hours before changing the appliance.

11. The client with an ileal conduit will be using a reusable appliance at home. The nurse should teach the client to clean the appliance routinely with which product?
☐ **1.** Baking soda.
☐ **2.** Soap.
☐ **3.** Hydrogen peroxide.
☐ **4.** Alcohol.

12. The nurse is evaluating the discharge teaching for a client who has an ileal conduit. Which of the following statements indicates that the client has correctly understood the teaching? Select all that apply.
☐ **1.** "If I limit my fluid intake, I will not have to empty my ostomy pouch as often."
☐ **2.** "I can place an aspirin tablet in my pouch to decrease odor."
☐ **3.** "I can usually keep my ostomy pouch on for 3 to 7 days before changing it."
☐ **4.** "I must use a skin barrier to protect my skin from urine."
☐ **5.** "I should empty my ostomy pouch of urine when it is full."

13. Which of the following solutions will be useful to help control odor in the urine collecting bag after it has been cleaned?
☐ **1.** Salt water.
☐ **2.** Vinegar.
☐ **3.** Ammonia.
☐ **4.** Bleach.

14. A female client who has a urinary diversion tells the nurse, "This urinary pouch is embarrassing. Everyone will know that I'm not normal. I don't see how I can go out in public anymore." The most appropriate nursing diagnosis for this client is:
☐ **1.** *Anxiety* related to the presence of a urinary diversion.
☐ **2.** *Deficient knowledge* about how to care for the urinary diversion.
☐ **3.** *Low self-esteem* related to feelings of worthlessness.
☐ **4.** *Disturbed body image* related to creation of a urinary diversion.

15. The nurse teaches the client with a urinary diversion to attach the appliance to a standard urine collection bag at night. The most important reason for doing this is to prevent:
☐ **1.** Urine reflux into the stoma.
☐ **2.** Appliance separation.
☐ **3.** Urine leakage.
☐ **4.** The need to restrict fluids.

16. The nurse teaches the client with an ileal conduit measures to prevent a urinary tract infection. Which of the following measures would be most effective?
☐ **1.** Avoid people with respiratory tract infections.
☐ **2.** Maintain a daily fluid intake of 2,000 to 3,000 ml.
☐ **3.** Use sterile technique to change the appliance.
☐ **4.** Irrigate the stoma daily.

17. The nurse evaluates the effectiveness of the client's postoperative plan of care. Which of the following would be an expected outcome for a client with an ileal conduit?
☐ **1.** The client verbalizes the understanding that his physical activity must be curtailed.
☐ **2.** The client states that he will place an aspirin in the drainage pouch to help control odor.
☐ **3.** The client demonstrates how to catheterize the stoma.
☐ **4.** The client states that he will empty the drainage pouch frequently throughout the day.

18. A nurse is planning care for a client who underwent a percutaneous needle biopsy of the kidney. What should the nurse plan to do immediately after the biopsy? Select all that apply.
☐ **1.** Assess the biopsy site.
☐ **2.** Take vital signs every hour.
☐ **3.** Assess urine for hematuria.
☐ **4.** Place the client in a prone position.
☐ **5.** Assess the client for chest pain.

The Client with Renal Calculi

19. A client has renal colic due to renal lithiasis. What is the nurse's first priority in managing care for this client?
☐ **1.** Do not allow the client to ingest fluids.
☐ **2.** Encourage the client to drink at least 500 ml of water each hour.
☐ **3.** Request the central supply department to send supplies for straining urine.
☐ **4.** Administer an opioid analgesic as prescribed.

20. A client is scheduled for an intravenous pyelogram (IVP) to visualize the urinary tract after I.V. injection of contrast material. The evening before the procedure, the nurse learns that the client has a sensitivity to shellfish. Which of the following courses of actions should the nurse take?
☐ **1.** Administer a cathartic to the client to empty the colon.
☐ **2.** Administer an antiflatulent to the client to relieve gas.
☐ **3.** Keep the client on nothing-by-mouth (NPO) status.
☐ **4.** Cancel the IVP and notify the physician.

21. A client is admitted to the hospital with a diagnosis of renal calculi. She is experiencing severe flank pain and complains of nausea. Her temperature is 100.6° F (38.1° C). Which of the following would be a *priority* outcome for this client?
☐ **1.** Prevention of urinary tract complications.
☐ **2.** Alleviation of nausea.
☐ **3.** Alleviation of pain.
☐ **4.** Maintenance of fluid and electrolyte balance.

22. The client is scheduled to have a kidney, ureter, and bladder (KUB) radiograph. Which of the following would be ordered to prepare the client for this radiograph?
☐ **1.** Fluid and food will be withheld the morning of the examination.
☐ **2.** A tranquilizer will be given before the examination.
☐ **3.** An enema will be given before the examination.
☐ **4.** No special preparation is required for the examination.

23. In addition to nausea and severe flank pain, a female client with renal calculi complains of pain in the groin and bladder. The nurse should determine that these symptoms most likely result from which of the following?
☐ **1.** Nephritis.
☐ **2.** Referred pain.
☐ **3.** Urine retention.
☐ **4.** Additional stone formation.

24. Which of the following nursing interventions is likely to provide the most relief from the pain associated with renal colic?
☐ **1.** Applying moist heat to the flank area.
☐ **2.** Administering meperidine (Demerol).
☐ **3.** Encouraging high fluid intake.
☐ **4.** Maintaining complete bed rest.

25. A client who has been diagnosed with renal calculi reports that the pain is intermittent and less colicky. Which of the following nursing actions is most important at this time?
☐ **1.** Report hematuria to the physician.
☐ **2.** Strain the urine carefully.
☐ **3.** Administer meperidine (Demerol) every 3 hours.
☐ **4.** Apply warm compresses to the flank area.

26. The client is scheduled for an intravenous pyelogram (IVP) to determine the location of the renal calculi. Which of the following measures would be most important for the nurse to include in pretest preparation?
☐ **1.** Ensuring adequate fluid intake on the day of the test.
☐ **2.** Preparing the client for the possibility of bladder spasms during the test.
☐ **3.** Checking the client's history for allergy to iodine.
☐ **4.** Determining when the client last had a bowel movement.

27. After an intravenous pyelogram (IVP), the nurse should anticipate incorporating which of the following measures into the client's plan of care?

☐ **1.** Maintaining bed rest.
☐ **2.** Encouraging adequate fluid intake.
☐ **3.** Assessing for hematuria.
☐ **4.** Administering a laxative.

28. The nurse finds a container with the client's urine specimen sitting on a counter in the bathroom. The client states that the specimen has been sitting in the bathroom for at least 2 hours. What would be the nurse's most appropriate action?

☐ **1.** Discard the urine and obtain a new specimen.
☐ **2.** Send the urine to the laboratory as quickly as possible.
☐ **3.** Add fresh urine to the collected specimen and send the specimen to the laboratory.
☐ **4.** Refrigerate the specimen until it can be transported to the laboratory.

29. A client has a ureteral catheter in place after renal surgery. A priority nursing action for care of the ureteral catheter would be to:

☐ **1.** Irrigate the catheter with 30 ml of normal saline every 8 hours.
☐ **2.** Ensure that the catheter is draining freely.
☐ **3.** Clamp the catheter every 2 hours for 30 minutes.
☐ **4.** Ensure that the catheter drains at least 30 ml/hour.

30. Which of the following interventions would be the most appropriate for preventing the development of a paralytic ileus in a client who has undergone renal surgery?

☐ **1.** Encourage the client to ambulate every 2 to 4 hours.
☐ **2.** Offer 3 to 4 oz of a carbonated beverage periodically.
☐ **3.** Encourage use of a stool softener.
☐ **4.** Continue I.V. fluid therapy.

31. The nurse is conducting a postoperative assessment of a client on the first day after renal surgery. Which of the following findings would be most important for the nurse to report to the physician?

☐ **1.** Temperature, 99.8° F (37.7° C).
☐ **2.** Urine output, 20 ml/hour.
☐ **3.** Absence of bowel sounds.
☐ **4.** A 2″ × 2″ area of serosanguineous drainage on the flank dressing.

32. A client with a history of renal calculi formation is being discharged after surgery to remove the calculus. What instructions should the nurse include in the client's discharge teaching plan?

☐ **1.** Increase daily fluid intake to at least 2 to 3 L.
☐ **2.** Strain urine at home regularly.
☐ **3.** Eliminate dairy products from the diet.
☐ **4.** Follow measures to alkalinize the urine.

33. Because a client's renal stone was found to be composed of uric acid, a low-purine, alkaline-ash diet was ordered. Incorporation of which of the following food items into the home diet would indicate that the client understands the necessary diet modifications?

☐ **1.** Milk, apples, tomatoes, and corn.
☐ **2.** Eggs, spinach, dried peas, and gravy.
☐ **3.** Salmon, chicken, caviar, and asparagus.
☐ **4.** Grapes, corn, cereals, and liver.

34. Allopurinol (Zyloprim), 200 mg/day, is prescribed for the client with renal calculi to take at home. The nurse should teach the client about which of the following adverse effects of this medication?

☐ **1.** Retinopathy.
☐ **2.** Maculopapular rash.
☐ **3.** Nasal congestion.
☐ **4.** Dizziness.

35. A client has been prescribed allopurinol (Zyloprim) for renal calculi that are caused by high uric acid levels. Assessment of which of the following would lead the nurse to suspect that the client is experiencing potential adverse effects of this drug? Select all that apply.

☐ **1.** Nausea.
☐ **2.** Rash.
☐ **3.** Constipation.
☐ **4.** Flushed skin.
☐ **5.** Bone marrow depression.

36. The client has a clinic appointment scheduled for 10 days after discharge. Which laboratory finding at that time would indicate that allopurinol (Zyloprim) has had a therapeutic effect?

☐ **1.** Decreased urine alkaline phosphatase level.
☐ **2.** Increased urine calcium excretion.
☐ **3.** Increased serum calcium level.
☐ **4.** Decreased serum uric acid level.

The Client with Acute Renal Failure

37. A hospitalized female client with early acute renal failure has anemia, tachycardia, hypotension, and shortness of breath. The physician has ordered 2 units of packed red blood cells (RBCs). Which of the following assessments should the nurse make before initiating the blood transfusion? Select all that apply.
☐ 1. Is there an I.V. access with the appropriate tubing and normal saline as the priming solution?
☐ 2. Has an informed consent been obtained for transfusion therapy?
☐ 3. Has blood typing and cross-matching been done with documentation in the client's medical record?
☐ 4. Have the client's vital signs been taken and documented in accordance with facility policy and procedure?
☐ 5. Is the second unit of blood in the medication room?
☐ 6. Does the client have an identification bracelet and red blood band?

38. A client is to receive a prescribed peritoneal dialysis treatment. To prepare for the procedure, what should the nurse do?
☐ 1. Assess the dialysis access for a bruit and thrill.
☐ 2. Insert an indwelling urinary catheter and drain all urine from the bladder.
☐ 3. Ask the client to turn toward the left side.
☐ 4. Warm the solution in the warmer.

39. A client has been admitted with acute renal failure. What should the nurse do? Select all that apply.
☐ 1. Elevate the head of the bed 30 to 45 degrees.
☐ 2. Take vital signs.
☐ 3. Establish an I.V. access site.
☐ 4. Call the admitting physician for orders.
☐ 5. Contact the hemodialysis unit.

40. Which of the following urinary symptoms is the most common initial manifestation of acute renal failure?
☐ 1. Dysuria.
☐ 2. Anuria.
☐ 3. Hematuria.
☐ 4. Oliguria.

41. A client developed shock after a severe myocardial infarction and has now developed acute renal failure. The client's family asks the nurse why the client has developed acute renal failure. The nurse should base the response on the knowledge that there was:
☐ 1. A decrease in the blood flow through the kidneys.
☐ 2. An obstruction of urine flow from the kidneys.
☐ 3. A blood clot formed in the kidneys.
☐ 4. Structural damage to the kidney resulting in acute tubular necrosis.

42. The client's blood urea nitrogen (BUN) concentration is elevated in acute renal failure. What is the likely cause of this finding?
☐ 1. Fluid retention.
☐ 2. Hemolysis of red blood cells.
☐ 3. Below-normal metabolic rate.
☐ 4. Reduced renal blood flow.

43. The client's serum potassium level is elevated in acute renal failure, and the nurse administers sodium polystyrene sulfonate (Kayexalate). This drug acts to:
☐ 1. Increase potassium excretion from the colon.
☐ 2. Release hydrogen ions for sodium ions.
☐ 3. Increase calcium absorption in the colon.
☐ 4. Exchange sodium for potassium ions in the colon.

44. If the client's serum potassium level continues to rise in acute renal failure, the nurse should be prepared for which of the following emergencies?
☐ 1. Cardiac arrest.
☐ 2. Pulmonary edema.
☐ 3. Circulatory collapse.
☐ 4. Hemorrhage.

45. A high-carbohydrate, low-protein diet is prescribed for the client with acute renal failure. The rationale for the high-carbohydrate diet is that carbohydrates will:
☐ 1. Act as a diuretic.
☐ 2. Reduce demands on the liver.
☐ 3. Help maintain urine acidity.
☐ 4. Prevent the development of ketosis.

46. The client with acute renal failure asks the nurse for a snack. Because the client's potassium level is elevated, which of the following snacks is most appropriate?
☐ 1. A gelatin dessert.
☐ 2. Yogurt.
☐ 3. An orange.
☐ 4. Peanuts.

47. In the oliguric phase of acute renal failure, the nurse should anticipate the development of which of the following complications?
☐ 1. Pulmonary edema.
☐ 2. Metabolic alkalosis.
☐ 3. Hypotension.
☐ 4. Hypokalemia.

48. The client in acute renal failure has an external cannula inserted in the forearm for hemodialysis. Which of the following nursing measures is appropriate for the care of this client?
☐ 1. Use the unaffected arm for blood pressure measurements.
☐ 2. Draw blood from the cannula for routine laboratory work.
☐ 3. Percuss the cannula for bruits each shift.
☐ 4. Inject heparin into the cannula each shift.

49. The nurse initiates the client's first hemodialysis treatment. The client develops a headache, confusion, and nausea. These symptoms indicate which of the following potential complications?
- ☐ **1.** Disequilibrium syndrome.
- ☐ **2.** Myocardial infarction.
- ☐ **3.** Air embolism.
- ☐ **4.** Peritonitis.

50. If disequilibrium syndrome occurs during dialysis, which of the following would be the *priority* nursing action?
- ☐ **1.** Administer oxygen per nasal cannula.
- ☐ **2.** Slow the rate of dialysis.
- ☐ **3.** Reassure the client that the symptoms are normal.
- ☐ **4.** Place the client in Trendelenburg's position.

51. The client receives heparin while on hemodialysis. The nurse explains the rationale supporting anticoagulation by making which of the following statements?
- ☐ **1.** "Regional anticoagulation is achieved by putting heparin in the dialysis machine and protamine sulfate, which reverses the anticoagulation, in the client."
- ☐ **2.** "You will receive warfarin sodium (Coumadin) to maintain anticoagulation between treatments."
- ☐ **3.** "Heparin does not enter the body, so there is no risk of bleeding."
- ☐ **4.** "Clotting time is seriously prolonged for several hours after each treatment."

52. Which of the following abnormal blood values would not be improved by dialysis treatment?
- ☐ **1.** Elevated serum creatinine level.
- ☐ **2.** Hyperkalemia.
- ☐ **3.** Decreased hemoglobin concentration.
- ☐ **4.** Hypernatremia.

53. The nurse teaches the client how to recognize signs and symptoms of infection in the shunt by telling the client to assess the shunt each day for:
- ☐ **1.** Absence of a bruit.
- ☐ **2.** Sluggish capillary refill time.
- ☐ **3.** Coolness of the involved extremity.
- ☐ **4.** Swelling at the shunt site.

54. The client with acute renal failure is recovering and asks the nurse, "Will my kidneys ever function normally again?" The nurse's response is based on knowledge that the client's renal status will most likely:
- ☐ **1.** Continue to improve over a period of weeks.
- ☐ **2.** Result in the need for permanent hemodialysis.
- ☐ **3.** Improve only if the client receives a renal transplant.
- ☐ **4.** Result in end-stage renal failure.

The Client with Urinary Tract Infection

55. A client has a urinary tract infection. The physician ordered nitrofurantoin (Macrodantin) to be taken four times each day. The client asks the nurse what she should do if she forgets a dose. What should the nurse tell the client?
- ☐ **1.** "You can wait and take the next dose when it is due."
- ☐ **2.** "Double the amount prescribed with your next dose."
- ☐ **3.** "Take the prescribed dose as soon as you remember it, and if it is very close to the time for the next dose, delay that next dose."
- ☐ **4.** "Take a lot of water with a double amount of your prescribed dose."

56. A nurse is assessing a client with a urinary tract infection who takes an antihypertensive drug. The nurse reviews the client's urinalysis results (shown in the chart below). Which actions should the nurse take?
- ☐ **1.** Encourage the client to increase fluid intake.
- ☐ **2.** Withhold the next dose of antihypertensive medication.
- ☐ **3.** Restrict the client's sodium intake.
- ☐ **4.** Encourage the client to eat at least half of a banana per day.

LABORATORY RESULTS

Test	Result
pH	6.8
Red blood cells	3 per high power field
Color	yellow
Specific gravity	1.030

57. A client has nephropathy. The physician orders that a 24-hour urine collection be done for creatinine clearance. Which of the following actions is necessary to ensure proper collection of the specimen?
- ☐ **1.** Collect the urine in a preservative-free container and keep it on ice.
- ☐ **2.** Inform the client to discard the last voided specimen at the conclusion of urine collection.
- ☐ **3.** Ask the client what his weight is before beginning the collection of urine.
- ☐ **4.** Request an order for insertion of an indwelling urinary catheter.

58. A client who weighs 207 lb is to receive 1.5 mg/kg of gentamicin sulfate (Garamycin) I.V. three times each day. How many milligrams of medication should the nurse administer for each dose? Round to the nearest whole number.

_____ mg

59. A 24-year-old female client comes to an ambulatory care clinic in moderate distress with a probable diagnosis of acute cystitis. Which of the following symptoms should the nurse expect the client to report during the assessment?
- ☐ 1. Fever and chills.
- ☐ 2. Frequency and burning on urination.
- ☐ 3. Flank pain and nausea.
- ☐ 4. Hematuria.

60. The client asks the nurse, "How did I get this urinary tract infection?" The nurse should explain that in most instances, cystitis is caused by:
- ☐ 1. Congenital strictures in the urethra.
- ☐ 2. An infection elsewhere in the body.
- ☐ 3. Urinary stasis in the urinary bladder.
- ☐ 4. An ascending infection from the urethra.

61. The nurse is instructing the unlicensed assistant on the correct technique for obtaining a clean-catch urine culture from a female client. Which of the following statements indicates that the assistant has understood the instructions?
- ☐ 1. "I will have the client completely empty her bladder into the specimen cup."
- ☐ 2. "I will need to catheterize the client to get the urine specimen."
- ☐ 3. "I will ask the client to clean her labia, void into the toilet, and then into the specimen cup."
- ☐ 4. "I will obtain the specimen in the afternoon after the client has had plenty of fluids."

62. The client, who is a newlywed, is afraid to discuss her diagnosis of cystitis with her husband. Which would be the nurse's best approach?
- ☐ 1. Arrange a meeting with the client, her husband, the physician, and the nurse.
- ☐ 2. Insist that the client talk with her husband because good communication is necessary for a successful marriage.
- ☐ 3. Talk first with the husband alone and then with both of them together to share the husband's reactions.
- ☐ 4. Spend time with the client addressing her concerns and then stay with her while she talks with her husband.

63. The nurse teaches a client who has cystitis methods to relieve her discomfort until the antibiotic takes effect. Which of the following responses by the client would indicate that she understands the nurse's instructions?
- ☐ 1. "I will place ice packs on my perineum."
- ☐ 2. "I will take hot tub baths."
- ☐ 3. "I will drink a cup of warm tea every hour."
- ☐ 4. "I will void every 5 to 6 hours."

64. The client with cystitis is given a prescription for phenazopyridine hydrochloride (Pyridium). The nurse should teach the client that this drug is used to treat urinary tract infections by:
- ☐ 1. Releasing formaldehyde and providing bacteriostatic action.
- ☐ 2. Potentiating the action of the antibiotic.
- ☐ 3. Providing an analgesic effect on the bladder mucosa.
- ☐ 4. Preventing the crystallization that can occur with sulfa drugs.

65. Before the client starts taking phenazopyridine hydrochloride (Pyridium), she should be taught about which of the drug's adverse effects?
- ☐ 1. Bright orange-red urine.
- ☐ 2. Incontinence.
- ☐ 3. Constipation.
- ☐ 4. Slight drowsiness.

66. A client has been prescribed nitrofurantoin (Macrodantin) for treatment of a lower urinary tract infection. Which of the following instructions should the nurse include when teaching the client how to take this medication? Select all that apply.
- ☐ 1. "Take the medication on an empty stomach."
- ☐ 2. "Your urine may become brown in color."
- ☐ 3. "Increase your fluid intake."
- ☐ 4. "Take the medication until your symptoms subside."
- ☐ 5. "Take the medication with an antacid to decrease gastrointestinal distress."

67. Nitrofurantoin (Macrodantin), 75 mg four times per day, has been prescribed for a client with a lower urinary tract infection. The medication comes in an oral suspension of 25 mg/5 ml. How many milliliters should the nurse administer for each dose?

_____ ml

68. Which of the following statements by the client would indicate that she is at high risk for a recurrence of cystitis?
- ☐ **1.** "I can usually go 8 to 10 hours without needing to empty my bladder."
- ☐ **2.** "I take a tub bath every evening."
- ☐ **3.** "I wipe from front to back after voiding."
- ☐ **4.** "I drink a lot of water during the day."

69. To prevent recurrence of cystitis, the nurse should plan to encourage the client to include which of the following measures in her daily routine?
- ☐ **1.** Wearing cotton underpants.
- ☐ **2.** Increasing citrus juice intake.
- ☐ **3.** Douching regularly with 0.25% acetic acid.
- ☐ **4.** Using vaginal sprays.

70. The nurse explains to the client the importance of drinking large quantities of fluid to prevent cystitis. To help her understand, the nurse should tell her to drink:
- ☐ **1.** Twice as much fluid as she usually drinks.
- ☐ **2.** At least 1 quart more than she usually drinks.
- ☐ **3.** A lot of water, juice, and other fluids throughout the day.
- ☐ **4.** At least 3,000 ml of fluids daily.

The Client with Pyelonephritis

71. A client seen in the physician's office was diagnosed with acute pyelonephritis. Which of the following instructions should the nurse provide to the client?
- ☐ **1.** "The bacteria that cause acute pyelonephritis reach the kidneys by means of an infection that progresses upward from lower in the urinary tract."
- ☐ **2.** "Taking bubble baths will decrease the likelihood of further episodes of pyelonephritis."
- ☐ **3.** "You should take antibiotics for the rest of your life to prevent urinary tract infections."
- ☐ **4.** "By decreasing your fluid intake, you will decrease the need for frequent urination."

72. Which of the following symptoms would most likely indicate pyelonephritis?
- ☐ **1.** Ascites.
- ☐ **2.** Costovertebral angle (CVA) tenderness.
- ☐ **3.** Polyuria.
- ☐ **4.** Nausea and vomiting.

73. Which of the following factors would put the client at increased risk for pyelonephritis?
- ☐ **1.** History of hypertension.
- ☐ **2.** Intake of large quantities of cranberry juice.
- ☐ **3.** Fluid intake of 2,000 ml/day.
- ☐ **4.** History of diabetes mellitus.

74. Which of the following groups of laboratory tests is most important for assessing the client's renal status?
- ☐ **1.** Serum sodium and potassium levels.
- ☐ **2.** Arterial blood gases and hemoglobin.
- ☐ **3.** Serum blood urea nitrogen (BUN) and creatinine levels.
- ☐ **4.** Urinalysis and urine culture.

75. The client with pyelonephritis asks the nurse, "How will I know whether the antibiotics are effectively treating my infection?" The nurse's most appropriate response would be which of the following?
- ☐ **1.** "After you take the antibiotics for 2 weeks, you'll not have any infection."
- ☐ **2.** "Your health care provider can tell by the color and odor of your urine."
- ☐ **3.** "Your health care provider will take a urine culture."
- ☐ **4.** "When your symptoms disappear, you'll know that your infection is gone."

76. The client with acute pyelonephritis wants to know the possibility of developing chronic pyelonephritis. The nurse's response is based on knowledge that which of the following disorders most commonly leads to chronic pyelonephritis?
- ☐ **1.** Acute pyelonephritis.
- ☐ **2.** Recurrent urinary tract infections.
- ☐ **3.** Acute renal failure.
- ☐ **4.** Glomerulonephritis.

The Client with Chronic Renal Failure

77. A client has chronic renal failure with persistent hypertension. The nurse's actions are guided by the knowledge that this hypertension is from which one of the following mechanisms?
- ☐ **1.** Activation of the aldosterone-estrogen system.
- ☐ **2.** Erythropoietin system.
- ☐ **3.** Prostaglandin synthesis inhibition.
- ☐ **4.** Renin-angiotensin-aldosterone system.

78. The nurse assesses the client who has chronic renal failure and notes the following: crackles in the lung bases, elevated blood pressure, and weight gain of 2 lb in 1 day. Based on these data, which of the following nursing diagnoses is appropriate?
- [ ] **1.** *Excess fluid volume* related to the kidney's inability to maintain fluid balance.
- [ ] **2.** *Ineffective breathing pattern* related to fluid in the lungs.
- [ ] **3.** *Ineffective tissue perfusion* related to interrupted arterial blood flow.
- [ ] **4.** *Ineffective therapeutic regimen management* related to lack of knowledge about therapy.

79. The nurse is caring for a hospitalized client who has chronic renal failure. Which of the following nursing diagnoses are most appropriate for this client? Select all that apply.
- [ ] **1.** *Excess fluid volume.*
- [ ] **2.** *Imbalanced nutrition: Less than body requirements.*
- [ ] **3.** *Activity intolerance.*
- [ ] **4.** *Impaired gas exchange.*
- [ ] **5.** *Pain.*

80. What is the primary disadvantage of using peritoneal dialysis for long-term management of chronic renal failure?
- [ ] **1.** The danger of hemorrhage is high.
- [ ] **2.** It cannot correct severe imbalances.
- [ ] **3.** It is a time-consuming method of treatment.
- [ ] **4.** The risk of contracting hepatitis is high.

81. The client with chronic renal failure complains of feeling nauseated at least part of every day. The nurse should explain that the nausea is the result of:
- [ ] **1.** Acidosis caused by the medications.
- [ ] **2.** Accumulation of waste products in the blood.
- [ ] **3.** Chronic anemia and fatigue.
- [ ] **4.** Excess fluid load.

82. The dialysis solution is warmed before use in peritoneal dialysis primarily to:
- [ ] **1.** Encourage the removal of serum urea.
- [ ] **2.** Force potassium back into the cells.
- [ ] **3.** Add extra warmth to the body.
- [ ] **4.** Promote abdominal muscle relaxation.

83. Which of the following assessments would be most appropriate for the nurse to make while the dialysis solution is dwelling within the client's abdomen?
- [ ] **1.** Assess for urticaria.
- [ ] **2.** Observe respiratory status.
- [ ] **3.** Check capillary refill time.
- [ ] **4.** Monitor electrolyte status.

84. During the client's dialysis, the nurse observes that the solution draining from the abdomen is consistently blood-tinged. The client has a permanent peritoneal catheter in place. Which interpretation of this observation would be correct?
- [ ] **1.** Bleeding is expected with a permanent peritoneal catheter.
- [ ] **2.** Bleeding indicates abdominal blood vessel damage.
- [ ] **3.** Bleeding can indicate kidney damage.
- [ ] **4.** Bleeding is caused by too-rapid infusion of the dialysate.

85. During dialysis, the nurse observes that the flow of dialysate stops before all the solution has drained out. The nurse should:
- [ ] **1.** Have the client sit in a chair.
- [ ] **2.** Turn the client from side to side.
- [ ] **3.** Reposition the peritoneal catheter.
- [ ] **4.** Have the client walk.

86. Which of the following nursing interventions should be included in the client's plan of care during dialysis therapy?
- [ ] **1.** Limit the client's visitors.
- [ ] **2.** Monitor the client's blood pressure.
- [ ] **3.** Pad the side rails of the bed.
- [ ] **4.** Keep the client on nothing-by-mouth (NPO) status.

87. What is the most potentially dangerous complication of peritoneal dialysis?
- [ ] **1.** Abdominal pain.
- [ ] **2.** Gastrointestinal bleeding.
- [ ] **3.** Peritonitis.
- [ ] **4.** Muscle cramps.

88. After completion of peritoneal dialysis, the nurse should expect the client to exhibit which of the following characteristics?
- [ ] **1.** Hematuria.
- [ ] **2.** Weight loss.
- [ ] **3.** Hypertension.
- [ ] **4.** Increased urine output.

89. Aluminum hydroxide gel (Amphojel) is prescribed for the client with chronic renal failure to take at home. What is the purpose of giving this drug to a client with chronic renal failure?
☐ **1.** To relieve the pain of gastric hyperacidity.
☐ **2.** To prevent Curling's stress ulcers.
☐ **3.** To bind phosphate in the intestine.
☐ **4.** To reverse metabolic acidosis.

90. The nurse teaches the client with chronic renal failure when to take aluminum hydroxide gel (Amphojel). Which of the following statements would indicate that the client understands the teaching?
☐ **1.** "I'll take it every 4 hours around the clock."
☐ **2.** "I'll take it between meals and at bedtime."
☐ **3.** "I'll take it when I have a sour stomach."
☐ **4.** "I'll take it with meals and bedtime snacks."

91. The client with chronic renal failure tells the nurse he takes magnesium hydroxide (milk of magnesia) at home for constipation. The nurse suggests that the client switch to psyllium hydrophilic mucilloid (Metamucil) because:
☐ **1.** Milk of magnesia can cause magnesium intoxication.
☐ **2.** Milk of magnesia is too harsh on the bowel.
☐ **3.** Metamucil is more palatable.
☐ **4.** Milk of magnesia is high in sodium.

92. In planning teaching strategies for the client with chronic renal failure, the nurse must keep in mind the neurologic impact of uremia. Which teaching strategy would be most appropriate?
☐ **1.** Providing all needed teaching in one extended session.
☐ **2.** Validating frequently the client's understanding of the material.
☐ **3.** Conducting a one-on-one session with the client.
☐ **4.** Using videotapes to reinforce the material as needed.

93. The nurse helps the client with chronic renal failure develop a home diet plan with the goal of helping the client maintain adequate nutritional intake. Which of the following diets would be most appropriate for a client with chronic renal failure?
☐ **1.** High-carbohydrate, high-protein.
☐ **2.** High-calcium, high-potassium, high-protein.
☐ **3.** Low-protein, low-sodium, low-potassium.
☐ **4.** Low-protein, high-potassium.

94. Sexual problems can be troublesome to clients with chronic renal failure. Which one of the following strategies would be most useful in helping a client cope with such a problem?
☐ **1.** Help the client to accept that sexual activity will be decreased.
☐ **2.** Suggest using alternative forms of sexual expression and intimacy.
☐ **3.** Tell the client to plan rest periods after sexual activity.
☐ **4.** Suggest that the client avoid sexual activity to prevent embarrassment.

95. A client with chronic renal failure has asked to be evaluated for a home continuous ambulatory peritoneal dialysis (CAPD) program. The nurse should explain that the major advantage of this approach is that it:
☐ **1.** Is relatively low in cost.
☐ **2.** Allows the client to be more independent.
☐ **3.** Is faster and more efficient than standard peritoneal dialysis.
☐ **4.** Has fewer potential complications than standard peritoneal dialysis.

96. The client asks whether her diet would change on continuous ambulatory peritoneal dialysis (CAPD). Which of the following would be the nurse's best response?
☐ **1.** "Diet restrictions are more rigid with CAPD because standard peritoneal dialysis is a more effective technique."
☐ **2.** "Diet restrictions are the same for both CAPD and standard peritoneal dialysis."
☐ **3.** "Diet restrictions with CAPD are fewer than with standard peritoneal dialysis because dialysis is constant."
☐ **4.** "Diet restrictions with CAPD are fewer than with standard peritoneal dialysis because CAPD works more quickly."

97. Which of the following is the most significant sign of peritoneal infection?
☐ **1.** Cloudy dialysate fluid.
☐ **2.** Swelling in the legs.
☐ **3.** Poor drainage of the dialysate fluid.
☐ **4.** Redness at the catheter insertion site.

The Client with Urinary Incontinence

98. When developing a plan of care for the client with stress incontinence, the nurse should take into consideration that stress incontinence is best defined as the involuntary loss of urine associated with:
- ☐ 1. A strong urge to urinate.
- ☐ 2. Overdistention of the bladder.
- ☐ 3. Activities that increase abdominal pressure.
- ☐ 4. Obstruction of the urethra.

99. Which of the following assessment data would most likely be related to a client's current complaint of stress incontinence?
- ☐ 1. The client's intake of 2 to 3 L of fluid per day.
- ☐ 2. The client's history of three full-term pregnancies.
- ☐ 3. The client's age of 45 years.
- ☐ 4. The client's history of competitive swimming.

100. The primary goal of nursing care for a client with stress incontinence is to:
- ☐ 1. Help the client adjust to the frequent episodes of incontinence.
- ☐ 2. Eliminate all episodes of incontinence.
- ☐ 3. Prevent the development of urinary tract infections.
- ☐ 4. Decrease the number of incontinence episodes.

101. The nurse is developing a teaching plan for a client with stress incontinence. Which of the following instructions should be included?
- ☐ 1. Avoid activities that are stressful and upsetting.
- ☐ 2. Avoid caffeine and alcohol.
- ☐ 3. Do not wear a girdle.
- ☐ 4. Limit physical exertion.

102. A client has urge incontinence. Which of the following signs and symptoms would the nurse expect to find in this client?
- ☐ 1. Inability to empty the bladder.
- ☐ 2. Loss of urine when coughing.
- ☐ 3. Involuntary urination with minimal warning.
- ☐ 4. Frequent dribbling of urine.

103. Which of the following interventions would be most appropriate for a client who has urge incontinence?
- ☐ 1. Have the client urinate on a timed schedule.
- ☐ 2. Provide a bedside commode.
- ☐ 3. Administer prophylactic antibiotics.
- ☐ 4. Teach the client intermittent self-catheterization technique.

Correct Answers and Rationales

The letter in parentheses after each rationale identifies the client need addressed in the item, including management of care (M), safety and infection control (S), health promotion and maintenance (H), psychosocial adaptation (P), basic care and comfort (C), pharmacological and parenteral therapies (D), reduction of risk potential (R), and physiological adaptation (A).

The Client with Cancer of the Bladder

1. **1, 4.** An adequate fluid intake aids in the prevention of urinary calculi and infection. Odor-producing foods can produce offensive odors that may impact the client's lifestyle and relationships. Lack of activity leads to urinary stasis, which promotes urinary calculi development and infection. Acidic urine helps prevent urinary tract infections. Tight clothing over the stoma obstructs blood circulation and urine flow. (R)

2. **1, 2, 3.** Dermatitis with alkaline encrustations may occur when alkaline urine comes in contact with exposed skin. Yeast infections (or fungal infections) are another common peristomal skin problem. If the stoma is irritated from rubbing, there will be bleeding. The nurse and client should avoid irritating the stoma. Adhesive solvent is used on a gauze pad to remove old adhesive and would not contact the stoma directly. Only a minimal amount of skin cement is applied to the faceplate and skin to secure the appliance over the stoma, so obstruction of the stoma by the cement would not be possible. (A)

3. **3.** Painless hematuria is the most common clinical finding in bladder cancer. Other symptoms include urinary frequency, dysuria, and urinary urgency, but these are not as common as hematuria. Suprapubic pain and urine retention do not occur in bladder cancer. (A)

4. **2.** Chills could indicate the onset of acute infection that can progress to septic shock. Dizziness would not be an anticipated symptom after a cystoscopy. Pink-tinged urine and bladder spasms are common after cystoscopy. (R)

5. **4.** Lower abdominal pain after a cystoscopy is frequently caused by bladder spasms. Warm water can help relax muscles. Ice is not effective in relieving spasms. Massage and ambulation may increase bladder irritability. (C)

6. **3.** An ileal conduit is a permanent urinary diversion in which a portion of the ileum is surgically resected and one end of the segment is closed. The ureters are surgically attached to this segment of the ileum, and the open end of the ileum is brought to the skin surface on the abdomen to form the stoma. The client must wear a pouch to collect the urine that continually flows through the conduit. The bladder is removed during the surgical procedure and the ileal conduit is not reversible. Diversion of urine to the sigmoid colon is called a *ureteroileosigmoidostomy*. An opening in the bladder that allows urine to drain externally is called a *cystostomy*. (R)

7. **2.** After pelvic surgery, there is an increased chance of thrombophlebitis owing to the pelvic manipulation that can interfere with circulation and promote venous stasis. Peritonitis is a potential complication of any abdominal surgery, not just pelvic surgery. Ascites is most frequently an indication of liver disease. Inguinal hernia may be caused by an increase in intra-abdominal pressure or a congenital weakness of the abdominal wall; ventral hernia occurs at the site of a previous abdominal incision. (R)

8. **4.** Mucus is secreted by the intestinal segment used to create the conduit and is a normal occurrence. The client should be encouraged to maintain a large fluid intake to help flush the mucus out of the conduit. Because mucus in the urine is expected, it is not necessary to change the appliance bag or to notify the physician. The mucus is not an indication of an infection, so a urine culture is not necessary. (R)

9. **4.** If the appliance becomes too full, it is likely to pull away from the skin completely or to leak urine onto the skin. A full appliance will not rupture the ileal conduit or interrupt urine production. Odor formation has numerous causes. (A)

10. **1.** Inserting a gauze wick into the stoma helps prevent urine leakage when changing the appliance. The stoma should not be sealed or suctioned. Oral fluids do not need to be avoided. (A)

11. **2.** A reusable appliance should be routinely cleaned with soap and water. (A)

12. **3, 4.** The client with an ileal conduit must learn self-care activities related to care of the stoma and ostomy appliances. The client should be taught to increase fluid intake to about 3,000 ml per day and should not limit intake. Adequate fluid intake helps to flush mucus from the ileal conduit. The ostomy appliance should be changed approximately every 3 to 7 days and whenever a leak develops. A skin barrier is essential to protecting the skin from the irritation of the urine. An aspirin should not be used as a method of odor control because it can be an irritant to the stoma and lead to ulceration. The ostomy pouch should be emptied when it is one-third to one-half

full to prevent the weight of the urine from pulling the appliance away from the skin. (R)

13. **2.** A distilled vinegar solution acts as a good deodorizing agent after an appliance has been cleaned well with soap and water. If the client prefers, a commercial deodorizer may be used. Salt solution does not deodorize. Ammonia and bleaching agents may damage the appliance. (C)

14. **4.** It is normal for clients to express fears and concerns about the body changes associated with a urinary diversion. Allowing the client time to verbalize concerns in a supportive environment and suggesting that she discuss these concerns with people who have successfully adjusted to ostomy surgery can help her begin coping with these changes in a positive manner. Although the client may be anxious about this situation and self-esteem may be diminished, the underlying problem is a disturbance in body image. There are no data to support a diagnosis of *Deficient knowledge*. (P)

15. **1.** The most important reason for attaching the appliance to a standard urine collection bag at night is to prevent urine reflux into the stoma and ureters, which can result in infection. Use of a standard collection bag also keeps the appliance from separating from the skin and helps prevent urine leakage from an overly full bag, but the primary purpose is to prevent reflux of urine. A client with a urinary diversion should drink 2,000 to 3,000 ml of fluid each day; it would be inappropriate to suggest decreasing fluid intake. (A)

16. **2.** Maintaining a fluid intake of 2,000 to 3,000 ml/day is likely to be most effective in preventing urinary tract infection. A high fluid intake results in high urine output, which prevents urinary stasis and bacterial growth. Avoiding people with respiratory tract infections will not prevent urinary tract infections. Clean, not sterile, technique is used to change the appliance. An ileal conduit stoma is not irrigated. (A)

17. **4.** It is important that the client empty the drainage pouch throughout the day to decrease the risk of leakage. The client does not normally need to curtail physical activity. Aspirin should never be placed in a pouch because aspirin can irritate or ulcerate the stoma. The client does not catheterize an ileal conduit stoma. (A)

18. **1, 3, 4.** The nurse should assess the biopsy site for bleeding and hematoma formation. The client should remain prone for 8 to 24 hours after the biopsy. A pressure dressing will aid in blood coagulation. Vital signs assessment should be taken every 5 to 15 minutes for the first hour and then less often if the client is stable. The urine does not need to be collected and kept on ice. The nurse should collect serial urine specimens to assess for hematuria. A renal biopsy does not put the client at increased risk for chest pain. (R)

The Client with Renal Calculi

19. 4. If infection or blockage caused by calculi is present, a client can experience sudden severe pain in the flank area, known as *renal colic.* Pain from a kidney stone is considered an emergency situation and requires analgesic intervention. Withholding fluids will make urine more concentrated and stones more difficult to pass naturally. Forcing large quantities of fluid may cause hydronephrosis if urine is prevented from flowing past calculi. Straining urine for small stones is important, but does not take priority over pain management. (M)

20. 4. Sensitivity to shellfish or iodine may cause an anaphylactic reaction to the contrast material, which contains iodine. Administering a cathartic or antiflatulent will not prevent an anaphylactic reaction to the contrast material. Keeping a client on NPO status for 8 hours before the procedure is part of the usual preparation for such a procedure to prevent aspiration of food or fluids if the client vomits when lying on the X-ray table. (R)

21. 3. The priority nursing goal for this client is to alleviate the pain, which can be excruciating. Prevention of urinary tract complications and alleviation of nausea are appropriate throughout the client's hospitalization, but relief of the severe pain is a priority. The client is at little risk for fluid and electrolyte imbalance. (A)

22. 4. A KUB radiographic examination ordinarily requires no preparation. It is usually done while the client lies supine and does not involve the use of radiopaque substances. (R)

23. 2. The pain associated with renal colic due to calculi is commonly referred to the groin and bladder in female clients and to the testicles in male clients. Nausea, vomiting, abdominal cramping, and diarrhea may also be present. Nephritis or urine retention is an unlikely cause of the referred pain. The type of pain described in this situation is unlikely to be caused by additional stone formation. (A)

24. 2. During episodes of renal colic, the pain is excruciating. It is necessary to administer opioid analgesics to control the pain. Application of heat, encouraging high fluid intake, and limitation of activity are important interventions, but they will not relieve the renal colic pain. (R)

25. 2. Intermittent pain that is less colicky indicates that the calculi may be moving along the urinary tract. Fluids should be encouraged to promote movement, and the urine should be strained to detect passage of the stone. Hematuria is to be expected from the irritation of the stone. Analgesics should be administered when the client needs them, not routinely. Moist heat to the flank area is helpful when renal colic occurs, but it is less necessary as pain is lessened. (A)

26. 3. A client scheduled for an IVP should be assessed for allergies to iodine and shellfish. Clients with such allergies may be allergic to the IVP dye and be at risk for an anaphylactic reaction. Adequate fluid intake is important after the examination. Bladder spasms are not common during an IVP. Bowel preparation is important before an IVP to allow visualization of the ureters and bladder, but checking for allergies is most important. (R)

27. 2. After an IVP, the nurse should encourage fluids to decrease the risk of renal complications caused by the contrast agent. There is no need to place the client on bed rest or administer a laxative. An IVP would not cause hematuria. (R)

28. 1. The appropriate action would be to discard the specimen and obtain a new one. Urine that is allowed to stand at room temperature will become alkaline, with multiplying bacteria. The specimen should be examined within 1 hour after urination. (R)

29. 2. The ureteral catheter should drain freely without bleeding at the site. The catheter is rarely irrigated, and any irrigation would be done by the physician. The catheter is never clamped. The client's total urine output (ureteral catheter plus voiding or indwelling urinary catheter output) should be 30 ml/hour. (R)

30. 1. Ambulation stimulates peristalsis. A client with paralytic ileus is kept on nothing-by-mouth status until peristalsis returns. Carbonated beverages will increase gas and distention but will not stimulate peristalsis. A stool softener will not stimulate peristalsis. I.V. fluid infusion is a routine postoperative order that does not have any effect on preventing paralytic ileus. (A)

31. 2. The decrease in urine output may reflect inadequate renal perfusion and should be reported immediately. Urine output of 30 ml/hour or greater is considered acceptable. A slight elevation in temperature is expected after surgery. Peristalsis returns gradually, usually the second or third day after surgery. Bowel sounds will be absent until then. A small amount of serosanguineous drainage is to be expected. (A)

32. 1. A high daily fluid intake is essential for all clients who are at risk for calculi formation because it prevents urinary stasis and concentration, which can cause crystallization. Depending on the composition of the stone, the client also may be instructed to institute specific dietary measures aimed at preventing stone formation. Clients may need to limit purine, calcium, or oxalate. Urine may need to be either alkaline or acid. There is no need to strain urine regularly. (C)

33. **1.** Because a high-purine diet contributes to the formation of uric acid, a low-purine diet is advocated. An alkaline-ash diet is also advocated because uric acid crystals are more likely to develop in acid urine. Foods that may be eaten as desired in a low-purine diet include milk, all fruits, tomatoes, cereals, and corn. Foods allowed on an alkaline-ash diet include milk, fruits (except cranberries, plums, and prunes), and vegetables (especially legumes and green vegetables). Gravy, chicken, and liver are high in purine. (C)

34. **2.** Allopurinol (Zyloprim) is used to treat renal calculi composed of uric acid. Adverse effects of allopurinol include drowsiness, maculopapular rash, anemia, abdominal pain, nausea, vomiting, and bone marrow depression. Clients should be instructed to report rashes and unusual bleeding or bruising. Retinopathy, nasal congestion, and dizziness are not adverse effects of allopurinol. (D)

35. **1, 2, 5.** Common adverse effects of allopurinol (Zyloprim) include gastrointestinal distress, such as anorexia, nausea, vomiting, and diarrhea. A rash is another potential adverse effect. A potentially life-threatening adverse effect is bone marrow depression. Constipation and flushed skin are not associated with this drug. (D)

36. **4.** By inhibiting uric acid synthesis, allopurinol (Zyloprim) decreases its excretion. The drug's effectiveness is assessed by evaluating for a decreased serum uric acid concentration. Allopurinol does not alter the level of alkaline phosphatase, nor does it affect urine calcium excretion or the serum calcium level. (D)

The Client with Acute Renal Failure

37. **1, 2, 3, 4, 6.** Before ordering and administering packed RBCs, the nurse should assess the I.V. site to make sure it has an 18G to 20G Angiocath. The nurse should also ensure that normal saline solution is used to prime the tubing to prevent RBCs from adhering to the tubing. The client must indicate informed consent for the procedure by signing the consent form. The client's blood must be typed to determine ABO blood typing and Rh factor and ensure that the client receives compatible blood. Crossmatching is done to detect the presence of recipient antibodies to the donor's minor antigens. Vital signs provide a baseline reference for continuous monitoring throughout the transfusion. An identification bracelet and red blood band are essential for client identification per facility policy. Two nurses must double check the client's identification with the client listed on the unit of RBCs. The transfusion should be started within 30 minutes of the time that the RBC unit is checked out of the blood bank. Thus, no blood should be kept in the medication room before transfusion. (S)

38. **4.** Solution for peritoneal dialysis should be warmed to body temperature in a warmer or with a heating pad; do not use the microwave. Cold dialysate increases discomfort. Assessment for a bruit and thrill is necessary with hemodialysis when the client has a fistula, graft, or shunt. An indwelling urinary catheter is not required for this procedure. The nurse should position the client in a supine or low Fowler's position. (R)

39. **1, 2, 3, 4.** Elevation of the head of the bed will promote ease of breathing. Respiratory manifestations of acute renal failure include shortness of breath, orthopnea, crackles, and the potential for pulmonary edema. Therefore, priority is placed on facilitation of respiration. The nurse should assess the vital signs because the pulse and respirations will be elevated. Establishing a site for I.V. therapy will become important because fluids will be administered I.V. in addition to orally. The physician will need to be contacted for further orders; there is no need to contact the hemodialysis unit. (A)

40. **4.** Oliguria is the most common initial symptom of acute renal failure. Anuria is rarely the initial symptom. Dysuria and hematuria are not associated with acute renal failure. (A)

41. **1.** There are three categories of acute renal failure: prerenal, intrarenal, and postrenal. Causes of prerenal failure occur outside the kidney and include poor perfusion and decreased circulating volume resulting from such factors as trauma, septic shock, impaired cardiac function, and dehydration. In this case of severe myocardial infarction, there was a decrease in perfusion of the kidneys caused by impaired cardiac function. An obstruction within the urinary tract, such as from kidney stones, tumors, or benign prostatic hypertrophy, is called *postrenal failure.* Structural damage to the kidney resulting from acute tubular necrosis is called *intrarenal failure.* It is caused by such conditions as hypersensitivity (allergic disorders), renal vessel obstruction, and nephrotoxic agents. (A)

42. **4.** Urea, an end product of protein metabolism, is excreted by the kidneys. Impairment in renal function caused by reduced renal blood flow results in an increase in the plasma urea level. Fluid retention, hemolysis of red blood cells, and lowered metabolic rate do not cause an elevated BUN value. (R)

43. **4.** Polystyrene sulfonate, a cation-exchange resin, causes the body to excrete potassium through the gastrointestinal tract. In the intestines, particularly the colon, the sodium of the resin is partially replaced by potassium. The potassium is then eliminated when the resin is eliminated with feces. Although the result is to increase potassium excretion, the specific method of action is the exchange of sodium ions for potassium ions. Polystyrene sulfonate does not release hydrogen ions or increase calcium absorption. (D)

44. **1.** Hyperkalemia places the client at risk for serious cardiac arrhythmias and cardiac arrest. Therefore, the nurse should carefully monitor the client for cardiac arrhythmias and be prepared to treat cardiac arrest when caring for a client with hyperkalemia. Increased potassium levels do not result in pulmonary edema, circulatory collapse, or hemorrhage. (D)

45. **4.** High-carbohydrate foods meet the body's caloric needs during acute renal failure. Protein is limited because its breakdown may result in accumulation of toxic waste products. The main goal of nutritional therapy in acute renal failure is to decrease protein catabolism. Protein catabolism causes increased levels of urea, phosphate, and potassium. Carbohydrates provide energy and decrease the need for protein breakdown. They do not have a diuretic effect. Some specific carbohydrates influence urine pH, but this is not the reason for encouraging a high-carbohydrate, low-protein diet. There is no need to reduce demands on the liver through dietary manipulation in acute renal failure. (C)

46. **1.** Gelatin desserts contain little or no potassium and can be served to a client on a potassium-restricted diet. Foods high in potassium include bran and whole grains; most dried, raw, and frozen fruits and vegetables; most milk and milk products; chocolate, nuts, raisins, coconut, and strong brewed coffee. (C)

47. **1.** Pulmonary edema can develop during the oliguric phase of acute renal failure because of decreased urine output and fluid retention. Metabolic acidosis develops because the kidneys cannot excrete hydrogen ions, and bicarbonate is used to buffer the hydrogen. Hypertension may develop as a result of fluid retention. Hyperkalemia develops as the kidneys lose the ability to excrete potassium. (A)

48. **1.** The unaffected arm should be used for blood pressure measurement. The external cannula must be handled carefully and protected from damage and disruption. In addition, a tourniquet or clamps should be kept at the bedside because dislodgment of the cannula would cause arterial hemorrhage. The arm with the cannula is not used for blood pressure measurement, I.V. therapy, or venipuncture. Patency is assessed by auscultating for bruits every shift. Heparin is not injected into the cannula to maintain patency. Because it is part of the general circulation, the cannula cannot be heparinized. (R)

49. **1.** Common symptoms of disequilibrium syndrome include headache, nausea and vomiting, confusion, and even seizures. Disequilibrium syndrome typically occurs near the end or after the completion of hemodialysis treatment. It is the result of rapid changes in solute composition and osmolality of the extracellular fluid. These symptoms are not related to cardiac function, air embolism, or peritonitis. (R)

50. **2.** If disequilibrium syndrome occurs during dialysis, the most appropriate intervention is to slow the rate of dialysis. The syndrome is believed to result from too-rapid removal of urea and excess electrolytes from the blood; this causes transient cerebral edema, which produces the symptoms. Administration of oxygen and position changes do not affect the symptoms. It would not be appropriate to reassure the client that the symptoms are normal. (R)

51. **1.** Regional anticoagulation can be achieved by infusing heparin in the dialyzer and protamine sulfate, its antagonist, in the client. Warfarin sodium (Coumadin) is not used in dialysis treatment. There is some risk of bleeding; however, clotting time is monitored carefully. The client's clotting time will not be seriously affected, although some rebound effect may occur. (D)

52. **3.** Dialysis has no effect on anemia. Because some red blood cells are injured during the procedure, dialysis aggravates a low hemoglobin concentration. Dialysis will clear metabolic waste products from the body and correct electrolyte imbalances. (R)

53. **4.** Signs and symptoms of an external access shunt infection include redness, tenderness, swelling, and drainage from around the shunt site. The absence of a bruit indicates closing of the shunt. Sluggish capillary refill time and coolness of the extremity indicate decreased blood flow to the extremity. (R)

54. **1.** The kidneys have a remarkable ability to recover from serious insult. Recovery may take 3 to 12 months. The client should be taught how to recognize the signs and symptoms of decreasing renal function and to notify the physician if such problems occur. In a client who is recovering from acute renal failure, there is no need for renal transplantation or permanent hemodialysis. Chronic renal failure develops before end-stage renal failure. (A)

The Client with Urinary Tract Infection

55. 3. Antibiotics have the maximum effect when a blood level of the medication is maintained. However, because nitrofurantoin (Macrodantin) is readily absorbed from the gastrointestinal tract and is primarily excreted in urine, toxicity may develop by doubling the dose. The client should not skip a dose if she realizes that she has missed one. Additional fluids, especially water, should be encouraged, but not forced to promote elimination of the antibiotic from the body. Adequate fluid intake aids in the prevention of urinary tract infections, in addition to an acidic urine. (D)

56. 1. The client's urine specific gravity is elevated. Specific gravity is a reflection of the concentrating ability of the kidneys. This level indicates that the urine is concentrated. By increasing fluid intake, the urine will become more dilute. Antihypertensives do not make urine more concentrated unless there is a diuretic component within them. The nurse should not hold a dose of antihypertensive medication. Sodium tends to pull water with it; by restricting sodium, less water, not more, will be present. Bananas do not aid in the dilution of urine. (R)

57. 1. All urine for creatinine clearance determination must be saved in a container with no preservatives and refrigerated or kept on ice. The first urine voided at the beginning of the collection is discarded, not the last. A self-report of weight may not be accurate. It is not necessary to have an indwelling urinary catheter inserted for urine collection. (R)

58. 141

$$1 \text{ kg} = 2.2 \text{ lb}$$

$$1 \text{ kg} : 2.2 \text{ lb} = X \text{ kg} : 207 \text{ lb}$$

$$2.2 \text{ lb} \times X \text{ kg} = 1 \text{ kg} \times 207 \text{ lb}$$

$$X \text{ kg} = \frac{1 \text{kg} \times \overset{94.1}{\cancel{207 \text{ lb}}}}{\underset{1}{\cancel{2.2 \text{ lb}}}}$$

$$X = 94.1 \text{ kg}$$

$$1.5 \text{ mg} \times 94.1 = 141.15 = 141 \text{ mg}.$$

(D)

59. 2. The classic symptoms of cystitis are severe burning on urination, urgency, and frequent urination. Systemic symptoms, such as fever and nausea and vomiting, are more likely to accompany pyelonephritis than cystitis. Hematuria may occur, but it is not as common as frequency and burning. (A)

60. 4. Although various conditions may result in cystitis, the most common cause is an ascending infection from the urethra. Strictures and urine retention can lead to infections, but these are not the most common cause. Systemic infections are rarely causes of cystitis. (A)

61. 3. The correct technique for a clean-catch urine culture specimen is to have the female client clean the labia from front to back, void into the toilet, and then void into the cup. The client does not need to fully empty her bladder into the cup. It is not necessary to catheterize the client to obtain the specimen. The first voided specimen of the day has the highest bacterial counts. (C)

62. 4. As newlyweds, the client and her husband need to develop a strong communication base. The nurse can facilitate communication by preparing and supporting the client. Given the situation, an interdisciplinary conference is inappropriate and would not promote intimacy for the client and her husband. Insisting that the client talk with her husband is not addressing her fears. Being present allows the nurse to facilitate the discussion of a difficult topic. Having the nurse speak first with the husband alone shifts responsibility away from the couple. (P)

63. 2. Hot tub baths promote relaxation and help relieve urgency, discomfort, and spasm. Applying heat to the perineum is more helpful than cold because heat reduces inflammation. Although liberal fluid intake should be encouraged, caffeinated beverages, such as tea, coffee, and cola, can be irritating to the bladder and should be avoided. Voiding at least every 2 to 3 hours should be encouraged because it reduces urinary stasis. (C)

64. 3. Phenazopyridine hydrochloride (Pyridium) is a urinary analgesic that works directly on the bladder mucosa to relieve the distressing symptoms of dysuria. Phenazopyridine does not have a bacteriostatic effect. It does not potentiate antibiotics or prevent crystallization. (D)

65. 1. The client should be told that phenazopyridine hydrochloride (Pyridium) turns the urine a bright orange-red, which may stain underwear. It can be frightening for a client to see orange-red urine without having been forewarned. Other common adverse effects associated with phenazopyridine include headaches, gastrointestinal disturbances, and rash. Phenazopyridine does not cause incontinence, constipation, or drowsiness. (D)

66. 2, 3. Clients who are taking nitrofurantoin (Macrodantin) should be instructed to take the medication with meals and to increase their fluid intake to minimize gastrointestinal distress. The urine may become brown in color. Although this change is harmless, clients need to be prepared for this color change. The client should be instructed to take the full prescription and not to stop taking the drug because symptoms have subsided. The medication should not be taken with antacids as this may interfere with the drug's absorption. (D)

67. 15

The following formula is used to calculate the correct dosage:

$$25 \text{ mg}/5 \text{ ml} = 75 \text{ mg}/X \text{ ml}$$

$$X = 15 \text{ ml.}$$

(D)

68. **1.** Stasis of urine in the bladder is one of the chief causes of bladder infection, and a client who voids infrequently is at greater risk for reinfection. A tub bath does not promote urinary tract infections as long as the client avoids harsh soaps and bubble baths. Scrupulous hygiene and liberal fluid intake (unless contraindicated) are excellent preventive measures, but the client also should be taught to void every 2 to 3 hours during the day. (R)

69. **1.** A woman can adopt several health-promotion measures to prevent the recurrence of cystitis, including avoiding too-tight pants, noncotton underpants, and irritating substances, such as bubble baths and vaginal soaps and sprays. Increasing citrus juice intake can be a bladder irritant. Regular douching is not recommended; it can alter the pH of the vagina, increasing the risk of infection. (H)

70. **4.** Instructions should be as specific as possible, and the nurse should avoid general statements such as "a lot." A specific goal is most useful. A mix of fluids will increase the likelihood of client compliance. It may not be sufficient to tell the client to drink twice as much as or 1 quart more than she usually drinks if her intake was inadequate to begin with. (C)

The Client with Pyelonephritis

71. **1.** Pyelonephritis usually begins with colonization and infection of the lower urinary tract via the ascending urethral route. Bubble baths and limiting fluid intake increase the risk of developing a urinary tract infection. Antibiotics should be used on a short-term basis because the risk of antibiotic resistance may lead to breakthrough infections with increasingly virulent pathogens. (H)

72. **2.** Common symptoms of pyelonephritis include CVA tenderness, burning on urination, urinary urgency or frequency, chills, fever, and fatigue. Ascites, polyuria, and nausea and vomiting are not indicative of pyelonephritis. (A)

73. **4.** A client with a history of diabetes mellitus, urinary tract infections, or renal calculi is at increased risk for pyelonephritis. Others at high risk include pregnant

women and people with structural alterations of the urinary tract. A history of hypertension may put the client at risk for kidney damage, but not kidney infection. Intake of large quantities of cranberry juice and a fluid intake of 2,000 ml/day are not risk factors for pyelonephritis. (R)

74. **3.** Serum BUN and creatinine are the tests most commonly used to assess renal function, with creatinine being the most reliable indicator. Nonrenal factors may affect BUN levels as well as serum sodium and potassium levels. Arterial blood gases and hemoglobin are not used to assess renal status. Urinalysis is a general screening test, and a urine culture is used to detect urinary tract infections. (A)

75. **3.** Antibiotics are usually prescribed for a 2- to 4-week period. A urine culture is needed to evaluate the effectiveness of antibiotic therapy. Urine must be examined microscopically to adequately determine the presence of bacteria; looking at the color of the urine or checking the odor is not sufficient. Symptoms usually disappear 48 to 72 hours after antibiotic therapy is started, but antibiotics may need to continue for up to 4 weeks. (D)

76. **2.** Chronic pyelonephritis is most commonly the result of recurrent urinary tract infections. Chronic pyelonephritis can lead to chronic renal failure. Single cases of acute pyelonephritis rarely cause chronic pyelonephritis. Acute renal failure is not a cause of chronic pyelonephritis. Glomerulonephritis is an immunologic disorder, not an infectious disorder. (A)

The Client with Chronic Renal Failure

77. **4.** Renin is important in the regulation of blood pressure; it is released from the juxtaglomerular apparatus of the nephron in response to decreased arterial blood pressure and extracellular fluid depletion. Renin catalyzes the splitting of angiotensinogen into angiotensin I, which is subsequently converted to angiotensin II. Angiotensin II stimulates the release of aldosterone, which causes sodium and water retention and subsequent hypertension. The aldosterone-estrogen system does not exist. Erythropoietin stimulates the production of red blood cells by the bone marrow. Prostaglandins have a vasodilating action, increasing renal blood flow and promoting sodium excretion. (A)

78. **1.** Crackles in the lungs, weight gain, and elevated blood pressure are indicators of excess fluid volume, a common complication in chronic renal failure. The client's fluid status should be monitored carefully for imbalances on an ongoing basis. Although the client has ineffective breathing, the primary cause is related to the renal failure.

There are no data to suggest ineffective tissue perfusion or lack of knowledge. (A)

79. **1, 2, 3.** Appropriate nursing diagnoses for clients with chronic renal failure include *Excess fluid volume* related to fluid and sodium retention; *Imbalanced nutrition: Less than body requirements* related to anorexia, nausea, and vomiting; and *Activity intolerance* related to fatigue. The nursing diagnoses of *Impaired gas exchange* and *Pain* are not commonly related to chronic renal failure. (A)

80. **3.** A disadvantage of peritoneal dialysis in long-term management of chronic renal failure is that it requires large blocks of time. The risk of hemorrhage or hepatitis is not high with peritoneal dialysis. Peritoneal dialysis is effective in maintaining a client's fluid and electrolyte balance. (R)

81. **2.** Nausea typically results from the chronic presence of retained waste products in the body. The client can control nausea most effectively by following the diet regimen strictly to avoid wide variations in blood values between treatments. Metabolic acidosis results from impaired excretion, not medications. Chronic anemia and fatigue as well as excess fluid are potential problems but do not cause nausea. (A)

82. **1.** The main reason for warming the peritoneal dialysis solution is that the warm solution helps dilate peritoneal vessels, which increases urea clearance. Warmed dialyzing solution also contributes to client comfort by preventing chilly sensations, but this is a secondary reason for warming the solution. The warmed solution does not force potassium into the cells or promote abdominal muscle relaxation. (R)

83. **2.** During dwell time, the dialysis solution is allowed to remain in the peritoneal cavity for the time ordered by the physician (usually 20 to 45 minutes). During this time, the nurse should monitor the client's respiratory status because the pressure of the dialysis solution on the diaphragm can create respiratory distress. The dialysis solution would not cause urticaria or affect circulation to the fingers. The client's laboratory values are obtained before beginning treatment and are monitored every 4 to 8 hours during the treatment, not just during the dwell time. (R)

84. **2.** Because the client has a permanent catheter in place, blood-tinged drainage should not occur. Persistent blood-tinged drainage could indicate damage to the abdominal vessels, and the physician should be notified. The bleeding is originating in the peritoneal cavity, not the kidneys. Too-rapid infusion of the dialysate can cause pain, not blood-tinged drainage. (R)

85. **2.** Fluid return with peritoneal dialysis is accomplished by gravity flow. Actions that enhance gravity flow include turning the client from side to side, raising the head of the bed, and gently massaging the abdomen. The client is usually confined to a recumbent position during the dialysis. The nurse should not attempt to reposition the catheter. (R)

86. **2.** Because hypotension is a complication associated with peritoneal dialysis, the nurse records intake and output, monitors vital signs, and observes the client's behavior. The nurse also encourages visiting and other diversional activities. A client on peritoneal dialysis does not need to be placed in a bed with padded side rails or kept on NPO status. (R)

87. **3.** Peritonitis is a serious risk associated with peritoneal dialysis. Aseptic technique should be maintained during the procedure. Minor abdominal cramping may occur with dialysis. Gastrointestinal bleeding is an extremely rare complication. Muscle cramps are not an anticipated complication of peritoneal dialysis but may be a complication of hemodialysis. (R)

88. **2.** Weight loss is expected because of the removal of fluid. The client's weight before and after dialysis is one measure of the effectiveness of treatment. Blood pressure usually decreases because of the removal of fluid. Hematuria would not occur after completion of peritoneal dialysis. Dialysis only minimally affects the damaged kidneys' ability to manufacture urine. (R)

89. **3.** A client in renal failure develops hyperphosphatemia that causes a corresponding excretion of the body's calcium stores, leading to renal osteodystrophy. To decrease this loss, aluminum hydroxide gel is prescribed to bind phosphates in the intestine and facilitate their excretion. Gastric hyperacidity is not necessarily a problem associated with chronic renal failure. Antacids will not prevent Curling's stress ulcers and do not affect metabolic acidosis. (D)

90. **4.** Aluminum hydroxide gel (Amphojel) is administered to bind the phosphates in ingested foods and must be given with or immediately after meals and snacks. There is no need for the client to take it on a 24-hour schedule. It is not administered to treat hyperacidity in clients with chronic renal failure and therefore is not prescribed between meals. (D)

91. **1.** Magnesium is normally excreted by the kidneys. When the kidneys fail, magnesium can accumulate and cause severe neurologic problems. Milk of magnesia is harsher than Metamucil, but magnesium toxicity is a more serious problem. A client may find both milk of magnesia and Metamucil unpalatable. Milk of magnesia is not high in sodium. (D)

92. **2.** Uremia can cause decreased alertness, so the nurse needs to validate the client's comprehension frequently. Because the client's ability to concentrate is limited, short lessons are most effective. If family members are present at the sessions, they can reinforce the material. Written materials that the client can review are superior to videotapes because clients may not be able to maintain alertness during the viewing of the videotape. (A)

93. **3.** Dietary management for clients with chronic renal failure is usually designed to restrict protein, sodium, and potassium intake. Protein intake is reduced because the kidney can no longer excrete the byproducts of protein metabolism. The degree of dietary restriction depends on the degree of renal impairment. The client should also receive a high-carbohydrate diet along with appropriate vitamin and mineral supplements. Calcium requirements remain 1,000 to 2,000 mg/day. (C)

94. **2.** Altered sexual functioning commonly occurs in chronic renal failure and can stress marriages and relationships. Altered sexual functioning can be caused by decreased hormone levels, anemia, peripheral neuropathy, or medication. The client should not decrease or avoid sexual activity but instead should modify it. The client should rest before sexual activity. (P)

95. **2.** The major benefit of CAPD is that it frees the client from daily dependence on dialysis centers, health care personnel, and machines for life-sustaining treatment. This independence is a valuable outcome for some people. CAPD is costly and must be done daily. Adverse effects and complications are similar to those of standard peritoneal dialysis. Peritoneal dialysis usually takes less time but cannot be done at home. (R)

96. **3.** Dietary restrictions with CAPD are fewer than those with standard peritoneal dialysis because dialysis is constant, not intermittent. The constant slow diffusion of CAPD helps prevent accumulation of toxins and allows for a more liberal diet. CAPD does not work more quickly, but more consistently. Both types of peritoneal dialysis are effective. (C)

97. **1.** Cloudy drainage indicates bacterial activity in the peritoneum. Other signs and symptoms of infection are fever, hyperactive bowel sounds, and abdominal pain. Swollen legs may indicate heart failure. Poor drainage of dialysate fluid is probably the result of a kinked catheter. Redness at the insertion site indicates local infection, not peritonitis. However, a local infection that is left untreated can progress to the peritoneum. (R)

The Client with Urinary Incontinence

98. **3.** Stress incontinence is the involuntary loss of urine during such activities as coughing, sneezing, laughing, or physical exertion. These activities increase abdominal and detrusor pressure. A strong urge to urinate is associated with urge incontinence. Overdistention of the bladder can lead to overflow incontinence. Obstruction of the urethra can lead to urine retention. (A)

99. **2.** The history of three pregnancies is most likely the cause of the client's current episodes of stress incontinence. The client's fluid intake, age, or history of swimming would not create an increase in intra-abdominal pressure. (R)

100. **4.** The primary goal of nursing care is to decrease the number of incontinence episodes and the amount of urine expressed in an episode. Behavioral interventions (e.g., diet and exercise) and medications are the nonsurgical management methods used to treat stress incontinence. Without surgical intervention, it may not be possible to eliminate all episodes of incontinence. Helping the client adjust to the incontinence is not treating the problem. Clients with stress incontinence are not prone to the development of urinary tract infection. (A)

101. **2.** Clients with stress incontinence are encouraged to avoid substances, such as caffeine and alcohol, that are bladder irritants. Emotional stressors do not cause stress incontinence. It is most commonly caused by relaxed pelvic musculature. Wearing girdles is not contraindicated. Although clients may want to limit physical exertion to avoid incontinence episodes, they should be encouraged to seek treatment instead of limiting their activities. (R)

102. **3.** A characteristic of urge incontinence is involuntary urination with little or no warning. The inability to empty the bladder is urine retention. Loss of urine when coughing occurs with stress incontinence. Frequent dribbling of urine is common in male clients after some types of prostate surgery or may occur in women after the development of a vesicovaginal or urethrovaginal fistula. (A)

103. **1.** Instructing the client to void at regularly scheduled intervals can help decrease the frequency of incontinence episodes. Providing a bedside commode does not decrease the number of incontinence episodes and does not help the client who leads an active lifestyle. Infections are not a common cause of urge incontinence, so antibiotics are not an appropriate treatment. Intermittent self-catheterization is appropriate for overflow or reflux incontinence, but not urge incontinence, because it does not treat the underlying cause. (A)

The Client with Reproductive Health Problems

- The Client with a Vaginal Infection
- The Client with Uterine Fibroids
- The Client with Breast Disease
- The Client with Benign Prostatic Hypertrophy
- The Client with a Sexually Transmitted Disease
- The Client with Cancer of the Cervix
- The Client Having Gynecological Surgery
- The Client with Testicular Disease
- The Client with Cancer of the Prostate
- The Client with Erectile Dysfunction
- Correct Answers and Rationales

The Client with a Vaginal Infection

1. A nurse is reviewing a client's chart and notes the Papanicolaou smear laboratory report indicates visualization of clue cells and a vaginal pH of 3.8. What should the nurse teach this client? Select all that apply.
- ☐ **1.** Seek care if the vaginal discharge has a fishy odor.
- ☐ **2.** Seek care if experiencing thick, white, adherent vaginal discharge.
- ☐ **3.** All vaginal infections are sexually transmitted infections.
- ☐ **4.** Do not douche unless instructed by a health care provider.
- ☐ **5.** Usually vaginal infections can be treated with over-the-counter preparations.

2. A nurse is discussing daily activities with a client. Which of the following activities puts the client at risk for altering the normal pH of her vagina?
- ☐ **1.** Consuming over 4 cups of coffee per day.
- ☐ **2.** Having sexual intercourse during the menstrual cycle.
- ☐ **3.** Douching unless instructed to do so by the health care provider.
- ☐ **4.** Using tampons during the menstrual cycle.

3. A client is prescribed oral metronidazole (Flagyl) for treatment of bacterial vaginosis. What should the nurse instruct the client to avoid during treatment and for 24 hours thereafter?
- ☐ **1.** Douching.
- ☐ **2.** Sexual intercourse.
- ☐ **3.** Hot tub baths.
- ☐ **4.** Alcohol consumption.

4. The nurse is teaching the pregnant client the importance of seeking treatment for suspected bacterial vaginosis during pregnancy because it has been associated with:
- ☐ **1.** Gestational diabetes.
- ☐ **2.** Placenta previa.
- ☐ **3.** Preterm labor.
- ☐ **4.** Pregnancy-induced hypertension.

5. Which treatment is recommended by the Centers for Disease Control and Prevention (CDC) for bacterial vaginosis in pregnancy?
- ☐ **1.** Vinegar douche.
- ☐ **2.** 100 g clindamycin (Cleocin) ovules intravaginally.
- ☐ **3.** 300 mg clindamycin P.O. twice a day for 7 days.
- ☐ **4.** 500 mg metronidazole (Flagyl) I.V.

6. Which of the following females is at greatest risk for bacterial vaginosis?
- ☐ **1.** A 75-year-old.
- ☐ **2.** A 52-year-old experiencing menopause.
- ☐ **3.** A 28-year-old.
- ☐ **4.** A 12-year-old experiencing menarche.

7. A nurse is assessing a client with vaginal discharge. Which of the following diseases are commonly associated with vaginal discharge? Select all that apply.
☐ **1.** Candidiasis.
☐ **2.** Bacterial vaginosis.
☐ **3.** Gonorrhea.
☐ **4.** Trichomoniasis.
☐ **5.** Syphilis.

8. A female client with which condition would be at increased risk for vulvovaginal candidiasis? Select all that apply.
☐ **1.** Uncontrolled diabetes.
☐ **2.** Immunosuppression due to cancer.
☐ **3.** Human immunodeficiency virus (HIV) infection.
☐ **4.** Hypertension.
☐ **5.** Asthma.

9. A client taking oral contraceptives is placed on a 10-day course of antibiotics for an infection. Which of the following instructions should the nurse include in the teaching plan?
☐ **1.** "Use a barrier method of birth control for the rest of your cycle."
☐ **2.** "You should stop taking the oral contraceptives while taking the antibiotic."
☐ **3.** "Call your health care provider for increased hunger or fluid retention."
☐ **4.** "Take the antibiotics 2 hours after the oral contraceptive."

10. A client is asking for information about using an intrauterine device (IUD). Which of the following questions asked by the nurse would provide pertinent information on whether or not a client is a candidate for an IUD?
☐ **1.** "Do you smoke?"
☐ **2.** "Do you have hypertension?"
☐ **3.** "How often do you have sex?"
☐ **4.** "Are you in a monogamous relationship?"

11. A nurse is caring for a 22-year-old female client with type 1 diabetes mellitus and toxic shock syndrome (TSS). Which of the following physician orders should the nurse perform first?
☐ **1.** Administer 5% dextrose in half-normal saline solution at 150 ml/hour I.V.
☐ **2.** Administer 50 mg of meperidine (Demerol) I.M. every 4 hours as needed for pain.
☐ **3.** Teach the client to use pads at night instead of tampons during her menstrual period.
☐ **4.** Administer 400 mg of ciprofloxacin (Cipro) I.V. every 12 hours infused over 1 hour.

The Client with Uterine Fibroids

12. A 39-year-old female client has been experiencing intermittent vaginal bleeding for several months. Her physician tells her that she has uterine fibroids and recommends an abdominal hysterectomy. The nurse is completing the routine admission assessment when the client expresses fear about the surgery. Which of the following statements offers the best guide for the nurse's response? The nurse should:
☐ **1.** Reassure the client of her physician's competence.
☐ **2.** Give the client opportunities to express her fears.
☐ **3.** Teach the client that fear impedes recovery.
☐ **4.** Change the subject of conversation to pleasantries when the client appears fearful.

13. A female with uterine fibroids presents with dysmenorrhea and menorrhagia. The nurse practitioner orders a complete blood count and blood chemistry. Which results should the nurse report? Select all that apply.
☐ **1.** Hemoglobin, 9.0 g/dl.
☐ **2.** Hematocrit, 27.1%.
☐ **3.** White blood cell count, 10,000 cells/mm³.
☐ **4.** Potassium, 4.0 mEq/L.
☐ **5.** Normocytic red blood cells.

14. The client having an abdominal hysterectomy is admitted the morning of surgery. Essential information the client needs before admission includes which of the following?
☐ **1.** What to wear to the hospital.
☐ **2.** What she can eat and drink before admission.
☐ **3.** The type of pain medication that will be prescribed postoperatively.
☐ **4.** Preoperative teaching about exercises at home.

15. The nurse is witnessing the client's signature on the informed surgical consent for an abdominal hysterectomy. It is important to ascertain that the client understands that with this surgical procedure she will have:
☐ **1.** Decreased libido.
☐ **2.** Infertility.
☐ **3.** Depression.
☐ **4.** Weight gain.

16. During the immediate postoperative period after an abdominal hysterectomy, the client requires catheterization because she is unable to void. When preparing to insert the catheter into the urinary meatus, the nurse locates the anatomic structures between the labia minora. Starting from the area nearer the pubic bone and moving downward toward the anus, in which order do the clitoris, vaginal opening, and urinary meatus lie?
☐ **1.** Clitoris, vaginal opening, urinary meatus.
☐ **2.** Urinary meatus, vaginal opening, clitoris.
☐ **3.** Vaginal opening, clitoris, urinary meatus.
☐ **4.** Clitoris, urinary meatus, vaginal opening.

17. The nurse is assigning tasks to the unlicensed assistive personnel (UAP) for a client with an abdominal hysterectomy on the first postoperative day. Which of the following cannot be delegated to the UAP?
- ☐ **1.** Taking vital signs.
- ☐ **2.** Recording intake and output.
- ☐ **3.** Giving perineal care.
- ☐ **4.** Assessing the incision site.

18. Which of the following physical sensations will the client who has had an abdominal hysterectomy most likely experience if she hyperventilates while performing deep-breathing exercises?
- ☐ **1.** Dyspnea.
- ☐ **2.** Dizziness.
- ☐ **3.** Blurred vision.
- ☐ **4.** Mental confusion.

19. The unlicensed assistive personnel (UAP) reports to the nurse that the client with an abdominal hysterectomy who returned from the recovery room 1 hour earlier has saturated the blue pad with bright red blood. The nurse should:
- ☐ **1.** Call the surgeon to report the bleeding.
- ☐ **2.** Ask the UAP to obtain vital signs while the nurse calls the surgeon.
- ☐ **3.** Ask the UAP to increase the flow of I.V. fluids to prevent shock.
- ☐ **4.** Assess the client again in 15 minutes before the nurse takes any further action.

20. Which nursing measure would most likely relieve postoperative gas pains after abdominal hysterectomy?
- ☐ **1.** Offering the client a hot beverage.
- ☐ **2.** Providing extra warmth.
- ☐ **3.** Applying a snugly fitting abdominal binder.
- ☐ **4.** Helping the client walk.

21. On the second postoperative day after an abdominal hysterectomy, the client develops a temperature of 100.4° F (38° C). The nurse's first action should be to:
- ☐ **1.** Increase the number of wound changes to minimize infection.
- ☐ **2.** Obtain a culture and sensitivity study of the urine to determine the source of infection.
- ☐ **3.** Ensure that the client takes at least 10 deep breaths every hour.
- ☐ **4.** Change the site of the client's I.V. fluid catheter to reduce the risk of infection.

22. The nurse in a rural hospital has just been notified that a client is being admitted from the emergency department with a nursing home–acquired pneumonia. The unit has four empty beds in semiprivate rooms. The room that would be most suitable for this client is the one with a:
- ☐ **1.** 60-year-old client admitted for investigation of transient ischemic attacks.
- ☐ **2.** 45-year-old client with an abdominal hysterectomy.
- ☐ **3.** 24-year-old client with non-Hodgkin's lymphoma.
- ☐ **4.** 55-year-old client with alcoholic cirrhosis.

23. The nurse is changing the dressing of a client after an abdominal hysterectomy. Which of the following nursing measures would be most appropriate if the dressing adheres to the client's incisional area?
- ☐ **1.** Pull off the dressing quickly and then apply slight pressure over the area.
- ☐ **2.** Lift an easily moved portion of the dressing and then remove it slowly.
- ☐ **3.** Moisten the dressing with sterile normal saline solution and then remove it.
- ☐ **4.** Remove part of the dressing and then remove the remainder gradually over a period of several minutes.

24. A priority nursing diagnosis for the postoperative client who experiences wound dehiscence after an abdominal hysterectomy would be:
- ☐ **1.** *Risk for infection.*
- ☐ **2.** *Excess fluid volume.*
- ☐ **3.** *Ineffective airway clearance.*
- ☐ **4.** *Imbalanced nutrition: Less than body requirements.*

25. The client with an abdominal hysterectomy is being prepared for discharge in the morning. The nurse knows from the admission psychosocial assessment that the client has a mentally retarded adult son whom she cares for at home. The nurse should discuss with the physician the need for referral to which of the following departments?
- ☐ **1.** Home health care.
- ☐ **2.** Social work.
- ☐ **3.** Pastoral care.
- ☐ **4.** Volunteer services.

26. Which of the following hormones is likely to be prescribed for the client experiencing hot flashes after an abdominal hysterectomy and removal of the ovaries and fallopian tubes?
- ☐ **1.** Estrogen.
- ☐ **2.** Thyroxine.
- ☐ **3.** Prolactin.
- ☐ **4.** Testosterone.

27. Which of the following nursing diagnoses would be most appropriate for the client being discharged from the hospital 3 days after an abdominal hysterectomy?

☐ **1.** *Imbalanced nutrition: Less than body requirements* related to nausea and vomiting.

☐ **2.** *Excess fluid volume* related to surgery.

☐ **3.** *Ineffective breathing pattern* related to postoperative pneumonia.

☐ **4.** *Ineffective coping* related to body image disturbance.

28. When preparing discharge instructions for a client after an abdominal hysterectomy, the nurse should first:

☐ **1.** Have the client watch an educational video.

☐ **2.** Assess the client's available social supports.

☐ **3.** Call the social worker to evaluate the client.

☐ **4.** Read the discharge instructions to the client.

29. Which of the following should the nurse include in the teaching plan about menopause for a client? Select all that apply.

☐ **1.** The average age of onset for menopause is 50 to 52 years.

☐ **2.** Follicle-stimulating hormone (FSH) and luteinizing hormone (LH) levels are elevated.

☐ **3.** Depression is very common as a result of menopause.

☐ **4.** Hot flashes, especially at night, can occur in about 80% of women.

☐ **5.** When periods become irregular, contraception is unnecessary.

The Client with Breast Disease

30. A postmenopausal woman is worried about pain in the upper outer quadrant of her left breast. The nurse's first course of action is to:

☐ **1.** Do a breast examination and report the results to the physician.

☐ **2.** Explain that pain is caused by hormonal fluctuations.

☐ **3.** Reassure the client that pain is not a symptom of breast cancer.

☐ **4.** Teach the client the correct procedure for breast self-examination (BSE).

31. The nurse teaches a female client that the best time in the menstrual cycle to examine the breasts is during the:

☐ **1.** Week that ovulation occurs.

☐ **2.** Week that menstruation occurs.

☐ **3.** First week after menstruation.

☐ **4.** Week before menstruation occurs.

32. A female with bilateral breast implants asks if she still needs to do breast examinations because she does not know what to feel for. Which of the following is the nurse's best response?

☐ **1.** "Have your partner assess your breasts on a regular basis."

☐ **2.** "I will show you the correct technique as I do the breast examination."

☐ **3.** "A breast examination is very difficult when you have had implant surgery."

☐ **4.** "You need to have a mammogram instead."

33. The client states that she has noticed that her bra fits more snugly at certain times of the month. She asks the nurse if this is a sign of breast disease. The nurse should base the reply to this client on the knowledge that:

☐ **1.** Benign cysts tend to cause the breasts to vary in size.

☐ **2.** It is normal for the breasts to increase in size before menstruation begins.

☐ **3.** A change in breast size warrants further investigation.

☐ **4.** Differences in breast size are related to normal growth and development.

34. A 76-year-old client tells the nurse that she has lived long and does not need mammograms. Which is the nurse's best response?

☐ **1.** "Having a mammogram when you are older is less painful."

☐ **2.** "The incidence of breast cancer increases with age."

☐ **3.** "We need to consider your family history of breast cancer first."

☐ **4.** "It will be sufficient if you perform breast examinations monthly."

35. After the surgeon's meeting with a client to obtain the client's informed consent for a modified radical mastectomy, the client asks the nurse many questions about breast reconstruction that the nurse finds difficult to answer. The nurse should:

☐ **1.** Inform the surgeon that the client has questions about reconstruction before she signs the consent.

☐ **2.** Inform the client that she should concentrate on recovering from the mastectomy first.

☐ **3.** Inform the client that she can have a consultation with the plastic surgeon in a few weeks.

☐ **4.** Inform the client she can ask the surgeon these questions later when the surgeon makes rounds.

36. During the admission workup for a modified radical mastectomy, the client is extremely anxious and asks many questions. Which of the following statements would offer the best guide for the nurse to answer questions raised by this apprehensive preoperative client? It is usually best to:
- ☐ 1. Tell the client as much as she wants to know and is able to understand.
- ☐ 2. Delay discussing the client's questions with her until she is convalescing.
- ☐ 3. Delay discussing the client's questions with her until her apprehension subsides.
- ☐ 4. Explain to the client that she should discuss her questions first with the physician.

37. A client asks the nurse, "Where is cancer usually found in the breast?" When responding to the client, the nurse uses a diagram of a left breast and indicates that most malignant tumors occur in which quadrant of the breast?
- ☐ 1. Upper outer quadrant.
- ☐ 2. Upper inner quadrant.
- ☐ 3. Lower outer quadrant.
- ☐ 4. Lower inner quadrant.

38. Atropine sulfate is included in the preoperative orders for a client undergoing a modified radical mastectomy. The primary reason for giving this drug preoperatively is that it:
- ☐ 1. Helps to promote general muscular relaxation.
- ☐ 2. Helps to decrease pulse and respiratory rates.
- ☐ 3. Helps to decrease nausea.
- ☐ 4. Helps to inhibit oral and respiratory secretions.

39. During the postoperative period after a modified radical mastectomy, the client confides in the nurse that she thinks she got breast cancer because she had an abortion and she did not tell her husband. The best response by the nurse is which of the following?
- ☐ 1. "Cancer is not a punishment; it is a disease."
- ☐ 2. "You might feel better if you confided in your husband."
- ☐ 3. "Tell me more about your feelings on this."
- ☐ 4. "I can have the social worker talk to you if you would like."

40. Postoperatively after a modified radical mastectomy, a client has an incisional drainage tube attached to Hemovac suction. The primary purpose of this tube is to:
- ☐ 1. Decrease intrathoracic pressure and facilitate breathing.
- ☐ 2. Increase collateral lymphatic flow toward the operative area.
- ☐ 3. Remove accumulated serum and blood in the operative area.
- ☐ 4. Prevent formation of adhesions between the skin and chest wall in the operative area.

41. Which of the following positions would be best for a client's right arm when she returns to her room after a right modified radical mastectomy with multiple lymph node excisions?
- ☐ 1. Across her chest wall.
- ☐ 2. At her side at the same level as her body.
- ☐ 3. In the position that affords her the greatest comfort without placing pressure on the incision.
- ☐ 4. On pillows, with her hand higher than her elbow and her elbow higher than her shoulder.

42. The client with breast cancer is prescribed tamoxifen (Nolvadex) 20 mg daily. The client states she does not like taking medicine and asks the nurse if the tamoxifen is really worth taking. The nurse's best response is which of the following?
- ☐ 1. "This drug is part of your chemotherapy program."
- ☐ 2. "This drug has been found to decrease metastatic breast cancer."
- ☐ 3. "This drug will act as an estrogen in your breast tissue."
- ☐ 4. "This drug will prevent hot flashes since you cannot take hormone replacement."

43. A client undergoing chemotherapy after a modified radical mastectomy asks the nurse questions about a breast prosthesis and wigs. After answering the questions directly, the nurse should also:
- ☐ 1. Provide a list of resources, including the local breast cancer support group.
- ☐ 2. Offer a referral to the social worker.
- ☐ 3. Call the home health care agency.
- ☐ 4. Contact the plastic surgeon.

44. A client is to have radiation therapy after a modified radical mastectomy. The client should be taught to care for the skin at the site of therapy by:
- ☐ 1. Washing the area with water.
- ☐ 2. Exposing the area to dry heat.
- ☐ 3. Applying an ointment to the area.
- ☐ 4. Using talcum powder on the area.

45. The nurse should teach a client that a normal local tissue response to radiation is:
☐ **1.** Atrophy of the skin.
☐ **2.** Scattered pustule formation.
☐ **3.** Redness of the surface tissue.
☐ **4.** Sloughing of two layers of skin.

46. The nurse refers a client who had a mastectomy to "Reach to Recovery." The primary purpose of the American Cancer Society's Reach to Recovery program is to:
☐ **1.** Foster rehabilitation in women who have had mastectomies.
☐ **2.** Raise funds to support early breast cancer detection programs.
☐ **3.** Provide free dressings for women who have had radical mastectomies.
☐ **4.** Collect statistics for research from women who have had mastectomies.

The Client with Benign Prostatic Hypertrophy

47. A 72-year-old male client is brought to the emergency department by his son. The client is extremely uncomfortable and has been unable to void for the past 12 hours. He has known for some time that he has an enlarged prostate but has wanted to avoid surgery. The best method for the nurse to use when assessing for bladder distention in a male client is to check for:
☐ **1.** A rounded swelling above the pubis.
☐ **2.** Dullness in the lower left quadrant.
☐ **3.** Rebound tenderness below the symphysis.
☐ **4.** Urine discharge from the urethral meatus.

48. During a client's urinary bladder catheterization, the nurse ensures that the bladder is emptied gradually. The best rationale for the nurse's action is that completely emptying an overdistended bladder at one time tends to cause:
☐ **1.** Renal failure.
☐ **2.** Abdominal cramping.
☐ **3.** Possible shock.
☐ **4.** Atrophy of bladder musculature.

49. The primary reason for lubricating the urinary catheter generously before inserting it into a male client is that this technique helps reduce:
☐ **1.** Spasms at the orifice of the bladder.
☐ **2.** Friction along the urethra when the catheter is being inserted.
☐ **3.** The number of organisms gaining entrance to the bladder.
☐ **4.** The formation of encrustations that may occur at the end of the catheter.

50. The primary reason for taping an indwelling catheter laterally to the thigh of a male client is to:
☐ **1.** Eliminate pressure at the penoscrotal angle.
☐ **2.** Prevent the catheter from kinking in the urethra.
☐ **3.** Prevent accidental catheter removal.
☐ **4.** Allow the client to turn without kinking the catheter.

51. The primary function of the prostate gland is to:
☐ **1.** Store underdeveloped sperm before ejaculation.
☐ **2.** Regulate the acidity and alkalinity of the environment for proper sperm development.
☐ **3.** Produce a secretion that aids the nourishment and passage of sperm.
☐ **4.** Secrete a hormone that stimulates the production and maturation of sperm.

52. Many older males with prostatic hypertrophy do not seek medical attention until urinary obstruction is almost complete. Investigations have found that the primary reason for this delay in seeking attention is that these males:
☐ **1.** Feel too self-conscious to seek help when reproductive organs are involved.
☐ **2.** Expect that it is normal to have to live with some urinary problems as they grow older.
☐ **3.** Fear that sexual indiscretions in earlier life may be the cause of their problem.
☐ **4.** Have little discomfort in relation to the amount of pathology because responses to pain stimuli fade with age.

53. The nurse anticipates that a client with prostatic hypertrophy will most likely report having experienced which of the following symptoms?
☐ **1.** Voiding at less frequent intervals.
☐ **2.** Difficulty starting the flow of urine.
☐ **3.** Painful urination.
☐ **4.** Increased force of the urine stream.

54. The nurse is reviewing the medication history of a client with benign prostatic hypertrophy (BPH). Which medication should be recognized as likely to aggravate BPH?
☐ **1.** Metformin (Glucophage).
☐ **2.** Buspirone (BuSpar).
☐ **3.** Inhaled ipratropium (Atrovent).
☐ **4.** Ophthalmic timolol (Timoptic).

55. A client is scheduled to undergo transurethral resection of the prostate. The procedure is to be done under spinal anesthesia. Postoperatively, the nurse should be particularly alert for early signs and symptoms of:
- [ ] **1.** Seizures.
- [ ] **2.** Cardiac arrest.
- [ ] **3.** Renal shutdown.
- [ ] **4.** Respiratory paralysis.

56. A common nursing diagnosis for a client in the immediate postoperative phase after transurethral resection of the prostate (TURP) is:
- [ ] **1.** *Ineffective peripheral tissue perfusion* related to deep vein thrombosis.
- [ ] **2.** *Acute pain* related to pain of bladder spasms.
- [ ] **3.** *Disturbed body image* related to disfiguring surgery.
- [ ] **4.** *Imbalanced nutrition: Less than body requirements.*

57. A client with benign prostatic hypertrophy (BPH) is being treated with terazosin (Hytrin) 2 mg at bedtime. The nurse should monitor the client's:
- [ ] **1.** Urine nitrites.
- [ ] **2.** White blood cell count.
- [ ] **3.** Blood pressure.
- [ ] **4.** Pulse.

58. A client underwent transurethral resection of the prostate (TURP), and a large three-way indwelling urinary catheter was inserted in the bladder with continuous bladder irrigation. In which of the following circumstances should the nurse increase the flow rate of the continuous bladder irrigation?
- [ ] **1.** When drainage is continuous but slow.
- [ ] **2.** When drainage appears cloudy and dark yellow.
- [ ] **3.** When drainage becomes bright red.
- [ ] **4.** When there is no drainage of urine and irrigating solution.

59. A client is to receive belladonna and opium suppositories, as needed, postoperatively after transurethral resection of the prostate (TURP). The nurse should give the client these drugs when he demonstrates signs of:
- [ ] **1.** A urinary tract infection.
- [ ] **2.** Urine retention.
- [ ] **3.** Frequent urination.
- [ ] **4.** Pain from bladder spasms.

60. A nursing assistant tells the nurse, "I think the client is confused. He keeps telling me he has to void, but that isn't possible because he has a catheter in place that is draining well." Which of the following responses would be most appropriate for the nurse to make?
- [ ] **1.** "His catheter is probably plugged. I'll irrigate it in a few minutes."
- [ ] **2.** "That's a common complaint after prostate surgery. The client only imagines the urge to void."
- [ ] **3.** "The urge to void is usually created by the large catheter, and he may be having some bladder spasms."
- [ ] **4.** "I think he may be somewhat confused."

61. A report on a urine culture indicates numerous white and red blood cells and a moderate amount of bacterial growth. The nurse evaluating these findings should deduce that the client most likely has a:
- [ ] **1.** Urethral stricture.
- [ ] **2.** Decreased renal filtration rate.
- [ ] **3.** Urinary tract infection (UTI).
- [ ] **4.** Prostate gland malignancy.

62. In discussing home care with a client after transurethral resection of the prostate (TURP), the nurse should teach the male client that dribbling of urine:
- [ ] **1.** Can be a chronic problem.
- [ ] **2.** Can persist for several months.
- [ ] **3.** Is an abnormal sign that requires intervention.
- [ ] **4.** Is a sign of healing within the prostate.

63. A priority nursing diagnosis for the client who is being discharged to home 3 days after transurethral resection of the prostate (TURP) would be:
- [ ] **1.** *Deficient fluid volume.*
- [ ] **2.** *Imbalanced nutrition: Less than body requirements.*
- [ ] **3.** *Impaired tissue integrity.*
- [ ] **4.** *Ineffective airway clearance.*

64. If a client's prostate enlargement is caused by a malignancy, which of the following blood examinations should the nurse anticipate to assess to determine whether metastasis has occurred?
- [ ] **1.** Serum creatinine level.
- [ ] **2.** Serum acid phosphatase level.
- [ ] **3.** Total nonprotein nitrogen level.
- [ ] **4.** Endogenous creatinine clearance time.

The Client with a Sexually Transmitted Disease

65. A home care nurse begins caring for a 25-year-old female client who has just been diagnosed with human immunodeficiency virus (HIV) infection. The client asks the nurse, "How could this have happened?" The nurse responds to the question based on the most frequent mode of HIV transmission, which is:
- ☐ 1. Hugging an HIV-positive sexual partner without using barrier precautions.
- ☐ 2. Inhaling cocaine.
- ☐ 3. Sharing food utensils with an HIV-positive person without proper cleaning of the utensils.
- ☐ 4. Having sexual intercourse with an HIV-positive person without using a condom.

66. A client with human immunodeficiency virus (HIV) infection is taking zidovudine (AZT). AZT is a drug that acts to:
- ☐ 1. Destroy the virus.
- ☐ 2. Enhance the body's antibody production.
- ☐ 3. Slow replication of the virus.
- ☐ 4. Neutralize toxins produced by the virus.

67. Women who have human papillomavirus (HPV) are at risk for development of:
- ☐ 1. Sterility.
- ☐ 2. Cervical cancer.
- ☐ 3. Uterine fibroid tumors.
- ☐ 4. Irregular menses.

68. Which of the following nursing diagnoses would most likely be a priority for a client with herpes genitalis?
- ☐ 1. *Insomnia.*
- ☐ 2. *Imbalanced nutrition: Less than body requirements.*
- ☐ 3. *Pain.*
- ☐ 4. *Ineffective breathing pattern.*

69. The primary reason that a herpes simplex virus (HSV) infection is a serious concern to a client with human immunodeficiency virus (HIV) infection is that it:
- ☐ 1. Is an acquired immunodeficiency virus (AIDS)–defining illness.
- ☐ 2. Is curable only after 1 year of antiviral therapy.
- ☐ 3. Leads to cervical cancer.
- ☐ 4. Causes severe electrolyte imbalances.

70. In educating a client about human immunodeficiency virus (HIV), the nurse should take into account the fact that the most effective method known to control the spread of HIV infection is:
- ☐ 1. Premarital serologic screening.
- ☐ 2. Prophylactic treatment of exposed people.
- ☐ 3. Laboratory screening of pregnant women.
- ☐ 4. Ongoing sex education about preventive behaviors.

71. A male client with human immunodeficiency virus (HIV) infection becomes depressed and tells the nurse: "I have nothing worth living for now." Which of the following statements would be the best response by the nurse?
- ☐ 1. "You are a young person and have a great deal to live for."
- ☐ 2. "You should not be too depressed; we are close to finding a cure for AIDS."
- ☐ 3. "You are right; it is very depressing to have HIV."
- ☐ 4. "Tell me more about how you are feeling about being HIV-positive."

72. The organism responsible for causing syphilis is classified as a:
- ☐ 1. Virus.
- ☐ 2. Fungus.
- ☐ 3. Rickettsia.
- ☐ 4. Spirochete.

73. The typical chancre of syphilis appears as:
- ☐ 1. A grouping of small, tender pimples.
- ☐ 2. An elevated wart.
- ☐ 3. A painless, moist ulcer.
- ☐ 4. An itching, crusted area.

74. When interviewing a client with newly diagnosed syphilis, the public health nurse should be aware that the spread of the disease can be controlled by:
- ☐ 1. Motivating the client to undergo treatment.
- ☐ 2. Obtaining a list of the client's sexual contacts.
- ☐ 3. Increasing the client's knowledge of the disease.
- ☐ 4. Reassuring the client that records are confidential.

75. Benzathine penicillin G, 2.4 million units I.M., is prescribed as treatment for an adult client with primary syphilis. The I.M. injection is administered in the:
- ☐ 1. Deltoid.
- ☐ 2. Upper outer quadrant of the buttock.
- ☐ 3. Quadriceps lateralis of the thigh.
- ☐ 4. Midlateral aspect of the thigh.

76. A priority nursing diagnosis for a client with primary syphilis is:
- [ ] 1. *Deficient knowledge* related to lack of information about the mode of transmission.
- [ ] 2. *Pain* related to cutaneous skin lesions on palms and soles.
- [ ] 3. *Ineffective tissue perfusion* related to a bleeding chancre.
- [ ] 4. *Disturbed body image* related to alopecia.

77. An 18-year-old female college student is seen at the university health center. She undergoes a pelvic examination and is diagnosed with gonorrhea. Which of the following responses by the nurse would be best when the client says that she is nervous about the upcoming pelvic examination?
- [ ] 1. "Can you tell me more about how you're feeling?"
- [ ] 2. "You're not alone. Most women feel uncomfortable about this examination."
- [ ] 3. "Do not worry about Dr. Smith. He's a specialist in female problems."
- [ ] 4. "We'll do everything we can to avoid embarrassing you."

78. When educating a female client with gonorrhea, the nurse should emphasize that for women gonorrhea:
- [ ] 1. Is often marked by symptoms of dysuria or vaginal bleeding.
- [ ] 2. Does not lead to serious complications.
- [ ] 3. Can be treated but not cured.
- [ ] 4. May not cause symptoms until serious complications occur.

79. Which of the following groups has experienced the greatest rise in the incidence of sexually transmitted diseases (STDs) over the past two decades?
- [ ] 1. Teenagers.
- [ ] 2. Divorced people.
- [ ] 3. Young married couples.
- [ ] 4. Older adults.

80. A 16-year-old sexually active male client comes to the clinic with a complaint of burning on urination and a milky discharge from the urethral meatus. Documentation on the client's chart should include which of the following information? Select all that apply.
- [ ] 1. History of unprotected sex (sex without a condom).
- [ ] 2. Length of time since symptoms presented.
- [ ] 3. History of fever or chills.
- [ ] 4. Presence of any enlarged lymph nodes on examination.
- [ ] 5. Names and phone numbers of all sexual contacts.
- [ ] 6. Allergies to any medications.

81. A 19-year-old male client is diagnosed with a chlamydial infection. Azithromycin (Zithromax) 1 g is ordered. The supply of azithromycin is in 250-mg tablets. How many tablets should the nurse administer?

_____ tablets

82. A female client with gonorrhea informs the nurse that she has had sexual intercourse with her boyfriend and asks the nurse, "Would he have any symptoms?" The nurse responds that in men the symptoms of gonorrhea include:
- [ ] 1. Impotence.
- [ ] 2. Scrotal swelling.
- [ ] 3. Urine retention.
- [ ] 4. Dysuria.

83. The nurse assesses the mouth and oral cavity of a client with human immunodeficiency virus (HIV) infection because the most common opportunistic infection initially presents as:
- [ ] 1. Herpes simplex virus (HSV) lesions on the lips.
- [ ] 2. Oral candidiasis.
- [ ] 3. Cytomegalovirus (CMV) infection.
- [ ] 4. Aphthae on the gingiva.

The Client with Cancer of the Cervix

84. A 45-year-old female client makes a clinic appointment for a routine gynecologic examination. The position of choice for a client undergoing a vaginal examination is the:
- [ ] 1. Sims position.
- [ ] 2. Lithotomy position.
- [ ] 3. Genupectoral position.
- [ ] 4. Dorsal recumbent position.

85. A client asks the nurse to explain the meaning of her abnormal Papanicolaou (Pap) smear result of atypical squamous cells. Which of the following concepts should the nurse include in the response?
- [ ] 1. An atypical Pap smear means that abnormal viral cells were found in the smear.
- [ ] 2. An atypical Pap smear means that cancer cells were found in the smear.
- [ ] 3. A positive Pap smear alone is not very important diagnostically because there are many false-positive results.
- [ ] 4. Abnormal cells in a Pap smear may be caused by various conditions that help identify a problem early.

86. Which of the following is a risk factor for cervical cancer?
☐ 1. Sexual experiences with one partner.
☐ 2. Sedentary lifestyle.
☐ 3. Obesity.
☐ 4. Adolescent pregnancy.

87. The American Cancer Society recommends that adult women follow which schedule for Papanicolaou (Pap) smear screening?
☐ 1. Annually for women in the high-risk category.
☐ 2. Annually if sexually active; every 5 years if sexually abstinent.
☐ 3. Every 3 years after one initial negative test.
☐ 4. Every 3 years until age 40 and annually thereafter.

88. A woman tells the nurse that she is always nervous about the pelvic examination and Papanicolaou (Pap) smear because "there's been a lot of cancer in my family." The nurse should be aware that a possible sign of cervical cancer is:
☐ 1. Pain.
☐ 2. Leg edema.
☐ 3. Urinary and rectal symptoms.
☐ 4. Light bleeding or watery vaginal discharge.

89. A 30-year-old female client asks the nurse about douching. What information should the nurse include in the teaching plan?
☐ 1. Douching during menstruation is safe.
☐ 2. Daily douching will decrease vaginal odor.
☐ 3. Perfumed douches are recommended to decrease odors.
☐ 4. Douching removes natural mucus and changes the balance of normal vaginal flora.

90. A 28-year-old female without health insurance is receiving treatment for cervical cancer. She is a single parent of two young children and is referred to the social worker. The client states to the nurse, "I feel overwhelmed and beyond help. What can the social worker do to help me?" Which responses by the nurse about the role of the social worker are most appropriate? Select all that apply.
☐ 1. "The social worker is a part of a multidisciplinary team that provides care for clients with cancer."
☐ 2. "The social worker can explain federal, state, and not-for-profit resources and programs to you."
☐ 3. "Based on your income and family situation, the social worker will help you in applying for various assistance programs."
☐ 4. "Your entire family will be included in the treatment plan. Your needs and those of your children will be assessed and determined so that referrals can be made to appropriate resources."
☐ 5. "As the client, you will not have choices about the programs and resources you utilize.

91. The husband of a client with cervical cancer says to the nurse, "The doctor told my wife that her cancer is curable. Is he just trying to make us feel better?" Which would be the nurse's most accurate response?
☐ 1. "When cervical cancer is detected early and treated aggressively, the cure rate is almost 100%."
☐ 2. "The 5-year survival rate is about 75%, which makes the odds pretty good."
☐ 3. "Saying a cancer is curable means that 50% of all women with the cancer survive at least 5 years."
☐ 4. "Cancers of the female reproductive tract tend to be slow-growing and respond well to treatment."

92. A client with suspected cervical cancer is undergoing a colposcopy with conization. The nurse gives instructions to the client about her menstrual periods, emphasizing that:
☐ 1. Her periods will return to normal after 6 months.
☐ 2. Her next two or three periods may be heavier and more prolonged than usual.
☐ 3. Her next two or three periods will be lighter than normal.
☐ 4. She may skip her next two periods.

93. A client with cervical cancer is undergoing internal radium implant therapy. A lead-lined container and a pair of long forceps are kept in the client's hospital room for:
☐ 1. Disposal of emesis or other bodily secretions.
☐ 2. Handling of the dislodged radiation source.
☐ 3. Disposal of the client's eating utensils.
☐ 4. Storage of the radiation dose.

94. The mother of a client who has a radium implant asks why so many nurses are involved in her daughter's care. She states, "The doctor said I can be in the room for up to 2 hours each day, but the nurses say they're restricted to 30 minutes." The nurse explains that this variation is based on the fact that nurses:
☐ 1. Touch the client, which increases their exposure to radiation.
☐ 2. Work with many clients and could carry infection to a client receiving radiation therapy, if exposure is prolonged.
☐ 3. Work with radiation on an ongoing basis, while visitors have infrequent exposure to radiation.
☐ 4. Are at greater risk from the radiation because they are younger than the mother.

95. A priority nursing diagnosis for a client with cervical cancer who has an internal radium implant would be:
- ☐ 1. *Pain* related to cervical tumor.
- ☐ 2. *Anxiety* related to self-care deficit from imposed immobility during radiation.
- ☐ 3. *Ineffective health maintenance* related to surgery.
- ☐ 4. *Insomnia* related to interruptions by health care personnel.

96. A client with human papillomavirus (HPV) infection is being treated by a colposcopy. The client asks the nurse if this procedure is really necessary. The nurse explains that the procedure to treat the warts is important because HPV can lead to:
- ☐ 1. Infertility.
- ☐ 2. Cervical cancer.
- ☐ 3. Pelvic inflammatory disease.
- ☐ 4. Rectal cancer.

97. Which of the following would be standard nursing care for a client with cervical cancer who has an internal radium implant in place?
- ☐ 1. Offer the bedpan every 2 hours.
- ☐ 2. Provide perineal care twice daily.
- ☐ 3. Check the position of the applicator hourly.
- ☐ 4. Offer a low-residue diet.

98. The nurse should carefully observe a client with internal radium implants for typical adverse effects associated with radiation therapy to the cervix. These effects include:
- ☐ 1. Severe vaginal itching.
- ☐ 2. Confusion.
- ☐ 3. High fever in the afternoon or evening.
- ☐ 4. Nausea and a foul vaginal discharge.

The Client Having Gynecological Surgery

99. The nurse-manager on a gynecologic surgical unit is addressing many complaints from the clients that they have to wait too long on the night shift for their pain medication. Which course of action should the nurse-manager take first?
- ☐ 1. Change the staffing schedule on nights to include a medication nurse.
- ☐ 2. Consult the nursing supervisor.
- ☐ 3. Consult the nurses on the evening shift about their evaluation of the night nurses regarding these complaints.
- ☐ 4. Complete a quality improvement study with the night nurses to document the waiting times for pain medication and other data, including staffing and patient acuity.

100. A nurse is reviewing the physician's admitting orders on a 52-year-old client scheduled for a dilatation and curettage. The nurse is unable to decipher the handwriting and determines the medication order reads either metoprolol succinate (Toprol) or topiramate (Topamax). What should the nurse do to focus on client safety?
- ☐ 1. Ask the client if she has hypertension.
- ☐ 2. Ask the client if she has migraines.
- ☐ 3. Call the physician to clarify the order.
- ☐ 4. Ask the pharmacist to interpret the order.

101. A client returned to the recovery room after a dilatation and curettage has the postoperative medication orders shown in the chart below. What should the nurse do next?
- ☐ 1. Ask the client to rate the intensity of her pain on a scale of 1 to 10 and administer the analgesia according to the intensity of the pain.
- ☐ 2. Administer the Demerol first because the client had surgery today.
- ☐ 3. Administer the Tylenol #3 first, and if it does not relieve the pain in 2 hours, administer the Demerol.
- ☐ 4. Administer the Motrin first and if it does not relieve the pain, administer the Demerol.

PRESCRIPTIONS

Rx   Meperidine (Demerol) 50 mg I.M. every 4 hours for severe pain

Acetaminophen (Tylenol #3) P.O. every 4 hours for pain

Ibuprofen (Motrin) 800 mg P.O. every 4 hours for pain.

102. A nurse on the gynecologic surgery unit observes a respiratory therapist (RT) take a medication cup with pills that was sitting in the medication room. What course of action should the nurse take?
- ☐ 1. Report the situation to the supervisor of respiratory therapy.
- ☐ 2. Tell the RT that you saw her take the pills from the medication room.
- ☐ 3. Report the situation to the nursing supervisor.
- ☐ 4. Tell the nurse who was administering medications not to leave pills out.

103. On the second day following an abdominal hysterectomy, a client reports she has had three brown, loose stools in moderate amount. The morning medications include an order for 100 mg of docusate sodium (Colace) daily. What should the nurse do next?
- ☐ **1.** Administer the Colace according to the physician's order.
- ☐ **2.** Ask the client if she is having gas pains or hunger.
- ☐ **3.** Withhold the medication and document withholding the medication on the medical record.
- ☐ **4.** Administer the Colace and instruct the client to avoid high-fiber foods.

The Client with Testicular Disease

104. A 28-year-old male is diagnosed with acute epididymitis. The nurse should expect to find that the signs and symptoms that caused the client to seek medical care are:
- ☐ **1.** Burning and pain on urination.
- ☐ **2.** Severe tenderness and swelling in the scrotum.
- ☐ **3.** Foul-smelling ejaculate.
- ☐ **4.** Foul-smelling urine.

105. A 20-year-old client is being treated for epididymitis. Teaching for this client should include the fact that epididymitis is commonly a result of a:
- ☐ **1.** Virus.
- ☐ **2.** Parasite.
- ☐ **3.** Sexually transmitted infection.
- ☐ **4.** Protozoon.

106. When teaching a client to perform testicular self-examination, the nurse explains that the examination should be performed:
- ☐ **1.** After intercourse.
- ☐ **2.** At the end of the day.
- ☐ **3.** After a warm bath or shower.
- ☐ **4.** After exercise.

107. The normal testes can be described as:
- ☐ **1.** Soft.
- ☐ **2.** Egg-shaped.
- ☐ **3.** Spongy.
- ☐ **4.** Lumpy.

108. A client has a testicular nodule that is highly suspicious for testicular cancer. A laboratory test that supports this diagnosis is:
- ☐ **1.** Decreased alpha fetoprotein (AFP).
- ☐ **2.** Decreased beta–human chorionic gonadotropin (hCG).
- ☐ **3.** Increased testosterone.
- ☐ **4.** Increased AFP.

109. Although the cause of testicular cancer is unknown, it is associated with a history of:
- ☐ **1.** Undescended testes.
- ☐ **2.** Sexual relations at an early age.
- ☐ **3.** Seminal vesiculitis.
- ☐ **4.** Epididymitis.

110. Risk factors associated with testicular malignancies include:
- ☐ **1.** African-American race.
- ☐ **2.** Residing in a rural area.
- ☐ **3.** Lower socioeconomic status.
- ☐ **4.** Age older than 40 years.

111. A client with a testicular malignancy undergoes a radical orchiectomy. A priority problem in the immediate postoperative period is:
- ☐ **1.** Bladder spasms.
- ☐ **2.** Urine elimination.
- ☐ **3.** Pain.
- ☐ **4.** Nausea.

112. A right orchiectomy is performed on a client with a testicular malignancy. The client expresses concerns regarding his sexuality. The nurse should base the response on the knowledge that the client:
- ☐ **1.** Is not a candidate for sperm banking.
- ☐ **2.** Should retain normal sexual drive and function.
- ☐ **3.** Will be impotent.
- ☐ **4.** Will have a change in secondary sexual characteristics.

113. A client diagnosed with seminomatous testicular cancer expresses fear and questions the nurse about his prognosis. The nurse should base the response on the knowledge that:
- ☐ **1.** Testicular cancer is almost always fatal.
- ☐ **2.** Testicular cancer has a cure rate of 90% when diagnosed early.
- ☐ **3.** Surgery is the treatment of choice for testicular cancer.
- ☐ **4.** Testicular cancer has a 50% cure rate when diagnosed early.

The Client with Cancer of the Prostate

114. A client asks the nurse why the prostate specific antigen (PSA) level is determined before the digital rectal examination. The nurse's best response is which of the following?
☐ 1. "It is easier for the client."
☐ 2. "A prostate examination can possibly decrease the PSA."
☐ 3. "A prostate examination can possibly increase the PSA."
☐ 4. "If the PSA is normal, the client will not have to undergo the rectal examination."

115. During a digital rectal examination, a key sign for prostate cancer is:
☐ 1. A hard prostate, localized or diffuse.
☐ 2. Abdominal pain.
☐ 3. A boggy, tender prostate.
☐ 4. A nonindurated prostate.

116. A client is undergoing a total prostatectomy for prostate cancer. The client asks questions about his sexual function. The best response by the nurse is which of the following?
☐ 1. "Loss of the prostate gland means that you will be impotent."
☐ 2. "Loss of the prostate gland means that you will be infertile and there will be no ejaculation. You can still experience the sensations of orgasm."
☐ 3. "Loss of the prostate gland means that you will have no loss of sexual function and drive."
☐ 4. "Loss of the prostate gland means that your erectile capability will return immediately after surgery."

117. A 65-year-old client has been told by the physician that his prostate cancer was graded at stage IIB. The client inquires if this means he is going to die soon. The best response by the nurse is which of the following?
☐ 1. "Prostate cancer at this stage is very slow growing."
☐ 2. "Prostate cancer at this stage is very fast growing."
☐ 3. "Prostate cancer at this stage has spread to the bone."
☐ 4. "Prostate cancer at this stage is difficult to predict."

118. A client with prostate cancer is treated with hormone therapy consisting of diethylstilbestrol (DES; Stilphostrol), 2 mg daily. The nurse should instruct the client that the medication can cause.
☐ 1. Tenderness of the scrotum.
☐ 2. Tenderness of the breasts.
☐ 3. Loss of pubic hair.
☐ 4. Decreased blood pressure.

The Client with Erectile Dysfunction

119. A male client complains of impotence. The nurse examines the client's medication regimen and is aware that a contributing factor to impotence could be:
☐ 1. Aspirin.
☐ 2. Antihypertensives.
☐ 3. Nonsteroidal anti-inflammatory drugs.
☐ 4. Anticoagulants.

120. A 65-year-old male client with erectile dysfunction (ED) asks the nurse, "Is all this just in my head? Am I crazy?" The best response by the nurse is based on the knowledge that:
☐ 1. ED is believed to be psychogenic in most cases.
☐ 2. More than 50% of the cases are attributed to organic causes.
☐ 3. Evaluation of nocturnal erections does not help differentiate psychogenic or organic causes.
☐ 4. ED is an uncommon problem among men older than age 65.

121. The nurse should teach the client with erectile dysfunction (ED) to alter his lifestyle to:
☐ 1. Avoid alcohol.
☐ 2. Follow a low-salt diet.
☐ 3. Decrease smoking.
☐ 4. Increase attempts at sexual intercourse.

Correct Answers and Rationales

The letter in parentheses after each rationale identifies the client need addressed in the item, including management of care (M), safety and infection control (S), health promotion and maintenance (H), psychosocial adaptation (P), basic care and comfort (C), pharmacological and parenteral therapies (D), reduction of risk potential (R), and physiological adaptation (A).

The Client with a Vaginal Infection

1. 1, 2, 4. Bacterial vaginosis is a clinical syndrome resulting from the replacement of the normal vaginal *Lactobacillus* species with overgrowth of anaerobic bacteria that cause a cluster of symptoms. Presence of a thick, white, adherent vaginal discharge with a fishy odor is evidence for bacterial vaginosis, and the client should seek treatment. The client should not douche unless under medical orders because douching can cause bacteria to ascend into the uterus. Bacterial vaginosis is not sexually transmitted, and it does not require treatment of the partner. Vaginal infections commonly require an examination and diagnostic assessment. (R)

2. 3. Douching may disrupt the normal flora of the vaginal lactobacilli and change the pH, which could result in overgrowth of other bacteria. Coffee, intercourse during menses, and tampons are not related to changes in vaginal pH or the incidence of bacterial vaginosis. (H)

3. 4. Metronidazole (Flagyl) interacts with alcohol and can cause a serious disulfiram (Antabuse)-type reaction, with severe, prolonged vomiting. The client should not douche unless following a medical order, but douching does not interact with Flagyl. Sexual intercourse and hot tub baths are not known to affect the incidence or treatment of bacterial vaginosis. (D)

4. 3. Bacterial vaginosis in pregnancy has been associated with premature delivery. Guidelines from the Centers for Disease Control and Prevention state that all pregnant women symptomatic for bacterial vaginosis should be treated and asymptomatic pregnant women who are at high risk for premature delivery should be evaluated for bacterial vaginosis. No other complications of pregnancy are known to be associated bacterial vaginosis. (R)

5. 3. Clindamycin P.O. is the recommended treatment for bacterial vaginosis in a pregnant client. Douching is contraindicated in pregnancy and is not an effective treatment for bacterial vaginosis. The use of topical agents for bacterial vaginosis in pregnancy is not recommended by the CDC. Studies have linked clindamycin creams with an increased risk of such adverse effects as premature delivery. I.V. administration of metronidazole (Flagyl) is not necessary and exposes the client to an unnecessary procedure and risk. (D)

6. 3. Bacterial vaginosis is the most common vaginal infection in reproductive-age women, and up to 50% of women may be asymptomatic. Bacterial vaginosis is not associated with menarche, menopause, or aging. Bacterial vaginosis is not usually transmitted sexually, and treatment of the male sex partner has not been beneficial in preventing recurrence of bacterial vaginosis. (H)

7. 1, 2, 4. According to the Centers for Disease Control and Prevention, the three most common diseases associated with vaginal discharge are candidiasis, bacterial vaginosis, and trichomoniasis. Candidiasis causes a white discharge that results in redness and itching. Bacterial vaginosis causes a thick, white, adherent discharge. Trichomoniasis causes a diffuse, yellow-green discharge and is a sexually transmitted infection. Gonorrhea and syphilis usually do not change vaginal discharge. (R)

8. 1, 2, 3. Candidiasis is classified by the Centers for Disease Control and Prevention as complicated or uncomplicated. Women with underlying medical conditions, such as uncontrolled diabetes and HIV infection or cancer-causing immunosuppression, correlate with an increasing severity of candidiasis. Hypertension and asthma are not related to immunosuppression or complicated candidiasis. (H)

9. 1. Antibiotics may decrease the effectiveness of oral contraceptives. The client should be instructed to continue the contraceptives and use a barrier method as a back-up method of birth control until the next menstrual cycle. The client should not stop taking her oral contraceptives and there is no indication for or benefit to taking the antibiotic 2 hours after the contraceptive. There is no incidence of the adverse effects of increased hunger and fluid retention with the interaction of antibiotic therapy and oral contraceptives. (D)

10. 4. Due to the increased risk of pelvic inflammatory disease, candidates for the IUD should be in a monogamous relationship. Smoking and hypertension are not contraindications for an IUD. The frequency of sexual relations will not affect IUD use. (D)

11. 1. Fluid losses can occur from vomiting, diarrhea, and fever and can lead to hypovolemic shock. The first nursing action is to treat the hypovolemic shock that accompanies toxic shock, so the I.V. fluids must be administered immediately. The fluid replacement is critical to avoid circulatory collapse. Pain medication and teaching can be implemented later. Antibiotics will be given because TSS is caused by a staphylococcal infection; however, fluid replacement is initiated first to treat life-threatening hypovolemic shock. (R)

The Client with Uterine Fibroids

12. 2. The best approach for a client who is fearful about having surgery is to allow the client opportunities to express her fears. Open-ended questions should elicit the client's individual and specific fears. This then gives the nurse the opportunity to provide clarification, information, and support and possibly to offer other resources. The other actions are not supportive and deny the client the opportunity to express her feelings. (P)

13. 1, 2. A woman with uterine fibroids and dysmenorrhea is at risk for iron deficiency anemia. The hemoglobin and hematocrit indicate the likelihood that the fibroids causing heavy menstrual blood loss have resulted in anemia. A hemoglobin of less than 12 g/dl in women is considered low. The white blood cell count and potassium levels are within normal parameters, and normocytic red blood cells are normal. (M)

14. 2. It is a priority that the client knows she will not be able to eat or drink for 8 hours before admission. A client who consumes food and fluid before receiving a general anesthetic is at risk for aspiration, which can lead to aspiration pneumonia, respiratory arrest, and even death. The clothing she should wear to the hospital and the type of medication she will receive are important, but not the priority. Information on exercise and resumption of normal activities can be included in the discharge teaching. (C)

15. **2.** The client needs to understand that with removal of the uterus she will no longer be able to bear children or have menstrual periods. The surgical procedure should not change her libido or sexual functioning. Research does not support the idea that hysterectomy contributes to depression or weight gain. Research demonstrates that women who have managed health problems for some time before the hysterectomy may actually have a more positive effect, with less worry about their health condition, contraception, or pregnancy. (M)

16. **4.** Starting from the area nearer the pubic bone and moving toward the anus, the anatomic order is clitoris, urinary meatus, and vaginal opening. (R)

17. **4.** The registered nurse is responsible for monitoring the surgical site for condition of the dressing, status of the incision, and signs and symptoms of complications. Unlicensed assistive personnel who have been trained to report abnormalities to the registered nurse supervising the care may take vital signs, record intake and output, and give perineal care. (M)

18. **2.** Hyperventilation occurs when the client breathes so rapidly and deeply that she exhales excessive amounts of carbon dioxide. A characteristic symptom of hyperventilation is dizziness. To avoid hyperventilation, the nurse should assist the client in the practice of slow, deep breathing in a regular breathing pattern. Dyspnea, blurred vision, and mental confusion are not associated with hyperventilation. (A)

19. **2.** The surgeon should be notified when a client who has had an abdominal hysterectomy develops vaginal bleeding that saturates a blue pad in 1 hour, and care should be managed so that other personnel can obtain vital signs while the nurse contacts the surgeon. The client may need to have I.V. fluids increased, but the surgeon needs to be notified first. Waiting 15 minutes while the client is having bright-red bleeding is an unsafe nursing action; the client may lose a large amount of blood. (M)

20. **4.** The discomfort associated with gas pains is likely to be relieved when the client ambulates. The gas will be more easily expelled with exercise. The anesthesia, analgesics, and immobility have altered normal peristalsis. Peristalsis will be stimulated by exercise. Offering a hot beverage, providing extra warmth, and applying an abdominal binder are not recommended and could aggravate the discomfort of postoperative gas pains. (A)

21. **3.** Elevated temperature on the second postoperative day is suggestive of a respiratory tract infection. Respiratory infections most often occur during the first 48 hours after surgery. The client's vital signs should be monitored closely, and abnormalities should be reported to the surgeon. Signs of infection, if present in the wound or urinary tract, are likely to occur later in the postoperative period. There is no indication that the I.V. catheter is the source of infection. (A)

22. **1.** The client with a possible transient ischemic attack is the only client who has not had surgery and is not immunocompromised. The client with a recent surgery and incision should not be exposed to a client with infection. Clients with cancer or alcoholic cirrhosis are very susceptible to infection, and it would not be safe to expose them to a client with a respiratory infection. (M)

23. **3.** When a dressing sticks to a wound, it is best to moisten the dressing with sterile normal saline solution and then remove it carefully. Trying to remove a dry dressing is likely to irritate the skin and wound. This may contribute to tension or tearing along the suture line. (M)

24. **1.** Dehiscence, the opening of a wound, places the client at an immediate increased risk for infection. The wound should be covered with sterile saline and reported to the surgeon immediately. The fluid and caloric needs of the client should be maintained by I.V. replacement. *Ineffective airway clearance* or *Imbalanced nutrition* could be an applicable diagnosis but not a priority diagnosis in this situation. *Excess fluid volume* is not an applicable diagnosis. (A)

25. **2.** The social worker will be able to coordinate respite care for the son and other community resources for this family. Home health care would provide care for the client herself, but respite care for the son is the priority need for this family. Pastoral care provides spiritual care. The volunteer department would not be responsible for coordination of care at the client's home. (M)

26. **1.** The primary ovarian hormone is estrogen. It may be prescribed for a woman whose ovaries, fallopian tubes, and uterus have been surgically removed, creating a "surgical menopause." Estrogen is prescribed at the lowest dose for the shortest period of time for the treatment of vasomotor symptoms. Thyroxine is synthesized by the thyroid gland and is unaffected by a hysterectomy. Prolactin is the hormone involved in the production of breast milk. Testosterone is the male hormone. (D)

27. **4.** Body image disturbance related to loss of female reproductive organs may lead to ineffective coping in some women. Therefore, interventions to address this problem should be incorporated into discharge planning. The nurse should address concerns regarding image, sexuality, and loss of fertility with the client. The other diagnoses are not expected problems 3 days after a hysterectomy. (P)

28. **2.** Assessment is the first step in planning client education. Assessing social support resources is a key aspect of discharge planning that begins when the client is admitted to the hospital. It is imperative to know what assistance and support the client has at home. Assessment includes obtaining data about any family or home responsibilities the client is concerned with during the recovery period. It is within the scope of nursing practice to provide discharge instructions. A social worker is not needed at this time. The nurse should assess the client's needs before determining whether using a video or reading instructions to the client is appropriate. (H)

29. **1, 2, 3.** The average age of menopause is 50 to 52 years, although some variation exists. With menopause, FSH and LH levels increase dramatically. Hot flashes occur in about 80% of women, from mild to very debilitating, with disruption of sleep patterns. Depression is not a normal expectation of menopause; if symptoms of depression arise, the woman should be assessed and treated. Contraception should be used until menses has ceased for a full year. (A)

The Client with Breast Disease

30. **1.** This complaint warrants the nurse's performing an examination and reporting the results to the physician. Hormone fluctuations do cause breast discomfort, but an examination must be done at this time to assess the breast. Although pain is not common with breast cancer, it can be a symptom. Teaching the client to perform BSE is important, but it is not the priority action in this case. (A)

31. **3.** It is generally recommended that the breasts be examined during the first week after menstruation. During this time, the breasts are least likely to be tender or swollen because estrogen is at its lowest level. Therefore, the examination will be more comfortable for the client. The examination may also be more accurate because the client is more likely to notice an actual change in her breast that is not simply related to hormonal changes. (H)

32. **2.** The client needs to become more confident and knowledgeable about the normal feel of the implants and her breast tissue. The best technique is for the nurse to demonstrate breast self-examination (BSE) to the client as the nurse conducts the clinical breast examination. Implant surgery does not exclude the need for monthly BSE. A mammogram is not a substitute for monthly BSE. (H)

33. **2.** The breasts may vary in size before menstruation because of breast engorgement caused by hormonal changes. A woman may then note that her bra fits more tightly than usual. Benign cysts do not cause variation in breast size. A change in breast size that does not follow hormonal changes could warrant further assessment. The breasts normally are about the same size, although some women have one breast slightly larger than the other. (H)

34. **2.** Advancing age in postmenopausal women has been identified as a risk factor for breast cancer. A 76-year-old client needs monthly breast self-examination and a yearly clinical breast examination and mammogram to comply with the screening schedule. While mammograms are less painful as breast tissue becomes softer, the nurse should advise the woman to have the mammogram. Family history is important, but only about 5% of breast cancers are genetic. (H)

35. **1.** If a client has questions the nurse cannot answer, it is best to delay the signing of the consent until the questions are clarified for the client. The surgeon should be notified, and the appropriate information or collaboration should be provided for the client before she signs the surgical consent. Telling her she should concentrate on recovery first ignores the client's questions and concerns. Frequently the plastic surgeon needs to be consulted at the beginning of the treatment because various surgical decisions depend on the future plans for breast reconstruction. (M)

36. **1.** An important nursing responsibility is preoperative teaching, and the most frequently recommended guide for teaching is to tell the client as much as she wants to know and is able to understand. Delaying discussion of issues about which the client has concerns is likely to aggravate the situation and cause the client to feel distrust. As a general guide, the client would not ask the question if she were not ready to discuss her situation. The nurse is available to answer the client's questions and concerns and should not delay discussing these with the client. (P)

37. **1.** About half of malignant breast tumors occur in the upper outer quadrant of the breast. For no known reason, cancer appears in the left breast more often than in the right breast. The upper outer quadrants of the breast, and especially the axillary area, should be covered thoroughly in the clinical breast examination and breast self-examination. (A)

38. **4.** Atropine sulfate, a cholinergic blocking agent, is given preoperatively to reduce secretions in the mouth and respiratory tract, which assists in maintaining the integrity of the respiratory system during general anesthesia. Atropine is not used to promote muscle relaxation, decrease nausea and vomiting, or decrease pulse and respiratory rates. It causes the pulse to increase. (D)

39. 3. The nurse should respond with an open-ended statement that elicits further exploration of the client's feelings. Women with cancer may feel guilt or shame. Previous life decisions, sexuality, and religious beliefs may influence a client's adjustment to a diagnosis of cancer. The nurse should not contradict the client's feelings of punishment or offer advice such as confiding in the husband. A social worker referral may be beneficial in the future, but is not the first response needed to elicit exploration of the client's feelings. (P)

40. 3. A drainage tube is placed in the wound after a modified radical mastectomy to help remove accumulated blood and fluid in the area. Removal of the drainage fluids assists in wound healing and is intended to decrease the incidence of hematoma, abscess formation, and infection. Drainage tubes placed in a wound do not decrease intrathoracic pressure, increase collateral lymphatic flow, or prevent adhesion formation. (R)

41. 4. Lymph nodes can be removed from the axillary area when a modified radical mastectomy is done, and each of the nodes is biopsied. To facilitate drainage from the arm on the affected side, the client's arm should be elevated on pillows with her hand higher than her elbow and her elbow higher than her shoulder. A sentinel node biopsy procedure is associated with a decreased risk of lymphedema because fewer nodes are excised. (A)

42. 2. Tamoxifen is an antiestrogen drug that has been found to be effective against metastatic breast cancer and to improve the survival rate. The drug causes hot flashes as an adverse effect. (D)

43. 1. Giving the client a list of community resources that could provide support and guidance assists the client to maintain her self-image and independence. The support group will include other women who have undergone similar therapies and can offer suggestions for breast products and wigs. Because the client is asking about specific resources, she does not need a referral to a social worker, home health agency, or plastic surgeon. (M)

44. 1. A client receiving radiation therapy should avoid lotions, ointments, and anything that may cause irritation to the skin, such as exposure to sunlight, heat, or talcum powder. The area may safely be washed with water if it is done gently and if care is taken not to injure the skin. (R)

45. 3. The most common reaction of the skin to radiation therapy is redness of the surface tissues. Dryness, tanning, and capillary dilation are also common. Atrophy of the skin, pustules, and sloughing of two layers would not be expected and should be reported to the radiologist. (R)

46. 1. The American Cancer Society's Reach to Recovery is a rehabilitation program for women who have had breast surgery. It is designed to meet their physical, psychological, and emotional needs. The Reach to Recovery program is implemented by women who have had breast cancer themselves. Many women benefit from this peer information and support. (P)

The Client with Benign Prostatic Hypertrophy

47. 1. The best way to assess for a distended bladder in either a male or female client is to check for a rounded swelling above the pubis. This swelling represents the distended bladder rising above the pubis into the abdominal cavity. Dullness does not indicate a distended bladder. The client might experience tenderness or pressure above the symphysis. No urine discharge is expected; the urine flow is blocked by the enlarged prostate. (R)

48. 3. Rapid emptying of an overdistended bladder may cause hypotension and shock due to the sudden change of pressure within the abdominal viscera. Previously, removing no more than 1,000 ml at one time was the standard of practice, but this is no longer thought to be necessary as long as the overdistended bladder is emptied slowly. (R)

49. 2. Liberal lubrication of the catheter before catheterization of a male reduces friction along the urethra and irritation and trauma to urethral tissues. Because the male urethra is tortuous, a liberal amount of lubrication is advised to ease catheter passage. The female urethra is not tortuous, and, although the catheter should be lubricated before insertion, less lubricant is necessary. Lubrication of the catheter will not decrease spasms. The nurse should use sterile technique to prevent introducing organisms. Crusts will not form immediately. Irrigating the catheter as needed will prevent clot and crust formation. (R)

50. 1. The primary reason for taping an indwelling catheter to a male client so that the penis is held in a lateral position is to prevent pressure at the penoscrotal angle. Prolonged pressure at the penoscrotal angle can cause a ureterocutaneous fistula. (R)

51. 3. The prostate gland is located below the bladder and surrounds the urethra. It serves one primary purpose: to produce a secretion that aids the nourishment and passage of sperm. The testicles store the sperm and produce testosterone to aid sperm production and maturation. The seminal vesicle regulates acidity and alkalinity. (A)

52. 2. Research shows that older men tend to believe it is normal to live with some urinary problems. As a result, these men often overlook symptoms and simply attribute them to aging. As part of preventive care for men older than age 40, the yearly physical examination should include palpation of the prostate via rectal examination. Prostate-specific antigen screening also is done annually to determine elevations or increasing trends in elevations. The nurse should teach male clients the value of early detection and adequate follow-up for the prostate. (R)

53. **2.** Signs and symptoms of prostatic hypertrophy include difficulty starting the flow of urine, urinary frequency and hesitancy, decreased force of the urine stream, interruptions in the urine stream when voiding, and nocturia. The prostate gland surrounds the urethra, and these symptoms are all attributed to obstruction of the urethra resulting from prostatic hypertrophy. Nocturia from incomplete emptying of the bladder is common. Straining and urine retention are usually the symptoms that prompt the client to seek care. Painful urination is generally not a symptom of prostatic hypertrophy. (A)

54. **3.** Ipratropium is a bronchodilator, and its anticholinergic effects can aggravate urine retention. Metformin and buspirone do not affect the urinary system; timolol does not have a systemic effect. (D)

55. **4.** If paralysis of vasomotor nerves in the upper spinal cord occurs when spinal anesthesia is used, the client is likely to develop respiratory paralysis. Artificial ventilation is required until the effects of the anesthesia subside. Seizures, cardiac arrest, and renal shutdown are not likely results of spinal anesthesia. (A)

56. **2.** The acute pain of bladder spasms frequently necessitates pharmacologic intervention, as ordered by the surgeon. Deep vein thrombosis is not common after TURP. The surgery is not disfiguring because no incision is made; the surgical entry is via the urethral meatus. The client resumes dietary intake shortly after the procedure because a general anesthetic was not administered. (A)

57. **3.** Terazosin is an antihypertensive drug that is also used in the treatment of BPH. Blood pressure must be monitored to ensure that the client does not develop hypotension, syncope, or orthostatic hypotension. The client should be instructed to change positions slowly. Urine nitrates, white blood cell count, and pulse rate are not affected by terazosin. (D)

58. **3.** The decision by the surgeon to insert a catheter after TURP or prostatectomy depends on the amount of bleeding that is expected after the procedure. During continuous bladder irrigation after a TURP or prostatectomy, the rate at which the solution enters the bladder should be increased when the drainage becomes brighter red. The color indicates the presence of blood. Increasing the flow of irrigating solution helps flush the catheter well so that clots do not plug it. There would be no reason to increase the flow rate when the return is continuous or when the return appears cloudy and dark yellow. Increasing the flow

would be contraindicated when there is no return of urine and irrigating solution. (D)

59. **4.** Belladonna and opium suppositories are prescribed and administered to reduce bladder spasms that cause pain after TURP. Bladder spasms frequently accompany urologic procedures. Antispasmodics offer relief by eliminating or reducing spasms. Antimicrobial drugs are used to treat an infection. Belladonna and opium do not relieve urine retention or urinary frequency. (D)

60. **3.** The indwelling urinary catheter creates the urge to void and can also cause bladder spasms. The nurse should ensure adequate bladder emptying by monitoring urine output and characteristics. Urine output should be at least 50 ml/hour. A plugged catheter, imagining the urge to void, and confusion are less likely reasons for the client's complaint. (R)

61. **3.** The presence of red and white blood cells and moderate bacteria in the urine is most typical of a UTI. Positive leukocyte esterase and nitrites are also significant for UTI. The pH increases with a UTI, becoming more alkaline. A urethral stricture, decreased renal filtration rate, or prostate malignancy would not be evident in the urinalysis. (R)

62. **2.** Dribbling of urine can occur for several months after TURP. The client should be informed that this is expected and is not an abnormal sign. The nurse should teach the client perineal exercises to strengthen sphincter tone. The client may need to use pads for temporary incontinence. The client should be reassured that continence will return in a few months and will not be a chronic problem. Dribbling is not a sign of healing, but is related to the trauma of surgery. (C)

63. **1.** *Deficient fluid volume* is a priority diagnosis because the client needs to drink a large amount of fluids to keep the urine clear. The urine should be almost without color. About 2 weeks after TURP, when desiccated tissue is sloughed out, a secondary hemorrhage could occur. The client should be instructed to call the surgeon or go to the emergency department if at any time the urine turns bright red. The client is not specifically at risk for nutritional problems after TURP. The client is not specifically at risk for impaired tissue integrity because there is no external incision, and the client is not specifically at risk for airway problems because the procedure is done under spinal anesthesia. (C)

64. **2.** The most specific examination to determine whether a malignancy extends outside of the prostatic capsule is a study of the serum acid phosphatase level. The level increases when a malignancy has metastasized. A prostate-specific antigen determination and a digital rectal examination are done when screening for prostate cancer. Serum creatinine level, total nonprotein nitrogen level, and endogenous creatinine clearance time give information about kidney function, not prostate malignancy. (R)

The Client with a Sexually Transmitted Disease

65. **4.** HIV infection is transmitted through blood and body fluids, particularly vaginal and seminal fluids. A blood transfusion is one way the disease can be contracted. Other modes of transmission are sexual intercourse with an infected partner and sharing I.V. needles with an infected person. Women now have the highest rate of newly diagnosed HIV infection. Many of these women have contracted HIV from unprotected sex with male partners. HIV cannot be transmitted by hugging, inhaling cocaine, or sharing utensils. (S)

66. **3.** Zidovudine (AZT) interferes with replication of HIV and thereby slows progression of HIV infection to acquired immunodeficiency syndrome (AIDS). There is no known cure for HIV infection. Today, clients are not treated with monotherapy but are usually on triple therapy due to a much-improved clinical response. Decreased viral loads with the drug combinations have improved the longevity and quality of life in clients with HIV/AIDS. AZT does not destroy the virus, enhance the body's antibody production, or neutralize toxins produced by the virus. (D)

67. **2.** Women who have HPV are much more likely to develop cervical cancer than women who have never had the disease. Cervical cancer is now considered a sexually transmitted disease. Regular examinations, including Papanicolaou tests, are recommended to detect and treat cervical cancer at an early stage. HPV does not cause sterility, uterine fibroid tumors, or irregular menses. (H)

68. **3.** Pain is a common problem in women with herpes genitalis. Analgesia may be prescribed for the pain along with antiviral therapy, such as valacyclovir (Valtrex), acyclovir (Zovirax), or famciclovir (Famvir). Clients commonly describe the pain as an intense burning. Urination can be very painful because of the burning sensation from herpes lesions in the perineal area. Sleep disturbances, nutritional deficits, and ineffective breathing patterns are not frequently associated with herpes genitalis. (A)

69. **1.** HSV infection is one of a group of disorders that, when diagnosed in the presence of HIV infection, are considered to be diagnostic for AIDS. Other AIDS-defining illnesses include Kaposi's sarcoma; cytomegalovirus of the liver, spleen, or lymph nodes; and *Pneumocystis carinii* pneumonia. HSV infection is not curable and does not cause severe electrolyte imbalances. Human papillomavirus can lead to cervical cancer. (A)

70. **4.** Education to prevent behaviors that cause HIV transmission is the primary method of controlling HIV infection. Behaviors that place people at risk for HIV infection include unprotected sexual intercourse and sharing of needles for I.V. drug injection. Educating clients about using condoms during sexual relations is a priority in controlling HIV transmission. (S)

71. **4.** The nurse should respond with a statement that allows the client to express his thoughts and feelings. After sharing feelings about their diagnosis, clients will need information, support, and community resources. Statements of encouragement or agreement do not provide an opportunity for the client to express himself. (P)

72. **4.** *Treponema pallidum*, the organism that causes syphilis, is classified as a spirochete because of its corkscrew appearance. There are more than 100 different types of sexually transmitted diseases (STDs) caused by various types of organisms. Viruses and bacteria are responsible for many common STDs. Fungi and rickettsia do not cause STDs. (S)

73. **3.** The chancre of syphilis is characteristically a painless, moist ulcer. The serous discharge is very infectious. Because the chancre is usually painless and disappears, the client may not be aware of it or may not seek care. The chancre does not appear as pimples or warts, and does not itch, thus making diagnosis difficult. (A)

74. **2.** An important aspect of controlling the spread of sexually transmitted diseases (STDs) is obtaining a list of the sexual contacts of an infected client. These contacts, in turn, should be encouraged to obtain immediate care. Many people with STDs are reluctant to reveal their sexual contacts, which makes controlling STDs difficult. Increasing clients' knowledge of the disease and reassuring clients that their records are confidential can motivate them to seek treatment, which does help to control the spread of the disease, but it is not as critical as information about the client's sexual contacts. (A)

75. **2.** Because of the large dose, the upper outer quadrant of the buttocks is the recommended site. The Centers for Disease Control and Prevention recommends benzathine penicillin G 2.4 million units I.M. in a single dose for adults with primary or secondary syphilis who are not allergic to penicillin. The deltoid and the quadriceps lateralis of the thigh are not large enough for the recommended dose. In infants and small children, the midlateral aspect of the thigh may be preferred. (D)

76. **1.** A client with primary syphilis is at risk for transmitting the disease to sexual partners if he or she is not knowledgeable about how the disease is spread. Cutaneous lesions on the palms and soles and alopecia are signs of secondary syphilis. Chancres do not bleed sufficiently to alter tissue perfusion. Chancres often disappear even without treatment. (A)

77. **1.** Asking the client to describe her nervousness gives her the opportunity to express her concerns. It also allows the nurse to understand her better and gives the nurse a base to respond to the client's stated fears, questions, or need for further information. Responses that make assumptions about the source of the concern or offer reinforcement are not supportive and block successful communication. (P)

78. **4.** Many women do not seek treatment because they are unaware that they have gonorrhea. They may be symptom-free or have only very mild symptoms until the disease progresses to pelvic inflammatory disease. Dysuria and vaginal bleeding are not present in gonorrhea. Gonorrhea can lead to very serious complications. It can be cured with the proper treatment. (A)

79. **1.** Statistics reveal that the incidence of STDs is rising more rapidly among teenagers than among any other age-group. Many reasons have been given for this trend, including a change in societal mores and increasing sexual activity among teenagers. During this developmental stage, teenagers may engage in high-risk sexual behaviors because they often are living in the present and feel that it won't happen to them. (H)

80. **1, 2, 3, 4, 6.** The client is suspected of having a sexually transmitted infection. Therefore, the client's sexual history, assessment, and examination must be documented, including symptoms (such as fever, chills, and enlarged glands) and their onset and duration. Allergies are critical to document for every client, but are especially noteworthy in this case because antibiotics will be ordered. If a sexually transmitted infection is confirmed, sexual contacts need to be treated. To protect privacy, the names and phone numbers should never be placed in the chart. The public health department will also assist in obtaining information and treating known sexual contacts. (S)

81. **4**

First, convert 1 g to milligrams:

$$1 \text{ g} = 1,000 \text{ mg}.$$

Next, divide the desired dose by the dose on hand:

$$1,000 \text{ mg} / 250 \text{ mg} = 4 \text{ tablets}.$$

(D)

82. **4.** Dysuria and a mucopurulent urethral discharge characterize gonorrhea in men. Gonococcal symptoms are so painful and bothersome for men that they usually seek treatment with the onset of symptoms. Impotence, scrotal swelling, and urine retention are not associated with gonorrhea. (A)

83. **2.** The most common opportunistic infection in HIV infection initially presents as oral candidiasis, or thrush. The client with HIV should always have an oral assessment. HSV and CMV are opportunistic infections that present later in acquired immunodeficiency syndrome. Aphthous stomatitis, or recurrent canker sores, is not an opportunistic infection, although the sores are thought to occur more often when the client is under stress. (H)

The Client with Cancer of the Cervix

84. **2.** Although other positions may be used, the preferred position for a vaginal examination is the lithotomy position. This position offers the best visualization. If the client is elderly and frail, staff members may need to support the client's flexed legs while the examiner conducts the examination and obtains the Papanicolaou smear. Positioning the client in the other positions will make visualization more difficult and may not be as comfortable for the client. (H)

85. **4.** The Pap smear identifies atypical cervical cells that may be present for various reasons. Cancer is the most common possible cause, but not the only one. The Pap smear does not show abnormal viral cells unless specific gene typing is done for human papillomavirus. An adequate smear provides accurate diagnostic data; the false-positive rate is only about 5%. (H)

86. **4.** Young age at first pregnancy is a risk factor for cervical cancer. Other risk factors include a family history of the disease, sexual experience with multiple partners, and a history of sexually transmitted disease (e.g., syphilis, human papillomavirus infection, gonorrhea). Cigarette smoking, promiscuous male partner, human immunodeficiency virus infection or other immunosuppression, and low socioeconomic status are other risk factors. Sexual relations with one partner, sedentary lifestyle, and obesity are not risk factors for cervical cancer. (H)

87. **1.** Annual screening is recommended for any woman in the high-risk category. When detected early, cervical cancer has an excellent prognosis. Most women who die of cervical cancer have never had a Pap test or have not had one in the last 5 years. Current American Cancer Society guidelines advocate Pap smears every 3 years after a pattern of three initial negative annual tests is established and the woman is deemed to be at low risk for development of cervical cancer. Sexual history and sexually transmitted infections are the primary criteria related to the frequency of Pap tests. (H)

88. **4.** In its early stages, cancer of the cervix is usually asymptomatic, which underscores the importance of regular Pap smears. A light bleeding or serosanguineous discharge may be apparent as the first noticeable symptom. Pain, leg edema, urinary and rectal symptoms, and weight loss are late signs of cervical cancer. (A)

89. **4.** The vagina naturally cleans itself, and douching is not recommended unless it is prescribed by a health care provider for a medical condition. Daily douching could destroy normal flora. Perfumed douches could trigger allergenic responses. Douching should be avoided during menses. (R)

90. **1, 2, 3, 4.** The social worker is part of the comprehensive, holistic health care team. Because the client does not have insurance and is a single parent, appropriate government and charity programs and potential resources need to be explained to the client. The needs of the client and the family members are included in the treatment plan. The client will have choices about whether or not she elects to participate in any of the assistance programs. (M)

91. **1.** When cervical cancer is detected early and treated aggressively, the cure rate approaches 100%. The incidence of cervical cancer has increased among African Americans, Native Americans, and Latinas, and these women often have a poorer prognosis because the cancer is not identified early. Papanicolaou smears and colposcopy have the potential to decrease mortality from invasive carcinoma when these screening and treatment programs are utilized by women. (A)

92. **2.** The client should be informed that her next two or three periods could be heavy and prolonged. The client is instructed to report any excessive bleeding. The nurse should reinforce the necessity for the follow-up check and the review of the biopsy results with the client. The client's periods will not be normal for 2 to 3 months. (R)

93. **2.** Dislodged radioactive materials should not be touched with bare or gloved hands. Forceps are used to place the material in the lead-lined container, which shields the radiation. Exposure to radiation can occur only by direct exposure to the encased radioactive substance; it cannot result from contact with emesis or urine or from touching the client. Disposal of eating utensils cannot lead to radiation exposure. Radioactive dose materials are kept only in the radiation department. (S)

94. **3.** The three factors related to radiation safety are time, distance, and shielding. Nurses on radiation oncology units work with radiation frequently and so must limit their contact. Nurses are physically closer to clients than are visitors, who are often asked to sit 6 feet away from the client. Touching the client does not increase the amount of radiation exposure. Aseptic technique and isolation prevent the spread of infection. Age is a risk factor for people in their reproductive years. (S)

95. **2.** A client can experience anxiety because she is immobilized on strict bed rest and cannot care for herself while the implant is in place. During an intracavity implant, the woman is kept flat in bed to prevent dislodgment of the radioactive substance. The implant may be left in place for 24 to 72 hours. Usually, the tumor is removed before implant insertion. *Ineffective health maintenance* and *Insomnia* are not priority nursing diagnoses. (P)

96. **2.** HPV infection, or genital warts, can lead to dysplastic changes of the cervix, referred to as cervical intraepithelial neoplasia. The development of cervical cancer remains the largest threat of all condyloma-associated neoplasias. Infertility, pelvic inflammatory disease, and rectal cancer are not complications of genital warts. (H)

97. **4.** Bowel movements can be difficult with the radium applicator in place. The purpose of the low-residue diet is to decrease bowel movements. The bowel is cleaned before therapy, and the woman is maintained on a low-residue diet during treatment to prevent bowel distention and defecation. To prevent dislodgment of the applicator, the client is maintained on strict bed rest and allowed only to turn from side to side. Perineal care is omitted during radium implant therapy, although any vaginal discharge should be reported to the physician. It is rare for the applicator to extrude, so this does not need to be checked every hour. (C)

98. **4.** Nausea, vomiting, and a foul vaginal discharge are common adverse effects of internal radiation therapy for cervical cancer. A foul-smelling discharge may develop from the destruction and sloughing of cells. Vaginal discharge may persist for some time. General signs and symptoms of radiation syndrome include nausea, vomiting, anorexia, and malaise. Vaginal itching, confusion, and high fever are not typical adverse effects of radiation therapy for cervical cancer. (S)

The Client Having Gynecological Surgery

99. **4.** To determine the cause of this problem, a quality improvement study should be conducted. Before implementing solutions to a complaint, the precise issues in the hospital system must be observed and documented. Consulting with the evening nurses may result in biased observations because the evening nurses are not conducting care under the same environment as the night nurses. Including a medication nurse is not the first step in understanding the problem and may be an unrealistic or expensive solution. The supervisor is not directly involved with the problem and should only be consulted if the problem cannot be solved by those involved. (M)

100. **3.** The nurse must clarify this order with the admitting physician to ensure medication accuracy and client safety. In health care settings without computerized medical records or computer prescribing, misinterpretation of handwriting remains a leading cause of medication errors. It is not safe practice to question the client regarding a diagnosis and assume the medication is correctly prescribed. The pharmacist will need clarification of the order as well. It is not the role of the pharmacist to interpret the order. (D)

101. **1.** The nurse must first assess the intensity of the client's pain before selecting the correct analgesia. A high score would necessitate administering the meperidine (Demerol). If the intensity rating is low, an oral analgesic would be appropriate. If acetaminophen (Tylenol #3) is given without assessing the intensity of the client's pain, the nurse must then wait 4 hours before administering another analgesic. (D)

102. **3.** The nurse should follow the line of authority or chain of command by reporting the observation immediately to the nursing supervisor. The nurse should not confront the person or the medication nurse because the line of authority for reporting incidents should be followed. The RT supervisor may subsequently be involved in the incident, but the nursing supervisor should initiate and follow the policy and procedure. (M)

103. **3.** The nurse should withhold administering docusate sodium (Colace), a stool softener, and document the rationale on the medical record. The nurse must assess the need for a medication even though it is ordered. Documentation of why the medication was withheld should be written in the medical record. The nurse is responsible for assessing contraindications and adverse effects of medications, and administering the medication when the client already has loose stools is unsafe. The assessment should also include auscultation of bowel sounds and inquiry about gas pains, but the stool softener should still be withheld. (D)

The Client with Testicular Disease

104. **2.** Epididymitis causes acute tenderness and pronounced swelling of the scrotum. Gradual onset of unilateral scrotal pain, urethral discharge, and fever are other key signs. Epididymitis is occasionally, but not routinely, associated with urinary tract infection. Burning and pain on urination and foul-smelling ejaculate or urine are not classic symptoms of epididymitis. (A)

105. **3.** Among men younger than age 35, epididymitis is most frequently caused by a sexually transmitted infection. Causative organisms are usually chlamydia or *Neisseria gonorrhoeae*. The other major form of epididymitis is bacterial, caused by the *Escherichia coli* or *Pseudomonas* organisms. The nurse should always include safe sex teaching for a client with epididymitis. The client should also be advised against anogenital intercourse because this is a mode of transmission of gram-negative rods to the epididymis. (R)

106. **3.** After a warm bath or shower, the testes hang lower and are both relaxed and in the ideal position for manual evaluation and palpation. (H)

107. **2.** Normal testes feel smooth, egg-shaped, and firm to the touch, without lumps. The surface should feel smooth and rubbery. The testes should not be soft or spongy to the touch. Testicular malignancies are usually nontender, nonpainful hard lumps. Lumps, swelling, nodules, or signs of inflammation should be reported to the physician. (H)

108. **4.** AFP and hCG are considered markers that indicate the presence of testicular disease. Elevated AFP and hCG and decreased testosterone are markers for testicular disease. Measurements of AFP, hCG, and testosterone are also obtained throughout the course of therapy to help measure the effectiveness of treatment. (A)

109. **1.** Cryptorchidism (undescended testes) carries a greatly increased risk for testicular cancer. Undescended testes occurs in about 3% of male infants, with an increased incidence in premature infants. Other possible causes of malignancy include chemical carcinogens, trauma, orchitis, and environmental factors. Testicular cancer is not associated with early sexual relations in men, even though cervical cancer is associated with early sexual relations in women. Testicular cancer is not associated with seminal vesiculitis or epididymitis. (H)

110. **2.** The incidence of testicular cancer is higher in men who live in rural rather than suburban areas. Testicular cancer is more common in white than black men. Men with higher socioeconomic status seem to have a greater incidence of testicular cancer. The exact cause of testicular cancer is unknown. Cancer of the testes is the leading cause of death from cancer in the 15- to 35-year-old age-group. (H)

111. **3.** Because of the location of the incision in the high inguinal area, pain is a major problem during the immediate postoperative period. The incisional area and discomfort caused by movement contribute to increased pain. Bladder spasms and elimination problems are more commonly associated with prostate surgery. Nausea is not a priority problem. (A)

112. **2.** Unilateral orchiectomy alone does not result in impotence if the other testis is normal. The other testis should produce enough testosterone to maintain normal sexual drive, functioning, and characteristics. Sperm banking before treatment is commonly recommended because radiation or chemotherapy can affect fertility. (P)

113. **2.** When diagnosed early and treated aggressively, testicular cancer has a cure rate of about 90%. Treatment of testicular cancer is based on tumor type, and seminoma cancer has the best prognosis. Modes of treatment include combinations of orchiectomy, radiation therapy, and chemotherapy. The chemotherapeutic regimen used currently is responsible for the successful treatment of testicular cancer. (A)

The Client with Cancer of the Prostate

114. **3.** Manipulation of the prostate during the digital rectal examination may falsely increase the PSA levels. The PSA determination and the digital rectal examination are both necessary as screening tools for prostate cancer, and both are recommended for all men older than age 50. Prostate cancer is the most common cancer in men and the second leading killer from cancer among men in the United States. Incidence increases sharply with age, and the disease is predominant in the 60- to 70-year-old age-group. (H)

115. **1.** On digital rectal examination, key signs of prostate cancer are a hard prostate, induration of the prostate, and an irregular, hard nodule. Accompanying symptoms of prostate cancer can include constipation, weight loss, and lymphadenopathy. Abdominal pain usually does not accompany prostate cancer. A boggy, tender prostate is found with infection (e.g., acute or chronic prostatitis). (H)

116. **2.** Loss of the prostate gland interrupts the flow of semen, so there will be no ejaculation fluid. The sensations of orgasm remain intact. The client needs to be advised that return of erectile capability is often disrupted after surgery, but within 1 year 95% of men have returned to normal erectile function with sexual intercourse. (A)

117. **1.** Clients who have stage IA or IIB prostate cancer have an excellent survival rate. Prostate cancer is usually slow growing, and many men who have prostate cancer do not die from it. A stage I or II tumor is confined to the prostate gland and has not spread to the extrapelvic region or bone. (A)

118. **2.** Diethylstilbestrol causes engorgement and tenderness of the breasts (gynecomastia). Stilbestrol is prescribed as palliative therapy for men with androgen-dependent prostatic carcinoma. An increase in blood pressure can occur. Tenderness of the scrotum and dramatic changes in secondary sexual characteristics should not occur. (D)

The Client with Erectile Dysfunction

119. **2.** Antihypertensives, especially beta blockers such as propranolol (Inderal), can cause impotence. When a male client complains of impotence, the nurse should always examine his medication regimen as a potential contributing factor. Aspirin, nonsteroidal anti-inflammatory drugs, and anticoagulants do not cause erectile dysfunction. (D)

120. **2.** ED is multifactorial in origin, and more than 50% of the cases can be attributed to organic causes, which include alteration in vascular supply, hormonal changes, neurologic dysfunction, medications, and associated systemic diseases, such as diabetes mellitus or alcoholism. The presence of nocturnal erections is the first evaluation to differentiate between organic and psychogenic causes. ED is a common problem among men older than age 65. (P)

121. **1.** Avoidance of alcohol can improve the outcome of therapy. Alcohol and smoking can affect a man's ability to have and maintain an erection. The client should be encouraged to follow a healthy diet, but no specific diet is associated with improvement of sexual function. The client should cease smoking, not just decrease smoking. Increasing attempts at intercourse without treatment will not facilitate improvement. The client should be reassured that ED is a common problem and that help is available. (R)

The Client with Neurologic Health Problems

The Client with a Head Injury

1. Following a craniotomy, a client has been admitted to the neurological intensive care unit. The nurse has established a goal to maintain intracranial pressure (ICP) within the normal range. What should the nurse do? Select all that apply.
- ☐ **1.** Encourage the client to cough and take deep breaths.
- ☐ **2.** Elevate the head of the bed 15 to 30 degrees.
- ☐ **3.** Contact the health care provider if ICP is greater than 20 mm Hg.
- ☐ **4.** Monitor neurologic status using the Glasgow Coma Scale.
- ☐ **5.** Stimulate the client with active range-of-motion exercises.

2. The nurse is monitoring a client with increased intracranial pressure (ICP). What indicators are the most critical for the nurse to monitor? Select all that apply.
- ☐ **1.** Systolic blood pressure.
- ☐ **2.** Urine output.
- ☐ **3.** Breath sounds.
- ☐ **4.** Cerebral perfusion pressure.
- ☐ **5.** Level of pain.

3. A nurse is assessing a client with increasing intracranial pressure. What is a client's mean arterial pressure (MAP) in mm Hg when blood pressure (BP) is 120/60 mm Hg?

_____ mm Hg

4. A client with a contusion has been admitted for observation following a motor vehicle accident when he was driving his wife to the hospital to deliver their child. The next morning, instead of asking about his wife and baby, he asked to see the football game on television that he thinks is starting in 5 minutes. He is agitated that the nurse will not turn on the television. What should the nurse do next? Select all that apply.
- ☐ **1.** Find a television so the client can view the football game.
- ☐ **2.** Determine if the client's pupils are equal and react to light.
- ☐ **3.** Ask the client if he has a headache.
- ☐ **4.** Arrange for the client to be with his wife and baby.
- ☐ **5.** Administer a sedative.

5. An unconscious client with multiple injuries arrives in the emergency department. Which nursing intervention receives the *highest* priority?
- ☐ **1.** Establishing an airway.
- ☐ **2.** Replacing blood loss.
- ☐ **3.** Stopping bleeding from open wounds.
- ☐ **4.** Checking for a neck fracture.

6. A client is at risk for increased intracranial pressure (ICP). Which of the following would be the priority for the nurse to monitor?
- ☐ **1.** Unequal pupil size.
- ☐ **2.** Decreasing systolic blood pressure.
- ☐ **3.** Tachycardia.
- ☐ **4.** Decreasing body temperature.

7. What should the nurse do first when a client with a head injury begins to have clear drainage from his nose?
- ☐ **1.** Compress the nares.
- ☐ **2.** Tilt the head back.
- ☐ **3.** Give the client tissues to collect the fluid.
- ☐ **4.** Administer an antihistamine for postnasal drip.

8. Which of the following respiratory patterns indicates increasing increased intracranial pressure in the brain stem?
- ☐ **1.** Slow, irregular respirations.
- ☐ **2.** Rapid, shallow respirations.
- ☐ **3.** Asymmetric chest excursion.
- ☐ **4.** Nasal flaring.

9. Which of the following nursing interventions is appropriate for a client with an increased intracranial pressure (ICP) of 20 mm Hg?
- ☐ **1.** Give the client a warming blanket.
- ☐ **2.** Administer low-dose barbiturates.
- ☐ **3.** Encourage the client to hyperventilate.
- ☐ **4.** Restrict fluids.

10. A client has signs of increased intracranial pressure (ICP). Which of the following is an *early* indicator of deterioration in the client's condition?
- ☐ **1.** Widening pulse pressure.
- ☐ **2.** Decrease in the pulse rate.
- ☐ **3.** Dilated, fixed pupils.
- ☐ **4.** Decrease in level of consciousness (LOC).

11. A nurse obtains a specimen of clear nasal drainage from a client with a head injury. Which of the following tests differentiates mucus from cerebrospinal fluid (CSF)?
- ☐ **1.** pH.
- ☐ **2.** Specific gravity.
- ☐ **3.** Glucose.
- ☐ **4.** Microorganisms.

12. The client has a sustained increased intracranial pressure (ICP) of 20 mm Hg. Which client position would be most appropriate?
- ☐ **1.** The head of the bed elevated 30 to 45 degrees.
- ☐ **2.** Trendelenburg's position.
- ☐ **3.** Left Sims position.
- ☐ **4.** The head elevated on two pillows.

13. The nurse administers mannitol (Osmitrol) to the client with increased intracranial pressure. Which parameter requires close monitoring?
- ☐ **1.** Muscle relaxation.
- ☐ **2.** Intake and output.
- ☐ **3.** Widening of the pulse pressure.
- ☐ **4.** Pupil dilation.

14. A client is being admitted with a spinal cord transection at C7. Which of the following assessments take priority upon the client's arrival? Select all that apply.
- ☐ **1.** Reflexes.
- ☐ **2.** Bladder function.
- ☐ **3.** Blood pressure.
- ☐ **4.** Temperature.
- ☐ **5.** Respirations.

15. The nurse is assessing a client for movement after halo traction placement for a C8 fracture. The nurse should document which of the following?
- ☐ **1.** The client's shoulders shrug against downward pressure of the examiner's hands.
- ☐ **2.** The client's arm pulls up from a resting position against resistance.
- ☐ **3.** The client's arm straightens out from a flexed position against resistance.
- ☐ **4.** The client's hand-grasp strength is equal.

16. Four days after surgery for internal fixation of a C3 to C4 fracture, a nurse is moving a client from the bed to the wheelchair. The nurse is checking the wheelchair for correct features for this client. Which of the following features of the wheelchair are appropriate for the needs of this client? Select all that apply.
- ☐ **1.** Back at the level of the client's scapula.
- ☐ **2.** Back and head that are high.
- ☐ **3.** Seat that is lower than normal.
- ☐ **4.** Seat with firm cushions.
- ☐ **5.** Chair controlled by the client's breath.

17. A male client with a head injury regains consciousness after several days. Which of the following nursing statements is most appropriate as the client awakens?
- ☐ **1.** "I'll get your family."
- ☐ **2.** "Can you tell me your name and where you live?"
- ☐ **3.** "I'll bet you're a little confused right now."
- ☐ **4.** "You are in the hospital. You were in an accident and unconscious."

18. A client who is regaining consciousness after a craniotomy becomes restless and attempts to pull out her I.V. line. Which nursing intervention protects the client without increasing her increased intracranial pressure (ICP)?
- ☐ **1.** Place her in a jacket restraint.
- ☐ **2.** Wrap her hands in soft "mitten" restraints.
- ☐ **3.** Tuck her arms and hands under the drawsheet.
- ☐ **4.** Apply a wrist restraint to each arm.

19. Which activity should the nurse encourage the client to avoid when there is a risk for increased intracranial pressure (ICP)?
- ☐ **1.** Deep breathing.
- ☐ **2.** Turning.
- ☐ **3.** Coughing.
- ☐ **4.** Passive range-of-motion (ROM) exercises.

20. Which of the following is most effective in assessing the client suspected of developing diabetes insipidus?
- ☐ **1.** Taking vital signs every 2 hours.
- ☐ **2.** Measuring urine output hourly.
- ☐ **3.** Assessing arterial blood gas values every other day.
- ☐ **4.** Checking blood glucose levels.

21. A client who had a serious head injury with increased intracranial pressure is to be discharged to a rehabilitation facility. Which of the following rehabilitation outcomes would be appropriate for the client? The client will:
- ☐ **1.** Exhibit no further episodes of short-term memory loss.
- ☐ **2.** Be able to return to his construction job in 3 weeks.
- ☐ **3.** Actively participate in the rehabilitation process as appropriate.
- ☐ **4.** Be emotionally stable and display pre-injury personality traits.

22. Which of the following describes decerebrate posturing?
- ☐ **1.** Internal rotation and adduction of arms with flexion of elbows, wrists, and fingers.
- ☐ **2.** Back hunched over, rigid flexion of all four extremities with supination of arms and plantar flexion of feet.
- ☐ **3.** Supination of arms, dorsiflexion of the feet.
- ☐ **4.** Back arched, rigid extension of all four extremities.

23. A client receiving vent-assisted mode ventilation begins to experience cluster breathing after recent intracranial occipital bleeding. Which action would be most appropriate?
- ☐ **1.** Count the rate to be sure that ventilations are deep enough to be sufficient.
- ☐ **2.** Notify the physician of the client's breathing pattern.
- ☐ **3.** Increase the rate of ventilations.
- ☐ **4.** Increase the tidal volume on the ventilator.

24. In planning the care for a client who has had a posterior fossa (infratentorial) craniotomy, which of the following is contraindicated when positioning the client?
- ☐ **1.** Keeping the client flat on one side or the other.
- ☐ **2.** Elevating the head of the bed to 30 degrees.
- ☐ **3.** Logrolling or turning as a unit when turning.
- ☐ **4.** Keeping the neck in a neutral position.

The Client with Seizures

25. Which of the following is contraindicated for a client with seizure precautions?
- ☐ **1.** Encouraging him to perform his own personal hygiene.
- ☐ **2.** Allowing him to wear his own clothing.
- ☐ **3.** Assessing oral temperature with a glass thermometer.
- ☐ **4.** Encouraging him to be out of bed.

26. A client who is unconscious from an overdose of an unknown drug is having generalized tonic-clonic seizures. Which of the following should the nurse expect to administer? Select all that apply.
- ☐ **1.** Dextrose 50%, 50 ml I.V. bolus.
- ☐ **2.** Flumazenil, 0.2 mg I.V.
- ☐ **3.** Thiamine, 100 mg I.V.
- ☐ **4.** Naloxone, 0.45 mg I.V.
- ☐ **5.** Regular insulin, 5 units I.V.

27. Which of the following will the nurse observe in the client in the ictal phase of a generalized tonic-clonic seizure?
- ☐ **1.** Jerking in one extremity that spreads gradually to adjacent areas.
- ☐ **2.** Vacant staring and abruptly ceasing all activity.
- ☐ **3.** Facial grimaces, patting motions, and lip smacking.
- ☐ **4.** Loss of consciousness, body stiffening, and violent muscle contractions.

28. It is the night before a client is to have a computed tomography (CT) scan of the head without contrast. Which statement by the nurse would be most appropriate?
- ☐ **1.** "You must shampoo your hair tonight to remove all oil and dirt."
- ☐ **2.** "You may drink fluids until midnight, but after that drink nothing until the scan is completed."
- ☐ **3.** "You will have some hair shaved to attach the small electrode to your scalp."
- ☐ **4.** "You will need to hold your head very still during the examination."

29. For breakfast on the morning a client is to have an electroencephalogram (EEG), the client is served a soft-boiled egg, toast with butter and marmalade, orange juice, and coffee. Which of the following should the nurse do?
☐ 1. Remove all the food.
☐ 2. Remove the coffee.
☐ 3. Remove the toast, butter, and marmalade only.
☐ 4. Substitute vegetable juice for the orange juice.

30. A 20-year-old who hit his head while playing football has a tonic-clonic seizure. Upon awakening from the seizure, the client asks the nurse, "What caused me to have a seizure? I've never had one before." Which cause should the nurse include in the response as a primary cause of tonic-clonic seizures in adults older than age 20?
☐ 1. Head trauma.
☐ 2. Electrolyte imbalance.
☐ 3. Congenital defect.
☐ 4. Epilepsy.

31. Which of the following should the nurse include in the teaching plan for a client with seizures who is going home with a prescription for gabapentin (Neurontin)?
☐ 1. Take all the medication until it is gone.
☐ 2. Notify the physician if vision changes occur.
☐ 3. Store gabapentin in the refrigerator.
☐ 4. Take gabapentin with an antacid to protect against ulcers.

32. What is the *priority* nursing intervention in the postictal phase of a seizure?
☐ 1. Reorient the client to time, person, and place.
☐ 2. Determine the client's level of sleepiness.
☐ 3. Assess the client's breathing pattern.
☐ 4. Position the client comfortably.

33. Which intervention is most effective in minimizing the risk of seizure activity in a client who is undergoing diagnostic studies after having experienced several episodes of seizures?
☐ 1. Maintain the client on bed rest.
☐ 2. Administer butabarbital sodium (phenobarbital) 30 mg P.O., three times per day.
☐ 3. Close the door to the room to minimize stimulation.
☐ 4. Administer carbamazepine (Tegretol) 200 mg P.O., twice per day.

34. What nursing assessments should be documented at the beginning of the ictal phase of a seizure?
☐ 1. Heart rate, respirations, pulse oximeter, and blood pressure.
☐ 2. Last dose of anticonvulsant and circumstances at the time.
☐ 3. Type of visual, auditory, and olfactory aura the client experienced.
☐ 4. Movement of the head and eyes and muscle rigidity.

35. Which clinical manifestation does the nurse expect in the client in the postictal phase of generalized tonic-clonic seizure?
☐ 1. Drowsiness.
☐ 2. Inability to move.
☐ 3. Paresthesia.
☐ 4. Hypotension.

36. A client with seizures asks the nurse how phenytoin sodium (Dilantin) will help. Based on knowledge of the drug's action, what is the nurse's best response?
☐ 1. It corrects the abnormal synthesis of norepinephrine in the body.
☐ 2. It depresses transmission of abnormal impulses in the spinal cord.
☐ 3. It reduces the responsiveness of neurons in the brain to abnormal impulses.
☐ 4. It interrupts the flow of abnormal impulses from peripheral neurons in the viscera to the brain.

37. When preparing to teach a client about phenytoin sodium (Dilantin) therapy, the nurse should urge the client not to stop the drug suddenly because:
☐ 1. Physical dependency on the drug develops over time.
☐ 2. Status epilepticus may develop.
☐ 3. A hypoglycemic reaction develops.
☐ 4. Heart block is likely to develop.

38. A client states that she is afraid she will not be able to drive again because of her seizures. Which response by the nurse would be best?
☐ 1. A person with a history of seizures can drive only during daytime hours.
☐ 2. A person with evidence that the seizures are under medical control can drive.
☐ 3. A person with evidence that seizures occur no more often than every 12 months can drive.
☐ 4. A person with a history of seizures can drive if he carries a medical identification card.

39. A client tells the nurse that he is unclear about what an aura is. The nurse's response indicates that an aura is:
- [ ] 1. A postictal state of amnesia.
- [ ] 2. An hallucination that occurs during a seizure.
- [ ] 3. A symptom that occurs just before a seizure.
- [ ] 4. A feeling of relaxation as the seizure begins to subside.

40. Which statement by a client with a seizure disorder taking topiramate (Topamax) indicates the client has understood the nurse's instruction?
- [ ] 1. "I will take the medicine before going to bed."
- [ ] 2. "I will drink 6 to 8 glasses of water a day."
- [ ] 3. "I will eat plenty of fresh fruits."
- [ ] 4. "I will take the medicine with a meal or snack."

41. Which clinical manifestation does the nurse assess as a typical reaction to long-term phenytoin sodium (Dilantin) therapy?
- [ ] 1. Weight gain.
- [ ] 2. Insomnia.
- [ ] 3. Excessive growth of gum tissue.
- [ ] 4. Deteriorating eyesight.

42. A 21-year-old female client takes clonazepam (Klonopin). What should the nurse ask this client about? Select all that apply.
- [ ] 1. Seizure activity.
- [ ] 2. Pregnancy status.
- [ ] 3. Alcohol use.
- [ ] 4. Cigarette smoking.
- [ ] 5. Intake of caffeine and sugary drinks.

The Client with a Stroke

43. A client is being monitored for transient ischemic attacks. She is oriented, can open her eyes spontaneously, and follows commands. What is her Glasgow Coma Scale score?

_____

44. The nurse is teaching a client about taking prophylactic warfarin sodium (Coumadin). Which statement indicates that the client understands how to take the drug? Select all that apply.
- [ ] 1. "The drug's action peaks in 2 hours."
- [ ] 2. "Maximum dosage is not achieved until 3 to 4 days after starting the medication."
- [ ] 3. "Effects of the drug continue for 4 to 5 days after discontinuing the medication."
- [ ] 4. "Protamine sulfate is the antidote for warfarin."
- [ ] 5. "I should have my blood levels tested periodically."

45. Regular oral hygiene is an essential intervention for the client who has had a stroke. Which of the following nursing measures is inappropriate when providing oral hygiene?
- [ ] 1. Placing the client on the back with a small pillow under the head.
- [ ] 2. Keeping portable suctioning equipment at the bedside.
- [ ] 3. Opening the client's mouth with a padded tongue blade.
- [ ] 4. Cleaning the client's mouth and teeth with a toothbrush.

46. A client arrives in the emergency department with an ischemic stroke and receives tissue plasminogen activator (t-PA) administration. Which is the priority nursing assessment?
- [ ] 1. Current medications.
- [ ] 2. Complete physical and history.
- [ ] 3. Time of onset of current stroke.
- [ ] 4. Upcoming surgical procedures.

47. During the first 24 hours after thrombolytic treatment for an ischemic stroke, the primary goal is to control the client's:
- [ ] 1. Pulse.
- [ ] 2. Respirations.
- [ ] 3. Blood pressure.
- [ ] 4. Temperature.

48. What is a priority nursing assessment in the first 24 hours after admission of the client with a thrombotic stroke?
- [ ] 1. Cholesterol level.
- [ ] 2. Pupil size and pupillary response.
- [ ] 3. Bowel sounds.
- [ ] 4. Echocardiogram.

49. What is a priority nursing intervention when suctioning an unconscious client to maintain cerebral perfusion?
- [ ] 1. Hyperoxygenate before and after suctioning.
- [ ] 2. Administer analgesics.
- [ ] 3. Provide oral hygiene.
- [ ] 4. Administer diuretics.

50. The nursing assessment of a client's functional status before and after a stroke is essential. Why is it so important?
- [ ] 1. The rehabilitation plan will be guided by it.
- [ ] 2. Functional status before the stroke will help predict outcomes.
- [ ] 3. It will help the client recognize his physical limitations.
- [ ] 4. The client can be expected to regain much of his functioning.

51. Which of the following techniques does the nurse avoid when changing a client's position in bed if the client has hemiparalysis?
- ☐ **1.** Rolling the client onto the side.
- ☐ **2.** Sliding the client to move up in bed.
- ☐ **3.** Lifting the client when moving the client up in bed.
- ☐ **4.** Having the client help lift off the bed using a trapeze.

52. Which nursing intervention has been found to be the most effective means of preventing plantar flexion in a client who has had a stroke with residual paralysis?
- ☐ **1.** Place the client's feet against a firm footboard.
- ☐ **2.** Reposition the client every 2 hours.
- ☐ **3.** Have the client wear ankle-high tennis shoes at intervals throughout the day.
- ☐ **4.** Massage the client's feet and ankles regularly.

53. The nurse is planning the care of a hemiplegic client to prevent joint deformities of the arm. What position would be inappropriate?
- ☐ **1.** Placing a pillow in the axilla so that the arm is away from the body.
- ☐ **2.** Placing a pillow under the slightly flexed arm so that the hand is higher than the elbow.
- ☐ **3.** Positioning the hands in a slightly pronated position.
- ☐ **4.** Positioning a roll in the hand so that the fingers are barely flexed.

54. For the client who is experiencing expressive aphasia, which nursing intervention is *most* helpful in promoting communication?
- ☐ **1.** Speaking loudly.
- ☐ **2.** Using a picture board.
- ☐ **3.** Writing directions so client can read them.
- ☐ **4.** Speaking in short sentences.

55. The nurse is teaching the family of a client with dysphagia about decreasing the risk of aspiration while eating. Which of the following strategies is inappropriate?
- ☐ **1.** Maintaining an upright position.
- ☐ **2.** Restricting the diet to liquids until swallowing improves.
- ☐ **3.** Introducing foods on the unaffected side of the mouth.
- ☐ **4.** Keeping distractions to a minimum.

56. Which food-related behaviors would the nurse observe in a client who has had a stroke that has left him with homonymous hemianopia?
- ☐ **1.** Increased preference for foods high in salt.
- ☐ **2.** Eating food on only half of the plate.
- ☐ **3.** Forgetting the names of foods.
- ☐ **4.** Inability to swallow liquids.

57. A nurse is teaching a client who had a stroke about ways to adapt to a visual disability. Which does the nurse identify as the primary safety precaution to use?
- ☐ **1.** Wear a patch over one eye.
- ☐ **2.** Place personal items on the sighted side.
- ☐ **3.** Lie in bed with the unaffected side toward the door.
- ☐ **4.** Turn the head from side to side when walking.

58. A client is experiencing mood swings after a stroke and often has episodes of tearfulness that are distressing to the family. Which is the best technique for the nurse to instruct family members to try when the client experiences a crying episode?
- ☐ **1.** Sit quietly with the client until the episode is over.
- ☐ **2.** Ignore the behavior.
- ☐ **3.** Attempt to divert the client's attention.
- ☐ **4.** Tell the client that this behavior is unacceptable.

59. The client who has had a stroke with residual physical handicaps becomes discouraged by his physical appearance. What attitude is best for the nurse to display to help the client overcome his negative self-concept?
- ☐ **1.** Helpfulness and sympathy.
- ☐ **2.** Concern and charity.
- ☐ **3.** Directives and firmness.
- ☐ **4.** Encouragement and patience.

60. When communicating with a client who has aphasia, which of the following nursing interventions is inappropriate?
- ☐ **1.** Present one thought at a time.
- ☐ **2.** Encourage the client not to write messages.
- ☐ **3.** Speak with normal volume.
- ☐ **4.** Make use of gestures.

61. What is the expected outcome of thrombolytic drug therapy for stroke?
- ☐ **1.** Increased vascular permeability.
- ☐ **2.** Vasoconstriction.
- ☐ **3.** Dissolved emboli.
- ☐ **4.** Prevention of hemorrhage.

The Client with Parkinson's Disease

62. A health care provider has ordered carbidopa-levodopa (Sinemet) four times per day for a client with Parkinson's disease. The client states that he wants "to end it all now that the Parkinson's disease has progressed." What should the nurse do? Select all that apply.
- ☐ 1. Explain that the new prescription for Sinemet will treat his depression.
- ☐ 2. Encourage the client to discuss his feelings as the Sinemet is being administered.
- ☐ 3. Contact the health care provider before administering the Sinemet.
- ☐ 4. Determine if the client is on antidepressants or monoamine oxidase (MAO) inhibitors.
- ☐ 5. Determine if the client is at risk for suicide.

63. Which of the following is an initial sign of Parkinson's disease?
- ☐ 1. Rigidity.
- ☐ 2. Tremor.
- ☐ 3. Bradykinesia.
- ☐ 4. Akinesia.

64. The nurse develops a teaching plan for a client newly diagnosed with Parkinson's disease. Which of the following topics that the nurse plans to discuss is the *most* important?
- ☐ 1. Maintaining a balanced nutritional diet.
- ☐ 2. Enhancing the immune system.
- ☐ 3. Maintaining a safe environment.
- ☐ 4. Engaging in diversional activity.

65. The nurse observes that a client's upper arm tremors disappear as he unbuttons his shirt. Which statement best guides the nurse's analysis of this observation about the client's tremors?
- ☐ 1. The tremors are probably psychological and can be controlled at will.
- ☐ 2. The tremors sometimes disappear with purposeful and voluntary movements.
- ☐ 3. The tremors disappear when the client's attention is diverted by some activity.
- ☐ 4. There is no explanation for the observation; it is probably a chance occurrence.

66. At what time of day should the nurse encourage a client with Parkinson's disease to schedule the most demanding physical activities to minimize the effects of hypokinesia?
- ☐ 1. Early in the morning, when the client's energy level is high.
- ☐ 2. To coincide with the peak action of drug therapy.
- ☐ 3. Immediately after a rest period.
- ☐ 4. When family members will be available.

67. Which goal is the most realistic and appropriate for a client diagnosed with Parkinson's disease?
- ☐ 1. To cure the disease.
- ☐ 2. To stop progression of the disease.
- ☐ 3. To begin preparations for terminal care.
- ☐ 4. To maintain optimal body function.

68. What is the primary goal collaboratively established by the client with Parkinson's disease, nurse, and physical therapist?
- ☐ 1. To maintain joint flexibility.
- ☐ 2. To build muscle strength.
- ☐ 3. To improve muscle endurance.
- ☐ 4. To reduce ataxia.

69. A client with Parkinson's disease is prescribed levodopa (L-dopa) therapy. Improvement in which of the following indicates effective therapy?
- ☐ 1. Mood.
- ☐ 2. Muscle rigidity.
- ☐ 3. Appetite.
- ☐ 4. Alertness.

70. A client is being switched from levodopa (L-dopa) to carbidopa-levodopa (Sinemet). The nurse should monitor for which of the following possible complications during medication changes and dosage adjustment?
- ☐ 1. Euphoria.
- ☐ 2. Jaundice.
- ☐ 3. Vital sign fluctuation.
- ☐ 4. Signs and symptoms of diabetes.

71. A new medication regimen is ordered for a client with Parkinson's disease. At which time should the nurse make certain that the medication is taken?
- ☐ 1. At bedtime.
- ☐ 2. All at one time.
- ☐ 3. Two hours before mealtime.
- ☐ 4. At the time scheduled.

72. A client with Parkinson's disease needs a long time to complete her morning hygiene, but she becomes annoyed when the nurse offers assistance and refuses all help. Which action is the nurse's best initial response in this situation?
- [ ] **1.** Tell the client firmly that she needs assistance and help her with her care.
- [ ] **2.** Praise the client for her desire to be independent and give her extra time and encouragement.
- [ ] **3.** Tell the client that she is being unrealistic about her abilities and must accept the fact that she needs help.
- [ ] **4.** Suggest to the client that if she insists on self-care, she should at least modify her routine.

73. A client with Parkinson's disease asks the nurse to explain to his nephew "what the doctor said the pallidotomy would do." The nurse's best response includes stating that the main goal for the client after pallidotomy is improved:
- [ ] **1.** Functional ability.
- [ ] **2.** Emotional stress.
- [ ] **3.** Alertness.
- [ ] **4.** Appetite.

The Client with Multiple Sclerosis

74. The nurse is teaching a client with bladder dysfunction from multiple sclerosis (MS) about bladder training at home. Which instructions should the nurse include in the teaching plan? Select all that apply.
- [ ] **1.** Restrict fluids to 1,000 ml/24 hours.
- [ ] **2.** Drink 400 to 500 ml with each meal.
- [ ] **3.** Drink fluids midmorning, midafternoon, and late afternoon.
- [ ] **4.** Attempt to void at least every 2 hours.
- [ ] **5.** Use intermittent catheterization as needed.

75. Which of the following is not a typical clinical manifestation of multiple sclerosis (MS)?
- [ ] **1.** Double vision.
- [ ] **2.** Sudden bursts of energy.
- [ ] **3.** Weakness in the extremities.
- [ ] **4.** Muscle tremors.

76. A client with multiple sclerosis (MS) is receiving baclofen (Lioresal). The nurse determines that the drug is effective when it achieves which of the following?
- [ ] **1.** Induces sleep.
- [ ] **2.** Stimulates the client's appetite.
- [ ] **3.** Relieves muscular spasticity.
- [ ] **4.** Reduces the urine bacterial count.

77. A client has had multiple sclerosis (MS) for 15 years and has received various drug therapies. What is the primary reason why the nurse has found it difficult to evaluate the effectiveness of the drugs that the client has used?
- [ ] **1.** The client exhibits intolerance to many drugs.
- [ ] **2.** The client experiences spontaneous remissions from time to time.
- [ ] **3.** The client requires multiple drugs simultaneously.
- [ ] **4.** The client endures long periods of exacerbation before the illness responds to a particular drug.

78. When the nurse talks with a client with multiple sclerosis who has slurred speech, which nursing intervention is contraindicated?
- [ ] **1.** Encouraging the client to speak slowly.
- [ ] **2.** Encouraging the client to speak distinctly.
- [ ] **3.** Asking the client to repeat indistinguishable words.
- [ ] **4.** Asking the client to speak louder when tired.

79. The right hand of a client with multiple sclerosis trembles severely whenever she attempts a voluntary action. She spills her coffee twice at lunch and cannot get her dress fastened securely. Which is the best legal documentation in nurses' notes of the chart for this client assessment?
- [ ] **1.** "Has an intention tremor of the right hand."
- [ ] **2.** "Right-hand tremor worsens with purposeful acts."
- [ ] **3.** "Needs assistance with dressing and eating due to severe trembling and clumsiness."
- [ ] **4.** "Slight shaking of right hand increases to severe tremor when client tries to button her clothes or drink from a cup."

80. A client with multiple sclerosis (MS) is experiencing bowel incontinence and is starting a bowel retraining program. Which strategy is inappropriate?
- [ ] **1.** Eating a diet high in fiber.
- [ ] **2.** Setting a regular time for elimination.
- [ ] **3.** Using an elevated toilet seat.
- [ ] **4.** Limiting fluid intake to 1,000 ml/day.

81. Which of the following is an inappropriate outcome to establish with a client who has multiple sclerosis (MS)? The client will:
- [ ] **1.** Develop joint mobility.
- [ ] **2.** Develop muscle strength.
- [ ] **3.** Develop cognition.
- [ ] **4.** Develop mood elevation.

82. The nurse is preparing a client with multiple sclerosis (MS) for discharge from the hospital to home. Which of the following instructions is appropriate?
- ☐ **1.** "You will need to accept the necessity for a quiet and inactive lifestyle."
- ☐ **2.** "Keep active, use stress reduction strategies, and avoid fatigue."
- ☐ **3.** "Follow good health habits to change the course of the disease."
- ☐ **4.** "Practice using the mechanical aids that you will need when future disabilities arise."

83. Which of the following is inappropriate for the nurse to include in the discharge plan for a client with multiple sclerosis who has an impaired peripheral sensation?
- ☐ **1.** Carefully test the temperature of bath water.
- ☐ **2.** Avoid kitchen activities because of the risk of injury.
- ☐ **3.** Avoid hot water bottles and heating pads.
- ☐ **4.** Inspect the skin daily for injury or pressure points.

84. Which intervention should the nurse suggest to help a client with multiple sclerosis avoid episodes of urinary incontinence?
- ☐ **1.** Limit fluid intake to 1,000 ml/day.
- ☐ **2.** Insert an indwelling urinary catheter.
- ☐ **3.** Establish a regular voiding schedule.
- ☐ **4.** Administer prophylactic antibiotics, as ordered.

85. A client with multiple sclerosis (MS) lives with her daughter and 3-year-old granddaughter. The daughter asks the nurse what she can do at home to help her mother. Which of the following measures would be most beneficial?
- ☐ **1.** Psychotherapy.
- ☐ **2.** Regular exercise.
- ☐ **3.** Day care for the granddaughter.
- ☐ **4.** Weekly visits by another person with MS.

The Unconscious Client

86. A client is brought to the emergency department unconscious. An empty bottle of aspirin was found in his car, and a drug overdose is suspected. Which of the following medications should the nurse have available for further emergency treatment?
- ☐ **1.** Vitamin K.
- ☐ **2.** Dextrose 50%.
- ☐ **3.** Activated charcoal powder.
- ☐ **4.** Sodium thiosulfate.

87. Several clients have come to the emergency department after a possible bioterrorist act of arsenic overexposure. The nurse should assess these clients for which signs or symptoms immediately following the poisoning? Select all that apply.
- ☐ **1.** Violent vomiting.
- ☐ **2.** Severe diarrhea.
- ☐ **3.** Abdominal pain.
- ☐ **4.** Sensory neuropathy.
- ☐ **5.** Persistent cough.

88. Which clinical manifestations should the nurse expect to assess in a client diagnosed with an overdose of a cholinergic agent. Select all that apply.
- ☐ **1.** Dry mucous membranes.
- ☐ **2.** Urinary incontinence.
- ☐ **3.** Central nervous system (CNS) depression.
- ☐ **4.** Seizures.
- ☐ **5.** Skin rash.

89. The wife and sister of a client who had attempted suicide with an overdose are distraught about his comatose condition and the possibility that he took an intentional drug overdose. Which of the following would be an appropriate initial nursing intervention with this family?
- ☐ **1.** Explain that because the client was found on hospital property, he was probably asking for help and did not intentionally overdose.
- ☐ **2.** Give the wife and sister a big hug and assure them that the client is in good hands.
- ☐ **3.** Encourage the wife and sister to express their feelings and concerns, and listen carefully.
- ☐ **4.** Allow the wife and sister to help care for the client by rubbing his back when he is turned.

90. Which of the following is a *priority* during the first 24 hours of hospitalization for a comatose client with suspected drug overdose?
- ☐ **1.** Educate regarding drug abuse.
- ☐ **2.** Minimize pain.
- ☐ **3.** Maintain intact skin.
- ☐ **4.** Increase caloric intake.

91. An unconscious intubated client does not have increased intracranial pressure. Which nursing intervention would be essential?
- ☐ **1.** Monitoring the oral temperature, keep the room temperature at 70° F (21.1° C), and place the client on a cooling blanket if the client's temperature is higher than 101° F (38.3° C).
- ☐ **2.** Cleaning the mouth carefully, applying a thin coat of petroleum jelly, and moving the endotracheal tube to the opposite side daily.
- ☐ **3.** Positioning the client in the supine position with the head to the side and slightly elevated on two pillows.
- ☐ **4.** Turning the client with a drawsheet and placing a pillow behind the back and one between the legs.

92. An unconscious client has been positioned on one side. The nurse monitors which of the following anatomic areas as a pressure point?
- ☐ **1.** Sacrum.
- ☐ **2.** Occiput.
- ☐ **3.** Ankles.
- ☐ **4.** Heels.

93. The client is placed in a right side-lying position. Which of the following positions is incorrect?
- ☐ **1.** The head is placed on a small pillow.
- ☐ **2.** The right leg is extended without pillow support.
- ☐ **3.** The left arm is rested on the mattress with the elbow flexed.
- ☐ **4.** The left leg is supported on a pillow with the knee flexed.

94. What is the intended outcome for the nursing intervention of performing passive range-of-motion (ROM) exercises on an unconscious client?
- ☐ **1.** Preservation of muscle mass.
- ☐ **2.** Prevention of bone demineralization.
- ☐ **3.** Increase in muscle tone.
- ☐ **4.** Maintenance of joint mobility.

95. When the nurse performs oral hygiene for an unconscious client, which nursing intervention is the *priority*?
- ☐ **1.** Keep a suction machine available.
- ☐ **2.** Place the client in a prone position.
- ☐ **3.** Wear sterile gloves while brushing the client's teeth.
- ☐ **4.** Use gauze wrapped around the fingers to clean the client's gums.

96. The nurse observes that the client's right eye does not close totally. Based on this finding, which nursing intervention is *most* appropriate?
- ☐ **1.** Make sure the client wears eyeglasses at all times.
- ☐ **2.** Place an eye patch over the completely closed right eye.
- ☐ **3.** Instill artificial tears once every shift.
- ☐ **4.** Clean the eyelid with a clean washcloth every shift.

97. Which sign is an early indicator of hypoxia in the unconscious client?
- ☐ **1.** Cyanosis.
- ☐ **2.** Decreased respirations.
- ☐ **3.** Restlessness.
- ☐ **4.** Hypotension.

98. When administering intermittent enteral feeding to an unconscious client, the nurse should:
- ☐ **1.** Heat the formula in a microwave.
- ☐ **2.** Place the client in a semi-Fowler's position.
- ☐ **3.** Obtain a sterile gavage bag and tubing.
- ☐ **4.** Weigh the client before administering the feeding.

99. The client is to receive 200 ml of tube feeding every 4 hours. When the nurse checks for the client's gastric residual before administering the next scheduled feeding and obtains 40 ml of gastric residual, what is the appropriate intervention?
- ☐ **1.** Withhold the tube feeding and notify the physician.
- ☐ **2.** Dispose of the residual and continue with the feeding.
- ☐ **3.** Delay feeding the client for 1 hour and then recheck the residual.
- ☐ **4.** Readminister the residual to the client and continue with the feeding.

100. Of the following nursing interventions for catheter care, which should have the *highest* priority?
- ☐ **1.** Cleaning the area around the urethral meatus.
- ☐ **2.** Clamping the catheter periodically to maintain muscle tone.
- ☐ **3.** Irrigating the catheter with several ounces of normal saline solution.
- ☐ **4.** Changing the location where the catheter is taped to the client's leg.

101. A client has been pronounced brain dead. Which findings should the nurse assess? Select all that apply.
- ☐ **1.** Decerebrate posturing.
- ☐ **2.** Nonreactive dilated pupils.
- ☐ **3.** Deep tendon reflexes.
- ☐ **4.** Absent corneal reflex.
- ☐ **5.** Blink reflex.

The Client in Pain

102. A 34-year-old Chinese man is admitted with multiple injuries from a motor vehicle accident. He complains of severe pain and requests frequent medication. One of the assistive nursing personnel expresses surprise, saying, "I thought Asian people were very stoic about pain." Which is the nurse's best response about pain?
- ☐ **1.** Expression and perception of pain vary widely from person to person.
- ☐ **2.** Tolerance of pain is about the same in all people.
- ☐ **3.** Tolerance of pain is determined by a person's genetic makeup.
- ☐ **4.** Pain perception is about the same in all people.

103. The nurse finds it difficult to relieve a client's pain satisfactorily. Which of the following measures should the nurse take into consideration when continuing efforts to promote comfort?
- ☐ **1.** Improve the nurse-client relationship.
- ☐ **2.** Enlist the help of the client's family.
- ☐ **3.** Allow the client additional time to work through his or her own responses to pain.
- ☐ **4.** Arrange to have the client share a room with a client who has little pain.

104. A client from China tells the nurse, "If I could be among my people, I could receive acupuncture for this pain." The nurse understands that acupuncture in the Asian culture is based on which theory?
- ☐ **1.** Elimination of evil spirits.
- ☐ **2.** Promotion of tranquility with a higher being.
- ☐ **3.** Restoration of the balance of energy.
- ☐ **4.** Blockade of nerve pathways to the brain.

105. The client's physician decides to change the analgesia medication from meperidine hydrochloride (Demerol) 75 mg I.M. every 4 hours as needed to meperidine hydrochloride by the oral route. What dosage of oral meperidine is required to provide an equivalent analgesic dose?
- ☐ **1.** 25 to 50 mg.
- ☐ **2.** 75 to 100 mg.
- ☐ **3.** 125 to 150 mg.
- ☐ **4.** 250 to 300 mg.

106. After administering meperidine hydrochloride (Demerol), the nurse determines its effectiveness as an analgesic was related to its ability to:
- ☐ **1.** Reduce the perception of pain.
- ☐ **2.** Decrease the sensitivity of pain receptors.
- ☐ **3.** Interfere with pain impulses traveling along sensory nerve fibers.
- ☐ **4.** Block the conduction of pain impulses along the central nervous system.

107. The nurse bases interventions to reduce pain on the gate-control theory of pain. This theory holds that a regulatory process controls impulses reaching the brain. Where is this regulatory process believed to be located?
- ☐ **1.** Brain stem.
- ☐ **2.** Cerebellum.
- ☐ **3.** Spinal cord.
- ☐ **4.** Hypothalamus.

108. A client is arousing from a coma and keeps saying, "Just stop the pain." The nurse responds based on the knowledge that the human body typically and automatically responds to pain first with attempts to:
- ☐ **1.** Tolerate the pain.
- ☐ **2.** Decrease the perception of pain.
- ☐ **3.** Escape the source of pain.
- ☐ **4.** Divert attention from the source of pain.

109. Ergotamine tartrate (Gynergen) is prescribed for a client's migraine headaches. The client's report of which of the following indicates effectiveness?
- ☐ **1.** Prevention of the migraine.
- ☐ **2.** Reduced severity of the developing migraine.
- ☐ **3.** Relief from the sleeplessness experienced in the past after a migraine.
- ☐ **4.** Relief from the vision problems experienced in the past after a migraine.

110. The client asks the nurse why she has migraine headaches. What is the nurse's best response?
- ☐ **1.** Migraine headaches are believed to be caused by dilation of the cranial arteries.
- ☐ **2.** Migraine headaches are believed to be caused by a temporary decrease in intracranial pressure.
- ☐ **3.** Migraine headaches are believed to be caused by irritation and inflammation of the openings of the sinuses.
- ☐ **4.** Migraine headaches are believed to be caused by sustained contraction of muscles around the scalp and face.

111. The nurse explains to the client with pain that the purpose of biofeedback is to enable him to exert control over his physiologic processes by:
- ☐ **1.** Regulating the body processes through electrical control.
- ☐ **2.** Shocking himself when an undesirable response is elicited.
- ☐ **3.** Monitoring the body processes for the therapist to interpret.
- ☐ **4.** Translating the signals of his body processes into observable forms.

112. The nurse explains to the client that the main reason a back rub is used as therapy to relieve pain is because the massage:
- ☐ **1.** Blocks pain impulses from the spinal cord to the brain.
- ☐ **2.** Blocks pain impulses from the brain to the spinal cord.
- ☐ **3.** Stimulates the release of endorphins.
- ☐ **4.** Distracts the client's focus on the source of the pain.

113. Nursing responsibilities for the client with a patient-controlled analgesia (PCA) system should include:
- ☐ **1.** Reassuring the client that pain will be relieved.
- ☐ **2.** Documenting the client's response to pain medication on a routine basis.
- ☐ **3.** Instructing the client to continue pressing the system's button whenever pain occurs.
- ☐ **4.** Titrating the client's pain medication until the client is free from pain.

114. A client has an epidural catheter inserted for postoperative pain management. The client rates his pain at 4 on a 0-to-5 pain scale. What should the nurse do first?
- ☐ **1.** Check the patient-controlled analgesia (PCA) pump function.
- ☐ **2.** Adjust the epidural catheter.
- ☐ **3.** Assess vital signs.
- ☐ **4.** Notify the physician.

115. When locating the ventrogluteal site before giving an I.M. injection, the nurse should place the palm on the client's:
- ☐ **1.** Iliac crest.
- ☐ **2.** Greater trochanter.
- ☐ **3.** Anterior superior iliac spine.
- ☐ **4.** Posterior superior iliac spine.

116. The nurse using healing touch affects a client's pain primarily through:
- ☐ **1.** Energy fields.
- ☐ **2.** Touch therapy.
- ☐ **3.** Massage.
- ☐ **4.** Hypnosis.

117. A client asks why the nurse does not give a 1.5-ml intramuscular injection into the upper arm. The nurse explains that the deltoid muscle is not used because the muscle:
- ☐ **1.** Is small.
- ☐ **2.** Is difficult to locate.
- ☐ **3.** Has many pain receptors.
- ☐ **4.** Has a poor blood supply.

Correct Answers and Rationales

The letter in parentheses after each rationale identifies the client need addressed in the item, including management of care (M), safety and infection control (S), health promotion and maintenance (H), psychosocial adaptation (P), basic care and comfort (C), pharmacological and parenteral therapies (D), reduction of risk potential (R), and physiological adaptation (A).

The Client with a Head Injury

1. 2, 3, 4. The nurse should maintain ICP by elevating the head of the bed and monitoring neurologic status. An ICP greater than 20 mm Hg indicates increased ICP, and the nurse should notify the health care provider. Coughing and range-of-motion exercises will increase ICP and should be avoided in the early postoperative stage. (A)

2. 1, 4. The nurse must monitor the systolic and diastolic blood pressure to obtain the mean arterial pressure (MAP), which represents the pressure needed for each cardiac cycle to perfuse the brain. The nurse must also monitor the cerebral perfusion pressure (CPP), which is obtained from the ICP and the MAP. The nurse should also monitor urine output, respirations, and pain; however, crucial measurements needed to maintain CPP are ICP and MAP. When ICP equals MAP, there is no CPP. (M)

3. 80

To obtain the MAP, use this formula:

$$MAP = [\text{systolic BP} + (2 \times \text{diastolic BP})] \div 3$$

$$MAP = [120 + (2 \times 60)] \div 3$$

$$MAP = 240 \div 3 = 80.$$

(M)

4. 2, 3. The nurse should determine if the client's pupils are equal and react to light, and ask the client if he has a headache. Confusion, agitation, and restlessness are subtle clinical manifestations of increased intracranial pressure (ICP). At this time, it is not appropriate for the nurse to find a television or arrange for the client to see his wife and baby. Administering a sedative at this time will obscure assessment of increased ICP. (M)

5. 1. The highest priority for a client with multiple injuries is to establish an open airway for effective ventilation and oxygenation. Unless the client has a patent airway, other care measures will be futile. Replacing blood loss, stopping bleeding from open wounds, and checking for a neck fracture are important nursing interventions to be completed after the airway and ventilation are established. (S)

6. 1. Increasing ICP causes unequal pupils as a result of pressure on the third cranial nerve. Increasing ICP causes an increase in the systolic pressure, which reflects the additional pressure needed to perfuse the brain. It increases the pressure on the vagus nerve, which produces bradycardia, and it causes an increase in body temperature from hypothalamic damage. (R)

7. 3. The clear drainage must be analyzed to determine whether it is nasal drainage or cerebrospinal fluid (CSF). The nurse should not give the client tissues because it is important to know how much leakage of CSF is occurring. Compressing the nares will obstruct the drainage flow. It is inappropriate to tilt the head back, which would allow the fluid to drain down the throat and not be collected for a sample. It is inappropriate to administer an antihistamine because the drainage may not be from post-nasal drip. (R)

8. 1. Neural control of respiration takes place in the brain stem. Deterioration and pressure produce irregular respiratory patterns. Rapid, shallow respirations, asymmetric chest movements, and nasal flaring are more characteristic of respiratory distress or hypoxia. (A)

9. 3. Normal ICP is 15 mm Hg or less for 15 to 30 seconds or longer. Hyperventilation causes vasoconstriction, which reduces cerebrospinal fluid and blood volume, two important factors for reducing a sustained ICP of 20 mm Hg. A cooling blanket is used to control the elevation of temperature because a fever increases the metabolic rate, which in turn increases ICP. High doses of barbiturates may be used to reduce the increased cellular metabolic demands. Fluid volume and inotropic drugs are used to maintain cerebral perfusion by supporting the cardiac output and keeping the cerebral perfusion pressure greater than 80 mm Hg. (A)

10. 4. A decrease in the client's LOC is an early indicator of deterioration of the client's neurologic status. Changes in level of consciousness, such as restlessness and irritability, may be subtle. Widening of the pulse pressure, decrease in the pulse rate, and dilated, fixed pupils occur later if the increased ICP is not treated. (A)

11. 3. The constituents of CSF are similar to those of blood plasma. An examination for glucose content is done to determine whether body fluid is mucus or CSF. CSF contains glucose; mucus does not. (R)

12. 1. The client's ICP is elevated, and the client should be positioned to avoid extreme neck flexion or extension. The head of the bed is usually elevated 30 to 45 degrees to drain the venous sinuses and thus decrease the ICP. Trendelenburg's position places the client's head lower than the body, which would increase ICP. The Sims position (side lying) and elevating the head on two pillows may extend or flex the neck, which increases ICP. (R)

13. 2. After administering mannitol, the nurse closely monitors intake and output because mannitol promotes diuresis and is given primarily to pull water from the extracellular fluid of the edematous brain. Mannitol can cause hypokalemia and may lead to muscle contractions, not muscle relaxation. Signs and symptoms, such as widening pulse pressure and pupil dilation, should not occur because mannitol serves to decrease ICP. (D)

14. 3, 4, 5. The nurse should assess the client for spinal shock, which is the immediate response to spinal cord transection. Hypotension occurs and the body loses core temperature to environmental temperature. The nurse must treat the client immediately to manage hypotension and hypothermia. The nurse should also ensure that there is an adequate airway and respirations; there may be respiratory compromise due to intercostal muscle involvement. Once the client is stable, the nurse should conduct a complete neurologic check. The nurse should take all precautions to keep the client's head, neck, and spine position in straight alignment. If the client is conscious, the nurse should briefly assess major reflexes, such as the Achilles, patellar, biceps, and triceps tendons, and sensation of the perineum for bladder function. (M)

15. 4. The correct motor function test for C8 is a hand-grasp check. The motor function check for C4 to C5 is shoulders shrugging against downward pressure of the examiner's hands. The motor function check for C5 to C6 is an arm pulling up from a resting position against resistance. The motor function check for C7 is an arm straightening out from a flexed position against resistance. (M)

16. 2, 3. The client with a C3 to C4 fracture has neck control but may tire easily using sore muscles around the incision area to hold up his head. Therefore, the head and neck of his wheelchair should be high. The seat of the wheelchair should be lower than normal to facilitate transfer from the bed to the wheelchair. When a client can use his hands and arms to move the wheelchair, the placement of the back to the client's scapula is necessary. This client cannot use his arms and will need an electric chair with breath, chin, or voice control to manipulate movement of the chair. A firm or hard cushion adds pressure to bony prominences; the cushion should instead be padded to reduce the risk of pressure ulcers. (C)

17. 4. It is important to first explain where a client is to orient him to time, person, and place. Offering to get his family and asking him questions to determine whether he is oriented are important, but the first comments should let the client know where he is and what happened to him. It is useful to be empathetic to the client, but making a comment such as "I'll bet you're a little confused" when he first awakens is not helpful and may cause him anxiety. (P)

18. 2. It is best for the client to wear mitts, which help prevent the client from pulling on the I.V. without causing additional agitation. Using a jacket or wrist restraint or tucking the client's arms and hands under the drawsheet restrict movement and add to feelings of being confined, all of which would increase her agitation and increase ICP. (A)

19. 3. Coughing is contraindicated for a client at risk for increased ICP because coughing increases ICP. Deep breathing can be continued. Turning and passive ROM exercises can be continued with care not to extend or flex the neck. (R)

20. 2. Diabetes insipidus results from deficiency of antidiuretic hormone (ADH). The condition may occur in conjunction with head injuries as well as with other disorders. In ADH deficiency, the client is extremely thirsty and excretes large amounts of highly diluted urine. Measuring the urine output to detect excess amount and checking the specific gravity of urine samples to determine urine concentration are appropriate measures to determine the onset of diabetes insipidus. The client may be tachycardic and hypotensive from fluid deficit; however, altered vital signs in a client with a head injury may occur for other reasons as well. Blood gas analysis and blood glucose levels will not reveal diabetes insipidus. (A)

21. 3. Recovery from a serious head injury is a long-term process that may continue for months or years. Depending on the extent of the injury, clients who are transferred to rehabilitation facilities most likely will continue to exhibit cognitive and mobility impairments as well as behavior and personality changes. The client would be expected to participate in the rehabilitation efforts to the extent he is capable. Family members and significant others will need long-term support to help them cope with the changes that have occurred in the client. (A)

22. 4. Decerebrate posturing occurs in clients with damage to the upper brain stem, midbrain, or pons and is demonstrated clinically by arching of the back, rigid extension of the extremities, pronation of the arms, and plantar flexion of the feet. Internal rotation and adduction of arms with flexion of elbows, wrists, and fingers describes decorticate posturing, which indicates damage to corticospinal tracts and cerebral hemispheres. (A)

23. 2. Cluster breathing consists of clusters of irregular breaths followed by periods of apnea on an irregular basis. A lesion in the upper medulla or lower pons is usually the cause of cluster breathing. Because the client had a bleed in the occipital lobe, which is just superior and posterior to the pons and medulla, clinical manifestations that indicate

a new lesion are monitored very closely in case another bleed ensues. The nurse should notify the physician immediately so that treatment can begin before respirations cease. The client is not obtaining sufficient oxygen and the depth of breathing is assisted by the ventilator. The health care provider will determine changes in the ventilator settings. (A)

24. 2. Elevating the head of the bed to 30 degrees is contraindicated for infratentorial craniotomies because it could cause herniation of the brain down onto the brain stem and spinal cord, resulting in sudden death. Elevation of the head of the bed to 30 degrees with the head turned to the side opposite the incision, if not contraindicated by the increased intracranial pressure, is used for supratentorial craniotomies. (A)

The Client with Seizures

25. 3. Temperatures are not assessed orally with a glass thermometer because the thermometer could break and cause injury if a seizure occurred. The client can perform personal hygiene. There is no clinical reason to discourage the client from wearing his own clothes. As long as there are no other limitations, the client should be encouraged to be out of bed. (A)

26. 1, 3, 4. Severe hypoglycemia causing irreversible brain damage can occur quickly in a client who is unconscious and experiencing a seizure. Therefore, unless a blood glucose level determination is rapidly available to rule out hypoglycemia, the nurse should expect to administer a bolus of dextrose 50%, 50 to 100 ml I.V. Thiamine is administered to clients who are malnourished or who abuse alcohol and would not be contraindicated in this client. Naloxone is administered to clients suspected of an opioid overdose to reverse comas or opioid-induced respiratory depression and is an appropriate order for this client. Flumazenil is administered to reverse benzodiazepine overdose, and it should not be given to a client with a seizure disorder. Insulin is administered for hyperglycemia. (D)

27. 4. A generalized tonic-clonic seizure involves both a tonic phase and a clonic phase. The tonic phase consists of loss of consciousness, dilated pupils, and muscular stiffening or contraction, which lasts about 20 to 30 seconds. The clonic phase involves repetitive movements. The seizure ends with confusion, drowsiness, and resumption of respiration. A partial seizure starts in one region of the cortex and may stay focused or spread (e.g., jerking in the extremity spreading to other areas of the body). An absence seizure usually occurs in children and involves a vacant stare with a brief loss of consciousness that often goes unnoticed. A complex partial seizure involves facial grimacing with patting and smacking. (A)

28. **4.** The client will be asked to hold the head very still during the examination, which lasts about 30 to 60 minutes. In some instances, food and fluids may be withheld for 4 to 6 hours before the procedure if a contrast medium is used because the radiopaque substance sometimes causes nausea. There is no special preparation for a CT scan, so a shampoo the night before is not required. The client may drink fluids until 4 hours before the scan is scheduled. Electrodes are not used for a CT scan, nor is the head shaved. (A)

29. **2.** Beverages containing caffeine, such as coffee, tea, and cola drinks, are withheld before an EEG because of the stimulating effects of the caffeine on the brain waves. A meal should not be omitted before an EEG because low blood sugar could alter brain wave patterns; the client can have the entire meal except for the coffee. (A)

30. **1.** Trauma is one of the primary causes of brain damage and seizure activity in adults. Other common causes of seizure activity in adults include neoplasms, withdrawal from drugs and alcohol, and vascular disease. Given the history of head injury, electrolyte imbalance is not the cause of the seizure. There is no information to indicate that the seizure is related to a congenital defect. Epilepsy is usually diagnosed in younger clients. (A)

31. **2.** Gabapentin (Neurontin) may impair vision. Changes in vision, concentration, or coordination should be reported to the physician. Gabapentin should not be stopped abruptly because of the potential for status epilepticus; this is a medication that must be tapered off. Gabapentin is to be stored at room temperature and out of direct light. It should not be taken with antacids. (D)

32. **3.** A priority for the client in the postictal phase (after a seizure) is to assess the client's breathing pattern for effective rate, rhythm, and depth. The nurse should apply oxygen and ventilation to the client as appropriate. Other interventions, to be completed after the airway has been established, include reorientation of the client to time, person, and place. Determining the client's level of sleepiness is useful, but it is not a priority. Positioning the client comfortably promotes rest but is of less importance than ascertaining that the airway is patent. (R)

33. **4.** Carbamazepine (Tegretol) is an anticonvulsant that helps prevent further seizures. Bed rest, sedation (phenobarbital), and providing privacy do not minimize the risk of seizures. (D)

34. **4.** During a seizure, the nurse should note movement of the client's head and eyes and muscle rigidity, especially when the seizure first begins, to obtain clues about the location of the trigger focus in the brain. Other important assessments would include noting the progression and duration of the seizure, respiratory status, loss of consciousness, pupil size, and incontinence of urine and stool. It is typically not possible to assess the client's pulse and blood pressure during a tonic-clonic seizure because the muscle contractions make assessment difficult to impossible. The last dose of anticonvulsant medication can be evaluated later. The nurse should focus on maintaining an open airway, preventing injury to the client, and assessing the onset and progression of the seizure to determine the type of brain activity involved. The type of aura should be assessed in the preictal phase of the seizure. (A)

35. **1.** The nurse should expect a client in the postictal phase to experience drowsiness to somnolence because exhaustion results from the abnormal spontaneous neuron firing and tonic-clonic motor response. An inability to move a muscle part is not expected after a tonic-clonic seizure because a lack of motor function would be related to a complication, such as a lesion, tumor, or stroke, in the correlating brain tissue. A change in sensation would not be expected because this would indicate a complication such as an injury to the peripheral nerve pathway to the corresponding part from the central nervous system. Hypotension is not typically a problem after a seizure. (A)

36. **3.** Exactly how phenytoin sodium helps control seizures is unclear. The most common theory is that it reduces the responsiveness of neurons in the brain to abnormal impulses—that is, it depresses neural activity. Dilantin does not influence norepinephrine or transmission of impulses in the spinal cord, nor does it interrupt the flow of abnormal impulses from peripheral neurons in the viscera to the brain. (D)

37. **2.** Anticonvulsant drug therapy should never be stopped suddenly; doing so can lead to life-threatening status epilepticus. Phenytoin sodium does not carry a risk of physical dependency or lead to hypoglycemia. Phenytoin has antiarrhythmic properties, and discontinuation does not cause heart block. (D)

38. **2.** Specific motor vehicle regulations and restrictions for people who experience seizures vary locally. Most commonly, evidence that the seizures are under medical control is required before the person is given permission to drive. Time of day is not a consideration when determining driving restrictions related to seizures. The amount of time a person has been seizure-free is a consideration for lifting driving restrictions; however, the time frame is usually 2 years. It is recommended, not required, that a person who is subject to seizures carry a card or wear an identification bracelet describing the illness to facilitate quick identification in the event of an emergency. (R)

39. **3.** An aura is a premonition of an impending seizure. Auras usually are of a sensory nature (e.g., an olfactory, visual, gustatory, or auditory sensation); some may be of a psychic nature. Evaluating an aura may help identify the area of the brain from which the seizure originates. Auras occur before a seizure, not during or after (postictal). They are not similar to hallucinations or amnesia or related to relaxation. (A)

40. **2.** Toxic effects of topiramate (Topamax) include nephrolithiasis, and clients are encouraged to drink 6 to 8 glasses of water a day to dilute the urine and flush the renal tubules to avoid stone formation. Topiramate is taken in divided doses because it produces drowsiness. Although eating fresh fruits is desirable from a nutritional standpoint, this is not related to the topiramate. The drug does not have to be taken with meals. (D)

41. **3.** A common adverse effect of long-term phenytoin therapy is an overgrowth of gingival tissues. Problems may be minimized with good oral hygiene, but in some cases, overgrown tissues must be removed surgically. Phenytoin does not cause weight gain, insomnia, or deteriorating eyesight. (D)

42. **1, 2, 3.** The nurse should assess the number and type of seizures the client has experienced since starting clonazepam monotherapy for seizure control. The nurse should also determine if the client might be pregnant because clonazepam crosses the placental barrier. The nurse should also ask about the client's use of alcohol because alcohol potentiates the action of clonazepam. Although the nurse may want to check on the client's diet or use of cigarettes for health maintenance and promotion, such information is not specifically related to clonazepam therapy. (D)

The Client with a Stroke

43. **15**

The Glasgow Coma Scale provides three objective neurologic assessments: spontaneity of eye opening, best motor response, and best verbal response on a scale of 3 to 15. The client who scores the best on all three assessments scores 15 points. (M)

44. **2, 3, 5.** The maximum dosage of warfarin sodium (Coumadin) is not achieved until 3 to 4 days after starting the medication, and the effects of the drug continue for 4 to 5 days after discontinuing the medication. The client should have his blood levels tested periodically to make sure that the desired level is maintained. Warfarin has a peak action of 9 hours. Vitamin K is the antidote for warfarin; protamine sulfate is the antidote for heparin. (D)

45. **1.** A helpless client should be positioned on the side, not on the back, with the head on a small pillow. A lateral position helps secretions escape from the throat and mouth, minimizing the risk of aspiration. It may be necessary to suction the client if he aspirates. Suction equipment should be nearby. It is safe to use a padded tongue blade, and the client should receive oral care, including brushing with a toothbrush. (R)

46. **3.** Studies show that clients who receive recombinant t-PA treatment within 3 hours after the onset of a stroke have better outcomes. The time from the onset of a stroke to t-PA treatment is critical. A complete physical and history is not possible when a client is receiving emergency care. Upcoming surgical procedures may need to be delayed because of the administration of t-PA, which is a priority in the immediate treatment of the current stroke. While the nurse should identify which medications the client is taking, it is more important to know the time of the onset to determine the course of action for administering t-PA. (D)

47. **3.** Control of blood pressure is critical during the first 24 hours after treatment because an intracerebral hemorrhage is the major adverse effect of thrombolytic therapy. Vital signs are monitored, and blood pressure is maintained as identified by the physician and specific to the client's ischemic tissue needs and risk of bleeding from treatment. The other vital signs are important, but the priority is to monitor blood pressure. (R)

48. **2.** It is crucial to monitor the pupil size and pupillary response to indicate changes around the cranial nerves. The cholesterol level is not a priority assessment, although it may be an assessment to be addressed for long-term healthy lifestyle rehabilitation. Bowel sounds need to be assessed because an ileus or constipation can develop, but this is not a priority in the first 24 hours, when the primary concerns are cerebral hemorrhage and increased intracranial pressure. An echocardiogram is not needed for the client with a thrombotic stroke without heart problems. (A)

49. **1.** It is a priority to hyperoxygenate the client before and after suctioning to prevent hypoxia and maintain cerebral perfusion. Analgesics are administered to provide pain relief. Oral hygiene provides asepsis and comfort. Diuretics help reduce intracranial pressure. (R)

50. **1.** The primary reason for the nursing assessment of a client's functional status before and after a stroke is to guide the plan. The assessment does not help to predict how far the rehabilitation team can help the client to recover from the residual effects of the stroke, only what plans can help a client who has moved from one functional level to another. The nursing assessment of the client's functional status is not a motivating factor. (A)

51. 2. Sliding a client on a sheet causes friction and is to be avoided. Friction injures skin and predisposes to pressure ulcer formation. Rolling the client is an acceptable method to use when changing positions as long as the client is maintained in anatomically neutral positions and her limbs are properly supported. The client may be lifted as long as the nurse has assistance and uses proper body mechanics to avoid injury to himself or herself or the client. Having the client help lift herself off the bed with a trapeze is an acceptable means to move a client without causing friction burns or skin breakdown. (R)

52. 3. The use of ankle-high tennis shoes has been found to be most effective in preventing plantar flexion (footdrop) because they add support to the foot and keep it in the correct anatomic position. Footboards stimulate spasms and are not routinely recommended. Regular repositioning and range-of-motion exercises are important interventions, but the client's foot needs to be in the correct anatomic position to prevent overextension of the muscle and tendon. Massaging does not prevent plantar flexion and, if rigorous, could release emboli. (R)

53. 3. When voluntary muscle control is lost, the flexor muscles, which are stronger, exert control over the extensor muscles. Folding the arms over the chest allows the flexor muscles to flex and exert control over the already weaker extensor muscles. It is better to extend the arms of the client to allow the extensor muscles to exert control over the flexor muscles and prevent contractures. Placing a pillow in the axilla so that the arm is away from the body keeps the arm abducted and prevents skin from touching skin, which leads to skin breakdown. Placing a pillow under the slightly flexed arm so that the hand is higher than the elbow prevents edema. Positioning a roll in the hand so that the fingers are barely flexed prevents the flexor muscles from overtaking the extensors. (R)

54. 2. Expressive aphasia is a condition in which the client understands what is heard or written but cannot say what he or she wants to say. A communication or picture board helps the client communicate with others in that the client can point to objects or activities that he or she desires. (A)

55. 2. A client with dysphagia (difficulty swallowing) commonly has the most difficulty ingesting thin liquids, which are easily aspirated. Liquids should be thickened to avoid aspiration. Maintaining an upright position while eating is appropriate because it minimizes the risk of aspiration. Introducing foods on the unaffected side allows the client to have better control over the food bolus. The client

should concentrate on chewing and swallowing; therefore, distractions should be avoided. (S)

56. 2. Homonymous hemianopia is blindness in half of the visual field; therefore, the client would see only half of his plate. Eating only the food on half of the plate results from an inability to coordinate visual images and spatial relationships. There may be an increased preference for foods high in salt after a stroke, but this would not be related to homonymous hemianopia. Forgetting the names of foods would be aphasia, which involves a cerebral cortex lesion. Being unable to swallow liquids is dysphagia, which involves motor pathways of cranial nerves IX and X, including the lower brain stem. (A)

57. 4. To expand the visual field, the partially sighted client should be taught to turn the head from side to side when walking. Neglecting to do so may result in accidents. This technique helps maximize the use of remaining sight. Covering an eye with a patch will limit the field of vision. Personal items can be placed within sight and reach, but most accidents occur from tripping over items that cannot be seen. It may help the client to see the door, but walking presents the primary safety hazard. (R)

58. 3. A client who has brain damage may be emotionally labile and may cry or laugh for no explainable reason. Crying is best dealt with by attempting to divert the client's attention. Ignoring the behavior will not affect the mood swing or the crying and may increase the client's sense of isolation. Telling the client to stop is inappropriate. (P)

59. 4. When offering emotional support to a client who is discouraged and has a negative self-concept because of physical handicaps, the nurse should display encouragement and patience. The client should be praised when he shows progress in his efforts to overcome handicaps. An attitude of helpfulness and sympathy allows the client to assume a role of someone not ordinary, someone who is not like others. Regardless of the handicap, the client still feels the same on the inside and has the same innate needs for his growth and developmental age-group. An attitude of concern and charity tends to make the client feel like a "charity case" or like someone who is given something free because of his "condition." The client feels unequal to his peers or unable to fulfill the role relationships that were obtained before the stroke. An attitude of directives and firmness is inappropriate because it implies that the client can do better if he just tries harder and leaves no room for softness in the approach to overcoming a negative self-concept. (P)

60. 2. The nurse should encourage the client to write messages or use alternative forms of communication to avoid frustration. Presenting one thought at a time decreases stimuli that may distract the client, as does speaking in a normal volume and tone. The nurse should ask the client to "show me" and should encourage the use of gestures to assist in getting the message across with minimal frustration and exhaustion for the client. (P)

61. 3. Thrombolytic enzyme agents are used for clients with a thrombotic stroke to dissolve emboli, thus reestablishing cerebral perfusion. They do not increase vascular permeability, cause vasoconstriction, or prevent further hemorrhage. (D)

The Client with Parkinson's Disease

62. 3, 4, 5. The nurse should contact the health care provider before administering Sinemet because this medication can cause further symptoms of depression. Suicide threats in clients with chronic illness should be taken seriously. The nurse should also determine if the client is on an MAO inhibitor because concurrent use with Sinemet can cause a hypertensive crisis. Sinemet is not a treatment for depression. Having the client discuss his feelings is appropriate when the prescription is finalized. (D)

63. 2. The first sign of Parkinson's disease is usually tremors. The client commonly is the first to notice this sign because the tremors may be minimal at first. Rigidity is the second sign, and bradykinesia is the third sign. Akinesia is a later stage of bradykinesia. (A)

64. 3. The primary focus is on maintaining a safe environment because the client with Parkinson's disease usually has a propulsive gait, characterized by a tendency to take increasingly quicker steps while walking. This type of gait commonly causes the client to fall or to have trouble stopping. The client should maintain a balanced diet, enhance the immune system, and enjoy diversional activities; however, safety is the primary concern. (R)

65. 2. Voluntary and purposeful movements often temporarily decrease or stop the tremors associated with Parkinson's disease. In some clients, however, tremors may increase with voluntary effort. Tremors associated with Parkinson's disease are not psychogenic but are related to an imbalance between dopamine and acetylcholine. Tremors cannot be reduced by distracting the client. (A)

66. 2. Demanding physical activity should be performed during the peak action of drug therapy. Clients should be encouraged to maintain independence in self-care activities to the greatest extent possible. Although some clients may have more energy in the morning or after rest, tremors are managed with drug therapy. (A)

67. 4. Helping the client function at his or her best is most appropriate and realistic. There is no known cure for Parkinson's disease. Parkinson's disease progresses in severity, and there is no known way to stop its progression. Many clients live for years with the disease, however, and it would not be appropriate to start planning terminal care at this time. (A)

68. 1. The primary goal of physical therapy and nursing interventions is to maintain joint flexibility and muscle strength. Parkinson's disease involves a degeneration of dopamine-producing neurons; therefore, it would be an unrealistic goal to attempt to build muscles or increase endurance. The decrease in dopamine neurotransmitters results in ataxia secondary to extrapyramidal motor system effects. Attempts to reduce ataxia through physical therapy would not be effective. (A)

69. 2. Levodopa is prescribed to decrease severe muscle rigidity. Levodopa does not improve mood, appetite, or alertness in a client with Parkinson's disease. (D)

70. 3. Vital signs should be monitored, especially during periods of adjustment. Changes, such as orthostatic hypotension, cardiac irregularities, palpitations, and light-headedness, should be reported immediately. The client may actually experience suicidal or paranoid ideation instead of euphoria. The nurse should monitor the client for elevated liver enzyme levels, such as lactate dehydrogenase, aspartate aminotransferase, alanine aminotransferase, blood urea nitrogen, and alkaline phosphatase, but the client should not be jaundiced. The client should not experience signs and symptoms of diabetes or a low serum glucose level, but the nurse should check the hemoglobin and hematocrit levels. (D)

71. 4. While the client is hospitalized for adjustment of medication, it is essential that the medications be administered exactly at the scheduled time, for accurate evaluation of effectiveness. For example, levodopa-carbidopa (Sinemet) is taken in divided doses over the day, not all at one time, for optimum effectiveness. (D)

72. 2. Ongoing self-care is a major focus for clients with Parkinson's disease. The client should be given additional time as needed and praised for her efforts to remain independent. Firmly telling the client that she needs assistance will undermine her self-esteem and defeat her efforts to be independent. Telling the client that her perception is unrealistic does not foster hope in her ability to care for herself. Suggesting that the client modify her routine seems to put the hospital or the nurse's time schedule before the client's needs. This will only decrease the client's self-esteem and her desire to try to continue self-care, which is obviously important to her. (P)

73. 1. The goal of a pallidotomy is to improve functional ability for the client with Parkinson's disease. This is a priority. The pallidotomy creates lesions in the globus pallidus to control extrapyramidal disorders that affect control of movement and gait. If functional ability is improved by the pallidotomy, the client may experience a secondary response of an improved emotional response, but this is not the primary goal of the surgical procedure. The procedure will not improve alertness or appetite. (C)

The Client with Multiple Sclerosis

74. 2, 3, 4, 5. Maintaining urinary function in a client with neurogenic bladder dysfunction from MS is an important goal. The client should ideally drink 400 to 500 ml with each meal; 200 ml midmorning, midafternoon, and late afternoon; and attempt to void at least every 2 hours to prevent infection and stone formation. The client may need to catheterize herself to drain residual urine in the bladder. Restricting fluids during the day will not produce sufficient urine. However, in bladder training for nighttime continence, the client may restrict fluids for 1 to 2 hours before going to bed. The client should drink at least 2,000 ml every 24 hours. (A)

75. 2. With MS, hyperexcitability and euphoria may occur, but because of muscle weakness, sudden bursts of energy are unlikely. Visual disturbances, weakness in the extremities, and loss of muscle tone and tremors are common symptoms of MS. (A)

76. 3. Baclofen is a centrally acting skeletal muscle relaxant that helps relieve the muscle spasms common in MS. Drowsiness is an adverse effect, and driving should be avoided if the medication produces a sedative effect. Baclofen does not stimulate the appetite or reduce bacteria in the urine. (D)

77. 2. Evaluating drug effectiveness is difficult because a high percentage of clients with MS exhibit unpredictable episodes of remission, exacerbation, and steady progress without apparent cause. Clients with MS do not necessarily have increased intolerance to drugs, nor do they endure long periods of exacerbation before the illness responds to a particular drug. Multiple drug use is not what makes evaluation of drug effectiveness difficult. (A)

78. 4. Asking a client to speak louder even when tired may aggravate the problem. Asking the client to speak slowly and distinctly and to repeat hard-to-understand words helps the client to communicate effectively. (P)

79. 4. The nurses' notes should be concise, objective, clearly stated, and relevant. This client trembles when she attempts voluntary actions, such as drinking a beverage or fastening clothing. This activity should be described exactly as it occurs so that others reading the note will have no doubt about the nurse's observation of the client's behavior. Identifying the "intentional" activity of daily living will help the interdisciplinary team individualize the client's

plan of care. Clarifying what is meant by "worsening" with a purposeful act will facilitate the inter-rater reliability of the team. It is better to state what the client did than to give vague nursing orders in the nurses' notes. (M)

80. 4. Limiting fluid intake is likely to aggravate rather than relieve symptoms when a bowel retraining program is being implemented. Furthermore, water imbalance, as well as electrolyte imbalance, tends to aggravate the signs and symptoms of MS. A diet high in fiber helps keep bowel movements regular. Setting a regular time each day for elimination helps train the body to maintain a schedule. Using an elevated toilet seat facilitates transfer of the client from the wheelchair to the toilet or from a standing to a sitting position. (A)

81. 3. MS is a progressive, chronic neurologic disease characterized by patchy demyelination throughout the central nervous system. This interferes with the transmission of electrical impulses from one nerve cell to the next. MS affects speech, coordination, and vision, but not cognition. Care for the client with MS is directed toward maintaining joint mobility, preventing deformities, maintaining muscle strength, rehabilitation, preventing and treating depression, and providing client motivation. (R)

82. 2. The nurse's most positive approach is to encourage a client with MS to keep active, use stress reduction strategies, and avoid fatigue because it is important to support the immune system while remaining active. A quiet, inactive lifestyle is not necessarily indicated. Good health habits are not likely to alter the course of the disease, although they may help minimize complications. Practicing using aids that will be needed for future disabilities may be helpful but also can be discouraging. (A)

83. 2. The client should not be instructed to avoid kitchen activities out of fear of injury; independence and self-care are also important. However, the client should meet with an occupational therapist to learn about assistive devices and techniques that can reduce injuries, such as burns and cuts, that are common in kitchen activities. A client with impaired peripheral sensation does not feel pain as readily as someone whose sensation is unimpaired; therefore, water temperatures should be tested carefully. The client should be advised to avoid using hot water bottles or heating pads. Because the client cannot rely on minor pain to alert him to damaged skin or sore spots, he should carefully inspect the skin daily to visualize any injuries that he cannot feel. (R)

84. 3. Maintaining a regular voiding pattern is the most appropriate measure to help the client avoid urinary incontinence. Fluid intake is not related to incontinence. Incontinence is related to the strength of the detrusor and urethral sphincter muscles. Inserting an indwelling catheter would be a treatment of last resort because of the increased risk of infection. If catheterization is required, intermittent self-catheterization is preferred because of its lower risk of infection. Antibiotics do not influence urinary incontinence. (A)

85. **2.** An individualized regular exercise program helps the client to relieve muscle spasms. The client can be trained to use unaffected muscles to promote coordination because MS is a progressive, debilitating condition. The data do not indicate that the client needs psychotherapy, day care for the granddaughter, or visits from other clients. (A)

The Unconscious Client

86. **3.** Activated charcoal powder is administered to absorb remaining particles of salicylate. Vitamin K is an antidote for warfarin sodium (Coumadin). Dextrose 50% is used to treat hypoglycemia. Sodium thiosulfate is an antidote for cyanide. (D)

87. **1, 2, 3.** When arsenic overexposure occurs, the symptoms include violent nausea, vomiting, abdominal pain, skin irritation, severe diarrhea, laryngitis, and bronchitis. Dehydration can lead to shock and death. After the acute phase, bone marrow depression, encephalopathy, and sensory neuropathy occur. A persistent cough is not a sign of arsenic exposure. (A)

88. **2, 3, 4.** An excess of cholinergic agents produce urinary and fecal incontinence, increased salivation, diarrhea, and diaphoresis. In a severe overdose, CNS depression, seizures and muscle fasciculations, bradycardia or tachycardia, weakness, and respiratory arrest due to respiratory muscle paralysis occur. Anticholinergics produce dry mucous membranes. Skin rash is not a sign of overdose with a cholinergic agent. (D)

89. **3.** The initial response to crisis is high anxiety. Anxiety must dissipate before a person can deal with the actual situation. Allowing family members to ventilate their feelings can help diffuse their anxiety. The reasons for the client's actions are unknown; assumptions must be validated before they become facts. Touch can be appropriate but not when it is used as false reassurance. Helping with the client's care is appropriate at a later time. (P)

90. **3.** Maintaining intact skin is a priority for the unconscious client. Unconscious clients need to be turned every hour to prevent complications of immobility, which include pressure ulcers and stasis pneumonia. The unconscious client cannot be educated at this time. Pain is not a concern. During the first 24 hours, the unconscious client will mostly likely be on nothing-by-mouth status. (R)

91. **2.** The nurse must clean the unconscious client's mouth carefully, apply a thin coat of petroleum jelly, and move the endotracheal tube to the opposite side daily to prevent dryness, crusting, inflammation, and parotiditis. The unconscious client's temperature should be monitored by a route other than the oral route (e.g., rectal, tympanic) because oral temperatures will be inaccurate. The client should be positioned in a lateral or semiprone position, not a supine position, to allow for drainage of secretions and for the jaw and tongue to fall forward. The client should not be dragged when turned, as may happen when a drawsheet is used. Care should be taken to lift the client's heels, buttocks, arms, and head off of the sheets when turning. Trochanter rolls, splints, foam boot aids, specialty beds, and so on—not just two pillows—should be used to keep the client in correct body position and to decrease pressure on bony prominences. (R)

92. **3.** Pressure points in the side-lying position include the ears, shoulders, ribs, greater trochanter, medial or lateral condyles, and ankles. The sacrum, occiput, and heels are pressure points in the supine position. (R)

93. **3.** The client is not in proper body alignment if, when in the right side-lying position, the client's left arm rests on the mattress with the elbow flexed. This positioning of the arm pulls the left shoulder out of good alignment, restricting respiratory movements. The arm should be supported on a pillow. The client's head also should be placed on a small pillow to keep it in alignment with the body. The right leg should be extended on the mattress without a pillow to avoid hyperrotation of the hip. A pillow should be placed between the left and right legs with the left knee flexed so that on no parts of the legs is skin touching skin. (A)

94. **4.** The goal of performing passive ROM exercises is to maintain joint mobility. Active exercise is needed to preserve bone and muscle mass. Passive ROM movements do not prevent bone demineralization or have a positive effect on the client's muscle tone. (A)

95. **1.** Maintaining a patent airway is the priority. Therefore, the nurse should keep suction equipment available to remove secretions. The client should be placed in a side-lying, not prone, position. Performing oral hygiene is a clean procedure; therefore, the nurse wears clean gloves, not sterile gloves. The nurse should never place any fingers in an unconscious client's mouth; the client may bite down. Padded tongue blades, swabs, or a toothbrush should be used instead; but maintaining the airway is the priority. (A)

96. **2.** When the blink reflex is absent or the eyes do not close completely, the cornea may become dry and irritated. Placing a patch over the completely closed eye is the most appropriate intervention to prevent eye injury. Having the client wear eyeglasses or cleaning the eyelid with a washcloth will not protect the cornea from dryness or irritation. Instilling artificial tears may be ordered to help prevent dryness and irritation; however, administration of artificial tears once per shift would be too infrequent to be of benefit. (A)

97. 3. Restlessness is an early indicator of hypoxia. The nurse should suspect hypoxia in the unconscious client who becomes restless. The most accurate method for determining the presence of hypoxia is to evaluate the pulse oximeter value or arterial blood gas values. Cyanosis and decreased respirations are late indicators of hypoxia. Hypertension, not hypotension, is a sign of hypoxia. (A)

98. 2. The client should be placed in a semi-Fowler's position to reduce the risk of aspiration. The formula should be at room temperature, not heated. Administering enteral tube feedings is a clean procedure, not a sterile one; therefore, sterile supplies are not required. Clients receiving enteral feedings should be weighed regularly, but not necessarily before each feeding. (R)

99. 4. Gastric residuals are checked before administration of enteral feedings to determine whether gastric emptying is delayed. A residual of less than 50% of the previous feeding volume is usually considered acceptable. In this case, the amount is not excessive and the nurse should reinstill the aspirate through the tube and then administer the feeding. If the amount of gastric residual is excessive, the nurse should notify the physician and withhold the feeding. Disposing of the residual can cause electrolyte and fluid losses. (R)

100. 1. Good catheter care, including meticulous cleaning of the area around the urethral meatus, is the highest priority for the client with an indwelling catheter. Clamping an indwelling catheter is not recommended. Irrigation of the catheter, which requires breaking the closed system, is not recommended. Manipulation of the catheter taped to the client's leg causes trauma to the urethral meatus, which can predispose the client to an infection and is also not recommended. (R)

101. 2, 3, 4. A client who is brain dead typically demonstrates nonreactive dilated pupils and nonreactive or absent corneal and gag reflexes. The client may still have spinal reflexes, such as deep tendon and Babinski reflexes, in brain death. Decerebrate or decorticate posturing would not be seen. Clients who are brain dead do not have a blink reflex. (A)

The Client in Pain

102. 1. Pain perception is an individual experience. Research indicates that pain tolerance and perception vary widely among individuals, even within cultures. (P)

103. 1. Experience has demonstrated that clients who feel confidence in the persons who are caring for them do not require as much therapy for pain relief as those who have less confidence. Without the client's confidence, developed in an effective nurse-client relationship, other interventions may be less effective. The client's family can be an important source of support, but it is the nurse who plans strategies for pain relief. The client may require time to adjust to the pain, but the nurse and client can collaborate to try to evaluate a variety of pain relief strategies. Arranging for the client to share a room with another client who has little pain may have negative effects on the client who has pain that is difficult to relieve. (C)

104. 3. Acupuncture, like acupressure and acumassage, is performed in certain Asian cultures to help restore the energy balance within the body. Pressure, massage, and fine needles are applied to "energy pathways" to help restore the body's balance. In the Western world, many researchers think that the gate-control theory of pain may be applicable to acupuncture, acumassage, and acupressure. The concept of evil spirits is not appropriate or relevant to the practice of acupuncture. Promoting tranquility with a higher being is not the purpose of acupuncture. Acupuncture does not block nerve pathways to the brain. (C)

105. 4. Although meperidine hydrochloride can be given orally, it is more effective when given intramuscularly. The equianalgesic dose of oral meperidine is up to four times the I.M. dose ($75 \times 4 = 300$). (D)

106. 1. Opioid analgesics relieve pain by reducing or altering the perception of pain. Meperidine hydrochloride does not decrease the sensitivity of pain receptors, interfere with pain impulses traveling along sensory nerve fibers, or block the conduction of pain impulses in the central nervous system. (D)

107. 3. According to the gate-control theory, the regulatory process that controls pain impulses reaching the brain most probably occurs in the spinal cord. (A)

108. 3. The client's innate responses to pain are directed initially toward escaping from the source of pain. Variations in tolerance and perception of pain are apparent only in conscious clients, and only conscious clients can employ distraction to help relieve pain. (A)

109. 1. Ergotamine tartrate is used to help abort a migraine attack. It should be taken as soon as prodromal symptoms appear. Reduced migraine severity and relief from sleeplessness and vision problems address symptoms that occur after the migraine has occurred and are not effects of ergotamine. (D)

110. **1.** Migraine headaches are believed to be caused by a vascular disturbance involving branches of the carotid artery, where vasoconstriction of blood vessels apparently occurs first. The extracranial and intracranial arteries then dilate, causing the headache. There is no temporary decrease in intracranial pressure. Sinusitis is not the cause of migraine headaches. Muscle contractions of the head and neck are commonly caused by stress and result in a tension headache. (A)

111. **4.** Biofeedback translates body processes into observable signs so that the client can develop some control over certain body processes. Biofeedback does not involve electrical stimulation. Use of unpleasant stimuli such as electrical shock is a form of aversion therapy. Biofeedback does not involve monitoring body processes for the therapist to interpret; rather, it is a self-directed, self-care activity that reinforces learning because the client can see the results of his actions. (P)

112. **1.** A back rub stimulates the large-diameter cutaneous fibers, which block transmission of pain impulses from the spinal cord to the brain. It does not block the transmission of pain impulses or stimulate the release of endorphins. A back rub may distract the client, but the physiologic process of fiber stimulation is the main reason a back rub is used as therapy for pain relief. (C)

113. **2.** It is essential that the nurse document the client's response to pain medication on a routine, systematic basis. Reassuring the client that pain will be relieved is often not realistic. A client who continually presses the PCA button may not be getting adequate pain relief, but through careful assessment and documentation, the effectiveness of pain relief interventions can be evaluated and modified. Pain medication is not titrated until the client is free from pain but rather until an acceptable level of pain management is reached. (D)

114. **1.** An epidural catheter is used for postoperative pain management to block the pain sensation below the point of insertion. If the client is rating pain high, the PCA pump may be malfunctioning, the catheter may have become misplaced, or the amount of medication may not be sufficient. The nurse should first check the PCA pump to determine if it is functioning properly. Assessing vital signs would be important to provide additional data about the possible cause of pain. The catheter placement, including removing the dressing or manipulating the catheter, and drug dosage are the responsibility of the physician, usually an anesthesiologist, who inserted the catheter. This person should be contacted if the PCA pump is functioning appropriately. The epidural catheter lies just above the dura of the spinal space. Infection, hypotension, and loss of mental alertness are just a few of the complications that can occur if the catheter is pushed through the dura. (D)

115. **2.** To locate the ventrogluteal site, the nurse places the palm on the client's greater trochanter for careful and correct identification to avoid tissue or nerve damage. The middle finger slides on the skin along the iliac crest while the palm is on the greater trochanter. The nurse places the index finger on the anterosuperior iliac spine. The posterior iliac spine is a landmark for locating the dorsogluteal site. (D)

116. **1.** The nurse using healing touch affects a client's pain primarily through assessing and directing the flow of energy fields. Healing touch can involve touching, but it does not have to involve body contact. Massage and hypnosis are not parts of healing touch. (A)

117. **1.** The deltoid muscle is small and is not used for injections greater than 1 ml. The muscle is easy to locate. It does not have excessive pain receptors. The deltoid muscle does have a good blood supply, just as the other muscles in the body have. (D)

The Client with Musculoskeletal Health Problems

- The Client with Rheumatoid Arthritis
- The Client with Osteoarthritis
- The Client with a Hip Fracture
- The Client with a Herniated Disk
- The Client with an Amputation due to Peripheral Vascular Disease
- The Client with Fractures
- The Client with a Femoral Fracture
- The Client with a Spinal Cord Injury
- Correct Answers and Rationales

The Client with Rheumatoid Arthritis

1. On a visit to the clinic, a client reports the onset of early symptoms of rheumatoid arthritis. Which of the following would the nurse *most* likely assess?
- ☐ **1.** Limited motion of joints.
- ☐ **2.** Deformed joints of the hands.
- ☐ **3.** Early morning stiffness.
- ☐ **4.** Rheumatoid nodules.

2. A client with rheumatoid arthritis states, "I can't do my household chores without becoming tired. My knees hurt whenever I walk. Which nursing diagnosis would be most appropriate?
- ☐ **1.** *Activity intolerance* related to fatigue and pain.
- ☐ **2.** *Self-care deficit* related to increasing joint pain.
- ☐ **3.** *Ineffective coping* related to chronic pain.
- ☐ **4.** *Disturbed body image* related to fatigue and joint pain.

3. After teaching the client about risk factors for rheumatoid arthritis, which of the following, if stated by the client as a risk factor, would indicate that the client needs additional teaching?
- ☐ **1.** History of Epstein-Barr virus infection.
- ☐ **2.** Female gender.
- ☐ **3.** Adults between the ages of 60 and 75.
- ☐ **4.** Positive testing for human leukocyte antigen (HLA)-DR4 allele.

4. A client is in the acute phase of rheumatoid arthritis. Which of the following should the nurse identify as lowest priority in the plan of care?
- ☐ **1.** Relieving pain.
- ☐ **2.** Preserving joint function.
- ☐ **3.** Maintaining usual ways of accomplishing tasks.
- ☐ **4.** Preventing joint deformity.

5. The nurse teaches a client about heat and cold treatments to manage arthritis pain. Which of the following client statements indicates that the client still has a knowledge deficit?
- ☐ **1.** "I can use heat and cold as often as I want."
- ☐ **2.** "With heat, I should apply it for no longer than 20 minutes at a time."
- ☐ **3.** "Heat-producing liniments can be used with other heat devices."
- ☐ **4.** "Ten to 15 minutes per application is the maximum time for cold applications."

6. The client with rheumatoid arthritis tells the nurse, "I have a friend who took gold shots and had a wonderful response. Why didn't my physician let me try that?" Which of the following responses by the nurse would be *most* appropriate?
- ☐ **1.** "It's the physician's prerogative to decide how to treat you. The physician has chosen what is best for your situation."
- ☐ **2.** "Tell me more about your friend's arthritic condition. Maybe I can answer that question for you."
- ☐ **3.** "That drug is used for cases that are worse than yours. It wouldn't help you, so don't worry about it."
- ☐ **4.** "Every person is different. What works for one client may not always be effective for another."

7. The teaching plan for the client with rheumatoid arthritis includes rest promotion. Which of the following would the nurse expect to instruct the client to avoid during rest periods?
- ☐ **1.** Proper body alignment.
- ☐ **2.** Elevating the part.
- ☐ **3.** Prone lying positions.
- ☐ **4.** Positions of flexion.

8. After teaching the client with rheumatoid arthritis about measures to conserve energy in activities of daily living involving the small joints, which of the following, if stated by the client, would indicate the need for additional teaching?

- ☐ 1. Pushing with palms when rising from a chair.
- ☐ 2. Holding packages close to the body.
- ☐ 3. Sliding objects.
- ☐ 4. Carrying a laundry basket with clinched fingers and fists.

9. After teaching the client with severe rheumatoid arthritis about prescribed methotrexate (Rheumatrex), which of the following statements indicates the need for further teaching?

- ☐ 1. "I will take my vitamins while I'm on this drug."
- ☐ 2. "I must not drink any alcohol while I'm taking this drug."
- ☐ 3. "I should brush my teeth after every meal."
- ☐ 4. "I will continue taking my birth control pills."

10. A 25-year-old client taking hydroxychloroquine (Plaquenil) for rheumatoid arthritis reports difficulty seeing out of her left eye. Correct interpretation of this assessment finding indicates which of the following?

- ☐ 1. Development of a cataract.
- ☐ 2. Possible retinal degeneration.
- ☐ 3. Part of the disease process.
- ☐ 4. A coincidental occurrence.

11. Postoperatively, a client's right leg is placed in a continuous passive motion (CPM) device. Which of the following should the nurse perform when caring for a client receiving CPM therapy?

- ☐ 1. Adjusting the settings as needed to prevent client discomfort.
- ☐ 2. Increasing the range-of-motion settings at least every 8 hours.
- ☐ 3. Maintaining proper positioning of the joint on the CPM machine.
- ☐ 4. Discontinuing the CPM therapy when range of motion increases to 90 degrees.

12. A client with rheumatoid arthritis tells the nurse, "I know it is important to exercise my joints so that I won't lose mobility, but my joints are so stiff and painful that exercising is difficult." Which of the following responses by the nurse would be most appropriate?

- ☐ 1. "You are probably exercising too much. Decrease your exercise to every other day."
- ☐ 2. "Tell the physician about your symptoms. Maybe your analgesic medication can be increased."
- ☐ 3. "Stiffness and pain are part of the disease. Learn to cope by focusing on activities you enjoy."
- ☐ 4. "Take a warm tub bath or shower before exercising. This may help with your discomfort."

13. Which of the following statements should the nurse include in the teaching session when preparing a client for arthrocentesis? Select all that apply.

- ☐ 1. "A local anesthetic agent may be injected into the joint site for your comfort."
- ☐ 2. "A syringe and needle will be used to withdraw fluid from your joint."
- ☐ 3. "The procedure, although not painful, will provide immediate relief."
- ☐ 4. "We'll want you to keep your joint active after the procedure to increase blood flow."
- ☐ 5. "You will need to wear a compression bandage for several days after the procedure."

The Client with Osteoarthritis

14. A client with osteoarthritis will undergo an arthrocentesis on his painful edematous knee. What should be included in the nursing plan of care? Select all that apply.

- ☐ 1. Explain the procedure.
- ☐ 2. Administer preoperative medication 1 hour before surgery.
- ☐ 3. Instruct the client to immobilize the knee for 2 days after the surgery.
- ☐ 4. Assess the site for bleeding.
- ☐ 5. Offer pain medication.

15. A postmenopausal client is scheduled for a bone-density scan. To plan for the client's test, what should the nurse communicate to the client?

- ☐ 1. Request that the client remove all metal objects on the day of the scan.
- ☐ 2. Instruct the client to consume foods and beverages with a high content of calcium for 2 days before the test.
- ☐ 3. Inform the client that she will need to ingest 600 mg of calcium gluconate by mouth for 2 weeks before the test.
- ☐ 4. Tell the client that she should report any significant pain to her physician at least 2 days before the test.

16. A physician orders a lengthy X-ray examination for a client with osteoarthritis. Which of the following actions by the nurse would demonstrate client advocacy?

- ☐ 1. Contact the X-ray department and ask the technician if the lengthy session can be divided into shorter sessions.
- ☐ 2. Contact the physician to determine if an alternative examination could be scheduled.
- ☐ 3. Provide a dose of acetaminophen (Tylenol).
- ☐ 4. Cancel the examination because of the hard X-ray table.

17. Which of the following should the nurse assess when completing the history and physical examination of a client diagnosed with osteoarthritis?
- ☐ 1. Anemia.
- ☐ 2. Osteoporosis.
- ☐ 3. Weight loss.
- ☐ 4. Local joint pain.

18. A client with osteoporosis needs education about diet and ways to increase bone density. Which of the following should be included in the teaching plan? Select all that apply.
- ☐ 1. Maintain a diet with adequate amounts of vitamin D, as found in fortified milk and cereals.
- ☐ 2. Choose good calcium sources, such as figs, broccoli, and almonds.
- ☐ 3. Use alcohol in moderation because a moderate intake has no known negative effects.
- ☐ 4. Try swimming as a good exercise to maintain bone mass.
- ☐ 5. Avoid the use of high-fat foods, such as avocados, salad dressings, and fried foods.

19. Which of the following statements indicates that the client with osteoarthritis understands the effects of capsaicin (Zostrix) cream?
- ☐ 1. "I always wash my hands right after I apply the cream."
- ☐ 2. "After I apply the cream, I wrap my knee with an elastic bandage."
- ☐ 3. "I keep the cream in the cabinet above the stove in the kitchen."
- ☐ 4. "I also use the same cream when I get a cut or a burn."

20. At which of the following times should the nurse instruct the client to take ibuprofen (Motrin), prescribed for left hip pain secondary to osteoarthritis, to minimize gastric mucosal irritation?
- ☐ 1. At bedtime.
- ☐ 2. On arising.
- ☐ 3. Immediately after a meal.
- ☐ 4. On an empty stomach.

21. When preparing a teaching plan for the client with osteoarthritis who is taking celecoxib (Celebrex), the nurse expects to explain that the major advantage of celecoxib over diclofenac (Voltaren) is that celecoxib is less likely to produce which of the following?
- ☐ 1. Hepatotoxicity.
- ☐ 2. Renal toxicity.
- ☐ 3. Gastrointestinal bleeding.
- ☐ 4. Nausea and vomiting.

22. The client diagnosed with osteoarthritis states, "My friend takes steroid pills for her rheumatoid arthritis. Why don't I take steroids for my osteoarthritis?" Which of the following is the best explanation?
- ☐ 1. Intra-articular corticosteroid injections are used to treat osteoarthritis.
- ☐ 2. Oral corticosteroids can be used in osteoarthritis.
- ☐ 3. A systemic effect is needed in osteoarthritis.
- ☐ 4. Rheumatoid arthritis and osteoarthritis are two similar diseases.

23. After teaching a group of clients with osteoarthritis about using regular exercise, which of the following client statements indicates effective teaching?
- ☐ 1. "Performing range-of-motion exercises will increase my joint mobility."
- ☐ 2. "Exercise helps to drive synovial fluid through the cartilage."
- ☐ 3. "Joint swelling should determine when to stop exercising."
- ☐ 4. "Exercising in the outdoors year-round promotes joint relaxation."

24. In preparation for total knee surgery, a 200-lb client with osteoarthritis must lose weight. Which of the following exercises should the nurse recommend as best if the client has no contraindications?
- ☐ 1. Weight lifting.
- ☐ 2. Walking.
- ☐ 3. Aquatic exercise.
- ☐ 4. Tai chi exercise.

25. A client needs preoperative teaching for a total hip replacement. With which intervention should the nurse initiate the teaching?
- ☐ 1. Teaching how to prevent hip flexion.
- ☐ 2. Demonstrating coughing and deep-breathing techniques.
- ☐ 3. Showing the client what an actual hip prosthesis looks like.
- ☐ 4. Assessing the client's fears about the procedure.

26. The client has just had a total knee replacement for severe osteoarthritis. Which of the following assessment findings should lead the nurse to suspect possible nerve damage?
- ☐ 1. Numbness.
- ☐ 2. Bleeding.
- ☐ 3. Dislocation.
- ☐ 4. Pinkness.

27. After surgery and insertion of a total joint prosthesis, a client develops severe sudden pain and an inability to move the extremity. The nurse correctly interprets these findings as indicating which of the following?
- ☐ 1. A developing infection.
- ☐ 2. Bleeding in the operative site.
- ☐ 3. Joint dislocation.
- ☐ 4. Glue seepage into soft tissue.

The Client with a Hip Fracture

28. A client in a double hip spica cast complains of being constipated. She has not had a bowel movement for the past 4 days. The surgeon cuts a window into the cast. Which of the following outcomes should the nurse anticipate?
- [ ] 1. The window will allow the nurse to palpate the superior mesenteric artery.
- [ ] 2. The window will allow the surgeon to manipulate the fracture site.
- [ ] 3. The window will allow the nurses to reposition the client.
- [ ] 4. The window will provide some relief from pressure due to abdominal distention as a result of constipation.

29. Which of the following would the nurse assess in a client with an intracapsular hip fracture?
- [ ] 1. Internal rotation.
- [ ] 2. Muscle flaccidity.
- [ ] 3. Shortening of the affected leg.
- [ ] 4. Absence of pain in the fracture area.

30. The nurse is developing the plan of care for an older adult client with a hip fracture. Which of the following chronic health problems would the nurse be least likely to assess in the client?
- [ ] 1. Hypertension.
- [ ] 2. Cardiac decompensation.
- [ ] 3. Pulmonary disease.
- [ ] 4. Multiple sclerosis.

31. When teaching a client with an extracapsular hip fracture scheduled for surgical internal fixation with the insertion of a pin, the nurse bases the teaching on the understanding that this surgical repair is the treatment of choice. Which of the following explains the reason?
- [ ] 1. Hemorrhage at the fracture site is prevented.
- [ ] 2. Neurovascular impairment risk is decreased.
- [ ] 3. The risk of infection at the site is lessened.
- [ ] 4. The client is able to be mobilized sooner.

32. A client with an extracapsular hip fracture returns to the nursing unit after internal fixation and pin insertion with a drainage tube at the incision site. Her husband asks, "Why does she have this tube inserted in her hip?" Which of the following responses would be best?
- [ ] 1. "The tube helps us to detect a wound infection early on."
- [ ] 2. "This way we won't have to irrigate the wound."
- [ ] 3. "Fluid won't be allowed to accumulate at the site."
- [ ] 4. "We have a way to administer antibiotics into the wound."

33. A client had a posterolateral total hip replacement 2 days ago. What should the nurse include in the client's plan of care? Select all that apply.
- [ ] 1. When using a walker, encourage the client to point the toes inward.
- [ ] 2. Position a pillow between the legs to maintain abduction.
- [ ] 3. Allow the client to be in the supine position or in the lateral position on the unoperated side.
- [ ] 4. Do not allow the client to bend down to tie or slip on shoes.
- [ ] 5. Place ice on the incision after physical therapy.

34. Which information should the nurse include when performing discharge teaching with a client who had an anterolateral approach for a total hip replacement? Select all that apply.
- [ ] 1. Avoid turning the toes or knee outward.
- [ ] 2. Use an abduction pillow between the legs when in bed.
- [ ] 3. Use an elevated toilet seat and shower chair.
- [ ] 4. Do not extend the operative leg backwards.
- [ ] 5. Restrict motion for 2 weeks after surgery.

35. The nurse is assessing a client for neurologic impairment after a total hip replacement. Which of the following would indicate impairment in the affected extremity?
- [ ] 1. Decreased distal pulse.
- [ ] 2. Inability to move.
- [ ] 3. Diminished capillary refill.
- [ ] 4. Coolness to the touch.

36. A client with a hip fracture has undergone surgery for insertion of a femoral head prosthesis. Which of the following activities should the nurse instruct the client to avoid?
- [ ] 1. Crossing the legs while sitting down.
- [ ] 2. Sitting on a raised commode seat.
- [ ] 3. Using an abductor splint while lying on the side.
- [ ] 4. Rising straight from a chair to a standing position.

37. The nurse advises the client who has had a femoral head prosthesis placement on the type of chair to sit in during the first 6 to 8 weeks after surgery. Which would be the correct type to recommend?
- [ ] 1. A desk-type swivel chair.
- [ ] 2. A padded upholstered chair.
- [ ] 3. A high-backed chair with armrests.
- [ ] 4. A recliner with an attached footrest.

38. The nurse is assessing the home environment of an elderly client who is using crutches during the postoperative recovery phase after hip pinning. Which of the following would pose the greatest hazard to the client as a risk for falling at home?
- [ ] 1. A 4-year-old cocker spaniel.
- [ ] 2. Scatter rugs.
- [ ] 3. Snack tables.
- [ ] 4. Rocking chairs.

The Client with a Herniated Disk

39. The nurse is observing a client who is recovering from back strain lift a box as shown below. What should the nurse do?
- [ ] 1. Praise the client for using correct body mechanics.
- [ ] 2. Suggest to the client that she put both knees on the floor before attempting to lift the box.
- [ ] 3. Advise the client to bend from the waist rather than stretching her back in this position.
- [ ] 4. Inform the client that she should keep her back straight by squatting with both knees parallel.

40. Which of the following activities should the nurse instruct the client with low back pain to avoid?
- [ ] 1. Keeping light objects below the level of the elbows when lifting.
- [ ] 2. Leaning forward while bending the knees.
- [ ] 3. Exceeding the prescribed exercise program.
- [ ] 4. Sleeping on the side with legs flexed.

41. A client is unable to get out of bed because of low back pain radiating down to his right heel and lateral foot. Which of the following categories of medication should the nurse anticipate that the physician will order?
- [ ] 1. Angiotensin-converting enzyme (ACE) inhibitors.
- [ ] 2. Beta-adrenergic blocking agents.
- [ ] 3. Nonsteroidal anti-inflammatory drugs (NSAIDs).
- [ ] 4. Barbiturates.

42. A client with a ruptured intervertebral disc at L4–5 stands with a flattened spine slightly tilted forward and slightly flexed to the affected side. The nurse interprets this finding as indicating which of the following?
- [ ] 1. Motor changes.
- [ ] 2. Postural deformity.
- [ ] 3. Alteration of reflexes.
- [ ] 4. Sensory changes.

43. Which of the following positions would be most comfortable for a client with a ruptured disc at L5–S1 right?
- [ ] 1. Prone.
- [ ] 2. Supine with the legs flexed.
- [ ] 3. High Fowler's.
- [ ] 4. Right Sims.

44. The client with a herniated intervertebral disc scheduled for a myelogram asks the nurse about the procedure. The nurse explains that radiographs will be taken of the client's spine after an injection of which of the following?
- [ ] 1. Sterile water.
- [ ] 2. Normal saline solution.
- [ ] 3. Liquid nitrogen.
- [ ] 4. Radiopaque dye.

45. Which of the following would be inappropriate to include when preparing a client for magnetic resonance imaging (MRI) to evaluate a ruptured disc?
- [ ] 1. Informing the client that the procedure is painless.
- [ ] 2. Taking a thorough history of past surgeries.
- [ ] 3. Checking for previous complaints of claustrophobia.
- [ ] 4. Starting an I.V. line at keep-open rate.

46. A client complaining of numbness from the back of his left buttock to the dorsum of his foot and big toe is scheduled to undergo a laminectomy. The operative consent form states, "a left lumbar laminectomy of L3–4." Which of the following should the nurse do next?
- [ ] 1. Have the client sign the consent form.
- [ ] 2. Call the surgeon.
- [ ] 3. Change the consent form.
- [ ] 4. Review the client's history.

47. Which of the following is a priority nursing diagnosis after a bilateral lumbar laminectomy at L5–S1?
- [ ] 1. *Impaired physical mobility* related to back pain.
- [ ] 2. *Imbalanced nutrition: Less than body requirements* related to postoperative status.
- [ ] 3. *Bowel incontinence* related to decreased physical activity.
- [ ] 4. *Disturbed body image* related to fear of disfiguring surgical scar.

48. Immediately after a lumbar laminectomy, the nurse administers ondansetron hydrochloride (Zofran) to the client as ordered. The nurse determines that the drug is effective when which of the following is controlled?
- [ ] 1. Muscle spasms.
- [ ] 2. Nausea.
- [ ] 3. Shivering.
- [ ] 4. Dry mouth.

49. After a laminectomy, the client states, "The physician said that I can do anything I want to." Which of the following client-stated activities indicates the need for further teaching?
☐ **1.** Drying the dishes.
☐ **2.** Sitting outside on firm cushions.
☐ **3.** Making the bed walking from side to side.
☐ **4.** Sweeping the front porch.

50. The nurse is developing the discharge teaching plan for a client after a lumbar laminectomy L4–5 who will be returning to work in 6 weeks. Which of the following actions should the nurse encourage the client to avoid?
☐ **1.** Placing one foot on a stepstool during prolonged standing.
☐ **2.** Sleeping on the back with support under the knees.
☐ **3.** Maintaining average body weight for height.
☐ **4.** Sitting whenever possible.

51. A male client, who had normal preoperative baseline data except for dysfunction associated with his operative diagnosis, underwent a spinal fusion yesterday. Which of the following nursing assessments should alert the nurse to the development of a possible complication?
☐ **1.** Lateral rotation of the head and neck.
☐ **2.** Clear yellowish fluid on the dressing.
☐ **3.** Use of the standing position to void.
☐ **4.** Nonproductive cough.

52. After a spinal fusion, a client is required to wear a back brace. Which of the following should the nurse expect to do before applying the brace?
☐ **1.** Have the client in bed lying on the side.
☐ **2.** Verify with the physician the position to use.
☐ **3.** Ask the client to stand with arms held out to the side.
☐ **4.** Encourage the client to sit in a straight chair.

53. After the nurse teaches a client about wearing a back brace after a spinal fusion, which of the following client statements indicates effective teaching?
☐ **1.** "I will apply lotion before putting on the brace."
☐ **2.** "I will be sure to pad the area around my iliac crest."
☐ **3.** "I can use baby powder under the brace to absorb perspiration."
☐ **4.** "I should wear a thin cotton undershirt under the brace."

54. The nurse develops a teaching plan for a client scheduled for a spinal fusion. Which of the following should the nurse expect to include?
☐ **1.** The client typically experiences more pain at the donor site than at the fusion site.
☐ **2.** The surgeon will apply a simple gauze dressing to the donor site.
☐ **3.** Neurovascular checks are unnecessary if the fibula is the donor site.
☐ **4.** The client's level of activity restriction is determined by the amount of pain.

55. A client who has had a lumbar laminectomy with a spinal fusion is sitting in a chair. In which position are his feet if he is complying with his postoperative instructions?
☐ **1.** On the floor with the feet flat.
☐ **2.** On a low footstool.
☐ **3.** In any comfortable position with legs uncrossed.
☐ **4.** On a high footstool so the feet are level with the chair seat.

56. The nurse develops a plan of care for a client in the initial postoperative period following a lumbar laminectomy. Which of the following activities is contraindicated?
☐ **1.** Assisting with her daily hygiene activities.
☐ **2.** Lying flat in bed.
☐ **3.** Walking in the hall.
☐ **4.** Sitting all afternoon in her room.

57. Which of the following exercises should the nurse advise the client to avoid after a lumbar laminectomy?
☐ **1.** Knee-to-chest lifts.
☐ **2.** Hip tilts.
☐ **3.** Sit-ups.
☐ **4.** Pelvic tilts.

The Client with an Amputation due to Peripheral Vascular Disease

58. Which of the following should the nurse identify as the least likely factor contributing to a client's peripheral vascular disease?
☐ **1.** Uncontrolled diabetes mellitus for 15 years.
☐ **2.** A 20-pack-year history of cigarette smoking.
☐ **3.** Current age of 39 years.
☐ **4.** A serum cholesterol concentration of 275 mg/dl.

59. A client has severe arterial occlusive disease and gangrene of the left great toe. Which of the following findings should the nurse expect to assess in the client's left leg and foot?
☐ **1.** Edema around the ankle.
☐ **2.** Loss of hair on the lower leg.
☐ **3.** Thin, soft toenails.
☐ **4.** Warmth in the foot.

60. A client with absent peripheral pulses and pain at rest is scheduled for an arterial Doppler study of the affected extremity. Which of the following should the nurse include when preparing the client for this test?
☐ **1.** Have the client sign a consent form for the procedure.
☐ **2.** Administer a pretest sedative as appropriate.
☐ **3.** Keep the client tobacco-free for 30 minutes before the test.
☐ **4.** Wrap the client's affected foot with a blanket.

61. The client with peripheral arterial disease says, "I've really tried to manage my condition well." Which of the following should the nurse determine as appropriate for this client?
☐ **1.** Resting with the legs elevated above the level of the heart.
☐ **2.** Walking slowly but steadily for 30 minutes twice a day.
☐ **3.** Minimizing activity as much and as often as possible.
☐ **4.** Wearing antiembolism stockings at all times when out of bed.

62. Which of the following should the nurse include in the teaching plan for a client with arterial insufficiency to the feet that is being managed conservatively?
☐ **1.** Daily lubrication of the feet.
☐ **2.** Soaking the feet in warm water.
☐ **3.** Applying antiembolism stockings.
☐ **4.** Wearing firm, supportive leather shoes.

63. A client says, "I hate the idea of being an invalid after they cut off my leg." Which of the following would be the nurse's most therapeutic response?
☐ **1.** "At least you will still have one good leg to use."
☐ **2.** "Tell me more about how you're feeling."
☐ **3.** "Let's finish the preoperative teaching."
☐ **4.** "You're lucky to have a wife to care for you."

64. The client asks the nurse, "Why can't the physician tell me exactly how much of my leg he's going to take off? Don't you think I should know that?" On which of the following should the nurse base the response?
☐ **1.** The need to remove as much of the leg as possible.
☐ **2.** The adequacy of the blood supply to the tissues.
☐ **3.** The ease with which a prosthesis can be fitted.
☐ **4.** The client's ability to walk with a prosthesis.

65. A client who has had an above-the-knee amputation develops a dime-sized bright red spot on the dressing after 45 minutes in the postanesthesia recovery unit. Which of the following actions would be most appropriate?
☐ **1.** Elevating the stump.
☐ **2.** Reinforcing the dressing.
☐ **3.** Calling the surgeon.
☐ **4.** Drawing a mark around the site.

66. A client in the postanesthesia care unit with a left below-the-knee amputation complains of pain in her left big toe. Which of the following should the nurse do first?
☐ **1.** Tell the client it is impossible to feel the pain.
☐ **2.** Show the client that the toes are not there.
☐ **3.** Explain to the client that her pain is real.
☐ **4.** Give the client the prescribed opioid analgesic.

67. The client with an above-the-knee amputation is to use crutches while his prosthesis is being adjusted. In which of the following exercises should the nurse instruct the client to best prepare him for using crutches?
☐ **1.** Abdominal exercises.
☐ **2.** Isometric shoulder exercises.
☐ **3.** Quadriceps setting exercises.
☐ **4.** Triceps stretching exercises.

68. The nurse teaches a client about using the crutches, instructing the client to support her weight primarily on which of the following body areas?
☐ **1.** Axillae.
☐ **2.** Elbows.
☐ **3.** Upper arms.
☐ **4.** Hands.

69. The client is to be discharged on a low-fat, low-cholesterol, low-sodium diet. Which of the following should be the nurse's first step in planning the dietary instructions?
☐ **1.** Determining the client's knowledge level about cholesterol.
☐ **2.** Asking the client to name foods that are high in fat, cholesterol, and salt.
☐ **3.** Explaining the importance of complying with the diet.
☐ **4.** Assessing the client's and family's typical food preferences.

The Client with Fractures

70. A client has a leg immobilized in traction. Which of the following activities demonstrated by the client would assist with preventing muscle atrophy?
☐ **1.** The client adducts the affected leg every 2 hours.
☐ **2.** The client rolls the affected leg away from the body's midline twice per day.
☐ **3.** The client performs isometric exercises to the affected extremity three times per day.
☐ **4.** The client asks the nurse to add a 5-lb weight to the traction for 30 minutes per day.

71. Three hours ago a client was thrown from a car into a ditch, and he is now admitted to the emergency department in a stable condition with vital signs within normal limits, alert and oriented with good coloring and an open fracture of the right tibia. For which signs and symptoms should the nurse be especially alert?
☐ **1.** Hemorrhage.
☐ **2.** Infection.
☐ **3.** Deformity.
☐ **4.** Shock.

72. The client with a fractured tibia has been taking methocarbamol (Robaxin). Which of the following should the nurse identify as the drug's primary effect?
- ☐ **1.** Killing of microorganisms.
- ☐ **2.** Reduction in itching.
- ☐ **3.** Relief of muscle spasms.
- ☐ **4.** Decrease in nervousness.

73. When developing a teaching plan for a client who is prescribed acetaminophen (Tylenol) for muscle pain, which information should the nurse expect to include? Select all that apply.
- ☐ **1.** The drug can be used if the person is allergic to aspirin.
- ☐ **2.** Acetaminophen does not affect platelet aggregation.
- ☐ **3.** This drug causes little or no gastric distress.
- ☐ **4.** Acetaminophen exerts a strong anti-inflammatory effect.
- ☐ **5.** The client should have the International Normalized Ratio (INR) checked regularly.

74. A client who has been taking carisoprodol (Soma) at home for a fractured arm is admitted with a blood pressure of 80/50 mg Hg, a pulse rate of 115 bpm, and respirations of 8 breaths/minute and shallow. The nurse correctly interprets these findings as indicating which of the following?
- ☐ **1.** Expected common adverse effects.
- ☐ **2.** Hypersensitivity reaction.
- ☐ **3.** Possible habituating effect.
- ☐ **4.** Hemorrhage from gastrointestinal irritation.

75. When admitting a client with a fractured extremity, the nurse should first focus the assessment on which of the following?
- ☐ **1.** The area proximal to the fracture.
- ☐ **2.** The actual fracture site.
- ☐ **3.** The area distal to the fracture.
- ☐ **4.** The opposite extremity for baseline comparison.

76. Which of the following client statements identifies a knowledge deficit about cast care?
- ☐ **1.** "I'll elevate the cast above my heart initially."
- ☐ **2.** "I'll exercise my joints above and below the cast."
- ☐ **3.** "I can pull out cast padding to scratch inside the cast."
- ☐ **4.** "I'll apply ice for 10 minutes to control edema for the first 24 hours."

77. Which of the following interventions would be least appropriate for a client who is in a double hip spica cast?
- ☐ **1.** Encouraging the intake of cranberry juice.
- ☐ **2.** Advising the client to eat large amounts of cheese.
- ☐ **3.** Establishing regular times for elimination.
- ☐ **4.** Having the client dangle at the bedside.

78. The nurse prepares a teaching plan for a client about crutch walking using a two-point gait pattern. Which of the following should the nurse include?
- ☐ **1.** Advance a crutch on one side and then advance the opposite foot; repeat on the opposite side.
- ☐ **2.** Advance a crutch on one side and simultaneously advance and bear weight on the opposite foot; repeat on the opposite side.
- ☐ **3.** Advance both crutches together and then follow by lifting both lower extremities to the level of the crutches.
- ☐ **4.** Advance both crutches together and then follow by lifting both lower extremities past the level of the crutches.

79. A client returned from surgery with a debrided open tibial fracture and a three-way drainage system. Which of the following should the nurse expect to assess?
- ☐ **1.** Results of culture and sensitivity testing of the wound.
- ☐ **2.** Presence of a pressure dressing over the wound.
- ☐ **3.** Complaints of increased pain from exposed nerve endings.
- ☐ **4.** Hypotension resulting from additional vessel bleeding.

80. A client who crashed her motorcycle suffered a tibial fracture that required casting. Approximately 5 hours later, the client begins to complain of increasing pain distal to the left tibial fracture despite the morphine injection administered 30 minutes previously. Which of the following should be the nurse's next assessment?
- ☐ **1.** Presence of a distal pulse.
- ☐ **2.** Pain with a pain rating scale.
- ☐ **3.** Vital sign changes.
- ☐ **4.** Potential for drug tolerance.

81. A client with a fracture develops compartment syndrome. Which of the following signs should alert the nurse to impending organ failure?
- ☐ **1.** Crackles.
- ☐ **2.** Jaundice.
- ☐ **3.** Generalized edema.
- ☐ **4.** Dark, scanty urine.

The Client with a Femoral Fracture

82. A client with a fractured right femur has not had any immunizations since childhood. Which of the following biologic products should the nurse administer to provide the client with passive immunity for tetanus?
- ☐ **1.** Tetanus toxoid.
- ☐ **2.** Tetanus antigen.
- ☐ **3.** Tetanus vaccine.
- ☐ **4.** Tetanus antitoxin.

83. After teaching the client with a femoral fracture about treatment with skeletal traction, which of the following, if stated by the client as a purpose, would indicate the need for additional teaching?
- ☐ **1.** To align injured bones.
- ☐ **2.** To provide long-term pull.
- ☐ **3.** To apply 25 lb of traction.
- ☐ **4.** To pull weight with a boot.

84. The nurse is planning care for the client with a femoral fracture who is in balanced suspension traction. Which of the following would the nurse be least likely to include in the plan of care?
- ☐ **1.** Use of a fracture bedpan.
- ☐ **2.** Checks for redness over the ischial tuberosity.
- ☐ **3.** Elevation of the head of bed no more than 25 degrees.
- ☐ **4.** Personal hygiene with a complete bed bath.

85. A client is in balanced suspension traction using a half-ring Thomas splint with a Pearson attachment that suspends the lower extremity and applies direct skeletal traction for a hip fracture. Which of the following nursing assessments would be inappropriate?
- ☐ **1.** Greater trochanter skin checks.
- ☐ **2.** Pin site inspection.
- ☐ **3.** Neurovascular checks proximal to the splint.
- ☐ **4.** Foot movement evaluation.

86. The client in balanced suspension traction is transported to surgery for closed reduction and internal fixation of his fractured femur. Which of the following should the nurse complete when transporting the client to the operating room?
- ☐ **1.** Transfer the client to a cart with manually suspended traction.
- ☐ **2.** Call the surgeon to request an order for temporarily removing the traction.
- ☐ **3.** Send the client on his bed with extra help to stabilize the traction.
- ☐ **4.** Remove the traction and send the client on a cart.

87. A client has a Pearson attachment on the traction setup. Which of the following is the purpose of this attachment?
- ☐ **1.** To support the lower portion of the leg.
- ☐ **2.** To support the thigh and upper leg.
- ☐ **3.** To allow attachment of the skeletal pin.
- ☐ **4.** To prevent flexion deformities in the ankle and foot.

88. Which of the following should lead the nurse to suspect that a client with a fracture of the right femur may be developing a fat embolus?
- ☐ **1.** Acute respiratory distress syndrome.
- ☐ **2.** Migraine-like headaches.
- ☐ **3.** Numbness in the right leg.
- ☐ **4.** Muscle spasms in the right thigh.

89. The client with a fractured femur is upset and agitated about her injury and its treatment. She says, "How can I stay like this for weeks? I can't even move!" Which of the following is the most appropriate nursing diagnosis?
- ☐ **1.** *Impaired physical mobility* related to traction.
- ☐ **2.** *Ineffective coping* related to prolonged immobility.
- ☐ **3.** *Deficient diversional activity* related to prolonged hospitalization.
- ☐ **4.** *Activity intolerance* related to impaired mobility.

90. The client asks the nurse what his activity limitations are while he is in Buck's traction. Which of the following responses by the nurse would be most appropriate?
- ☐ **1.** "You can sit up whenever you want."
- ☐ **2.** "You must lie flat on your back most of the time."
- ☐ **3.** "You can turn your body."
- ☐ **4.** "You must lie on your stomach."

91. Because a client has a Thomas splint, the nurse would need to assess the client regularly for which of the following?
- ☐ **1.** Signs of skin pressure in the groin area.
- ☐ **2.** Evidence of decreased breath sounds.
- ☐ **3.** Skin breakdown behind the heel.
- ☐ **4.** Urine retention.

92. The client has a nursing diagnosis of *Self-care deficit* related to the confinement of traction. Which of the following would indicate a successful outcome for this diagnosis?
- ☐ **1.** The client assists as much as possible in his care, demonstrating increased participation over time.
- ☐ **2.** The client allows the nurse to complete his care in an efficient manner without interfering.
- ☐ **3.** The client allows his wife to assume total responsibility for his care.
- ☐ **4.** The client allows his wife to complete his care to promote feelings of usefulness.

93. The client who had an open femoral fracture was discharged to her home where she developed fever, night sweats, chills, restlessness, and restrictive movement of the fractured leg. Which of the following reflects the best interpretation of these findings?
- ☐ **1.** Pulmonary emboli.
- ☐ **2.** Osteomyelitis.
- ☐ **3.** Fat emboli.
- ☐ **4.** Urinary tract infection.

94. Antibiotics are not producing the desired outcome for a client with osteomyelitis. Which of the following is the most likely interpretation?
- ☐ **1.** Formation of scar tissue interfering with absorption.
- ☐ **2.** Development of pus leading to ischemia.
- ☐ **3.** Production of bacterial growth by avascular tissue.
- ☐ **4.** Antibiotics not being instilled directly into the bone.

The Client with a Spinal Cord Injury

95. A client who fell during a rock-climbing trip is alert and conscious but unable to move her arms or legs on command. When planning to move a person with a possible spinal cord injury, which of the following should be the priority concern?
☐ **1.** Wrapping and supporting the extremities, which can be easily injured.
☐ **2.** Moving the person gently to help reduce pain.
☐ **3.** Immobilizing the head and neck to prevent further injury.
☐ **4.** Cushioning the back with pillows to ensure comfort.

96. The nurse is taking care of a client with a spinal cord injury. The extent of the client's injury is shown below. Which of the following findings is expected when assessing this client?
☐ **1.** Inability to move his arms.
☐ **2.** Loss of sensation in his hands and fingers.
☐ **3.** Dysfunction of bowel and bladder.
☐ **4.** Difficulty breathing.

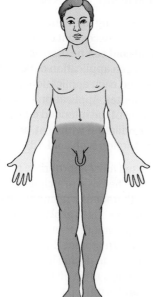

97. When the client has a cord transection at T4, which of the following is the primary focus of the nursing assessment?
☐ **1.** Renal status.
☐ **2.** Vascular status.
☐ **3.** Gastrointestinal function.
☐ **4.** Biliary function.

98. When assessing the client with a cord transection above T5 for possible complications, which of the following should the nurse expect as least likely to occur?
☐ **1.** Diarrhea.
☐ **2.** Paralytic ileus.
☐ **3.** Stress ulcers.
☐ **4.** Intra-abdominal bleeding.

99. The nurse is planning to teach the client with spinal cord injury and intermittent nasogastric suctioning about interventions to protect her integumentary system. Which of the following should the nurse include?
☐ **1.** Eat enough calories to maintain desired weight.
☐ **2.** Stay in cool environments to avoid sweating.
☐ **3.** Stay in warm environments to avoid chilling.
☐ **4.** Eat low-sodium foods to avoid edema.

100. Which of the following should the nurse use as the best method to assess for the development of deep vein thrombosis in a client with a spinal cord injury?
☐ **1.** Homans' sign.
☐ **2.** Pain.
☐ **3.** Tenderness.
☐ **4.** Leg girth.

101. During the period of spinal shock, the nurse should expect the client's bladder function to be which of the following?
☐ **1.** Spastic.
☐ **2.** Normal.
☐ **3.** Atonic.
☐ **4.** Uncontrolled.

102. After 1 month of therapy, the client in spinal shock begins to experience muscle spasms in his legs. He calls the nurse in excitement to report the leg movement. Which of the following responses by the nurse would be the most accurate?
☐ **1.** "These movements indicate that the damaged nerves are healing."
☐ **2.** "This is a good sign. Keep trying to move all the affected muscles."
☐ **3.** "The return of movement means that eventually you should be able to walk again."
☐ **4.** "The movements occur from muscle reflexes that can't be initiated or controlled by the brain."

103. The client with a spinal cord injury asks the nurse why the dietitian has recommended that she decrease her total daily intake of calcium. Which of the following responses by the nurse would provide the most accurate information?
☐ **1.** "Excessive intake of dairy products makes constipation more common."
☐ **2.** "Immobility increases calcium absorption from the intestine."
☐ **3.** "Lack of weight bearing causes demineralization of the long bones."
☐ **4.** "Dairy products likely will contribute to weight gain."

104. As a first step in teaching a woman with a spinal cord injury and quadriplegia about her sexual health, the nurse assesses her understanding of her current sexual functioning. Which of the following statements by the client indicates a good understanding of her sexual functioning?

☐ 1. "I won't be able to have sexual intercourse until the urinary catheter is removed."

☐ 2. "I can participate in sexual activity but might not experience orgasm."

☐ 3. "I can't have sexual intercourse because it causes hypertension, but other sexual activity is okay."

☐ 4. "I should be able to participate in sexual activity, but I will be infertile."

105. A client with a spinal cord injury who has been active in sports and outdoor activities talks almost obsessively about his past activities. In tears, one day he asks the nurse, "Why can't I stop talking about these things? I know those days are gone forever." Which of the following responses by the nurse conveys the best understanding of the client's behavior?

☐ 1. "Be patient. It takes time to adjust to such a massive loss."

☐ 2. "Talking about the past is a form of denial. We have to help you focus on today."

☐ 3. "Reviewing your losses is a way to help you work through your grief and loss."

☐ 4. "It's a simple escape mechanism to go back and live again in happier times."

Correct Answers and Rationales

The letter in parentheses after each rationale identifies the client need addressed in the item, including management of care (M), safety and infection control (S), health promotion and maintenance (H), psychosocial adaptation (P), basic care and comfort (C), pharmacological and parenteral therapies (D), reduction of risk potential (R), and physiological adaptation (A).

The Client with Rheumatoid Arthritis

1. 3. Initially, most clients with early symptoms of rheumatoid arthritis complain of early morning stiffness or stiffness after sitting still for a while. Later symptoms of rheumatoid arthritis include limited joint range of motion; deformed joints, especially of the hand; and rheumatoid nodules. (A)

2. 1. Based on the client's complaints, the most appropriate nursing diagnosis would be *Activity intolerance* related to fatigue and pain. Nursing interventions would focus on helping the client conserve energy and decrease episodes of fatigue. Although the client may develop a self-care deficit related to the activity intolerance and increasing joint pain, the client is voicing concerns about household chores and difficulty around the house and yard, not self-care issues. Over time, the client may develop ineffective coping or body image disturbance as the disorder becomes chronic with increasing pain and fatigue. (C)

3. 3. Rheumatoid arthritis is a disorder of adults between the ages of 20 and 55, not 60 and 75. Research has found that rheumatoid arthritis occurs in clients who have had infectious disease such as the Epstein-Barr virus. Female gender is a risk factor because rheumatoid arthritis occurs three times more often in women than in men. The genetic link, specifically HLA-DR4, has been found in 65% of clients with rheumatoid arthritis. (R)

4. 3. Maintaining usual ways of accomplishing tasks would be the lowest priority during the acute phase. Rather, the focus is on developing less stressful ways of accomplishing routine tasks. Pain relief is a high priority during the acute phase because pain is typically severe and interferes with the client's ability to function. Preserving joint function and preventing joint deformity are high priorities during the acute phase to promote an optimal level of functioning and reduce the risk of contractures. (A)

5. 3. Heat-producing liniment can produce a burn if used with other heat devices that could intensify the heat reaction. Heat and cold can be used as often as the client desires. However, each application of heat should not exceed 20 minutes, and each application of cold should not exceed 10 to 15 minutes. Application for longer periods results in the opposite of the intended effect: vasoconstriction instead of vasodilation with heat, and vasodilation instead of vasoconstriction with cold. (R)

6. 4. The nurse's most appropriate response is one that is therapeutic. The basic principle of therapeutic communication and a therapeutic relationship is honesty. Therefore, the nurse needs to explain truthfully that each client is different and that there are various forms of arthritis and arthritis treatment. To state that it is the physician's prerogative to decide how to treat the client implies that the client is not a member of his or her own health care team and is not a participant in his or her care. The statement also is defensive, which serves to block any further communication or questions from the client about the physician. Asking the client to tell more about the friend presumes that the client knows correct and complete information, which is not a valid assumption to make. The nurse does not know about the client's friend and should not make statements about another client's condition. Stating that the drug is for cases that are worse than the client's demonstrates that the nurse is making assumptions that are not necessarily valid or appropriate. Also, telling the client not to worry ignores the underlying emotions associated with the question, totally discounting the client's feelings. (P)

7. 4. Positions of flexion should be avoided to prevent loss of functional ability of affected joints. Proper body alignment during rest periods is encouraged to maintain correct muscle and joint placement. Lying in the prone position is encouraged to avoid further curvature of the spine and internal rotation of the shoulders. (A)

8. 4. Carrying a laundry basket with clinched fingers and fists is not an example of conserving energy of small joints. The laundry basket should be held with both hands opened as wide as possible and with outstretched arms so that pressure is not placed on the small joints of the fingers. When rising from a chair, the palms should be used instead of the fingers so as to distribute weight over the larger area of the palms. Holding packages close to the body provides greater support to the shoulder, elbow, and wrist joints because muscles of the arms and hands are used to stabilize the weight against the body. This decreases the stress and weight or pull on small joints such as the fingers. Objects can be slid with the palm of the hand, which distributes weight over the larger area of the palms instead of stressing the small joints of the fingers to pick up the weight of the object to move it to another place. (C)

9. 1. Because some over-the-counter vitamin supplements contain folic acid, the client should avoid self-medication with vitamins while taking methotrexate, a folic acid antagonist. Because methotrexate is hepatotoxic, the client should avoid the intake of alcohol, which could increase the risk for hepatotoxicity. Methotrexate can cause bone marrow depression, placing the client at risk for infection. Therefore, meticulous mouth care is essential to minimize the risk of infection. Contraception should be used during methotrexate therapy and for 8 weeks after the therapy has been discontinued because of its effect on mitosis. Methotrexate is considered teratogenic. (D)

10. 2. Difficulty seeing out of one eye, when evaluated in conjunction with the client's medication therapy regimen, leads to the suspicion of possible retinal degeneration. The possibility of an irreversible retinal degeneration caused by deposits of hydroxychloroquine (Plaquenil) in the layers of the retina requires an ophthalmologic examination before therapy is begun and at 6-month intervals. Although cataracts may develop in young adults, they are less likely, and damage from the hydroxychloroquine is the most obvious at-risk factor. Eyesight is not affected by the disease process of rheumatoid arthritis. (D)

11. 3. The nurse must frequently evaluate the positioning of the client's leg to prevent misalignment and development of possible contractures. Initially the client may experience some discomfort when using a CPM machine. If the client cannot tolerate the discomfort, the physician should be notified to obtain an order to adjust the settings. The settings for the machine are determined by the physician and cannot be changed without an order. Although the optimal degree of flexion is 90 degrees, therapy will continue until the individual regains the maximal degree of flexion in the knee as determined by the physician. (R)

12. 4. Superficial heat applications, such as tub baths, showers, and warm compresses, can be helpful in relieving pain and stiffness. Exercises can be performed more comfortably and more effectively after heat applications. The client with rheumatoid arthritis must balance rest with exercise every day, not every other day. Typically, large doses of analgesics, which can lead to hepatotoxic effects, are not necessary. Learning to cope with the pain by refocusing is inappropriate. (C)

13. 1, 2, 5. An arthrocentesis is performed to aspirate excess synovial fluid, pus, or blood from a joint cavity to relieve pain or to diagnosis inflammatory diseases such as rheumatoid arthritis. A local agent may be used to decrease the pain of the needle insertion through the skin and into the joint cavity. Aspiration of the fluid into the syringe can be very painful because of the size and inflammation of the joint. Usually a steroid medication is injected locally to alleviate the inflammation; a compression bandage is applied to help decrease swelling; and the client is asked to rest the joint for up to 24 hours afterwards to help relieve the pain and promote rest to the inflamed joint. The client may experience pain during this time until the inflammation begins to resolve and swelling decreases. (R)

The Client with Osteoarthritis

14. 1, 4, 5. To prepare a client for an arthrocentesis, the nurse should tell the client that a local anesthetic administered by the physician will decrease discomfort. There may be bleeding after the procedure, so the nurse should check the dressing. The client may experience pain. The nurse should offer pain medication and evaluate outcomes for pain relief. Because a local anesthetic is used, the client will not require preoperative medication. The client will rest the knee for 24 hours and then should begin range-of-motion and muscle strengthening exercises. (M)

15. 1. Metal will interfere with the test. Metallic objects within the examination field, such as jewelry, earrings, and dental amalgams, may inhibit organ visualization and can produce unclear images. Ingesting foods and beverages days before the test will not affect bone mineral status. Short-term calcium gluconate intake will also not influence bone mineral status. The client may already have had chronic pain as a result of a bone fracture or from osteoporosis. (M)

16. 1. Shorter sessions will allow the client to rest between the sessions. Changing the physician's order to a different examination will not provide the information needed for this client's treatment. Acetaminophen is a nonopioid analgesic and an antipyretic, not an anti-inflammatory agent. Thus, it would not help this client avoid the adverse effects of a lengthy X-ray examination. Although the X-ray table is hard, there are other options for making the client comfortable, rather than canceling the examination. (M)

17. **4.** Osteoarthritis is a degenerative joint disease with local manifestations such as local joint pain, unlike rheumatoid arthritis, which has systemic manifestation such as anemia and osteoporosis. Weight loss occurs in rheumatoid arthritis, whereas most clients with osteoarthritis are overweight. (A)

18. **1, 2, 3.** A diet with adequate amounts of vitamin D aids in the regulation, absorption, and subsequent utilization of calcium and phosphorus, which are necessary for the normal calcification of bone. Figs, broccoli, and almonds are very good sources of calcium. Moderate intake of alcohol has no known negative effects on bone density but excessive alcohol intake does reduce bone density. Swimming, biking, and other non–weight-bearing exercises do not maintain bone mass. Walking and running, which are weight-bearing exercises, do maintain bone mass. The client should eat a balanced diet but does not need to avoid the use of high-fat foods. (R)

19. **1.** Capsaicin cream, which produces analgesia by preventing the reaccumulation of substance P in the peripheral sensory neurons, is made from the active ingredients of hot peppers. Therefore, clients should wash their hands immediately after applying capsaicin cream if they do not wear gloves, to avoid possible contact between the cream and mucous membranes. Clients are instructed to avoid wearing tight bandages over areas where capsaicin cream has been applied because swelling may occur from inflammation of the arthritis in the joint and lead to constriction on the peripheral neurovascular system. Capsaicin cream should be stored in areas between 59° F and 86° F (15° C and 30° C). The cabinet over the stove in the kitchen would be too warm. Capsaicin cream should not come in contact with irritated and broken skin, mucous membranes, or eyes. Therefore it should not be used on cuts or burns. (D)

20. **3.** Drugs that cause gastric irritation, such as ibuprofen, are best taken after or with a meal, when stomach contents help minimize the local irritation. Taking the medication on an empty stomach at any time during the day will lead to gastric irritation. Taking the drug at bedtime with food may cause the client to gain weight, possibly aggravating the osteoarthritis. When the client arises, he is stiff from immobility and should use warmth and stretching until he gets food in his stomach. (D)

21. **3.** The major advantage of celecoxib, the new generation of cyclooxygenase-2 (COX-2) inhibitors, over diclofenac, a COX-1 inhibitor, is that celecoxib is less likely to produce gastrointestinal problems, such as ulcers and bleeding. There is no evidence of less hepatotoxicity, renal toxicity, or nausea and vomiting with COX-2 inhibitors. (D)

22. **1.** Corticosteroids are used for clients with osteoarthritis to obtain a local effect. Therefore, they are given only via intra-articular injection. Oral corticosteroids are avoided because they can cause an acceleration of osteoarthritis. Rheumatoid arthritis and osteoarthritis are two different diseases. (D)

23. **2.** Weight-bearing exercise plays a very important role in stimulating regeneration of cartilage, which lacks blood vessels, by driving synovial fluid through the joint cartilage. Joint mobility is increased by weight-bearing exercises, not range-of-motion exercises, because surrounding muscles, ligaments, and tendons are strengthened. Pain is an early sign of degenerative joint bone problems. Swelling may not occur for some time after pain, if at all. Osteoarthritic pain is worsened in cold, damp weather; therefore, exercising outdoors is not recommended year round in all settings. (H)

24. **3.** When combined with a weight loss program, aquatic exercise would be best because it cushions the joints and allows the client to burn off calories. Aquatic exercise promotes circulation, muscle toning, and lung expansion, which promote healthy preoperative conditioning. Weight lifting and walking are too stressful to the joints, possibly exacerbating the client's osteoarthritis. Although tai chi exercise is designed for stretching and coordination, it would not be the best exercise for this client to help with weight loss. (A)

25. **4.** Before implementing a teaching plan, the nurse should determine the client's fears about the procedure. Only then can the client begin to hear what the nurse has to share about the individualized teaching plan designed to meet the client's needs. In the preoperative period, the client needs to learn how to correctly prevent hip flexion and to demonstrate coughing and deep breathing. However, this teaching can be effective only after the client's fears have been assessed and addressed. Although the client may appreciate seeing what a hip prosthesis looks like, so as to understand the new body part, this is not a necessity. (P)

26. **1.** The nurse should suspect nerve damage if numbness is present. However, whether the damage is short-term and related to edema or long-term and related to permanent nerve damage would not be clear at this point. The nurse needs to continue to assess the client's neurovascular status, including pain, pallor, pulselessness, paresthesia, and paralysis (the five P's). Bleeding would suggest vascular damage or hemorrhage. Dislocation would suggest malalignment. Pink color would suggest adequate circulation to the area. Numbness would suggest neurologic damage. (R)

27. **3.** The joint has dislocated when the client with a total joint prosthesis develops severe sudden pain and an inability to move the extremity. Clinical manifestations of an infection would include inflammation, redness, erythema, and possibly drainage and separation of the wound. Bleeding could be external (e.g., blood visible from the wound or on the dressing) or internal and manifested by signs of shock (e.g., pallor, coolness, hypotension, tachycardia). The seepage of glue into soft tissue would have occurred in the operating room, when the glue is still in the liquid form. The glue dries into the hard, fixed form before the wound is closed. (R)

The Client with a Hip Fracture

28. **4.** The hip spica cast is used for treatment of femoral fractures; it immobilizes the affected extremity and the trunk securely. It extends from above the nipple line to the base of the foot of both extremities in a double hip spica. Constipation, possible due to lack of mobility, can cause abdominal distention or bloating. When the spica cast becomes too tight due to distention, the cast will compress the superior mesenteric artery against the duodenum. The compression produces abdominal pain, abdominal pressure, nausea, and vomiting. The nurse should assess the abdomen for decreased bowel sounds, not the superior mesenteric artery. The surgeon cannot manipulate a fracture through a small window in a double hip spica cast. The nurse cannot use the window to aid in repositioning because the window opening can break and cause cast disruption. (R)

29. **3.** With an intracapsular hip fracture, the affected leg is shorter than the unaffected leg because of the muscle spasms and external rotation. The client also experiences severe pain in the region of the fracture. (A)

30. **4.** Multiple sclerosis would be the least likely chronic health problem for an older client with a hip fracture. Typically, multiple sclerosis is considered a severe crippling disorder of young clients. Hypertension is a common chronic health problem in older clients. Cardiac decompensation is common in older clients; it arises from cardiac musculature changes and age-related changes in the heart. This comorbid condition can complicate the treatment and care when the older client experiences a hip fracture. Pulmonary disease commonly arises from age-related changes in the respiratory system. These comorbid conditions can complicate the treatment and care when the older client experiences a hip fracture. (R)

31. **4.** Insertion of a pin for the internal fixation of an extracapsular fractured hip provides good fixation of the fracture. The fracture site is stabilized and fractured bone ends are well approximated. As a result, the client is able to be mobilized sooner, thus reducing the risks of complications related to immobility. Internal fixation with a pin insertion does not prevent hemorrhage or decrease the risk of neurovascular impairment, potential complications associated with any joint or bone surgery. It does not lessen the client's risk of infection at the site. (R)

32. **3.** The primary purpose of the drainage tube is to prevent fluid accumulation in the wound. Fluid, when it accumulates, creates dead space. Elimination of the dead space by keeping the wound free of fluid greatly enhances wound healing and helps prevent abscess formation. Although the characteristics of the drainage from the tube, such as a change in color or appearance, may suggest a possible infection, this is not the tube's primary purpose. The drainage tube does not eliminate the need for wound irrigation or provide a way to instill antibiotics into the wound. (R)

33. **2, 3, 4, 5.** A client who has had a posterolateral total hip replacement should not adduct the hip joint, which would lead to dislocation of the ball out of the socket; therefore, the client should be encouraged to keep the toes pointed slightly outward when using a walker. An abduction pillow should be kept between the legs to keep the hip joint in an abducted position. The client should rotate between lying supine and lateral on the unoperated side, but not on the operated side. Ice is used to reduce swelling on the operative side. The client should not flex the operated hip beyond a 90-degree angle, such as when bending down to tie or slip on shoes. Doing so could lead to joint dislocation. (R)

34. **1, 3, 4.** A client who has had a total hip replacement via an anterolateral approach has almost the opposite precautions as those for a client who has had a total hip replacement through the posterolateral approach. The hip joint should not be actively abducted. The client should avoid turning the toes or knee outward. The client should keep the legs side by side without a pillow or wedge. The client should use an elevated toilet seat and shower chair and should not extend the operative leg backwards. The client should perform range-of-motion exercises as directed by the physical therapist. (R)

35. **2.** Being unable to move the affected leg suggests neurologic impairment. A decrease in the distal pulse, diminished capillary refill, and coolness to touch of the affected extremity suggest vascular compromise. (R)

36. **1.** Any activity or position that causes flexion, adduction, or internal rotation of greater than 90 degrees should be avoided until the soft tissue surrounding the prosthesis has stabilized, at approximately 6 weeks. Crossing the legs while sitting down can lead to dislocation of the femoral head from the hip socket. Sitting on a raised commode seat prevents hip flexion and adduction. Using an abductor splint while side-lying keeps the hip joint in abduction, thus preventing adduction and possible dislocation. Rising straight from a chair to a standing position is acceptable for this client because this action avoids hip flexion, adduction, and internal rotation of greater than 90 degrees. (R)

37. **3.** A high-backed straight chair with armrests is recommended to help keep the client in the best possible alignment after surgery for a femoral head prosthesis placement. Use of this type of chair helps to prevent dislocation of the prosthesis from the socket. A desk-type swivel chair, padded upholstered chair, or recliner should be avoided because it does not provide for good body alignment and can cause the overly flexed femoral head to dislocate. (R)

38. **2.** Although pets and furniture, such as snack tables and rocking chairs, may pose a problem, scatter rugs are the single greatest hazard in the home, especially for elderly people who are unsure and unsteady with walking. Falls have been found to account for almost half the accidental deaths that occur in the home. The risk of falls is further compounded by the client's need for crutches. (S)

The Client with a Herniated Disk

39. **1.** The client is using correct body mechanics for lifting because she is keeping her back as straight as possible and is holding the box close to her body. She is using her large leg muscles to lift the box. She is using a broad base of support by placing her feet as wide apart as possible. The other suggestions would cause the client to put a strain on her back. (R)

40. **3.** The client with low back pain should not exceed the prescribed exercises even though they may think, "If this will make me well, double will make me well quicker." When exceeding prescribed exercise programs, the client's muscle may be unconditioned and easily tired, leading to injury and increased pain. To use proper body mechanics when lifting light objects, the client should bring the item close to the center of gravity, which occurs when the object is kept below the level of the elbows. Leaning forward while bending the knees allows for the muscles of the thigh to be used instead of those of the lower back. Sleeping on the side with the legs flexed is appropriate because the spine is kept in a neutral position without twisting or pulling on muscles. (R)

41. **3.** For the client who has back pain radiating down to his right heel and lateral foot, suggesting radiculopathy of a herniated disc at L5–S1, typically the physician would order NSAIDs, oral analgesics, and muscle relaxants. ACE inhibitors are indicated for clients with hypertension and those with heart failure unresponsive to conventional therapy. Beta blockers are indicated for clients with cardiovascular disorders, such as hypertension and angina, and also for migraine prophylaxis. Barbiturates are central nervous system depressants; they are indicated for clients with seizures or insomnia and for those being prepared for surgery. (D)

42. **2.** Standing with a flattened spine slightly tilted forward and slightly flexed to the affected side indicates a postural deformity. Motor changes would include findings such as hypotonia or muscle weakness. Absent or diminished reflexes related to the level of herniation would indicate alteration in reflexes. Sensory changes would include findings such as paresthesia and numbness related to the specific tract of the herniation. (A)

43. **2.** A supine position with the client's legs flexed is the most comfortable position because it allows for the disc to recess off of the nerve, thus alleviating the pressure and pain. The prone position causes hyperextension of the spine and increased pressure of the disc on the nerve root on the right. A ruptured disc at L5–S1 right is a term commonly used in the analysis of a history and physical examination, magnetic resonance image, or myelogram to identify a ruptured disc compressing the right nerve root exiting the L5–S1 spinous process, as opposed to the central area or the left nerve root of that spinous process. If the ruptured area of the disc were in the central area of the

spinous process, the prone position and hyperextension might relieve the disc pressure on the nerve. A high Fowler's or sitting position increases the pressure of the disc on the nerve root because of gravity, as does a right Sims position. (A)

44. **4.** Myelography, used to determine the exact location of a herniated disk, involves the use of a radiopaque dye (usually an iodized oil, but in some instances a water-soluble compound). In some instances, air is used for an air-contrast study. (R)

45. **4.** An I.V. line is not required for an MRI. If a client has an I.V. line, it is usually converted to an intermittent infusion device, such as a saline lock, to avoid infiltration during transport of the client and completion of the procedure. When a contrast agent is used, the client is moved out of the cylinder, the contrast material is injected, and the client is moved back in. An MRI scan is painless. Typically the staff positions the client with pillows, blankets, earplugs, and music, to ensure client comfort, before the procedure is started. A history of past surgeries is important, especially if the surgery involved implantation of any metallic devices (e.g., implants, clips, pacemakers). Additionally, the nurse needs to assess for hearing aids, electronic devices, shrapnel, bra hooks, necklaces, jewelry, credit cards, zippers, or any type of metal that the magnet of the MRI unit would attract. Although open MRI units are now available, they are not in widespread use. Therefore, the nurse needs to determine whether the client is claustrophobic because the unit is a closed cylinder in which the client hears pops of noise. A number of clients develop claustrophobia that causes the procedure to be cancelled. If the client is claustrophobic, the procedure may need to be rescheduled after an open MRI unit is located or made available. (R)

46. **2.** Based on the client's complaints, the nurse should call the surgeon to verify the location of the surgery. The client's complaints indicate radiculopathy of L4 to L5, but the consent form states L3 to L4. Radiculopathy of L3 to L4 involves pain radiating from the back to the buttocks to the posterior thigh to the inner calf. The nurse must act as a client advocate and not ask the client to sign the consent until the correct procedure is identified and confirmed on the consent. The nurse has no legal authority or responsibility to change the consent. The history is a source of information, but when the client is coherent and the history is contradictory, the physician should be contacted to clarify the situation. Ultimately, it is the surgeon's responsibility to identify the site of surgery specified on the surgical consent form. (M)

47. **1.** *Impaired physical mobility* related to back pain, muscle spasms, and tissue manipulation is a priority after a laminectomy because based on individual factors, such as the length of time of the disease and previous scarring or injury to the muscles or nerves before the surgery, spasms and pain can be quite severe. *Imbalanced nutri-*

tion: Less than body requirements related to inability to eat in the supine position is not a priority nursing diagnosis because the client is encouraged to take fluids as soon as the gag reflex returns, no nausea is present, and bowel sounds begin to return. *Bowel incontinence* related to decreased physical activity is not a priority nursing diagnosis because the client is encouraged to sit up and to ambulate to the bathroom with assistance as soon as the anesthesia wears off. *Disturbed body image* related to fear of disfiguring surgical scar should also not be a priority nursing diagnosis because the laminectomy incision is commonly small, possibly as small as 1 inch for a lumbar laminectomy L5–S1 bilateral. (A)

48. 2. Ondansetron hydrochloride (Zofran) is a selective serotonin receptor antagonist that acts centrally to control the client's nausea in the postoperative phase. It does not control muscle spasms, shivering, or dry mouth. (D)

49. 4. Sweeping causes a twisting motion, which should be avoided because twisting can cause undue stress on the recently ruptured disc site, muscle spasms, and a potential recurrent disc rupture. Although the client should not bend at the waist, such as when washing dishes at the sink, the client can dry dishes because no bending is necessary. The client can sit in a firm chair that keeps the back anatomically aligned. The client should not twist and pull, so when making the bed, the client should pull the covers up on one side and then walk around to the other side before trying to pull the covers up there. (A)

50. 4. After a lumbar laminectomy L4–5, a client who is returning to work should avoid sitting whenever possible. If the client must sit, he or she should sit only in chairs that allow the knees to be higher than the hips and support the arms to maintain correct body alignment and reduce undue stress on the spine. Maintaining good body postures is most important after a lumbar laminectomy L4–5. By 6 weeks after the surgery, the client should have regained stamina. To maintain correct body posture, the client should also place one foot on a stepstool during prolonged standing. Sleeping on the back with a support under the knees is effective in maintaining correct body posture. Maintaining an average weight for height is important in maintaining a healthy back because carrying extra weight causes undue stress on back muscles. (A)

51. 2. Clear yellowish fluid on the dressing may be cerebrospinal fluid (CSF). This fluid must be tested for glucose to determine whether it is CSF. If so, the client is at great risk for an infection of the central nervous system, which has a high mortality rate. The client should be able to laterally rotate the head and neck, which is above the surgical site in the spinal column. During the nursing postoperative neuromuscular-vascular assessment of movement of the head and neck, the nurse should find results consistent with the preoperative baseline status. Using the standing position to void is normal for a male

client. Coughing is the body's defense mechanism to help clear the lungs of the anesthetic agents and to ventilate the lungs in response to a sustained deep inspiration for ventilation of the lower lobes of the lungs. A frequent cough could place a strain on the incision site and should be avoided. Also, a productive cough of thick, yellow sputum would indicate the complication of a respiratory infection. (R)

52. 2. The nurse should verify with the surgeon the preferred position to use before applying the brace. Traditionally, the client who had a spinal fusion was asked to lie on the side and logroll onto the brace. Now physicians also have clients stand and sit for the brace application. Therefore, the nurse needs to verify the surgeon's preference. (R)

53. 4. The client should wear a thin cotton undershirt under the brace to prevent the brace from abrading directly against the skin. The cotton material also aids in absorbing any moisture, such as perspiration, that could lead to skin irritation and breakdown. Applying lotion is not recommended before applying the brace because further skin breakdown can result (related to the collection of moisture where microorganisms can grow) and irritants from the lotion can cause further irritation. Applying extra padding (e.g., to the iliac crests) is not recommended because the padding can become wrinkled, producing more pressure sites and skin breakdown. Use of baby or talcum powder is not recommended because the irritation from the talcum also can cause irritation and skin breakdown. (R)

54. 1. Typically, the donor site causes more pain than the fused site does because inflammation, swelling, and venous oozing around the nerve endings in the donor site, where the subcutaneous tissue was removed, occur during the first 24 to 48 hours postoperatively. After surgery, the surgeon applies a pressure dressing to the donor site to compress the veins that were transected for the removal of subcutaneous tissue but that did not stop oozing blood after surgical cauterization during the surgical procedure. Pressure on a transected vein, which is low pressure, stops the oozing and loss of blood from the venous site. When the donor site is the fibula, neurovascular checks must be performed every hour to ensure adequate neurologic function of and circulation to the area. The surgeon, not the degree or amount of pain, specifies activity restrictions. (A)

55. 1. A client who has had back surgery should place his feet flat on the floor to avoid strain on the incision. Placing the feet on a low or high footstool or in any other position of comfort with the legs uncrossed increases the pressure on the suture line and increases the inflammation around the involved nerve root, thereby increasing the risk of possible rerupture of the disc site. (R)

56. 4. After a lumbar laminectomy, a client should not sit for prolonged periods in a chair because of the increased pressure against the nerve root and incision site. Assisting with daily hygiene is an appropriate activity during the initial postoperative period because, as with any surgical procedure, the client needs to return to her optimal level of functioning as soon as possible. There is no limitation on the client's participation in daily hygiene activities except for her individual response of pain, nausea, vomiting, or weakness. Lying flat in bed is appropriate because it does not cause stress on the spinal column where the laminectomy was performed and the disc tissue was removed. Positions that should be avoided are those that would cause twisting and flexion of the spine. Walking in the hall is an acceptable activity. It promotes good postoperative ventilation, circulation, and return of peristalsis, which are needed for all surgical clients. In addition, walking provides the postoperative lumbar laminectomy client an opportunity to build up endurance and muscle strength and to promote circulation to the operative and incision sites for healing without twisting or stressing them. (A)

57. 3. Sit-ups are not recommended for the client who has had a lumbar laminectomy because these exercises place too great a stress on the back. Knee-to-chest lifts, hip tilts, and pelvic tilt exercises are recommended to strengthen back and abdominal muscles. (R)

The Client with an Amputation due to Peripheral Vascular Disease

58. 3. Typically, peripheral vascular disease is considered to be a disorder affecting older adults. Therefore, an age of 39 years would not be considered as a risk factor contributing to the development of peripheral vascular disease. Uncontrolled diabetes mellitus is considered a risk factor for peripheral vascular disease because of the macroangiopathic and microangiopathic changes that result from poor blood glucose control. Cigarette smoking is a known risk factor for peripheral vascular disease. Nicotine is a potent vasoconstrictor. Serum cholesterol levels greater than 200 mg/dl are considered a risk factor for peripheral vascular disease. (H)

59. 2. The client with severe arterial occlusive disease and gangrene of the left great toe would have lost the hair on the leg due to decreased circulation to the skin. Edema around the ankle and lower leg would indicate venous insufficiency of the lower extremity. Thin, soft toenails (i.e., not thickened and brittle) are a normal finding. Warmth in the foot indicates adequate circulation to the extremity. Typically, the foot would be cool to cold if a severe arterial occlusion were present. (A)

60. 3. The client should be tobacco-free for 30 minutes before the test to avoid false readings related to the vasoconstrictive effects of smoking on the arteries. Because this test is noninvasive, the client does not need to sign a consent form. The client should receive an opioid analgesic, not a sedative, to control the pain as the blood pressure cuffs are inflated during the Doppler studies to determine the ankle-to-brachial pressure index. The client's ankle should not be covered with a blanket because the weight of the blanket on the ischemic foot will cause pain. A bed cradle should be used to keep even the weight of a sheet off the affected foot. (R)

61. 2. Slow, steady walking is a recommended activity for the client with peripheral arterial disease because it stimulates the development of collateral circulation needed to ensure adequate tissue oxygenation. The client with peripheral arterial disease should not minimize activity. Activity is necessary to foster the development of collateral circulation. Elevating the legs above the heart is an appropriate strategy for reducing venous congestion. Wearing antiembolism stockings promotes the return of venous circulation, which is important for clients with venous insufficiency. However, their use in clients with peripheral arterial disease may cause the disease to worsen. (A)

62. 1. Daily lubrication, inspection, cleaning, and patting dry of the feet should be performed to prevent cracking of the skin and possible infection. Soaking the feet in warm water should be avoided because soaking can lead to maceration and subsequent skin breakdown. Additionally, the client with arterial insufficiency typically experiences sensory changes, so the client may be unable to detect water that is too warm, thus placing the client at risk for burns. Antiembolism stockings, appropriate for clients with venous insufficiency, are inappropriate for clients with arterial insufficiency and could lead to a worsening of the condition. Footwear should be roomy, soft, and protective and allow air to circulate. Therefore, firm, supportive leather shoes would be inappropriate. (R)

63. 2. Encouraging the client who will be undergoing amputation to verbalize his feelings is the most therapeutic response. Asking the client to tell more about how he is feeling helps to elicit information, providing insight into his view of the situation and also providing the nurse with ideas to help him cope. The nurse should avoid value-laden responses, such as, "At least you will still have one good leg to use," that may make the client feel guilty or hostile, thereby blocking further communication. Furthermore, stating that the client still has one good leg ignores his expressed concerns. The client has verbalized feelings of helplessness by using the term "invalid." The nurse needs to focus on this concern and not try to complete the teaching first before discussing what is on the client's mind. The client's needs, not the nurse's needs, must be met first. It is inappropriate for the nurse to assume to know the relationship between the client and his wife or the roles they now must assume as dependent client and caregiver. Additionally, the response about the client's wife caring for him may reinforce the client's feelings of helplessness as an invalid. (P)

64. **2.** The level of amputation often cannot be accurately determined until during surgery, when the surgeon can directly assess the adequacy of the circulation of the residual limb. From a moral, ethical, and legal viewpoint, the surgeon attempts to remove as little of the leg as possible. Although a longer residual limb facilitates prosthesis fitting, unless the stump is receiving a good blood supply the prosthesis will not function properly because tissue necrosis will occur. Although the client's ability to walk with a prosthesis is important, it is not a determining factor in the decision about the level of amputation required. Blood supply to the tissue is the primary determinant. (A)

65. **4.** The priority action is to draw a mark around the site of bleeding to determine the rate of bleeding. Once the area is marked, the nurse can determine whether the bleeding is increasing or decreasing by the size of the area marked. Because the spot is bright red, the bleeding is most likely arterial in origin. Once the rate and source of bleeding are identified, the surgeon should be notified. The stump is not elevated because adhesions may occur, interfering with the ability to fit a prosthesis. The dressing would be reinforced if the bleeding is determined to be of venous origin, characterized by slow oozing of darker blood that ceases with the application of a pressure dressing. Typically, operative dressings are not changed for 24 hours. Therefore, the dressing is reinforced to prevent organisms from penetrating through the blood-soaked areas of the initial postoperative dressing. (A)

66. **4.** The nurse's first action should be to administer the prescribed opioid analgesic to the client, because this phenomenon is phantom sensation and interventions should be provided to relieve it. Pain relief is the priority. Phantom sensation is a real sensation. It is incorrect and inappropriate to tell a client that it is impossible to feel the pain. Although it does relieve the client's apprehensions to be told that phantom sensations are a real phenomenon, the client needs prompt treatment to relieve the pain sensation. Usually phantom sensation will go away. However, showing the client that the toes are not there does nothing to provide the client with relief. (A)

67. **4.** Use of crutches requires significant strength from the triceps muscles. Therefore, efforts are focused on strengthening these muscles in anticipation of crutch walking. Bed and wheelchair push-ups are excellent exercises targeted at the triceps muscles. Abdominal exercises, range-of-motion and isometric exercises of the shoulders, and quadriceps and gluteal setting exercises are not helpful in preparing for crutch walking. (R)

68. **4.** When using crutches, the client is taught to support her weight primarily on the hands. Supporting body weight on the axillae, elbows, or upper arms must be avoided to prevent nerve damage from excessive pressure. (R)

69. **4.** Before beginning dietary instructions and interventions, the nurse must first assess the client's and family's food preferences, such as pattern of food intake, life style, food preferences, and ethnic, cultural, and financial influences. Once this information is obtained, the nurse can begin teaching based on the client's current knowledge level and then building on this knowledge base. (A)

The Client with Fractures

70. **3.** Isometric contractions increase the tension within a muscle but do not produce movement. Repeated isometric contractions make muscles grow larger and stronger. Adduction of the leg puts work onto the hip joint as well as altering the pull of traction. Rolling the leg, or *external rotation,* alters the pull of traction. Additional weight should not be added to traction unless ordered by the physician; it will not prevent muscle atrophy. (R)

71. **2.** Because of the degree of contamination of the open fracture and the time that has passed since the accident, the risk of infection is very high. Therefore, the nurse should be especially alert for signs and symptoms of possible existing infection or early signs of infection, such as debris in the wound site, temperature abnormalities, results of laboratory studies (such as complete blood cell count and wound culture and sensitivities), or heat or redness around or in the wound. Because the client's vital signs and cardiovascular status are stable at this time, hemorrhage is not the primary concern. The client is talking coherently at this point, so his mentation does not suggest that he is in shock. However, assessment for signs and symptoms of hemorrhage and shock would certainly be ongoing. The fracture would be corrected by surgery as soon as possible, thereby minimizing the risk of deformity. (A)

72. **3.** Methocarbamol is a muscle relaxant and acts primarily to relieve muscle spasms. It has no effect on microorganisms, does not reduce itching, and has no effect on nervousness. (D)

73. **1, 2, 3.** Acetaminophen is an alternative for a client who is allergic to aspirin. It does not affect platelet aggregation and the client does not need to have coagulation studies (such as INR). Acetaminophen causes little or no gastric distress. Acetaminophen exerts no anti-inflammatory effects. (D)

74. **3.** Hypotension, tachycardia, and depressed respirations are signs of high levels of ingestion of muscle relaxants, and the client may be developing a habit of taking this drug for a prolonged period. The potential for abuse should be considered when large doses of a muscle relaxant such as carisoprodol are taken for prolonged periods. Expected common adverse effects would include drowsiness, fatigue, lassitude, blurred vision, headache, ataxia, weakness, and gastrointestinal upset. Hemorrhage from gastrointestinal irritation is not associated with this drug. Hypersensitivity reactions would be manifested by pruritus and rashes. (D)

75. 3. The nursing assessment is first focused on the region distal to the fracture for neurovascular injury or compromise. When a nerve or blood vessel is severed or obstructed at the actual fracture site, innervation to the nerve or blood flow to the vessel is disrupted below the site; therefore, the area distal to the fracture site is the area of compromised neurologic input or vascular flow and return, not the area above the fracture site or the fracture site itself. The nurse may assess the opposite extremity at the area proximal to the fracture site for a baseline comparison of pulse quality, color, temperature, size, and so on, but the comparison would be made after the initial neurovascular assessment. (A)

76. 3. Clients should not pull out cast padding to scratch inside the cast because of the hazard of skin breakdown and subsequent potential for infection. Clients are encouraged to elevate the casted extremity above the level of the heart to reduce edema and to exercise or move the joints above and below the cast to promote and maintain flexibility and muscle strength. Applying ice for 10 minutes during the first 24 hours helps to reduce edema. (R)

77. 2. The client in a double hip spica cast should avoid eating foods that can be constipating, such as cheese. Rather, fresh fruits and vegetables should be encouraged and the client should be encouraged to drink at least 2,500 ml/day. Drinking cranberry juice, which helps keep urine acidic, thereby avoiding the development of renal calculi, is encouraged. The client should be encouraged to establish regular times for elimination to promote regularity in bowel and bladder habits. The client will develop orthostatic hypotension unless the circulatory system is reconditioned slowly through dangling and standing exercises. (A)

78. 2. A two-point gait involves partial weight bearing on each foot, with each crutch advancing simultaneously with the opposing leg. Advancing a crutch on one side and then advancing the opposite foot, and repeating on the opposite side, illustrates the four-point gait. When the client advances both crutches together and follows by lifting both lower extremities to the same level as the crutches, the gait is called a "swing to" gait. When the client advances both crutches together and follows by lifting both lower extremities past the level of the crutches, the gait is called a "swing through" gait. The "swing through" gait is often used by paraplegic clients because it allows them to place weight on their legs while the crutches are moved one stride ahead. (R)

79. 1. The wound was left open with a three-way drainage system in place to irrigate the debrided wound with normal saline or an antibiotic. Before the debridement, a sample of the wound would be taken for culture and sensitivity testing so that an organism-specific antibiotic could be administered to prevent possible serious sequelae of osteomyelitis. Therefore, the nurse should assess the results of the culture and sensitivity report. A pressure dressing would not be applied to an open wound. Rather, a wet-to-dry dressing most likely would be used. There should not be increased pain related to the exposure of nerve endings in the subcutaneous tissue of the wound that was left open to the environment. The bleeding of vessels should be controlled as it would have been if the wound had been closed. Therefore, additional vessel bleeding should not be a problem. (A)

80. 1. The nurse should assess the client's ability to move her toes and for the presence of distal pulses, including a neurovascular assessment of the area below the cast. Increasing pain unrelieved by usual analgesics and occurring 4 to 12 hours after the onset of casting or trauma may be the first sign of compartment syndrome, which can lead to permanent damage to nerves and muscles. Although the nurse can use a pain rating scale or assess for changes in vital signs to objectively assess the client's pain, the client's complaints suggest early and important signs of compartment syndrome requiring immediate intervention. The nurse should not confuse these signs with the potential for drug tolerance. This assessment might be appropriate once the suspicion of compartment syndrome has been ruled out. (A)

81. 4. The client with compartment syndrome may release myoglobin from damaged muscle cells into the circulation. This becomes trapped in the renal tubules, resulting in dark, scanty urine, possibly leading to acute renal failure. Crackles may suggest respiratory complications; jaundice suggests liver failure; and generalized edema may suggest heart failure. However, these are not associated with compartment syndrome. (R)

The Client with a Femoral Fracture

82. 4. Passive immunity for tetanus is provided in the form of tetanus antitoxin or tetanus immune globulin. An antitoxin is an antibody to the toxin of an organism. Administering tetanus toxoid, antigen, or vaccine would provide active immunity by stimulating the body to produce its own antibodies. (D)

83. 4. Skeletal traction is not used to pull weight with a boot. Skeletal traction involves the insertion of a wire or a pin into the bone to maintain a pull of 5 to 45 lb on the area, promoting proper alignment of the fractured bones over a long term. (R)

84. 4. The client with a femoral fracture in balanced suspension traction should not be given a complete bed bath. Rather, the client is encouraged to participate in self-care and movement in bed, such as with a trapeze triangle. Use of a fracture bedpan is appropriate. A fracture bedpan is lower, and it is easier for the client to move on and off the bedpan without altering the line of traction. Checking for areas of redness or pressure over all areas in contact with the traction or bed, including the ischial tuberosity, is important to prevent possible skin breakdown. The client should be positioned so that the feet do not press against the footboard. Therefore, elevating the head of the bed no more than 25 degrees is recommended to keep the client from moving down in the bed. (R)

85. 3. Neurovascular checks should be performed distal or past the site of the splint, not proximal or above the site of the splint, at least every 4 hours. An injury or compromise to the peripheral nervous innervation or blood flow will reflect a change on the site of the splint after the pathway from the heart and brain. Checking the skin over the greater trochanter is appropriate because the half-ring of the Thomas splint can slide around the greater trochanter area where the traction is applied; it should be checked routinely along with other areas at high risk for pressure necrosis, such as the fibular head, ischial tuberosity, malleoli, and hamstring tendons. Inspecting the pin site is appropriate because any drainage or redness might indicate an infection in the bone in which the pin is inserted. Immediate treatment is imperative to avoid osteomyelitis and possible loss of the limb. Evaluation of the foot for movement is important to obtain neuromuscular-vascular data for assessment in comparison with the baseline data of the affected extremity and with the opposite extremity to detect any compromise of the client's condition. (R)

86. 3. The nurse should send the client to the operating room on his bed with extra help to keep the traction from moving to maintain the femur in the proper alignment before surgery. Transferring the client to a cart with manually suspended traction is inappropriate because doing so places the client at risk for additional trauma to the surrounding neurovascular and soft tissues, as would removing the traction. The surgeon need not be called because the decision about transferring the client is an independent nursing action. (R)

87. 1. The Pearson attachment supports the lower leg and provides increased stability in the overall traction set-up. It also makes it easier to maintain correct alignment. It does not support the thigh and upper leg or prevent flexion deformities in the ankle and foot. It is not attached to the skeletal pin. (R)

88. 1. Fat emboli usually result in symptoms of acute respiratory distress syndrome, such as apprehension, chest pain, cyanosis, dyspnea, tachypnea, tachycardia, and decreased partial pressure of arterial oxygen resulting from poor oxygen exchange. Migraine-like headaches are not a symptom of a fat embolism, but mental confusion, memory loss, and a headache from poor oxygen exchange may be seen with central nervous system involvement. Numbness in the right leg is a peripheral neurovascular response that most likely is related to the femoral fracture. Muscle spasms in the right thigh are a symptom of a neuromuscular response affecting the local muscle around the femoral fracture site. (R)

89. 2. Based on the client's statements, *Ineffective coping* is the most appropriate nursing diagnosis because the client is voicing frustration about the current situation and her inability to move. The nurse should seek ways to help the client adjust to and cope with her present state of immobility. Emphasis should be placed on what the client can do to care for herself, such as participating in her daily care and exercises to maintain muscle strength, to help her maintain some control over her situation. The data do not support a diagnosis of *Impaired mobility, Deficient diversional activities,* or *Activity intolerance.* (P)

90. 1. The client can sit up in bed, remaining in the supine position so that an even, sustained amount of traction is maintained under the bandage used in the Buck's traction. Maintenance of even, sustained traction decreases the chance that the bandage or traction strap might slip and cause compression or stress on the nerves or vascular tracts, resulting in permanent damage. The client does not have to remain flat but may adjust the head of the bed to varying degrees of elevation while remaining in the supine position. The client should not turn his body to another position because the bandage may slip. (R)

91. 1. The nurse should assess for signs of skin pressure in the groin area because the Thomas splint, which is a half-ring that slips over the thigh and suspends the lower extremity in direct skeletal traction, may cause discomfort, pressure, or skin irritation in the groin. The nurse always assesses respirations as part of routine vital signs, but assessing for evidence of decreased breath sounds is not a routine assessment related directly to the Thomas splint. The head of the bed can be elevated to facilitate breathing, but not more than 25 degrees, to avoid continually moving the client toward the foot of the bed from the weight of the traction. The nurse always assesses for pressure areas on dependent parts, but assessing for skin breakdown behind the heel is not a routine assessment related directly to the Thomas splint, in which the heel is free of any contact with padding or metal parts of the Pearson attachment for the balanced suspension traction. The client who is in a Thomas splint is able to use a bedpan to urinate, especially the fracture bedpan for a female client and the urinal for a male. Urine retention should not be a special assessment directly related to the Thomas splint, but it may be a client-specific assessment. (R)

92. 1. The client's assisting as much as possible in his care and increasing participation over time indicate that the client has accomplished self-care by gaining a sense of control. If the client lets the nurse complete his care without interfering, his behavior would indicate passivity, possibly from denial or depression. If the client allows his wife to assume total responsibility for his care or to complete his care, he still has a self-care deficit and a successful outcome has not been reached. (C)

93. 2. Fever, night sweats, chills, restlessness, and restrictive movement of the fractured leg are clinical manifestations of osteomyelitis, which is a pyogenic bone infection caused by bacteria (usually staphylococci), a virus, or a fungus. The bone is inaccessible to macrophages and antibodies for protection against infections, so an infection in this site can become serious quickly. The client with a pulmonary or fat embolus would develop symptoms of pulmonary compromise, such as shortness of breath, chest pain, angina, and mental confusion. Signs and symptoms of urinary tract infection would include pain over the suprapubic, groin, or back region with fever and chills, with no restrictive movement of the leg. (R)

94. 1. With osteomyelitis, scar tissue forms because of the continuing presence of the infecting organism, usually *Staphylococcus aureus.* Subsequently, pus and bacteria collect to form avascular tissue. This scar tissue does not absorb the antibiotics. The scar tissue or devitalized (dead) tissue must be scraped from the bone so that antibiotic irrigation can be instituted to clear up the chronic osteomyelitis. (A)

The Client with a Spinal Cord Injury

95. 3. The priority concern is to immobilize the head and neck to prevent further trauma when a fractured vertebra is unstable and easily displaced. Although wrapping and supporting the extremities is important, it does not take priority over immobilizing the head and neck. Pain usually is not a significant consideration with this type of injury. Cushioning is contraindicated. The neck should be kept in a neutral position and immobilized. Flexion of the neck is avoided. (S)

96. 3. This client has a spinal cord injury of the sacral region of the spinal cord and will have bladder and bowel dysfunction, as well as loss of sensation and muscle control below the injury. The other options are true of a client who has quadriplegia. (A)

97. 2. Although assessment of renal status, gastrointestinal function, and biliary function is important, with the spinal cord transection at T4 the client's vascular status is the primary focus of the nursing assessment because the sympathetic feedback system is lost and the client is at risk for hypotension and bradycardia. (A)

98. 1. The client with a spinal cord transection above T5 is least likely to develop diarrhea. Rather, constipation due to atonia would be possible. The client with a spinal cord transection above T5 is at risk for development of a paralytic ileus because the sympathetic nerve innervation to the vagus nerve, which dominates all the vessels and organs below T5 (e.g., the intestinal tract), has been disrupted and therefore so has movement or peristalsis. The client is at risk for development of stress ulcers because the sympathetic nerve innervation to the stomach has been disrupted, which results in an excessive release of hydrochloric acid in the stomach, allowing contact of hydrochloric acid with the stomach mucosa. The client does not feel subjective signs of stress ulcers (e.g., pain, guarding, tenderness) and therefore is at increased risk for bleeding because complications of an ulcer can develop before early diagnosis. (R)

99. 1. The client should eat enough calories to maintain her desired weight, a positive nitrogen balance, and enough protein to help decrease the rate of muscle atrophy and prevent skin breakdown and infection. The client with a spinal cord injury does not have poikilothermy, the ability to adjust body temperature to the environmental temperature. The client should add additional clothes or coverage below the level of transection in cool environments. The client does not sweat below the level of transection and should be sensitive to the possibility of overheating in extremely hot climates and the need for sprinkling or moving into an air-conditioned environment. The client with intermittent nasogastric suctioning is at risk for development of metabolic alkalosis and an electrolyte imbalance that leads to decreased tissue perfusion; therefore, the client needs to increase the sodium and potassium in her diet, not decrease the sodium. (R)

100. 4. Measuring the leg girth is the most appropriate method because the usual signs, such as a positive Homans' sign, pain, and tenderness, are not present. Other means of assessing for deep vein thrombosis in a client with a spinal cord injury are through a Doppler examination and impedance plethysmography. (R)

101. 3. During the period of spinal shock, the bladder is completely atonic and will continue to fill passively unless the client is catheterized. The bladder will not go into spasms or cause uncontrolled urination. Bladder function will not be normal during the period of spinal shock. (R)

102. 4. The movements occur from muscle reflexes and cannot be initiated or controlled by the brain. After the period of spinal shock, the muscles gradually become spastic owing to an increased sensitivity of the lower motor neurons. It is an expected occurrence and does not indicate that healing is taking place or that the client will walk again. The movement is not voluntary and cannot be brought under voluntary control. (A)

103. 3. Long-bone demineralization is a serious consequence of the loss of weight bearing. An excessive calcium load is brought to the kidneys, and precipitation may occur, predisposing to stone formation. Excessive intake of dairy products may promote constipation. However, this is not the most accurate reason for decreasing calcium intake. Immobility does not increase calcium absorption from the intestine. Dairy products do not necessarily contribute to weight gain. (C)

104. **2.** The woman with spinal cord injury can participate in sexual activity but might not experience orgasm. Cessation in the nerve pathway may occur in spinal cord injury, but this does not negate the client's mental and emotional needs to creatively participate with her partner in a sexual relationship and to reach orgasm. An indwelling urinary catheter may be left in place during intercourse and need not be removed because the indwelling urinary catheter is placed in the urethra, which is not the channel used for sexual intercourse. There are no contraindications, such as hypertension, to sexual activity in a woman with spinal cord injury. Sexual intercourse is allowed, and hypertension should be manageable. Because a spinal cord injury does not affect fertility, the client should have access to family planning information so that an unplanned pregnancy can be avoided. (C)

105. **3.** Spinal cord injury represents a physical loss; grief is the normal response to this loss. Working through grief entails reviewing memories and eventually letting go of them. The process may take as long as 2 years. Telling the client to be patient and that adjustment takes time is a clichéd type of response, one that is not empathetic or responsive to the client's needs. Telling the client to focus on today does not allow time for the grief process, which is necessary for the client to work through and adjust to the loss. The client is not escaping but is reminiscing on what is lost, to work through the grieving process. (P)

The Client with Cancer

The Client at Risk for Cancer

1. Which of the following clients is at highest risk for colorectal cancer?
- [ ] **1.** The client who smokes.
- [ ] **2.** The client who eats a vegetarian diet.
- [ ] **3.** The client who has been treated for Crohn's disease for 20 years.
- [ ] **4.** The client who has a family history of lung cancer.

2. A 21-year-old client undergoes bone marrow aspiration at the clinic to establish a diagnosis of possible lymphoma. Which statement made by the client demonstrates proper understanding of discharge teaching? Select all that apply.
- [ ] **1.** "I will take Tylenol for pain."
- [ ] **2.** "I do not need to inspect the puncture site."
- [ ] **3.** "I will not be able to play basketball for the next 2 days."
- [ ] **4.** "I will take aspirin if I have pain."
- [ ] **5.** "I can apply an ice pack or a cold compress to the puncture site."

3. A nurse is conducting a cancer risk screening program. Which of the following clients is at greatest risk for skin cancer?
- [ ] **1.** 45-year-old physician.
- [ ] **2.** 15-year-old high school student.
- [ ] **3.** 30-year-old butcher.
- [ ] **4.** 60-year-old mountain biker.

4. Which of the following would be considered an iatrogenic cause of cancer?
- [ ] **1.** Ionizing radiation from radon.
- [ ] **2.** Ionizing radiation from uranium ore.
- [ ] **3.** X-rays used to treat a tumor.
- [ ] **4.** Ultraviolet radiation from the sun.

5. An epidemiologic study or investigation is to be conducted on workers in uranium mines who are currently free of any cancer. Subjects are to be monitored over a 5-year period, and the incidence rates of certain types of cancers are to be determined. This study design illustrates what kind of research study?
- [ ] **1.** Prospective study.
- [ ] **2.** Historical retrospective study.
- [ ] **3.** Retrospective study.
- [ ] **4.** Historical prospective study.

6. Carcinogenesis is irreversible in which of the following stages?
- [ ] **1.** Progression stage.
- [ ] **2.** Promotion stage.
- [ ] **3.** Initiation stage.
- [ ] **4.** Regression stage.

7. Cancer prevalence is defined as:
- [ ] **1.** The likelihood cancer will occur in a lifetime.
- [ ] **2.** The number of persons with cancer at a given point in time.
- [ ] **3.** The number of new cancers in a year.
- [ ] **4.** All cancer cases more than 5 years old.

8. Which of the following groups would benefit most from education regarding potential risk factors for melanoma?
- [ ] **1.** Adults older than age 35.
- [ ] **2.** Senior citizens who have been repeatedly exposed to the effects of ultraviolet A and ultraviolet B rays.
- [ ] **3.** Parents with children.
- [ ] **4.** Employees of a chemical factory.

9. A nurse is providing education in a community setting about general measures to avoid excessive sun exposure. Which of the following recommendations is appropriate?
- ☐ 1. Apply sunscreen only after going into the water.
- ☐ 2. Avoid peak exposure hours from 9 a.m. to 1 p.m.
- ☐ 3. Wear loosely woven clothing for added ventilation.
- ☐ 4. Apply sunscreen with a sun protection factor (SPF) of 15 or more before sun exposure.

10. A 29-year-old woman is concerned about her personal risk factors for malignant melanoma. She is upset because her 49-year-old sister was recently diagnosed with the disease. After gathering information about the client's history of sun exposure, the nurse's best response would be to explain that:
- ☐ 1. Some melanomas have a familial component and she should seek medical advice.
- ☐ 2. Her personal risk is low because most melanomas occur at age 60 or later.
- ☐ 3. Her personal risk is low because melanoma does not have a familial component.
- ☐ 4. She should not worry because she did not experience severe sunburn as a child.

11. A nurse is palpating a female client's breast while assessing for breast disease. In the illustration below, indicate the area of the breast in which tumors are most commonly found.

12. While being educated by the nurse about breast self-examination, a client asks what the rationale is for moving her arms in different positions while standing in front of a mirror. The nurse explains that these positions are used to:
- ☐ 1. Increase the examiner's comfort during procedure.
- ☐ 2. More easily diagnose any masses.
- ☐ 3. Determine whether there is any nipple discharge with movement.
- ☐ 4. Emphasize any change in shape or contour of the breast.

13. A 17-year-old, sexually active female client is seen in the family planning clinic and requests hormonal contraceptives. Before examination, the nurse should explain the importance of regular Papanicolaou (Pap) smears. This recommendation is based on the current screening guidelines of the American Cancer Society for Pap smears, which state that:
- ☐ 1. Pap smears are recommended every other year.
- ☐ 2. If four consecutive annual Pap smears are negative, the client should schedule repeat Pap smears every 3 years.
- ☐ 3. The initial Pap smear should be done at age 21 or earlier if the woman is sexually active.
- ☐ 4. If four consecutive smears are negative, the client should request a colposcopy.

14. A client with a family history of cancer asks the nurse what the single most important risk factor is for cancer. Which of the following risk factors should the nurse discuss?
- ☐ 1. Family history.
- ☐ 2. Lifestyle choices.
- ☐ 3. Age.
- ☐ 4. Menopause or hormonal events.

15. Experimental and epidemiologic evidence suggests that a high-fat diet increases the risk of several cancers. Which of the following cancers is linked to a high-fat diet?
- ☐ 1. Ovarian.
- ☐ 2. Lung.
- ☐ 3. Colon.
- ☐ 4. Liver.

16. A 42-year-old female highway construction worker is concerned about her cancer risks. She reveals that she has been married for 18 years, has two children, smokes one pack of cigarettes per day, and drinks one to two beers with her husband after work almost every day. She is 30 lb overweight, eats fast food often, and rarely eats fresh fruits and vegetables. Her mother was diagnosed with breast cancer 2 years ago. Her father and an aunt both died of lung cancer. She had a basal cell carcinoma removed from her cheek 3 years earlier. What behavioral changes should the nurse instruct this client to make first?
- ☐ 1. Decrease fat in the diet, decrease alcohol consumption, and use sunscreen every day.
- ☐ 2. Decrease intake of salt-cured food, lose weight, and stop smoking.
- ☐ 3. Stop drinking beer, decrease fiber in the diet, and use sun protection.
- ☐ 4. Stop smoking, use sun protection, and lose weight.

17. A nurse who is teaching smoking cessation programs to healthy adult smokers is participating in what type of prevention activity?
- ☐ 1. Primary.
- ☐ 2. Secondary.
- ☐ 3. Tertiary.
- ☐ 4. Nonspecific.

18. The incidence and risk of cancer increase when smoking is combined with:
☐ **1.** Asbestos exposure and alcohol consumption.
☐ **2.** Ultraviolet radiation exposure and alcohol consumption.
☐ **3.** Asbestos exposure and ultraviolet radiation exposure.
☐ **4.** Alcohol consumption and human papillomavirus (HPV) infection.

19. A 60-year-old male comes to the clinic with complaints of hoarseness. What information will be helpful in determining his risk for head and neck cancer?
☐ **1.** Patterns of medication use and history of alcohol consumption.
☐ **2.** Exposure to sun and family history of head and neck cancers.
☐ **3.** Exposure to wood dust and a high-fat diet.
☐ **4.** History of tobacco use and alcohol consumption.

20. A 42-year-old female is interested in making dietary changes to reduce her risk of colon cancer. What dietary selections should the nurse suggest?
☐ **1.** Croissant, granola and peanut butter squares, whole milk.
☐ **2.** Bran muffin, skim milk, stir-fried broccoli.
☐ **3.** Granola, bagel with cream cheese, cauliflower salad.
☐ **4.** Oatmeal, raisin cookies, baked potato with sour cream, turkey sandwich.

21. Which of the following is an environmental factor that increases the risk of cancer?
☐ **1.** Gender.
☐ **2.** Nutrition.
☐ **3.** Immunologic status.
☐ **4.** Age.

22. A client at risk for lung cancer asks why he is scheduled for a computed tomography (CT) scan as part of his initial workup. The nurse's best response is which of the following?
☐ **1.** "CT is far superior to magnetic resonance imaging for evaluating lymph node metastasis."
☐ **2.** "CT is noninvasive and readily available."
☐ **3.** "CT is useful for distinguishing small differences in tissue density and detecting nodal involvement."
☐ **4.** "CT can distinguish a malignant from a nonmalignant adenopathy."

23. Lifestyle influences that are considered risk factors for colorectal cancer include:
☐ **1.** A diet low in vitamin C.
☐ **2.** A high dietary intake of artificial sweeteners (Aspartame).
☐ **3.** A high-fat, low-fiber diet.
☐ **4.** Multiple sex partners.

24. The development of a culturally sensitive health education program for the socioeconomically disadvantaged requires the nurse to:
☐ **1.** Locate the program at an existing government facility.
☐ **2.** Integrate folk beliefs and traditions into the content.
☐ **3.** Prepare materials in the primary language of the program sponsor.
☐ **4.** Exclude community leaders from initial planning efforts.

The Client with Pain

25. The nurse-manager on the oncology unit wants to address the issue of correct documentation on the effectiveness of the analgesia medication within 30 minutes after administration. What should the nurse-manager do first?
☐ **1.** Change the policy of documentation to 45 minutes.
☐ **2.** Consult the pharmacist.
☐ **3.** Consult the nurses on the evening shift where documentation of analgesia is the greatest problem.
☐ **4.** Complete a brief quality improvement study and chart audit to document the rate of adherence to the policy and the pattern of documentation over shifts.

26. A client is transferred to his room from the intensive care unit after a craniotomy for treatment of a malignant brain tumor in the occipital region. The nurse should question which of these orders?
☐ **1.** 400 mg of ibuprofen (Motrin).
☐ **2.** 500 mg of naproxen (Naprosyn).
☐ **3.** Morphine sulfate.
☐ **4.** Acetaminophen (Tylenol).

27. A 62-year-old female is taking long-acting morphine 120 mg every 12 hours for pain from metastatic breast cancer. She can have 20 mg of immediate-release morphine every 3 to 4 hours as needed for breakthrough pain. The physician should be notified if the client uses more than how many breakthrough doses of morphine in 24 hours?
☐ **1.** Seven.
☐ **2.** Four.
☐ **3.** Two.
☐ **4.** One.

28. In addition to acetaminophen, which drugs are recommended from step 1 of the World Health Organization (WHO) analgesic ladder for the treatment of mild to moderate cancer-related pain?
☐ **1.** Oxycodone.
☐ **2.** Nonsteroidal anti-inflammatory drugs (NSAIDs).
☐ **3.** Codeine.
☐ **4.** Propoxyphene.

29. Assessment of a client taking a nonsteroidal anti-inflammatory drug (NSAID) for pain management should include specific questions regarding which of the following systems?
☐ **1.** Gastrointestinal.
☐ **2.** Renal.
☐ **3.** Pulmonary.
☐ **4.** Cardiac.

30. Which of the following best describes a client's response to chronic pain?
☐ **1.** Elevated vital signs, physical inactivity, facial grimacing, and periods of anxiety.
☐ **2.** Normal vital signs, physical inactivity, and normal facial expressions.
☐ **3.** Normal vital signs, normal facial expressions, and moaning.
☐ **4.** Elevated vital signs, grimacing, and depression.

31. Which of the following terms describes the condition of a client who requires an increase in dosage to maintain adequate analgesia?
☐ **1.** Pseudoaddiction.
☐ **2.** Physical dependence.
☐ **3.** Psychological dependence.
☐ **4.** Drug tolerance.

32. A client with lung cancer is being cared for by his wife at home. His pain is increasing in severity. The nurse recognizes that teaching has been effective when the wife does which of the following? Select all that apply.
☐ **1.** Administers long-acting or sustained-release oral pain formula (OxyContin) regularly around-the-clock.
☐ **2.** Administers immediate-release medication (oxycodone) for breakthrough pain.
☐ **3.** Avoids long-acting opioids due to her concern about addiction.
☐ **4.** Uses music for distraction as well as heat or cold in combination with medications.
☐ **5.** Substitutes acetaminophen (Tylenol) to avoid tolerance to the medications.
☐ **6.** Has her husband use a pain rating scale to measure the effectiveness at reaching his individual pain goal.

33. A client is experiencing severe pain from advanced cancer disease. The client's son is concerned about the drugs the client has taken and wonders which are the best. The nurse tells him that, overall, the drug of choice to treat advanced cancer pain is:
☐ **1.** methadone (Dolophine).
☐ **2.** oxycodone.
☐ **3.** morphine sulfate.
☐ **4.** hydromorphone (Dilaudid).

34. A 52-year-old male was discharged from the hospital for cancer-related pain. His pain appeared to be well controlled on the I.V. morphine. He was switched to oral morphine when discharged 2 days ago. He now reports his pain as an 8 on a 10-point scale and wants the I.V. morphine. Which of the following represents the most likely explanation for the client's reports of inadequate pain control?
☐ **1.** He is addicted to the I.V. morphine.
☐ **2.** He is going through withdrawal from the I.V. opioid.
☐ **3.** He is physically dependent on the I.V. morphine.
☐ **4.** He is undermedicated on the oral opioid.

35. A nurse is assessing a client with bone cancer pain. Which of the following components of a thorough pain assessment is most significant for this client?
☐ **1.** Intensity.
☐ **2.** Cause.
☐ **3.** Aggravating factors.
☐ **4.** Location.

36. A 48-year-old client with cancer has been receiving 10 mg of I.V. morphine while hospitalized. In order to give an equivalent dose of oral morphine, the nurse should be sure the physician has ordered which of the following doses?
☐ **1.** 25 mg.
☐ **2.** 30 mg.
☐ **3.** 40 mg.
☐ **4.** 10 mg.

37. Which of the following reasons explains why meperidine (Demerol) is not recommended for chronic cancer-related pain?
☐ **1.** It has a high potential for abuse.
☐ **2.** It has agonist-antagonist properties.
☐ **3.** It must be given intramuscularly to be effective.
☐ **4.** It contains a metabolite that causes seizures.

38. A 60-year-old female with chronic cancer pain has been receiving opiates for 4 months. She rated her pain as an 8 on a 10-point scale before starting the opioid medication. She has just had a thorough examination with no new evidence of increased disease, yet her pain is close to 8 again. The most likely explanation for her increasing pain is:
☐ **1.** Development of an addiction to the opioids.
☐ **2.** Tolerance to the opioid.
☐ **3.** Withdrawal from the opioid.
☐ **4.** Placebo effect has decreased.

39. The nurse teaches the client with chronic cancer pain about optimal pain control. Which of the following recommendations is most effective for pain control?

☐ 1. Get used to some pain and use a little less medication than needed to keep from being addicted.

☐ 2. Take prescribed analgesics on an around-the-clock schedule to prevent recurrent pain.

☐ 3. Take analgesics only when pain returns.

☐ 4. Take enough analgesics around the clock so that you can sleep 12 to 16 hours a day to block the pain.

The Client Who Is Receiving Chemotherapy

40. The nurse is caring for a 78-year-old male with lung cancer who is receiving chemotherapy. The client states he is not eating well but otherwise feels healthy. Which meal suggestion would be best for this client?

☐ 1. Cereal with milk and strawberries.

☐ 2. Toast, gelatin dessert, and cookies.

☐ 3. Broiled chicken, green beans, and cottage cheese.

☐ 4. Steak and french fries.

41. A nurse is assessing a female who is receiving her second administration of chemotherapy for breast cancer. When obtaining this client's health history, what is the most important information the nurse should obtain?

☐ 1. "Has your hair been falling out in clumps?"

☐ 2. "Have you had nausea or vomiting?"

☐ 3. "Have you been sleeping at night?"

☐ 4. "Do you have your usual energy level?"

42. A 68-year-old male has been receiving monthly doses of chemotherapy for treatment of stage III colon cancer. He comes to the clinic for his fourth monthly dose. Which laboratory result should be reported to the oncologist before the next dose of chemotherapy is administered? Select all that apply.

☐ 1. Hemoglobin of 14.5 g/dl.

☐ 2. Platelet count of 40,000/mm³.

☐ 3. Blood urea nitrogen (BUN) level of 12 mg/dl.

☐ 4. White blood cell count of 2,300/mm³.

☐ 5. Temperature of 101.2° F (38.4° C).

☐ 6. Urine specific gravity of 1.020.

43. A nurse is checking the laboratory results of a 52-year-old client with colon cancer admitted for further chemotherapy. The client has lost 30 lb (13.6 kg) since initiation of the treatment. Which laboratory result should be reported?

☐ 1. Blood glucose level of 95 mg/dl.

☐ 2. Total cholesterol level of 182 mg/dl.

☐ 3. Hemoglobin level of 12.3 mg/dl.

☐ 4. Albumin level of 2.8 g/dl.

44. The nurse is teaching a 17-year-old client and the client's family about what to expect with high-dose chemotherapy and the effects of neutropenia. What should the nurse teach as the most reliable early indicator of infection in a neutropenic client?

☐ 1. Fever.

☐ 2. Chills.

☐ 3. Tachycardia.

☐ 4. Dyspnea.

45. A nurse is caring for a client who is undergoing chemotherapy. Current laboratory values are noted on the chart below. Which action would be most appropriate for the nurse to implement?

☐ 1. Wearing a protective gown and particulate respiratory mask when completing treatments.

☐ 2. Washing hands before and after entering the room.

☐ 3. Restricting visitors.

☐ 4. Contacting the physician for an order for hematopoietic factors such as erythropoietin (Epogen, Procrit).

LABORATORY RESULTS	
Test	**Result**
Hemoglobin	12.0 mg/dl
Hematocrit	34%
Platelet count	108,000/mm³
White blood cell (WBC) count	1,600/mm³
Absolute neutrophil count (ANC)	less than 1,000/mm³

46. A client informs the nurse that she is using an herbal therapy while receiving chemotherapy. Which of the following actions should the nurse take?

☐ 1. Determine what substances the client is using and make sure that the physician is aware of all therapies the client is using.

☐ 2. Guide the client in the decision-making process to select either Western or alternative medicine.

☐ 3. Encourage the client to seek alternative modalities that do not require the ingestion of substances.

☐ 4. Recommend that the client stop using the alternative medicines immediately.

47. A 58-year-old male is going to have chemotherapy for lung cancer. He asks the nurse how the chemotherapeutic drugs will work. The most accurate explanation the nurse can give is which of the following?

☐ 1. "Chemotherapy affects all rapidly dividing cells."

☐ 2. "The molecular structure of the DNA is altered."

☐ 3. "Cancer cells are susceptible to drug toxins."

☐ 4. "Chemotherapy encourages cancer cells to divide."

48. A 56-year-old client is receiving chemotherapy that has the potential to cause pulmonary toxicity. Which of the following symptoms indicates a toxic response to the chemotherapy?
- [ ] 1. Decrease in appetite.
- [ ] 2. Drowsiness.
- [ ] 3. Spasms of the diaphragm.
- [ ] 4. Cough and shortness of breath.

The Client Who Is Receiving Radiation Therapy

49. A female receiving radiation therapy for lung cancer complains to the radiation oncology nurse that she is having difficulty sleeping. What should the nurse do?
- [ ] 1. Suggest the client stop watching television before bed.
- [ ] 2. Assess the client's usual sleep patterns, amount of sleep, and bedtime rituals.
- [ ] 3. Tell the client sleeplessness is expected with radiation therapy.
- [ ] 4. Suggest that the client stop drinking coffee until the therapy is completed.

50. A 56-year-old female is currently receiving radiation therapy to the chest wall for recurrent breast cancer. She calls her health care provider to report that she has pain while swallowing and burning and tightness in her chest. Which of the following complications of radiation therapy is most likely responsible for her symptoms?
- [ ] 1. Hiatal hernia.
- [ ] 2. Stomatitis.
- [ ] 3. Radiation enteritis.
- [ ] 4. Esophagitis.

51. A 48-year-old female is receiving radiation therapy for treatment of breast cancer. She reports to the clinic today complaining of apathy, impaired concentration, and feeling tired all the time even though she is sleeping more and more. These complaints suggest symptoms of:
- [ ] 1. Advanced breast cancer.
- [ ] 2. Fatigue.
- [ ] 3. Hypocalcemia.
- [ ] 4. Radiation pneumonitis.

52. A 36-year-old female is scheduled to receive external radiation therapy and a cesium implant for cancer of the cervix. Which of the following statements would be most accurate to include in the teaching plan about the potential effects of radiation therapy on sexuality?
- [ ] 1. "You can have sexual intercourse while the implant is in place."
- [ ] 2. "You may notice some vaginal dryness after treatment is completed."
- [ ] 3. "You may notice some vaginal relaxation after treatment is completed."
- [ ] 4. "You will continue to have normal menstrual periods during treatment."

53. The nurse caring for a client who is receiving external beam radiation therapy for treatment of lung cancer should anticipate that the client will have which of the following?
- [ ] 1. Diarrhea.
- [ ] 2. Improved energy level.
- [ ] 3. Dysphagia.
- [ ] 4. Normal white blood cell count.

The Client Who Requires Symptom Management

54. A client with bladder cancer has lost a large amount of blood from the tumor in his urine. The blood loss is estimated at approximately 500 ml. Because his hemoglobin is 8.0 g/dl, the physician orders a unit of packed blood cells. To administer the packed red blood cells, the nurse should:
- [ ] 1. Attach the packed cells to the existing 19G I.V. of normal saline solution using Y tubing.
- [ ] 2. Start an additional 22G I.V. site because the packed blood cells must be given in a separate line.
- [ ] 3. Attach the packed blood cells to the existing 22G I.V. of 5% dextrose using Y tubing.
- [ ] 4. Start an additional I.V. access device with a 22G Intracath.

55. A nurse is caring for a client 24 hours after he has undergone an abdominal-perineal resection for a bowel tumor. The client's wife asks if she can bring him some of his favorite home-cooked Italian minestrone soup. What would be an appropriate action by the nurse?
- [ ] 1. Auscultate for bowel sounds.
- [ ] 2. Ask the client if he feels hunger or gas pains.
- [ ] 3. Consult the dietician.
- [ ] 4. Encourage the wife to bring the soup.

56. A registered nurse (RN) instructs the unlicensed assistive personnel (UAP) to check the urine intake and output (I&O) on clients on the oncology unit at the end of the 8-hour shift. It is important for the nurse to instruct the UAP to do what?
- [ ] 1. Ask the clients if they are thirsty when calculating the I&O.
- [ ] 2. Report back to the nurse immediately if any client has an output less than 240 ml.
- [ ] 3. Document the I&O results on the medical records.
- [ ] 4. Write the I&O results down for the nurse to give report to the next shift.

57. When assessing the client with lung cancer who is dyspneic, the nurse observes which of the following behaviors?
- [ ] 1. Euphoria.
- [ ] 2. Anger.
- [ ] 3. Anxiety.
- [ ] 4. Laziness.

58. A nurse in charge of the oncology outpatient office is making follow-up phone calls. Place the options below in the order of priority that the nurse should return the calls.

> **1.** The client receiving chemotherapy who complains of a loss of appetite.

> **2.** The client who underwent a mastectomy 2 weeks ago who called for information on the Reach for Recovery program.

> **3.** The client receiving spinal radiation for bone cancer metastases who complains of urinary incontinence.

> **4.** The client with colon cancer who has questions about a high-fiber diet.

>

>

>

>

59. Which of the following nursing interventions would be most helpful in making the respiratory effort of a client with metastatic lung cancer more efficient?
- [ ] **1.** Teaching the client diaphragmatic breathing techniques.
- [ ] **2.** Administering cough suppressants as ordered.
- [ ] **3.** Teaching and encouraging pursed-lip breathing.
- [ ] **4.** Placing the client in a low semi-Fowler's position.

60. Which of the following should be included in the teaching plan for a cancer client who is experiencing thrombocytopenia? Select all that apply.
- [ ] **1.** Use an electric razor.
- [ ] **2.** Use a soft-bristle toothbrush.
- [ ] **3.** Avoid frequent flossing for oral care.
- [ ] **4.** Include an over-the-counter nonsteroidal anti-inflammatory (NSAID) daily for pain control.
- [ ] **5.** Monitor temperature daily.
- [ ] **6.** Report bleeding, such as nosebleed, petechiae, or melena, to a health care professional.

61. A 28-year-old client with cancer is afraid of experiencing a febrile reaction associated with blood transfusions. He asks the nurse if this will happen to him. The nurse's best response is which of the following?
- [ ] **1.** "Febrile reactions are caused when antibodies on the surface of blood cells in the transfusion are directed against antigens of the recipient."
- [ ] **2.** "Febrile reactions can usually be prevented by administering antipyretics and antihistamines before the start of the transfusion."
- [ ] **3.** "Febrile reactions are rarely immune-mediated reactions and can be a sign of hemolytic transfusion."
- [ ] **4.** "Febrile reactions primarily occur within 15 minutes after initiation of the transfusion and can occur during the blood transfusion."

62. A 56-year-old male client is admitted to the oncology unit for dyspnea. He recently had a pneumonectomy for treatment of lung cancer. The client has not had other cancer treatment therapies. The increased dyspnea is most likely caused by:
- [ ] **1.** Fibrotic changes in lung parenchyma.
- [ ] **2.** Pneumonia or bronchitis.
- [ ] **3.** Anemia related to myelosuppression.
- [ ] **4.** Pericardial effusion.

63. Which of the following has been associated with fatigue from cancer chemotherapy?
- [ ] **1.** Decreased quality of life.
- [ ] **2.** Increased risk of infection.
- [ ] **3.** Improved disease prognosis.
- [ ] **4.** Increased pain.

64. When the nurse is teaching the client and family how to manage possible nausea and vomiting at home, which of the following should be discussed?
- [ ] **1.** Eating frequent, small meals throughout the day.
- [ ] **2.** Eating three normal meals a day.
- [ ] **3.** Eating only cold foods with no odor.
- [ ] **4.** Limiting the amount of fluid intake.

65. A terminally ill 82-year-old client in hospice care is experiencing nausea and vomiting because of a partial bowel obstruction. Conservative management of the nausea and vomiting may be achieved with the use of:
- [ ] **1.** A nasogastric (NG) suction tube.
- [ ] **2.** I.V. antiemetics.
- [ ] **3.** Osmotic laxatives.
- [ ] **4.** A clear liquid diet.

66. A 62-year-old male is dying from metastatic lung cancer, and all treatments have been discontinued. The client's breathing pattern is labored, with gurgling sounds. The client's wife asks the nurse, "Can't you do something to help with his breathing?" Which of the following is the nurse's best response in this situation?

☐ 1. Direct the unlicensed personnel to assess the client's vital signs and provide oral care.

☐ 2. Suction the client so that the client's wife knows all interventions were performed.

☐ 3. Reposition the client, elevate the head of the bed, and provide a cool compress.

☐ 4. Explain to the wife that dying clients do not need suctioning.

67. A 40-year-old female is losing most of her hair as a result of chemotherapy. Which of the following statements best explains chemotherapy-induced alopecia?

☐ 1. "The new growth of hair will be gray."

☐ 2. "The hair loss is temporary."

☐ 3. "New hair growth will always be the same texture and color as it was before chemotherapy."

☐ 4. "The client should avoid use of wigs when possible."

68. A 62-year-old male with a history of chronic obstructive pulmonary disease (COPD) and metastatic carcinoma of the lung has not responded to radiation therapy and is being admitted to the hospice program. Initial client assessment will most likely reveal that the client has:

☐ 1. Ascites.

☐ 2. Pleural friction rub.

☐ 3. Dyspnea.

☐ 4. Peripheral edema.

69. The nurse is working with a client who has cancer to improve the client's independence in activities of daily living after radiation therapy. Which of the following is an appropriate nursing intervention?

☐ 1. Refer the client to a community support group after discharge from the rehabilitation unit.

☐ 2. Make certain that a family member is present for the rehabilitation sessions.

☐ 3. Provide positive reinforcement for skills achieved.

☐ 4. Inform the client of rehabilitation plans made by the rehabilitation team.

70. When teaching about prevention of infection to a client with a long-term venous catheter, the nurse can document that the client has understood discharge instructions when the client states which of the following?

☐ 1. "I will not remove the dressing until I return to the clinic next week."

☐ 2. "My husband or I will do the dressing changes three times per week, exactly the way you showed us."

☐ 3. "I will monitor my temperature once each weekday."

☐ 4. "I know it is very important to wash my hands after irrigating the catheter."

71. When caring for a client with a central venous line, which of the following nursing actions should be implemented in the plan of care for chemotherapy administration? Select all that apply.

☐ 1. Verify patency of the line by the presence of a blood return at regular intervals.

☐ 2. Inspect the insertion site for swelling, erythema, or drainage.

☐ 3. Administer a cytotoxic agent to keep the regimen on schedule even if blood return is not present.

☐ 4. If unable to aspirate blood, reposition the client and encourage the client to cough.

☐ 5. Contact the health care provider about verifying placement if the status is questionable.

72. Indicate on the illustration the area that correctly identifies the position of the distal tip of a central line that is inserted into the subclavian vessel.

73. A 58-year-old client with pancreatic cancer, who has been bed-bound for 3 weeks, has just returned from having a left subclavian, long-term, tunneled catheter inserted for administration of analgesics. The nurse has not yet received radiographic results for confirmation of placement. The client becomes restless and dyspneic and complains of chest pain radiating to the middle of his back. Physical assessment reveals tachycardia and absent breath sounds in the left lung. The nurse suspects that the client is experiencing:

☐ 1. An air embolus.

☐ 2. A pneumothorax.

☐ 3. A pulmonary embolus.

☐ 4. A myocardial infarction.

74. In setting goals for a client with advanced liver cancer who has poor nutrition, the nurse determines that which of the following is a realistic desired outcome for the client? The client will:

☐ 1. Have normalized albumin levels.

☐ 2. Return to ideal body weight.

☐ 3. Gain 1 lb every 2 weeks.

☐ 4. Maintain current weight.

75. The nurse administers a bolus tube feeding to a client with cancer. Which of the following nursing interventions is most appropriate to decrease the risk of aspiration?

☐ **1.** Place the client on bed rest with the head of the bed elevated to 60 degrees for 2 hours.

☐ **2.** Place the client on the left side with the head of the bed at 45 degrees for 15 minutes.

☐ **3.** Assist the client out of bed to sit upright in a chair for 1 hour.

☐ **4.** Ask the client to rest in bed with the head of the bed elevated to 30 degrees for 20 minutes.

76. A client with colon cancer had a left hemicolectomy 3 weeks previously. The client is still having difficulty maintaining an adequate oral intake to meet metabolic needs for optimal healing. Which of the following nutritional support methods should the nurse anticipate for the client?

☐ **1.** Total parenteral nutrition through a central catheter.

☐ **2.** I.V. infusion of dextrose.

☐ **3.** Nasogastric feeding tube with protein supplement.

☐ **4.** Jejunostomy for high caloric feedings.

77. A client with colon cancer undergoes surgical removal of a segment of colon and creation of a sigmoid colostomy. What assessments by the nurse indicate the client is developing complications within the first 24 hours? Select all that apply.

☐ **1.** Coarse breath sounds auscultated bilaterally at the bases.

☐ **2.** Dusky appearance of the stoma.

☐ **3.** No drainage in the ostomy appliance.

☐ **4.** Temperature greater than 101.2° F (38.5° C).

☐ **5.** Decreased bowel sounds.

78. A client with stomach cancer is admitted to the oncology unit after vomiting for 3 days. Physical assessment findings include irregular pulse, muscle twitching, and complaints of prickling sensations in the fingers and hands. Laboratory results include a potassium level of 2.9 mEq/L, a pH of 7.46, and a bicarbonate level of 29 mEq/L. The client is experiencing:

☐ **1.** Respiratory alkalosis.

☐ **2.** Respiratory acidosis.

☐ **3.** Metabolic alkalosis.

☐ **4.** Metabolic acidosis.

79. A 32-year-old female meets with the nurse on her first office visit since undergoing a left mastectomy. When asked how she is doing, the woman says her appetite is still not good, she is not getting much sleep because she doesn't go to bed until her husband is asleep, and she is really anxious to get back to work. Which of the following nursing interventions should the nurse explore to support the client's current needs?

☐ **1.** Call the physician to discuss allowing the client to return to work earlier.

☐ **2.** Suggest that the client learn relaxation techniques for help with her insomnia.

☐ **3.** Perform a nutritional assessment to assess for anorexia.

☐ **4.** Ask open-ended questions about sexuality issues related to her mastectomy.

80. Which of the following client situations would require the most intensive nursing interventions for immobility?

☐ **1.** A 38-year-old woman receiving internal radiation therapy for cervical cancer.

☐ **2.** A 7-year-old boy with leukemia hospitalized for induction of high-dose chemotherapy.

☐ **3.** A 75-year-old man with metastatic prostate cancer hospitalized for a pathologic fracture of the femur.

☐ **4.** A 6-month-old undergoing surgery for placement of a central venous catheter.

81. Immobility affects several body systems because of a reduction in the amount of weight-bearing and physical activity. Which of the following is most indicative of the changes that can occur with immobility?

☐ **1.** Cardiovascular workload increases, lung expansion increases.

☐ **2.** Cardiovascular workload decreases, lung expansion increases.

☐ **3.** Cardiovascular workload increases, metabolism decreases.

☐ **4.** Metabolism increases, lung expansion decreases.

82. A 52-year-old client with lung cancer is calling the outpatient center with complaints of a low-grade fever (100.6° F [38.1° C]), nonproductive cough, and increasing fatigue. He completed the radiation therapy to the mass in his right lung and mediastinum 10 weeks ago and has a follow-up appointment to see the physician in 2 weeks. What is the most appropriate response by the telephone triage nurse?
☐ 1. Advise the client to take two acetaminophen tablets every 4 to 6 hours for 2 days and call back if his temperature increases to 101° F (38.3° C) or greater.
☐ 2. Advise the client that this is an expected side effect of the radiation therapy and to keep his appointment in 2 weeks.
☐ 3. Advise the client to come to the office to be examined today.
☐ 4. Advise the client to go to the nearest emergency department.

83. A 52-year-old African-American woman has a history of breast cancer. She has developed recurrent pleural effusions. Before a scheduled thoracentesis for palliation of symptoms, the nurse should anticipate which of the following orders?
☐ 1. Arterial blood gases.
☐ 2. Electrocardiogram (ECG).
☐ 3. White blood cell (WBC) count with differential.
☐ 4. Posterior and lateral view (radiographs) of chest.

84. *Impaired spontaneous ventilation* is a nursing diagnosis most likely applicable to which of the following client populations?
☐ 1. Clients with lymphatic malignancies who are undergoing chemotherapy.
☐ 2. Clients with hematopoietic malignancies who are undergoing chemotherapy.
☐ 3. Clients with head and neck malignancies who are undergoing surgery.
☐ 4. Clients with brain tumors who are undergoing radiation.

85. A 58-year-old male has just had a sclerosing agent instilled after chest tube drainage of a pleural effusion. The nurse should instruct the client to:
☐ 1. Lie still to prevent a pneumothorax.
☐ 2. Sit upright with arms on an overhead table to promote lung expansion.
☐ 3. Change position frequently to distribute the agent.
☐ 4. Lie on the side where the thoracentesis was done to hold pressure on the chest tube site.

86. After surgery for head and neck cancer, a 67-year-old male has a permanent tracheostomy. One of the most important long-term interventions the nurse can teach the client and his family is to emphasize the importance of:
☐ 1. Providing tracheostomy site care.
☐ 2. Addressing the psychosocial issues related to tracheostomy.
☐ 3. Observing for early signs and symptoms of skin breakdown around the tracheostomy site.
☐ 4. Using humidifiers to prevent thick, tenacious secretions.

87. Which of the following signs and symptoms should the nurse expect to find in a client with malignant pleural effusions?
☐ 1. Hiccups, anxiety.
☐ 2. Cough, weight gain.
☐ 3. Peripheral edema, temperature of 99° F (37.2° C).
☐ 4. Chest pain, dyspnea.

88. A 56-year-old female is undergoing a thoracentesis. Which of the following outcomes of the procedure is *least* likely?
☐ 1. Treatment of recurrent malignant effusion.
☐ 2. Diagnosis of underlying disease.
☐ 3. Palliation of symptoms.
☐ 4. Relief of acute respiratory distress.

89. Which of the following signs and symptoms is associated with anemia?
☐ 1. Decreased salivation.
☐ 2. Bradycardia.
☐ 3. Cold intolerance.
☐ 4. Nausea.

90. The nurse is assisting the physician with a thoracentesis for a client with suspected lung cancer. If the client has a malignant effusion, the nurse should expect the fluid to be:
☐ 1. Milky white.
☐ 2. Straw-colored.
☐ 3. Turbid.
☐ 4. Bloody.

91. Many oncology clients are at risk for development of a hypercoagulable state and thrombosis. Laboratory tests to monitor for these complications include:
☐ 1. Carcinoembryonic antigen (CEA).
☐ 2. Alpha-fetoprotein (AFP).
☐ 3. Prothrombin time (PT) and partial thromboplastin time (PTT).
☐ 4. Complete blood count (CBC) with differential.

92. One of the most serious blood coagulation complications for individuals with cancer and for those undergoing cancer treatments is disseminated intravascular coagulation (DIC). The most common cause of this bleeding disorder is:
- ☐ **1.** Underlying liver disease.
- ☐ **2.** Brain metastasis.
- ☐ **3.** I.V. heparin therapy.
- ☐ **4.** Sepsis.

93. A nurse is assessing a 42-year-old client who has been receiving chemotherapy. The client has a platelet count of 22,000 cells/mm³ and has petechiae on the lower extremities. The nurse should advise the client to:
- ☐ **1.** Increase the amount of iron in the client's diet.
- ☐ **2.** Apply lotion to the lower extremities.
- ☐ **3.** Elevate the legs.
- ☐ **4.** Consult the oncologist.

94. A nurse is teaching a 62-year-old female who has had a left modified radical mastectomy with axillary node dissection about lymphedema. The nurse should tell the client that lymphedema occurs:
- ☐ **1.** If all cancer cells are not removed.
- ☐ **2.** In older women.
- ☐ **3.** At any time after surgery or not at all.
- ☐ **4.** Only with radical mastectomy.

95. Formation of blood clots or thrombi is a complication that can occur in clients with long-term vascular access devices. To prevent or minimize the risk of thrombus formation, prophylactic administration of daily medication may be used. What medication should the nurse expect to be ordered?
- ☐ **1.** Urokinase.
- ☐ **2.** Vitamin B₁₂.
- ☐ **3.** Warfarin sodium (Coumadin).
- ☐ **4.** Acetaminophen (Tylenol).

96. The client with lymphedema has an increased risk of cellulitis and lymphangitis because of:
- ☐ **1.** Fragility of the capillaries.
- ☐ **2.** Myelosuppression of the bone marrow.
- ☐ **3.** Stagnation of accumulated fluid.
- ☐ **4.** Increased use of the extremity.

97. A 38-year-old female client with a history of breast-conserving surgery, axillary node dissection, and radiation therapy calls the clinic to report that her arm is red, warm to touch, and slightly swollen. Which of the following actions should the nurse suggest?
- ☐ **1.** Apply warm compresses to the affected arm.
- ☐ **2.** Elevate the arm on two pillows.
- ☐ **3.** See the physician immediately.
- ☐ **4.** Schedule an appointment within 2 to 3 weeks.

98. The nurse is assessing a 42-year-old client with cancer. He has lost 1 lb in 4 weeks. He is taking ondansetron (Zofran) for nausea. He has a temperature of 101° F (38.3° C). The fever is indicative of:
- ☐ **1.** Inadequate nutrition.
- ☐ **2.** New resistance to current antiemetic therapy.
- ☐ **3.** Expected response to chemotherapy treatment.
- ☐ **4.** Infection.

99. A pneumonectomy is a surgical procedure sometimes indicated for treatment of non-small-cell lung cancer. A pneumonectomy involves removal of:
- ☐ **1.** An entire lung field.
- ☐ **2.** A small, wedge-shaped lung surface.
- ☐ **3.** One lobe of a lung.
- ☐ **4.** One or more segments of a lung lobe.

100. Many biologic response modifiers (BRMs) have expected adverse effects of fever and chills or a flulike syndrome. These adverse effects typically:
- ☐ **1.** Are controlled with antipyretics.
- ☐ **2.** Last 24 to 72 hours.
- ☐ **3.** Increase in intensity with continued therapy.
- ☐ **4.** Have a biphasic pattern.

101. A 36-year-old male with lymphoma presents with signs and symptoms of impending septic shock 9 days after chemotherapy. The nurse should expect which of the following to be present?
- ☐ **1.** Flushing, decreased oxygen saturation, mild hypotension.
- ☐ **2.** Low-grade fever, chills, tachycardia.
- ☐ **3.** Elevated temperature, oliguria, hypotension.
- ☐ **4.** High-grade fever, normal blood pressure, increased respirations.

102. An appropriate nursing intervention for a client with fatigue related to cancer treatment includes teaching the client to:
- ☐ **1.** Increase fluid intake.
- ☐ **2.** Minimize naps or periods of rest during day.
- ☐ **3.** Conserve energy by prioritizing activities.
- ☐ **4.** Limit dietary intake of high-fiber foods.

103. The nurse is aware that the most common issue associated with sleep disturbances in the hospitalized client with cancer is:
- ☐ **1.** Social.
- ☐ **2.** Nutritional.
- ☐ **3.** Cultural.
- ☐ **4.** Psychological.

104. Which of the following represents the most appropriate nursing intervention for a client with pruritus caused by cancer or the treatments?
- ☐ **1.** Administration of antihistamines.
- ☐ **2.** Steroids.
- ☐ **3.** Silk sheets.
- ☐ **4.** Medicated cool baths.

105. The nurse is caring for a client with cancer who has intractable dyspnea. The nurse is aware that the physician may order which of the following types of drugs to relieve the dyspnea?
- ☐ 1. Mucolytic agents.
- ☐ 2. Antidepressants.
- ☐ 3. Opioids.
- ☐ 4. Diuretics.

106. A 62-year-old female has experienced a flare-up of pruritus. Which of the client's actions could be the cause of the flare-up?
- ☐ 1. Wearing clothes made from 100% cotton.
- ☐ 2. Sleeping in a cool, humidified room.
- ☐ 3. Increasing fluid intake to at least 3,000 ml per day.
- ☐ 4. Daily baths with a deodorant soap.

107. Which of the following variables is *most* important to assess when determining the impact of the cancer diagnosis and treatment modalities on a long-term survivor's quality of life?
- ☐ 1. Occupation and employability.
- ☐ 2. Functional status.
- ☐ 3. Evidence of disease.
- ☐ 4. Individual values and beliefs.

108. A 68-year-old female with breast cancer complains of abdominal bloating and cramping with no bowel movement for 5 days. She says she usually has a bowel movement every day after her morning coffee. Bowel sounds are present in all four quadrants. She received 80 mg of doxorubicin hydrochloride (Adriamycin)10 days ago. The nurse should expect to administer which of the following?
- ☐ 1. A Fleet enema to stimulate peristalsis.
- ☐ 2. A soapsuds enema until clear.
- ☐ 3. An oral cathartic until the client has a bowel movement; then evaluate the need for daily stool softeners.
- ☐ 4. A daily stool softener for constipation and a mild opioid for abdominal discomfort.

109. An 82-year-old elderly, alert, and oriented female with metastatic lung cancer is admitted to the medical-surgical unit for treatment of heart failure. She was given 80 mg of furosemide (Lasix) in the emergency department. Although the client is ambulatory, the unlicensed assistive personnel are concerned about urinary incontinence because the client is frail and in a strange environment. The nurse should instruct the unlicensed personnel to assist with implementing the nursing plan of care by:
- ☐ 1. Ordering adult diapers for the client so she will not have to worry about incontinence.
- ☐ 2. Requesting an indwelling urinary catheter to avoid incontinence.
- ☐ 3. Padding the bed with extra absorbent linens.
- ☐ 4. Placing a commode at the bedside and instructing the client in its use.

110. A cancer client has diarrhea and a nursing diagnosis of *Impaired skin integrity* related to the frequent diarrhea. Which of the following nursing interventions is appropriate for this diagnosis?
- ☐ 1. Discourage sitz baths because they promote bacterial growth.
- ☐ 2. Apply zinc oxide ointment to the rectal area after each bowel movement to protect the skin.
- ☐ 3. Apply a skin-barrier dressing daily to the rectal area to form a protective barrier.
- ☐ 4. Clean the rectal area with unscented soap and water after each bowel movement, rinse well, and pat dry.

111. Which of the following statements is most accurate regarding the long-term toxic effects of cancer treatments on the immune system?
- ☐ 1. Clients with persistent immunologic abnormalities after treatment are at a much greater risk for infection than clients with a history of splenectomy.
- ☐ 2. The use of radiation and combination chemotherapy can result in more frequent and more severe immune system impairment.
- ☐ 3. Long-term immunologic effects have been studied only in clients with breast and lung cancer.
- ☐ 4. The helper T cells recover more rapidly than the suppressor T cells, which results in positive helper cell balance that can last 5 years.

112. The nurse should expect single-donor platelets to be ordered for which of the following clients?
- ☐ 1. A client who is receiving multiple platelet transfusions.
- ☐ 2. A client who is deficient in coagulation factors.
- ☐ 3. A client whose platelet count is greater than 50,000/mm³.
- ☐ 4. A client who is refractory to random-donor platelets.

The Client Who Is Coping with Loss, Grief, Bereavement, and Spiritual Distress

113. A client is newly diagnosed with cancer and is beginning a treatment plan. Which of the following nursing interventions will be most effective in helping the client cope?
- ☐ 1. Assume decision making for the client.
- ☐ 2. Encourage strict compliance with all treatment regimens.
- ☐ 3. Inform the client of all possible adverse treatment effects.
- ☐ 4. Identify available resources.

114. A daughter is concerned that her mother is in denial when discussing her diagnosis of breast cancer because she sometimes says that breast cancer isn't that serious and changes the subject. The nurse informs the daughter that denial can be a healthy defense mechanism if it is used:

☐ 1. To permit her mother to seek unconventional treatments.

☐ 2. When making decisions about her care.

☐ 3. Alone and not in combination with other defense mechanisms.

☐ 4. To allow her mother to continue in her role as a mother.

115. A 45-year-old single mother of three teenaged boys has metastatic breast cancer. Her parents live 750 miles away and have only been able to visit twice since her initial diagnosis 14 months ago. The progression of her disease has forced the client to consider high-dose chemotherapy. She is concerned about her children's welfare during the treatment. When assessing the client's present support systems, the nurse will be most concerned about the potential problems with:

☐ 1. Denial as a primary coping mechanism.

☐ 2. Support systems and coping strategies.

☐ 3. Decision-making abilities.

☐ 4. Transportation and money for the boys.

116. Which of the following characteristics displayed by the wife of a 36-year-old man with pancreatic cancer suggests that she may be at risk for negative bereavement outcomes?

☐ 1. She is preparing for her husband's death.

☐ 2. Her high socioeconomic status.

☐ 3. Her strong family support.

☐ 4. She blames herself for her husband's cancer.

117. Which of the following factors assists a person to achieve positive bereavement outcomes?

☐ 1. Young age.

☐ 2. History of anxiety.

☐ 3. History of depression.

☐ 4. Higher socioeconomic status.

118. Which of the following nursing interventions will be *most* effective when caring for a client who is experiencing powerlessness?

☐ 1. Make certain that all staff members focus only on the client's capabilities.

☐ 2. Encourage family members to become more responsible for the client's care.

☐ 3. Request a referral to a psychologist.

☐ 4. Include the client in decision making whenever possible.

119. During the initial stage of adaptation to the diagnosis of cancer and its treatment, the nurse can facilitate the client's adaptation by:

☐ 1. Encouraging the client to maintain her usual role.

☐ 2. Facilitating family-related disagreements and conflicts.

☐ 3. Supporting the client in her use of denial as a coping strategy.

☐ 4. Arranging transportation and child care on treatment days.

120. The son of a 78-year-old client with metastatic prostate cancer is asking the nurse about the purpose of hospice care. Which of the following statements by the nurse best describes hospice care?

☐ 1. "Hospice care uses a team approach to direct hospice activity."

☐ 2. "Clients and their families are the focus of care."

☐ 3. "The client's physician coordinates all the care."

☐ 4. "All hospice clients will die at home."

121. A client's husband expresses concern that his dying wife keeps saying, "I have to go to the store." Which of the following statements by the nurse will be most effective in assisting the husband to understand the dying process?

☐ 1. "Many dying clients are restless and can be treated with sedatives."

☐ 2. "The client may be fighting death and you should leave her alone."

☐ 3. "Comments related to going somewhere or leaving on a trip are common in dying clients."

☐ 4. "Decreased circulation and lack of oxygen to the brain often causes delirium."

122. The wife of a terminally ill client asks the nurse, "Why is he having frequent bowel movements if he is not eating?" Which of the following responses by the nurse informs the wife about the client's condition?

☐ 1. "I know he is having frequent loose stools and it is distressing for you, but that's just the way it is."

☐ 2. "I don't know when the bowels will shut down, but they will eventually."

☐ 3. "The pain medication will eventually help to slow the process of bowel function."

☐ 4. "The intestines still produce some waste products even when a person is not eating."

123. The nurse formulates a nursing diagnosis of *Spiritual distress* related to advanced cancer disease. An appropriate goal for the client would be to:

☐ 1. Start attending church or chapel services once a week.

☐ 2. Call a chaplain and set up an appointment for spiritual guidance.

☐ 3. Reflect on past accomplishments.

☐ 4. Participate in spiritual activities of the client's choice.

124. A 72-year-old client with cancer needs assistance with paying her hospital bills. The nurse should refer the client to a:
- ☐ **1.** Bank representative.
- ☐ **2.** Social worker.
- ☐ **3.** Loan officer.
- ☐ **4.** Representative of the hospital billing department.

125. The family members caring for a 72-year-old client who is near death from colon cancer are concerned about dehydration. What should the nurse tell them about dehydration at end of life?
- ☐ **1.** The physician will make the decision regarding hydration therapy.
- ☐ **2.** Dehydration may prolong the dying process.
- ☐ **3.** Hydration is used only in extreme situations of dehydration.
- ☐ **4.** Dehydration is expected during the dying process.

126. Which of the following actions should the nurse plan to do *first* when caring for a client who is experiencing spiritual distress?
- ☐ **1.** Make a referral to a member of the clergy.
- ☐ **2.** Explain the major beliefs of different religions.
- ☐ **3.** Suggest reading material.
- ☐ **4.** Help the client explore his or her own values and beliefs.

127. A nurse is caring for a client at home on hospice care for terminal renal cancer. People are calling the nurse to inquire about the client's condition. Which of the following is a correct response made by the nurse?
- ☐ **1.** "Please call the oncologist."
- ☐ **2.** "The client is in a coma now."
- ☐ **3.** "Please call the client's sister for an update on her condition."
- ☐ **4.** "The client is not expected to live much longer."

128. The nursing team on an oncology unit consists of a registered nurse (RN), a licensed vocational nurse (LVN-LPN), and an unlicensed assistive personnel (UAP). Which client is most appropriate for the registered nurse?
- ☐ **1.** A 52-year-old client with lung cancer admitted for acute dyspnea.
- ☐ **2.** A 45-year-old client receiving tube feedings.
- ☐ **3.** A 28-year-old client being evaluated for a bone marrow transplant.
- ☐ **4.** A 65-year-old client diagnosed with endometrial cancer who underwent an abdominal hysterectomy 3 days ago.

129. A 42-year-old client with breast cancer is concerned that her husband is depressed by her diagnosis. Which of the following changes in her husband's behavior may confirm her fears?
- ☐ **1.** Increased decisiveness.
- ☐ **2.** Problem-focused coping style.
- ☐ **3.** Increase in social interactions.
- ☐ **4.** Disturbance in his sleep patterns.

130. The most appropriate advice for the hospice nurse to give a woman whose husband died 3 months ago and her three young children would be to:
- ☐ **1.** Seek group counseling support for the three children.
- ☐ **2.** Request individual counseling and medication to manage depression.
- ☐ **3.** Remind her gently that bereavement care before death minimizes grieving.
- ☐ **4.** Continue her bereavement support through hospice.

131. Which of the following interventions will be most effective in improving transcultural communications with oncology clients and their families?
- ☐ **1.** Use touch to show concern and caring for the client.
- ☐ **2.** Focus attention on verbal communication skills only.
- ☐ **3.** Establish a rapport and listen to their concerns.
- ☐ **4.** Maintain eye contact at all times.

132. A client with cancer verbalizes that he is afraid he won't be able to cope with all the issues that will arise. The nurse can best support the coping behaviors of a client with cancer by:
- ☐ **1.** Helping the client identify available resources.
- ☐ **2.** Encouraging compliance with treatment regimens.
- ☐ **3.** Relieving the client of decision making as much as possible.
- ☐ **4.** Assisting the client to prepare for adverse treatment effects.

133. The "I Can Cope," "CanSurmount," and "Reach to Recovery" programs are all designed to help cancer clients:
- ☐ **1.** Choose treatment centers.
- ☐ **2.** Find financial help.
- ☐ **3.** Obtain home health care.
- ☐ **4.** Cope with cancer.

134. A 56-year-old cancer survivor feels guilty at the "I Can Cope" meetings. The nurse can help him manage his feelings of guilt by pointing out that:
- ☐ **1.** He is really angry at the terminally ill clients in the group.
- ☐ **2.** He is experiencing very volatile emotions.
- ☐ **3.** This is a spiritual response to his illness.
- ☐ **4.** This is a normal reaction when surviving a life-threatening experience.

135. A 68-year-old client with colon cancer experiences an increase in his feelings of anxiety and depression and has suicidal ideation. He appears to be in great distress. The nurse realizes that he is at which stage in his disease?
- ☐ **1.** Initiation of definitive treatment.
- ☐ **2.** End of his first course of treatment.
- ☐ **3.** End stage of his disease.
- ☐ **4.** Recurrence of the disease.

136. A 57-year-old client has difficulty with mobility after cancer treatment therapies and states, "Why should I bother trying to get better? It doesn't seem to make any difference what I do." The nurse responds by helping the client establish reasonable activity goals, choose her own foods from the menu, and make choices about her daily activities. These interventions represent the nurse's attempt to address which of the following nursing diagnoses?
- ☐ 1. *Ineffective coping.*
- ☐ 2. *Powerlessness.*
- ☐ 3. *Risk prone health behavior.*
- ☐ 4. *Complicated grieving.*

137. The nurse is aware that a 65-year-old widower whose only son is 500 miles away is at higher risk for psychosocial distress because the client:
- ☐ 1. Has been successful in dealing with stress all his life.
- ☐ 2. Does not have to deal with other stressors right now.
- ☐ 3. Is able to use denial as a coping mechanism.
- ☐ 4. Perceives he has minimal social support.

138. A client with a diagnosis of cancer is frequently disruptive and challenges the nurse. This behavior is probably caused by:
- ☐ 1. Uncertainty and an underlying fear of recurrence.
- ☐ 2. The usual trajectory of a short-term illness.
- ☐ 3. A history of a behavioral illness.
- ☐ 4. The one-time crisis from learning of the diagnosis.

139. A 42-year-old husband and father of a 7-year-old girl and a 10-year-old boy is concerned about what he should tell his children regarding his wife's impending death from aggressive breast cancer. The nurse should:
- ☐ 1. Refer the family to pastoral care services.
- ☐ 2. Encourage the husband to come to terms with his own grief first.
- ☐ 3. Suggest that the children be told nothing until after death occurs.
- ☐ 4. Begin education about strategies for communication with his children.

140. While talking to her husband, who is caring for their children, a 52-year-old client slams the phone down. She begins to cry and states that she is feeling guilty for being hospitalized. Which of the following interventions will best support the client emotionally?
- ☐ 1. Call the physician and ask for a psychiatry consultation.
- ☐ 2. Call the physician and request an antidepressant medication.
- ☐ 3. Sit with the client and help her acknowledge and discuss her feelings.
- ☐ 4. Sit with the client and encourage her to see the good side of the situation.

141. A 56-year-old female who is receiving radiation therapy tells the nurse that she feels inadequate as a wife and mother because she can no longer carry out her usual duties with the same energy as before. What recommendations should the nurse make to help the client cope with this situation?
- ☐ 1. Suggest that she reassign all household chores to other members of the family.
- ☐ 2. Suggest that she prioritize her activities and ask for help from friends and family.
- ☐ 3. Suggest that she ignore the household chores during the crisis period.
- ☐ 4. Tell her not to worry so much because everyone gets a little tired at this phase of the therapy.

142. A 66-year-old female who is usually meticulous about her appearance and dress arrives today for her 23rd day of radiation therapy. She appears disheveled and emotionally labile, and her responses to the usual questions are a little inappropriate. Her heart rate is 124 bpm, her respirations are 32 breaths/minute, and her skin is cold and clammy. These findings would suggest that the client has early signs of which of the following conditions?
- ☐ 1. Schizophrenia.
- ☐ 2. Panic disorder.
- ☐ 3. Depression.
- ☐ 4. Delirium.

143. A client has undergone surgical resection for lung cancer. Which of the following nursing interventions will promote adaptation and rehabilitation?
- ☐ 1. Arranging a visit from a member of the American Cancer Society Lost Chord Club.
- ☐ 2. Planning a progressive activity regimen with the client.
- ☐ 3. Teaching tracheostomy care.
- ☐ 4. Planning a vigorous exercise program.

144. Which of the following activities indicates that the client with cancer is adapting well to body image changes?
- ☐ 1. The client names his brother as the person to call if he is experiencing suicidal ideation.
- ☐ 2. The client discusses changes in body structure and function.
- ☐ 3. The client discusses the date of his return to work.
- ☐ 4. The client serves as a volunteer in a client-to-client visitation program.

The Client Who Is Experiencing Problems with Sexuality

145. A 36-year-old female is complaining of increased vaginal dryness during sexual intercourse. She has received chemotherapy in the past and has menopausal symptoms due to ovarian suppression. An appropriate nursing intervention would be to instruct the client on the use of:
☐ **1.** Vaginal dilators.
☐ **2.** Nightly douches.
☐ **3.** Water-soluble vaginal lubricants.
☐ **4.** Relaxation techniques.

146. A 49-year-old male with a tracheostomy tube confides to the nurse during a clinic visit that he is beginning to avoid sexual activity because of the increased tracheostomy secretions. Which of the following statements by the nurse will be *most* helpful to the client?
☐ **1.** "Use a scopolamine patch to decrease secretions."
☐ **2.** "Avoid fluid intake 2 hours before sexual activity."
☐ **3.** "Place a thin piece of gauze over the tracheostomy."
☐ **4.** "Wash the tracheostomy area with deodorizing antibacterial soap before sexual activity."

147. A 52-year-old client is scheduled for a total abdominal hysterectomy for cervical cancer. Discussion regarding the client's feelings and the potential impact of this procedure on her sexuality should include which of the following questions?
☐ **1.** "All women experience sexual problems with this surgical procedure. Do you have any questions?"
☐ **2.** "When can I schedule an appointment with you and your partner to discuss any issues either of you may have regarding sexuality?"
☐ **3.** "Do you anticipate any problems with sex related to your scheduled hysterectomy?"
☐ **4.** "Most women have concerns about their sexuality after this type of surgery. Do you have any concerns or questions?"

148. A young man with early-stage testicular cancer is scheduled for a unilateral orchiectomy. The client confides to the nurse that he is concerned about what effects the surgery will have on his sexual performance. Which of the following responses by the nurse provides accurate information about sexual performance after an orchiectomy?
☐ **1.** "Most impotence resolves in a couple of months."
☐ **2.** "You could have early ejaculation with this type of surgery."
☐ **3.** "We will refer you to a sex therapist because you will probably notice erectile dysfunction."
☐ **4.** "Because your surgery does not involve other organs or tissues, you'll likely not notice much change in your sexual performance."

149. A young female client is receiving chemotherapy and mentions to the nurse that she and her husband are using a diaphragm for birth control. Which of the following is most important for the nurse to discuss?
☐ **1.** Inconvenience of the diaphragm.
☐ **2.** Transmission of sexually transmitted diseases.
☐ **3.** Body changes related to hormones.
☐ **4.** Infection control.

150. To promote comfort and optimal respiratory expansion for a client with chronic obstructive pulmonary disease during sexual intimacy, the nurse can suggest that the couple:
☐ **1.** Use a waterbed.
☐ **2.** Use pillows to raise the affected partner's head and upper torso.
☐ **3.** Have the affected partner assume a dependent position.
☐ **4.** Limit the duration of the sexual activity.

Ethical and Legal Issues Related to Clients with Cancer

151. A registered nurse is assigning care on the oncology unit and assigns the client with Kaposi's sarcoma and human immunodeficiency virus (HIV) infection to the licensed vocational nurse (LVN-LPN). The LVN-LPN states that she does not want to care for this client. How should the nurse respond?
☐ **1.** "I will assign this client to another nurse."
☐ **2.** "I will help you take care of this client so you are confident with his care."
☐ **3.** "You seem worried about this assignment."
☐ **4.** "I will review blood and body fluid precautions with you."

152. In an attempt to call public attention to the cancer survivor's needs, a bill of rights was put forth by the:
☐ **1.** American Cancer Society.
☐ **2.** National Coalition of Cancer Survivors.
☐ **3.** National Cancer Institute.
☐ **4.** National Hospice Organization.

153. A 32-year-old teacher is concerned that she will lose her job if she requests a leave of absence to care for her father who is getting daily treatment for colon cancer in a city 300 miles away. Which legislative measure will likely protect her job during an extended illness?
☐ **1.** Family Leave Act of 1993.
☐ **2.** Americans with Disabilities Act of 1990.
☐ **3.** Medicare Coverage for Catastrophic Illness Act of 1988.
☐ **4.** Rehabilitation Act of 1973.

154. A 62-year-old woman thinks her husband's rehabilitation needs have been unmet by his employer after his diagnosis and treatment of colon cancer. The nurse should give her information about:
- ☐ 1. The Americans With Disabilities Act of 1990.
- ☐ 2. Title V of the Rehabilitation Act of 1973.
- ☐ 3. The Civil Rights Act of 1964.
- ☐ 4. The Patient Self-Determination Act of 1991.

155. A client and nurse have established a goal for the client to be more autonomous. Which of the following situations indicates that the goal has been met?
- ☐ 1. The physician directs the client's care.
- ☐ 2. The nurse provides the client with the facts and then allows the client to reach an unassisted decision.
- ☐ 3. The nurse respects a client's choice not to know particular information.
- ☐ 4. The health care team makes health and treatment decisions.

End-of-Life Care

156. The family of a hospitalized client demonstrates understanding of the teaching about advance directives when they make which of the following statements? Select all that apply.
- ☐ 1. "Advance directives give instructions about future medical care and treatment."
- ☐ 2. "If people are not capable of communicating their wishes, health care providers and family together can agree on measures or actions that will be taken."
- ☐ 3. "Ethics experts agree that the family is the sole deciding factor when the client is competent."
- ☐ 4. "Medical power-of-attorney gives primarily financial access to the designee."
- ☐ 5. "Medical power-of-attorney or durable power-of-attorney for health care is a document that lists who can make health care decisions should a person be unable to make an informed decision for himself or herself."
- ☐ 6. "Advance directives give details about the client's past medical history."

157. The nurse can be an important advocate for the client who is considering an alternative method of cancer treatment. Which of the following statements best demonstrates the nurse as client advocate?
- ☐ 1. The nurse will provide the information about standard therapies.
- ☐ 2. The nurse will monitor blood tests as indicated by the alternative therapy.
- ☐ 3. The nurse will document the client's desire to try an alternative therapy.
- ☐ 4. The nurse will allow the client to make health care choices on her own but will assist in ensuring the client is fully informed when making those decisions.

158. After completing the nursing assessment for a client and family entering the palliative care program, the nurse should expect to develop a teaching plan that includes an understanding of which of the following as goals or outcomes of this type of care? Select all that apply.
- ☐ 1. Alteration in the family's usual coping strategies.
- ☐ 2. Achievement of a dignified and respectful death.
- ☐ 3. Improvement in the client's quality of life.
- ☐ 4. Provision of comfort during the dying process.
- ☐ 5. Provision of support for client and family.
- ☐ 6. Advocation for prolonging life while curing the disease.

159. When a 62-year-old client and his family receive the initial diagnosis of colon cancer, the nurse can act as an advocate by:
- ☐ 1. Helping them maintain a sense of optimism and hopefulness.
- ☐ 2. Determining their understanding of the results of the diagnostic testing.
- ☐ 3. Listening carefully to their perceptions of what their needs are.
- ☐ 4. Providing them with written materials about the cancer site and its treatment.

160. A client who is dying of acquired immunodeficiency syndrome (AIDS) is admitted to the inpatient psychiatric unit because he attempted suicide. His close friend recently died of AIDS. The client begins to talk about his feelings related to his illness and the loss of his friend. He begins to cry. Which of the following responses by the nurse would be *most* appropriate?
- ☐ 1. Give the client some tissues and tell him it is okay to cry.
- ☐ 2. Tell the client to stop crying and that everything will be okay.
- ☐ 3. Sort the client's mail to distract the client.
- ☐ 4. Change the subject.

161. A 79-year-old male client is admitted again for heart failure and kidney failure. After completing his admission, the nurse is talking with the client's wife, who expresses several concerns. She says, "I know he doesn't want to die in a hospital, but it is so hard for me to take care of him at home. He said he doesn't want any more treatment, but I'm not ready to let him go. We have so many arrangements to decide before he dies." Which of the following statements by the nurse to the client's wife would be most appropriate? Select all that apply.

☐ **1.** "He's not going to die that soon judging by his current symptoms."

☐ **2.** "What are your fears about your husband dying?"

☐ **3.** "I can imagine that it is hard for you to care for him at home."

☐ **4.** "What do you and your husband know about advance directives?"

☐ **5.** "We can discuss types of hospice and home care available."

☐ **6.** "What kind of arrangements do you think need to be made before he dies?"

162. A terminally ill client's husband tells the nurse, "I wish we had taken that trip to Europe last year. We just kept putting it off, and now I'm furious that we didn't go." The nurse interprets the husband's statement as indicating which of the following stages of adaptation to dying?

☐ **1.** Anger.

☐ **2.** Denial.

☐ **3.** Bargaining.

☐ **4.** Depression.

163. The nurse who usually is most effective when caring for a dying client and helping the family deal with death is one who has participated in which of the following activities?

☐ **1.** Contemplating his or her own death and mortality.

☐ **2.** Attending continuing education classes on death and dying.

☐ **3.** Providing compassionate and physical care while remaining distant emotionally.

☐ **4.** Viewing dying people as distinct populations of people in need of comfort.

164. Which of the following philosophies should the nurse most likely integrate into the plan of care for a client and family to help them best cope during the final stages of the client's illness?

☐ **1.** Living each day as it comes as fully as possible.

☐ **2.** Reliving the pleasant memories of days gone by.

☐ **3.** Expecting the worst and being grateful when it does not happen.

☐ **4.** Planning ahead for the remaining good times that will be spent together.

165. A 13-year-old boy admitted to the hospital for the third time is diagnosed as having acute lymphatic leukemia. The liaison psychiatric nurse is asked by the team leader to help the nursing staff work more effectively with this terminally ill child and his family. One of the nurses says to the liaison nurse, "Whenever I go to the client's room, I feel that I have to smile and act happy even though I want to cry when I see him." Which of the following responses by the liaison nurse would be *most* appropriate?

☐ **1.** "Call me when you feel that way. We can talk it over at the time."

☐ **2.** "Try not to show emotion, such as crying. You'll upset the client."

☐ **3.** "Keep smiling. The client and his parents need all the support they can get."

☐ **4.** "Tell the client you feel bad because he is ill and cry, too, if it seems appropriate."

166. A client who is in the end-stages of cancer is increasingly prone to outbursts concerning her chemotherapy treatments. Which of the following approaches by the nurse would likely be most helpful in gaining her cooperation?

☐ **1.** Telling the client how the treatment can be expected to help her.

☐ **2.** Describing the probable effect on her body that missing a treatment would have.

☐ **3.** Asking her to be "a good client" and not make the treatment any harder for herself.

☐ **4.** Promising to give her a backrub if she does not make a fuss about the treatment.

167. A 10-year-old client suspects that he will not live. However, others talk about only pleasant matters with him and maintain a persistently cheerful facade around him. The nurse anticipates that the client will most likely feel which of the following as a result of such behavior?

☐ **1.** Relief.

☐ **2.** Isolation.

☐ **3.** Hopefulness.

☐ **4.** Independence.

168. The young sister of a client with leukemia asks, "Can you check my blood? When my sister got the measles, so did I. And I think I have this, too." Which of the following by the nurse would be *inappropriate*?

☐ **1.** Asking the client's physician to take a sample of the sister's blood.

☐ **2.** Explaining to the sister that leukemia is not a communicable disease.

☐ **3.** Discussing the sister's concern with her parents.

☐ **4.** Telling the sister's parents about a group for siblings of clients with terminal illness.

169. When talking with the nurse, the 15-year-old brother of a client with leukemia says, "We used to play pretty rough games together. Maybe some of the bruises he got when I tackled him caused this." Which of the following would be the nurse's *best* response?
- ☐ 1. "Don't feel guilty. You didn't cause your brother's illness."
- ☐ 2. "I can see you're worried. Let's talk about how people get leukemia."
- ☐ 3. "Here is some information about leukemia for you to read."
- ☐ 4. "Lots of people worry about things like this. It isn't your fault."

170. During the nursing shift report, the team leader lists tasks and routines completed for a terminally ill client. Which of the following kinds of behavior is the nurse *most* likely demonstrating when emphasizing the technical aspects of caring for a dying client?
- ☐ 1. Tactful behavior.
- ☐ 2. Efficient behavior.
- ☐ 3. Objective behavior.
- ☐ 4. Defensive behavior.

Correct Answers and Rationales

The letter in parentheses after each rationale identifies the client need addressed in the item, including management of care (M), safety and infection control (S), health promotion and maintenance (H), psychosocial adaptation (P), basic care and comfort (C), pharmacological and parenteral therapies (D), reduction of risk potential (R), and physiological adaptation (A).

The Client at Risk for Cancer

1. 3. Clients over age 50 who have a history of inflammatory bowel disease are at risk for colon cancer. The client who smokes is at high risk for lung cancer. While the exact cause is not always known, other risk factors for colon cancer are a diet high in animal fats, including a large amount of red meat and fatty foods with low fiber, and the presence of colon cancer in a first-generation relative. (R)

2. 1, 3, 5. Acetaminophen (Tylenol) is a safer analgesic than aspirin in order to avoid bleeding. Contact sports or trauma to the site should be avoided. Cool compresses should limit swelling and bruising. The puncture site should be inspected every 2 hours for bleeding or bruising during the first 24 hours. (R)

3. 4. Basal cell carcinoma occurs most commonly in sun-exposed areas of the body. The incidence of skin cancer is highest in older people who live in the mountains or spend outdoor leisure time at higher altitudes. (H)

4. 3. Only treatment-related X-rays are iatrogenic. The others are agents that occur in the physical environment naturally. (R)

5. 1. Prospective studies begin with an examination of presumed causes and go forward in time to observe presumed effects. Data about miners with exposure to uranium (the presumed cause) are collected over time to evaluate the incidence of cancer (the presumed effect). This is representative of a prospective study. Historical studies critically evaluate existing data to test hypotheses or answer questions about the causes or effects of past events. Retrospective studies begin with the effect (e.g., cancer) and then attempt to link the effect to a presumed cause that occurred in the past. (H)

6. 1. Progression is the change in a tumor from the preneoplastic state or low degree of malignancy to a rapidly growing tumor; it cannot be reversed. Promotion is reversible. Initiation is at first reversible (through repair of damaged DNA) and later irreversible. Regression is not a recognized stage of carcinogenesis. (H)

7. 2. The word *prevalence* in a statistical setting is defined as the number of cases of a disease present in a specified population at a given time. (H)

8. 3. Sun damage is a cumulative process. Parents should be taught to apply sunscreen and teach their children to use sunscreen at an early age. Although preventive education is always valuable, serious sunburns in childhood are associated with an increased risk of melanoma. Adults and senior citizens have already been exposed to the harmful effects of the sun and, although they, too, should use sunscreen, they are not the group that will most benefit from intervention. Exposure to chemicals is not a risk factor for melanoma. (H)

9. 4. A sunscreen with an SPF of 15 or higher should be worn on all sun-exposed skin surfaces. It should be applied before sun exposure and reapplied after being in the water. Peak sun exposure usually occurs from 10 a.m. to 2 p.m. Tightly woven clothing, protective hats, and sunglasses are recommended to decrease sun exposure. Suntanning parlors should be avoided. (H)

10. 1. Malignant melanoma may have a familial basis, especially in families with dysplastic nevi syndrome. First-degree relatives should be monitored closely. Malignant melanoma occurs most often in the 20- to 45-year-old age-group. Severe sunburn as a child does increase the risk; however, this client is at increased risk because of her family history. (H)

11. The upper outer quadrant is the area of the breast in which most breast tumors are found. This area should be palpated thoroughly. Although breast tumors can be found in any area of the breast, including the nipple, the tumors are most often in the upper outer quadrant. (H)

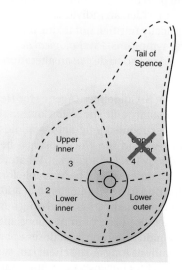

12. **4.** All arm positions, except when the arms are relaxed by the sides, will accentuate skin changes. When the arms are raised over the head, visualization of the underside of the breasts is easier. When the hands are placed on the hips and arms are pressed forward, the breast tissue is pushed outward, which accentuates dimpling and puckering. Breast self-examination is not an uncomfortable procedure. Although masses may be seen on inspection, palpation is a more important maneuver for detecting masses. Nipple discharge is assessed by gently squeezing the nipples. (H)

13. **3.** The American Cancer Society guidelines (2004) state that a Pap smear and pelvic examination should be done 3 years after a woman first has vaginal intercourse, but no later than 21 years of age. Annual Pap smears are recommended only for clients at risk and not for the general female population. After three or more consecutive annual examinations with normal findings, the Pap smear may be performed less frequently at the discretion of the physician. Colposcopy is indicated for an abnormal Pap smear, not a negative Pap smear. (H)

14. **3.** Because more than 50% of the cancers occur in people who are older than age 65, the single most important factor in determining risk would be age. (H)

15. **3.** Evidence suggests that a high-fat diet increases the risk of several cancers, including breast, colon, and prostate cancers. Ovarian, lung, and liver cancers have not been linked to a high-fat diet. (H)

16. **4.** The client is at increased risk for development of lung, skin, or breast cancer. Consequently, the most urgent changes in behavior should include smoking cessation, protection from the sun, and weight loss. Decreasing alcohol consumption is certainly desirable, as is improving overall nutritional intake (e.g., eating low-fat foods, increasing fiber) but is not the most urgent behavior change for this client. (H)

17. **1.** Primary cancer prevention targets healthy individuals and includes steps to avoid factors that might lead to the development of disease. Secondary prevention includes identification of high-risk groups with precursor states of disease. Early detection, screening, and treatment of early stages of disease are included in this category. Tertiary cancer prevention focuses on rehabilitation to assist individuals in achieving an optimal level of functioning. It includes minimizing the effect of cancer and preventing complications. "Nonspecific" is not a category of prevention activities. (H)

18. **1.** Asbestos and alcohol, when combined with smoking, produce a synergistic effect and result in increased cancer risk and incidence. Ultraviolet radiation exposure is associated with skin cancer. HPV exposure is associated with cervical cancer. However, the risks of contracting these types of cancer are not markedly increased when combined with smoking. (H)

19. **4.** Although exposure to the sun increases the risk of skin cancers and family history is significant in the development of some types of cancer, heavy tobacco use and alcohol intake have a synergistic effect and increase the risk and incidence of head and neck cancers. Patterns of medication use, exposure to wood dust, and a high-fat diet are not associated with an increased risk and incidence of head and neck cancers. (H)

20. **2.** High-fiber, low-fat diets are recommended to reduce the risk of colon cancer. Stir-frying, poaching, steaming, and broiling are all low-fat methods to prepare foods. Croissants are made of refined flour. They are also high in fat, as are peanut butter squares and whole milk, granola, cream cheese, and sour cream. (H)

21. **2.** Environmental factors include place of residence, nutrition, occupation, personal habits, iatrogenic factors, and physical environment. Gender, immunologic status, and age are individual factors. (H)

22. **3.** CT scanning is the standard noninvasive method used in a workup for lung cancer because it can distinguish small differences in tissue density and can detect nodal involvement. CT is comparable to magnetic resonance imaging in evaluating lymph node metastasis. CT is noninvasive and usually available, but these are not the main reasons for its use. CT can distinguish malignancy in some situations only. (A)

23. 3. A high-fat, low-fiber diet is a risk factor for colorectal cancer. A diet low in vitamin C, use of artificial sweeteners, and multiple sex partners are not considered risk factors for colorectal cancer. (H)

24. 2. Strategies to reach the socioeconomically disadvantaged should include incorporating the folk beliefs and traditions of the target population into the program. Identification of a centrally located building with available access by the target population, use of materials in the native or primary language of the target population, and involvement by the community leaders will also help the program succeed. (H)

The Client with Pain

25. 4. To determine the cause of this problem, a quality improvement study should be conducted. Before implementing solutions to a problem, the precise issues in the hospital system must be observed and documented. The Joint Commission requirements mandate documentation of the effectiveness of analgesia within 30 minutes after administration. It is not the pharmacist's role to provide consultation about documentation of drugs administered by nurses. Consulting the evening nurses may be helpful, but this is a systems issue of the entire unit and involves every registered nurse administering analgesia. (M)

26. 3. Administration of morphine sulfate is contraindicated because morphine causes respiratory depression. It may also increase intracranial pressure if the client is not ventilating properly, which could result in an accumulation of CO_2, a potent vasodilator. Ibuprofen, naproxen, and acetaminophen are not likely to mask symptoms of increased intracranial pressure or impact respiratory status. (D)

27. 1. Around-the-clock dosing is mandatory to achieve a steady state of analgesia. The rescue dose for breakthrough pain is administered over and above the regularly scheduled medication. If three to four analgesic doses are required every 24 hours, the sustained-release around-the-clock dose should be increased to include the amount used for previous breakthrough pain while maintaining a dose for future breakthrough pain. (C)

28. 2. Step 1 includes nonopioids, such as acetaminophen or NSAIDs. Opioid analgesics are not part of step 1 of the WHO ladder. Mild opioids, such as oxycodone, codeine, and propoxyphene, and adjuvant therapy are included in step 2. (D)

29. 1. The most common toxicities from NSAIDs are gastrointestinal disorders (nausea, epigastric pain, ulcers, bleeding, diarrhea, and constipation). Renal dysfunction, pulmonary complications, and cardiovascular complications from NSAIDs are much less common. (D)

30. 2. In the client with chronic pain, physiologic adaptation results in minimal changes in behavior and vital signs. Elevated vital signs, grimacing, and moaning are characteristic responses to acute pain. (C)

31. 4. *Tolerance* is a reduced responsiveness to the effect of any drug, which necessitates larger doses to achieve an equivalent effect of the initial dose. *Pseudoaddiction* is a term used to describe the iatrogenic syndrome of drug-seeking behavior that develops as a direct consequence of inadequate pain management. *Physical dependence* refers to the state in which an individual must take the substance to feel physically normal; not taking the drug results in withdrawal symptoms. *Psychological dependence* refers to an individual's need to derive an alteration in mood from a substance. (C)

32. 1, 2, 4, 6. Guidelines (Agency for Healthcare Research and Quality and The Joint Commission) recommend use of scheduled long-acting opioids (MS Contin, OxyContin). Around-the-clock dosing is necessary to achieve a steady level of analgesia. Whatever the route or frequency, an order should be available for "breakthrough" pain medication to be administered in addition to the regularly scheduled medication. Oral drug administration is the route of choice for economy, safety, and ease of use. Even severe pain requiring high doses of opioids can be managed orally as long as the client can swallow medication and has a functioning gastrointestinal system. Tolerance occurs due to the need for increasing doses to achieve the same pain relief and will not be avoided with the use of Tylenol. Addiction is a complex condition in which the drug is used for psychological effect and not analgesia. Nurses need to educate families about the appropriate use of opioids and assure them that addiction is not a concern when managing cancer pain. Nonpharmacologic methods are useful as an adjunct to assist in pain control. Self-report is the best assessment of pain and is an individual response. (D)

33. 3. Morphine sulfate is the drug of choice to treat severe cancer pain. Methadone, oxycodone, and hydromorphone are not as effective as morphine in controlling severe cancer pain. (D)

34. 4. Most cancer clients with inadequate pain control while taking an oral opioid after being switched from I.V. administration have been undermedicated. Equianalgesic conversions should be made to provide estimates of the equivalent dose needed for the same level of relief as provided by the I.V. dose. There is research to suggest that cancer clients do not become addicted to opioids when dosed adequately. There is no evidence to suggest that the client is physically addicted or is having withdrawal symptoms. (D)

35. 1. Intensity is indicative of the severity of pain and is important for evaluating the efficacy of pain management. The cause and location of the pain cannot be managed but the intensity of the pain can be controlled. The nurse and client can collaborate to reduce aggravating factors; however, the goal will ultimately be to reduce the intensity of the pain. (C)

36. **2.** There is a 1:3 ratio with equianalgesic dosing of I.V. to oral morphine; therefore, the physician should order three times the I.V. dose. (D)

37. **4.** Normeperidine is a potent long-acting metabolite, which can cause central nervous system (CNS) stimulation and seizures. Meperidine is a short-acting drug and must be given in more frequent intervals and may require increased dosages for effectiveness. Mixed agonist-antagonists act competitively at different pain receptor sites. It is generally accepted by cancer pain experts that opioid agonist-antagonist drugs have very limited usefulness in cancer pain management because of their tendency to induce opioid withdrawal and cause severe CNS adverse effects. Meperidine does not have a higher potential for abuse than other opioids. There are other routes of meperidine administration, so the route of administration is not the limiting factor. (D)

38. **2.** Tolerance to an opioid occurs when a larger dose of the analgesic is needed to provide the same level of pain control. The risk of addiction is low with opioids to treat cancer pain. There are no data to support that this client is experiencing withdrawal. Although the client may have experienced a placebo effect at one time, placebo effects tend to diminish over time, especially in regard to chronic cancer pain. (D)

39. **2.** The regular administration of analgesics provides a consistent serum level of medication, which can help prevent breakthrough pain. Therefore, taking the prescribed analgesics on a regular schedule is the best way to manage chronic cancer-related pain. There is little risk for the client with cancer-related pain to become addicted. Sleeping 12 to 16 hours a day would not allow the client to participate in usual daily activities or preferred activities. (D)

The Client Who Is Receiving Chemotherapy

40. **3.** Carbohydrates are the first substance used by the body for energy. Proteins are needed to maintain muscle mass, repair tissue, and maintain osmotic pressure in the vascular system. Fats, in a small amount, are needed for energy production. Chicken, green beans, and cottage cheese are the best selection to provide a nutritionally well-balanced diet of carbohydrate, protein, and a small amount of fat. Cereal with milk and strawberries as well as toast, gelatin dessert, and cookies have a large amount of carbohydrates and not enough protein. Steak and french fries provide some carbohydrates and a good deal of protein; however, they also provide a large amount of fat. (H)

41. **2.** Chemotherapy agents typically cause nausea and vomiting when not controlled by antiemetic drugs. Antineoplastic drugs attack rapidly growing normal cells, such as in the gastrointestinal tract. These drugs also stimulate the vomiting center in the brain. Hair loss, loss of energy, and sleep are important aspects of the health history, but not as critical as the potential for dehydration and electrolyte imbalance caused by nausea and vomiting. (D)

42. **2, 4, 5.** Chemotherapy causes bone marrow suppression and risk of infection. A platelet count of 40,000/mm^3 and a white blood cell count of 2,300/mm^3 are low. A temperature of 101.2° F (38.4° C) is high and could indicate an infection. Further assessment and examination should be performed to rule out infection. The BUN, hemoglobin, and specific gravity values are normal. (R)

43. **4.** The nurse must recognize that an albumin level of 2.8 g/dl indicates catabolism and potential for malnutrition. Normal albumin is 3.5 to 5.0 g/dl; less than 3.5 indicates malnutrition. The other laboratory results are normal. (R)

44. **1.** Fever is an early sign requiring clinical intervention to identify potential causes. Chills and dyspnea may or may not be observed. Tachycardia can be an indicator in a variety of clinical situations when associated with infection; it usually occurs in response to an elevated temperature or change in cardiac function. (R)

45. **2.** Chemotherapy causes myelosuppression with a decrease in red blood cells (RBCs), WBCs, and platelets. This client's data demonstrate neutropenia, placing the client at risk for infection. An ANC of 500 to 1,000/mm^3 indicates a moderate risk of infection; an ANC of less than 500/mm^3 indicates severe neutropenia and a high risk of infection. When the WBC count is low and immature WBCs are present, normal phagocytosis is impaired. Precautions are implemented to protect the client from life-threatening infections. These may be instituted when ANC is less than 1,000/mm^3. Hand washing is the single best way to avoid the spread of infection. It is not necessary to wear a gown and mask to take care of this client. It is also not necessary to restrict visitors; however, the client's visitors should be screened to avoid exposing the client to possible infections. Epogen or Procrit are used for stimulating RBCs, not WBCs. Granulocyte colony-stimulating factors or granulocyte macrophage colony-stimulating factors are useful for treating neutropenia. (S)

46. **1.** The role of the nurse is to assess what substances or medications the client is using and to document and inform other members of the health care team. It is very important to encourage the client to keep the physician informed of all therapeutic agents, medications, and supplements she is using, to avoid adverse interactions. It is not appropriate for the nurse to suggest that the client choose either Western or alternative therapies or to discourage the client's use of alternative therapies. The nurse should remain objective about the client's treatment choices and respect her autonomy. (R)

47. 1. There are many mechanisms of action for chemotherapeutic agents, but most affect the rapidly dividing cells—both cancerous and noncancerous. Cancer cells are characterized by rapid cell division. Chemotherapy slows cell division. Not all chemotherapeutic agents affect molecular structure. All cells are susceptible to drug toxins, but not all chemotherapeutic agents are toxins. (D)

48. 4. Cough and shortness of breath are significant symptoms because they may indicate decreasing pulmonary function secondary to drug toxicity. Decrease in appetite, difficulty in thinking clearly, and spasms of the diaphragm may occur as a result of chemotherapy; however, they are not indicative of pulmonary toxicity. (A)

The Client Who Is Receiving Radiation Therapy

49. 2. The nurse should first assess the client's usual sleep patterns, hours of sleep required before treatment, and usual bedtime routine. Refraining from watching television before bedtime and avoiding caffeine intake are reasonable suggestions and sleeplessness is an adverse effect of radiation therapy. However, assessment is required before any of these options should be suggested. (H)

50. 4. Difficulty in swallowing, pain, and tightness in the chest are signs of esophagitis, which is a common complication of radiation therapy of the chest wall. Hiatal hernia is a herniation of a portion of the stomach into the esophagus. The client could experience burning and tightness in the chest secondary to a hiatal hernia, but not pain when swallowing. Also, hiatal hernia is not a complication of radiation therapy. Stomatitis is an inflammation of the oral cavity characterized by pain, burning, and ulcerations. The client with stomatitis may experience pain with swallowing, but not burning and tightness in the chest. Radiation enteritis is a disorder of the large and small bowel that occurs during or after radiation therapy to the abdomen, pelvis, or rectum. Nausea, vomiting, abdominal cramping, the frequent urge to have a bowel movement, and watery diarrhea are the signs and symptoms. (A)

51. 2. Impaired concentration, apathy, and feelings of tiredness despite more sleep all suggest fatigue. Fatigue is a common complaint of individuals receiving radiation therapy. There are no data to suggest advanced breast cancer, hypocalcemia, or radiation pneumonitis. (A)

52. 2. Radiation fields that include the ovaries usually result in premature menopause. Vaginal dryness will occur without estrogen replacement. There should be no sexual intercourse while the implant is in place. Cesium is a radioactive isotope used for therapeutic irradiation of cancerous tissue. There is no documentation to support vaginal relaxation after treatment. Because the client will have premature menopause, she will not have normal menstrual periods. (A)

53. 3. Radiation-induced esophagitis with dysphagia is particularly common in clients who receive radiation to the chest. The anatomic location of the esophagus is posterior to the mediastinum and is within the field of primary treatment. Diarrhea may occur with radiation to the abdomen. Decreased energy level and decreased white blood cell count are potential complications of radiation therapy. (R)

The Client Who Requires Symptom Management

54. 1. The packed cells should be administered using a central catheter or 19G needle. Y tubing is used and the normal saline solution is used to keep the vein open when the blood transfusion is complete. Blood is not compatible with dextrose because dextrose may cause blood coagulation. Blood products should be given with normal saline solution. A blood filter must be used for all blood products to filter out sediment from stored blood products. It is not necessary to add another I.V. access. (D)

55. 1. The nurse should perform a thorough assessment of the abdomen and auscultate for bowel sounds in all four quadrants. Clients who have gastrointestinal surgery may have decreased peristalsis for several days after surgery. The nurse should check the abdomen for distention and check with the client and the medical record regarding the passage of flatus or stool. Consulting a dietician would be inappropriate because the client must be kept on nothing-by-mouth status until bowel sounds are present. The nurse should explain to the wife that it is too soon after surgery for her husband to eat. (R)

56. 2. The RN is responsible for describing to the UAP when to report to the RN a result that indicates a potential client problem with dehydration. The RN must assess and interpret results, but must give concrete feedback to the UAP on what is an expected situation or a specific result to report back to the RN. Urine output should be at least 30 ml/hour, or 240 ml over the 8-hour shift. Dehydrated clients may be thirsty and the UAP can ask if the client is thirsty and offer water if permitted. However, because urine output is the critical indicator of dehydration, the UAP should document I&O and give results outside the normal range to the nurse. The nurse is specifically assessing dehydration and should request to receive this information. (M)

57. 3. Anxiety is a common response in the dyspneic client and may be intensified with a diagnosis of cancer. The anxiety is usually caused by fear of choking or cessation of breathing. Labored respirations and lack of energy are not associated with euphoria, and they usually prevent angry behavior. Lack of energy associated with the disease should not be mistaken for laziness. (P)

58.

> **3.** The client receiving spinal radiation for bone cancer metastases who complains of urinary incontinence.

> **1.** The client receiving chemotherapy who complains of a loss of appetite.

> **4.** The client with colon cancer who has questions about a high-fiber diet.

> **2.** The client who underwent a mastectomy 2 weeks ago who called for information on the Reach for Recovery program.

Using Maslow's hierarchy of needs to set priorities, the nurse should first call the client with bone cancer metastases to the spine because this client is at risk for compression, damage, or severing of the spinal cord. The nurse should evaluate the client immediately for urinary incontinence, paralysis, difficulty ambulating, and possible weakness or loss of motor function. The nurse should next call the client with loss of appetite to assess weight loss and suggest ways to increase the appetite. The client with colon cancer requires assistance with diet planning, also a physiologic need, but this client is not at high risk for weight loss. Lastly, the nurse should obtain information on Reach to Recovery and return the call to the client with a mastectomy. The needs of this client are the least urgent. (R)

59. 3. For clients with obstructive versus restrictive disorders, extending exhalation through pursed-lip breathing will make the respiratory effort more efficient. The usual position of choice for this client is the upright position, leaning slightly forward to allow greater lung expansion. Teaching diaphragmatic breathing techniques will be more helpful to the client with a restrictive disorder. Administering cough suppressants will not help respiratory effort. A low semi-Fowler's position does not encourage lung expansion. Lung expansion is enhanced in the upright position. (C)

60. 1, 2, 3, 6. Thrombocytopenia places the client at risk for bleeding. Therefore, electric razors will reduce the potential for skin nicks and bleeding. Oral hygiene should be provided with a soft toothbrush and with minimal friction to gently clean without trauma. Clients should be instructed to read labels on all over-the-counter medications and avoid medication such as aspirin or NSAIDs due to their effect on platelet adhesiveness. Clients should evaluate mucous membranes, skin, stools, or other sources of potential bleeding. Monitoring temperature may be an important part of assessment but is focused on neutropenia instead of the problem of thrombocytopenia. (R)

61. 2. The administration of antipyretics and antihistamines before initiation of the transfusion in the frequently transfused client can decrease the incidence of febrile reactions. Febrile reactions are immune-mediated and are caused by antibodies in the recipient that are directed against antigens present on the granulocytes, platelets, and lymphocytes in the transfused component. They are the most common transfusion reactions and may occur with onset, during transfusion, or hours after transfusion is completed. (D)

62. 2. After surgical resection, functional lung tissue is lost, resulting in chronic difficulty meeting the body's demand for oxygen, and thus the dyspnea. Increased dyspnea may indicate an additional respiratory stress, such as pneumonia or bronchitis. Fibrotic changes usually are a result of radiation therapy. There is no indication that the client has received myelosuppressive therapy to cause anemia. Pericardial effusions would be more likely to result from chemotherapy or radiation. (A)

63. 1. Negative outcomes due to fatigue may include diminished quality of life, loss of self-esteem, depression, caregiver strain and fatigue, social isolation, decreased functional status, and poor disease prognosis. Increased risk of infection is not related to fatigue but is related to immunosuppression secondary to chemotherapy. Fatigue does not indicate an improved prognosis. It does not cause increased pain. Cancer pain is caused by many factors, including bone metastasis, nerve compression, infiltration of the tumor into normal structures, and ischemia. (P)

64. 1. Dietary suggestions to reduce adverse effects of cancer and cancer therapies include a soft, bland diet low in fat and sugar. Frequent, small meals are usually better tolerated. It is not necessary to restrict the diet to cold foods. Fluid intake should be encouraged to avoid dehydration. (C)

65. 4. The use of diet modification is a conservative approach to treat the terminally ill or hospice clients who have nausea and vomiting related to bowel obstruction. Osmotic laxatives would be harder for the client to tolerate. An NG tube is more aggressive and invasive. I.V. antiemetics are also invasive. The hospice philosophy involves comfort and palliative care for the terminally ill. (C)

66. 3. Repositioning the client, elevating the head of the bed, and providing a cool compress are comfort interventions consistent with the concept of palliative care of the dying. Directing the unlicensed personnel to assess vital signs focuses on the dying process, not the client. Suctioning may not benefit the client and is considered invasive and uncomfortable. Telling the wife an intervention is not needed discounts her judgment and concerns. (C)

67. 2. Alopecia from chemotherapy is temporary. The new hair will not be necessarily gray, but the texture and color of new hair growth may be different. Clients who will be receiving chemotherapy should be encouraged to purchase a wig while they still have hair so that they can match the color and texture of their hair. Loss of hair, or alopecia, is a serious threat to self-esteem and should be addressed quickly before treatment. (D)

68. **3.** Dyspnea is a distressing symptom in clients with advanced cancer including metastatic carcinoma of the lung, previous radiation therapy, and coexisting COPD. Ascites does occur in clients with metastatic carcinoma; however, in the client with COPD and lung cancer, dyspnea is a more common finding. A pleural friction rub is usually associated with pneumonia, pleurisy, or pulmonary infarct. (A)

69. **3.** The positive reinforcement builds confidence and facilitates achievement of rehabilitation goals. Community support may or may not be applicable after discharge. Although family support is an important component of rehabilitation, reinforcing the skills the client has acquired is of greater importance when regaining independence. Rehabilitation plans should include the client, family, or both. (P)

70. **2.** The most important intervention for infection control is to continue meticulous catheter site care. Dressings are to be changed two to three times per week depending on institutional policies. Temperature should be monitored at least once a day in someone with a vascular access device. Hand washing before and after irrigation or any manipulation of the site is a must for infection prevention. (S)

71. **1, 2, 4, 5.** A major concern with I.V. administration of cytotoxic agents is vessel irritation or extravasation. The Oncology Nursing Society and hospital guidelines require frequent reevaluation of blood return when administering vesicant or nonvesicant chemotherapy due to the risk of extravasation. These guidelines apply to peripheral and central venous lines. The nurse should also assess the insertion site for signs of infiltration, such as swelling and redness. In addition, central venous lines may be long-term venous access devices. Thus, difficulty drawing or aspirating blood may indicate the line is against the vessel wall or may indicate the line has occlusion. Having the client cough or move position may change the status of the line if it is temporarily against a vessel wall. Occlusion warrants more thorough evaluation via X-ray study to verify placement if the status is questionable and may require a declotting regimen (Abbokinase). The nurse should not administer any drug if the I.V. line is not open or does not have an adequate blood return. (D)

72. The distal tip of a central line lies in the superior vena cava or right atrium. (D)

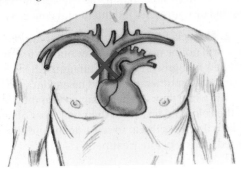

73. **2.** The client is exhibiting signs and symptoms of a pneumothorax from the insertion of the subclavian venous catheter. Although it is possible that the client suffered an air embolus during the procedure, and the client is at risk for pulmonary emboli because of his immobility, absent breath sounds immediately after insertion of a subclavian line are strongly suggestive of a pneumothorax. Unilateral absent breath sounds are not associated with a myocardial infarction. (A)

74. **4.** An appropriate and realistic outcome would be for the client to maintain current weight or not lose weight. It is unrealistic to expect that the client with advanced liver cancer will have normal albumin levels or will be able to gain weight. (C)

75. **3.** As long as the client is able to get out of bed, the preferred position and time frame for preventing aspiration after a bolus tube feeding is sitting upright out of bed in a chair for 30 to 60 minutes. Placing the client on the right, not the left, side may facilitate gastric emptying, but this is not the preferred position. Elevating the bed 30 degrees decreases the risk of aspiration, but this elevation must be maintained for at least 45 to 60 minutes. (C)

76. **1.** Total parenteral nutrition solutions supply the body with sufficient amounts of dextrose, amino acids, fats, vitamins, and minerals to meet metabolic needs. Clients who are unable to tolerate adequate quantities of foods and fluids and those who have had extensive bowel surgery may not be candidates for enteral feedings. The nurse would anticipate total parenteral nutrition via central catheter to promote wound healing. I.V. dextrose does not supply all the nutrients required to promote wound healing. (D)

77. **1, 2, 4.** Elevated temperature in the first 24 hours along with coarse breath sounds may indicate a respiratory complication or the result of general anesthesia. Use of incentive spirometry and increasing activity would be key interventions. A healthy stoma will be beefy red. A dusky appearance of the stoma indicates decreased blood supply and is of concern. It is not uncommon to have decreased bowel sounds initially after gastrointestinal surgery. In addition, it usually will take time for the ostomy to function. (R)

78. **3.** The client is experiencing metabolic alkalosis caused by loss of hydrogen and chloride ions from excessive vomiting. This is shown by a pH of 7.46 (normal is 7.35 to 7.45) and an elevated bicarbonate level of 29 mEq/L (normal is 22 to 26 mEq/L). Respiratory alkalosis, which results from hyperventilation, is characterized by a low carbon dioxide (CO_2) level due to blowing off CO_2 (normal is 35 to 45 mm Hg) with hyperventilation. Respiratory acidosis is characterized by a decreased pH, which is a result of CO_2 retention. A decreased bicarbonate level and a decreased pH characterize metabolic acidosis, which can result from various pathophysiologic states. (A)

79. **4.** The content of the client's comments suggests that she is avoiding intimacy with her husband by waiting until he is asleep before going to bed. Addressing sexuality issues is appropriate for a client who has undergone a mastectomy. Rushing her return to work may debilitate her and add to her exhaustion. Suggesting that she learn relaxation techniques for help with her insomnia is appropriate; however, the nurse must first address the psychosocial and sexual issues that are contributing to her sleeping difficulties. A nutritional assessment may be useful, but there is no indication that she has anorexia. (P)

80. **3.** Although each client listed is at some risk of complication secondary to immobility, the 75-year-old man is in need of intensive interventions. Contributing factors include his age, pain management, extended bed rest, and the potential for preexisting nutritional deficits. (M)

81. **3.** Immobility sets up the tissue to atrophy and protein catabolism to increase, which results in a decreased metabolic rate. Cardiovascular workload increases because of venous stasis. Lung expansion decreases because there is less gas exchange. (R)

82. **3.** The client is exhibiting early symptoms of pulmonary toxicity as a result of the radiation therapy. These are not expected adverse effects of radiation. He needs to be examined to differentiate between an infection and radiation pneumonitis. Suggesting that the client take acetaminophen and call back in 2 days is inappropriate. These signs and symptoms are not indicative of a true emergency, but the client should be seen before his next scheduled office visit. (R)

83. **4.** Orders should include X-rays to see whether the fluid moves freely and is amenable to removal by thoracentesis. Fluid loculation is a risk of repeated thoracentesis. A platelet count may be necessary if the client is at risk for bleeding tendencies. Arterial blood gases or an ECG is not required before a thoracentesis. An abnormal WBC count may not necessarily preclude the procedure and is not required before thoracentesis. (R)

84. **3.** Surgery for head and neck malignancies often causes edema of the upper airway that can result in difficulty breathing and the need for a tracheostomy. Clients undergoing chemotherapy or radiation may have impaired gas exchange from suppression of red blood cells. However, they will still have spontaneous ventilation. (R)

85. **3.** Changing positions frequently aids in distributing the agent to the pleura for sealing. The majority of the pleural fluid is drained, and the lung should already be re-expanded before instillation of the sclerosing agent. A pressure dressing is applied to the chest tube exit site, and it is not necessary to lie on that side to hold pressure on the area. (R)

86. **4.** Providing adequate humidification for the client with a tracheostomy is essential. The client no longer has the functions of the nose for warming, moistening, or filtering the air when breathing through the tracheostomy site. Providing tracheostomy site care, addressing the psychosocial issues, and observing for early signs and symptoms of skin breakdown around the tracheostomy site are also important; however, using humidifiers to prevent thick, tenacious secretions is the most important recommendation for long-term management and the prevention of pulmonary infection. (R)

87. **4.** A malignant pleural effusion is an accumulation of excessive fluid within the pleural space that occurs when cancer cells irritate the pleural membrane. Dyspnea can result from the increased pressure that may contribute to increased anxiety and fear of suffocation. Pain is a consequence of the pleural irritation. Cough is related to the atelectasis of the bronchi and inability to clear the airways. Hiccups are usually associated with pericardial effusions. Weight gain and peripheral edema may occur with peritoneal effusion. (A)

88. **1.** The thoracentesis is less likely to be successful as a treatment for recurrent pleural effusion because the fluid accumulates rapidly. Thoracentesis is usually successful for diagnosis of underlying disease, palliation of symptoms, and acute respiratory distress. Alleviation of the symptoms and distress is usually short-term in recurrent effusions. (R)

89. **3.** Cold intolerance may be associated with anemia because of the diminished oxygen supply to the peripheral circulation. Decreased salivation is not necessarily associated with anemia. Tachycardia may be expected in severe anemia. Clients with anemia are usually not nauseated. (A)

90. **4.** A bloody effusion is strong indication of a malignancy. Milky fluid suggests a chylous process from lymphatic obstruction. Straw-colored fluid is considered normal. Turbid fluid may indicate an infection. (A)

91. **3.** The PT and PTT are blood tests that measure factors involved in the clotting process and can give a fair indication if there is a clotting deficit. CEA and AFP are tumor markers associated with malignancies and are not used to evaluate a hypercoagulable state. A platelet count may be used in the evaluation of a hypercoagulable state, but it is not always included in the CBC and would need to be ordered separately. (R)

92. **4.** Bacterial endotoxins released from gram-negative bacteria activate the Hageman factor or coagulation factor XII. This factor inhibits coagulation via the intrinsic pathway of homeostasis, as well as stimulating fibrinolysis. Liver disease can cause multiple bleeding abnormalities resulting in chronic, subclinical DIC; however, sepsis is the most common cause. Brain metastasis is not related to DIC. I.V. heparin therapy is sometimes used to treat clients with DIC, but this treatment is controversial. It does not cause DIC but can result in bleeding tendencies if the therapeutic dose is exceeded. (A)

93. **4.** Petechiae are tiny purplish, hemorrhagic spots visible under the skin. Petechiae usually appear when platelets are depleted. Bleeding gums or oozing of blood may accompany the petechiae, and the client should seek medical assistance immediately. Increasing iron in the diet will not improve the platelet count. Lotion will not treat the petechiae. Elevating the legs will not cause the petechiae to disappear. (A)

94. **3.** Lymphedema after breast cancer surgery is the accumulation of lymph tissue in the tissues of the upper extremity extending down from the upper arm. It may occur at any time after surgery in women of any age. It is caused by the interruption or removal of lymph channels and nodes after axillary node dissection. Removal results in less efficient filtration of lymph fluid and a pooling of lymph fluid in the tissues on the affected side. Treatments or interventions should be instituted as soon as lymphedema is noted to prevent or reduce further progression. Range-of-motion exercises, elevation, and avoidance of injury in the affected arm are important when completing client teaching. Lymphoma is not caused by failure to remove all cancer cells. Lymphedema can occur after any surgery that disrupts lymph flow, not just radical mastectomy. (R)

95. **3.** Low-dose administration of warfarin prophylactically appears to prevent or decrease the incidence of thrombus formation because of a mild anticoagulation effect. Urokinase is not used prophylactically but is used to treat massive pulmonary emboli, vascular thromboses, or occluded I.V. catheters. Vitamin B_{12} is used to treat pernicious anemia, and neither it nor acetaminophen affects thrombus formation. (D)

96. **3.** Infection may occur in a client with lymphedema because of the stagnant accumulated fluid, which becomes an excellent medium for bacteria growth. Capillary permeability, not fragility, increases fluid in lymphedema. Myelosuppression is not related to lymphedema, only to a neoplastic disease or sequela to treatment of neoplastic disease. Increased use of the extremity may also cause increased accumulation of fluid, but it is not a direct cause of cellulitis and lymphangitis. (R)

97. **3.** Redness, warmth, and swelling are all signs of infection. Treatment with antibiotics is usually indicated. Infection usually increases fluid accumulation and could worsen the lymphedema. Warm compresses could also increase fluid accumulation. Elevation will not treat the infection. It is critical that the client not delay treatment. (R)

98. **4.** Fever is most commonly related to infection. In a neutropenic client, fever frequently occurs in the absence of the usual clinical signs and symptoms of infection. Inadequate nutrition or antiemetic therapy resistance would not result in fever. Fever is not usually expected with most chemotherapy drugs. (A)

99. **1.** A pneumonectomy is the removal of an entire lung field. A wedge resection refers to removal of a wedge-shaped section of lung tissue. A lobectomy is the removal of one lobe. Removal of one or more segments of a lung lobe is called a partial lobectomy. (R)

100. **1.** The fever and chills associated with the administration of BRMs tend to be predictable and usually respond very well to antipyretics. They usually diminish in 8 to 12 hours after each administration. The symptoms tend to decrease in intensity with continued therapy. There is no biphasic pattern associated with these adverse effects. (D)

101. **2.** Nine days after chemotherapy, one would expect the client to be immunocompromised. The clinical signs and symptoms of shock reflect changes in cardiac function, vascular resistance, cellular metabolism, and capillary permeability. Low-grade fever, tachycardia, and chills may be early signs of shock. The client with signs and symptoms of impending septic shock may not have decreased oxygen saturation levels. Oliguria and hypotension are late signs of shock. Urine output can be initially normal or increased. (D)

102. **3.** Prioritizing physical activities helps to conserve energy, which promotes adaptation to fatigue. The client should learn to take short naps or short rest periods during the day for additional energy conversation. Increased fluid intake is important but may interrupt rest periods by causing frequent urination. Limiting intake of high-fiber foods can add to constipation, which may be a problem because of inactivity in fatigued clients. (C)

103. **4.** Most hospitalized persons are at risk for sleep disturbances. Psychological issues (such as anxiety and depression) and pain are related to sleep deprivation. Social, nutritional, and cultural issues are not necessarily associated with sleep disturbances. (P)

104. **4.** Nursing interventions to decrease the discomfort of pruritus include those that prevent vasodilation, decrease anxiety, and maintain skin integrity and hydration. Medicated baths with salicylic acid or colloidal oatmeal can be soothing as a temporary relief. The use of antihistamines or topical steroids depends on the cause of the pruritus, and these agents should be used with caution. Using silk sheets is not a practical intervention for the hospitalized client with pruritus. (C)

105. **3.** Opioids can be effective in controlling intractable dyspnea and are considered safe, even though an adverse side effect may be decreased respiratory rate. Mucolytic agents, antidepressants, and diuretics do not affect dyspnea. (D)

106. **4.** Use of deodorant or fragrant soaps is drying to the skin. Cotton clothing gives the least irritation to skin. A cool, humidified environment adds to the client's comfort as well as providing hydration for skin comfort. Fluid intake of 3,000 ml per day is recommended for adequate hydration. (C)

107. **4.** Individuals with cancer have various cultural values and beliefs that help them cope with the cancer experience. Quality of life cannot be evaluated solely by quantifiable factors such as employability, functional status, or evidence of disease. It must be evaluated by the survivors within the context of their subjective and individual values and beliefs. (P)

108. **3.** Constipation lasting 3 days or longer is unusual in this client and warrants immediate action. However, because the client had chemotherapy with doxorubicin (Adriamycin) 10 days ago, she is susceptible to infection and should avoid rectal medications and treatments. Abdominal discomfort secondary to constipation will be relieved after the client has a bowel movement; an opioid would contribute to the constipation. (D)

109. **4.** A bedside commode should be near the client for easy, safe access. Measurement of urine output is also important in a client with heart failure. Putting diapers on an alert and oriented individual would be demeaning and inappropriate. Indwelling catheters are associated with increased risk of infection and are not a solution to possible incontinence. There is no reason to think that the client would not be able to use the bedside commode. (S)

110. **4.** The rectal area needs to be cleaned and gently dried after each bowel movement to prevent skin breakdown and inhibit growth of bacteria. Sitz baths are appropriate because they promote comfort. Zinc oxide ointment does form a protective skin barrier, but it makes it difficult to thoroughly clean the perirectal area of feces and increases the risk of infection, as do skin-barrier dressings. (S)

111. **2.** Studies of long-term immunologic effects in clients treated for leukemia, Hodgkin's disease, and breast cancer reveal that combination treatments of chemotherapy and radiation can cause overall bone marrow suppression, decreased leukocyte counts, and profound immunosuppression. Persistent and severe immunologic impairment may follow radiation and chemotherapy (especially multiagent therapy). There is no evidence of greater risk of infection in clients with persistent immunologic abnormalities. Suppressor T cells recover more rapidly than the helper T cells. (D)

112. **1.** Clients who receive multiple platelet transfusions may form antibodies against many foreign antigens, thereby decreasing platelet response. Single-donor platelets are drawn from a single donor, decreasing the number of possible foreign antigens and increasing platelet response for long-term therapy. Platelets do not contain coagulation factors in clinically significant amounts. Clients with a platelet count greater than 50,000/mm³ are not at risk for bleeding. Human leukocyte antigen–matched platelets are used when clients become refractory to single-donor and random-donor platelets. (D)

The Client Who Is Coping with Loss, Grief, Bereavement, and Spiritual Distress

113. **4.** Identifying available resources for the client and family represents a respectful effort to make options available and encourages the client to become involved in treatment decisions. Assuming decision making for the client may foster dependence. Encouraging strict compliance with all treatment regimens may increase anxiety and limit the client's options and treatment choices. Informing the client of all possible adverse treatment effects may increase anxiety and fear by focusing on adverse outcomes too soon. (P)

114. **4.** Denial is a defense mechanism used to shut out a situation that is too frightening or threatening to tolerate. In this case, denial allows the client to vacillate between acceptance of the illness and its treatment and denial of the actual or potential seriousness of the disease. This may allow the client more psychological freedom to maintain her current roles in the family and elsewhere. Denial can be harmful if the client ignores standard medical therapies in favor of unconventional treatments. Denial is not helpful when it interferes with a client's willingness to seek treatment or make decisions about care. Using any one defense mechanism exclusively usually reflects maladaptive coping. Other defense mechanisms that may be used include regression, humor, and sublimation. (P)

115. **2.** The client's resources for coping with the emotional and practical needs of herself and her family need to be assessed because usual coping strategies and support systems are often inadequate in especially stressful situations. The nurse may be concerned with the client's use of denial, decision-making abilities, and ability to pay for transportation; however, the client's support systems will be of more importance in this situation. (P)

116. **4.** Variables that are most predictive of negative bereavement outcomes include anger and self-reproach, low socioeconomic status, lack of preparation for death, and lack of family support. Making preparations suggests that she is coping with her husband's approaching death. (P)

117. **4.** Having a higher socioeconomic status helps a person achieve healthy bereavement. Younger people are at higher risk for negative bereavement outcomes. Having a history of depressive illness or anxiety is a risk factor for negative bereavement outcomes. (P)

118. **4.** Focusing on the client's physical capabilities is important, but powerlessness reflects a perceived lack of control over the current situation and the belief that one's actions will not affect the outcome. Participation in decision making is key to getting the client involved and feeling more in control of his own care. Apathy and dependence on others are characteristics of powerlessness. Encouraging others to take responsibility for the client's care will increase his feelings of powerlessness. A referral to a psychologist is not necessarily indicated. The nurse should implement strategies to involve the client in decisions about his care and evaluate the response to this intervention before suggesting a referral. (P)

119. **1.** Maintaining role function has been found to be a supportive source of normalcy and positive self-esteem for the client and family during the cancer experience. Facilitating family-related disagreements and conflicts is not the nurse's role. Supporting the client in her use of denial as a coping strategy will not help facilitate the client's adaptation to the diagnosis. Arranging transportation and child care on treatment days may be helpful but does not necessarily facilitate adaptation to the diagnosis. (P)

120. **2.** The most important central component of hospice care is focus of care on the client as well as the family or significant other. The team approach and the physician's coordination of the hospice team are important, but they are not the focus. Not all hospice clients want to die at home. (C)

121. **3.** Mental changes and decreased level of consciousness are common in the dying process. Comments that allude to travel, trips, or going somewhere are also common. Suggesting that the client be sedated ignores the husband's question about what his wife is experiencing. Suggesting that the client is fighting death and that the husband should leave her alone is inappropriate and denies the husband time to spend with his wife. Although decreased circulation and lack of oxygen may cause delirium, delirium is not the norm in the dying process. (P)

122. **4.** It is important to give factual information to answer a loved one's questions and concerns. Stating, "That's just the way it is," is unprofessional and uncaring. Saying, "I don't know when the bowels will shut down, but they will eventually," projects an uncaring attitude and does not address the wife's concern for her husband or her need for information. Although it may be true that the pain medication will slow bowel function, this does not provide the wife with the information she is seeking. (P)

123. **4.** It is important to allow the client to choose his or her own form of spiritual support. The dying client who is weakened by disease may not be able to attend services. The client must be consulted before referral to a chaplain is made. Reflection on past accomplishments may be comforting to the client, but it does not directly address spiritual concerns. (P)

124. **2.** A social worker can provide information for supportive services and can help the client with financial concerns. A bank representative, loan officer, or someone from the hospital billing department may be needed; however, it is most appropriate for the social worker to first assess the client's needs. (P)

125. **4.** Dehydration is an expected event within the dying process. Hydration may be used in any situation of dehydration as long as it is within the client and family's wishes. Rehydrating the client may actually prolong the dying process. Decisions about treatment are made with the family. (C)

126. **4.** The nurse must first allow the client to explore his or her own beliefs and values before making referrals, explaining various religious beliefs, or suggesting appropriate reading material. (P)

127. **3.** The family is in the best position to give the information they elect to disclose to friends and community members. The hospice nurse and the oncologist must maintain client confidentiality. Therefore, disclosing any information about the client's condition would be inappropriate. (M)

128. **1.** Ongoing assessment by the RN is required to evaluate the client with dyspnea to monitor for potential deterioration of the respiratory status. If the RN is the care provider, she will have greater interaction with the individual client. The RN is responsible for assessment of all the clients. The other clients would not be considered unstable, and maintaining a patent airway is always the priority in providing care. Care for the other clients could be assigned safely, according to the abilities of the LVN-LPN and UAP. (M)

129. **4.** Depression can be a mixture of affective responses (feelings of worthlessness, hopelessness, sadness), behavioral responses (appetite changes, withdrawal, sleep disturbances, lethargy), and cognitive responses (decreased ability to concentrate, indecisiveness, suicidal ideation). Increased decisiveness, problem-solving ability, and increased social interactions are reflective of adaptive coping. (P)

130. **4.** Bereavement support after death usually continues for about 1 year or as needed at little or no cost to the remaining family. Mutual support groups by nonprofessionals are usually free or inexpensive but are not necessarily appropriate for young children. Professional individual counseling and medication are expensive, and medication may not be appropriate for young children. To remind someone of what she should have done before the death is not helpful at this time. (P)

131. **3.** It is important to establish rapport with the client and family by listening to verbal and nonverbal concern and showing respect for cultural differences. The use of touch or eye contact is culture-specific and cannot be generalized as an intervention for all individuals with cancer. Miscommunication between individuals of different cultures is often caused by language differences, rules of communication, age, and gender. (P)

132. **1.** Helping the client to identify available resources allows the client respect and time to make informed decisions and encourages him to become actively involved with treatment options. Encouraging compliance with treatment regimens discourages the client from becoming actively involved in his treatment and diminishes coping ability. Relieving the client of decision making as much as possible is not appropriate and encourages feelings of helplessness and powerlessness. Assisting the client to prepare for adverse treatment effects may foster hopelessness and increase anxiety by focusing on adverse outcomes too soon. (P)

133. **4.** These American Cancer Society–sponsored groups are designed to educate clients and their families experiencing cancer about the disease and methods of coping positively with it. These are self-help and support groups monitored by professionals and cancer survivors who have undergone a training course that helps them to facilitate small groups. (P)

134. **4.** Many cancer survivors question why they are doing so well and others are not. Often they express feeling guilty when they hear that others are not doing well. Suggesting that the client does not know how to describe his own emotions is inappropriate and may discourage him from expressing his feelings. Although the client may be experiencing volatile emotions, this is not the likely source of his feelings of guilt. Guilt about doing well after cancer treatment is not a spiritual response to illness. (P)

135. **4.** The recurrence of the disease is found to be the most distressing time, and clients may experience anxiety, depression, and suicidal ideation. Clients may feel a decrease in their anxiety and depression with the initiation of definitive treatment or at the end of their first course of treatment. Clients in the end stage of the disease may feel all of these emotions; however, when clients have been free from cancer for some time and learn that there is a recurrence, they often experience a sharp increase in their feelings of distress. (P)

136. **2.** Powerlessness is a subjective experience of helplessness and apathy that can be threatening to one's competency and result in increased dependence on others. Effective nursing interventions will provide opportunities for the client to be involved in decision making and to regain a sense of control. Ineffective coping may also be a response to altered mobility, but the nursing interventions would be directed toward enhancing coping skills. Impaired adjustment is characterized by statements or actions suggesting that the client has not accepted the change in her health status. Complicated grieving is characterized by sadness, reliving past experiences, and expressions of distress about the loss. (P)

137. **4.** The person who has minimal social support, has not been successful in dealing with stressors, and has multiple other stressors is at greater risk for psychosocial distress. Being successful in dealing with stress all his life would decrease the client's risk for psychosocial distress. Not having to deal with other stressors would be helpful in managing the current stressful situation. The denial coping mechanism, if used for short periods, can decrease the risk for psychosocial distress. (P)

138. **1.** Cancer clients report that the lifelong fear of recurrence is one of the most disruptive aspects of the disease. The trajectory of the disease is unpredictable and can be intertwined with many short- and long-term illnesses related to cancer and the treatment modalities. A diagnosis of cancer challenges the individual and the family with a series of crises rather than a time-limited episode. There are no data to indicate that the client has an underlying behavioral disorder. (P)

139. **4.** Without clear, consistent communication, the parent-child relationship may become strained during the illness and subsequent death of a parent. A great number of parents do not know how to communicate with their children, especially about difficult emotional topics at a time when they are also under great emotional stress. The nurse should begin by providing information and developmentally appropriate books about the grieving process for children. Referral to pastoral care services may be appropriate; however, the nurse's direct intervention of beginning education about strategies for communication will be of immediate and long-term benefit. The grieving process cannot be rushed for the husband, nor should an opportunity for the father and children to communicate and grieve together be delayed. Excluding children from participating in the grieving ritual is not shielding them from the sorrow and sadness. (P)

140. **3.** Acknowledgment and discussion of the client's feelings begin the establishment of a therapeutic relationship between nurse and client. It also acknowledges the seriousness of the current situation and validates the client's feelings. Psychiatric help and antidepressant medication may be options if the depression is severe and prolonged. Encouraging a client to see the good or positive side of a situation minimizes the client's feelings. (P)

141. **2.** Individuals who are experiencing fatigue need to prioritize their activities and ask for assistance from others. It is best not to take away all of the client's activities because her role as wife and mother is obviously important to her and to her sense of self-worth. Suggesting that she ignore the household chores or telling her not to worry because everyone gets tired disregards the client's feelings and is not appropriate. (C)

142. **4.** Tachycardia, tachypnea, moist or clammy skin, and disorientation are classic symptoms of delirium. Clients with panic disorder do not exhibit disorientation. Clients with depression exhibit a flat affect, apathy, and sleep disturbances. Clients with schizophrenia have thought disorders such as hallucinations or delusions. (A)

143. **2.** A progressive activity regimen may be prescribed to increase pulmonary function after surgical lung resection. Rehabilitation should include walking and some stair climbing as tolerated. Vigorous exercise is usually not recommended initially. Joining the Lost Chord Club and learning tracheostomy care are appropriate for the client who has undergone a laryngectomy. (P)

144. **4.** Serving as a volunteer in a client-to-client program represents reintegration with constructive channeling of energies, which indicates a higher level of adaptation than attention to safety, knowledge, or planned activity. (P)

The Client Who Is Experiencing Problems with Sexuality

145. **3.** Water-soluble lubricants used during sexual intercourse can augment reduced natural vaginal lubrication caused by ovarian dysfunction and decreased circulating estrogen related to chemotherapy. The use of vaginal dilators, relaxation techniques, or nightly douches would not increase vaginal lubrication. Frequent douching can disrupt the normal vaginal environment. (H)

146. **3.** Placing a thin piece of gauze over the tracheostomy during sexual activity will help to contain the secretions and yet allow ventilation. Although a scopolamine patch may depress the salivary and bronchial secretions, it is not recommended for long-term use and would not be indicated in this situation. Avoiding fluids before sexual activity is not recommended to decrease secretions. Washing the tracheostomy area with any deodorizing soap may cause skin irritation and place the client at risk for infection. (H)

147. **4.** This question introduces some basic information and allows for support for the client who may be experiencing some sexuality concerns. Not all women experience sexual problems after undergoing a hysterectomy. Assuming that the client will want to schedule an appointment with her partner is inappropriate and may embarrass her. Simply asking the client whether she expects to have problems with sex is too abrupt and does not provide any information. (P)

148. **4.** Although there may not be a big change in sexual function with a unilateral orchiectomy, the loss of a gonad and testosterone may result in decreased libido and sterility. Sperm banking may be an option worth exploring if the number and motility of the sperm are adequate. Remember, the population most affected by testicular cancer is generally young men ages 15 to 34, and in this crucial stage of life, sexual anxieties may be a large concern. (P)

149. **4.** The risk of becoming neutropenic during chemotherapy is very high. Therefore, an inserted foreign object such as a diaphragm may be a nidus for infection. Although the nurse may wish to inform the client about the ease with which various contraceptive modalities may be used, the focus of this discussion should be on preventing an infection, which can be fatal for the neutropenic client. There are no data to suggest the client is at risk for acquiring a sexually transmitted disease. The client will not be experiencing body changes directly related to hormonal changes. (S)

150. **2.** Raising the upper torso for the affected partner facilitates respiratory function. The use of a waterbed may be helpful for the sensation of movement but it does not promote respiratory expansion. A dependent position may compromise respiratory expansion, even though energy may be conserved. Duration of sexual activity is not necessarily related to exertion. (H)

Ethical and Legal Issues Related to Clients with Cancer

151. **3.** The registered nurse assigning care should first give the LVN-LPN the opportunity to explore his concerns and fears about caring for a client with HIV infection. Reassigning care for this client, assisting with care, and reviewing precautions do not address the present concern or create an environment that will generate useful knowledge regarding future assignments for client care. (M)

152. **1.** The American Cancer Society wrote *The Cancer Survivors' Bill of Rights*. These rights address medical care, personal life adjustment, job opportunities, and insurance coverage. (M)

153. **1.** The Family Leave Act of 1993 ensures that family caregivers who must take a leave of absence or decrease their hours during the treatment or recovery phase of an illness will not lose their jobs. The Americans with Disabilities Act of 1990 prohibits employment discrimination against persons with disabilities or those who are perceived to have disabilities; it has an indirect economic impact for cancer victims and their families. The Medicare Coverage for Catastrophic Illness Act of 1988 provides increased coverage for clients with a catastrophic illness. The Rehabilitation Act of 1973 prohibits discrimination on the basis of handicap under any program or activity receiving federal financial assistance. (M)

154. **1.** The Americans with Disabilities Act of 1990 requires equal opportunity in selection, testing, and hiring of qualified applicants with disabilities. Under this act, anyone who has had cancer is considered disabled. This law prohibits discrimination against workers with disabilities and is similar to the Civil Rights Act of 1964 and Title V of the Rehabilitation Act of 1973. The Patient Self-Determination Act addresses the rights of clients in regard to making health care decisions and the use of advance directives. (M)

155. **3.** The goal of client autonomy is to respect the client's choice not to know particular information. The client's best interests should be determined by the client after he or she receives all the necessary information and in conjunction with other people of the client's choice, including family, physicians, and other health care personnel. The client's best interests are not totally directed by the physician or the health care team. (M)

End-of-Life Care

156. **1, 2, 5.** In 1991, the Omnibus Reconciliation Act became effective. This Patient Self-Determination Act requires all institutions that participate in Medicare to provide information about and the right to initiate advance directives. Advance directives are written statements of person's wishes related to health care if they are unable to decide for themselves. These documents relate to current or future health care and not past medical history. Competent adults are responsible for their own health care decisions and their own right to accept or refuse treatment. Advance directives are used when the person cannot make the decision. Medical power-of-attorney is a term used to describe the person who makes health care decisions should someone be unable to make informed decisions for himself or herself. The focus is not primarily financial access. (M)

157. **4.** The advocacy role of the nurse implies that the nurse will ensure that the client's wishes are being respected and that she is making informed decisions. Therefore, the nurse will assist in ensuring that the client is fully informed. The other interventions are appropriate for the nurse but are not related to client advocacy. The client may not understand or have all the necessary information for standard therapy. A client who is taking an alternative therapy should be monitored for adverse effects. If a client is taking an alternative therapy, it is essential for the physician to know so that the therapy can be incorporated into the client's treatment plan and to ensure that there are no incompatibilities with other therapies or medications. (M)

158. **2, 3, 4, 5.** End-of-life care is the term currently used for issues related to death and dying. End-of-life care focuses on physical and psychosocial needs at the end of life for the client and client's family. Palliative care is health care aimed at symptom management rather than curative treatment for diseases. Goals would include providing comfort and support for the client and family and improving the client's quality of life. Grief counseling is a component and efforts would be to enhance the coping of all involved and not to alter usual coping methods. (M)

159. **3.** The best nursing advocacy intervention is listening carefully to the client's and family's perceptions of their needs. Studies have demonstrated that these needs are not necessarily what the nurse thinks they are. Intervening without listening carefully may result in a lack of responsiveness to the real needs. Helping the client and family maintain a sense of optimism and hopefulness is appropriate but is not necessarily advocacy. Determining the client's and family's understanding of the results of the diagnostic testing and providing written materials about the cancer site and its treatment are examples of the nurse's role as educator. (P)

160. **1.** The nurse would give the client a tissue and tell him it's okay to cry to convey acceptance and empathy. He needs to know that it is natural to have tremendous feelings of loss and sadness. Telling the client to stop crying, busying oneself in the client's room, and changing the subject are not helpful to the client because they ignore his needs and inhibit the expression of emotion. (P)

161. **2, 3, 4, 5, 6.** With serious, chronic, and terminal illnesses, it is important to help clients and families address fears, difficulties with home care, advance directives, hospice and home care options, and final arrangements. Predicting the length of life for this client is not appropriate at admission. (P)

162. **1.** The client's husband is experiencing anger, much of which stems from feelings of guilt about not taking the trip. During the stage of denial, the husband is more likely to deny the client's diagnosis and prognosis. During the stage of bargaining, the husband would offer to do certain things in exchange for more time before the client dies. In the stage of depression, the husband is likely to make few or no comments and to act dejected. (P)

163. **1.** Nurses who have contemplated or examined their own feelings about death and dying are usually more effective when caring for the dying client and family. Many authorities consider self-examination of one's own finiteness essential before one can successfully meet the needs of a dying client. Continuing education classes on death and dying do not ensure that the nurse truly understands and comprehends death and mortality. Remaining emotionally distant is not helpful for dying clients who need emotional support. Viewing the dying as a separate population is a way of distancing oneself from them. (P)

164. **1.** When supporting the friends or family of a terminally ill client, it is best to focus on the present. This can be accomplished by living each day to its fullest. Friends and families also want to know what to expect and want someone to listen to them as they express grief over the approaching death. Focusing on the past can interfere with enjoying the present. Expecting the worst interferes with focusing on day-to-day positive experiences. Planning ahead is inappropriate because of uncertainty when the length of life is unknown. (P)

165. **4.** Clients often sense a nurse's feelings. Therefore, when the nurse becomes emotionally upset while caring for a terminally ill child, it is best for her to share her emotions with the child when it seems appropriate. It is also acceptable to cry. It is of little help to the client or the nurse who is upset if the nurse waits until a later time when she can speak to someone about the situation. Trying to smile or not to show emotion is inappropriate. Children are very aware of someone's incongruent mood and behavior. (P)

166. **1.** The best course of action when the client has outbursts concerning her treatments is to tell her how the treatment can be expected to help her. Describing the effect on her body if she misses a treatment is a negative approach and may be threatening to the client. The client is likely to feel angry if told to be a "good client" during treatments. Offering to give the client a backrub if she does not fuss does not give her the information to which she is entitled. It also negatively reinforces the behavior. (P)

167. **2.** Children are aware of and show anxieties about death at an earlier age than was once thought, and they recognize false cheerfulness. They tend to experience isolation and loneliness when those around them are trying to hide or mask the truth. They are then left to face the realities of death alone. Children do not experience relief or hopefulness when others are falsely cheerful. Independence is promoted by offering the child realistic choices about care at the end of life. (H)

168. **1.** Taking a blood sample is an unnecessary, invasive procedure that would not directly address the child's fear. Leukemia is not considered a communicable disease. Providing an age-appropriate explanation and alerting the parents to the sibling's concern and the resources available to assist siblings to deal with the terminal illness are all appropriate interventions. (P)

169. **2.** A response that acknowledges the brother's concern and provides him with information is most helpful. Therefore, telling the brother that the nurse sees that he is worried and then following this up with a discussion about leukemia is most appropriate. Providing reassurance or information without acknowledging the expressed concern is not as helpful as acknowledging the concern and providing the information. Although acknowledging his worry is appropriate, more importantly, he needs factual information about the disease. (P)

170. **4.** The nurse caring for a terminally ill client who reports only tasks and routines completed for the client is probably behaving defensively. This behavior does not convey compassion and caring for the client. It is likely that this nurse has not come to grips with death and dying. Tactful behavior respects the client's needs. Efficient care will prevent unnecessary disturbance for the client. When caring for a terminally ill client, the nurse can remain objective while providing comprehensive nursing care to this client. (P)

TEST
14

The Client Having Surgery

■ The Client Who Is Preparing for Surgery

■ The Client Who Is Receiving or Recovering from Anesthesia

■ The Client Who Has Had Surgery

■ Legal and Ethical Issues Associated with Surgery

■ Correct Answers and Rationales

The Client Who Is Preparing for Surgery

1. A client is admitted on the day of surgery for an arthroscopy of the left knee. Which nursing activities should be completed to avoid wrong-site surgery? Select all that apply.

☐ **1.** Ask the surgeon preoperatively to mark with a permanent marker the correct knee for the surgical site.

☐ **2.** Verbally ask the client to state his name, surgical site, and procedure.

☐ **3.** Verify the correct client with the correct operative site by medical records and radiographic diagnostic reports.

☐ **4.** Call a "time-out" in the operating room to have the surgeon verify the correct knee before making the incision.

☐ **5.** Show the client an anatomic model of the surgery site.

2. During preadmission testing for same-day surgery, a client states that she has added a lot of garlic to her diet to help control her blood pressure. The nurse should further inquire about which of the following?

☐ **1.** The type of surgery the client is having.

☐ **2.** What her blood pressure has been running.

☐ **3.** The amount of garlic she is eating.

☐ **4.** Her preference for the type of anesthesia.

3. What action should this nurse take to avoid spreading nosocomial infections?

☐ **1.** Remove the face mask.

☐ **2.** Remove the hair covering.

☐ **3.** Wash her hands before tying the strings on the mask.

☐ **4.** Tie the dangling strings of the mask around her neck.

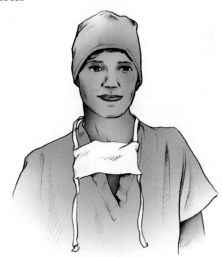

4. The client is to have surgery on his fourth metatarsal. Identify the correct site on the illustration below.

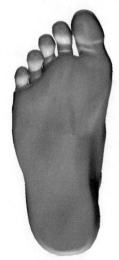

5. The nurse is reviewing the chart of a 55-year-old male client who is scheduled for a lumbar laminectomy. Which nursing assessment finding should the nurse report to the surgeon?

☐ **1.** Pimple on the lower back.
☐ **2.** Abnormal electrocardiogram (ECG).
☐ **3.** Hearing aid.
☐ **4.** Allergy to iodine.

6. The client tells the preoperative nurse that she cannot hear without her hearing aid and asks to wear it to surgery and recovery. What is the nurse's *best* response?

☐ **1.** Explain to the client that it is policy not to take personal items to surgery because they may be lost or broken.
☐ **2.** Tell the client that she will bring the hearing aid to the postanesthesia care unit so that she can have it as soon as she wakes up.
☐ **3.** Explain to the client that she will have a premedication that will make her sleepy before she goes to surgery and she won't need to hear.
☐ **4.** Call the surgery unit to explain the client's concern and ask if she can wear her hearing aid to surgery.

7. The client is to take nothing by mouth after 4 a.m. The nurse recognizes that the client has deficient knowledge when he states that he:

☐ **1.** Ate a gelatin dessert at 3:30 a.m.
☐ **2.** Brushed his teeth at 4:00 a.m. but did not swallow.
☐ **3.** Held a cold washcloth against his lips.
☐ **4.** Smoked a cigarette at 6:00 a.m.

8. The nurse should suspect that a client who reports an allergy to shellfish is also allergic to:

☐ **1.** All other seafood.
☐ **2.** Iodine skin preparations.
☐ **3.** Caffeine.
☐ **4.** Alcohol-based skin preparations.

9. The surgeon orders cefazolin (Ancef) 1 g to be given I.V. at 7:30 a.m. when the client's surgery is scheduled at 8:00 a.m. What is the primary reason to start the antibiotic exactly at 7:30 a.m.?

☐ **1.** Legally the medication has to be given at the ordered time.
☐ **2.** The antibiotic is most effective in preventing infection if it is given 30 to 60 minutes before the operative incision is made.
☐ **3.** The postoperative dose of Ancef needs to be started exactly 8 hours after the preoperative dose of Ancef.
☐ **4.** The peak and titer levels are needed for antibiotic therapy.

10. Which of the following is the best way for the nurse to begin the preoperative interview?

☐ **1.** Walk in and ask, "Are you Mrs. Smith?"
☐ **2.** Walk in, sit down, and take the client's blood pressure.
☐ **3.** Walk in, sit down, maintain eye contact, and introduce yourself.
☐ **4.** Walk in and ask the client her name.

11. A client who is to receive general anesthesia has a serum potassium level of 5.8 mEq/L. What should be the nurse's *first* response?

☐ **1.** Call the surgeon.
☐ **2.** Send the client to surgery.
☐ **3.** Make a note on the front of the chart.
☐ **4.** Notify the anesthesiologist.

12. The intraoperative nurse asks the client whether he has any allergies. The client responds, "Doesn't anyone communicate with anyone? I have been asked that question over and over!" What is the nurse's *best* response?

☐ **1.** "I'm sorry! I just have to ask that question for the record."
☐ **2.** "It's an important question and we just have to check."
☐ **3.** "You will hear it again and again as you go through surgery."
☐ **4.** "This question is asked for verification and safety with each new phase of treatment."

13. For which of the following preoperative clients should the nurse assess the glucose level? Select all that apply.

☐ **1.** A client with diabetes mellitus controlled by diet.
☐ **2.** A client with a high stress response to surgery.
☐ **3.** A client receiving corticosteroids for the past 3 months.
☐ **4.** A client with a family history of diabetes receiving dextrose 5% in lactated Ringer's solution (D_5LR) I.V. fluids.
☐ **5.** A client who consumes a high carbohydrate diet.

14. On the day of surgery, a diabetic client who takes insulin on a sliding scale is ordered to have nothing by mouth and all medications withheld. Her 6 a.m. glucose level is 300 mg/dl. What is the correct initial nursing action regarding the client's high blood glucose level?

☐ **1.** Withhold all medications as ordered.
☐ **2.** Administer the insulin dose dictated by the sliding scale.
☐ **3.** Call the physician for specific orders based on the glucose level.
☐ **4.** Notify the surgery department.

15. The nurse is preparing a preoperative teaching plan for a client who is undergoing a bilateral breast reduction. On which component of the care plan should the nurse expect to spend the most time?
- ☐ **1.** Reduction of risk potential.
- ☐ **2.** Physiologic adaptation.
- ☐ **3.** Psychosocial integrity.
- ☐ **4.** Health promotion and maintenance.

16. A client is scheduled to have an elective mandibular osteotomy to correct a mandibular fracture sustained in an accident 6 months earlier. Which statement by the client indicates to the nurse maladaptive coping?
- ☐ **1.** "I will be glad to have my jaw fixed because my wife thinks I do not look like myself."
- ☐ **2.** "I am somewhat afraid to have the surgery but feel OK about it."
- ☐ **3.** "My wife will help me, but I don't think I will need that much help."
- ☐ **4.** "I am ready to get this over with."

17. The nurse is assessing a client's nutritional status preoperatively. Which of the following observations would indicate poor nutrition in a 5-foot 7-inch female client who is 21 years of age?
- ☐ **1.** Poor posture.
- ☐ **2.** Brittle nails.
- ☐ **3.** Dull expression.
- ☐ **4.** Weight of 128 lb (58.1 kg).

18. A 92-year-old male client who is independent and lives alone has an inguinal hernia repair. Which teaching method is the best approach to use for his postoperative and discharge teaching plans?
- ☐ **1.** Explaining all the instructions to him.
- ☐ **2.** Demonstrating the instructions to him.
- ☐ **3.** Explaining all the instructions to a family member.
- ☐ **4.** Writing the instructions down for him.

19. A client is admitted for an arthroscopy of the right shoulder through same-day surgery. Which nurse is responsible for starting the client's discharge planning?
- ☐ **1.** Preadmission nurse.
- ☐ **2.** Preoperative nurse.
- ☐ **3.** Intraoperative nurse.
- ☐ **4.** Postoperative nurse.

20. The nurse is preparing to administer a premedication. Which of the following actions should the nurse take first?
- ☐ **1.** Have the family present.
- ☐ **2.** Ensure that the preoperative shave is completed.
- ☐ **3.** Have the client empty his bladder.
- ☐ **4.** Make sure the client is covered with a warm blanket.

21. A preoperative client states that she is afraid of surgery because her cousin died in surgery when having her tonsils removed. What is the nurse's *best* response?
- ☐ **1.** Reassure the client that technology has changed over the last 10 years.
- ☐ **2.** Encourage the client to further express her concerns.
- ☐ **3.** Explain to the client that it is normal to be afraid.
- ☐ **4.** Ask the client if anyone else in her family has had trouble when they had surgery.

22. An allergy to which of the following would be least likely in clients who are at risk for latex allergies?
- ☐ **1.** Avocados.
- ☐ **2.** Apples.
- ☐ **3.** Kiwi.
- ☐ **4.** Peaches.

23. Which of the following clients is more at risk for latex allergies?
- ☐ **1.** A woman who is admitted for her seventh surgery.
- ☐ **2.** A man who works as a sales clerk.
- ☐ **3.** A man with well-controlled type 2 diabetes.
- ☐ **4.** A woman who is having laser surgery.

24. After the nurse applies gloves to insert an I.V. catheter, the client begins to rub her eyes and wipe away nasal drainage. Which of the following should the nurse complete first?
- ☐ **1.** Distract the client's attention.
- ☐ **2.** Assess the client for pain.
- ☐ **3.** Remove the catheter and assess the client's vital signs.
- ☐ **4.** Increase the rate of administration of I.V. fluids.

25. When evaluating a client's preoperative cognitive-perceptual pattern, which of the following questions should the nurse ask the client?
- ☐ **1.** "Do you have difficulty swallowing?"
- ☐ **2.** "Do you need special equipment to walk?"
- ☐ **3.** "Do you smoke?"
- ☐ **4.** "Do you wear glasses?"

26. When attempting to check the pupils of a client scheduled to receive general anesthesia, the nurse notices that the client has trouble tilting his head back. Which of the following does the nurse recognize as the primary concern related to this finding?
- ☐ **1.** The client has limited movement of his neck.
- ☐ **2.** The client is at risk for postoperative neck pain.
- ☐ **3.** The client is at risk for difficult intubation.
- ☐ **4.** The ability to assess the client's pupils is limited.

27. The nurse is teaching a client deep-breathing exercises to expand collapsed alveoli and prevent postoperative atelectasis and pneumonia. Which of the following steps should be included? Select all that apply.

☐ **1.** Splint or support the incision to promote maximal comfort.

☐ **2.** Inhale slowly through the nostrils; exhale through pursed lips.

☐ **3.** Hold the breath for about 5 seconds to expand the alveoli.

☐ **4.** Repeat this breathing method 5 to 10 times hourly.

☐ **5.** Close one nostril while inhaling.

28. The nurse receives the preoperative blood work report for a client who is scheduled to undergo surgery. Which of the following laboratory findings should be reported to the surgeon?

☐ **1.** Red blood cells, 4.5 million/mm^3.

☐ **2.** Creatinine, 2.6 mg/dl.

☐ **3.** Hemoglobin, 12.2 g/dl.

☐ **4.** Blood urea nitrogen, 15 mg/dl.

29. A client will receive I.V. midazolam hydrochloride (Versed) during surgery. Which of the following should the nurse determine as a therapeutic effect?

☐ **1.** Amnesia.

☐ **2.** Nausea.

☐ **3.** Mild agitation.

☐ **4.** Blurred vision.

30. Which nursing intervention is *most* essential when administering I.V. midazolam hydrochloride (Versed)?

☐ **1.** Assessing the blood pressure.

☐ **2.** Monitoring the pulse oximeter.

☐ **3.** Encouraging slow, deep breaths.

☐ **4.** Explaining relaxation techniques.

31. When the nurse administers I.V. midazolam hydrochloride (Versed), the client demonstrates signs of an overdose. Which of the following interventions should the nurse be prepared to implement first?

☐ **1.** Ventilate with an oxygenated Ambu bag.

☐ **2.** Shock with ECG paddles.

☐ **3.** Administer 0.5 ml 1:1000 epinephrine.

☐ **4.** Titrate flumazenil (Romazicon).

32. Metoclopramide (Reglan) is ordered as a premedication for a client about to undergo a gastroduodenoscopy. The nurse expects which of the following as the primary therapeutic effect?

☐ **1.** Increased gastric pH.

☐ **2.** Increased gastric emptying.

☐ **3.** Reduced anxiety.

☐ **4.** Inhibited respiratory secretions.

33. What therapeutic outcome does the nurse expect for a client who has received a premedication of glycopyrrolate (Robinul)?

☐ **1.** Increased heart rate.

☐ **2.** Increased respiratory rate.

☐ **3.** Decreased secretions.

☐ **4.** Decreased amnesia.

34. Atropine sulfate (Atropine) is contraindicated in all but which one of the following clients?

☐ **1.** A client with diabetes.

☐ **2.** A client with glaucoma.

☐ **3.** A client with urine retention.

☐ **4.** A client with bowel obstruction.

35. After the nurse has administered droperidol (Inapsine), care is taken to move the client slowly based on the knowledge of droperidol's effect on the:

☐ **1.** Central nervous system.

☐ **2.** Respiratory system.

☐ **3.** Cardiovascular system.

☐ **4.** Psychoneurologic system.

36. A client has been ordered to receive enoxaparin (Lovenox) 6 hours before the scheduled time of her laparoscopic vaginal assisted hysterectomy. Which of the following effects does the nurse recognize as an intended therapeutic action of the enoxaparin?

☐ **1.** Increase in red blood cell production.

☐ **2.** Reduction of postoperative thrombi.

☐ **3.** Decrease in postoperative bleeding.

☐ **4.** Promotion of tissue healing.

37. During the preoperative interview, the nurse obtains information about the client's medication history. Which of the following is *not* necessary to record about the client?

☐ **1.** Current use of medications, herbs, and vitamins.

☐ **2.** Over-the-counter medication use in the last 6 weeks.

☐ **3.** Steroid use in the last year.

☐ **4.** Use of all drugs taken in the last 18 months.

38. When the nurse is conducting a preoperative interview with a client who is having a vaginal hysterectomy, the client states that she forgot to tell her doctor that she had a total hip replacement 3 years ago. The nurse communicates this information to the perioperative nurse because:

☐ **1.** The prosthesis may cause a problem with the electrosurgical unit used to control bleeding.

☐ **2.** The client should not have her hip externally rotated when she is positioned for the procedure.

☐ **3.** The perioperative nurse can inform the rest of the team about the total hip replacement.

☐ **4.** There is not enough time to notify the surgeon and note this finding on the history and physical information before the procedure.

39. The nurse learns that a client who is scheduled for a tonsillectomy has been taking 40 mg of oral prednisone daily for the last week for poison ivy on his leg. What is the nurse's *best* action?
- [ ] 1. Document the prednisone with current medications.
- [ ] 2. Notify the surgeon of the poison ivy.
- [ ] 3. Notify the anesthesiologist of the prednisone administration.
- [ ] 4. Send the client to surgery.

40. A client who is scheduled for an open cholecystectomy has a 20-pack-year history of smoking. For which postoperative complication is the client most at risk?
- [ ] 1. Deep vein thrombosis.
- [ ] 2. Atelectasis and pneumonia.
- [ ] 3. Delayed wound healing.
- [ ] 4. Prolonged immobility.

41. In planning a client's perioperative teaching, the nurse includes an explanation of the circulating nurse as the person who:
- [ ] 1. Passes instruments to the surgeon.
- [ ] 2. Answers the phone in surgery.
- [ ] 3. Provides the nursing process during surgery.
- [ ] 4. Ensures sterility of supplies.

42. The family cannot go with the surgical client past the doors that separate the public from the restricted area of the operating room suite. These traffic control measures are designed to:
- [ ] 1. Protect the privacy of clients.
- [ ] 2. Prevent electrical sparks that could ignite the anesthetic gases.
- [ ] 3. Separate the family from the surgical team while they are working on the client.
- [ ] 4. Provide for an aseptic environment to prevent infection.

43. Which of the following clients is most at risk for potential hazards from the surgical experience?
- [ ] 1. A 68-year-old client.
- [ ] 2. A 50-year-old client.
- [ ] 3. A 30-year-old client.
- [ ] 4. A 13-year-old client.

44. Which pediatric surgery client should not play with a balloon?
- [ ] 1. A child having her 15th laser surgery for a hemangioma.
- [ ] 2. A child having a tonsillectomy.
- [ ] 3. A child having an inguinal hernia repair.
- [ ] 4. A child having an orchiopexy.

45. In which of the following clients is an autotransfusion possible?
- [ ] 1. The client who has cancer.
- [ ] 2. The client who is in danger of cardiac arrest.
- [ ] 3. The client with a contaminated wound.
- [ ] 4. The client with a ruptured bowel.

46. The nurse teaches a client who had cystoscopy about the urge to void when the procedure is over. What other teaching should be included?
- [ ] 1. Ignore the urge to void.
- [ ] 2. Force fluids.
- [ ] 3. Ask for the bedpan.
- [ ] 4. Ring for assistance to the bathroom.

47. Which of the following nursing interventions is most important in preventing postoperative complications?
- [ ] 1. Progressive diet planning.
- [ ] 2. Pain management.
- [ ] 3. Bowel and elimination monitoring.
- [ ] 4. Early ambulation.

The Client Who Is Receiving or Recovering from Anesthesia

48. A client who had a gastrectomy has been in the postanesthesia recovery room for 30 minutes when his vital signs suddenly change. The nurse checks the recovery room record (shown below). In addition to notifying the physician, what other action should the nurse take immediately?
- [ ] 1. Administer dantrolene.
- [ ] 2. Elevate the head of the bed 30 degrees.
- [ ] 3. Administer a bolus of I.V. fluids.
- [ ] 4. Insert an indwelling urinary catheter.

VITAL SIGNS			
Date **Time**	06/30/07 1:45 p.m.	06/30/07 2:00 p.m.	06/30/07 2:15 p.m.
Pulse	70	82	90
Respiration	12	14	20
Blood pressure	100/60	110/70	140/90
Temperature	98° F (36.7° C)	99° F (37.2° C)	102° F (38.9° C)

49. A client has been in the position shown below for surgery. The nurse should document that the client has been in which of the following positions?
- [ ] **1.** Reverse Trendelenburg.
- [ ] **2.** Low Fowler's.
- [ ] **3.** High lithotomy.
- [ ] **4.** Prone.

50. A client arrives from surgery to the postanesthesia care unit. Which of the following respiratory assessments should the nurse complete *first*?
- [ ] **1.** Oxygen saturation.
- [ ] **2.** Respiratory rate.
- [ ] **3.** Breath sounds.
- [ ] **4.** Airway flow.

51. The nurse assesses vital signs on a client who has had epidural anesthesia. For which of the following should the nurse assess next?
- [ ] **1.** Bladder distention.
- [ ] **2.** Headache.
- [ ] **3.** Postoperative pain.
- [ ] **4.** Ability to move the legs.

52. When assessing a client who has had spinal anesthesia, which of the following would the nurse expect to find?
- [ ] **1.** The client feels pain before moving the legs.
- [ ] **2.** Blood pressure was significantly increased.
- [ ] **3.** Sensation returned to toes but not to the perineal area.
- [ ] **4.** The client complained of a headache while in the lying position.

53. The nurse in the postanesthesia care unit notes that one of the client's pupils is larger than the other. Which of the following actions should the nurse perform next?
- [ ] **1.** Rate the client on the Glasgow Coma Scale.
- [ ] **2.** Administer oxygen.
- [ ] **3.** Check the client's baseline data.
- [ ] **4.** Call the surgeon.

54. The surgical floor receives a new postoperative client from the postanesthesia care unit. Assessment reveals a patent airway and stable vital signs. What is the nurse's next action?
- [ ] **1.** Checking the dressing for signs of bleeding.
- [ ] **2.** Emptying any peri-incisional drains.
- [ ] **3.** Assessing the client's pain level.
- [ ] **4.** Assessing the client's bladder.

55. When preparing a teaching plan for an adult client about general anesthesia induction, which explanation would be most appropriate?
- [ ] **1.** "Your premedication will put you to sleep."
- [ ] **2.** "You will breathe in an inhalant anesthetic mixed with oxygen through a facial mask and receive intravenous medication to make you sleepy."
- [ ] **3.** "You will receive intravenous medication to make you sleepy."
- [ ] **4.** "You will breathe in medication through a facial mask to make you sleepy."

56. Which explanation would be most appropriate for a child when teaching him about general anesthesia induction?
- [ ] **1.** "You will be given an injection before you go to surgery to make you sleepy."
- [ ] **2.** "You will breathe in oxygen through a facial mask and receive intravenous medication to make you sleepy."
- [ ] **3.** "You will receive intravenous medication to make you sleepy."
- [ ] **4.** "You will breathe in medication through a facial mask to make you sleepy."

57. A client with impaired cardiac functioning is at risk during anesthesia induction with thiopental sodium (Sodium Pentothal) because this drug causes:
- [ ] **1.** Bradycardia.
- [ ] **2.** Complete muscle relaxation.
- [ ] **3.** Hypotension.
- [ ] **4.** Tachypnea.

58. The nurse anticipates that a client who has received propofol (Diprivan) as the induction and maintenance agent for general anesthesia will most likely experience:
- [ ] **1.** Minimal nausea and vomiting.
- [ ] **2.** Hypotension.
- [ ] **3.** Slow induction of anesthesia.
- [ ] **4.** Small tremors of the skeletal muscles.

59. What is the main reason desflurane (Suprane) and sevoflurane (Ultane), volatile liquid anesthesia agents, are used for surgical clients who go home the day of surgery?
- [ ] **1.** These agents are better tolerated.
- [ ] **2.** These agents are predictable in their cardiovascular effects.
- [ ] **3.** These agents are nonirritating to the respiratory tract.
- [ ] **4.** These agents are rapidly eliminated.

60. A 250-lb male client recovering from general anesthesia has the following assessment findings: pulse, 150 bpm; blood pressure, 90/50 mm Hg; respiratory rate, 28 breaths/minute; tympanic temperature, 99.8° F (37.7° C); and rigid muscles. The nurse determines that the client is:

☐ 1. Recovering as expected from the anesthesia and continues monitoring him.

☐ 2. Exhibiting the effects of excessive blood loss experienced in the operating room and increases the rate of his I.V. infusion.

☐ 3. In the early stages of malignant hyperthermia and obtains emergency medications and notifies the anesthesiologist.

☐ 4. In pain and offers him pain medication.

61. The nurse is assessing a client recovering from anesthesia. Which of the following signs or symptoms is an early indicator of hypoxemia?

☐ 1. Somnolence.

☐ 2. Restlessness.

☐ 3. Chills.

☐ 4. Urgency.

62. The nurse is to administer flumazenil (Mazicon) I.V. for reversal of sedation. Which of the following interventions should be included in the care plan? Select all that apply.

☐ 1. Administer the medication as a 2-mg bolus.

☐ 2. Give the medication undiluted in incremental doses.

☐ 3. Be alert for shivering and hypotension.

☐ 4. Use only a free-flowing I.V. line in a large vein.

☐ 5. Monitor the client's level of consciousness.

63. An 80-year-old client had spinal anesthesia for a transurethral resection of the prostate and received 4,000 ml of room temperature isotonic bladder irrigation. He now has continuous irrigation through a three-way indwelling urinary catheter. Which postoperative nursing intervention is most important to include in his plan of care?

☐ 1. Empty the catheter drainage bag.

☐ 2. Cover the client with warm blankets.

☐ 3. Hang new bags of irrigation.

☐ 4. Turn the client.

64. Which of the following clients is expected to retain anesthetic agents longest?

☐ 1. A client who is 6 feet 2 inches tall and weighs 250 lb.

☐ 2. A client who is 5 feet 4 inches tall and weighs 110 lb.

☐ 3. A client who is 5 feet 1 inch tall and weighs 200 lb.

☐ 4. A client who is 5 feet 7 inches tall and weighs 145 lb.

65. An awake postoperative client received an intravenous regional nerve block (Bier block) in the arm that is now casted and elevated on a pillow. What action should the nurse encourage the client to avoid until sensation returns?

☐ 1. Holding the operated arm close to the face.

☐ 2. Holding the operated arm with the unoperated arm.

☐ 3. Using the unoperated arm.

☐ 4. Using pain medication.

66. The physician ordered I.V. naloxone (Narcan) to reverse the respiratory depression from morphine administration. Which of the following interventions would be most appropriate after administration of the naloxone?

☐ 1. Check respirations in 5 minutes because naloxone is immediately effective in relieving respiratory depression.

☐ 2. Check respirations in 30 minutes because the effects of morphine will have worn off by then.

☐ 3. Monitor respirations frequently for 4 to 6 hours because the client may need repeated doses of naloxone.

☐ 4. Monitor respirations each time the client receives morphine sulfate 10 mg I.M.

67. The nurse monitors the surgical client closely for which clinical manifestation with the administration of naloxone (Narcan)?

☐ 1. Dizziness.

☐ 2. Biliary colic.

☐ 3. Bleeding.

☐ 4. Urine retention.

68. The nurse anticipates that the client who has received epidural anesthesia is at decreased risk for a spinal headache because:

☐ 1. A 17G needle is used.

☐ 2. A subarachnoid injection is made.

☐ 3. A noncutting needle is used.

☐ 4. A faster onset occurs.

69. Which of the following systems is not blocked by spinal anesthesia?

☐ 1. The sympathetic nervous system.

☐ 2. The sensory system.

☐ 3. The parasympathetic nervous system.

☐ 4. The motor system.

70. The nurse is to administer midazolam (Versed) 2.5 mg. This medication is available in a 5 mg/ml vial. What amount should the nurse administer?

☐ 1. 0.5 ml.

☐ 2. 0.25 ml.

☐ 3. 0.45 ml.

☐ 4. 0.75 ml.

71. A client in the postanesthesia care unit is being actively rewarmed with an external warming device. How often should the nurse monitor the client's body temperature?
- ☐ **1.** Every 5 minutes.
- ☐ **2.** Every 10 minutes.
- ☐ **3.** Every 15 minutes.
- ☐ **4.** Every 20 minutes.

The Client Who Has Had Surgery

72. Eight hours after surgery, a client has a distended bladder and is unable to void. Which of the following interventions is contraindicated?
- ☐ **1.** Facilitate voiding by normal position.
- ☐ **2.** Pour running water over perineum.
- ☐ **3.** Insert an indwelling urinary catheter.
- ☐ **4.** Insert a straight catheter every 4 hours.

73. A client who had open heart surgery is being transported to the intensive care unit (ICU) for postoperative recovery from anesthesia. The nurse in the ICU is assessing the client's level of consciousness. When asked, the client can give his name but is not sure about where he is or the time of day. What should the nurse do?
- ☐ **1.** Notify the surgeon.
- ☐ **2.** Rub the client's sternum to arouse the client.
- ☐ **3.** Encourage the client's wife to orient the client.
- ☐ **4.** Tell the client where he is and the time of day.

74. A nurse is assessing a client when she returns from same-day surgery for a dilatation and curettage. The nurse checks preoperative vital signs at 8:30 a.m. to compare them with the current vital signs at 10:30 p.m. (see the chart below). What should the nurse do first?
- ☐ **1.** Call the physician for pain medication.
- ☐ **2.** Cover the client with warmed blankets.
- ☐ **3.** Administer oxygen at 4 L/minute.
- ☐ **4.** Increase the I.V. fluid rate.

VITAL SIGNS		
	8:30 AM	10:30 PM
Pulse	80	90
Respirations	16	20
Blood pressure	90/60	100/80
Temperature	99.5	97

75. A client returns to the medical-surgical floor from the postanesthesia recovery room after a colon resection for adenocarcinoma. The client has comorbidities of stage 2 hypertension and a previous myocardial infarction. The first set of postoperative vital signs recorded are pulse rate of 110 bpm, respiration rate of 20/minute, blood pressure of 130/86 mm Hg, and temperature of 98° F (36.7° C). The surgeon calls to ask if the client needs a unit of packed red blood cells. The nurse's response should be based on which data? Select all that apply.
- ☐ **1.** Cyanotic mucous membrane.
- ☐ **2.** Warm, dry skin.
- ☐ **3.** Vital sign changes.
- ☐ **4.** Oxygen saturation.
- ☐ **5.** Intake and output.

76. A client had a colectomy 8½ hours ago. She has received 1,500 ml of dextrose 5% in water with normal saline solution. The client has just used a patient-controlled analgesia pump to administer morphine for pain, has been repositioned for comfort, and has stable pulse rate, respirations, and blood pressure. What should the nurse do next?
- ☐ **1.** Check that the family is comfortable.
- ☐ **2.** Assess vital signs following the use of morphine.
- ☐ **3.** Dim the lights in the room.
- ☐ **4.** Increase nasal oxygen from 2 to 3 L.

77. A client who had an esophageal hernia repair 4 hours ago has a pulse rate of 90 bpm, respiration rate of 16/minute, blood pressure of 130/80 mm Hg, pulse oximeter of 91, and a temperature of 100.4° F (38° C). What should the nurse do first?
- ☐ **1.** Obtain a culture of the incision.
- ☐ **2.** Notify the surgeon to obtain an antibiotic order.
- ☐ **3.** Offer pain medication.
- ☐ **4.** Assist the client to a sitting position to take deep breaths.

78. Which of the following activities should the nurse encourage the unlicensed assistive personnel to assist with in the care of postoperative clients? Select all that apply.
- ☐ **1.** Empty and measure indwelling urinary catheter collection bags.
- ☐ **2.** Reposition clients for pain relief.
- ☐ **3.** Teach clients the proper use of the incentive spirometer.
- ☐ **4.** Tell the nurse if clients report they are having pain.
- ☐ **5.** Assess I.V. insertion site for redness.

79. A client had a total abdominal hysterectomy and bilateral oophorectomy for ovarian carcinoma yesterday. She received 2 mg of morphine sulfate I.V. by patient-controlled analgesia (PCA) 10 minutes ago. The nurse was assisting her from the bed to a chair when the client felt dizzy and fell into the chair. The nurse should:

☐ **1.** Discontinue the PCA pump.
☐ **2.** Administer oxygen.
☐ **3.** Take the client's blood pressure.
☐ **4.** Assist the client back to bed.

80. A nurse is instructing a client who had abdominal surgery that day to do deep-breathing exercises. In which order should the nurse teach the client to perform diaphragmatic breathing and coughing?

1. Inhale through the nose.
2. Cough deeply from the lungs.
3. Exhale through pursed lips.
4. Splint the incisional site.

81. A very elderly, drowsy client with fragile skin is being transferred from the surgery cart to the bed. How should the nurse plan to direct the transfer to prevent skin shearing?

☐ **1.** With two people at each side using a drawsheet.
☐ **2.** With two people, one at each side using a drawsheet, and one person at the head.
☐ **3.** With two people using a roller and a drawsheet.
☐ **4.** With two people, one at each side using a drawsheet, one person at the head, and one person at the feet.

82. The postoperative nursing assessment of a client's ability to swallow fluids before providing oral fluids is based on the type of anesthesia given. Which of the following clients would not have delayed fluid restrictions?

☐ **1.** The client who has undergone a bronchoscopy under local anesthesia.
☐ **2.** The client who has undergone a transurethral resection of a bladder tumor under general anesthesia.
☐ **3.** The client who has undergone a repair of carpal tunnel syndrome under local anesthesia.
☐ **4.** The client who has undergone an inguinal herniorrhaphy with spinal and intravenous conscious sedation.

83. A client is admitted to the surgical floor after having bowel surgery. The nurse observes that the client's urine output has decreased from 50 to 20 ml/hour. Which of the following is the most likely cause?

☐ **1.** Bowel obstruction.
☐ **2.** Adverse effect of opioid analgesics.
☐ **3.** Hemorrhage.
☐ **4.** Hypertension.

84. A client who had a left thoracoscopy sustained an injury secondary to the surgery position. Which of the following injuries would the client demonstrate?

☐ **1.** Footdrop.
☐ **2.** Knee swelling and pain.
☐ **3.** Tingling in the arm.
☐ **4.** Absence of the Achilles reflex.

85. Which of the following is most likely to cause the client to experience postoperative nausea and vomiting?

☐ **1.** Total hip replacement.
☐ **2.** Mitral valve repair.
☐ **3.** Abdominal hysterectomy.
☐ **4.** Mastectomy of the left breast.

86. The nurse is planning to teach incisional care to a client before discharge. Which of the following instructions should be included?

☐ **1.** Do not touch your incision before your next appointment.
☐ **2.** Clean your incision three times a day with hydrogen peroxide and water.
☐ **3.** Do not be concerned about uneven lumps under the suture lines.
☐ **4.** If the staples don't come out by themselves before your next appointment, the surgeon will remove them.

87. The nurse is removing the client's staples from an abdominal incision when the client sneezes and the incision splits open, exposing the intestines. Which of the following actions should the nurse take next?

☐ **1.** Press the emergency alarm to call the resuscitation team.
☐ **2.** Cover the abdominal organs with sterile dressings moistened with sterile normal saline.
☐ **3.** Have all visitors and family leave the room.
☐ **4.** Call the surgeon to come to the client's room immediately.

88. On the fourth day after surgery, a client has a postoperative wound infection. Which of the following should the nurse expect to assess? Select all that apply.

☐ **1.** Total white blood count (WBC) 10,000/mm³.
☐ **2.** Redness and swelling beyond the incision line.
☐ **3.** Temperature of 102° F (38.9° C).
☐ **4.** 89% segmented neutrophils.
☐ **5.** Incisional pain greater than on day 2.

89. Which of the following should be included in the plan of care for a client with a surgical wound that requires a wet-to-dry dressing?
- [ ] **1.** Place a dry dressing in the wound.
- [ ] **2.** Use Burrow's solution to wet the dressing.
- [ ] **3.** Pack the wet dressing tightly into the wound.
- [ ] **4.** Cover the wet packing with a dry sterile dressing.

90. The nurse empties a Jackson-Pratt drainage bulb. Which of the following nursing interventions ensures correct functioning of the drain?
- [ ] **1.** Irrigating it with normal saline.
- [ ] **2.** Connecting it to low intermittent suction.
- [ ] **3.** Compressing it and then plugging it to establish suction.
- [ ] **4.** Connecting it to a drainage bag and clamping it off.

91. Which of the following interventions should the nurse implement for pulmonary emboli prophylaxis?
- [ ] **1.** Have the client perform leg exercises every hour while awake.
- [ ] **2.** Encourage the client to cough and deep-breathe.
- [ ] **3.** Massage the calves of the client's legs.
- [ ] **4.** Have the client wear antiembolism stockings when out of bed.

92. The nurse assesses a client who has just received morphine sulfate. The client's blood pressure is 90/50 mm Hg; pulse rate, 58 bpm; respiration rate, 4 breaths/minute. What drug should the nurse prepare to administer?
- [ ] **1.** Flumazenil (Romazicon).
- [ ] **2.** Naloxone hydrochloride (Narcan).
- [ ] **3.** Doxacurium (Nuromax).
- [ ] **4.** Remifentanil (Ultiva).

93. A client is being discharged from same-day surgery. Which of the following statements indicates that the client has deficient knowledge?
- [ ] **1.** "My husband is taking the day off from work to drive me home."
- [ ] **2.** "I can drive myself home after surgery."
- [ ] **3.** "I am taking a taxi home and my daughter will meet me at home."
- [ ] **4.** "My son will be here at noon to take me home."

94. The nurse is teaching a client who has had a laparoscopic cholecystectomy about postoperative pain management. Which of the following statements indicates that the client has deficient knowledge?
- [ ] **1.** "My pain is related to the gas used to distend my abdominal cavity."
- [ ] **2.** "My diet should include eating bland foods until the gas clears up."
- [ ] **3.** "My pain is related to the large incision and manipulation."
- [ ] **4.** "My pain should be relieved by walking to eliminate the gas."

95. The initial postoperative assessment is completed on a client who had an arthroscopy of the knee. Assessment of which of the following parameters is not necessary every 15 minutes during the first postoperative hour?
- [ ] **1.** Vital signs including pulse oximeter.
- [ ] **2.** Pain rating of the operative site.
- [ ] **3.** Urine output.
- [ ] **4.** Neurovascular check distal to the operative site.

96. After surgery, a client was treated for postoperative nausea and vomiting and now is experiencing hypotension and tachycardia. Which of the following medications would be most likely associated with these findings?
- [ ] **1.** Ondansetron hydrochloride (Zofran).
- [ ] **2.** Droperidol (Inapsine).
- [ ] **3.** Prochlorperazine (Compazine).
- [ ] **4.** Promethazine (Phenergan).

97. When an epidural catheter is used for postoperative pain management, the nurse should:
- [ ] **1.** Assess but not disturb the epidural dressing.
- [ ] **2.** Change the epidural dressing daily.
- [ ] **3.** Change the epidural dressing daily only if it is wet.
- [ ] **4.** Use strict aseptic technique when handling the epidural catheter.

98. The nurse understands that the client who has epidural pain management postoperatively can ambulate because:
- [ ] **1.** The analgesia is periodically administered through the epidural catheter.
- [ ] **2.** A low concentration of analgesia is used with the catheter.
- [ ] **3.** The analgesia from the epidural catheter bathes the spinal fluid.
- [ ] **4.** The epidural medication affects the sympathetic and motor function.

99. A surgical client develops pruritus and urticaria during the administration of an I.V. antibiotic. Which of the following types of reaction is this client most likely experiencing?
- [ ] **1.** Type I—anaphylactic reaction.
- [ ] **2.** Type II—cytotoxic and cytolytic reaction.
- [ ] **3.** Type III—immune-complex reaction.
- [ ] **4.** Type IV—delayed hypersensitivity reaction.

100. A postoperative client who is coughing, short of breath, and complaining of a feeling of doom exhibits the following: Blood pressure of 80/60 mm Hg; pulse rate of 120 bpm; and respiration rate, 24 breaths/minute. Which pathophysiologic condition should the nurse associate with these manifestations?
- [ ] **1.** Malignant hyperthermia.
- [ ] **2.** Anaphylaxis.
- [ ] **3.** Contact dermatitis.
- [ ] **4.** Cell-mediated response.

101. A 2-day postoperative hospitalized client continues to take hydrocodone 7.5 mg and acetaminophen 500 mg (Lortab 7.5/500). What should the nurse ask the client before administering the pain medication?
- ☐ 1. "Where is your pain located?"
- ☐ 2. "Have you emptied your bladder?"
- ☐ 3. "How long has it been since your last dose?"
- ☐ 4. "Is your pain better than before you had surgery?"

102. A client wakes up in the postanesthesia care unit and sees a drain with bright red fluid in it exiting from her total hip incision. She asks the nurse, "Is this the way it is supposed to be?" Which of the following represents the nurse's best response?
- ☐ 1. "The drainage is blood and fluid that must be drained out for healing."
- ☐ 2. "Don't worry about it. I will explain it when you are more awake."
- ☐ 3. "This blood is being kept sterile and will be given back to you."
- ☐ 4. "I will give you something to make you sleep so you will not worry."

103. A client has a Jackson-Pratt drainage tube in place the first day after surgical repair of a ruptured diverticulum. The client asks the nurse the purpose of the drain. What is the nurse's best response?
- ☐ 1. "The drainage tube is used to prevent infection in the peritoneal cavity."
- ☐ 2. "The drainage tube is used to prevent bleeding into the peritoneal cavity."
- ☐ 3. "The drainage tube is used to prevent pressure on the bladder."
- ☐ 4. "The drainage tube is used to prevent pressure on the gallbladder."

104. A client who had a cholecystectomy with a biliary drainage tube in place asks the nurse what the drainage should look like. Which of the following qualities should the nurse describe as normal?
- ☐ 1. Pinkish red.
- ☐ 2. Dark yellow-orange.
- ☐ 3. Clear.
- ☐ 4. Green.

105. A client is to be discharged from same-day surgery 7 hours after his inguinal hernia repair. Which of the following indicates this client is ready to be discharged?
- ☐ 1. The client voids 500 ml of urine.
- ☐ 2. The client tolerates eating a hamburger.
- ☐ 3. The client is pain-free.
- ☐ 4. The client walks in the hallway unassisted.

106. A client is eligible for patient-controlled analgesia (PCA) when:
- ☐ 1. A family member is able to assist with self-dosing.
- ☐ 2. There is a court-appointed advocate to assist with self-dosing.
- ☐ 3. The client has the ability to self-dose.
- ☐ 4. There is a nurse to assist with self-dosing.

107. How often should the postoperative client's temperature be assessed during the first 24 hours after surgery?
- ☐ 1. Every 2 hours.
- ☐ 2. Every 4 hours.
- ☐ 3. Every 6 hours.
- ☐ 4. Every 8 hours.

108. A nurse is assessing a surgical client's blood pressure 8 hours after surgery. The client's blood pressure before surgery was 120/80 mm Hg and on admission to the postsurgical nursing unit, it was 110/80 mm Hg. The client's blood pressure is now 90/70 mm Hg. What should the nurse do first?
- ☐ 1. Notify the health care provider.
- ☐ 2. Elevate the head of the bed.
- ☐ 3. Administer pain medication.
- ☐ 4. Check the intake and output record.

109. A client has been positioned in the lithotomy position under general anesthesia for a pelvic procedure. In which anatomic area may the client expect to experience postoperative discomfort?
- ☐ 1. Shoulders.
- ☐ 2. Thighs.
- ☐ 3. Legs.
- ☐ 4. Feet.

110. Which of the following nursing interventions does not aid in meeting the goal of clear breath sounds?
- ☐ 1. Offering pain relief before having the client cough.
- ☐ 2. Providing a minimum of 1,500 ml of fluid per day.
- ☐ 3. Monitoring breath sounds.
- ☐ 4. Assisting with early ambulation.

111. Which of the following is not a sign of thromboembolism?
- ☐ 1. Redness.
- ☐ 2. Swelling.
- ☐ 3. Coolness.
- ☐ 4. Edema.

112. The nurse is teaching the client about deep-breathing techniques. Which of the following client statements indicates the need for additional education?
- ☐ 1. "I will use my incentive spirometer every hour while I'm awake."
- ☐ 2. "I should place my hands lightly over my lower ribs and upper abdomen."
- ☐ 3. "I should get into a comfortable position before doing my breathing exercises."
- ☐ 4. "I should take four deep breaths and then cough deeply from the lungs."

113. A client has had a nasogastric tube connected to low intermittent suction. The client is at risk for which of the following complications?
- ☐ 1. Confusion.
- ☐ 2. Muscle cramping.
- ☐ 3. Edema.
- ☐ 4. Tremors.

Legal and Ethical Issues Associated with Surgery

114. On admission to same-day surgery, the nurse reviews the chart to verify the client's identification documentation. Which of the following is most important?
- ☐ 1. Admitting record.
- ☐ 2. Addressograph labels.
- ☐ 3. Identification bracelet.
- ☐ 4. Location of family.

115. Which of the following items of documentation is not required for the nurse to have on the chart before the client is transported to the operating suite?
- ☐ 1. Operative consent.
- ☐ 2. History and physical information.
- ☐ 3. Laboratory test results.
- ☐ 4. Anesthesia note.

116. A 15-year-old client needs life-saving emergency surgery, but his relatives live an hour away from the hospital and cannot sign the consent form. What is the nurse's best response?
- ☐ 1. Send the client to surgery without the consent.
- ☐ 2. Call the family for a consent over the telephone and have another nurse listen as a witness.
- ☐ 3. No action is necessary in this case because consent is not needed.
- ☐ 4. Have the family sign the consent form as soon as they arrive.

117. A client is being prepared to have a craniotomy for a brain tumor. As a client advocate, the nurse is evaluating the client's understanding of the informed consent before witnessing the client's signature on the operative consent form. Which of the following indicates that the nurse needs to contact the surgeon for further communication with the client?
- ☐ 1. "We talked about the effect of my diabetes on healing."
- ☐ 2. "The surgeon explained how the craniotomy was done."
- ☐ 3. "There are no major risks from this surgery."
- ☐ 4. "I will die if the tumor is not removed from my brain."

118. The nurse should ask all clients age 65 or older who are having surgery which question?
- ☐ 1. "Do you have Medicare Part A to help pay for the hospital reimbursement?"
- ☐ 2. "Do you have an advance directive such as a health care proxy or living will?"
- ☐ 3. "Do you have extra coverage to help pay for medications?"
- ☐ 4. "Do you have Medicare Part B to help pay for your expenses?"

119. The client's identification armband was removed to start an I.V. line as a part of the preoperative preparation. The transport team has arrived to transport the client to the operating room. The nurse notices that the client's identification band is not on his wrist. What is the nurse's best response?
- ☐ 1. Send the removed armband with the chart and the client to the operating room.
- ☐ 2. Place a new identification armband on the client's wrist before transport.
- ☐ 3. Tape the cut armband back onto the client's wrist.
- ☐ 4. Send the client without an armband because she can verbally identify herself.

120. When a client cannot read or write but is of sound mind, the nurse should read the consent to the client in the presence of two witnesses and:
- ☐ 1. Have the client's next-of-kin sign the consent.
- ☐ 2. Have the client put an "X" on the signature line.
- ☐ 3. Have a court appoint a guardian for the client.
- ☐ 4. Have a hospital quality management coordinator sign for the client.

Correct Answers and Rationales

The letter in parentheses after each rationale identifies the client need addressed in the item, including management of care (M), safety and infection control (S), health promotion and maintenance (H), psychosocial adaptation (P), basic care and comfort (C), pharmacological and parenteral therapies (D), reduction of risk potential (R), and physiological adaptation (A).

The Client Who Is Preparing for Surgery

1. **2, 3, 4.** The root cause of wrong-site surgery involves a breakdown in communication between the client and family and the health care team. Information retrieved from the client in the preoperative assessment, such as the client's name, surgical site, and procedure, should be verbally assessed and verified with medical records and radiographic diagnostic reports. This information should be compiled in a checklist that the intraoperative team can recheck, avoid unnecessary distraction and delay in the operating room. The nurse in the operating room is responsible for calling a "time-out" so that every surgical team member can double-check the correct site of surgery, verify the site using the operative consent form, and mark the operative site on the client. The client should mark the operative site in the preoperative period, not the surgeon, in order to avoid any miscommunication about the correct site of surgery. Showing the client an anatomic model will assist the client in understanding the location of the surgery, but it will not prevent anyone from identifying the wrong site on the client. (S)

2. **3.** Garlic has anticoagulant properties and may pose a problem with bleeding if enough has been taken too close to surgery. Therefore, the nurse must obtain more quantifiable details about the client's statement. The nurse should check the surgical procedure, anesthesia preference, and blood pressure status with the client. However, the part of the client's statement that needs further investigation concerns intake of an herb with anticoagulant properties before a surgical procedure. (D)

3. **1.** The nurse should remove the face mask. The face mask contains nasal and oral droplets, which are easily transmitted to the hands as the mask dangles when left hanging around the neck. When a face mask is not worn over the mouth and nose, it should be completely removed. (S)

4.

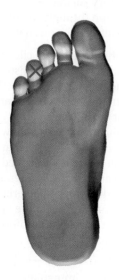

5. **1.** A pimple close to the incision site may be reason for the surgeon to cancel the surgical procedure because it increases the risk of infection. If the client had an abnormal ECG, the nurse would notify the anesthesiologist who will be administering the anesthesia. The anesthesiologist is the decision maker regarding the implications of the anesthesia on the cardiac system. The surgical team should be notified of the client's hearing disability, but the surgeon, who has already met the client, does not need to be notified. The surgical team should be notified of the client's allergy to iodine and it should be documented in all the appropriate places, but the surgeon would not need to be notified in advance of the surgical procedure. (S)

6. **4.** When a client has a concern, it is important to decrease her stress as much as possible. The nurse should call the operating room and inform the intraoperative nurse. A special container with correct identification can be prepared so that when the client is anesthetized and her hearing aid is removed, it will not be lost or broken. It

is usual policy not to send personal belongings to surgery because they are easily broken or lost in the transfer of an anesthetized client with higher priority needs, but special needs do exist. In some instances the nurse does bring a client's personal belongings to the postanesthesia care unit, but in this case the item involves the client's ability to communicate. Because the trend is to use little premedication, clients are more alert and may want to talk with their surgical team before going to sleep. Decreasing the client's anxieties preoperatively affects the amount of medication used to induce the client and her overall psychological and physiologic status. Telling the client that she won't need to hear is insensitive. (C)

7. **4.** The client has deficient knowledge if he smoked a cigarette after 4 a.m. because, even though he did not have anything to eat or drink, smoking has increased the production of gastric hydrochloric acid, which can increase the risk of aspiration in an anesthetized client. A gelatin dessert is a clear liquid and is acceptable. Comfort measures, such as brushing the teeth without swallowing or holding a cold washcloth against the lips, are acceptable for a client who is to have nothing by mouth. (R)

8. **2.** Clients who are allergic to shellfish are allergic to iodine skin preparations (Iodophor and Betadine) or any other products containing iodine, such as dyes. Clients who are allergic to shellfish do not necessarily have an allergy to any other substances or seafood. (R)

9. **2.** The antibiotic is most effective in preventing infection, according to research, if it is given 30 to 60 minutes before the operative incision is made. When the surgeon orders the antibiotic to be given at a specific time related to the scheduled time of the surgical procedure, it is imperative that the antibiotic is given on time. Legally, the nurse considers 30 minutes on either side of the scheduled time to be acceptable for administering medications; however, in this situation, giving the antibiotic 30 minutes too soon can make the prophylactic antibiotic ineffective. The postoperative dose of antibiotic is not timed according to the preoperative dose. Peak and titer levels are measured for some antibiotics, but in this case the primary reason is to have the antibiotic infused before the time of the incision. (R)

10. **3.** Nurses should provide the preoperative client individual and sincere attention by meeting the client at eye level and introducing themselves by name and role. The nurse should ask the client to tell her full name rather than asking if she is Mrs. Smith because there might be another client by that name on the schedule. Nurses should not start the physical assessment or ask the client's name without first identifying themselves and their role out of courtesy and to relieve the client's anxiety in the new environment of the surgical experience. (P)

11. **4.** The nurse should notify the anesthesiologist because a serum potassium level of 5.8 mEq/L places the client at risk for arrhythmias when under general anesthesia. The surgeon may be notified; however, the anesthesiologist will make the decision about whether to proceed with surgery. The nurse should not automatically send a client with abnormal laboratory findings to surgery because the procedure may be canceled. Once the client is inside the operating room and sterile supplies have opened up for the procedure, the client is usually charged. The nurse should call ahead of time to communicate the abnormal laboratory result instead of placing a note on the front of the chart. A note would not be seen until after the client has been transported to the operating room and the supplies have been opened. (R)

12. **4.** Clients should be made aware that some questions are asked for verification and safety with each new phase of treatment. (P)

13. **1, 2, 3.** Clients who have diabetes mellitus controlled by diet, those with a high stress response to surgery, or those who have been on steroid treatment for the last 3 months should have their serum glucose level assessed. A client with a family history of diabetes receiving D_5LR I.V. fluids does not need to have the serum glucose level checked unless other clinical manifestations are present. The client who has a high carbohydrate diet should be able to metabolize the glucose unless there are other health problems. (R)

14. **3.** The nurse should notify the physician directly for specific orders based on the client's glucose level. The nurse cannot ignore the elevated glucose level. The surgical experience is stressful and the client needs specific insulin coverage during the perioperative period. The nurse should not administer the insulin without checking with the surgeon because there are specific orders to withhold all medications. It is not necessary to notify the surgery department unless the physician cancels the surgery. (D)

15. **3.** Psychosocial integrity issues, including coping mechanisms, situational role changes, and body image changes, are more common in a client who undergoes elective cosmetic surgical procedures. Reduction of risk potential, physiologic adaptation, and health promotion and maintenance are greater needs for clients who are undergoing surgical correction of functional, anatomic, or physiologic defects in nonelective surgical procedures. (P)

16. **1.** A client should not elect surgery to meet someone else's needs. The nurse should encourage the client to share his feelings and his perception of the deformity and to clarify his reasons for electing to have the surgery. It is normal to be somewhat afraid, and it is good if a client says he feels "OK" about the surgery. The fact that a client believes that his wife will help him after surgery and that he will also be relatively independent reflects appropriate adaptation. It is a common feeling among preoperative clients that they are ready to "get this over with," indicating that the waiting period is stressful. (P)

17. **2.** Brittle nails indicate poor nutrition. Poor posture indicates that the client does not stand up straight and use her muscles to support herself. A dull expression reflects the client's affect and emotional status. The client's weight of 128 lb is within normal range. (H)

18. **4.** The Joint Commission requires that discharge instructions be written for the postoperative client. The nurse will review all instructions orally and will demonstrate any skill. Clients need to be given discharge instructions orally and in written form because of stress, medications, and the volume of material to be learned. Explaining all the instructions to a family member is important but does not replace the need for written instructions. (H)

19. **1.** The preadmission nurse, the first person in contact with the client, starts the discharge planning for the client undergoing surgery. All nurses involved with the client, from preadmission through postoperative recovery, should continue to reinforce the discharge plan. (H)

20. **3.** The nurse should have the client empty his bladder before the premedication is administered. This will be more comfortable and safe for the client. The purpose of the premedication is to decrease anxiety and promote a relaxed state. The client must have an empty bladder before being transferred to the operating room, where he will be immobilized and receive I.V. fluids. The family does not have to be present, but it is usually desired. Shaving the operative area is not generally recommended because it can cause small nicks that harbor bacteria. If the client must be shaved, it is usually done in the operating room holding area. The client should be comfortable at all times and offered a warm blanket whenever he is cool, before or after the premedication. (C)

21. **4.** The nurse should immediately think of the congenital metabolic tendency for malignant hyperthermia, which occurs in the presence of certain kinds of anesthetics. Whenever a preoperative client states that a family member has had problems with anesthesia or surgery, the nurse should inquire about the nature of the problems and whether other family members have had similar problems. Reassuring the client that technology has changed will do little to affect her fears and misses the opportunity to evaluate the risk for malignant hyperthermia. Encouraging the client to further express her concerns and reassuring her that her feelings are normal are important, but missing a familial tendency of malignant hyperthermia could be fatal. (R)

22. **2.** Clients who are allergic to apples are not known to be at risk for latex allergies. Clients who are allergic to avocados, kiwi, peaches, guava, bananas, water chestnuts, hazelnuts, tomatoes, potatoes, grapes, and apricots are at risk for latex allergies. (H)

23. **1.** Clients who have had long-term multiple exposures to latex products, such as would occur with six previous surgeries and recoveries, are at increased risk for latex allergies. The nurse should explore what types of surgeries these were, how involved the client's recoveries were, and whether signs of latex allergies have occurred in the past. Working as a sales clerk, having type 2 diabetes, or undergoing laser surgery does not expose a client to latex or increase the risk of latex allergy. (H)

24. **3.** The nurse should assess the vital signs of the client who exhibits urticaria, rhinitis, and conjunctivitis a few seconds after coming in contact with rubber gloves, a plastic catheter, plastic I.V. tubing, and a plastic I.V. solution bag. The nurse should recognize that these symptoms indicate that a type I allergic reaction is occurring, that the client is responding to the latex, and that the reaction can proceed into anaphylactic shock. The client does not need to be distracted or assessed for pain. Increasing the rate of administration of I.V. fluids is not the correct next action. (A)

25. **4.** The nurse would ask the client whether he wears glasses to evaluate his preoperative cognitive-perceptual pattern. Asking about the client's swallowing pattern would evaluate his nutritional-metabolic pattern. Asking about his need for special equipment to walk would evaluate his activity-exercise pattern. Asking the client about his history of smoking would evaluate his health perception–health management pattern. (A)

26. **3.** The client is at risk for a difficult intubation because the neck must be hyperextended to pass the endotracheal tube. Assessment of the pupils should not be limited. If the client is positioned appropriately during surgery, there is no risk of postoperative neck pain or limited neck movement. (R)

27. **1, 2, 3, 4.** Splinting the incision is important to avoid stress on the surgical site and to promote comfort so that the client will adhere to the plan of care. Inhaling and exhaling are important to bring in adequate oxygen and clear out carbon dioxide. However, closing one nostril when inhaling would be inappropriate and ineffective. The most important step is asking the client to hold the inhaled breath for about 5 seconds, which keeps the alveoli expanded. This step should be stressed the most. Repeating the exercise 5 to 10 times hourly is the second most important point to emphasize in this teaching plan. (R)

28. **2.** The nurse should call the surgeon for a serum creatinine level of 2.6 mg/dl, which is higher than the normal range of 0.5 to 1.0 mg/dl. An elevated serum creatinine value indicates that the kidneys are not filtering effectively and has important implications for the surgical client because many anesthesia and analgesia medications need to be filtered out through the renal system. The red blood cell count, hemoglobin level, and blood urea nitrogen level are within normal limits and do not need to be reported to the surgeon. (R)

29. **1.** Midazolam hydrochloride causes antegrade amnesia or decreased ability to remember events that occurred around the time of sedation. Nausea, mild agitation, and blurred vision are adverse effects of Versed. (D)

30. **3.** The client should be encouraged to take slow, deep breaths because midazolam hydrochloride is a respiratory depressant. The nurse should assess the client's blood pressure, monitor the pulse oximeter, and keep the client calm and relaxed, but the client will slip into very shallow, ineffective breathing if not encouraged to deep-breathe. (D)

31. **1.** The nurse should have an Ambu bag in the client's room because midazolam hydrochloride can lead to respiratory arrest if it is administered too quickly. The client does not need to be shocked back into a normal rhythm or to receive epinephrine unless cardiac compromise developed after the respiratory arrest. The client would receive titrated dosing of flumazenil to reverse the Versed, but first the nurse should ventilate the client. (D)

32. **2.** Metoclopramide is an antiemetic given because of its gastric emptying ability, which is necessary in gastrointestinal procedures. It does not increase gastric pH, reduce anxiety, or inhibit respiratory secretions. (D)

33. **3.** Glycopyrrolate is an anticholinergic given for its ability to reduce oral and respiratory secretions before general anesthesia. Increased heart rate and respiratory rate would be adverse effects of the drug. Amnesia should not be an effect of the drug. (D)

34. **1.** The nurse can administer atropine sulfate, an anticholinergic, to a client with diabetes. Atropine is contraindicated in clients with glaucoma because it increases intraocular pressure. It is contraindicated in clients with urine retention because it relaxes smooth muscle in the urinary tract and can exacerbate the problem. It is contraindicated in clients with gastrointestinal obstruction because it relaxes smooth muscle in the gut and may worsen the obstruction. (D)

35. **3.** Because droperidol causes tachycardia and orthostatic hypotension, the client should be moved slowly after receiving this medication. Inapsine produces a tranquilizing effect and does affect the central nervous, respiratory, or psychoneurologic system, but the primary reason for moving the client slowly is the potential cardiovascular effects of hypotension. (D)

36. **2.** Research findings have shown that enoxaparin and low-dose heparin given 6 to 12 hours preoperatively reduce the incidence of deep vein thrombosis and pulmonary emboli by 60% in clients who are at risk for deep vein thrombosis, such as those who are placed in the lithotomy position. Lovenox has no effect on red blood cell production, postoperative bleeding, or tissue healing. (D)

37. **4.** The nurse does not need to ask about all drugs used in the last 18 months unless the client is still taking them. The nurse does need to know all drugs the client is currently taking, including herbs and vitamins, over-the-counter medications such as aspirin taken in the past 6 weeks, the amount of alcohol consumed, and use of illegal drugs, because these can interfere with the anesthetic and analgesic agents. Steroid use is of concern because it can suppress the adrenal cortex for up to 1 year, and supplemental steroids may need to be administered in times of stress such as surgery. (R)

38. **2.** The nurse should notify the surgery department and document the past surgery in the chart in the preoperative notes so that the client's hip is not externally rotated and the hip dislocated while she is in the lithotomy position. The prosthesis should not be a problem as long as the perioperative nurse places the grounding pad away from the prosthesis site. The perioperative nurse will inform the rest of the team, but the primary reason to inform the perioperative nurse is related to safe positioning of the client. The surgeon can hand-write an addendum to the history and initial and date the entry. The history and physical information can then be retyped at a later date. (R)

39. **3.** The nurse should notify the anesthesiologist because supplemental prednisone suppresses the adrenal cortex's natural ability to produce increased corticosteroids in times of stress such as surgery. The anesthesiologist may need to order supplemental steroid coverage during the perioperative period. The nurse should document the prednisone with current medications, but it is a priority to inform the anesthesiologist. Because the poison ivy is not in the surgical field, the surgeon does not need to be called regarding the skin disruption. (D)

40. **2.** The client who has a significant cigarette smoking history and an operative manipulation close to the diaphragm (the gallbladder is against the liver) is at increased risk for atelectasis and pneumonia. Postoperatively this client will be reluctant to deep-breathe because of pain, in addition to having residual lung damage from smoking. Therefore, the client is at greater-than-average risk for pulmonary complications. The client does not have an increased risk of prolonged immobility (unless slowed by a respiratory problem), deep vein thrombosis (as long as the client performs leg exercises), or delayed wound healing (as long as the client maintains appropriate nutrition). (R)

41. **3.** The circulating nurse is a registered nurse who uses the nursing process (assessment, planning, implementation, and evaluation of client care) during the surgical procedure. The scrub role (passing instruments to the surgeon) can be assumed by a registered nurse or a surgical technologist. Personnel who are not scrubbed can answer the phone. The entire surgical team ensures the sterility of supplies. (M)

42. **4.** The purpose of separating the public from the restricted-attire area of the operating room is to provide an aseptic environment and prevent contamination of the environment by organisms. The client's privacy is protected, but the main purpose is infection control. (S)

43. **1.** The 68-year-old client is at greater risk because an older adult client is more likely to have comorbid conditions, a less-effective immune system, and less collagen in the integumentary system. (A)

44. **1.** The child having her 15th laser procedure for a hemangioma should not have a balloon unless it is latex free because this child has had numerous exposures to latex thus far. If she has not already developed some sensitivity, the nurse should help the family be aware of latex products to avoid when possible. A client who is having a tonsillectomy, inguinal hernia repair, or orchiopexy is probably having surgery for the first time and has not been exposed to latex, although it is a good practice to use latex-free products whenever possible and to inquire about past exposure. (S)

45. **2.** An autotransfusion is acceptable for the client who is in danger of cardiac arrest. An autotransfusion cannot be collected from a client who has cancer, a contaminated wound, or contamination from *Escherichia coli* because of a ruptured bowel. (D)

46. **2.** After a scope or catheter has been inserted into the urethra, the mucosal membrane is irritated and the client feels the need to void even though the bladder may not be full. The nurse should encourage the client to force fluids to make the urine dilute. The client should not ignore the urge to void. The client should be encouraged to use the bathroom; there is no need to use the bedpan. The client does not need assistance to the bathroom because this procedure does not require any anesthesia except a topical anesthetic for the male client. (C)

47. **4.** Early ambulation is the most significant general nursing measure to prevent postoperative complications and has been advocated for more than 40 years. Walking the client increases vital capacity and maintains normal respiratory functioning, stimulates circulation, prevents venous stasis, improves gastrointestinal and genitourinary function, increases muscle tone, and increases wound healing. The client should maintain a healthy diet, manage pain, and have regular bowel movements. However, early ambulation is the most important intervention. (R)

The Client Who Is Receiving or Recovering from Anesthesia

48. **1.** The client is demonstrating signs of malignant hyperthermia. Unless the body is cooled and the influx of calcium into the muscle cells is reversed, lethal cardiac arrhythmia and hypermetabolism occur. The client's body temperature can rise as high as 109° F (42.8° C) as body muscles contract. Dantrolene, an I.V. skeletal muscle relaxant, is used to reverse muscle rigidity. Elevating the head of the bed will not reverse the hyperthermia. Adding fluids and inserting an indwelling urinary catheter are not immediately beneficial steps in reversing the progression of malignant hyperthermia. (M)

49. **3.** The client is in the lithotomy position. The reverse Trendelenburg position is when the client is lying supine with the head lower than the rest of the body. A low Fowler's position is when the client is sitting up at a 30- to 45-degree angle. The prone position is when the client is lying face down. (M)

50. **4.** Airway flow is always the first assessment. Once the nurse establishes that the client has a patent airway, the pulse oximeter is applied to measure the oxygen saturation, the respiratory rate is counted, and the breath sounds are auscultated bilaterally. (A)

51. **1.** The last area to regain sensation is the perineal area, and the nurse should check the client for a distended bladder. The client has received a large volume of I.V. fluids since the epidural was inserted, and the client may not feel the urge to void or may be unable to void. In that case, the nurse should obtain an order to catheterize the client before the bladder becomes so distended as to cause bladder spasms. The nurse should assess for a spinal headache, postoperative pain, and the client's ability to move after determining whether the bladder is distended. (R)

52. **1, 3.** With spinal anesthesia, the fibers of the autonomic nervous system are blocked in a specific order: touch, pain, motor, pressure, and proprioception. Recovery from the block of the spinal anesthesia occurs in reverse order so that the client will experience return of motor function before pain is felt; thus, the legs will move before pain is felt. When the autonomic nervous system is blocked, vasodilation occurs and hypotension, not hypertension occurs. Sensation returns starting at the toes, then, in order, the feet, legs, and abdomen, so the client will feel sensation to the toes before the perineal area. Spinal fluid is lost from the dura when the client is in the upright position as gravity pushed the fluids through the hole made by the spinal needle. A spinal headache is a severe headache that occurs while in the upright position, but is relieved in the lying position. (A)

53. **3.** The nurse should check the client's baseline data to ascertain whether the client's pupil has always been enlarged or this is a new finding. The preoperative assessment is valuable as the baseline for comparison of all subsequent assessments made throughout the perioperative period. The nurse may determine that a more involved neurologic examination is indicated or may choose to assess other signs using the Glasgow Coma Scale, administer oxygen, or call the surgeon, but the nurse still needs to know the baseline data before proceeding. (A)

54. **1.** The nurse should check the dressing for signs of bleeding to establish a baseline for future assessments of the dressing and to verify that there is no obvious sign of hemorrhage. The nurse does not need to empty peri-incisional drains at this time. All drains should have been emptied and reconstituted by the postanesthesia care nurse before the client was transferred to the surgical floor. Assessing the client's pain level and assessing the bladder are important; however, it is more important to assess the surgical site for bleeding because hemorrhage is a life-threatening complication of any surgical procedure. (A)

55. **2.** Adult clients are induced for general anesthesia by breathing in an inhalant anesthetic mixed with oxygen through a facial mask and receiving intravenous medication to make them sleepy. Clients are not induced with the premedication. Clients usually are not induced with the intravenous infusion or the mask alone. (C)

56. **4.** Children are induced for general anesthesia by giving them medication through a facial mask to make them sleepy. Children are not induced with a injection. Children usually are not induced by use of a facial mask with I.V. administration started while they are still awake. (C)

57. **3.** Sodium pentothal, a short-acting barbiturate, can cause hypotension, which may be especially problematic for the client with impaired cardiac functioning. Sodium pentothal does not cause bradycardia, complete muscle relaxation, hypertension, or tachypnea. (D)

58. **1.** Propofol, a nonbarbiturate anesthetic, causes less nausea and vomiting because of a direct antiemetic action. It does not cause hypotension or skeletal muscle movement, and it does not act slowly. (D)

59. **4.** Desflurane and sevoflurane are volatile liquid anesthesia agents that are used for outpatient surgeries primarily because they are rapidly eliminated. They have the added benefits of being better tolerated and nonirritating to the respiratory tract, and they have predictable cardiovascular effects. However, rapid elimination is an important consideration for outpatient procedures. (D)

60. **3.** A heart rate of 150 bpm or greater, hypotension, and muscle rigidity are early signs of malignant hyperthermia. The nurse should quickly assemble emergency supplies and personnel because malignant hyperthermia is potentially and rapidly fatal in more than 50% of cases. Rapid, extreme rise in temperature is a late sign. Another factor influencing the analysis is that the client has a large body frame, and having large, bulky muscles is a risk factor for malignant hyperthermia. The client's vital signs are well out of the range of normal; analysis of the data and swift intervention are indicated. Excessive blood loss is unlikely and the data do not support this conclusion. Although clients do have changes in vital signs when in acute pain, the nurse would expect the client to be hypertensive, not hypotensive. (A)

61. **2.** One of the earliest signs of hypoxia is restlessness and agitation. Decreased level of consciousness and somnolence are later signs of hypoxia. Chills can be related to the anesthetic agent used but are not indicative of hypoxia. Urgency is not related to hypoxia. (A)

62. **2, 3, 4, 5.** Flumazenil should be administered in small quantities such as 0.2 mg over 15 to 30 seconds but never as a bolus. Flumazenil may be given undiluted in incremental doses. Adverse effects of flumazenil may include shivering and hypotension. The nurse should monitor the client's level of consciousness while recovering from sedation. Flumazenil should be administered through a free-flowing I.V. line in a large vein because extravasation causes local irritation. (D)

63. **2.** It is important for the nurse to cover this client with warm blankets because he is at high risk for hypothermia secondary to age, spinal anesthesia, placement in a lithotomy position in the cool operating room for 1.5 hours, instillation of 4,000 ml of room temperature bladder irrigation, and ongoing bladder irrigation. Spinal anesthesia causes vasodilation, which results in heat loss from the core to the periphery. The nurse will empty the catheter drainage bag and hang new bags of irrigation as needed, but the client's potential for hypothermia should be addressed first. The client will not be turned at this time. (R)

64. **3.** The client who is 5 feet 1 inch tall and weighs 200 lb would be expected to retain the anesthetic agents longer because adipose tissue absorbs the drug before the desired systemic effect is reached for anesthesia maintenance. Nursing interventions are aimed at encouraging the obese client to turn, cough, and deep-breathe despite feeling sleepy and tired. The sooner this client ambulates, the sooner the retained anesthesia will be worked out of the adipose tissue. (R)

65. **1.** The nurse should encourage the client to avoid holding his operated arm, the arm with the intravenous regional nerve block (Bier block), close to her face because she has no motor control over it. With the cast in place she could hit herself in the eye, nose, or mouth and cause soft-tissue damage. It is acceptable for the client to hold the operated arm with the unoperated arm or to use the unoperated arm. The nurse should administer the analgesic before the intravenous regional anesthetic completely wears off so that the pain does not peak before pain medication is administered. (R)

66. **3.** The nurse should monitor the client's respirations closely for 4 to 6 hours because naloxone has a shorter duration of action than opioids. The client may need repeated doses of naloxone to prevent or treat a recurrence of the respiratory depression. Naloxone is usually effective in a few minutes; however, its effects last only 1 to 2 hours and ongoing monitoring of the client's respiratory rate will be necessary. The client's dosage of morphine will be decreased or a new drug will be ordered to prevent another instance of respiratory depression. (D)

67. **3.** Abnormal coagulation test results have been associated with naloxone (Narcan), and the nurse should monitor surgical clients closely for bleeding. Dizziness, biliary colic, and urine retention are not associated with naloxone. (D)

68. **3.** The client who receives epidural anesthesia is at decreased risk for a headache because a noncutting needle is used instead of a side angle-cutting needle. The epidural needle is a 25G to 27G needle, which is much smaller than a 17G needle. The injection made for an epidural is an extradural, not a subarachnoid, injection as for spinal anesthesia. The onset of spinal anesthesia is faster because a larger dose of medication is usually administered. (A)

69. **3.** Spinal anesthesia does not cause parasympathetic blockage. The spinal anesthetic agent usually is injected into the L2 subarachnoid space, where it produces sympathetic, sensory, and motor blockade. (D)

70. **1.** Multiply 2.5 mg/5 mg by the unknown X mg/1 ml. Cross-multiply to get $5X = 2.5$ ml. Divide both sides of the equation by 5 to get $X = 0.5$ ml. (D)

71. **3.** In order to prevent burns, the nurse should assess the client's temperature every 15 minutes when using an external warming device. (S)

The Client Who Has Had Surgery

72. **3.** An indwelling urinary catheter increases the risk of urinary tract infection because microbes ascend the catheter and travel to the bladder. The nurse should try to facilitate the client's ability to void by using the sitting position for a woman or the standing position for a man and by running warm water over the perineum. If such conservative methods fail, the nurse should obtain an order to catheterize the client every 4 hours using a small French straight catheter until the client can void on his or her own. (R)

73. **4.** The first cognitive response that returns after anesthesia is orientation to person. The nurse assesses this by asking the client his name. Orientation to place and time usually occurs after orientation by the nurse because of confusion from anesthesia and waking in an unfamiliar place. The nurse can then continue to assess and document the client's cognitive ability to remember information. The nurse does not need to notify the surgeon. The client's cognitive response is normal. It is not necessary to ask the wife to reorient the client; however, she can continue to talk to him and help him regain consciousness. (A)

74. **2.** The client's body temperature dropped 2.5° F from the preoperative to postoperative phase. The client lost heat during the preoperative period. The client has not had time to regain the heat she has lost and should not be discharged postoperatively until her postoperative vital signs, which include body temperature, are closer to her preoperative vital signs. The client's pulse rate, respiratory rate, and blood pressure have compensated according to the client's hypothermic state and will reflect changes as the client warms up. There are no indications that the client needs more pain medication, oxygen, or I.V. fluids. (A)

75. **1, 3, 4, 5.** When assessing a postoperative client for perfusion and the manifestation of shock, nursing assessment should include an inspection for cyanotic mucous membranes; cold, moist, pale skin; and the level of oxygen saturation in relation to hemoglobin. The nurse should also compare the client's postoperative vital signs with his preoperative vital signs to determine how much physiologic stress has occurred during the intraoperative period. A client who is perfusing well would have warm, dry skin. A client well hydrated would have good skin turgor. The nurse would also assess fluid status using the intake and output record. If hemoglobin and hematocrit were available, the values would be included in the assessment. (M)

76. **3.** The nurse is helping the client manage her pain and comfort level. The nurse has completed her assessment of the client and should now dim the lights and create a quiet environment. Such nonpharmacologic measures as adjusting the light level in the room facilitate pain management. Decreasing stimulation from the environment, such as brightness to the optic nerve, promotes the client's ability to relax skeletal muscles and fall asleep. It is too soon to reassess vital signs. Checking that the family is comfortable is important but is not the next thing to do for this client. Increasing the oxygen flow rate is not indicated, and if needed should have been done before repositioning the client. (M)

77. **4.** When a postoperative client has a temperature elevation to greater than 100° F (37.8° C) in the first 24 hours after surgery, the temperature elevation is usually related to atelectasis. Because this client had upper abdominal surgery with manipulation around the diaphragm, the client is more prone to guarding the operative site and shallow breathing. Encouraging the client to take deep breaths and use incentive spirometry are appropriate measures to prevent atelectasis and pulmonary infection. The nurse must assist the client in filling the alveoli in the lower posterior lobes of the lungs. An incentive spirometer is a good visual biofeedback instrument that the client had practiced with preoperatively. Changing the client's position from lying to sitting for deep breathing will expand alveoli in the lower posterior lobes. There is no indication that a surgical wound infection is occurring. An antibiotic is not indicated at this time. Pain medication will decrease

respirations and the client is not indicating pain at the moment. (A)

78. **1, 2, 4.** Nurses can delegate to the unlicensed assistive personnel (UAP) to observe clients and promote their comfort following surgery, and to empty and measure urinary catheter drainage bags. UAPs cannot teach clients; that is the responsibility of the registered nurse or respiratory therapist. UAPs cannot assess I.V. insertion sites, which is the responsibility of a registered nurse. (M)

79. **3.** The nurse should take the client's blood pressure. She is likely experiencing orthostatic hypotension. The PCA pump does not need to be discontinued because, as soon as the blood pressure stabilizes, the pain medication can be resumed. Administering oxygen is not necessary unless the oxygen saturation also drops. The client should sit in the chair until the blood pressure stabilizes. (D)

80.

4. Splint the incisional site.
1. Inhale through the nose.
3. Exhale through pursed lips.
2. Cough deeply from the lungs.

The client must first splint the incision to avoid increased intolerable pain or he may not cooperate with the pulmonary ventilation. The next step is to inhale oxygen to expand the alveoli for a few seconds and then exhale carbon dioxide in successive steps 5 to 10 times. The client should try to cough on the end of the exhalation to remove retained secretions from the larger airways. (R)

81. **4.** The nurse should plan for two people, one at each side using a drawsheet, one person at the head, and one person at the feet to transfer an elderly, drowsy client with fragile skin to avoid shearing of the integumentary system. Using only two or three people allows for dragging of some part of the client, which leads to shearing of the dependent part. (S)

82. **3.** The client who has not had the gag reflex anesthetized is the client who had a repair of the carpal tunnel syndrome under local anesthesia because the area being anesthetized was the tissue in the wrist. The client who had a bronchoscopy received a local anesthetic on the vocal cords, and the nurse should check the gag reflex or ability to swallow before administering fluids. Clients who had general anesthesia or intravenous conscious sedation received medication for central nervous system sedation, and the nurse should assess the level of consciousness and ability to swallow before administering fluids. (R)

83. **3.** When the urine output is less than 30 ml/hour, the nurse should assess for potential causes such as hypovolemia or hemorrhage. The nurse should assess and evaluate the client's vital signs, intake and output, dressing, and available laboratory values and notify the physician. Bowel obstruction, although possible after surgery, is characterized most notably by abdominal distention and absent bowel sounds, not decreased urine output. The nurse would not expect the client to have hypertension, but rather hypotension. (A)

84. **3.** A client who had a left thoracoscopy is placed in the lateral position, in which the most common injury is an injury to the brachial plexus. Numbness and tingling in the arm suggests a brachial plexus injury. There is no undue pressure on the ankles or knees during thoracic surgery. (A)

85. **3.** Although any client may experience nausea and vomiting secondary to anesthetics or postoperative analgesics, the client who has had manipulation of the abdominal organs is more prone to postoperative nausea and vomiting than the client who has had a procedure such as a total joint replacement, open heart surgery, or a mastectomy. (A)

86. **3.** The nurse should inform the client that as the incision heals uneven lumps might appear under the incision line because the collagen is growing new tissue at different rates. Eventually, the lumps will even out and the tissue will be smooth. The client can touch the incision with clean hands as needed to perform incisional care. The client should not clean the incision with hydrogen peroxide because it may dry out the natural skin oils. The surgeon will remove the staples for the client. (R)

87. **2.** When a wound eviscerates (abdominal organs protruding through the opened incision), the nurse should cover the open area with a sterile dressing moistened with sterile normal saline and then cover it with a dry dressing. The surgeon should then be notified to take the client back to the operating room to close the incision under general anesthesia. The nurse should not press the emergency alarm because this is not a cardiac or respiratory arrest. The nurse should have the visitors and family leave the room to decrease the chance of airborne contamination, but the primary focus should be on covering the wound with a moist, sterile covering. (S)

88. **2, 3, 4.** WBC count should be above normal (4,500 to 11,000/mm³) with an acute infection or inflammatory response such as a postoperative wound infection. Redness and swelling beyond the incision line is expected with a wound infection. An elevated temperature such as 102° F (38.9° C) on the third to fourth postoperative day indicates an infection process rather than an inflammatory process. An elevation in the segmented neutrophils demonstrates that the most mature WBCs have responded to the invading bacteria at the incision site, which is an expected response. Typically, postoperative pain begins to lessen by the 4th day. (A)

89. **4.** A wet-to-dry dressing should be able to dry out between dressing changes. Thus, the dressing should be moist, not dry, when applied. As the moist dressing dries, the wound will be debrided of necrotic tissue, exudate, and so forth. Normal saline is most commonly used to moisten the sponge; Burrow's solution will irritate the wound. The sponge should not be packed into the wound tightly because the circulation to the site could be impaired. The moist sponge should be placed so that all surfaces of the wound are in contact with the dressing. Then the sponge is covered and protected by a dry sterile dressing to prevent contamination from the external environment. (S)

90. **3.** After emptying a Jackson-Pratt drainage bulb, the nurse should compress the bulb, plug it to establish suction, and then document the amount and type of drainage emptied. Irrigating a Jackson-Pratt drain is inappropriate because it could contaminate the wound. The Jackson-Pratt drain is not usually connected to wall suction. The purpose of the Jackson-Pratt drain is to remove bloody drainage from the deep tissues of the incision; clamping the drain would be counterproductive. (R)

91. **1.** Performing leg exercises, including ankle pumping, ankle rotation, and quadriceps setting exercises, will help prevent stasis of blood in the lower extremities, which can lead to blood clot formation. Encouraging the client to cough and deep-breathe is an important postoperative intervention; however, it is directed at preventing pneumonia, not pulmonary emboli. The nurse should not massage the calves because a deep vein thrombus could dislodge and travel to the pulmonary vasculature. Antiembolism stockings should be worn continuously during the postoperative period. (A)

92. **2.** Naloxone hydrochloride is the antidote for morphine sulfate. The signs of overdose on morphine sulfate are a respiration rate of 2 to 4 breaths/minute, bradycardia, and hypotension. Flumazenil is the antidote for midazolam. Doxacurium is a nondepolarizing muscle relaxant. Remifentanil is an opioid used as an anesthetic adjunct. (D)

93. **2.** The client admitted for same-day surgery should not drive home after the surgical procedure because it is unsafe. Even without an anesthetic, the surgical event can be more stressful than anticipated. It is acceptable to have someone arrive after the surgery has started to take the client home. A taxi is permissible but not desirable. (R)

94. **3.** The client has deficient knowledge when stating that pain from a laparoscopic cholecystectomy is related to a large incision and manipulation of tissue. The nurse should explain that there are four puncture sites for the incision and that gas is used to distend the abdominal cavity to keep the abdominal organs away from the operative site. There is no real manipulation of tissue to produce pain. The pain that clients do experience from this procedure is related to the gas, which irritates the diaphragm. The client should start on clear liquids and advance to bland foods until the gas is gone. Walking helps to eliminate the gas from the abdominal cavity within 12 to 24 hours after surgery. (R)

95. 3. The urine output does not have to be checked every 15 minutes for a client who has had an arthroscopy because this client probably does not have a catheter in place. If the client voids, the output would be recorded. Assessments every 15 minutes during the first hour would include vital signs, pulse oximeter values, and pain to monitor the client's comfort level and check for compartment syndrome. Neurovascular checks distal to the operative site are especially vital because a tourniquet was used proximal to the operative site during the surgical procedure and because edema may develop during the postoperative period. (R)

96. 2. Hypotension and tachycardia are common adverse effects of droperidol and should be monitored closely by the nurse. Hypotension and tachycardia are not common adverse effects of ondansetron hydrochloride, prochlorperazine, or promethazine. (D)

97. 1. The nurse should assess but not disturb the epidural dressing because the catheter can be easily dislodged and organisms can easily be transmitted into the central nervous system. The nurse should not have to change the dressing at all if a waterproof dressing is applied over the epidural site. Even with strict aseptic technique, a drain into a sterile cavity is a direct route for transmission of organisms and places a client at increased risk of infection. (D)

98. 2. The client who has epidural pain management postoperatively can ambulate because a low concentration of local analgesia causes sensory blockage only. The catheter is placed so that constant pain management plus patient-controlled administration of an analgesic dose can block sensory innervation. Motor function should not be affected since the catheter is placed above the dura lining the spinal fluid. If the catheter would move through the dura sac, spinal analgesia would occur, affecting motor function as well as sympathetic nervous system function. (D)

99. 1. The client who develops pruritus and urticaria while receiving an I.V. antibiotic has clinical manifestations of a type I (anaphylactic) reaction. The greatest number of anaphylactic reactions in surgical clients is related to use of I.V. antibiotics. An example of a type II (cytotoxic and cytolytic) reaction would be clumping of incompatible blood in a hemolytic blood transfusion reaction. Clinical manifestation of a type III (immune-complex) reaction depends on the number of complexes and location in the body; common sites are the kidneys, skin, joints, blood vessels, and lungs. Clinical manifestations of type IV (delayed hypersensitivity) reactions include papules, vesicles, and bullae. (A)

100. 2. Hypotension, tachycardia, bronchospasm, and pulmonary edema are clinical manifestations of anaphylaxis. These symptoms are not seen in malignant hyperthermia, contact dermatitis, or cell-mediated responses. (A)

101. 1. The nurse should ask the location of the client's pain because Lortab is an opioid, which can be constipating. By the third day, many clients become constipated and are feeling distended, with sharp, cramping pain due to gas, which is treated with ambulation, not more opioids. The client's emptying his bladder should not affect his pain level. The nurse should look at the client's chart to determine when the client's last dose of pain medication was administered, rather than asking the client. The client's statement regarding his pain level before the surgery is not relevant to whether the nurse should administer the Lortab. (A)

102. 1. Blood and serous fluid is drained from the operative site to prevent hematoma formation or a collection of fluid that could become a site for infection. This also minimizes postoperative swelling, which can be painful. A simple explanation such as this is appropriate because the client is just waking up from surgery. Blood from the operative site can be collected through an autotransfusion system so that it can be transfused to the client during or immediately after surgery. However, strict guidelines about volume of blood lost, how quickly the device fills, and how long the blood has been out of the client's body govern whether the blood can be transfused. Therefore, although it is possible that the drainage system to which the client refers is an autotransfusion system, it is more likely that the client has a simple Hemovac drain. It is incorrect to tell a client not to worry about something even if she is in the drowsy state of awakening from anesthesia. It is inappropriate to ignore the client and give her something to make her drowsy instead of addressing his concerns. (P)

103. 1. The purpose of the Jackson-Pratt drainage tube is to drain off the purulent drainage from the sterile peritoneal cavity and prevent peritonitis. A Jackson-Pratt drain cannot prevent bleeding. The Jackson-Pratt drain has no effect on pressure on the bladder. There is no reason to be concerned about pressure on the gallbladder. (R)

104. 2. Biliary drainage tubes (T tubes) are placed in the common bile duct and drain bile, which is dark yellow-orange. Serosanguineous drainage is thin and pinkish red. Bile is not clear and is not green unless it comes in contact with gastric fluid. (R)

105. **1.** Urinary elimination in the first 8 hours postoperatively is a requirement before the client who has had an inguinal hernia repair can be discharged from same-day surgery. Ingestion of fluids without nausea and vomiting is important, but eating solid foods is not a requirement for discharge from same-day surgery. Being completely pain-free is an unrealistic expectation for the time frame and is not a requirement for leaving same-day surgery. However, the client should be comfortable and his pain should be controlled. It is not a requirement for the client to ambulate in the hallway, but the client should be able to sit up and go to the bathroom without assistance. (R)

106. **3.** The ability to self-dose is a requirement for the client to use PCA. Having a family member or court-appointed advocate present is not a requirement for initiating PCA. The nurse teaches the client about how to use PCA and monitors effectiveness of the pain medication; however, it is not necessary for the nurse to assist with the dosing. (D)

107. **2.** The client's body temperature should be assessed every 4 hours during the first 24 hours because the client is still at risk for hypothermia or malignant hyperthermia. The client does not need to be checked every 2 hours unless indicated by an abnormal finding. (R)

108. **1.** The client's systolic blood pressure is dropping and the pulse pressure is narrowing, indicating impending shock. The nurse should notify the surgeon. Elevating the head of the bed will not increase the blood pressure. Administering pain medication could cause the blood pressure to drop further. The intake and output record may indicate decreased urine output related to shock but the nurse should first contact the health care provider. (R)

109. **1.** The client who has been positioned in the lithotomy position under general anesthesia may experience discomfort in the shoulders postoperatively because the client is placed in the Trendelenburg position to expose the perineal area. The client's weight is then shifted toward the shoulders and the client experiences muscle soreness postoperatively. (C)

110. **2.** The client should drink a minimum of 2,500 ml of fluid per day (not 1,500 ml) to keep secretions liquefied and easier to cough up and eliminate from the upper respiratory tract. The client should use pain medication before coughing. The nurse should monitor the client's breath sounds and temperature to detect early signs of infection. The nurse should assist with early ambulation. (R)

111. **3.** The client with thromboembolism does not have coolness. The client with thromboembolism has redness, swelling, increased warmth along the vein, edema, and pain and may have hemoptysis, chest pain, tachycardia, dyspnea, and restlessness. (A)

112. **3.** The client should sit in an upright position when doing breathing exercises to allow for full chest expansion of both lungs and all fields and bases. Using an incentive spirometer every hour while awake is appropriate and allows the client visual feedback. Placing his hands lightly over the lower ribs and upper abdomen allows the client to see muscles of inspiration and expiration and is appropriate. Coughing deeply from the lungs after four deep breaths allows the client to effectively cough up secretions. (R)

113. **2.** Muscle cramping is a sign of hypokalemia. Potassium is an electrolyte lost with nasogastric suctioning. Confusion is seen with hypercalcemia. Edema is seen with protein deficit or fluid volume overload. Tremors are seen with hypomagnesemia. (R)

Legal and Ethical Issues Associated with Surgery

114. **3.** The most critical piece of information is the client identification bracelet. Misidentification of clients can result in serious harm to the client. The nurse also needs the admitting records and Addressograph labels as part of verifying the client's identification. The location of the family is not included in verifying identification. (R)

115. **4.** The nurse is not is not required to have the anesthesia note on the chart before the client is transported to the operating room suite. The anesthesia record is on the chart after the surgical procedure is completed and is a good source of client information. The operative consent, history and physical information, and laboratory test results should be on the chart before the client is transported to the operating suite. (M)

116. **2.** When the client cannot sign the operative consent and it is a true life-saving emergency, consent may be obtained over the telephone from the client's next-of-kin or guardian. The surgeon must obtain the telephone consent, but if it is a true life-saving emergency the surgeon often is already in surgery, so the nurse makes the telephone call and another nurse witnesses the call. Some institutions have a special consent form for emergency surgery. Consent can be waived in situations in which no family is available; however, if the family can be reached by telephone before surgery, verbal consent is legally required. (M)

117. **3.** There are risks with both the surgical procedure and the general anesthesia required for a craniotomy. The risks involved in the procedure are a part of the informed consent. Other information that is part of an informed consent includes potential complications, expected benefits, inability of the surgeon to predict results, irreversibility of the procedure (if applicable), and other available treatments. Talking about the effects of the diabetes on healing, explaining how the craniotomy is performed, and explaining the consequences of declining treatment (e.g., death if the tumor is not removed) represent appropriate actions to provide information to the client. (M)

118. **2.** All health care facilities reimbursed under Medicare and Medicaid are required under the 1991 Patient Self-Determination Act to recognize clients' advance directives such as health care proxies or living wills. Advance directives are an important part of perioperative care and should be respected by all health care professionals caring for the client. The nurse should not be involved in specific questions regarding how the client is going to pay for health care services except as an advocate addressing the client's psychosocial needs. (M)

119. **2.** The client must have an identification bracelet properly secured on her person before being transported to the operating room to ensure correct identification. It is incorrect to send the client without a properly secured identification bracelet. The perioperative nurse must verify the client's identification by checking for the same name on the chart, armband, and schedule and by the client's statement. The preoperative nurse may be asked to physically identify the client and obtain a new armband. (M)

120. **2.** When the client cannot read or write, the consent can be read to the client and the client can sign in the presence of two witnesses. The client (not the next-of-kin) should always sign for himself unless he is a minor or not of sound mind. The court does not appoint a guardian for a person of sound mind just because he cannot read or write. Hospital personnel would not and could not sign a consent form for a client. (M)

The Client with Health Problems of the Eyes, Ears, Nose, and Throat

- The Client with Cataracts
- The Client with a Retinal Detachment
- The Client with Glaucoma
- The Client with Adult Macular Degeneration
- The Client Undergoing Nasal Surgery
- The Client with a Hearing Disorder
- The Client with Ménière's Disease
- The Client with Cancer of the Larynx
- Correct Answers and Rationales

The Client with Cataracts

1. The nurse is observing a student nurse administer eyedrops, as shown in the figure below. What should the nurse instruct the student to do?
☐ 1. Move the dropper to the inner canthus.
☐ 2. Have the client raise her eyebrows.
☐ 3. Administer the drops in the center of the lower lid.
☐ 4. Have the client squeeze both eyes after administering the drops.

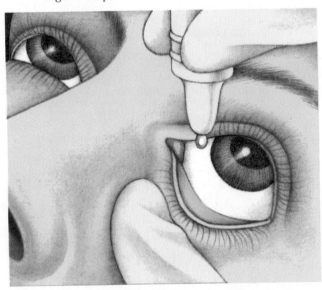

2. A client is having a cataract removed and will use eyeglasses after the surgery. What should the nurse instruct the client about? Select all that apply.
☐ 1. Images will appear to be one-third larger.
☐ 2. Look through the center of the glasses.
☐ 3. The changes will be immediate.
☐ 4. Use handrails when climbing stairs.
☐ 5. Stay out of the sun for 2 weeks.

3. A client is admitted to outpatient surgery for a cataract extraction on the right eye. The client asks the nurse, "What causes cataracts in old people?" Which of the following statements should form the basis for the nurse's response? Cataracts most commonly are a result of:
☐ 1. Chronic systemic disease.
☐ 2. The aging process.
☐ 3. Injuries sustained early in life.
☐ 4. The prolonged use of drugs.

4. A client asks, "What does the lens of my eye do?" The nurse should explain that the lens of the eye:
☐ 1. Produces aqueous humor.
☐ 2. Holds the rods and cones.
☐ 3. Focuses light rays onto the retina.
☐ 4. Regulates the amount of light entering the eye.

5. The client with a cataract tells the nurse that she is afraid of being awake during eye surgery. Which of the following responses by the nurse would be the most appropriate?
☐ 1. "Have you ever had any reactions to local anesthetics in the past?"
☐ 2. "What is it that disturbs you about the idea of being awake?"
☐ 3. "By using a local anesthetic, you won't have nausea and vomiting after the surgery."
☐ 4. "There's really nothing to fear about being awake. You'll be given a medication that will help you relax."

6. A client with a cataract would most likely complain of which symptoms?
☐ 1. Halos and rainbows around lights.
☐ 2. Eye pain and irritation that worsens at night.
☐ 3. Blurred and hazy vision.
☐ 4. Eye strain and headache when doing close work.

7. A client is scheduled for removal of a cataract of the right eye. Before surgery, the nurse is to instill drops of phenylephrine hydrochloride (Neo-Synephrine) into the client's right eye. This preparation acts in the eye to produce:

☐ **1.** Dilation of the pupil and blood vessels.

☐ **2.** Dilation of the pupil and constriction of blood vessels.

☐ **3.** Constriction of the pupil and constriction of blood vessels.

☐ **4.** Constriction of the pupil and dilation of blood vessels.

8. A short time after cataract surgery, the client complains of nausea. Which of the following represents the nurse's best course of action?

☐ **1.** Instruct the client to take a few deep breaths until the nausea subsides.

☐ **2.** Explain that this is a common feeling that will pass quickly.

☐ **3.** Tell the client to call the nurse promptly if vomiting occurs.

☐ **4.** Medicate the client with an antiemetic, as ordered.

9. Which of the following is a potential complication following cataract surgery? Select all that apply.

☐ **1.** Acute bacterial endophthalmitis.

☐ **2.** Retrobulbar hemorrhage.

☐ **3.** Rupture of the posterior capsule.

☐ **4.** Suprachoroidal hemorrhage.

☐ **5.** Vision loss.

10. The client is discharged on the day of the cataract surgery. Which of the following nursing diagnoses would be most appropriate for the client at this time?

☐ **1.** *Deficient diversional activity* related to activity limitations after surgery.

☐ **2.** *Chronic pain* related to postoperative incisional discomfort.

☐ **3.** *Risk for injury* related to limited vision after surgery.

☐ **4.** *Feeding self-care deficit* related to inability to see food.

11. After returning home, a client who has had cataract surgery will need to continue to instill eyedrops in the affected eye. The client is instructed to apply slight pressure against the nose at the inner canthus of the eye after instilling the eyedrops. The rationale that supports applying pressure is that it:

☐ **1.** Prevents the medication from entering the tear duct.

☐ **2.** Prevents the drug from running down the client's face.

☐ **3.** Allows the sensitive cornea to adjust to the medication.

☐ **4.** Facilitates distribution of the medication over the eye surface.

12. Which of the following activities should be avoided to achieve the goal of decreasing intraocular pressure after eye surgery?

☐ **1.** Lying supine.

☐ **2.** Coughing.

☐ **3.** Deep breathing.

☐ **4.** Ambulation.

13. After cataract removal surgery, the client is instructed to report any complaints of a sharp pain in the operative eye because this could indicate which of the following postoperative complications?

☐ **1.** Detached retina.

☐ **2.** Prolapse of the iris.

☐ **3.** Extracapsular erosion.

☐ **4.** Intraocular hemorrhage.

The Client with a Retinal Detachment

14. A client is admitted through the emergency department with a diagnosis of detached retina in the right eye. As the nurse completes the admission history, the client reports that before the physician patched his eye, he saw many spots, or "floaters." The nurse should explain to the client that these spots were caused by:

☐ **1.** Pieces of the retina floating in the eye.

☐ **2.** Blood cells released into the eye by the detachment.

☐ **3.** Contamination of the aqueous humor.

☐ **4.** Spasms of the retinal blood vessels traumatized by the detachment.

15. A client with detachment of the retina asks the nurse why it is necessary to patch both of her eyes. The nurse's reply should be based on the knowledge that eye patches serve to:

☐ **1.** Reduce rapid eye movements.

☐ **2.** Decrease the irritation caused by light entering the damaged eye.

☐ **3.** Protect the injured eye from infection.

☐ **4.** Rest the eyes to promote healing.

16. The client with retinal detachment in the right eye is extremely apprehensive. He states, "I'm afraid of going blind. It would be so hard to live that way." What factor should the nurse consider before responding to his statement?

☐ **1.** Repeat surgery is impossible, so if this procedure fails, vision loss is inevitable.

☐ **2.** The surgery will only delay blindness in the right eye, but vision is preserved in the left eye.

☐ **3.** More and more services are available to help newly blind people adapt to daily living.

☐ **4.** Optimism is justified because surgical treatment has a 90% to 95% success rate.

17. Which of the following statements would provide the best guide for activity during the rehabilitation period for a client who has been treated for retinal detachment?
- ☐ 1. Activity is resumed gradually, and the client can resume her usual activities in 5 to 6 weeks.
- ☐ 2. Activity level is determined by the client's tolerance; she can be as active as she wishes.
- ☐ 3. Activity level will be restricted for several months, so she should plan on being sedentary.
- ☐ 4. Activity level can return to normal and may include regular aerobic exercises.

18. Which of the following goals would be a priority for a client who has undergone surgery for retinal detachment?
- ☐ 1. Control pain.
- ☐ 2. Prevent an increase in intraocular pressure.
- ☐ 3. Promote a low-sodium diet.
- ☐ 4. Maintain a darkened environment.

19. Scleral buckling, a procedure used to treat retinal detachment, involves:
- ☐ 1. Removing the torn segment of the retina and stitching down the remaining segment.
- ☐ 2. Replacing the torn segment of the retina with a strip of retina from a donor.
- ☐ 3. Stitching the retina firmly to the optic nerve to give it support.
- ☐ 4. Creating a splint to hold the retina together until a scar can form and seal off the tear.

The Client with Glaucoma

20. A client with glaucoma is to receive 3 gtt of acetazolamide (Diamox) in the left eye. What should the nurse do?
- ☐ 1. Ask the client to close his right eye while administering the drug in the left eye.
- ☐ 2. Have the client look up while the nurse administers the eyedrops.
- ☐ 3. Have the client lift his eyebrows while the nurse positions the hand with the dropper on the client's forehead.
- ☐ 4. Wipe the eyes with a tissue following administration of the drops.

21. A client who has been treated for chronic open-angle glaucoma (COAG) for 5 years asks the clinic nurse, "How does glaucoma damage my eyesight?" The nurse's reply should be based on the knowledge that COAG:
- ☐ 1. Results from chronic eye inflammation.
- ☐ 2. Causes increased intraocular pressure.
- ☐ 3. Leads to detachment of the retina.
- ☐ 4. Is caused by decreased blood flow to the retina.

22. Which of the following signs or symptoms is most commonly experienced by clients with chronic open-angle glaucoma (COAG)?
- ☐ 1. Eye pain.
- ☐ 2. Excessive lacrimation.
- ☐ 3. Colored light flashes.
- ☐ 4. Decreasing peripheral vision.

23. Miotics are frequently used in the treatment of glaucoma. The nurse should understand that miotics work by:
- ☐ 1. Paralyzing ciliary muscles.
- ☐ 2. Constricting intraocular vessels.
- ☐ 3. Constricting the pupil.
- ☐ 4. Relaxing ciliary muscles.

24. Which of the following should the nurse provide as part of the information to prepare the client for tonometry?
- ☐ 1. Oral pain medication will be given before the procedure.
- ☐ 2. It is a painless procedure with no adverse effects.
- ☐ 3. Blurred or double vision may occur after the procedure.
- ☐ 4. Medication will be given to dilate the pupils before the procedure.

25. A client uses timolol maleate (Timoptic) eyedrops. The expected outcome of this beta-adrenergic blocker is to control glaucoma by:
- ☐ 1. Constricting the pupils.
- ☐ 2. Dilating the canals of Schlemm.
- ☐ 3. Reducing aqueous humor formation.
- ☐ 4. Improving the ability of the ciliary muscle to contract.

26. The nurse observes the client while he instills his eyedrops. The client says, "I just try to hit the middle of my eyeball so the drops don't run out of my eye." The nurse explains to the client that the method he is now using may cause:
- ☐ 1. Scleral staining.
- ☐ 2. Corneal injury.
- ☐ 3. Excessive lacrimation.
- ☐ 4. Systemic drug absorption.

27. The client with glaucoma is scheduled for a hip replacement. Which of the following orders would require clarification or correction before the nurse carries it out?
- ☐ 1. Administer morphine sulfate.
- ☐ 2. Administer atropine sulfate.
- ☐ 3. Teach deep-breathing exercises.
- ☐ 4. Teach leg lifts and muscle-setting exercises.

28. Which of the following clinical manifestations should the nurse associate with acute angle-closure glaucoma?
- [ ] **1.** Gradual loss of central vision.
- [ ] **2.** Acute light sensitivity.
- [ ] **3.** Loss of color vision.
- [ ] **4.** Sudden eye pain.

29. A client has been diagnosed with an acute episode of angle-closure glaucoma. The nurse plans the client's nursing care with the understanding that acute angle-closure glaucoma:
- [ ] **1.** Frequently resolves without treatment.
- [ ] **2.** Is typically treated with sustained bed rest.
- [ ] **3.** Is a medical emergency that can rapidly lead to blindness.
- [ ] **4.** Is most commonly treated with steroid therapy.

The Client with Adult Macular Degeneration

30. When assessing an older adult with macular degeneration the nurse should expect to find:
- [ ] **1.** Loss of central vision.
- [ ] **2.** Loss of peripheral vision.
- [ ] **3.** Total blindness.
- [ ] **4.** Blurring of vision.

31. A 75-year-old male client has a history of macular degeneration. While he is in the hospital, the priority nursing goal will be:
- [ ] **1.** To provide education regarding community services for clients with adult macular degeneration (AMD).
- [ ] **2.** To provide health care related to monitoring his eye condition.
- [ ] **3.** To promote a safe, effective care environment.
- [ ] **4.** To improve vision.

32. When admitting a blind female client to the hospital, the nurse should:
- [ ] **1.** Ask the client to have someone with her at all times.
- [ ] **2.** Encourage her to stay in bed until the nurse can assist.
- [ ] **3.** Orient the client to the room environment by providing opportunity to touch the objects.
- [ ] **4.** Allow time for the client to orient to the environment.

33. Although all of the following measures might be useful in reducing the visual disability of a client with adult macular degeneration (AMD), which measure should the nurse teach the client primarily as a safety precaution?
- [ ] **1.** Wear a patch over one eye.
- [ ] **2.** Place personal items on the sighted side.
- [ ] **3.** Lie in bed with the unaffected side toward the door.
- [ ] **4.** Turn the head from side to side when walking.

34. The nurse is assessing a client with macular degeneration. Identify the illustration that best depicts what clients with this disorder typically see.

The Client Undergoing Nasal Surgery

35. A 27-year-old female is admitted for elective nasal surgery for a deviated septum. Which of the following would be an important initial clue that bleeding was occurring even if the nasal drip pad remained dry and intact?
- [ ] **1.** Complaints of nausea.
- [ ] **2.** Repeated swallowing.
- [ ] **3.** Rapid respiratory rate.
- [ ] **4.** Feelings of anxiety.

36. The client is ready for discharge after surgery for a deviated septum. Which of the following discharge instructions would be appropriate?
- [ ] **1.** Avoid activities that elicit Valsalva's maneuver.
- [ ] **2.** Take aspirin to control nasal discomfort.
- [ ] **3.** Avoid brushing the teeth until the nasal packing is removed.
- [ ] **4.** Apply heat to the nasal area to control swelling.

37. Which of the following statements would indicate to the nurse that the client who has undergone repair of her nasal septum has understood the discharge instructions?
- [ ] **1.** "I should not shower until my packing is removed."
- [ ] **2.** "I will take stool softeners and modify my diet to prevent constipation."
- [ ] **3.** "Coughing every 2 hours is important to prevent respiratory complications."
- [ ] **4.** "It is important to blow my nose each day to remove the dried secretions."

The Client with a Hearing Disorder

38. A 75-year-old client who has been taking furosemide (Lasix) regularly for 4 months tells the nurse that he is having trouble hearing. What would be the nurse's best response to this statement?
☐ **1.** Tell the client that because he is 75 years old, it is inevitable that his hearing should begin to deteriorate.
☐ **2.** Have the client immediately report the hearing loss to his physician.
☐ **3.** Schedule the client for audiometric testing and a hearing aid.
☐ **4.** Tell the client that the hearing loss is only temporary; when his system adjusts to the furosemide, his hearing will improve.

39. The nurse has been assigned to a client who is hearing impaired and reads speech. Which of the following strategies should the nurse incorporate when communicating with the client? Select all that apply.
☐ **1.** Avoiding being silhouetted against strong light.
☐ **2.** Not blocking out the person's view of the speaker's mouth.
☐ **3.** Facing the client when talking.
☐ **4.** Having bright light behind so the individual can see.
☐ **5.** Ensuring the client is familiar with the subject material before discussing.
☐ **6.** Talking to the client while doing other nursing procedures.

40. Which of the following best describes the effect of a hearing aid for a client with sensorineural hearing loss?
☐ **1.** It makes sounds louder and clearer.
☐ **2.** It has no effect on hearing.
☐ **3.** It makes sounds louder but not clearer.
☐ **4.** It improves the client's ability to separate words from background noises.

41. A client states that she was told she has sensorineural hearing loss and asks the nurse what this means. The nurse's response is based on the knowledge that sensorineural hearing loss results from which of the following conditions?
☐ **1.** Presence of fluid and cerumen in the external canal.
☐ **2.** Sclerosis of the bones of the middle ear.
☐ **3.** Damage to the cochlear or vestibulocochlear nerve.
☐ **4.** Emotional disturbance resulting in a functional hearing loss.

42. A 65-year-old male complains of hearing loss and a sensation of fullness in both ears. The nurse examines his ears with the understanding that a common cause of hearing loss in older adults is related to:
☐ **1.** Accumulation of cerumen in the external canal.
☐ **2.** Accumulation of cerumen in the internal canal.
☐ **3.** External otitis.
☐ **4.** Exostosis.

43. The best method to remove cerumen from a client's ear involves:
☐ **1.** Inserting a cotton-tipped applicator into the external canal.
☐ **2.** Irrigating the ear gently.
☐ **3.** Using aural suction.
☐ **4.** Using a cerumen curette.

44. To prepare the irrigation solution used for removal of cerumen, the nurse uses:
☐ **1.** Normal saline.
☐ **2.** Sterile water.
☐ **3.** Antiseptic solution.
☐ **4.** Warm tap water.

45. A 26-year-old client has a history of chronic otitis media. Which of the following procedures is the most common surgical intervention for chronic otitis media?
☐ **1.** Ossiculoplasty.
☐ **2.** Tympanoplasty.
☐ **3.** Mastoidectomy.
☐ **4.** Myringotomy.

46. A client is about to have a tympanoplasty. She is asking the nurse what the surgical procedure involves. The nurse begins the conversation by:
☐ **1.** Assessing what the client's physician has told her.
☐ **2.** Describing the surgical procedure.
☐ **3.** Educating the client that the procedure will close the perforation and prevent recurrent infection.
☐ **4.** Informing the client that the procedure will improve her hearing.

47. A 50-year-old male has been taking aspirin regularly for 6 months to prevent a heart attack. He informs the nurse that he has noticed a constant "ringing" in both ears. How should the nurse respond to the client's comment?
☐ **1.** Tell the client that "ringing" in the ears is associated with the aging process.
☐ **2.** Inform the client he needs a Weber test done.
☐ **3.** Schedule the client for audiometric testing.
☐ **4.** Explain to the client that the "ringing" may be related to the aspirin he has been taking for his heart.

The Client with Ménière's Disease

48. The classic triad of symptoms associated with Ménière's disease is vertigo, tinnitus, and:
- ☐ **1.** Headache.
- ☐ **2.** Otitis media.
- ☐ **3.** Fluctuating hearing loss.
- ☐ **4.** Vomiting.

49. A client has vertigo. Which of the following actions would be most appropriate for the nursing diagnosis of *Risk for injury* related to altered immmobility and gait disturbances? Select all that apply.
- ☐ **1.** The client assumes safe position when dizzy.
- ☐ **2.** The client experiences no falls.
- ☐ **3.** The client performs vestibular/balance exercises.
- ☐ **4.** The client demonstrates family involvement.
- ☐ **5.** The client keeps head still when dizzy.

50. The client with Ménière's disease is instructed to modify his diet. The nurse should explain that the most frequently recommended diet modification for Ménière's disease is:
- ☐ **1.** Low sodium.
- ☐ **2.** High protein.
- ☐ **3.** Low carbohydrate.
- ☐ **4.** Low fat.

51. Which of the following statements by the client would indicate that she understands the expected course of Ménière's disease?
- ☐ **1.** "The disease process will gradually extend to the eyes."
- ☐ **2.** "Control of the episodes is usually possible, but a cure is not yet available."
- ☐ **3.** "Continued medication therapy will cure the disease."
- ☐ **4.** "Bilateral deafness is an inevitable outcome of the disease."

52. The potential for injury during an attack of Ménière's disease is great. The nurse should instruct the client to take which immediate action when experiencing vertigo?
- ☐ **1.** "Place your head between your knees."
- ☐ **2.** "Concentrate on rhythmic deep breathing."
- ☐ **3.** "Close your eyes tightly."
- ☐ **4.** "Assume a reclining or flat position."

53. The wife of a client with Ménière's disease expresses concern because her husband has curtailed family activities and evenings out. Based on this information, which of the following would be the most appropriate nursing diagnosis?
- ☐ **1.** *Social isolation* related to attacks of vertigo and hearing loss.
- ☐ **2.** *Anxiety* related to concern about progressive hearing loss.
- ☐ **3.** *Self-care deficit* related to labyrinth dysfunction.
- ☐ **4.** *Disturbed sensory perception* related to labyrinth dysfunction.

54. The nurse should anticipate that all of the following drugs may be used in the attempt to control the symptoms of Ménière's disease *except:*
- ☐ **1.** Antihistamines.
- ☐ **2.** Antiemetics.
- ☐ **3.** Diuretics.
- ☐ **4.** Glucocorticoids.

55. A client with Ménière's disease continues to have disabling attacks of vertigo and elects to have a labyrinthectomy. A priority nursing diagnosis for the client before surgery is:
- ☐ **1.** *Deficient diversional activity* related to inability to participate secondary to vertigo.
- ☐ **2.** *Risk for injury* related to vertigo.
- ☐ **3.** *Powerlessness* related to inability to influence effects of disease process
- ☐ **4.** *Social isolation* related to hearing loss.

The Client with Cancer of the Larynx

56. After a total laryngectomy, the client has a feeding tube. The primary rationale for tube feedings is to:
- ☐ **1.** Meet the fluid and nutritional needs of the client.
- ☐ **2.** Prevent aspiration.
- ☐ **3.** Prevent fistula formation.
- ☐ **4.** Maintain an open airway.

57. Complications associated with a tracheostomy tube include:
- ☐ **1.** Decreased cardiac output.
- ☐ **2.** Damage to the laryngeal nerve.
- ☐ **3.** Pneumothorax.
- ☐ **4.** Acute respiratory distress syndrome (ARDS).

58. A priority goal for the hospitalized client who 2 days earlier had a total laryngectomy with creation of a new tracheostomy would be to:
- ☐ **1.** Decrease secretions.
- ☐ **2.** Instruct the client in caring for the tracheostomy.
- ☐ **3.** Relieve anxiety related to the tracheostomy.
- ☐ **4.** Maintain a patent airway.

Correct Answers and Rationales

The letter in parentheses after each rationale identifies the client need addressed in the item, including management of care (M), safety and infection control (S), health promotion and maintenance (H), psychosocial adaptation (P), basic care and comfort (C), pharmacological and parenteral therapies (D), reduction of risk potential (R), and physiological adaptation (A).

The Client with Cataracts

1. 3. The student has positioned the dropper and the client correctly to prevent injury to the client's eye. The student should administer the drops in the center of the lower lid. Following administration of the eyedrops, the client should blink her eyes to distribute the medication; squeezing or rubbing her eyes might cause the medication to drip out of the eye. (S)

2. 1, 2, 4. The use of glasses following cataract surgery does not totally restore binocular vision. Glasses will cause images to appear larger and peripheral vision will be distorted; the client should look through the center of the glasses and turn his or her head to view objects in the periphery. The client should also use caution when walking or climbing stairs until he or she has adjusted to the change in vision. Changes in vision following cataract surgery are not immediate and the nurse can instruct the client to be patient while adjusting to the changes. The client does not need to stay out of the sun, but should wear dark glasses to prevent discomfort from photophobia. (A)

3. 2. Senile cataracts are related to the aging process. The second most common cause of cataracts is a history of eye injury. Systemic diseases (e.g., diabetes) and systemic syndromes (e.g., Down syndrome) as well as ingestion of injurious or toxic substances (e.g., alcohol, cigarette smoke, naphthalene, corticosteroids) are associated with cataract development; however, cataracts in older clients are related to the aging process. (H)

4. 3. The lens of the eye is suspended on the suspensory ligaments. The ligaments influence the tension on the lens and thereby focus light rays onto the retina. Accommodation is the ability of the lens to adjust to near and far objects. The ciliary bodies secrete aqueous humor. The retina contains the rods and cones. The iris regulates the amount of light entering the eye. (A)

5. 2. The nurse should give a client who seems fearful of surgery an opportunity to express her feelings. Only after identifying the client's concerns can the nurse intervene appropriately. Asking the client about previous reactions to local anesthetics may be warranted, but it does not address the client's concerns in this instance. Telling the client that she will not have nausea or vomiting ignores

the client's feelings of fear and does not provide any data about the client's feelings. More data would help the nurse plan care. Telling the client that there is nothing to be afraid of minimizes her feelings and does not address her concerns. Premature explanations and clichés do not provide needed assessment data and ignore the client's feelings. (P)

6. 3. A client with a cataract usually complains of dimness, blurring, and/or hazy vision. Typically, light scattering occurs and is related to the degree of opacity of the lens. Opacity of the lens blocks light rays from reaching the retina. Halos and rainbows are usually associated with glaucoma. Eye pain and irritation are not associated with cataracts. Eye strain and headache when doing close work is associated with refractive errors. (H)

7. 2. Instilled in the eye, phenylephrine hydrochloride (Neo-Synephrine) acts as a mydriatic, causing the pupil to dilate. It also constricts small blood vessels in the eye. (D)

8. 4. A prescribed antiemetic should be administered as soon as the client complains of nausea following a cataract extraction. Vomiting can increase intraocular pressure, which should be avoided after eye surgery because it can cause complications. Deep breathing is unlikely to relieve nausea. Postoperative nausea may be common; however, it doesn't necessarily pass quickly and can lead to vomiting. Telling the client to call only if vomiting occurs ignores the client's need for comfort and intervention to prevent complications. (D)

9. 1, 5. Acute bacterial endophthalmitis can occur in about 1 out of 1,000 cases. Organisms that are typically involved include *Staphylococcus epidermidis*, *S. aureus*, and *Pseudomonas* and *Proteus* species. Vision loss is one result of acute bacterial infection. In addition, vision loss can be the result of malposition of the intraocular lens implant or opacification of the posterior capsule. Retrobulbar hemorrhage is a complication that may occur right before surgery and is a result of retrobulbar infiltration of anesthetic agents. Rupture of the posterior capsule and suprachoroidal hemorrhage are both complications that can result during surgery. (A)

10. 3. Safety of the client is the major concern on the return home. The home environment should be assessed for safety hazards, and steps to decrease potential hazards should be implemented. Arrangements for home care, if necessary, should be made before surgery. The client is usually able to return to the activities of daily living rapidly, so a deficiency of diversional activities or a feeding self-care deficit would not typically be anticipated. Oral pain medication should control the client's discomfort. (S)

11. 1. Applying pressure against the nose at the inner canthus of the closed eye after administering eyedrops prevents the medication from entering the lacrimal (tear) duct. If the medication enters the tear duct, it can enter the nose and pharynx, where it may be absorbed and cause toxic symptoms. Eyedrops should be placed in the eye's lower conjunctival sac. Applying pressure will not prevent the drug from running down the face as long as the drops are instilled in the eye. Pressure does not affect the cornea or facilitate distribution of the medication over the eye surface. (D)

12. **2.** Coughing is contraindicated after cataract extraction because it increases intraocular pressure. Other activities that are contraindicated because they increase intraocular pressure include turning to the operative side, sneezing, crying, and straining. Lying supine, ambulating, and deep breathing do not affect intraocular pressure. (A)

13. **4.** Sudden, sharp pain after eye surgery should suggest to the nurse that the client may be experiencing intraocular hemorrhage. The physician should be notified promptly. Detached retina and prolapse of the iris are usually painless. Extracapsular erosion is not characterized by sharp pain. (A)

The Client with a Retinal Detachment

14. **2.** The spots, or floaters, commonly reported by clients with retinal detachment are blood cells released into the vitreous humor by the detachment. Floaters are not caused by pieces of retina, contamination, or spasms. (A)

15. **1.** Patching the eyes helps decrease random eye movements that could enlarge and worsen retinal detachment. Although clients with eye injuries frequently are light-sensitive, and preventing infection is important, the specific goal is to reduce rapid eye movements. Resting the eye is an indirect way of stating the objective. (A)

16. **4.** Untreated retinal detachment results in increasing detachment and eventual blindness, but 90% to 95% of clients can be successfully treated with surgery. If necessary, the surgical procedure can be repeated about 10 to 14 days after the first procedure. Many more services are available for newly blind people, but ideally this client will not need them. Surgery does not delay blindness. (A)

17. **1.** The scarring of the retinal tear needs time to heal completely. Therefore, resumption of activity should be gradual; the client may resume her usual activities in 5 to 6 weeks. Successful healing should allow the client to return to her previous level of functioning. (C)

18. **2.** After surgery to correct a detached retina, prevention of increased intraocular pressure is the priority goal. Control of pain with analgesics is the second goal. Following a low-sodium diet or maintaining a darkened environment is not a goal for this client. (A)

19. **4.** A choroidal scar will form a permanent seal to close the hole or tear in the retina. A scleral buckle serves as a splint to bring the two retinal layers in contact with each other until a scar can form. Loss of a portion of the retina or loss of the whole retina would interfere with sight. Retinal transplants are not performed. The retina is never stitched to the optic nerve. (A)

The Client with Glaucoma

20. **2.** The client should look up while the nurse instills the eyedrops. The client will need to keep both eyes open while the nurse administers the drug. If the client raises his eyebrows while the nurse's hand is positioned on the eyebrows, the movement of the forehead may cause the dropper to move and injure the eye. The client should gently blink his eyes after the eyedrops have been instilled. Using a tissue to wipe the eyes could remove some of the medication; excess fluid can be removed with a cotton ball. (D)

21. **2.** In COAG, there is an obstruction to the outflow of aqueous humor, leading to increased intraocular pressure. The increased intraocular pressure eventually causes destruction of the retina's nerve fibers. This nerve destruction causes painless vision loss. The exact cause of glaucoma is unknown. Glaucoma does not lead to retinal detachment. (A)

22. **4.** Although COAG is usually asymptomatic in the early stages, peripheral vision gradually decreases as the disorder progresses. Eye pain is not a feature of COAG but is common in clients with angle-closure glaucoma. Excessive lacrimation is not a symptom of COAG; it may indicate a blocked tear duct. Flashes of light is a common symptom of retinal detachment. (A)

23. **3.** A miotic agent constricts the pupil and contracts ciliary musculature. These effects widen the filtration angle and permit increased outflow of aqueous humor. Miotics also cause vasodilation of the intraocular vessels, where intraocular fluids leave the eye, also increasing aqueous humor outflow. Mydriatics cause cycloplegia, or paralysis of the ciliary muscle. (D)

24. **2.** Tonometry, which measures intraocular pressure, is a simple, noninvasive, and painless procedure that requires no particular preparation or postprocedure care and carries no adverse effects. It is not necessary to dilate the pupils for tonometry. (R)

25. **3.** Timolol maleate (Timoptic) is commonly administered to control glaucoma. The drug's action is not completely understood, but it is believed to reduce aqueous humor formation, thereby reducing intraocular pressure. Timolol does not constrict the pupils; miotics are used for pupillary constriction and contraction of the ciliary muscle. Timolol does not dilate the canal of Schlemm. (D)

26. **2.** The cornea is sensitive and can be injured by eyedrops falling onto it. Therefore, eyedrops should be instilled into the lower conjunctival sac of the eye to avoid the risk of corneal damage. The drops do not cause scleral staining or excessive lacrimation. Systemic absorption occurs when eyedrops enter the tear ducts. (D)

27. **2.** Atropine sulfate causes pupil dilation. This action is contraindicated for the client with glaucoma because it increases intraocular pressure. The drug does not have this effect on intraocular pressure in people who do not have glaucoma. Morphine causes pupil constriction. Deep-breathing exercises will not affect glaucoma. The client should resume taking all medications for glaucoma immediately after surgery. (D)

28. **4.** Acute angle-closure glaucoma produces abrupt changes in the angle of the iris. Clinical manifestations include severe eye pain, colored halos around lights, and rapid vision loss. Gradual loss of central vision is associated with macular degeneration. The loss of color vision, or achromatopsia, is a rare symptom that occurs when a stroke damages the fusiform gyrus. It most often affects only half of the visual field. (A)

29. **3.** Acute angle-closure glaucoma is a medical emergency that rapidly leads to blindness if left untreated. Treatment typically involves miotic drugs and surgery, usually iridectomy or laser therapy. Both procedures create a hole in the periphery of the iris, which allows the aqueous humor to flow into the anterior chamber. Bed rest does not affect the progression of acute angle-closure glaucoma. Steroids are not a treatment for acute angle-closure glaucoma; in fact, they are associated with the development of glaucoma. (A)

The Client with Adult Macular Degeneration

30. **1.** Macular degeneration generally involves loss of central vision. Gradual blurring of vision can occur as the disease progresses and may result in blindness; however, loss of central vision is the most common finding. Tiny yellowish spots, known as drusen, develop beneath the retina. Loss of peripheral vision is characteristic of glaucoma. (A)

31. **3.** AMD generally affects central vision. Confusion may result related to the changes in the environment and the inability to see the environment clearly. Therefore, providing safety is the priority goal in the care of this client. Educating him regarding community resources or monitoring his AMD may have been done at an earlier date or can be done after assessing his knowledge base and experience with the disease process. Improving his vision may not be possible. (S)

32. **3.** The priority goal of care for a client with limited eyesight is safety and preventing injury. The initial action is to orient the client to a new environment. Taking time to identify the objects and where they are located in the room can achieve this goal. It is unrealistic to have someone stay with the client at all times or for the client to stay in bed until the nurse can assist her. (M)

33. **4.** To expand the visual field, the partially sighted client should be taught to turn the head from side to side when walking. Neglecting to do so may result in accidents. This technique helps maximize the use of remaining sight. A patch does not address the problem of hemianopsia. Appropriate client positioning and placement of personal items will increase the client's ability to cope with the problem but will not affect safety. (S)

34. In macular degeneration the center vision is blackened out and only the outer visual fields are clear. (A)

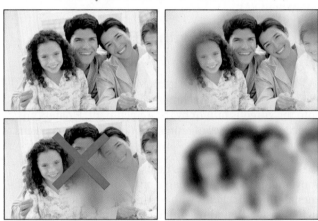

The Client Undergoing Nasal Surgery

35. **2.** Because of the dense packing, it is relatively unusual for bleeding to be apparent through the nasal drip pad. Instead, the blood runs down the throat, causing the client to swallow frequently. The back of the throat can be assessed with a flashlight. An accumulation of blood in the stomach may cause nausea and vomiting, but is not an initial sign of bleeding. Increased respiratory rate occurs in shock and is not an early sign of bleeding in the client after nasal surgery. Feelings of anxiety are not indicative of nasal bleeding. (A)

36. **1.** The client should be instructed to avoid any activities that cause Valsalva's maneuver (e.g., straining at stool, vigorous coughing, exercise) to reduce stress on suture lines and bleeding. The client should not take aspirin because of its antiplatelet properties, which may cause bleeding. Oral hygiene is important to rid the mouth of old dried blood and to enhance the client's appetite. Cool compresses, not heat, should be applied to decrease swelling and control discoloration of the area. (R)

37. **2.** Constipation can cause straining during defecation, which can induce bleeding. Showering is not contraindicated. The client should take measures to prevent coughing. The client should avoid blowing her nose for 48 hours after the packing is removed. Thereafter, she should blow her nose gently using the open-mouth technique to minimize bleeding in the surgical area. (A)

The Client with a Hearing Disorder

38. **2.** Furosemide may cause ototoxicity. The nurse should tell the client to promptly report the hearing loss, dizziness, or tinnitus, to help prevent permanent ear damage. Hearing loss is not inevitable, and it is inappropriate to make assumptions about the cause of symptoms without a thorough evaluation. The client's system will not "adjust," and hearing loss will not resolve. (D)

39. **1, 2, 3, 5.** When working with a client who is hearing impaired and speech reads, the presenter must face the person directly and devote full attention to the communication process. In addition, it will be useful for the client that the speaker not be to silhouetted against strong light, that the speaker's mouth not be blocked from the client's view, and that there are no objects in the mouth of the speaker. Finally, it is recommended that the presenter provide the client with the needed information to study before reviewing. This will provide the client with the ability to use contextual clues in speech reading. (C)

40. **3.** Hearing aids have limited use for clients with sensorineural hearing loss because these clients experience problems with sound discrimination as well as volume. A hearing aid can make sound louder but not necessarily clearer. The hearing aid cannot help the client distinguish spoken words from background noises. (C)

41. **3.** A sensorineural hearing loss results from damage to the cochlear or vestibulocochlear nerve. Presence of fluid and cerumen in the external canal or sclerosis of the bones of the middle ear results in a conductive hearing loss. Hearing loss resulting from an emotional disturbance is called a psychogenic hearing loss. (A)

42. **1.** Cerumen (ear wax) commonly gets impacted in older clients in the external canal. Otalgia is the "fullness" sensation or pain that an older client may experience when the cerumen becomes impacted. External otitis is an inflammation of the outer ear and would not explain the symptoms the client is experiencing. Exostosis is a bony growth that arises from the surface of a bone and would not explain the symptoms the client is experiencing. (H)

43. **2.** Irrigation is the first strategy to loosen cerumen. Successful removal of the cerumen involves gentle irrigation behind the impacted cerumen. The flow of the water must be behind the impaction to remove the cerumen from the canal. A cotton-tipped applicator or other device is not appropriate because it can cause damage to the eardrum. Use of aural suction or a cerumen curette is appropriate only if the impacted cerumen cannot be removed by irrigation. (R)

44. **1.** Normal saline is the solution that is generally used to irrigate the ear. Sterile water will cause tissue damage. An antiseptic solution is not typically used unless an infection is present. Warm tap water may cause tissue damage. (D)

45. **2.** Tympanoplasty involves surgical reconstruction of the tympanic membrane and is done to reestablish middle ear function, close perforations, and prevent recurrent infection. Ossiculoplasty is reconstruction of the bones of the middle ear. It is sometimes performed concurrently with tympanoplasty, but it is not as common as tympanoplasty. Mastoidectomy is done to remove a cholesteatoma, a cystlike mass that can occur in the middle ear secondary to infection. It also is not as common as tympanoplasty. Myringotomy involves making an incision in the tympanic membrane to relieve pressure and drain fluid from the ear. Myringotomy is more common with acute otitis media than chronic otitis media. (R)

46. **1.** The nurse should first assess the client's knowledge base. Working within the framework of the client's knowledge and educational level, the nurse then can describe the procedure and its benefits. (R)

47. **4.** Tinnitus (ringing in the ears) is an adverse effect of aspirin. Aspirin contains salicylate, which is an ototoxic drug that can induce reversible hearing loss and tinnitus. The nurse should encourage the client to inform the physician of the symptom. Tinnitus is not a function of aging. The Weber test and audiometric testing are useful for determining hearing loss but are not necessarily helpful in the management or diagnosis of drug-induced tinnitus. (D)

The Client with Ménière's Disease

48. **3.** Ménière's disease involves the inner ear and is characterized by episodes of acute vertigo, tinnitus, and fluctuating, progressive hearing loss. The severe vertigo can lead to nausea and vomiting, but vomiting is not considered one of the classic triad of symptoms. Headache is not associated with Ménière's disease. Otitis media is an inflammation of the middle ear. (A)

49. 1, 2, 3, 5. Assessment of vertigo, including history, onset, description of attacks, duration, frequency, and associated ear symptoms, is important. Vestibular/balance therapy or exercises should be taught and practiced. The client needs to be instructed to sit down when dizzy and decrease the amount of head movement. The client will benefit from recognizing whether he or she experiences an "aura" before an attack so appropriate action can be taken. Finally, it is recommended that the client keep the eyes open and look straight ahead when lying down. These expected outcomes will prevent the problem of injury. Family involvement is essential when dealing with a client experiencing vertigo but is not applicable for this particular nursing diagnosis. (R)

50. 1. A low-sodium diet is frequently an effective mechanism for reducing the frequency and severity of the disease episodes. About three-quarters of clients with Ménière's disease respond to treatment with a low-salt diet. A diuretic may also be ordered. Other dietary changes, such as high protein, low carbohydrate, and low fat, do not have an effect on Ménière's disease. (C)

51. 2. There is no cure for Ménière's disease, but the wide range of medical and surgical treatments allows for adequate control in many clients. The disease often worsens, but it does not spread to the eyes. The hearing loss is usually unilateral. (A)

52. 4. The client needs to assume a safe and comfortable position during an attack, which may last several hours. The client's location when the attack occurs may dictate the most reasonable position. Ideally, the client should lie down immediately in a reclining or flat position to control the vertigo. The danger of a serious fall is real. Placing the head between the knees will not help prevent a fall and is not practical because the attack may last several hours. Concentrating on breathing may be a useful distraction, but it will not help prevent a fall. Closing the eyes does not help prevent a fall. (S)

53. 1. A client with Ménière's disease may curtail social activities out of fear of embarrassment from having a dizzy spell in public. This seems likely in this situation, based on the wife's information, but would need to be validated by the client. However, the wife may be a more reliable source of information about social isolation than the client. There are no data to suggest nursing diagnoses of *Anxiety, Self-care deficit,* or *Disturbed sensory perception.* (P)

54. 4. A wide variety of medications may be used in an attempt to control Ménière's disease, including antihistamines, antiemetics, tranquilizers, and diuretics. Glucocorticoids play no significant role in disease treatment. (D)

55. 2. The client's *Risk for injury* related to vertigo is the highest priority nursing diagnosis preoperatively. The client should be instructed how to manage attacks of vertigo safely. *Deficient diversional activity* related to inability to participate secondary to vertigo is an appropriate nursing diagnosis, but it is not a priority. *Powerlessness* related to inability to influence effects of the disease process is a possible diagnosis, but more data are required before making such a diagnosis. *Social isolation* related to hearing loss is a possible diagnosis for the client after surgery. The client retains the ability to hear with Ménière's disease; however, total hearing loss is a possible complication of labyrinthectomy. (A)

The Client with Cancer of the Larynx

56. 1. The goal of postoperative care is to maintain physiologic integrity. Therefore, inserting a feeding tube is a strategy to ensure the fluid and nutritional needs of the client as the surgical site is healing. The feeding tube does help prevent aspiration by preventing ingested fluid from leaking through the wound into the trachea before healing occurs; however, the primary rationale is to meet the client's nutritional and fluid needs. A tracheoesophageal fistula is a rare complication of total laryngectomy and may occur if radiation therapy has compromised wound healing. A feeding tube does not help maintain an open airway. (R)

57. 2. Tracheostomy tubes carry several potential complications, including laryngeal nerve damage, bleeding, and infection. Tracheostomy tubes alone do not affect cardiac output or cause acute respiratory distress. The tube is inserted in the trachea, not the lung, so there is no risk of pneumothorax. (A)

58. 4. The main goal for a client with a new tracheostomy is to maintain a patent airway. A fresh tracheostomy frequently causes bleeding and excess secretions, and clients may require frequent suctioning to maintain patency. Decreasing secretions may be a component of a client's care after laryngectomy and tracheostomy, and relieving anxiety is always an important goal; however, the primary goal is to maintain a patent airway. Instruction in care of a tracheostomy is a priority later in the client's recovery. (A)

TEST 16

The Client with Health Problems of the Integumentary System

- The Client with Burns
- The Client with General Problems of the Integumentary System
- The Client with Skin Cancer
- Correct Answers and Rationales

The Client with Burns

1. There has been a fire in an apartment building. All residents have been evacuated, but many are burned. Which clients should be transported to a burn center for treatment? Select all that apply.

☐ **1.** An 8-year-old with third-degree burns over 10% of his body surface area (BSA).

☐ **2.** A 20-year-old who inhaled the smoke of the fire.

☐ **3.** A 50-year-old diabetic with first- and second-degree burns on his left forearm (about 5% of his BSA).

☐ **4.** A 30-year-old with second-degree burns on the back of his left leg.

☐ **5.** A 40-year-old with second-degree burns on his right arm (about 10% of his BSA).

2. The nurse in the immediate care clinic is assessing an 80-year-old client who lives with his son's family and has scald burns on his hands and both forearms (first- and second-degree burns on 10% of his body surface area). What should the nurse do first?

☐ **1.** Clean the wounds with warm water.

☐ **2.** Apply antibiotic cream.

☐ **3.** Refer the client to a burn center.

☐ **4.** Cover the burns with a sterile dressing.

3. The nurse assesses the client for fluid shifting. Fluid shifts that occur during the emergent phase of a burn injury are caused by fluid moving:

☐ **1.** From the vascular to the interstitial space.

☐ **2.** From the extracellular to the intracellular space.

☐ **3.** From the intracellular to the extracellular space.

☐ **4.** From the interstitial to the vascular space.

4. A client is admitted to the hospital after sustaining burns to the chest, abdomen, right arm, and right leg. The shaded areas in the illustration below indicate the burned areas on the client's body. Using the "rule of nines," the nurse would determine that about what percentage of the client's body surface has been burned?

☐ **1.** 18%.

☐ **2.** 27%.

☐ **3.** 45%.

☐ **4.** 64%.

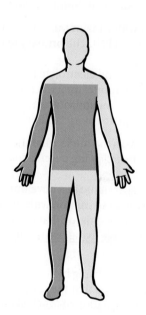

5. The nurse should recognize that fluid shift in a client with a burn injury results from an increase in the:
☐ **1.** Permeability of capillary walls.
☐ **2.** Total volume of intravascular plasma.
☐ **3.** Total volume of circulating whole blood.
☐ **4.** Permeability of the kidney tubules.

6. A priority nursing diagnosis for a client with burns during the emergent period would be:
☐ **1.** *Excess fluid volume.*
☐ **2.** *Imbalanced nutrition: Less than body requirements.*
☐ **3.** *Risk for injury* (falling).
☐ **4.** *Risk for infection.*

7. Which of the following activities should the nurse include in the plan of care for a client with burn injuries to be carried out about one-half hour before the daily whirlpool bath and dressing change?
☐ **1.** Soak the dressing.
☐ **2.** Remove the dressing.
☐ **3.** Administer an analgesic.
☐ **4.** Slit the dressing with blunt scissors.

8. The client with a major burn injury receives total parenteral nutrition (TPN). The primary reason for this therapy is to help:
☐ **1.** Correct water and electrolyte imbalances.
☐ **2.** Allow the gastrointestinal tract to rest.
☐ **3.** Provide supplemental vitamins and minerals.
☐ **4.** Ensure adequate caloric and protein intake.

9. The client asks the nurse what the word *eschar* means. Which of the following descriptions by the nurse best defines eschar?
☐ **1.** "Eschar is scar tissue in a developmental stage."
☐ **2.** "Eschar is crust formation without a blood supply."
☐ **3.** "Eschar is burned tissue that has become infected."
☐ **4.** "Eschar is visible living tissue with a rich blood supply."

10. An advantage of using biologic burn grafts such as porcine (pigskin) grafts is that they appear to help:
☐ **1.** Encourage formation of tough skin.
☐ **2.** Promote the growth of epithelial tissue.
☐ **3.** Provide for permanent wound closure.
☐ **4.** Facilitate development of subcutaneous tissue.

11. Which of the following factors would have the *least* influence on the survival and effectiveness of a burn victim's porcine grafts?
☐ **1.** Absence of infection in the wounds.
☐ **2.** Adequate vascularization in the grafted area.
☐ **3.** Immobilization of the area being grafted.
☐ **4.** Use of analgesics as necessary for pain relief.

12. The nurse should plan to begin rehabilitation efforts for the burn client:
☐ **1.** Immediately after the burn has occurred.
☐ **2.** After the client's circulatory status has been stabilized.
☐ **3.** After grafting of the burn wounds has occurred.
☐ **4.** After the client's pain has been eliminated.

13. When an individual is burned, there is massive cell destruction resulting in a disruption of the normal homeostasis of the body. The nurse anticipates that the client will be susceptible to which of the following in the early phase of burn care?
☐ **1.** Hypernatremia.
☐ **2.** Hyponatremia.
☐ **3.** Metabolic alkalosis.
☐ **4.** Hyperkalemia.

14. Endotracheal or tracheostomy tubes are placed in clients who have experienced:
☐ **1.** Electrical burns of the hands and arms causing arrhythmias.
☐ **2.** Thermal burns to the head, face, and airway resulting in hypoxia.
☐ **3.** Chemical burns on the chest and abdomen.
☐ **4.** Secondhand smoke inhalation.

15. A newly burned client is admitted to the unit. The nurse measures the client's urine output on an hourly basis, anticipating fluid balance problems related to fluid shifts. Which of the following hourly urine output rates will alert the nurse to potential problems?
☐ **1.** 20 ml/hour.
☐ **2.** 30 ml/hour.
☐ **3.** 50 ml/hour.
☐ **4.** 100 ml/hour.

16. After the initial phase of the burn injury, the client's plan of care will focus primarily on:
☐ **1.** Helping the client maintain a positive self-concept.
☐ **2.** Promoting hygiene.
☐ **3.** Preventing infection.
☐ **4.** Educating the client regarding care of the skin grafts.

17. The burned client needs fluid replacement because massive amounts of fluid are lost. The rate at which I.V. fluids are infused is based on the burn client's:
☐ **1.** Lean muscle mass and body surface area (BSA) burned.
☐ **2.** Total body weight and BSA burned.
☐ **3.** Total BSA and BSA burned.
☐ **4.** Height and weight and BSA burned.

18. The nurse is caring for a client with a burn injury and understands that stress reactions can result in hyper-secretion of gastric acids. Therefore, the nurse must assess the client for signs and symptoms of which of the following potential complications?
- ☐ **1.** Paralytic ileus.
- ☐ **2.** Gastric distention.
- ☐ **3.** Hiatal hernia.
- ☐ **4.** Curling's ulcer.

19. In the acute phase of burn injury, which pain medication would most likely be given to the client to decrease the perception of the pain?
- ☐ **1.** Oral analgesics such as ibuprofen (Motrin) or acetaminophen (Tylenol).
- ☐ **2.** Intravenous opioids.
- ☐ **3.** Intramuscular opioids.
- ☐ **4.** Oral antianxiety agents such as lorazepam (Ativan).

The Client with General Problems of the Integumentary System

20. The nurse is assessing a hospitalized older client for the presence of pressure ulcers. The nurse notes that the client has a $1'' \times 1''$ area on his sacrum in which there is skin breakdown as far as the dermis. What should the nurse note on the chart?
- ☐ **1.** Stage I pressure ulcer.
- ☐ **2.** Stage II pressure ulcer.
- ☐ **3.** Stage III pressure ulcer.
- ☐ **4.** Stage IV pressure ulcer.

21. The nurse is assessing an older adult's skin. The assessment will involve inspecting the skin for color, pigmentation, and vascularity. The critical component in the nurse's assessment is noting the:
- ☐ **1.** Similarities from one side to the other.
- ☐ **2.** Changes from the normal expected findings.
- ☐ **3.** Appearance of age-related wrinkles.
- ☐ **4.** Skin turgor.

22. Which of the following changes are associated with normal aging?
- ☐ **1.** The outer layer of skin is replaced with new cells every 3 days.
- ☐ **2.** Subcutaneous fat and extracellular water decrease.
- ☐ **3.** The dermis becomes highly vascular and assists in the regulation of body temperature.
- ☐ **4.** Collagen becomes elastic and strong.

23. Which of the following should the nurse expect to assess as normal skin changes in an elderly client? Select all that apply.
- ☐ **1.** Diminished hair on scalp and pubic areas.
- ☐ **2.** Dusky rubor of left lower extremity.
- ☐ **3.** Solar lentigo.
- ☐ **4.** Wrinkles.
- ☐ **5.** Xerosis.
- ☐ **6.** Yellow pigmentation.

24. The nurse will anticipate which of the following problems that can result for the older adult undergoing abdominal surgery?
- ☐ **1.** Increased scarring.
- ☐ **2.** Decreased melanin and melanocytes.
- ☐ **3.** Decreased healing.
- ☐ **4.** Increased immunocompetence.

25. Health maintenance and promotion activities are especially important for the older adult. Which of the following activities reflects a health maintenance activity for an otherwise healthy older adult?
- ☐ **1.** Drinks 1,500 ml of fluids per day.
- ☐ **2.** Consumes a balanced diet of 1,200 calories per day.
- ☐ **3.** Walks briskly for 10 minutes three times per week.
- ☐ **4.** Sleeps at least 8 hours each night.

26. Which of the following characteristics would put a client at the *greatest* risk for impaired wound healing after abdominal surgery?
- ☐ **1.** Age 75 years.
- ☐ **2.** Age 30 years, with poorly controlled diabetes.
- ☐ **3.** Age 55 years, with myocardial infarction.
- ☐ **4.** Age 60 years, with peripheral vascular disease.

27. An 82-year-old female has several ecchymotic areas on her left arm. The bruises are probably caused by:
- ☐ **1.** Elder abuse.
- ☐ **2.** Self-inflicted injury.
- ☐ **3.** Increased capillary fragility and permeability.
- ☐ **4.** Increased blood supply to the skin.

28. A 90-year-old male complains of feeling cold in his room even though the thermostat is set at 75° F (24° C). The client probably feels cold because older adults have:
- ☐ **1.** Increased cellular cohesion.
- ☐ **2.** Increased moisture content of the stratum corneum.
- ☐ **3.** Slower cellular renewal time.
- ☐ **4.** Decreased ability to thermoregulate.

29. Palpation of the skin provides the nurse useful information regarding:
- ☐ **1.** Bruising of the skin.
- ☐ **2.** Color of the skin.
- ☐ **3.** Hair distribution.
- ☐ **4.** Turgor of the skin.

30. A priority nursing diagnosis for an adult female who has pruritus and is continuously scratching the affected areas and demonstrates agitation and anxiety regarding the itching sensation would be:
- ☐ **1.** *Risk for infection* related to pruritus.
- ☐ **2.** *Ineffective health maintenance* related to lack of knowledge of the disease process.
- ☐ **3.** *Impaired skin integrity* related to dehydration from the treatment medications.
- ☐ **4.** *Social isolation* related to poor self-image.

31. An older adult client in stage 2 of Parkinson's disease is being discharged with cellulitis of the right lower extremity. Which of the following nursing diagnoses will guide the discharge teaching? Select all that apply.
- [ ] 1. *Ineffective tissue perfusion* related to decreased cardiac output.
- [ ] 2. *Impaired skin integrity* related to barrier changes of the skin.
- [ ] 3. *Risk for injury* related to environmental hazards.
- [ ] 4. *Impaired verbal communication related* to dysarthria.
- [ ] 5. *Activity intolerance* related to painful lower extremity.

32. The nurse finds an unlicensed assistive personnel massaging the reddened bony prominences of a client on bed rest. The correct action by the nurse is to:
- [ ] 1. Reinforce the aide's use of this intervention over the bony prominences.
- [ ] 2. Explain that massage is effective because it improves blood flow to the area.
- [ ] 3. Inform the aide that massage is even more effective when combined with lotion during the massage.
- [ ] 4. Instruct the aide that massage is contraindicated because it decreases blood flow to the area.

33. A stage II pressure ulcer is characterized by:
- [ ] 1. Redness in the involved area.
- [ ] 2. Muscle spasms in the involved area.
- [ ] 3. Pain in the involved area.
- [ ] 4. Tissue necrosis in the involved area.

34. An alert and oriented elderly client is admitted to the hospital for treatment of cellulitis of the left shoulder after an arthroscopy. Which fall prevention strategy is most appropriate for this client?
- [ ] 1. Keep all the lights on in the room at all times.
- [ ] 2. Use a nightlight in the bathroom.
- [ ] 3. Keep all four side rails up at all times.
- [ ] 4. Place the client in a room with a camera monitor.

35. Prevention of skin breakdown and maintenance of skin integrity among older clients is important because they are at greater risk secondary to:
- [ ] 1. Altered balance.
- [ ] 2. Altered protective pressure sensation.
- [ ] 3. Impaired hearing ability.
- [ ] 4. Impaired visual acuity.

The Client with Skin Cancer

36. Which of the following factors places a client at greatest risk for skin cancer?
- [ ] 1. Fair skin and history of chronic sun exposure.
- [ ] 2. Caucasian race and history of hypertension.
- [ ] 3. Dark skin and family history of skin cancer.
- [ ] 4. Dark skin and history of hypertension.

37. A nurse is providing teaching to a client about skin cancer. Which of the following should the nurse explain are risk factors for skin cancer? Select all that apply.
- [ ] 1. Increasing age.
- [ ] 2. Exposure to chemical pollutants.
- [ ] 3. Long-term exposure to the sun.
- [ ] 4. Increased pigmentation.
- [ ] 5. Genetics.
- [ ] 6. Immunosuppression.

38. Malignant melanoma is a result of:
- [ ] 1. A lesion arising from a mole.
- [ ] 2. A lesion arising from epidermal basal cells.
- [ ] 3. A tumor arising from squamous cells.
- [ ] 4. A tumor arising in cells producing melanin.

39. In planning an educational presentation for a client with malignant melanoma, the nurse understands that the prognosis of the client depends on:
- [ ] 1. The amount of ulceration of the lesion.
- [ ] 2. The age of the client.
- [ ] 3. The location of the lesion on the body.
- [ ] 4. The thickness of the lesion.

Correct Answers and Rationales

The letter in parentheses after each rationale identifies the client need addressed in the item, including management of care (M), safety and infection control (S), health promotion and maintenance (H), psychosocial adaptation (P), basic care and comfort (C), pharmacological and parenteral therapies (D), reduction of risk potential (R), and physiological adaptation (A).

The Client with Burns

1. **1, 2, 3.** Clients who should be transferred to a burn center include children under age 10 or adults over age 50 with second- and third-degree burns on 10% or greater of their body surface area (BSA), clients between ages 11 and 49 with second- and third-degree burns over 20% of their BSA, clients of any age with third-degree burns on more than 5% of their BSA, clients with smoke inhalation, and clients with chronic diseases, such as diabetes and heart or kidney disease. (M)

2. **3.** The nurse should have the client transported to a burn center. The client's age and the extent of the burns require care by a burn team and the client meets triage criteria for referral to a burn center. Because of the age of the client and the extent of the burns, the nurse should not treat the burn. Scald burns are not at high risk for infection and do not need to be cleaned, covered, or treated with antibiotic cream at this time. (A)

3. 1. In a burn injury, the injured capillaries dilate, and there is increased capillary permeability at the site of the burn. Plasma seeps out into the burned tissue, moving from the vascular space into the interstitial space. (A)

4. 3. According to the rule of nines, this client has sustained burns on about 45% of the body surface. The right arm is calculated as being 9%, the right leg is 18%, and the anterior trunk is 18%, for a total of 45%. (A)

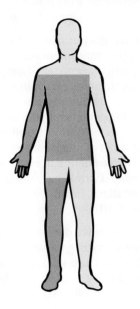

5. 1. When a burn occurs, the capillaries and small vessels dilate, and cell damage causes the release of a histamine-like substance. This substance causes the capillary walls to become more permeable, and significant quantities of fluid are lost. The initial fluid derangement after a burn is a shift from the plasma to the interstitial fluid shift. The intravascular plasma and circulating whole blood shift from vascular spaces to interstitial spaces during the first 24 to 36 hours, causing decreased vascular volume and the risk of shock. Renal function may be altered as a result of decreased blood flow secondary to blood loss; however, burns do not cause increased permeability of the kidney tubules. (A)

6. 4. Infection is a priority problem for the burned victim because of the loss of skin integrity and alteration in body defenses. Excess fluid or imbalanced nutrition is not a priority during the emergent period. A risk for falling is not a priority for this client because the client would be on bed rest and most likely in a critical care unit. (A)

7. 3. Removing dressings from severe burns exposes sensitive nerve endings to the air, which is painful. The client should be given a prescribed analgesic about one-half hour before the dressing change to promote comfort. The other activities are done as part of the whirlpool and dressing change process and not one-half hour beforehand. (R)

8. 4. Nutritional support with sufficient calories and protein is extremely important for a client with severe burns because of the loss of plasma protein through injured capillaries and an increased metabolic rate. Gastric dilation and paralytic ileus commonly occur in clients with severe burns, making oral fluids and foods contraindicated. Water and electrolyte imbalances can be corrected by administration of I.V. fluids with electrolyte additives, although TPN typically includes all necessary electrolytes. Resting the gastrointestinal tract may help prevent paralytic ileus, and TPN provides vitamins and minerals; however, the primary reason for starting TPN is to provide the protein necessary for tissue healing. (D)

9. 2. Eschar is a crust of dead tissue, heavily contaminated with bacteria and without a blood supply. Eschar has also been defined as devitalized skin. (A)

10. 2. Biologic dressings such as porcine grafts serve many purposes for a client with severe burns. They enhance the growth of epithelial tissues, minimize the overgrowth of granulation tissue, prevent loss of water and protein, decrease pain, increase mobility, and help prevent infection. They do not encourage growth of tougher skin, provide for permanent wound closure, or facilitate growth of subcutaneous tissue. (A)

11. 4. Analgesic administration to keep a burn victim comfortable is important but is unlikely to influence graft survival and effectiveness. Absence of infection, adequate vascularization, and immobilization of the grafted area promote an effective graft. (A)

12. 2. Rehabilitation efforts are implemented as soon as the client's condition is stabilized. Early emphasis on rehabilitation is important to decrease complications and to help ensure that the client will be able to make the adjustments necessary to return to an optimal state of health and independence. It is not possible to completely eliminate the client's pain; pain control is a major challenge in burn care. (C)

13. 4. Immediately after a burn, excessive potassium from cell destruction is released into the extracellular fluid. Hyponatremia is a common electrolyte imbalance in the burn client that occurs within the first week after being burned. Metabolic acidosis usually occurs as a result of the loss of sodium bicarbonate. (R)

14. 2. Airway management is the priority in caring for a burn client. Tracheostomy or endotracheal intubation is anticipated when significant thermal and smoke inhalation burns occur. Clients who have experienced burns to the face and neck usually will be compromised within 1 to 2 hours. Electrical burns of the hands and arms, even with cardiac arrhythmias, or a chemical burn of the chest and abdomen is not likely to result in the need for intubation. Secondhand smoke inhalation does influence an individual's respiratory status but does not require intubation unless the individual has an allergic reaction to the smoke. (A)

15. **2.** The acceptable range for urine output is greater than 30 ml/hour. Less than 30 ml/hour may indicate poor renal perfusion resulting from a hypovolemic state or myoglobin blocking the renal tubules, or both. Increased urine output of 100 ml/hour or more usually occurs after the first 48 hours of a burn. (R)

16. **3.** The inflammatory response begins when a burn is sustained. As a result of the burn, the immune system becomes impaired. There is a decrease in immunoglobulins, changes in white blood cells, alterations of lymphocytes, and decreased levels of interleukin. The human body's protective barrier, the skin, has been damaged. As a result, the burn client becomes vulnerable to infections. Education and interventions to maintain a positive self-concept would be appropriate during the rehabilitation phase. Promoting hygiene helps the client feel comfortable; however, the primary focus is on reducing the risk for infection. (S)

17. **2.** During the first 24 hours, fluid replacement for an adult burn client is based on total body weight and BSA burned. Lean muscle mass considers only muscle mass; replacement is based on total body weight. Total surface area is estimated by taking into account the individual's height and weight. Height is not a common variable used in formulas for fluid replacement. (A)

18. **4.** Curling's ulcer, or gastrointestinal ulceration, occurs in about half of the clients with a burn injury. The incidence of ulceration appears proportional to the extent of the burns and the ulceration is believed to be caused by hypersecretion of gastric acid and compromised gastrointestinal perfusion. Paralytic ileus and gastric distention do not result from hypersecretion of gastric acid and stress. Hiatal hernia is not necessarily a potential complication of a burn injury. (A)

19. **2.** The severe pain experienced by burn clients requires opioid analgesics. In addition, opioids such as morphine sedate and alleviate apprehension. Oral analgesics such as ibuprofen or acetaminophen are unlikely to be strong enough to effectively manage the intense pain experienced by the client who is severely burned. Because of the altered tissue perfusion from the burn injury, intravenous medications are preferred. Antianxiety agents are not effective against pain. (D)

The Client with General Problems of the Integumentary System

20. **2.** Stage I pressure ulcers appear as nonblanching macules that are red in color. Stage II ulcers have breakdown of the dermis. Stage III ulcers have full-thickness skin breakdown. In stage IV ulcers, the bone, muscle, and supporting tissue are involved. The nurse should immediately initiate plans to relieve the pressure, ensure good nutrition, and protect the area from abrasion. (R)

21. **2.** Noting changes from the normal expected findings is the most important component when assessing an older client's integumentary system. Comparing one extremity with the contralateral extremity (i.e., comparing one side with the other) is an important assessment step; however, the most important component is noting changes from an expected normal baseline. Noting wrinkles related to age is not of much consequence unless the client is admitted for cosmetic surgery to reduce the appearance of age-related wrinkling. Noting skin turgor is an assessment of fluid status, not an assessment of the integumentary system. (H)

22. **2.** With age, there is a decreased amount of subcutaneous fat, muscle laxity, degeneration of elastic fibers, and collagen stiffening. The outer layer of skin is almost completely replaced every 3 to 4 weeks. The vascular supply diminishes with age. Collagen thins and diminishes with age. (H)

23. **1, 3, 4, 5.** Skin changes associated with aging include the following: Diminished hair on scalp and pubic areas, solar lentigo (liver spots), wrinkles, and xerosis (dryness). Dusky rubor of the left lower extremity may indicate the individual has a venous stasis problem in the affected extremity and is generally associated with "unsuccessful aging." Yellow pigmentation of the skin that may be associated with liver inflammation is generally known as jaundice. (H)

24. **3.** Normal aging consists of decreased proliferative capacity of the skin. Decreased collagen synthesis slows capillary growth, impairs phagocytosis among older clients, and results in slow healing. Increased scarring is not a result of age-related skin changes. Both melanin and melanocytes give color to the skin and hair but are increased with aging. There is a decrease in the immunocompetence of the aging client. (H)

25. **1.** Drinking at least six 8-oz glasses of fluid per day helps the client stay well hydrated. Maintaining optimal fluid balance is important for all body systems. Caloric intake varies according to an individual's size and activity level. An intake of 1,200 calories per day may be insufficient for some older clients. Walking 10 minutes per day is useful, but an otherwise healthy older client should try to walk 20 minutes per day. It is important to get adequate rest; however, the amount of sleep needed varies with the individual. (H)

26. **2.** Poorly controlled diabetes is a serious risk factor for postoperative wound infection. Other factors that delay wound healing include advanced age, nutritional deficiencies (vitamin C, protein, zinc), inadequate blood supply, use of corticosteroid, infection, mechanical friction on the wound, obesity, anemia, and poor general health. (R)

27. **3.** The aging process involves increased capillary fragility and permeability. Older clients have a decreased amount of subcutaneous fat. Therefore, there is an increased incidence of bruiselike lesions caused by collection of extravascular blood in the loosely structured dermis. In addition, older clients do not always realize that injury has occurred because of a diminished awareness of pain, touch, and peripheral vibration. There are no data to support elder abuse or self-inflicted bruises. Blood supply to the skin declines with aging. (H)

28. **4.** Older clients have a decreased thermoregulation that is related to decreased blood supply and reabsorption of body fat. As a result, older adults are at risk for hypothermia. Cellular cohesion and moisture content diminish with age and cellular renewal time is slowed; however, these do not result in impaired thermoregulation. (H)

29. **4.** Assessment of the integumentary system includes both inspection and palpation. Palpation involves assessing temperature, turgor, moisture, and texture. Observing bruises and color and detecting hair distribution are inspection. (H)

30. **1.** *Risk for infection* related to pruritus is the priority nursing diagnosis because it has been documented that the client continues to scratch the affected areas. Satisfactory control of the itching sensation and discomfort associated with scratching may relieve the agitation and anxiety. More information is required regarding the knowledge level of the client and her disease process, but learning cannot take place when an individual's attention is distracted with pruritus. Impaired skin integrity is a potential problem if the client continues to scratch the affected areas and destroys the skin, but the risk of infection deserves priority attention because of the client's anxiety. There are no data to support that the client has a poor self-image. (R)

31. **2, 3.** Usual aging is associated with dry skin; however, seborrhea (oily skin and dandruff) is one result of the biochemical changes associated with Parkinson's disease. The client with Parkinson's disease has a higher risk of skin breakdown due to the moist and oily skin. To maintain skin integrity, a client with Parkinson's disease needs frequent skin care and aeration of the skin. Gait instability in a client with Parkinson's disease is a result of muscle rigidity, change in the center of gravity, and gait shuffling. Because of these changes in gait and balance, the client is at higher risk for injuries in the environment, such as hitting furniture or obstacles in the client's path. As a result, the environment should be evaluated for potential injury or falls. Tissue perfusion and verbal communication are not problems typically associated with Parkinson's disease. The client should not experience activity intolerance from the cellulitis or Parkinson's disease. (D)

32. **4.** Massaging areas that are reddened due to pressure is contraindicated because it further reduces blood flow to the area. The UAP should not massage the bony prominences or use lotion on the area. Massage does improve circulation and blood flow to muscle areas; however, because the area is reddened, the client is at risk for further skin breakdown. (M)

33. **3.** A stage II skin breakdown involves epidermal sloughing and pain. Redness without blanching is noted in stage I. Stage III involves tissue necrosis with subcutaneous involvement. Stage IV involves muscle or bone destruction. Muscle spasms are not a criterion used in the staging process. (A)

34. **2.** Many falls occur when older clients attempt to get to the bathroom at night. The risk is even greater in an unfamiliar environment. Use of a nightlight in the bathroom enables the older adult client to see the way to the bathroom. Keeping the lights on in the room at all times may contribute to sensory overload and prevent adequate rest. Raised side rails paradoxically contribute to falls when the older client tries to climb over them to get to the bathroom. The upper side rails may be raised, but it is not recommended that all four side rails be elevated. Camera monitoring can be used but does nothing to prevent a fall. (S)

35. **2.** Pressure ulcers usually occur over bony prominences. An alteration in the protective pressure sensation results from a decline in the number of Meissner's and pacinian corpuscles. Older adults do have altered balance that may result in falls, but not skin breakdown. Impaired hearing and vision do not contribute to pressure ulcers. (R)

The Client with Skin Cancer

36. **1.** Caucasians who have fair skin and a high exposure to ultraviolet light are at increased risk for malignant neoplasms of the skin. The other risk factors include exposure to tar and arsenicals and family history. History of hypertension is a coronary artery disease risk factor. Clients with dark skin have increased melanin and are not as prone to skin cancer. (H)

37. **1, 2, 3, 5, 6.** Risk factors associated with skin cancer include: Age, exposure to chemical pollutants, exposure to the sun, genetics, and immunosuppression. As individuals age, the risk of developing skin cancer increases. Long-time exposure to the sun and exposure to chemical pollutants (nitrates, coal, tar, etc.) increases the risk of skin cancer. Individuals who have less skin pigmentation (i.e., fair, blue-eyed people) have a higher risk of skin cancer because they tend to incur sunburns rather than tan. Family history plays a role in cancer. Regardless, immunosuppressed individuals are at a higher risk for the development of any type of cancer, as the body's defenses are not functioning properly. (H)

38. **4.** Malignant melanoma is a lesion or tumor that arises from melanin-producing cells. Although malignant melanoma may begin in a mole, not all lesions arising in moles are melanomas and melanomas can develop from flat areas of melanin. Lesions arising from the basal cells are called basal cell carcinomas. Lesions arising from squamous cells are called squamous cell carcinomas. (R)

39. **4.** Tumor or lesion thickness is the predictive factor for survival. Cutaneous melanoma that is confined to the epidermis has a high cure rate. Asymmetry, border, color, and diameter are known as the "ABCDs" of melanoma. Thus, the amount of ulceration, age, and location are not clearly associated with the prognosis. (H)

Responding to Emergencies, Mass Casualties, and Disasters

- Emergencies
- Mass Casualties
- Disasters
- Correct Answers and Rationales

Emergencies

1. A rescuer is called to a neighbor's home after a 56-year-old man collapses. After quickly assessing the victim, the rescuer determines that the victim is unresponsive. What can the rescuer do to determine unresponsiveness?
- ☐ **1.** Call the victim's name and gently shake the victim.
- ☐ **2.** Perform the chin-tilt to open the victim's airway.
- ☐ **3.** Feel for any air movement from the victim's nose or mouth.
- ☐ **4.** Watch the victim's chest for respirations.

2. Proper hand placement for chest compressions during cardiopulmonary resuscitation (CPR) is essential to reduce the risk of which complication?
- ☐ **1.** Gastrointestinal bleeding.
- ☐ **2.** Myocardial infarction.
- ☐ **3.** Emesis.
- ☐ **4.** Rib fracture.

3. The American Heart Association (AHA) guidelines urge greater availability of automated external defibrillators (AEDs) and people trained to use them. AEDs are used in cardiac arrest situations for:
- ☐ **1.** Early defibrillation in cases of atrial fibrillation.
- ☐ **2.** Cardioversion in cases of atrial fibrillation.
- ☐ **3.** Pacemaker placement.
- ☐ **4.** Early defibrillation in cases of ventricular fibrillation.

4. Indicate on the illustration below where the nurse would place the other electrode of the automated external defibrillator (AED) on a victim who has collapsed and does not have a pulse.

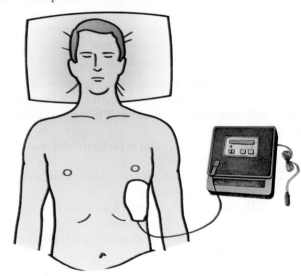

5. A client is admitted to the emergency department after being found in a daze walking away from her burning car after an accident. She was not injured in the accident, but the other driver died. She states, "I can't handle it anymore. There's no point to it all." The crisis nurse recommends hospital admission based on the identification of which priority nursing diagnosis?
- ☐ **1.** *Ineffective coping* related to burning of the car as evidenced by walking around in a daze.
- ☐ **2.** *Decisional conflict* related to burning of the car as evidenced by a lack of knowledge of what to do next.
- ☐ **3.** *Disturbed thought processes* related to causing a death as evidenced by the inability to think clearly.
- ☐ **4.** *Risk for suicide* related to the traumatic events of an accident as evidenced by statements of helplessness and hopelessness.

Mass Casualties

6. Thirty people are injured in a train derailment. Which client should be transported to the hospital first?
- [ ] **1.** A 20-year-old who is unresponsive and has a high injury to his spinal cord.
- [ ] **2.** An 80-year-old who has a compound fracture of the arm.
- [ ] **3.** A 10-year-old with a laceration on his leg.
- [ ] **4.** A 25-year-old with a sucking chest wound.

7. An explosion at a chemical plant produces flames and smoke. More than 20 persons have burn injuries. Which victims should be transported to a burn center? Select all that apply.
- [ ] **1.** The victim with chemical spills on both arms.
- [ ] **2.** The victim with third-degree burns of both legs.
- [ ] **3.** The victim with first-degree burns of both hands.
- [ ] **4.** The victim in respiratory distress.
- [ ] **5.** The victim who inhaled smoke.

8. An apartment fire spreads to seven apartment units. Victims suffer burns, minor injuries, and broken bones from jumping from windows. Which client should be transported first?
- [ ] **1.** A woman who is 5 months pregnant with no apparent injuries.
- [ ] **2.** A middle-aged man with no injuries who has rapid respirations and coughs.
- [ ] **3.** A 10-year-old with a simple fracture of the humerus who is in severe pain.
- [ ] **4.** A 20-year-old with first-degree burns on her hands and forearms.

9. There is a shooting in a shopping mall. Three victims with gunshot wounds are brought to the emergency department. What should the nurse do to preserve forensic evidence? Select all that apply.
- [ ] **1.** Cut around blood stains to remove clothing.
- [ ] **2.** Place each item of clothing in a separate paper bag.
- [ ] **3.** Hang wet clothing to dry.
- [ ] **4.** Refrain from documenting client statements.
- [ ] **5.** Place bullets in a sterile container.

10. A client who was a victim of a gunshot wound was treated in the emergency department and died. What should the nurse direct the unlicensed assistive personnel (UAP) to do during postmortem care? Select all that apply.
- [ ] **1.** Remove all tubes and I.V. lines.
- [ ] **2.** Cover the body with a sheet.
- [ ] **3.** Notify the family.
- [ ] **4.** Transport the body to the morgue.
- [ ] **5.** Notify the chaplain.

11. An airplane crash results in mass casualties. The nurse is directing personnel to tag all victims. Which information should be placed on the tag? Select all that apply.
- [ ] **1.** Triage priority.
- [ ] **2.** Identifying information when possible (such as name, age, and address).
- [ ] **3.** Medications and treatments administered.
- [ ] **4.** Presence of jewelry.
- [ ] **5.** Next of kin.

12. A car accident involves four vehicles on a remote interstate. The nearest emergency department is 15 minutes away. Which victim should be transported by helicopter to the nearest hospital?
- [ ] **1.** 10-year-old with a simple fracture of the femur who is crying and cannot find his parents.
- [ ] **2.** Middle-aged woman with cold, clammy skin and a heart rate of 120 bpm who is unconscious.
- [ ] **3.** Middle-aged man with severe asthma and a heart rate of 120 bpm who is having difficulty breathing.
- [ ] **4.** 70-year-old man with a severe headache who is conscious.

13. A small airplane crashes in a neighborhood of 10 houses. One of the victims appears to have a cervical spine injury. What should first-aid for this victim include? Select all that apply.
- [ ] **1.** Establish an airway with the jaw-thrust maneuver.
- [ ] **2.** Immobilize the spine.
- [ ] **3.** Logroll the victim to a side-lying position.
- [ ] **4.** Elevate the feet 6″ (15.2 cm).
- [ ] **5.** Place a cervical collar around the neck.

14. Thirty-two children are brought to the emergency department after a school bus accident. Two children were killed along with the three people in the car that caused the crash. Before the victims arrive, in addition to ensuring that the hospital staff are prepared for the emergency, which step should the nurse anticipate carrying out?
- [ ] **1.** Calling the nearest crisis response team.
- [ ] **2.** Alerting the news media.
- [ ] **3.** Notifying the hospital volunteer office.
- [ ] **4.** Calling the school to inform teachers of the accident.

Disasters

15. A suspected outbreak of anthrax has been transmitted by skin exposure. A client is admitted to the emergency department with lesions on his hands. The physician prescribes antibiotics and sends the client home. What should the nurse instruct the client to do? Select all that apply.

- ☐ **1.** Take the prescribed antibiotics for 60 days.
- ☐ **2.** Avoid contact with other members of his family during the treatment period.
- ☐ **3.** Wear a mask for 60 days.
- ☐ **4.** Expect the skin lesions to clear up within 1 to 2 weeks.
- ☐ **5.** Wash his hands frequently.

16. A severe acute respiratory syndrome (SARS) epidemic is suspected in a community of 10,000 people. As clients with SARS are admitted to the hospital, what type of precautions should the nurse institute?

- ☐ **1.** Enteric precautions.
- ☐ **2.** Hand-washing precautions.
- ☐ **3.** Reverse isolation.
- ☐ **4.** Standard precautions.

17. Several clients who work in the same building are brought to the emergency department. They all complain of similar clinical manifestations, including fever, headache, a rash over the entire body, and abdominal pain with vomiting and diarrhea. Upon initial assessment, the nurse finds that each client has low blood pressure and has developed petechiae in the area where the blood pressure cuff was inflated. Which isolation precautions should the nurse initiate?

- ☐ **1.** Contact isolation with double-gloving and shoe covers.
- ☐ **2.** Respiratory isolation with positive pressure rooms.
- ☐ **3.** Enteric precautions.
- ☐ **4.** Reverse isolation.

18. Several clients come to the emergency department with suspected contamination by the Ebola virus. What should the nurse do? Select all that apply.

- ☐ **1.** Call in extra staff to assist with the possibility of more clients with the same condition.
- ☐ **2.** Isolate all the suspected clients in the emergency department in one area.
- ☐ **3.** Call housekeeping for diluted household bleach.
- ☐ **4.** Restrict visitors from the emergency department.
- ☐ **5.** Quarantine all contacts.

19. A number of clients have come to the emergency department after a possible bioterrorist act of arsenic overexposure. The nurse should assess these clients for which signs or symptoms immediately following the poisoning? Select all that apply.

- ☐ **1.** Violent vomiting.
- ☐ **2.** Severe diarrhea.
- ☐ **3.** Abdominal pain.
- ☐ **4.** Sensory neuropathy.
- ☐ **5.** Persistent cough.

Correct Answers and Rationales

The letter in parentheses after each rationale identifies the client need addressed in the item, including management of care (M), safety and infection control (S), health promotion and maintenance (H), psychosocial adaptation (P), basic care and comfort (C), pharmacological and parenteral therapies (D), reduction of risk potential (R), and physiological adaptation (A).

Emergencies

1. 1. Calling the victim's name and gently shaking the victim is used to establish unresponsiveness. The head-tilt, chin-lift maneuver is used to open the victim's airway. Feeling for any air movement from the victim's nose or mouth indicates whether the victim is breathing on his own. The rescuer can watch the victim's chest for respirations to see if the victim is breathing. (A)

2. 4. Proper hand placement during chest compressions is essential to reduce the risk of rib fractures, which may lead to pneumothorax and other internal injuries. Gastrointestinal bleeding and myocardial infarction are generally not considered complications of CPR. Although the victim may vomit during CPR, this is not associated with poor hand placement, but rather with distention of the stomach. (A)

3. 4. AEDs are used for early defibrillation in cases of ventricular fibrillation. The AHA places major emphasis on early defibrillation for ventricular fibrillation and use of the AED as a tool to increase sudden cardiac arrest survival rates. (R)

4. One electrode is placed to the right of the upper sternum just below the right clavicle. The other is placed, as shown, over the fifth or sixth intercostal space at the left anterior axillary line. (R)

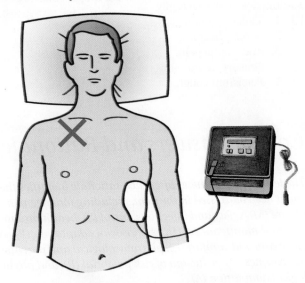

5. **4.** The client is demonstrating helplessness and hopelessness during a crisis, as evidenced by her statement, "I can't handle it. There is no point to it." Feelings of helplessness and hopelessness are common factors associated with suicidal ideation. Therefore, the client must be hospitalized to ensure safety to herself. Ineffective coping affects interventions. Not knowing what to do next reflects a request for help in making a decision. However, these diagnoses have less priority when compared with the client's risk for suicide. Disturbed thought processes would be evidenced by delusions, such as "The devil set my car on fire," not just the inability to think clearly. (P)

Mass Casualties

6. **4.** During a disaster, the nurse must make difficult decisions about which persons to treat first. The guidelines for triage offer general priorities for immediate, delayed, minimal, and expectant care. The client with a sucking chest wound needs immediate attention and will likely survive. The 80-year-old is classified as delayed; emergency response personnel can immobilize the fracture and cover the wound. The 10-year-old has minimal injuries and can wait to be treated. The client with a spinal cord injury is not likely to survive and should not be among the first to be transported to the health care facility. (M)

7. **1, 2, 3, 5.** Victims with chemical burns, second- and third-degree burns over more than 20% of their body surface area, and those with inhalation injuries should be transported to a burn center. The victim with first-degree burns of his hands can be treated with first-aid on the scene and referred to a health care facility. (M)

8. **2.** The man with respiratory distress and coughing should be transported first because he is probably experiencing smoke inhalation. The pregnant woman is not in imminent danger or likely to have a precipitous delivery. The 10-year-old is not at risk for infection and could be treated in an outpatient facility. First-degree burns are considered less urgent. (M)

9. **2, 3.** Preserving forensic evidence is essential for investigative purposes following injuries that may be caused by criminal intent. The nurse should put each item of clothing in a separate paper bag and label it; wet clothing should be hung to dry. The nurse should not cut or otherwise unnecessarily handle clothing, particularly clothing with such evidence as blood or body fluids. The nurse should document carefully the client's description of the incident and use quotes around the client's exact words where possible. The documentation will become a part of the client's record and can be subpoenaed for subsequent investigation. The nurse should not handle bullets from the client because they are an important piece of forensic evidence. (M)

10. **2, 4.** The UAP can cover the body and transport it to the morgue. Deaths by gunshot wound are considered reportable deaths. All evidence in a reportable death, including tubes and I.V. lines, should remain intact until the coroner has been contacted. The health care provider should be the one to notify the family. The nurse should be the one to notify the chaplain. (M)

11. **1, 2, 3.** Tracking victims of disasters is important for casualty planning and management. All victims should receive a tag, securely attached, that indicates the triage priority, any available identifying information, and what care, if any, has been given along with time and date. Tag information should be recorded in a disaster log and used to track victims and inform families. It is not necessary to document the presence of jewelry or next of kin. (M)

12. **2.** The middle-aged woman is likely in shock. She is classified as a triage level I, requiring immediate care. The child with moderate trauma is classified as triage level III (urgent and should be treated within 30 minutes). The man with asthma and the man with the severe headache are classified as triage level II (emergent), and can be transported by ambulance and reach the hospital within 15 minutes. (M)

13. **1, 2.** The victim of a neck injury should be immobilized and moved as little as possible. It is also important to ensure an open airway; this can be accomplished with the jaw-thrust maneuver, which does not require tilting the head. The victim should not be rolled to a side-lying position nor have his feet elevated. Both actions can cause additional injury to the spinal cord. Placing a cervical collar causes movement of the spinal column and should not be done as a first-aid measure. (M)

14. **1.** The children and their families are at risk for experiencing a crisis. Disaster teams are available for crisis intervention in such emergencies. Usually the news media monitors emergency radio frequencies and most likely are aware of the accident already. Although volunteers may help in some ways, they are not responsible for crisis intervention. Calling the school might be done, but the emergency issues take precedence. (P)

Disasters

15. **1, 4.** Anthrax is treated with antibiotics and the client must continue the prescription for 60 days, even if symptoms do not persist. The client may have skin lesions at the point of contact, with macula or papule formation; the eschar will fall off in 1 to 2 weeks. Clients with anthrax are not contagious; the client does not need to follow isolation procedures at home. Anthrax from skin exposure is not transmitted by respiratory contact and the client does not need to wear a mask. (S)

16. **4.** Transmission of SARS can be contained by following standard (universal) precautions, which include masks, gowns, eye protection, hand washing, and safe disposal of needles and sharps. The disease is spread by the respiratory, not enteric, route. Hand washing alone is not sufficient to prevent transmission. Reverse isolation (protection of the client) is not sufficient to prevent transmission. (S)

17. **1.** The nurse should institute treatment for hemorrhagic fever viruses, including contact isolation with double-gloving and shoe covers, strict hand hygiene, and protective eyewear. The nurse should start respiratory isolation with negative pressure rooms, not positive pressure rooms. Enteric precautions are not needed because the virus is spread by droplet and contact. Reverse isolation protects the client; in this situation, the health care team also needs protection. (R)

18. **2, 3, 4.** The nurse should isolate all the suspected clients in the emergency department in one area and restrict visitors from the emergency department to minimize exposure to others. The nurse should also obtain diluted household bleach (1:100) to decontaminate areas suspected of coming in contact with the virus. There is no indication at this time that extra staff is needed, so the nurse should not call in extra staff, to minimize exposure to health care workers. It is not necessary to quarantine contacts until a diagnosis is confirmed. In addition, it is the role of the public health officer to issue the quarantine if needed. (S)

19. **1, 2, 3.** When arsenic overexposure occurs, the signs and symptoms include violent nausea, vomiting, abdominal pain, skin irritation, severe diarrhea, laryngitis, and bronchitis. Dehydration can lead to shock and death. After the acute phase, bone marrow depression, encephalopathy, and sensory neuropathy occur. (A)

The Nursing Care of Clients with Psychiatric Disorders and Mental Health Problems

TEST 1

Mood Disorders

- The Client with Major Depression
- The Client with Bipolar Disorder, Manic Phase
- The Client with Suicidal Ideation and Suicide Attempt
- Correct Answers and Rationales

The Client with Major Depression

1. The client is receiving 6 mg of selegiline transdermal system (Emsam) every 24 hours for major depression. The nurse should judge teaching about Emsam to be effective when the client makes which statement?

- ☐ 1. "I need to avoid using the sauna at the gym."
- ☐ 2. "I can cut the patch and use a smaller piece."
- ☐ 3. "I need to wait until the next day to put on a new patch if it falls off."
- ☐ 4. "I might gain at least 10 lb from Emsam."

2. A client has been taking 30 mg of duloxetine hydrochloride (Cymbalta) twice daily for 2 months because of depression and vague aches and pains. While interacting with the nurse, the client discloses a pattern of drinking a 6-pack of beer daily for the past 10 years to help with sleep. What should the nurse do first?

- ☐ 1. Refer the client to the dual diagnosis program at the clinic.
- ☐ 2. Share the information at the next interdisciplinary treatment conference.
- ☐ 3. Report the client's beer consumption to the physician.
- ☐ 4. Teach the client relaxation exercises to perform before bedtime.

3. A client was admitted to the inpatient unit 3 days ago with a flat affect, psychomotor retardation, anorexia, hopelessness, and suicidal ideation. The physician prescribed 75 mg of venlafaxine extended release (Effexor XR) to be given every morning. The client interacted minimally with the staff and spent most of the day in his room. As the nurse enters the unit at the beginning of the evening shift, the client is smiling and cheerfully greets the nurse. He appears to be relaxed and joins the group for community meeting before supper. What should the nurse interpret as the most likely cause of the client's behavior?

- ☐ 1. The Effexor is helping the client's symptoms of depression significantly.
- ☐ 2. The client's sudden improvement calls for close observation by the staff.
- ☐ 3. The staff can decrease their observation of the client.
- ☐ 4. The client is nearing discharge due to the improvement of his symptoms.

4. The nurse is conducting an intake interview with an Asian American female in the outpatient clinic with complaints of sadness, physical and mental fatigue, anxiety, and sleep disturbance. Prior to the client's time with the physician, it is important for the nurse to obtain information about the client's use of which of the following? Select all that apply.
- [ ] **1.** Tea.
- [ ] **2.** Herbal medicine.
- [ ] **3.** Breathing exercise.
- [ ] **4.** Massage.
- [ ] **5.** Folk healer.

5. The client is taking 50 mg of lamotrigine (Lamictal) daily for bipolar depression. The client shows the nurse a rash on his arm. What should the nurse do?
- [ ] **1.** Report the rash to the physician.
- [ ] **2.** Explain that the rash is a temporary adverse effect.
- [ ] **3.** Give the client an ice pack for his arm.
- [ ] **4.** Question the client about recent sun exposure.

6. The nurse is reviewing the laboratory report with the client's lithium level taken that morning prior to administering the 5 p.m. dose of lithium. The lithium level is 1.8 mEq/L. What should the nurse do?
- [ ] **1.** Administer the 5 p.m. dose of lithium.
- [ ] **2.** Hold the 5 p.m. dose of lithium.
- [ ] **3.** Give the client 8 oz (236 ml) of water with the lithium.
- [ ] **4.** Give the lithium after the client's supper.

7. A nurse is conducting a psychoeducational group for family members of clients hospitalized with depression. Which family member's statement indicates a need for additional teaching?
- [ ] **1.** "My husband will slowly feel better as his medicine takes effect over the next 2 to 4 weeks."
- [ ] **2.** "My wife will need to take her antidepressant medicine and go to group to stay well."
- [ ] **3.** "My son will only need to attend outpatient appointments when he starts to feel depressed again."
- [ ] **4.** "My mother might need help with grocery shopping, cooking, and cleaning for a while."

8. A client diagnosed with major depression with psychotic features is experiencing mood congruent delusions. Which delusion would the client most likely experience?
- [ ] **1.** "My stomach is rotting."
- [ ] **2.** "They are talking about me."
- [ ] **3.** "I am Superman."
- [ ] **4.** "The FBI will find me."

9. The 16-year-old client is prescribed 10 mg of paroxetine (Paxil) at bedtime for major depression. The nurse should monitor the client closely for which adverse effect?
- [ ] **1.** Headache.
- [ ] **2.** Nausea.
- [ ] **3.** Fatigue.
- [ ] **4.** Agitation.

10. A client has an Axis I diagnosis of major depression. Which of the following features is most crucial for the nurse to assess?
- [ ] **1.** Sleep disturbance.
- [ ] **2.** Feelings of worthlessness.
- [ ] **3.** Difficulty with concentration.
- [ ] **4.** Suicidal ideation.

11. A client who has had three episodes of recurrent endogenous depression within the past 2 years states to the nurse, "I want to know why I'm so depressed." Which of the following statements by the nurse is most helpful?
- [ ] **1.** "I know you'll get better with the right medication."
- [ ] **2.** "Let's discuss possible reasons underlying your depression."
- [ ] **3.** "Your depression is most likely caused by a brain chemical imbalance."
- [ ] **4.** "Members of your family seem very supportive of you."

12. A client diagnosed with major depression spends most of the day lying in bed with the sheet pulled over his head. Which of the following approaches by the nurse is most therapeutic?
- [ ] **1.** Wait for the client to begin the conversation.
- [ ] **2.** Initiate contact with the client frequently.
- [ ] **3.** Sit outside the client's room.
- [ ] **4.** Question the client until he responds.

13. The client exhibits a flat affect, psychomotor retardation, and depressed mood. The nurse attempts to engage the client in an interaction but the client does not respond to the nurse. Which of the following responses by the nurse is most appropriate?
- [ ] **1.** "I'll sit here with you for 15 minutes."
- [ ] **2.** "I'll come back a little bit later to talk."
- [ ] **3.** "I'll find someone else for you to talk with."
- [ ] **4.** "I'll get you something to read."

14. After a few minutes of conversation, a female client who is depressed wearily asks the nurse, "Why pick me to talk to? Go talk to someone else." Which of the following replies by the nurse is best?
- [ ] **1.** "I'm assigned to care for you today, if you'll let me."
- [ ] **2.** "You have a lot of potential, and I'd like to help you."
- [ ] **3.** "I'll talk to someone else later."
- [ ] **4.** "I'm interested in you and want to help you."

15. A client is receiving paroxetine (Paxil) 20 mg every morning. After taking the first three doses, the client tells the nurse that the medication upsets his stomach. Which of the following instructions should the nurse give to the client?
- ☐ **1.** "Take the medication an hour before breakfast."
- ☐ **2.** "Take the medication with some food."
- ☐ **3.** "Take the medication at bedtime."
- ☐ **4.** "Take the medication with 4 oz of orange juice."

16. The physician orders fluoxetine (Prozac) orally every morning for a 72-year-old client with depression. Which transient adverse effect of this drug requires immediate action by the nurse?
- ☐ **1.** Nausea.
- ☐ **2.** Dizziness.
- ☐ **3.** Sedation.
- ☐ **4.** Dry mouth.

17. Which of the following statements by a client taking trazodone (Desyrel) as prescribed by the physician indicates to the nurse that further teaching about the medication is needed?
- ☐ **1.** "I will continue to take my medication after a light snack."
- ☐ **2.** "Taking Desyrel at night will help me to sleep."
- ☐ **3.** "My depression will be gone in about 5 to 7 days."
- ☐ **4.** "I won't drink alcohol while taking Desyrel."

18. A 62-year-old female client with severe depression and psychotic symptoms is scheduled for electroconvulsive therapy (ECT) tomorrow morning. The client's daughter asks the nurse, "How painful will the treatment be for Mom?" The nurse should correctly respond by saying which of the following?
- ☐ **1.** "Your mother will be given something for pain before the treatment."
- ☐ **2.** "The physician will make sure your mother doesn't suffer needlessly."
- ☐ **3.** "Your mother will be asleep during the treatment and will not be in pain."
- ☐ **4.** "Your mother will be able talk to us and tell us if she's in pain."

19. A client with sleep disturbances, feelings of worthlessness, fatigue, and an inability to concentrate was let go from her place of employment a month ago. While interacting with the nurse, the client states, "My boss was wonderful! He was understanding and a really nice man." The nurse interprets this statement as which defense mechanism?
- ☐ **1.** Repression.
- ☐ **2.** Suppression.
- ☐ **3.** Intellectualization.
- ☐ **4.** Reaction formation.

20. During a group session, a client who is depressed tells the group that he lost his job. Which of the following responses by the nurse is best?
- ☐ **1.** "It must have been very upsetting for you."
- ☐ **2.** "Would you tell us about your job."
- ☐ **3.** "You'll find another job when you're better."
- ☐ **4.** "You were probably too depressed to work."

21. During an interaction with the nurse, a client states, "My husband has supported me every time I've been hospitalized for depression. He'll leave me this time. I'm an awful wife and mother. I'm no good. Nothing I do is right." Based on this information, which of the following nursing diagnoses should the nurse identify when developing the client's plan of care?
- ☐ **1.** *Impaired social interaction* related to unsatisfactory relationships as evidenced by withdrawal.
- ☐ **2.** *Chronic low self-esteem* related to lack of self-worth as evidenced by negative statements.
- ☐ **3.** *Risk for self-directed violence* related to feelings of guilt as evidenced by statements of suicidal ideation.
- ☐ **4.** *Ineffective coping* related to hospitalizations as evidenced by impaired judgment.

22. A male client who is very depressed exhibits psychomotor retardation, a flat affect, and apathy. The nurse observes the client to be in need of grooming and hygiene. Which of the following nursing actions is most appropriate?
- ☐ **1.** Explaining the importance of hygiene to the client.
- ☐ **2.** Asking the client if he is ready to shower.
- ☐ **3.** Waiting until the client's family can participate in the client's care.
- ☐ **4.** Stating to the client that it's time for him to take a shower.

23. A client who is depressed states, "I'm an awful person. Everything about me is bad. I can't do anything right." Which of the following responses by the nurse is most therapeutic?
- ☐ **1.** "Everybody around here likes you."
- ☐ **2.** "I can see many good qualities in you."
- ☐ **3.** "Let's discuss what you've done correctly."
- ☐ **4.** "You were able to bathe today."

24. When developing the teaching plan for the family of a client with severe depression who is to receive electroconvulsive therapy (ECT), which of the following should the nurse include?
- ☐ **1.** Some temporary confusion and disorientation immediately after a treatment is common.
- ☐ **2.** During an ECT treatment session, the client is at risk for aspiration.
- ☐ **3.** Clients with severe depression usually do not respond to ECT.
- ☐ **4.** The client will not be able to breathe independently during a treatment.

25. Which of the following comments indicates that a client understands the nurse's teaching about sertraline (Zoloft)?
- ☐ **1.** "Zoloft will probably cause me to gain weight."
- ☐ **2.** "This medicine can cause delayed ejaculations."
- ☐ **3.** "Dry mouth is a permanent side effect of Zoloft."
- ☐ **4.** "I can take my medicine with St. John's wort."

26. The client with recurring depression will be discharged from the psychiatric unit. Which suggestion to the family is best to help them prepare for the client's return home?
- ☐ **1.** Discourage visitors while the client is at home.
- ☐ **2.** Provide for a schedule of activities outside the home.
- ☐ **3.** Involve the client in usual at-home activities.
- ☐ **4.** Encourage the client to sleep as much as possible.

27. A client with major depression is to be discharged home tomorrow. When preparing the client's discharge plan, which of the following areas is most important for the nurse to review with the client?
- ☐ **1.** Future plans for going back to work.
- ☐ **2.** A conflict encountered with another client.
- ☐ **3.** Results of psychological testing.
- ☐ **4.** Medication management with outpatient follow-up.

28. A client with major depression and psychotic features is admitted involuntarily to the hospital. He will not eat because his "bowels have turned to jelly," which the client states is punishment for his wickedness. The client requests to leave the hospital. The nurse denies the request because commitment papers have been initiated by the physician. Which of the following should the nurse identify as a criterion for the client to be legally committable?
- ☐ **1.** Evidence of psychosis.
- ☐ **2.** Being gravely disabled.
- ☐ **3.** Risk of harm to self or others.
- ☐ **4.** Diagnosis of mental illness.

29. The client who has been taking venlafaxine (Effexor) 25 mg P.O. three times a day for the past 2 days states, "This medicine isn't doing me any good. I'm still so depressed." Which of the following responses by the nurse is most appropriate?
- ☐ **1.** "Perhaps we'll need to increase your dose."
- ☐ **2.** "Let's wait a few days and see how you feel."
- ☐ **3.** "It takes about 2 to 4 weeks to receive the full effects."
- ☐ **4.** "It's too soon to tell if your medication will help you."

30. The client states to the nurse, "I take citalopram (Celexa) 40 mg every day like my physician prescribed. I have also been taking St. John's wort 750 mg daily for the past 2 weeks." Which of the following would lead the nurse to suspect that the client is developing serotonin syndrome? Select all that apply.
- ☐ **1.** Confusion.
- ☐ **2.** Restlessness.
- ☐ **3.** Headache.
- ☐ **4.** Constipation.
- ☐ **5.** Diaphoresis.
- ☐ **6.** Ataxia.

31. When teaching the client with atypical depression about foods to avoid while taking phenelzine (Nardil), which of the following should the nurse include?
- ☐ **1.** Roasted chicken.
- ☐ **2.** Salami.
- ☐ **3.** Fresh fish.
- ☐ **4.** Hamburger.

32. A client is taking phenelzine (Nardil) 15 mg P.O. three times a day. The nurse is about to administer the 1 p.m. dose when the client complains of a throbbing headache. Which of the following should the nurse do first?
- ☐ **1.** Give the client an analgesic ordered p.r.n.
- ☐ **2.** Call the physician to report the symptom.
- ☐ **3.** Administer the client's next dose of phenelzine.
- ☐ **4.** Obtain the client's vital signs.

33. A female client with severe depression and weight loss has not eaten since admission to the hospital 2 days ago. Which of the following approaches should the nurse include when developing this client's plan of care to ensure that she eats?
- ☐ **1.** Serving the client her meal trays in her room.
- ☐ **2.** Sitting with the client and spoon-feeding if required.
- ☐ **3.** Calling the family to bring the client food from home.
- ☐ **4.** Explaining the importance of nutrition in recovery.

34. After administering a prescribed medication to a client who becomes restless at night and has difficulty falling asleep, which of the following nursing actions is most appropriate?
- ☐ **1.** Sitting quietly with the client at the bedside until the medication takes effect.
- ☐ **2.** Engaging the client in interaction until the client falls asleep.
- ☐ **3.** Reading to the client with the lights turned down low.
- ☐ **4.** Encouraging the client to watch television until the client feels sleepy.

35. Which of the following behaviors exhibited by a client with depression should lead the nurse to determine that the client is ready for discharge?
- [ ] **1.** Interactions with staff and peers.
- [ ] **2.** Sleeping for 4 hours in the afternoon and 4 hours at night.
- [ ] **3.** Verbalization of feeling in control of self and situations.
- [ ] **4.** Statements of dissatisfaction over not being able to perform at work.

36. The client with major depression and suicidal ideation has been taking bupropion (Wellbutrin) 100 mg P.O. four times daily for 5 days. Assessment reveals the client to be somewhat less withdrawn, able to perform activities of daily living with minimal assistance, and eating 50% of each meal. At this time, the nurse should monitor the client specifically for which of the following behaviors?
- [ ] **1.** Seizure activity.
- [ ] **2.** Suicide attempt.
- [ ] **3.** Visual disturbances.
- [ ] **4.** Increased libido.

37. Which of the following outcomes should the nurse include as an outcome in the initial plan of care for a client who is exhibiting psychomotor retardation, withdrawal, minimal eye contact, and unresponsiveness to the nurse's questions?
- [ ] **1.** The client will initiate interactions with peers.
- [ ] **2.** The client will participate in milieu activities.
- [ ] **3.** The client will discuss adaptive coping techniques.
- [ ] **4.** The client will interact with the nurse.

38. When preparing a teaching plan for a client about imipramine (Tofranil), which of the following substances should the nurse tell the client to avoid while taking the medication?
- [ ] **1.** Caffeinated coffee.
- [ ] **2.** Sunscreen.
- [ ] **3.** Alcohol.
- [ ] **4.** Artificial tears.

39. The client with depression who is taking imipramine (Tofranil) states to the nurse, "My doctor wants me to have an electrocardiogram (ECG) in 2 weeks, but my heart is fine." Which of the following responses by the nurse is most appropriate?
- [ ] **1.** "It's routine practice to have ECGs periodically because there is a slight chance that the drug may affect the heart."
- [ ] **2.** "It's probably a precautionary measure because I'm not aware that you have a cardiac condition."
- [ ] **3.** "Try not to worry too much about this. Your doctor is just being very thorough in monitoring your condition."
- [ ] **4.** "You had an ECG before you were prescribed imipramine and the procedure will be the same."

40. The laboratory calls the nurse stating that a client's imipramine (Tofranil) level is within the therapeutic range. The nurse interprets this as indicating that the client's serum concentration is within which of the following ranges?
- [ ] **1.** 50 to 149 mg/ml.
- [ ] **2.** 150 to 250 mg/ml.
- [ ] **3.** 251 to 350 mg/ml.
- [ ] **4.** 351 to 450 mg/ml.

41. When assessing a client who is receiving tricyclic antidepressant therapy, which of the following should alert the nurse to the possibility that the client is experiencing anticholinergic effects?
- [ ] **1.** Tremors and cardiac arrhythmias.
- [ ] **2.** Sedation and delirium.
- [ ] **3.** Respiratory depression and convulsions.
- [ ] **4.** Urine retention and blurred vision.

42. A client with depression who is taking doxepin (Sinequan) 100 mg P.O. at bedtime complains of dizziness on arising. Which of the following suggestions is most appropriate?
- [ ] **1.** "Try taking a hot shower."
- [ ] **2.** "Get up slowly and dangle your feet before standing."
- [ ] **3.** "Stay in bed until you are feeling better."
- [ ] **4.** "You need to limit the fluids you drink."

43. The physician orders mirtazapine (Remeron) 30 mg P.O. at bedtime for a client diagnosed with depression. The nurse is responsible for which of the following?
- [ ] **1.** Giving the medication as ordered.
- [ ] **2.** Questioning the physician's order.
- [ ] **3.** Requesting to give the medication in the morning.
- [ ] **4.** Giving the medication in three divided doses.

44. A client taking mirtazapine (Remeron) is very disheartened about a 20-lb weight gain over the past 6 months. The client states, "I stopped taking my antidepressant 5 days ago. I don't want to get depressed again, but I feel awful about my weight." Which of the following responses by the nurse is most therapeutic?
- [ ] **1.** "Let's talk about your diet, exercise plan, and daily activities."
- [ ] **2.** "Your depression is much better now, so your medication is helping you."
- [ ] **3.** "Look at all the positive things that have happened since you've gotten better."
- [ ] **4.** "I hear how difficult this is for you and will help you talk with your doctor about it."

45. When developing a teaching plan for a client about the medications prescribed for depression, which of the following components is most important for the nurse to include?
- [ ] **1.** Pharmacokinetics of the medication.
- [ ] **2.** Current research related to the medication.
- [ ] **3.** Management of common adverse effects.
- [ ] **4.** Dosage regulation and adjustment.

46. The client with severe major depression has been taking imipramine (Tofranil) 100 mg P.O. at bedtime for the past 5 days. To evaluate the therapeutic efficacy of the antidepressant, which of the following should the nurse expect to improve first?
- ☐ **1.** Suicidal ideation.
- ☐ **2.** Agitation.
- ☐ **3.** Concentration.
- ☐ **4.** Mood.

47. A client taking paroxetine (Paxil) 40 mg P.O. every morning tells the nurse that her mouth "feels like cotton." Which of the following statements by the client should necessitate further assessment by the nurse?
- ☐ **1.** "I'm sucking on ice chips."
- ☐ **2.** "I'm using sugarless gum."
- ☐ **3.** "I'm sucking on sugarless candy."
- ☐ **4.** "I'm drinking lots of water."

48. The client with depression has been consistent with taking 12.5 mg of paroxetine (Paxil) extended release daily. The nurse judges the client to be benefiting from this drug therapy when the client demonstrates which of the following behaviors? Select all that apply.
- ☐ **1.** Takes 2-hour evening naps daily.
- ☐ **2.** Completes homework assignments.
- ☐ **3.** Decreases pacing.
- ☐ **4.** Increases somatization.
- ☐ **5.** Verbalizes feelings of anger.

49. A female client whose Axis I diagnosis is major depression has sleep and appetite disturbances, a flat affect, and psychomotor retardation and is withdrawn. The client has been taking amoxapine (Asendin) 50 mg three times daily for the past 5 days. Which of the following is most important to report to the next shift?
- ☐ **1.** The client's flat affect.
- ☐ **2.** The client's having a visitor.
- ☐ **3.** The client's sleeping from 11 p.m. to 6 a.m.
- ☐ **4.** The client's spending the evening in her room.

50. Which of the following should the nurse expect to identify as a good predictor of a client's favorable response to the choice of an antidepressant?
- ☐ **1.** The drug's side effect profile.
- ☐ **2.** The client's age at diagnosis.
- ☐ **3.** The cost of the medication.
- ☐ **4.** A favorable response by a family member.

51. For a client with dysthymic disorder, which of the following approaches should the nurse expect to implement?
- ☐ **1.** Antidepressant therapy.
- ☐ **2.** Electroconvulsive therapy.
- ☐ **3.** Psychotherapeutic approach.
- ☐ **4.** Psychoanalysis.

The Client with Bipolar Disorder, Manic Phase

52. The client with acute mania has been admitted to the inpatient unit voluntarily. The nurse approaches the client with medication to be taken orally as ordered by the physician. The client states, "I don't need that stuff." Which response by the nurse is best?
- ☐ **1.** "You can't refuse to take this medication."
- ☐ **2.** "If you don't take it orally, I'll give you a shot."
- ☐ **3.** "The medication will help you feel calmer."
- ☐ **4.** "I'll get you some written information about the medication."

53. A nurse observes a male client who is hyperactive and intrusive sitting very close to a female client with his arm around her shoulders. The nurse hears the male client verbalize a sexually explicit joke. The nurse approaches the client and asks him to walk down the hallway. Which of the following statements by the nurse should benefit the client?
- ☐ **1.** "She will not want to be around you with that kind of talk."
- ☐ **2.** "Telling sexual jokes and touching others is not permitted here."
- ☐ **3.** "You need to be careful about what you say to other people."
- ☐ **4.** "I think a time-out in your room would be appropriate now."

54. A client states to a nurse, "Hey sweetie, you're looking good today." Which of the following responses by the nurse is best?
- ☐ **1.** "Thank you for being so kind and thoughtful."
- ☐ **2.** "I know you are only teasing me."
- ☐ **3.** "My name is Molly, and I am a nurse on the unit today."
- ☐ **4.** "I am not here to receive compliments from clients."

55. A client with acute mania fails to respond to a nurse's interventions to decrease his agitation. The nurse attempted to defuse the client's anger and the client refuses to participate in interventions that would lower anxiety. Which action should the nurse take next?
- ☐ **1.** Seclude the client.
- ☐ **2.** Restrain the client.
- ☐ **3.** Medicate the client.
- ☐ **4.** Control the client.

56. The client with mania is irritable and insulting to a nursing assistant. The nursing assistant states, "I can't believe Mark is so rude. Shouldn't he be overly happy?" Which of the following responses by the nurse should help the nursing assistant understand the client's behavior?
- [ ] **1.** "It's our responsibility to listen to him even though we might not like what he's saying."
- [ ] **2.** "We must reprimand Mark for doing that because there is no reason for him to behave like that."
- [ ] **3.** "I will go and speak to him about his behavior and make sure he understands that he needs to control what he is saying."
- [ ] **4.** "I know it's difficult but Mark is a client whose irritable mood is a symptom of his mania."

57. Which milieu activity should the nurse recommend to a client with acute mania? Select all that apply.
- [ ] **1.** Scheduled rest periods.
- [ ] **2.** Relaxation exercises.
- [ ] **3.** Listening to soft music.
- [ ] **4.** Watching television.
- [ ] **5.** Aerobic exercises.

58. A nurse is assessing a client with hypomania. Which symptom is least likely to be evident in this client?
- [ ] **1.** Expansive mood.
- [ ] **2.** Auditory hallucinations.
- [ ] **3.** Heightened energy.
- [ ] **4.** Increased self-esteem.

59. The client with acute mania is prescribed 600 mg of lithium (Lithium Carbonate) P.O. three times per day. The physician also orders 5 mg of haloperidol (Haldol) P.O. at bedtime. Which action should the nurse take?
- [ ] **1.** Administer the medication as ordered.
- [ ] **2.** Question the physician about the order.
- [ ] **3.** Administer the Haldol, but not the lithium.
- [ ] **4.** Consult with the nursing supervisor before administering the medications.

60. The client with an Axis I diagnosis of bipolar disorder, manic phase, states to the nurse, "I'm the Queen of England. Bow before me." The nurse interprets this statement as important to document as which of the following areas of the mental status examination?
- [ ] **1.** Psychomotor behavior.
- [ ] **2.** Mood and affect.
- [ ] **3.** Attitude toward the nurse.
- [ ] **4.** Thought content.

61. The client is laughing and telling jokes to a group of clients. Suddenly, the client is in tears and talks about a death in the family. A moment later, the client is laughing and joking again. The nurse interprets this behavior as indicative of which of the following?
- [ ] **1.** Flat affect.
- [ ] **2.** Blunted affect.
- [ ] **3.** Labile affect.
- [ ] **4.** Normal affect.

62. A client with acute mania exhibits euphoria, pressured speech, and flight of ideas. The client has been talking to the nurse nonstop for 5 minutes and lunch has arrived on the unit. Which of the following should the nurse do next?
- [ ] **1.** Excuse self while telling the client to come to the dining room for lunch.
- [ ] **2.** Tell the client he needs to stop talking because it's time to eat lunch.
- [ ] **3.** Do not interrupt the client but wait for him to finish talking.
- [ ] **4.** Walk away and approach the client in a few minutes before the food gets cold.

63. A female client with acute mania brings six suitcases and three shopping bags of personal belongings on admission to the unit. When informed that some of the suitcases and bags need to be returned home with her husband because of a lack of storage space, the client begins to use profanity against the nurse. Which of the following responses by the nurse is most therapeutic?
- [ ] **1.** "You're acting inappropriately."
- [ ] **2.** "I won't tolerate your talking to me like that."
- [ ] **3.** "Swearing and profanity are unacceptable here."
- [ ] **4.** "We don't want to put you in seclusion yet."

64. The husband of a client who is experiencing acute mania and is swearing and using profanity apologizes to the nurse for his wife's behavior. Which of the following replies by the nurse is most therapeutic?
- [ ] **1.** "This must be difficult for you."
- [ ] **2.** "It's okay. We've heard worse."
- [ ] **3.** "How long has she been like this?"
- [ ] **4.** "She needs some medication."

65. The nurse overhears a client with acute mania who is euphoric and flirtatious attempting to be sexually inappropriate with other clients by talking about a sexual exploit to a group of clients seated at a table. Which of the following should the nurse do next?
- [ ] **1.** Continue walking down the hall, ignoring the conversation.
- [ ] **2.** Speak to the client later in private while saying nothing at this time.
- [ ] **3.** Tell the client others may not want to hear about sex, and invite him to play a game of ping-pong.
- [ ] **4.** Inform the client that if he continues to talk about sex no one will want to be around him.

66. The client with acute mania states to the nurse, "I'm the prince of peace and can save the world. Those against me will find me and take me to another world. They will come. I know it." The client is beginning to scan the room and starts to repeat his delusion. Which of the following responses by the nurse is most therapeutic?
- [ ] **1.** "Describe the people who will come."
- [ ] **2.** "The staff and I will protect you."
- [ ] **3.** "You are not the prince of peace. Your name is Joe."
- [ ] **4.** "Let's walk around the unit for a while."

67. A client with bipolar disorder, manic phase, is scheduled for a chest radiograph. Before taking the client to the radiology department, which of the following is most appropriate for the nurse to do?
- [ ] **1.** Give a thorough explanation of the procedure.
- [ ] **2.** Explain the procedure in simple terms.
- [ ] **3.** Call security to be on standby for possible problems.
- [ ] **4.** Cancel the appointment until the client can go unescorted.

68. A client exhibiting euphoria, hyperactivity, and distractibility cannot remain seated at mealtimes long enough to eat an adequate amount of food. When developing the client's plan of care, the nurse anticipates providing the client with "finger food" to eat while moving about the unit. Which of the following foods should the nurse expect to include in the client's plan of care?
- [ ] **1.** Bacon, lettuce, and tomato sandwich.
- [ ] **2.** Cheeseburger.
- [ ] **3.** Ice cream cone.
- [ ] **4.** Cut-up vegetables.

69. The client with bipolar disorder, manic phase, appears at the nurse's station wearing a transparent shirt, miniskirt, high heels, 10 bracelets, and 8 necklaces. Her makeup is overdone and she is not wearing underwear. A pair of inverted underpants is on her head. Which of the following should be the nurse's best response?
- [ ] **1.** Tell the client to dress appropriately while out of her room.
- [ ] **2.** Ask the client to put on hospital pajamas until she can dress appropriately.
- [ ] **3.** Instruct the client to go to her room and change clothes.
- [ ] **4.** Escort the client to her room and assist with choosing appropriate attire.

70. A client diagnosed with bipolar disorder, acute mania, states to the nurse, "Where is my son? I love Lucy. Rain, rain, go away. Dogs eat dirt." The nurse interprets these statements as indicating which of the following?
- [ ] **1.** Echolalia.
- [ ] **2.** Flight of ideas.
- [ ] **3.** Neologism.
- [ ] **4.** Clang associations.

71. The client with mania is skipping up and down the hallway practically running into other clients. Which of the following activities should the nurse expect to include in the client's plan of care?
- [ ] **1.** Leading a group activity.
- [ ] **2.** Watching television.
- [ ] **3.** Reading the newspaper.
- [ ] **4.** Cleaning the dayroom tables.

72. A client admitted to the unit with bipolar disorder, manic phase, is accompanied by his wife. The wife states that her husband has been overly energetic and happy, talking constantly, purchasing many unneeded items, and sleeping about 4 hours a night for the past 5 days. When completing the client's daily assessment, the nurse should be especially alert for which of the following findings?
- [ ] **1.** Exhaustion.
- [ ] **2.** Vertigo.
- [ ] **3.** Gastritis.
- [ ] **4.** Bradycardia.

73. The wife of a client with bipolar disorder, manic phase, states to the nurse, "He's acting so crazy. What did he do to get this way?" The nurse bases her response on the understanding of which of the following about this disorder?
- [ ] **1.** It is caused by underlying psychological difficulties.
- [ ] **2.** It is caused by disturbed family dynamics in the client's early life.
- [ ] **3.** It is the result of an imbalance of chemicals in the brain.
- [ ] **4.** It is the result of a genetic inheritance from someone in the family.

74. A client with acute mania has been taking lithium (Lithium Carbonate) 600 mg P.O. three times daily for 14 days. The nurse analyzes the client's serum lithium level, noting that it is therapeutic when the level is within which of the following ranges?
- [ ] **1.** 0.5 to 1.5 mEq/L.
- [ ] **2.** 1.6 to 2.5 mEq/L.
- [ ] **3.** 2.6 to 3.2 mEq/L.
- [ ] **4.** 3.3 to 4.0 mEq/L.

75. The client with bipolar disorder, manic phase, who is receiving lithium (Lithium Carbonate) 600 mg P.O. three times daily complains about being thirsty, feeling nauseous, and having slight shakiness of the hands. The nurse interprets these findings as indicating which of the following?
- [ ] **1.** An allergic reaction.
- [ ] **2.** Lithium toxicity.
- [ ] **3.** Common side effects.
- [ ] **4.** A drug interaction.

76. The physician orders determination of the serum lithium level tomorrow for a client with bipolar disorder, manic phase, who has been receiving lithium 300 mg P.O. three times daily for the past 5 days. At which of the following times should the nurse plan to have the blood specimen obtained?
- [ ] **1.** Before bedtime.
- [ ] **2.** After lunch.
- [ ] **3.** Before breakfast.
- [ ] **4.** During the afternoon.

77. A client will be discharged on lithium carbonate 600 mg three times daily. When teaching the client and his family about lithium therapy, the nurse determines that teaching has been effective if the client and family state that they will notify the prescribing health care provider immediately if which of the following occur? Select all that apply.
- [ ] 1. Nausea.
- [ ] 2. Muscle weakness.
- [ ] 3. Vertigo.
- [ ] 4. Fine hand tremor.
- [ ] 5. Vomiting.
- [ ] 6. Anorexia.

78. After the nurse teaches a client with bipolar disorder about lithium therapy, which of the following client statements indicates the need for additional teaching?
- [ ] 1. "It's important to keep using a regular amount of salt in my diet."
- [ ] 2. "It's okay to double my next dose of lithium if I forget a dose."
- [ ] 3. "I should drink about 8 to 10 eight-ounce glasses of water each day."
- [ ] 4. "I need to take my medicine at the same time each day."

79. A client with acute mania is to receive lithium carbonate 600 mg P.O. three times daily and 2 mg of haloperidol (Haldol) P.O. at bedtime. What should the nurse do?
- [ ] 1. Refuse to give the medications as ordered.
- [ ] 2. Give the lithium only.
- [ ] 3. Request a decreased dosage of lithium.
- [ ] 4. Give the medications as ordered.

80. After the nurse teaches a client about bipolar disorder, which of the following statements indicates that the client has developed insight about her condition?
- [ ] 1. "I enjoy feeling high. I don't need much sleep then and get really creative."
- [ ] 2. "My medicine really helped me. I know I won't need it in about another week."
- [ ] 3. "I'm cured now. I was really wild for a while even though I got into trouble."
- [ ] 4. "I know I'm getting sick when I don't need much sleep and start buying things."

81. During morning community meeting, a client with bipolar disorder, manic phase, interrupts others to the point where no one can finish their statements. Which of the following responses by the nurse is most appropriate?
- [ ] 1. "Please stop interrupting others. You can speak when it's your turn."
- [ ] 2. "Stop talking. It's time for you to leave the meeting."
- [ ] 3. "If you can't control yourself, we'll have to take action."
- [ ] 4. "Please behave like an adult. Your behavior is childish."

82. The physician orders valproic acid (Depakene) for a client with bipolar disorder who has achieved limited success with lithium carbonate (Lithane). Which of the following should the nurse anticipate including in the client's medication teaching plan?
- [ ] 1. Follow-up blood tests are unnecessary.
- [ ] 2. The tablet can be crushed if necessary.
- [ ] 3. Drowsiness and upset stomach are common side effects.
- [ ] 4. Consumption of a moderate amount of alcohol is safe.

83. The client with bipolar disorder, manic phase, has a valproic acid (Depakote) level of 15 µg/ml. Which of the following client behaviors should the nurse judge to be due to this level of valproic acid? Select all that apply.
- [ ] 1. Irritability.
- [ ] 2. Grandiosity.
- [ ] 3. Anhedonia.
- [ ] 4. Hypersomnia.
- [ ] 5. Flight of ideas.

84. The client with rapid-cycling bipolar disorder who is about to receive his 5 p.m. dose of carbamazepine (Tegretol) complains of a sore throat and chills. Which of the following should the nurse do next?
- [ ] 1. Administer the dose of carbamazepine.
- [ ] 2. Give the client acetaminophen (Tylenol) ordered p.r.n.
- [ ] 3. Report the symptoms to the physician in the morning.
- [ ] 4. Call the physician to report the symptoms.

85. A client's wife states, "I don't know what to do sometimes. It's so hard having a husband with a mental illness like bipolar disorder." After talking with the client's wife about her feelings and difficulties, which of the following actions is most appropriate?
- [ ] 1. Suggest that the wife see her physician.
- [ ] 2. Give the wife information about a support group.
- [ ] 3. Recommend that the wife talk with her close friend.
- [ ] 4. Have the wife share her feelings with her husband.

86. The client with bipolar disorder is approaching discharge after being hospitalized with her first episode of acute mania. The client's husband asks the nurse what he can do to help her. Which of the following recommendations for the husband should the nurse anticipate including in the teaching plan?
- [ ] 1. Help the client to be free from worry and anxiety.
- [ ] 2. Communicate openly and offer support.
- [ ] 3. Relieve the client of all responsibilities.
- [ ] 4. Remind the client to control her symptoms.

87. The client with bipolar disorder states to the nurse, "I guess the medication does help me after all. When I stopped taking it, I started to have trouble sleeping and my thoughts were racing." Which of the following replies by the nurse is therapeutic?
- [ ] 1. "I'm happy you realize that you started to get symptoms when you stopped your medication."
- [ ] 2. "Although it took a long time, you finally do understand that you need your medication."
- [ ] 3. "Why didn't you go to the community mental health center for help?"
- [ ] 4. "Didn't your family tell you that you were getting sick again?"

88. A client who is acutely manic and very anxious begins to pace, bump into furniture, and preach loudly. Which of the following is most appropriate for the nurse to do?
- [ ] 1. Walk with the client until he calms down.
- [ ] 2. Tell the client to go to his room.
- [ ] 3. Ask the client to sit in on a group therapy session.
- [ ] 4. Administer haloperidol (Haldol) ordered p.r.n.

89. The client with bipolar disorder, manic phase, has a nursing diagnosis of *Impaired social interaction.* The nurse judges that further intervention is needed for this diagnosis when the client demonstrates which behaviors? Select all that apply.
- [ ] 1. Interrupting group activities.
- [ ] 2. Changing clothes several times a day.
- [ ] 3. Jogging through the hallway.
- [ ] 4. Believing he is a famous king.
- [ ] 5. Stating others on the unit are stealing his socks.

90. The client with bipolar disorder, manic phase, states, "You're looking good. I'm taking you out to dinner." Which of the following replies by the nurse is most therapeutic?
- [ ] 1. "I don't want to go out to dinner."
- [ ] 2. "I can't go out to dinner with you."
- [ ] 3. "It doesn't matter how I look, the answer is no."
- [ ] 4. "I'm Chris Smith, a nurse working on this unit."

91. After the nurse administers haloperidol (Haldol) 5 mg P.O. to a client with acute mania, the client refuses to lie down on her bed, runs out on the unit, pushes clients in her vicinity out of the way, and screams threatening remarks to the staff. Which of the following should the nurse do next?
- [ ] 1. Follow the client and ask her to calm down.
- [ ] 2. Tell the client to lie down on the sofa in the community room.
- [ ] 3. Seclude the client and use restraints if necessary.
- [ ] 4. Tell the staff to ignore the client's remarks.

92. As the nurse is turning off the television, a client with bipolar disorder, manic phase, says, "I want the television on so I can watch the late show. I'm not tired and you can't tell me what to do. I want it on!" Which of the following responses by the nurse is most therapeutic?
- [ ] 1. "I'll let you watch television just this once. Don't tell anyone about this."
- [ ] 2. "I'll turn the television off when you get sleepy. Don't ask me to do this again."
- [ ] 3. "Television hours are from 7 to 10 p.m. It's 10 p.m., and the television goes off so everyone can sleep."
- [ ] 4. "The television goes off at 10 p.m. I've been telling you this for the past three evenings."

The Client with Suicidal Ideation and Suicide Attempt

93. The nurse manager in the emergency department (ED) is conducting an in-service for the nursing staff about screening clients for suicide. One of the nurses states, "Questioning adolescents about suicide will only increase their thinking about self-harm and they would not admit it to me anyhow." How should the nurse manager respond?
- [ ] 1. "You could be correct. Let's assess only adults because they'll be more honest."
- [ ] 2. "We will limit the assessment to adolescents with psychiatric diagnoses."
- [ ] 3. "It's a myth that talking about suicide leads to suicide attempts. Adolescents will disclose suicidal thoughts when asked directly."
- [ ] 4. "If you think the adolescent is not telling you the truth, you can question the parents."

94. When developing appropriate assignments for the staff, which of the following clients should the nurse manager judge to be at highest risk for suicide completion?
- [ ] 1. An 85-year-old Caucasian man who lives alone after his wife's death.
- [ ] 2. A 34-year-old single Hispanic woman who has recently been diagnosed with cancer.
- [ ] 3. A 15-year-old African American woman whose boyfriend broke up with her.
- [ ] 4. A 52-year-old Asian man who was terminated from his job because of downsizing.

95. When assessing a client for suicidal risk, which of the following methods of suicide should the nurse identify as most lethal?
- [ ] 1. Aspirin overdose.
- [ ] 2. Use of a gun.
- [ ] 3. Head-banging.
- [ ] 4. Wrist-cutting.

96. The nurse manager overhears two staff members talking in the snack room. One of the staff members states, "Her superficial cuts are just a means of getting our attention. She never should have been admitted. I hope she's out of here soon." Which of the following responses by the nurse manager is most appropriate?
- ☐ 1. "It's our job to help her no matter how we feel about her or what she did. She'll be discharged soon."
- ☐ 2. "I won't tolerate that kind of discussion from my staff. Now, it is time for you to go back to work."
- ☐ 3. "I know it's hard to understand, but we need to do the best we can even though she'll be back."
- ☐ 4. "No matter what the intent, all suicidal behavior is serious and deserves our serious consideration."

97. The history of a female client who has just been admitted to the unit and is very depressed reveals a weight loss of 10 lb in 2 weeks, sleeping 3 hours a night, and poor hygiene. The client states, "I'm no good to anyone. Everyone would be better off without me." Which of the following questions should the nurse ask first?
- ☐ 1. "What do you mean?"
- ☐ 2. "Are you thinking about hurting yourself?"
- ☐ 3. "Doesn't your family care about you?"
- ☐ 4. "What happened to make you think that?"

98. When developing the plan of care for a client with suicidal ideation, which of the following should the nurse anticipate as the priority?
- ☐ 1. Self-esteem.
- ☐ 2. Sleep.
- ☐ 3. Hygiene.
- ☐ 4. Safety.

99. Which of the following questions should the nurse ask to best determine the seriousness of a client's suicidal ideation?
- ☐ 1. "How are you planning on harming yourself?"
- ☐ 2. "Have you made out a will?"
- ☐ 3. "Does your family know you're here?"
- ☐ 4. "How long have you been thinking about harming yourself?"

100. The nursing assistant states to the nurse, "My client talks about how awful and useless she is. Sometimes she sounds angry for no reason. I'm tired of listening to her." Which of the following responses by the nurse is most appropriate?
- ☐ 1. "I'll switch your assignment to someone who's less depressed and less tiring."
- ☐ 2. "It's important for you to listen to her because she needs to verbalize how she is feeling."
- ☐ 3. "Don't worry about it. I know you haven't done anything to make her angry."
- ☐ 4. "Clients with depression are hard to deal with, but don't take what they say seriously."

101. A client states, "I'm so tired of living and just want to end it all." Which of the following responses is most therapeutic?
- ☐ 1. "I'll walk with you to your room so that you can get some rest."
- ☐ 2. "Perhaps after your son visits you'll feel better about things."
- ☐ 3. "You're in a lot of pain now but you will feel better. I'm here to help you."
- ☐ 4. "You are very depressed right now and want to die but you need to focus on life."

102. When developing staff assignments for the unit, the nurse manager should determine that which of the following clients needs one-to-one staff supervision?
- ☐ 1. The client who is sometimes preoccupied with death.
- ☐ 2. The client who tries to elope from the unit but is ambivalent about suicide.
- ☐ 3. The client who is impulsive and holds her breath until she faints.
- ☐ 4. The client who cannot sign a no-harm contract because of hallucinations.

103. A client who was recently discharged from the psychiatric unit telephones the unit to speak to the nurse. The client states that she took her children to the neighbors' house and has turned on the gas to kill herself. She is home alone and gives the nurse her address. Which of the following actions should the nurse do next?
- ☐ 1. Refer the caller to a 24-hour suicide hotline.
- ☐ 2. Tell the caller that another nurse will telephone the police.
- ☐ 3. Ask the caller whether she telephoned her physician.
- ☐ 4. Instruct the caller to telephone her family for help.

104. An adolescent walks into the clinic and tells the nurse she wants to die because her boyfriend broke up with her. The client states "I'll show him. He'll be sorry." The nurse interprets the client's statements as an expression of which of the following underlying themes?
- ☐ 1. Sadness.
- ☐ 2. Escape.
- ☐ 3. Loneliness.
- ☐ 4. Retaliation.

105. The client has been hospitalized for major depression and suicidal ideation. Which of the following statements indicates to the nurse that the client is improving?
- ☐ 1. "I couldn't kill myself because I don't want to go to hell."
- ☐ 2. "I don't think about killing myself as much as I used to."
- ☐ 3. "I'm of no use to anyone anymore."
- ☐ 4. "I know my kids don't need me anymore since they're grown."

106. The client states to the nurse at the outpatient clinic, "I don't feel ready to go back to work. It's only been a week since I left the hospital." Assessment reveals a flat affect, disheveled appearance, poor posture, and minimal eye contact during interaction. The nurse asks the client whether he is thinking about harming himself. The client tells the nurse he has a loaded revolver at home and will probably use it. Which of the following should the nurse do next?

☐ **1.** Tell the client to go and remove the gun from his home.

☐ **2.** Ask the client to call the nurse every hour when he gets home.

☐ **3.** Ask the client to promise not to harm himself.

☐ **4.** Initiate plans for hospitalization immediately.

107. The widow of a client who successfully completed suicide tearfully says, "I feel guilty because I'm so angry at him for killing himself. It must have been what he wanted." After assisting the widow with dealing with her feelings, which of the following is most helpful?

☐ **1.** Referring her to a group for survivors of suicide.

☐ **2.** Encouraging her to receive counseling from a chaplain.

☐ **3.** Providing her with the local suicide hotline number.

☐ **4.** Suggesting she receive individual therapy by the nurse.

108. The husband of a client to be discharged from the hospital after an episode of major depression and a suicide attempt asks, "What can I do if she tries to kill herself again?" Which of the following responses is most appropriate?

☐ **1.** "Don't worry. She'll be okay as long as she takes her medication."

☐ **2.** "She told me she wants to live so I don't think she'll try again."

☐ **3.** "Let's talk about some behavioral clues and resources that can help."

☐ **4.** "Tell her about your concern and just take care of her."

109. A client with depression is exhibiting a brighter affect, ability to attend to hygiene and grooming tasks, and beginning participation in group activities. The nurse asks the client to identify three of her strengths. After much hesitation and thinking, the client can state she is usually a nice person, a good cook, and a hard worker. Which of the following should the nurse do next?

☐ **1.** Ask the client to identify an additional three strengths.

☐ **2.** Volunteer the client to lead the cooking group later in the day.

☐ **3.** Educate the client about the importance of medication.

☐ **4.** Praise the client for identifying and sharing her strengths.

110. The friend of a client with depression and suicidal ideation asks the nurse, "How should I act around her?"" Which of the following responses by the nurse is best?

☐ **1.** "Try to cheer her up."

☐ **2.** "Be caring and genuine."

☐ **3.** "Control your expressions."

☐ **4.** "Avoid asking how she's feeling."

111. A client with depression and suicidal ideation voices feelings of self-doubt and powerlessness and is very dependent on the nurse for most aspects of her care. According to Erikson's stages of growth and development, the nurse determines the client to be manifesting problems in which of the following stages?

☐ **1.** Trust versus mistrust.

☐ **2.** Autonomy versus shame/doubt.

☐ **3.** Initiative versus guilt.

☐ **4.** Industry versus inferiority.

112. A 68-year-old client has improved with medication and treatment and no longer experiences suicidal ideation. She can manage her diabetic care and understands her diet requirements. She will be discharged to live alone in her apartment. Visits by which of the following individuals are most important for the nurse to arrange before the client's discharge?

☐ **1.** Psychiatric home care nurse.

☐ **2.** Medical social worker.

☐ **3.** Clergy.

☐ **4.** Unit volunteer.

113. A client who overdosed on barbiturates is being transferred to the inpatient psychiatric unit from the intensive care unit. The nurse receiving the client should anticipate which of the following as a priority?

☐ **1.** Nutrition.

☐ **2.** Sleep.

☐ **3.** Safety.

☐ **4.** Hygiene.

114. A client is brought to the psychiatric unit from the emergency department (ED) escorted by ED staff and a security officer. The client's shoulder is bandaged and his arm is in a sling because of a self-inflicted gunshot wound to his shoulder. Later, the client's wife follows with a bag of her husband's belongings. Which of the following nursing actions is most appropriate at this time?

☐ **1.** Tell the wife to take her husband's things home because he is suicidal.

☐ **2.** Instruct the wife to unpack the bag and put her husband's things in the dresser.

☐ **3.** Ask the wife whether the bag contains anything dangerous.

☐ **4.** Inspect the bag and its contents in the presence of the client and his wife.

115. A suicidal client is placed in the seclusion room and given lorazepam (Ativan) because she tried to harm herself by banging her head against the wall. After 10 minutes, the client starts to bang her head against the wall in the seclusion room. Which of the following should the nurse do next?
☐ **1.** Tell the client to stop doing that and act like a responsible adult.
☐ **2.** Place the client in leather restraints.
☐ **3.** Call the physician for additional medication orders.
☐ **4.** Instruct a staff member to sit in the room with the client.

116. A client lives in a group home and visits the community mental health center regularly. During one visit with the nurse, the client states, "The voices are telling me to hurt myself again." Which of the following questions by the nurse is most important to ask?
☐ **1.** "When do you hear the voices?"
☐ **2.** "Are you going to hurt yourself?"
☐ **3.** "How long have you heard the voices?"
☐ **4.** "Why are the voices starting again?"

117. A 20-year-old client diagnosed with paranoid schizophrenia is recovering from his first psychotic break. Before discharge from the hospital, the client becomes depressed and states, "I don't want this illness. I'm about to begin my junior year in college." The nurse determines that the client is planning for the future and is not at risk for self-harm. Which of the following areas should the nurse plan to help the client with in relation to his illness and continuation in college?
☐ **1.** Disturbed thought processes.
☐ **2.** Disturbed sensory perception.
☐ **3.** Communication strategies.
☐ **4.** Coping abilities.

118. The nurse is teaching two nursing assistants who are new to the inpatient unit about caring for a client who is suicidal. The nurse determines that additional teaching is needed when which of the following statements is made?
☐ **1.** "I need to check the client precisely at 15-minute intervals."
☐ **2.** "Documenting suicide checks is absolutely necessary."
☐ **3.** "Clients on one-to-one suicide precautions can never be left alone."
☐ **4.** "All clients using razors must be supervised by staff."

119. Which of the following activities should the nurse recommend to the client on an inpatient unit when thoughts of suicide occur?
☐ **1.** Keeping track of feelings in a journal.
☐ **2.** Reading a magazine.
☐ **3.** Talking with the nurse.
☐ **4.** Playing a card game with other clients.

120. Which of the following amounts should the nurse expect to give a client being treated with imipramine (Tofranil) on an outpatient basis for recurring depression and suicidal ideation?
☐ **1.** A 30-day supply.
☐ **2.** A 21-day supply.
☐ **3.** A 14-day supply.
☐ **4.** A 7-day supply.

121. The client with recurrent depression and suicidal ideation states to the nurse, "I can't afford this medicine anymore. I know I'll be okay without it." Which of the following is most appropriate for the nurse to do at this time?
☐ **1.** Inform the physician of the client's statement.
☐ **2.** Ask the social worker to find assistance for the client.
☐ **3.** Schedule a follow-up appointment in 3 months.
☐ **4.** Ask the client whether a family member could help.

Correct Answers and Rationales

The letter in parentheses after each rationale identifies the client need addressed in the item, including management of care (M), safety and infection control (S), health promotion and maintenance (H), psychosocial adaptation (P), basic care and comfort (C), pharmacological and parenteral therapies (D), reduction of risk potential (R), and physiological adaptation (A).

The Client with Major Depression

1. 1. Selegiline transdermal system is the first transdermal monoamine oxidase inhibitor. The client on Emsam needs to avoid exposing the application site to external sources of direct heat, such as saunas, heating lamps, electric blankets, heating pads, heated water beds, and prolonged direct sunlight because heat increases the amount of selegiline that is absorbed, resulting in elevated serum levels of selegiline. Cutting the patch and using a smaller piece will result in a decreased amount of medication absorption, most likely leading to a worsening of the symptoms of depression. The client should apply a new patch as soon as possible if one falls off to ensure an adequate amount of medication absorption. Emsam is not associated with significant weight gain, although a weight gain of 1 to 2 lb (2.2 to 4.4 kg) is possible. (D)

2. 3. The nurse should report the client's beer consumption to the physician. Duloxetine should not be administered to a client with renal or hepatic insufficiency because the medication can elevate liver enzymes and, together with substantial alcohol use, can cause liver injury. Referring the client to the dual diagnosis program, sharing information at the next interdisciplinary treatment conference, and teaching the client relaxation exercises are helpful interventions for the nurse to implement. However, reporting the findings to the physician is most important. (D)

3. 2. The client's sudden improvement and decrease in anxiety most likely indicates that the client is relieved because he has made the decision to kill himself and may now have the energy to complete the suicide. Symptoms of severe depression do not suddenly abate because most antidepressants work slowly and take 2 to 4 weeks to provide a maximum benefit. The client will improve slowly due to the medication. The sudden improvement in symptoms does not mean the client is nearing discharge and decreasing observation of the client compromises the client's safety. (P)

4. 1, 2, 5. It is important for the nurse to obtain information about the client's use of tea, herbal medicine, and a folk healer because the information is critical to the safe prescription of psychotropic medication. Breathing exercises, massage, and acupuncture are also traditional therapies used by the Asian American population, but do not interfere with the use of medications. (D)

5. 1. The nurse should immediately report the rash to the physician because lamotrigine can cause Stevens-Johnson syndrome, a toxic epidermal necrolysis. The rash is not a temporary adverse effect. Giving the client an ice pack and questioning the client about recent sun exposure are irresponsible nursing actions because of the possible seriousness of the rash. (D)

6. 2. The nurse should hold the 5 p.m. dose of lithium because a level of 1.8 mEq/L can cause adverse reactions, including diarrhea, vomiting, drowsiness, muscle weakness, and lack of coordination, which are early signs of lithium toxicity. The nurse should report the lithium level to the physician, including any symptoms of toxicity. Administering the 5 p.m. dose of lithium, giving the client the lithium with 8 oz (236 ml) of water, or giving it after supper would result in an increase of the lithium level, thus increasing the risk of lithium toxicity. (D)

7. 3. Additional teaching is needed for the family member who states her son will only need to attend outpatient appointments when he starts to feel depressed again. Compliance with medication and outpatient follow-up are key in preventing relapse and rehospitalization. The statements expressing expectations of feeling better as medication takes effect, needing medicine and group therapy to stay well, and needing help with grocery shopping, cooking, and cleaning for a while indicate the families' understanding of depression, medication, and follow-up care. (P)

8. 1. "My stomach is rotting," is a somatic delusion congruent with a depressed mood. "They are talking about me," is a delusion of reference. "I am Superman," is a delusion of grandeur. "The FBI will find me," is a paranoid delusion. (P)

9. 4. The nurse closely monitors the client taking paroxetine for the development of agitation, which could lead to self-harm in the form of a suicide attempt. Headache, nausea, and fatigue are transient adverse effects of paroxetine. (D)

10. 4. The nurse must continually assess the client for suicidal ideation because the client with a mental health disorder, especially schizophrenia, depression, and alcoholism, is at a higher risk for suicide than the general adult population. Death of a psychiatric client by suicide is particularly important to the nurse because of her responsibility for assessment and intervention. Although sleep disturbances, feelings of worthlessness, and difficulty with concentration are associated with major depression, assessment of suicidal ideation is essential. Feelings of worthlessness may contribute to the client's potential for suicidal ideation. (P)

11. 3. Endogenous depression (depression coming from within the person) is biochemical in nature. The biologic theory of depression indicates a neurotransmitter imbalance involving serotonin, norepinephrine, and possibly dopamine. Reactive depression is caused by the occurrence of something happening outside the body, such as the death of a loved one or another significant loss. Stating that the client will improve with the right medication or that family members seem supportive does not address the client's immediate concerns of not knowing the cause of the depression. Discussing possible reasons for the client's depression is nontherapeutic because the depression is endogenous and biochemically based. (P)

12. 2. The nurse should initiate brief, frequent contacts throughout the day to let the client know that he is important to the nurse. This will positively affect the client's self-esteem. The nurse's action conveys acceptance of the client as a worthwhile person and provides some structure to the seemingly monotonous day. Waiting for the client to begin the conversation with the nurse is not helpful because the depressed client resists interaction and involvement with others. Sitting outside of the client's room is not productive and not necessary in this situation. If the client were actively suicidal, then a one-on-one client-to-staff assignment would be necessary. Questioning the client until he responds would overwhelm him because he could not meet the nurse's expectations to interact. (P)

13. 1. The most appropriate action is for the nurse to remain with the client even if the client does not engage in conversation with the nurse. A client with severe depression may be unable to engage in an interaction with the nurse because the client feels worthless and lacks the necessary energy to do so. However, the nurse's presence conveys acceptance and caring, thus helping to increase the client's self-worth. Telling the client that the nurse will come back later, stating that the nurse will find someone else for the client to talk with, or telling the client that the nurse will get her something to read conveys to the client that she is not important, reinforcing the client's negative view of herself. Additionally, such statements interfere with the client's development of a sense of security and trust in the nurse. (P)

14. 4. The nurse tells the client that the nurse is interested in her to increase the client's sense of importance, worth, and self-esteem. Also, stating that the nurse wants to help conveys to the client that she is worthwhile and important. Telling the client that the nurse is assigned to care for her is impersonal and implies that the client is being uncooperative. Telling the client that the nurse is there because the client has potential for improvement will not help the client with low self-esteem because most people develop a sense of self-worth through accomplishment. Simply saying that the client has a lot of potential will not convince her that she is worthwhile. Telling the client that the nurse will talk to someone else later is not client-focused and does not address the client's question or concern. (P)

15. 2. Nausea and gastrointestinal upset is a common, but usually temporary, side effect of paroxetine (Paxil). Therefore, the nurse would instruct the client to take the medication with food to minimize nausea and stomach upset. Other more common side effects are dry mouth, constipation, headache, dizziness, sweating, loss of appetite, ejaculatory problems in men, and decreased orgasms in women. Taking the medication an hour before breakfast would most likely lead to further gastrointestinal upset. Taking the medication at bedtime is not recommended because Paxil can cause nervousness and interfere with sleep. Because orange juice is acidic, taking the medication with it, especially on an empty stomach, may lead to nausea or increase the client's gastrointestinal upset. (D)

16. 2. The presence of dizziness could indicate orthostatic hypotension, which may cause injury to the client from falling. Nausea, sedation, and dry mouth do not require immediate intervention by the nurse. (D)

17. 3. Symptom relief can occur during the 1st week of therapy, with optimal effects possible within 2 weeks. For some clients, 2 to 4 weeks is needed for optimal effects. The client's statement that the depression will be gone in 5 to 7 days indicates to the nurse that clarification and further teaching is needed. Trazodone should be taken after a meal or light snack to enhance its absorption. Trazodone can cause drowsiness, and therefore the major portion of the drug should be taken at bedtime. The depressant effects of central nervous system depressants and alcohol may be potentiated by this drug. (D)

18. 3. The nurse should explain that ECT is a safe treatment and that the client is given an ultra–short-acting anesthetic to induce sleep before ECT and a muscle relaxant to prevent musculoskeletal complications during the convulsion, which typically lasts 30 to 60 seconds to be therapeutic. Atropine is given before ECT to inhibit salivation and respiratory tract secretions and thereby minimize the risk of aspiration. Medication for pain is not necessary and is not given before or during the treatment. Some clients experience a headache after the treatment and may request and be given an analgesic such as acetaminophen (Tylenol). Telling the daughter that the physician will ensure that the client does not suffer needlessly would not provide accurate information about ECT. This statement also implies that the client will have pain during the treatment, which is untrue. (R)

19. 4. Reaction formation is a conscious behavior that is the opposite of an unconscious feeling. The client compliments her boss when, unconsciously, she most likely does not like him because he fired her. Repression refers to the unconscious forgetting of painful ideas, events, or conflicts. For example, a car accident victim cannot remember details about the accident but at the time was aware of what had happened. Suppression refers to the voluntary exclusion of anxiety-producing feelings, ideas, and situations from awareness. For example, a client states that he doesn't want to talk about his impending divorce. Intellectualization occurs when the client uses only logical explanations without feelings or an affective component. For example, a client talks about her son's recent bout with leukemia and subsequent death as being mercifully short while at the same time not displaying signs of sadness. (P)

20. 1. By stating, "It must have been very upsetting for you," the nurse conveys empathy to the client by recognizing the underlying meaning of a painful occurrence. The nurse's statement invites the client to verbalize feelings and thoughts and lets the client know that the nurse is listening to and respects the client. Telling the client to talk about the job disregards the client's feelings and is nontherapeutic for the depressed client because of underlying feelings of worthlessness and guilt that are commonly present. Telling the client that he will find another job when he is better or that he was probably too depressed to work is inappropriate because it disregards the client's feelings and may promote additional feelings of failure and inadequacy in the client. (P)

21. 2. The client's negative thinking and statements are directly related to the psychopathology of depression. The client's views and feelings about herself reflect low self-esteem. Although *Impaired social interaction, Risk for self-directed violence,* and *Ineffective coping* are possible nursing diagnoses, there are insufficient data to support these diagnoses. Further assessment is needed to identify supportive data. (P)

22. **4.** The client with depression is preoccupied, has decreased energy, and cannot make decisions, even simple ones. Therefore, the nurse presents the situation, "It's time for a shower," and assists the client with personal hygiene to preserve his dignity and self-esteem. Explaining the importance of good hygiene to the client is inappropriate because the client may know the benefits of hygiene but is too fatigued and preoccupied to pay attention to self-care. Asking the client if he is ready for a shower is not helpful because the client with depression commonly cannot make even simple decisions. This action also reinforces the client's feeling about not caring about showering. Waiting for the family to visit to help with the client's hygiene is inappropriate and irresponsible on the part of the nurse. The nurse is responsible for making basic decisions for the client until the client can make decisions for himself. (P)

23. **4.** By saying, "You were able to bathe today," the nurse is pointing out a visible accomplishment or strength, thereby increasing the client's feelings of self-worth and self-esteem. Stating that "everybody around here likes you" or discussing what the client has done correctly is inappropriate because although the client may agree with the nurse, the client still may be depressed. Stating that the nurse sees many good qualities in the client is not helpful because a person's feeling of self-worth is generally determined by accomplishments. Intellectual understanding does not help the client with severe depression. Additionally, the nurse cannot talk a client out of depression because major depression is endogenous and biochemical in nature. Medication should restore the neurotransmitter balance and relieve the depression. (P)

24. **1.** The family needs to be informed that some confusion and disorientation will occur as the client emerges from anesthesia immediately after ECT, to lessen their fear and anxiety about the procedure. The nurse will assist the client with reorientation (time, person, and place) and will give clear, simple instructions. The client may need to lie down after ECT because of the effects of the anesthesia. Informing the family that there is a danger of aspiration during ECT is inappropriate and unnecessary. The risk of aspiration occurring during ECT is minimal because food and fluids are withheld for 6 to 8 hours before the treatment. In addition, the client receives atropine to inhibit salivation and respiratory tract secretions. Telling the family that the client will not be able to breathe independently during ECT may frighten them unnecessarily. If asked, the nurse should inform the family that the anesthesiologist mechanically ventilates the client with 100% oxygen immediately before the treatment. The client with severe depression responds to ECT. Usually, ECT is used for those who are severely depressed and not responding to pharmacotherapy and for those who are highly suicidal. (P)

25. **2.** Sertraline, like other selective serotonin reuptake inhibitors (SSRIs), can cause decreased libido and sexual dysfunction such as delayed ejaculation in men and an inability to achieve orgasm in women. SSRIs do not typically cause weight gain but may cause loss of appetite and weight loss. Dry mouth is a possible side effect, but it is temporary. The client should be told to take sips of water, suck on ice chips, or use sugarless gum or candy. St. John's wort should not be taken with SSRIs because a severe reaction could occur. (D)

26. **3.** It is best to involve the client in usual at-home activities as much as the client can tolerate them. Discouraging visitors may not be in the client's best interest because visits with supportive significant others will help reinforce supportive relationships, which are important to the client's self-worth and self-esteem. Providing for a schedule of activities outside the home may be overwhelming for the client initially. Involving the client in planning for outside activities would be appropriate. Encouraging the client to sleep as much as possible is nontherapeutic and promotes withdrawal from others. (P)

27. **4.** Medication management with outpatient follow-up is of vital importance to discuss with the client before discharge. The nurse teaches and clarifies any questions related to medication and outpatient treatment. The client also has the opportunity to voice feelings related to medication and treatment. The goal is to assist the client in making a successful transition from hospital to home with optimal functioning outside the hospital for as long as possible. The nurse may also need to assist with decreasing any anxiety the client may have related to discharge. Discussing future plans for returning to work or employment is not as immediate a concern as assisting with medication and treatment compliance. Noncompliance with medication is a primary cause of relapse in a client with a psychiatric disorder. Reviewing a conflict the client had encountered with another client is not appropriate or therapeutic at this time unless the client brings it to the nurse's attention. The conflict should have been dealt with and resolved when it occurred. Reviewing the results of psychological testing is the responsibility of the physician if he chooses. (P)

28. **2.** Criteria for commitment include being gravely disabled and posing a harm to self or others. This client is not threatening to harm himself in the form of suicide or to harm others. The client is gravely disabled because of his inability to care for himself—namely, not eating because of his delusion. Evidence of psychosis or psychotic symptoms or diagnosis of a mental illness alone does not make the client legally eligible for commitment. (M)

29. **3.** The client needs to be informed of the time lag involved with antidepressant therapy. Although improvement in the client's symptoms will occur gradually over the course of 1 to 2 weeks, typically it takes 2 to 4 weeks to get the full effects of the medication. This information will help the client be compliant with medication and will also help in decreasing any anxiety the client has about not feeling better. The client's dose may not need to be increased; it is too early to determine the full effectiveness of the drug. Additionally, such a statement may increase the client's anxiety and diminish self-worth. Telling the client to wait a few days discounts the client's feelings and is inappropriate. Although it is too soon to tell whether the medication will be effective, telling this to the client may cause the client undue distress. This statement is somewhat negative because it is possible that the medication will not be effective, possibly further compounding the client's anxiety about not feeling better. (D)

30. **1, 2, 3, 5, 6.** Serotonin syndrome can occur if a selective serotonin reuptake inhibitor is combined with a monoamine oxidase inhibitor, a tryptophan-serotonin precursor, or St. John's wort. Signs and symptoms of serotonin syndrome include mental status changes, such as confusion, restlessness or agitation, headache, diaphoresis, ataxia, myoclonus, shivering, tremor, diarrhea, nausea, abdominal cramps, and hyperreflexia. Constipation is not associated with serotonin syndrome. (D)

31. **2.** Phenelzine is a monoamine oxidase inhibitor (MAOI). MAOIs block the enzyme monoamine oxidase, which is involved in the decomposition and inactivation of norepinephrine, serotonin, dopamine, and tyramine (a precursor to the previously stated neurotransmitters). Foods high in tyramine—those that are fermented, pickled, aged, or smoked—must be avoided because, when they are ingested in combination with MAOIs, a hypertensive crisis occurs. Some examples include salami, bologna, dried fish, sour cream, yogurt, aged cheese, bananas, pickled herring, caffeinated beverages, chocolate, licorice, beer, Chianti, and alcohol-free beer. (D)

32. **4.** The nurse should first take the client's vital signs because the client could be experiencing a hypertensive crisis, which requires prompt intervention. Signs and symptoms of a hypertensive crisis include occipital headache, a stiff or sore neck, nausea, vomiting, sweating, dilated pupils and photophobia, nosebleed, tachycardia, bradycardia, and constricting chest pain. Giving this client an analgesic without taking his vital signs first is inappropriate. After the client's vital signs have been obtained, then the nurse would call the physician to report the client's complaints and vital signs. Administering the client's next dose of phenelzine before taking his vital signs could result in a dangerous situation if the client is experiencing a hypertensive crisis. (D)

33. **2.** A depressed client commonly is not interested in eating because of the psychopathology of the disorder. Therefore, the nurse must take responsibility to ensure that the client eats, including spoon-feeding the client (placing the food on the spoon, putting the food near the client's mouth, and asking her to eat) if necessary. Serving the client her tray in her room does not ensure that she will eat. Calling the family to bring the client food from home usually is allowed, but it is still the nurse's responsibility to ensure that the client eats. Explaining the importance of nutrition in recovery is not helpful. The client may intellectually know that eating is important but may not be interested in eating or want to eat. (P)

34. **1.** To promote adequate rest (6 to 8 hours per night) and to eliminate hyposomnia, the nurse should sit with the client at the bedside until the medication takes effect. The presence of a caring nurse provides the client with comfort and security and helps to decrease the client's anxiety. Engaging the client in interaction until the client falls asleep, reading to the client, or encouraging the client to watch television may be too stimulating for the client, consequently increasing rather than decreasing the client's restlessness. (P)

35. **3.** The client who verbalizes feeling in control of self and situations no longer feels powerless to affect an outcome but realizes that one's actions can have an impact on self and situations. It is common for the client with depression to feel powerless to affect an outcome and to feel a lack of control over a situation. Although interacting with staff and peers is a positive action, the client could be conversing in a negative or nontherapeutic manner. Sleeping 4 hours in the afternoon and 4 hours at night is evidence of symptomatology and does not indicate improvement or recovery. Verbalizing dissatisfaction over not being able to perform at work indicates that the client is most likely focusing on shortcomings and powerlessness. (P)

36. **2.** The nurse must monitor the client for a suicide attempt at this time when the client is starting to feel better because the depressed client may now have enough energy to carry out an attempt. Bupropion inhibits dopamine reuptake; it is an activating antidepressant and could cause agitation. Although bupropion lowers the seizure threshold, especially at doses greater than 450 mg per day, and visual disturbances and increased libido are possible adverse effects, the nurse must closely monitor the client for suicide attempt. As the client with major depression begins to feel better, the client may have enough energy to carry out an attempt. (P)

37. **4.** In the initial plan of care, the most appropriate outcome would be that the client will interact with the nurse. First, the client would begin interacting with one individual, the nurse. The nurse would gradually assist the client to engage in interactions with other clients in one-on-one contacts, progressing toward informal group gatherings and eventually taking part in structured group activities. The client needs to experience success according to the client's level of tolerance. Initiating interactions with peers occurs when the client can gain a measure of confidence and self-esteem instead of feeling intimidated or unduly anxious. Discussing adaptive coping techniques is an outcome the client may be able to reach when symptoms are not as severe and the client can concentrate on improving coping skills. (P)

38. **3.** Imipramine, a tricyclic antidepressant, in combination with alcohol will produce additive central nervous system depression. Although caffeinated coffee is safe to use when the client is taking imipramine, it is not recommended for a client with depression who may be experiencing sleep disturbances. Imipramine may cause photosensitivity so the client would be instructed to use sunscreen and protective clothing when exposed to the sun. Reduced lacrimation may occur as a side effect of imipramine. Therefore, the use of artificial tears may be recommended. (D)

39. **1.** Telling the client that ECGs are done routinely for all clients taking imipramine, a tricyclic antidepressant, is an honest and direct response. Additionally, it provides some reassurance for the client. Commonly, a client with depression will ruminate, leading needlessly to increased anxiety. Tricyclic antidepressants may cause tachycardia, ECG changes, and cardiotoxicity. Telling the client that it's probably a precautionary measure because the nurse is not aware of a cardiac condition instills doubt and may cause undue anxiety for the client. Telling the client not to worry because the doctor is very thorough dismisses the client's concern and does not give the client adequate information. Explaining that the client had an ECG before initiating therapy with imipramine and that the procedure will be the same does not answer the client's question. (D)

40. **2.** The therapeutic serum concentration level for imipramine is 150 to 250 mg/ml. At the upper limit of the therapeutic range, serious cardiac and central nervous system effects may begin to develop. (D)

41. **4.** Anticholinergic effects, which result from blockage of the parasympathetic (craniosacral) nervous system, include urine retention, blurred vision, dry mouth, and constipation. Tremors, cardiac arrhythmias, and sexual dysfunction are possible side effects, but they are caused by increased norepinephrine availability. Sedation and delirium are not anticholinergic effects. Sedation may be a therapeutic effect because many clients with depression experience agitation and insomnia. Delirium, typically not a side effect, would indicate toxicity, especially in elderly clients. Respiratory depression, convulsions, ataxia, agitation, stupor, and coma indicate tricyclic antidepressant toxicity. (D)

42. **2.** Doxepin and other tricyclic antidepressants may cause postural hypotension, especially in the morning. Postural hypotension occurs because the tricyclic antidepressant inhibits the body's natural vasoconstrictive reaction when a person stands. The nurse regularly monitors the client's vital signs, both lying and standing. The nurse should instruct the client to rise slowly and dangle his feet before standing. Advising the client to take a hot shower is detrimental to the client's safety. Heat causes vasodilation, which could further exacerbate the dizziness, placing the client at risk for falls and subsequent injury. Telling the client to stay in bed until he is feeling better is not helpful and is impractical. The client with depression would rather stay in bed and withdraw from others. Placing the client on fluid restriction is detrimental to the client with depression whose fluid and food intake may be inadequate. (D)

43. **1.** The nurse should give the medication as ordered. Mirtazapine is given once daily, preferably at bedtime to minimize the risk of injury resulting from postural hypotension and sedative effects. The usual dosage ranges from 15 to 45 mg. There is no reason to question the physician's order. The nurse should administer the medication as ordered. Requesting to give the medication in three divided doses is inappropriate and demonstrates the nurse's lack of knowledge about the drug. (D)

44. **4.** Stating, "I hear how difficult this is for you and will help you talk with your doctor about it," conveys empathy and is focused on the client's request. Offering to talk to the physician with the client lends support and forms a therapeutic alliance with the client. The client who has stopped taking medication must be taken seriously because medication noncompliance is an issue here and could result in a recurrence of symptoms of depression, leading to many adverse effects. Discussing the client's diet, exercise, and daily activities may not be helpful at this point because the client has stopped taking the medication. Pointing out that the medication has helped the client or telling the client that positive things have happened since the depression improved may be true, but these responses do not focus on the client's feelings and needs at the present time. (P)

45. 3. Compliance with medication therapy is crucial for the client with depression. Medication noncompliance is the primary cause of relapse among psychiatric clients. Therefore, the nurse needs to teach the client about managing common adverse effects to promote compliance with medication. Teaching the client about the medication's pharmacokinetics may help the client to understand the reason for the drug. However, teaching about how to manage common adverse effects to promote compliance is crucial. Current research about the medication is more important to the nurse than to the client. Teaching about dosage regulation and adjustment of medication may be helpful, but typically the physician, not the client, is the person in charge of this aspect. (D)

46. 2. Client manifestations such as sleep, appetite, or psychomotor disturbances (agitation and anxiety) should improve first with pharmacologic therapy. Cognitive symptoms of depression, such as low self-esteem, guilt, pessimism, suicidal thought, lack of concentration, and indecision tend to improve more slowly. Disturbances in the client's ability to concentrate take longer to improve. The client's depressed mood may be the last symptom to show improvement. (D)

47. 4. Dry mouth is a common, temporary side effect of paroxetine. The nurse needs to further assess the client's water intake when the client states she is drinking lots of water. Excessive intake of water could be harmful to the client and could lead to electrolyte imbalance. Dry mouth is caused by the medication, and drinking a lot of water will not eliminate it. Sucking on ice chips or using sugarless gum or candy is appropriate to ease the discomfort of dry mouth associated with paroxetine. (D)

48. 2, 3, 5. Symptoms of depression include depressed mood, anhedonia, appetite disturbance, sleep disturbance, psychomotor disturbance, fatigue, feelings of worthlessness, excessive or inappropriate guilt, decreased concentration, and recurrent thoughts of death or suicide. Paroxetine is a selective serotonin reuptake inhibitor antidepressant that also can be used to treat anxiety. Improved concentration, verbalization of feelings, and decreased agitation or pacing are signs of improvement. Taking 2-hour evening naps daily is still a sign of fatigue or lack of energy, and the increased use of somatization (bodily complaints) could be signs of continued symptoms of depression. (D)

49. 3. The most important behavior to report to the next shift is that the client was able to sleep from 11 p.m. to 6 a.m. This indicates that improvement in the symptoms of depression is occurring as a result of pharmacologic therapy. The nurse would expect to observe improvement in sleep, appetite, and psychomotor behavior first before improvement in cognitive symptoms. The client's flat affect is still a symptom of depression. The fact that the client had a visitor is not as important as changes in the client's behavior. Spending the evening in the room is a continuation of the client's withdrawn behavior and is important to report but not as important as the improvement in sleep. (P)

50. 4. A favorable response by a family member to a medication and a previous response to medication are good predictors of a favorable client response to a medication because the illness is genetic and hereditary. Although the side effects of the drug, the client's age at diagnosis, and the cost of the medication are important factors to consider when choosing antidepressant therapy, this information does not necessarily predict how a client will respond to a specific drug. (D)

51. 3. Dysthymia is a less severe, chronic depression diagnosed when a client has had a depressed mood for more days than not for at least 2 years. The client with dysthymic disorder benefits from psychotherapeutic approaches that assist the client in reversing the negative self-image, negative feelings about the future, and poor self-esteem that are typically part of the clinical presentation. Antidepressant therapy usually is not prescribed for the client with dysthymic disorder unless the client experiences an episode of major depression. Electroconvulsive therapy is appropriate treatment for severe depression, not dysthymic disorder. Psychoanalysis is an inappropriate treatment for dysthymic disorder. (M)

The Client with Bipolar Disorder, Manic Phase

52. 3. The nurse should concisely explain the benefit of the medication to the client to increase the possibility of compliance. The client has the right to refuse treatment, which in this instance is the medication. If the client was under involuntary commitment and the hospital had received a court order to treat, the client would have to comply with taking the medication and the physician would usually order the medication to be give intramuscularly if the oral medication was refused. The nurse would not threaten the client by stating that a shot will be given when there is no physician order and court order to treat. Giving written medication information to a client with acute mania is poor nursing judgment because a client with acute mania cannot benefit from written information due to his impaired ability to focus and concentrate. (M)

53. 2. The nurse clearly informs the client about behavior that is unacceptable on the unit, such as voicing jokes with sexual content and touching others. Setting limits on behavior provides safety and security to the client and conveys to the client that he is worthy of help. Saying "she will not want to be around you with that kind of talk" and "you need to be careful about what you say to others" does not clearly inform the client about behaviors that are unacceptable and implies that the client can control behaviors if he chooses. A time-out in the client's room does not inform the client about the inappropriateness of his behaviors and could be interpreted by the client as punitive as well as diminishing his self-esteem. (P)

54. **3.** The nurse states her identity and purpose for being on the unit to clarify any misperception by the client. Saying "thank you for being so kind," "I know you are only teasing me," or "I am not here to receive compliments from clients" are nontherapeutic statements and do not clarify the nurse's identity and purpose. (P)

55. **3.** The nurse should medicate the client who does not respond to verbal interventions and whose anxiety is escalating. This will reduce the client's anxiety and agitation and prevent harm or injury to the client and others. Seclusion, restraint, and controlling the client are a last resort and require a physician's order and close assessment for when the orders can be discontinued. (P)

56. **4.** The nurse should help the nursing assistant understand the client's behavior by stating that his irritable mood is a symptom of mania. Not all clients with mania are euphoric or have an expansive mood. Saying, "It's our responsibility to listen to him even though we might not like what he's saying" does not help the nursing assistant understand the client with mania. Reprimanding the client for his behavior or asking him to control his behavior are inappropriate actions and show poor nursing judgment and a lack of understanding of the manic client. (P)

57. **1, 2, 3, 5.** Scheduled rest periods, relaxation exercises, and listening to soft music are activities that reduce environmental stimuli for the client who is hyperactive, talkative, easily distracted, irritable, and angry. Aerobic exercise is also beneficial to discharge some of the client's need to be active. Watching television is not therapeutic because it would stimulate the client with acute mania. (P)

58. **2.** Symptoms of hypomania are less severe than those of mania and include elevated, expansive, or irritable mood, increased self-esteem, decreased need for sleep, distractibility, increase in goal-directed activity, flight of ideas or racing thoughts, and excessive involvement in pleasurable activities. The client with hypomania remains in contact with reality and does not have delusions or hallucinations. Usually, the episode is not severe enough to cause major problems at home, work, or school. (P)

59. **1.** The nurse should administer the medication as ordered. Lithium has a clinical response lag time of 1 to 2 weeks. Haloperidol is prescribed temporarily to produce a neuroleptic effect until the lithium starts to produce a clinical response. Haldol is usually discontinued when the lithium starts to take effect. (D)

60. **4.** The client's statement, "I'm the Queen of England. Bow before me," is an example of a grandiose delusion and refers to thought content of the mental status examination. Examples of psychomotor behavior to be documented would include excited, typically exaggerated and repetitive physical movements and excessive talking and gesturing. Mood is a subjective state, and affect is an observable expression of emotion. Mood is what a client tells you she is feeling, and affect is what you see the client feeling. For example, the client may state that she feels sad or happy in reference to mood. Affect refers to the display of physical emotion, commonly described as "appropriate" or "flat." Attitude toward the nurse refers to the client's behavior in the presence of the nurse during the mental status examination (pleasant and cooperative, irritable and guarded). (P)

61. **3.** The client is exhibiting a labile affect or an affect that quickly changes (for example, from happy to sad). A flat affect refers to an absence of facial expression or an expression that does not change even though the topic of what the client is verbalizing changes. An example would be a client maintaining a flat affect or absence of expression while talking about a party, a television show, and a sad event. A blunted affect is an incomplete expression. For example, the corner of the mouth can indicate a hint of a smile. Normal affect is one that changes appropriately with the topic of conversation. (P)

62. **1.** The nurse would excuse herself, showing respect and regard for the client, while telling the client to come to the dining room for lunch. Acutely manic clients need clear, concise comments and directions. Telling the client that he needs to stop talking because it's lunchtime is disrespectful and does not give the client directions for what he needs to do. Using the familiar skill of waiting without interrupting until the person pauses would not be effective with the very talkative, manic client. Walking away and approaching the client after a few minutes before the food gets cold is not helpful because the client would probably continue talking. (P)

63. **3.** By stating to the client, "Swearing and profanity is unacceptable here," the nurse is setting limits in a nonpunitive manner for behavior that is inappropriate or threatening to other clients and staff. Setting limits helps the client regain self-control, prevents alienation from others, and preserves self-esteem. It is common for the irritable manic client to misperceive the nurse's and other's statements and intentions, feel threatened, and respond in a manner that is out of character for the client when not in a manic phase. Stating that the client is acting very inappropriately, that the nurse will not tolerate the client's swearing and profanity, or threatening to put the client in seclusion is threatening and punitive and thus nontherapeutic. (P)

64. **1.** Stating that this must be difficult for the husband conveys empathy and understanding and offers him the opportunity to voice his feelings to the nurse. Telling the husband that it is okay and that the nurse has heard worse is inappropriate and minimizes the impact of the wife's illness on the husband. Asking about the length of the client's illness or telling the husband that his wife needs some medication ignores the husband's feelings, thereby minimizing his self-respect. (P)

65. **3.** Telling the client that others may not want to hear about sex and inviting him to play a game of ping-pong with the nurse informs the client that even though his behavior is unacceptable, the nurse considers him worthy of help. The client's thoughts and actions are out of control, and directing him to an activity with the nurse is an appropriate way of regaining control. The nurse is responsible for providing safety and security to this client and others on the unit. Continuing to walk down the hall while ignoring the conversation does nothing to meet the needs of this or other clients. Doing so also diminishes trust in the nurse. Speaking to the client later in private while saying nothing at the time allows the client to continue his provocative behavior instead of focusing his energy toward productive activity. Informing the client that if he continues to talk about sex, no one will want to be around him is not helpful because his behavior is a symptom of his illness and the statement diminishes his self-worth. (P)

66. **4.** The nurse suggests an activity such as walking around the unit to distract the client from the paranoid grandiose delusion that could result in loss of control. This action interrupts the client's anxious state and helps to redirect energy and focus on an activity based in reality. The focus must be on the underlying need or feeling of the delusion and not on the content. Asking the client to describe the people who will come challenges the client and forces the client to cling to the delusion. Stating that the nurse and staff will protect the client conveys agreement with the client's belief system, reinforcing the client's delusion. Telling the client that he is not the prince of peace and repeating his name challenges the client and his present belief system. Doing so may lead to decreased trust in the nurse and an aggressive response, or it may force the client to defend his beliefs. (P)

67. **2.** The nurse needs to explain the procedure in simple terms because the client in a manic phase has difficulty concentrating, is easily distracted, and can misinterpret what the nurse states. Giving a thorough explanation of the procedure is not helpful and can confuse the client. Calling security to be on standby is inappropriate. If the nurse judges that the client might elope or become agitated, the nurse should schedule the appointment for another time. Canceling the appointment until the client can go unescorted is impractical and may not follow unit or hospital policy and the client's treatment plan. (P)

68. **2.** The nurse needs to provide the client who cannot sit long enough to eat adequate amounts of "finger foods," or food that can be held and eaten while moving. High-protein and high-carbohydrate foods, such as a cheeseburger or peanut butter sandwich, are best for the hyperactive client to help maintain body weight. A bacon, lettuce, and tomato sandwich would not provide the client with adequate protein and carbohydrates. Additionally, this type of sandwich is difficult to carry around and can be dropped easily. An ice cream cone, although high in calories, would not provide the client with adequate protein. Cut-up vegetables are a poor selection because, although they are high in vitamins, they are low in protein, which is necessary for building and repairing body cells and tissues, and low in carbohydrates, which are needed for energy. (C)

69. **4.** The nurse escorts the client to her room and assists with choosing appropriate attire to preserve the client's dignity and self-esteem and prevent ridicule from others on the unit. It is common for a client with bipolar disorder, manic phase, to exhibit poor judgment, provocative behavior, and hyperactivity. The client in the manic phase commonly dresses inappropriately and changes clothes many times throughout the day. The nurse needs to assist the client with hygiene, grooming, and proper attire until her judgment improves. Telling the client to dress appropriately while out of her room may be perceived by the client as an attack. Additionally, the client may be incapable of making that decision. Asking the client to put on hospital pajamas until she can dress appropriately is punitive and demeaning. Because of the client's cognitive difficulties, the client may not understand the instructions to go to her room to change clothes. Additionally, the client may become distracted by stimuli on the unit and may not reach her room. (P)

70. **2.** Flight of ideas is a speech pattern of rapid transition from topic to topic, usually without finishing one idea. It is common in mania. Echolalia refers to the repetition of words heard. For example, when the nurse states, "It is time for bed," the client responds, "Bed, bed, bed, bed." Neologism is a word invented by the client. For example, the client states, "The beefocles are brewing." Clang association is the use of rhyming words. For example, the client states, "Let's eat lunch, bunch, munch, crunch." (P)

71. **4.** The client with mania is very active and needs to have this energy channeled in a constructive task such as cleaning or tidying the dayroom. Because the client is distracted easily and can concentrate only for short periods, the successful completion of a helpful task would give the nurse the opportunity to thank the client for the help, thereby enhancing the client's self-esteem. Leading a group activity is too stimulating for the client. Participating in this type of activity also may cause the client to be disruptive. Watching television or reading the newspaper would be inappropriate for the client who cannot sit for a period of time. (P)

72. **1.** The client in the manic phase experiences insomnia, as evidenced by his sleeping only for about 4 hours a night for the past 5 days. The client experiencing an acute manic episode is not capable of judging the need for sleep. Therefore, the nurse should assess the amount of rest the client is receiving daily to prevent exhaustion. The development of vertigo, gastritis, or bradycardia typically does not result from acute mania. (P)

73. **3.** Bipolar disorder is a biochemical disorder caused by an imbalance of neurotransmitters in the brain. Manic episodes seem to be related to excessive levels of norepinephrine, serotonin, and dopamine. Psychopharmacologic therapy aims to restore the balance of neurotransmitters. In the past, it was thought that bipolar disorder may have been caused by early psychodynamics or disturbed families, but the current view emphasizes the role of biology. Bipolar disorder could be genetic or inherited from someone in the family, but it is best for the client and family to understand the disease concept related to neurotransmitter imbalance. This understanding also helps them to refrain from placing blame on anyone. Siblings and close relatives have a higher incidence of bipolar disorder and mood disorders in general when compared with the general population. (P)

74. **1.** It takes 10 to 21 days to achieve a lithium level within the therapeutic range. During an acute manic episode, the normal therapeutic range is 0.5 to 1.5 mEq/L and the maintenance margin is 0.6 to 1.2 mEq/L. With a level of 1.6 to 3.2 mEq/L, the client would be exhibiting signs and symptoms of toxicity. A level of 3.3 to 4.0 mEq/L is extremely high and toxic. (D)

75. **3.** Lithium is associated with some common side effects, including thirst, nausea, mild hand tremors, dry mouth, headache, and taste distortion. These side effects usually are transient, subsiding in approximately 6 weeks. An allergic reaction may be manifested by headache, fever, or rash. If the reaction is severe, signs and symptoms of anaphylaxis occur. Lithium toxicity is manifested by coarse hand tremors, vomiting, diarrhea, sedation, muscle weakness, vertigo, blurred vision, and dilute urine. The symptoms described do not indicate a drug interaction. The client is taking only lithium. Drug interactions (thiazide diuretics) could increase the risk of toxicity by decreasing renal clearance of lithium. (D)

76. **3.** Because lithium reaches peak blood levels in 1 to 3 hours, blood specimens for serum lithium concentration determinations are usually drawn before the first dose of lithium in the morning (which is usually 8 to 12 hours after the previous dose) or before breakfast. Stat lithium levels can be drawn at any time, usually when toxicity is suspected. (D)

77. **2, 3, 5.** Serious side effects that may indicate lithium toxicity include muscle weakness, vertigo, vomiting, extreme hand tremor, and sedation. The prescribing health care provider should be notified immediately when these symptoms occur. When lithium is initiated, mild or transient side effects can occur, such as nausea, fine hand tremor, anorexia, increased thirst and urination, and diarrhea or constipation. (D)

78. **2.** The therapeutic and toxic range of lithium is very narrow. If the client forgets to take a scheduled dose of lithium, the client needs to wait until the next scheduled time to take it, because taking twice the amount of lithium can cause lithium toxicity. The client needs to maintain a regular diet and regular salt intake. Lithium and sodium are eliminated from the body through the kidneys. An increase in salt intake leads to decreased plasma lithium levels because lithium is excreted more rapidly. A decrease in salt intake leads to increased plasma lithium levels. The client needs to drink 8 to 10 eight-ounce glasses of water daily to maintain fluid balance and decrease thirst. Decreased water intake can lead to an increase in the lithium level, and consequently a risk of toxicity. Lithium must be taken on a regular basis at the same time each day to ensure maximum therapeutic effect. (D)

79. **4.** Lithium commonly is combined with an antipsychotic agent, such as haloperidol, or a benzodiazepine such as lorazepam (Ativan). Antipsychotic agents, such as Haldol, are prescribed to produce a neuroleptic effect until the lithium, which has a clinical response lag time of 1 to 2 weeks, produces a clinical response. After a clinical response is achieved, the antipsychotic agent usually is discontinued. Additionally, the dosages of each drug listed are appropriate. Therefore, the nurse would administer the drugs as ordered. (D)

80. **4.** The client's statement, "I know I'm getting sick when I don't need much sleep and start buying things," indicates insight into her illness because the client recognizes symptoms that can lead to relapse. The statement, "I enjoy feeling high; I don't need much sleep then and get really creative," gives no indication that the client recognizes the detrimental effects of bipolar disorder. The statements about not needing medicine in another week or being cured indicate the client's lack of understanding about the chronic nature of the disorder. The client is not cured from bipolar disorder, but symptoms of the disorder are usually managed when she is stabilized on medication. Medication may be needed by the client for many years or throughout her life. (P)

81. **1.** For this client, the nurse needs to set limits on the client's intrusive, interruptive behavior by saying, "Please stop interrupting others; you can speak when it's your turn." This statement also clearly points out to the client the specific unacceptable behavior. The nurse helps the client to attain control and helps the other clients become more tolerant of the situation. Saying, "Stop talking; it's time for you to leave the meeting," is not helpful because it leaves the client unaware of what has happened or the behavior that is unacceptable. Also, such a statement may seem punitive. The statement, "If you can't control yourself, we'll have to take action," is threatening to the client and diminishes the client's self-worth. Using the statement, "Please behave like an adult. Your behavior is childish," is demeaning and scolding to the client, thereby diminishing the client's self-esteem. (P)

82. **3.** Depakene, an anticonvulsant agent, is used as a mood stabilizer in the client with bipolar disorder. Common side effects include drowsiness and gastrointestinal upset. The client needs to be cautioned not to drive or perform tasks requiring alertness and to take the medication with food or milk or eat frequent, small meals. Blood tests are required to evaluate the serum level (usually 50 to 100 µg/ml) and to check for possible hematologic effects. Depakene can cause changes in liver function and blood dyscrasias. The tablet must be swallowed whole and not chewed or crushed to prevent irritation of the mouth and throat. Alcohol as well as over-the-counter drugs and sleep-inducing agents must be avoided to prevent oversedation. (D)

83. **1, 2, 5.** The therapeutic level of valproic acid is 50 to 100 µg/ml. A level of 15 µg/ml is not considered therapeutic. Therefore, the client would be manifesting symptoms of mania. Irritability, euphoria, grandiosity, pressured speech, flight of ideas, distractibility, and a decreased need for sleep are some characteristics of a manic episode. Anhedonia and hypersomnia are related to a depressive illness and not mania. (D)

84. **4.** The nurse should call the physician to report symptoms of a sore throat, fever, and chills because these symptoms may be signs of serious adverse effects of the medication, including potentially fatal hematologic, cardiovascular, and hepatic complications. Giving the dose of carbamazepine is contraindicated in this situation. Giving the acetaminophen ordered p.r.n. would be inappropriate and potentially detrimental to the client's health. Waiting until morning to report the client's symptoms is a serious error in judgment. (D)

85. **2.** The nurse's most appropriate action is to give the wife information about a support group in her area. The National Alliance for the Mentally Ill (NAMI) has affiliates in every state and many locales. NAMI has separate groups for consumers and family members and offers a 12-week program for family members or caregivers called *Family to Family.* The program is psychoeducational in nature, and participants learn, share, and support each other. Family members need and want education and support. Suggesting that the wife see a physician is not necessary in this situation. She needs support and education. Recommending that she talk with her close friend may be helpful if she so chooses. However, this is not as helpful as attending a support group. Here the wife can learn, share, obtain support from, and provide support to others with similar situations. Having the wife share her feelings with her husband may or may not be appropriate or helpful to her or her husband. The husband may be unable to help his wife with adaptive coping, and therefore the client's self-esteem could be diminished. (P)

86. **2.** The nurse should encourage the husband to support and communicate openly with his wife to maintain effective family-client interactions. During any illness, open communication and support helps the relationship between husband and wife. It is unrealistic for any individual to be free from anxiety or worry and impossible for the husband to be able to control what his wife may think or feel. Relieving the client of all responsibilities is unrealistic and not helpful. The client needs to resume activities as soon as she can manage them. Reminding his wife to control her symptoms is not appropriate and indicates that the husband needs further teaching about this condition. (P)

87. **1.** The statement, "I'm happy you realize that you started to get symptoms when you stopped your medication," praises the client for realistic self-appraisal and development of insight. Positive reinforcement by the nurse strengthens insight and promotes good judgment in the client. The statements, "Although it took a long time, you finally do understand that you need your medication" and "Why didn't you go to the community mental health center for help?" blame the client and diminish the client's self-worth. When clients begin to experience symptoms of relapse, they may not realize what is happening to them and may not have the judgment to seek help. The statement, "Didn't your family tell you that you were getting sick again?" blames the family and makes an unfair assumption. (P)

88. **4.** The nurse should administer haloperidol ordered p.r.n. to the acutely manic and anxious client to help calm him and reduce the risk of violent or destructive behavior. The manic client is beginning to exhibit behaviors that may escalate and lead to loss of control, thereby causing the client to be a danger to self or others. Walking with the client is not helpful because his current anxiety is too high and his pacing is not helping him. Telling the client to go to his room is not helpful, because the client is exhibiting a high level of anxiety and hyperactivity and will be unable to stay in his room. Asking the client to sit in on a group therapy session is not helpful because the client cannot sit for a period of time. The client would be disruptive to the members of the group and his behavior could lead to increased anxiety in the other clients. (P)

89. **1, 2.** *Impaired social interaction* refers to behaviors that are insufficient, excessive, or ineffective for social exchange. Interrupting group activities, changing clothes several times a day, engaging in insulting and sexually provocative dialogue, and blaming others are some behaviors of the client with mania indicating a problem with social interaction. Jogging through the hallway puts the client at risk for injury. Believing he is a famous king and stating others on the unit are stealing his socks indicate altered thought processes. (P)

90. 4. The nurse should state her name and purpose on the unit to clarify her identity and to counteract other beliefs the client may have. Stating that the nurse doesn't want to or can't go out to dinner is not therapeutic because it fails to clarify the client's misperceptions or erroneous beliefs, as is the statement, "It doesn't matter how I look, the answer is no." (P)

91. 3. The client is visibly out of control, and other measures have not helped. Therefore, the nurse needs to seclude the client and use restraints if necessary to protect the client and others from harm. Following the client and asking her to calm down or telling the client to lie down on the sofa is not helpful because the client's level of anxiety is too high for her to attempt to calm down on her own and she cannot control her behavior. Telling the staff to ignore the client's remarks is not helpful because the client needs external means of control to protect the client, other clients on the unit, and the staff. Safety is the priority. (S)

92. 3. When the client in a manic state attempts to manipulate the nurse or demands privileges, the nurse must restate the unit rules in a calm and matter-of-fact manner. "The television hours are from 7 to 10 p.m. It is 10 p.m., and the television goes off so everyone can sleep," is the most therapeutic response because it restates the rules and is nonthreatening. During a manic phase, the client is impulsive and has difficulty concentrating. The client needs consistency and structure from the staff. The statement, "I'll let you watch television just this once; don't tell anyone about this," allows the client to manipulate the nurse, as does "I'll turn the television off when you get sleepy. Don't ask me to do this again." In addition, the last portion of the statement is a threat. The statement, "The television goes off at 10 p.m.; I've been telling you this for the past three evenings," is inappropriate because it is authoritative and demeaning to the client. (P)

The Client with Suicidal Ideation and Suicide Attempt

93. 3. Assessing for suicide risk in the ED is important because suicidal clients can be discharged without being assessed for suicide potential. Many visitors to the ED are there for comprehensive health care needs and lack primary care providers. It is a myth that talking about suicide will cause young people to think about suicide, and evidence exists that they will talk about suicide if asked directly. Assessing adults only because they will be more honest is an incorrect assumption. Limiting the assessment of suicide risk only to adolescents with psychiatric diagnoses falsely assumes that other young people are not at risk for suicide. Questioning the parents about their adolescent's suicide risk may be an unreliable method because the parents may not be aware that suicide risk is present. (P)

94. 1. High-risk factors that have been related to suicide include hopelessness, Caucasian race, male gender, advanced age, living alone, previous suicide attempts, family history of suicide attempts, family history of substance abuse, general medical illnesses, psychosis, and substance abuse. The highest suicide rate is among people over the age of 65, particularly Caucasian males age 85 and over. Psychiatric diagnosis is considered to be the most reliable factor for suicide, especially for those with depression, schizophrenia, and substance disorders. Therefore, an 85-year-old Caucasian male who lives alone after his wife's death is at high risk for suicide completion. (M)

95. 2. A crucial factor in determining the lethality of a method is the amount of time that occurs between initiating the method and the delivery of the lethal impact of the method. Lethal methods of suicide include using a gun, jumping from a high place, hanging, drowning, carbon monoxide poisoning, and overdose with certain drugs, such as central nervous system depressants, alcohol, and barbiturates. The more detailed the suicide plan, the more lethal and accessible the method, and the more effort exerted to block rescue, the greater the chance is for the suicide to be completed. Impulsive attempts at suicide even with rescuers in sight may be lethal depending on the method. Less lethal methods may include overdosing on aspirin and wrist cutting. Head-banging is a self-injurious behavior that requires intervention and is not to be taken lightly; however, it is not considered a lethal method of suicide. (P)

96. 4. The statement, "No matter what the intent, all suicidal behavior is serious and deserves our serious consideration," is most appropriate because it provides accurate information for the staff. Superficial cuts may be termed *suicide gestures*. Nevertheless, they still are a cry for help and may indicate ambivalence about dying. Clients have accidentally and unintentionally killed themselves because previous attempts were not taken seriously, they acted on impulse, or rescue attempts were foiled. Stating, "It's our job to help her no matter how we feel about her or what she did; she'll be discharged soon," is inappropriate because it does not provide the staff members with accurate information. Stating, "I won't tolerate that kind of discussion from my staff; now it is time for you to go back to work," is authoritarian and punitive. Additionally, it does not help the staff members gain insight. Stating, "I know it's hard to understand, but we need to do the best we can even though she'll be back," voices agreement with the staff's bias and lack of knowledge. As such, this statement is inappropriate. (M)

97. 2. On hearing the client's statement, the nurse must ask the client directly if she plans to kill herself. It is erroneous to think that talking to the client about suicide will drive her to it. Asking directly about suicidal intent is absolutely necessary. Commonly, doing so provides the client with a sense of relief. In addition, the nurse conveys concern for and a sense of worth to the client, thus enabling appropriate planning for care. Asking "What do you mean?" is an indirect method of inquiry that provides the client with the opportunity to evade the nurse's intent. Asking, "Doesn't your family care about you?" shows poor judgment on the nurse's part and is demeaning to the client. Asking, "What happened to make you think that?" conveys a lack of knowledge of psychopathology. (P)

98. 4. For the client with suicidal ideation, client safety is the priority. The nurse protects the client from self-harm or self-destruction. Although self-esteem, sleep, and hygiene are common areas that require intervention for a client with suicidal ideation, ensuring the client's safety is the most immediate and serious concern. (S)

99. 1. To determine the seriousness of the suicidal ideation, the nurse must ask directly about the intent and the plan. The nurse needs to determine whether the client has a concrete plan and will act on his thoughts. Then the nurse assesses the lethality of the method, immediacy, means to complete suicide, and possibility of rescue. Asking the client, "Have you made out a will?" is not as important and does not necessarily imply that he is planning self-harm. Many individuals have made out wills without planning self-harm. Asking the client, "Does your family know you're here?" provides no information about the client's intent and plan. Asking the client, "How long have you been thinking about harming yourself?" does provide information that the client is thinking about self-harm. However, it does not provide information about the client's immediate intent and plan. (P)

100. 2. The nurse's best response is to teach the nursing assistant about the appropriate intervention and why it is important for the client. Staff members need to be client-focused and to understand why a specific intervention is important and appropriate. Telling the assistant that the assignment will be switched or not to worry about it is not appropriate because it does not teach the nursing assistant about the client's illness and appropriate client care. The statement, "Clients who are depressed are hard to deal with, but don't take what they say seriously," does not help the staff member understand why listening is important and may jeopardize the client's safety. (M)

101. 3. The most therapeutic response is for the nurse to state, "You're in a lot of pain now but you will feel better and I'm here to help you." The client with active suicidal ideation believes that the solution to his problems is suicide. This statement by the nurse conveys empathy and hope to the client that he will get better and offers the nurse's help in doing so. The statement, "I'll walk with you to your room so that you can get some rest," is inappropriate because it focuses only on the client's use of the word tired, not the underlying feeling or intent of the statement. The statement about feeling better after the client's son visits is inappropriate because the nurse does not recognize the client's suicidal behavior and does not convey an understanding of the psychopathology of depression. The statement, "You are very depressed right now and want to die but you need to think about life," is inappropriate because it will not change the way the client is thinking or feeling. It also minimizes the client's feelings. (P)

102. 4. One-to-one staff supervision is needed for the client who is unwilling or cannot sign a no-harm contract because of an impairment in reality testing due to hallucinations, delusions, dementia, or delirium. Other high-risk clients include those with constant suicidal thoughts, past attempts with high lethality, high risk of elopement, available access to a planned method, and severe depression. The client who is sometimes preoccupied with death or who tries to elope but is ambivalent about suicide is not at high risk for suicide and therefore does not need one-to-one supervision, nor does the client who is impulsive and holds her breath until she faints. This client may be seeking attention and not intending self-harm in the form of suicide. Furthermore, fainting is not a lethal method of suicide. (M)

103. 2. The immediate priority is to save the caller's life. Therefore, the nurse should tell the caller that another nurse will telephone the police. The immediate goal is to rescue the caller because the suicide attempt has begun. Referring the caller to a 24-hour suicide hotline or instructing the caller to telephone her family for help may be appropriate as part of discharge planning. Asking the caller whether she has telephoned her physician is not appropriate. The nurse is responsible for notifying the physician. (P)

104. 4. The statement refers to the suicidal client's wish to use her own death to retaliate or get even with her boyfriend. Loss of self-esteem, abandonment, and relief from pain as well as helplessness, hopelessness, and loneliness are other themes commonly expressed by individuals who are suicidal. For example, a person fails out of college and wants to kill herself; a child loses both parents in a car accident and attempts suicide; or a person with cancer who is terminally ill desires to kill herself because of unbearable physical and psychic pain. (P)

105. **2.** The statement, "I don't think about killing myself as much as I used to," indicates a lessening of suicidal ideation and improvement in the client's condition. The statement, "I couldn't kill myself because I don't want to go to hell," indicates that the client will not attempt suicide but could still be thinking about death. The statements, "I'm of no use to anyone anymore," and "I know my kids don't need me anymore since they're on their own," indicate that the client feels worthless and may be experiencing suicidal ideation. (P)

106. **4.** Based on the client's statement, the nurse must initiate plans for hospitalization immediately because the client has suicidal ideation with a definite plan, lethal method, and immediate access to the method. (P)

107. **1.** The survivor of suicide, in this situation, would be referred to a group for survivors of suicide to help her with her feelings and to work through the grief reaction. This group provides support and understanding of what the individual is experiencing by members who are experiencing similar reactions, including anger and guilt. Depression and unresolved grief can occur when the survivor does not receive appropriate help. Counseling by a chaplain or individual therapy by the nurse may be appropriate in addition to referral to the group. Giving the survivor the suicide hotline number would be appropriate if the survivor herself were thinking about suicide. (P)

108. **3.** The most appropriate response is to discuss the behavioral clues and resources because it provides the husband with important information that he needs to cope with his wife's condition. Family members are commonly afraid of future suicidal activity and need helpful information and resources to turn to in a crisis. Telling the husband not to worry minimizes the husband's concern and is not necessarily true. Additionally, past suicide attempts need to be considered when evaluating the client's future risk of suicide. The statement, "She told me she wants to live so I don't think she'll try again," ignores the husband's request and concerns. Additionally, there is no way for the nurse to know whether the client will attempt suicide again. The statement, "Tell her about your concern and just take care of her," is not helpful because the husband needs information and resources to turn to should a crisis develop. (P)

109. **4.** After the client identifies and shares her strengths, the nurse praises the client for her ability to evaluate herself in a positive manner. Doing so promotes self-esteem and offers hope for improvement. Asking the client to identify an additional three strengths or volunteering the client to lead the cooking group could be too overwhelming for the client at this time and may increase her anxiety and feelings of worthlessness. Although educating the client about the importance of medication is important, doing so at another time would be more appropriate. (P)

110. **2.** The best response would be for the nurse to advise the visitor to be caring and genuine to the client as a friend normally would. Family and friends are commonly afraid or at a loss about how to act or what to say to someone with a mental illness or to someone who may voice thoughts of self-harm. The statement, "Try to cheer her up," is inappropriate because the client may feel overwhelmed and thus become more despondent when she cannot meet or match the cheerful demeanor. The statement, "Control your expressions," is inappropriate because the client is not helped when interactions are not natural and genuine. The statement, "Avoid asking how she's feeling," is inappropriate because it conveys a lack of interest in and concern for the client. (P)

111. **2.** The client with feelings of self-doubt, inability to control her life, and dependency is manifesting problems evident in autonomy versus shame/doubt. Because of illness, regression has occurred and the client's behaviors affect how the nurse will intervene with the client. With trust versus mistrust, some behaviors reflecting problems include suspiciousness, projection of blame, and withdrawal from others. With initiative versus guilt, some behaviors reflecting problems include excessive guilt, reluctance to show emotions, and passivity. With industry versus inferiority, some behaviors reflecting problems include feelings of being unworthy, poor work history, and inadequate problem-solving skills. (P)

112. **1.** The nurse should arrange for a psychiatric home care nurse to visit the client and follow her care. The psychiatric home care nurse will help the client manage her psychiatric disorder, medications for her mental illness and diabetes, diabetic care, and nutrition. A medical social worker may be involved with the client's care after discharge to help with interactions among agencies, and visits by clergy may be helpful, but a psychiatric home care nurse would be most important to help the client manage the many needs associated with her illness. A unit volunteer would be unable to manage the many needs of the client. (M)

113. **3.** Client safety is the priority to prevent further self-harm. Nutrition, sleep, and hygiene are important concerns, but they are secondary to safety. (S)

114. **4.** The nurse inspects the bag and its contents in the presence of the client and his wife so that they know what is allowed on the unit and what should be returned home and why. The nurse is responsible for the client's safety and that of the other clients and staff. Telling the wife to take her husband's things home because he is suicidal diminishes the client's self-worth and is inaccurate. Instructing the wife to unpack the bag and put her husband's things away is inappropriate because it is the nurse's responsibility to manage safety issues pertaining to the client and the unit. Asking the wife whether the bag contains anything dangerous would be poor judgment on the part of the nurse because the wife would not be knowledgeable about the safety factors. (P)

115. 2. The nurse and staff should place the client in leather restraints to protect her from further self-harm. The client's behavior is out of control and necessitates external controls for her safety. Telling the client to stop and act like a responsible adult is ineffective and not therapeutic. Calling the physician for additional medication orders is not appropriate because the lorazepam (Ativan) given by the nurse may take effect if the client remains still. The nurse is responsible for judging whether additional medication is needed later. Instructing a staff member to sit in the room with the client is unsafe for the client and the staff member. (S)

116. 2. The nurse needs to ask the client whether he is going to hurt himself to determine the client's ability to cope with the voices and to assess the client's impulse control. The nurse's assessment will then determine the course of action to take regarding the client's safety. Asking when the client hears the voices and how long the client has heard them is important but not as important as determining whether the client will act on what the voices are saying. Asking "Why are the voices starting again?" would be inappropriate because the client may not know why and may not be able to answer the nurse. (S)

117. 4. The nurse needs to focus on the client's strengths and successful coping strategies to reinforce strengths and teach adaptive coping behaviors to manage his illness and life in college. It is not uncommon for a young man diagnosed with schizophrenia to become depressed when he realizes the impact the illness could have on his life, his hopes, and his ability to succeed and reach his goals. There are no data to support a problem involving disturbed thought processes, disturbed sensory perceptions, or communication strategies at this time. (P)

118. 1. Clients on 15-minute suicide checks must be observed by a staff member every 15 minutes. However, the staff member must stagger the timing of the check so that the client cannot predict the precise time. The staff member could check the client at 10 minutes and then at 8 minutes, and so on, to protect the client from self-harm. The nurse would further explain the necessity of this procedure to help the staff understand its importance. Documenting that suicide checks have been done is absolutely necessary. Clients on one-to-one suicide precautions can never be left alone. All clients using razors must be supervised by staff. (M)

119. 3. Talking with a staff member when suicidal thoughts occur is an important part of contracting for safety. The nurse or another staff member can then assess whether the client will act on the thoughts and assist the client with methods of coping when suicidal ideation occurs. Writing in a journal, reading, or playing games with others does not allow the client to verbalize suicidal thoughts to the nurse. (S)

120 4. Because the client has a history of recurring depression and suicidal ideation, the nurse would give the client a 7-day supply of imipramine to prevent possible overdose. Giving the client a 14-, 21-, or 30-day supply of medication would provide the client with enough medication to complete a suicide attempt. Tricyclic antidepressants are associated with a higher rate of death than are selective serotonin reuptake inhibitors. (D)

121. 2. Because the client is in danger of noncompliance with the medication due to financial concerns, the nurse should contact the social worker to assist with locating available resources for the client to ensure continuation of the medication needed for the recurrent illness. The client needs to continue the medications with no interruptions to minimize the chance of decompensation. Although the physician is the person responsible for ordering the client's medication, routinely the physician is not involved in finding financial assistance for the client's medication needs. The client needs the medication at the present time. Three months is too long to wait for a follow-up appointment. The client could be severely depressed and could even attempt suicide. A family member's assistance may not be a sufficient or a permanent means of financial help for the client in terms of medication needs. (M)

Schizophrenia, Other Psychoses, and Cognitive Disorders

The Client with Paranoid Schizophrenia

1. A newly admitted client describes her mission in life as one of saving her son by eliminating the "provocative sluts" of the world. There are several attractive young women on the unit. What should the nurse do first?

- ☐ **1.** Ask the client for her definition of "provocative sluts."
- ☐ **2.** Ask the young female clients on the unit to dress less provocatively.
- ☐ **3.** Ask the client to discuss her concerns in the next group session.
- ☐ **4.** Ask the client to inform the staff if she has negative thoughts about other clients.

2. A young client diagnosed with paranoid schizophrenia is talking with the nurse. "You know, when I thought everyone was out to get me, I liked staying in my apartment all the time. Now, I'd like to get out and do things again." What is the best initial response by the nurse?

- ☐ **1.** "With whom do you want to do things?"
- ☐ **2.** "What activities did you enjoy in the past?"
- ☐ **3.** "What kind of transportation do you use?"
- ☐ **4.** "How much money can you spend?"

3. A client is becoming agitated during a discussion group. She states, "I know that all of you hate me." She leaves the group and goes to her room. Which action by the nurse is most therapeutic for the client?

- ☐ **1.** After group, ask the client to talk to the nurse about her concerns.
- ☐ **2.** Ask the client to return to group and share her feelings.
- ☐ **3.** Explain to group members about the client's problems.
- ☐ **4.** Ask the group members to apologize to the client individually.

4. A client who was diagnosed with undifferentiated schizophrenia 8 years ago is admitted to a unit because of increasingly severe mood swings. His diagnosis is changed to schizoaffective disorder. He asks the nurse, "So now what? My risperidone (Risperdal) is just not doing the job." How should the nurse respond?

- ☐ **1.** "The doctor will probably increase the dosage of your Risperdal."
- ☐ **2.** "With your mood swings, you may need to take a mood stabilizer along with your Risperdal."
- ☐ **3.** "The doctor will have to see how severe your mood swings are before he decides what to do."
- ☐ **4.** "If you are not suicidal, nothing will be done about your moods."

5. A client who is neatly dressed and clutching a leather briefcase tightly in his arms scans the adult inpatient unit on his arrival at the hospital and backs away from the window. The client requests that the nurse move away from the window. The nurse recognizes that doing as the client requested is contraindicated for which of the following reasons?

- ☐ **1.** The action will make the client feel that the nurse is humoring him.
- ☐ **2.** The action indicates nonverbal agreement with the client's false ideas.
- ☐ **3.** The client will then think that he will have his way when he wishes.
- ☐ **4.** The nurse will be demonstrating a lack of composure over the situation.

6. Which of the following nursing diagnoses should the nurse identify for the client reporting thoughts of being followed by foreign agents who are after his secret papers?

☐ **1.** *Disturbed sensory perception: Visual* related to increased anxiety, as evidenced by inappropriate responses.

☐ **2.** *Disturbed thought processes* related to increased anxiety, as evidenced by delusional thinking.

☐ **3.** *Impaired verbal communication* related to disordered thinking, as evidenced by loose associations.

☐ **4.** *Social isolation* related to mistrust, as evidenced by withdrawal behaviors.

7. A client is brought to the emergency department by the police after threatening to kill her ex-husband. She states emphatically, "The police should bring him in, not me. He's paranoid about my dating and has been stalking us for weeks. He's probably off his medicines. His case manager and the police won't do anything." Which are the most urgent priorities for helping this client? Select all that apply.

☐ **1.** Ask about the marital problems leading to the divorce.

☐ **2.** Assess her risk for harm to herself and others.

☐ **3.** Obtain the name of her ex-husband's case manager.

☐ **4.** Ask the police about the client's reports of stalking by her ex-husband.

☐ **5.** Request a psychiatric consult for the client.

☐ **6.** Interview the client about her current situation and her immediate needs.

8. During a conversation with the nurse, the client suddenly jumps up, begins pacing, and wrings her hands. Which of the following should the nurse do next?

☐ **1.** Take the client for a walk to help reduce her restlessness.

☐ **2.** Change the subject of conversation to the weather.

☐ **3.** Share observations about the client's appearing anxious.

☐ **4.** Leave after pointing out that the client doesn't appear to want to talk.

9. When assessing an aggressive client, which of the following behaviors warrants the nurse's most prompt reporting and use of safety precautions?

☐ **1.** Crying when talking about his divorce.

☐ **2.** Starting a petition to delay bedtime.

☐ **3.** Declining attendance at a daily group therapy session.

☐ **4.** Naming another client as his adversary.

10. When developing the plan of care for a client receiving haloperidol (Haldol), which of the following medications would the nurse anticipate administering if the client developed extrapyramidal adverse effects?

☐ **1.** Lorazepam (Ativan).

☐ **2.** Benztropine mesylate (Cogentin).

☐ **3.** Paroxetine (Paxil).

☐ **4.** Olanzapine (Zyprexa).

11. The parents of a 20-year-old female client diagnosed with paranoid schizophrenia admitted 4 days ago are attending a family psychoeducation group in the hospital. Which of the following statements by the mother indicates that she understands her daughter's illness and management?

☐ **1.** "I know that I'll have to do everything for my daughter when she comes home."

☐ **2.** "Tasks as simple as getting out of bed and showering in the morning may be difficult for her."

☐ **3.** "I know that visits from her friends at home should be discouraged for a while."

☐ **4.** "She won't experience a relapse as long as she takes her prescribed medication."

12. While conducting a home visit for a client diagnosed with paranoid schizophrenia discharged 1 week ago, the client's mother tearfully states, "I can hardly sleep because I'm so worried about my daughter. I'm afraid to leave her alone in the house. What if something should happen while I'm gone?" Which of the following problems related to the caregiver would be the most inclusive one for the nurse to incorporate into the client's plan of care?

☐ **1.** Caregiver role strain.

☐ **2.** Anxiety.

☐ **3.** Fear.

☐ **4.** Disturbed sleep pattern.

13. When conducting a mental status examination with a newly admitted client who has an Axis I diagnosis of paranoid schizophrenia, the client states, "I'm being followed; it's not safe. They're monitoring my every move." In which of the following areas of the mental status examination should the nurse document this information?

☐ **1.** Thought content.

☐ **2.** Quality of speech.

☐ **3.** Insight.

☐ **4.** Judgment.

14. The wife of a client diagnosed with paranoid schizophrenia visits 2 days after her husband's admission and states to the nurse, "Why isn't he eating? He's still talking about his food being poisoned." Which of the following appraisals by the nurse is most accurate?

☐ **1.** The wife's inquiry is reasonable.

☐ **2.** Education about her husband's medications is needed.

☐ **3.** Her expectations of her husband are realistic.

☐ **4.** An increase in the client's medication is indicated.

15. A client states that she hears God's voice telling her that she has sinned and needs to be punished. Which of the following nursing diagnoses is most appropriate?
- ☐ **1.** *Disturbed sensory perception* related to guilt as evidenced by auditory hallucinations.
- ☐ **2.** *Social isolation* related to mistrust, as evidenced by withdrawal behaviors.
- ☐ **3.** *Disturbed thought processes* related to increased anxiety as evidenced by delusional thinking.
- ☐ **4.** *Impaired verbal communication* related to disordered thinking as evidenced by loose associations.

16. A client is complaining about blurred vision after 4 days of taking haloperidol (Haldol), benztropine (Cogentin), quetiapine (Seroquel), and buspirone (BuSpar). Which of the following medications should the nurse suspect as the most likely cause of this adverse effect?
- ☐ **1.** Buspirone.
- ☐ **2.** Quetiapine.
- ☐ **3.** Haloperidol.
- ☐ **4.** Benztropine.

17. When developing the plan of care for a client who is staying in his room because he perceives that staff want to harm him, which of the following outcomes is most appropriate?
- ☐ **1.** Within 2 days the client will complete his activities of daily living.
- ☐ **2.** Within 3 days the client will participate in recreation with other clients.
- ☐ **3.** Within 4 days the client will demonstrate an absence of verbal aggression.
- ☐ **4.** Within 5 days the client will seek out staff to talk about feelings.

18. In addition to experiencing paranoid delusions, a client is withdrawn, unkempt, and unmotivated to get out of bed. Which of the following medications would the nurse expect to be most beneficial for the client's symptoms?
- ☐ **1.** Haloperidol (Haldol).
- ☐ **2.** Chlorpromazine (Thorazine).
- ☐ **3.** Olanzapine (Zyprexa).
- ☐ **4.** Trihexyphenidyl (Artane).

19. A pregnant client in her third trimester is started on chlorpromazine (Thorazine) 25 mg four times daily. Which of the following instructions is most important for the nurse to include in the client's teaching plan?
- ☐ **1.** "Don't drive because there's a possibility of seizures occurring."
- ☐ **2.** "Avoid going out in the sun without a sunscreen with a sun protection factor of 25."
- ☐ **3.** "Stop the medication immediately if constipation occurs."
- ☐ **4.** "Tell your doctor if you experience an increase in blood pressure."

20. A client reports that men in blue clothes keep looking in her window and talking about her. Which of the following responses by the nurse is most appropriate?
- ☐ **1.** "Those men are groundskeepers. They're talking about their work, not you."
- ☐ **2.** "Don't take things so personally. Not everyone who is talking is talking about you."
- ☐ **3.** "Let's not pay attention to the men. Let's play cards instead."
- ☐ **4.** "I'll close the drapes so you can't see the men."

21. When preparing the teaching plan for a client who is to start clozapine (Clozaril), which of the following is crucial to include?
- ☐ **1.** Description of akathisia and drug-induced parkinsonism.
- ☐ **2.** Measures to relieve episodes of diarrhea.
- ☐ **3.** The importance of reporting insomnia.
- ☐ **4.** An emphasis on the need for weekly blood tests.

22. A client is sitting in the corner of the dayroom cocking his head to one side as if he hears something, but no one is nearby. The nurse suspects he is having auditory hallucinations. Which of the following questions should the nurse ask first?
- ☐ **1.** "Are you seeing someone other than me?"
- ☐ **2.** "What are you hearing right now?"
- ☐ **3.** "What is going on with you right now?"
- ☐ **4.** "Do you want to go to the recreation room?"

23. A client who is newly diagnosed with paranoid schizophrenia tells the nurse, "The aliens are telling me that I'm defective and need to be eliminated." Which of the following responses by the nurse is most appropriate initially?
- ☐ **1.** "I know those voices are real to you, but I don't hear them."
- ☐ **2.** "You are having hallucinations as a result of your illness."
- ☐ **3.** "I want you to agree to tell staff when you hear these voices."
- ☐ **4.** "Your medications will help control these voices you are hearing."

24. When administering antipsychotics to a client with paranoid schizophrenia, the nurse understands that the newer atypical antipsychotics, such as olanzapine (Zyprexa) and risperidone (Risperdal), are more effective than the older medications in treating the negative symptoms of schizophrenia because of which of the following?
- ☐ **1.** Serotonin and gamma-aminobutyric acid (GABA) levels are not affected.
- ☐ **2.** Dopamine and serotonin receptors are blocked.
- ☐ **3.** GABA and norepinephrine levels are increased.
- ☐ **4.** Norepinephrine and dopamine receptors are blocked.

25. An outpatient client who has a history of paranoid schizophrenia and chronic alcohol dependency has been taking risperidone (Risperdal) for several months. She reports that she stopped drinking 4 days ago. The client is very frightened by the tactile hallucinations of bugs crawling under her skin. Which of the following factors would the nurse incorporate into the plan of care when explaining the tactile hallucinations?

☐ **1.** Alcohol intoxication.

☐ **2.** Ineffectiveness of risperidone.

☐ **3.** Alcohol withdrawal.

☐ **4.** Interaction of alcohol and risperidone.

26. A client with a long history of paranoid schizophrenia is readmitted voluntarily after missing his last two injections of haloperidol decanoate (Haldol Decanoate). He reports, "I'm not sleeping much and my friend says I smell from not showering. God is telling me to protect myself from others. My parents are sick and tired of me and my illness. They wish I were dead." Which of the following admission notes by the nurse contains assumptions and potentially false accusations? Select all that apply.

☐ **1.** Client has been noncompliant with his medications, causing decreased sleep and activities of daily living, increased auditory hallucinations, and paranoid delusions about his parents harming him.

☐ **2.** Client has missed two injections of Haldol Decanoate and was admitted voluntarily. He reports he has decreased sleep and showering and that he hears God's voice telling him to protect himself from others. He stated, "My parents are sick and tired of me and my illness. They wish I were dead."

☐ **3.** Client has missed two doses of Haldol Decanoate. He's not sleeping and showering. Has a strained relationship with his parents and delusions that they want him dead. Voluntary admission to restart Haldol Decanoate.

☐ **4.** Client admitted for noncompliance with Haldol Decanoate injections, sleep disturbance, poor hygiene, auditory hallucinations, and suspiciousness of his parents. Needs to be monitored for suicidal and homicidal ideation.

☐ **5.** Client admitted because of hallucinations and delusions. His parents may be abusing him. He states he has not taken his medications for 2 days.

27. A newly admitted client diagnosed with paranoid schizophrenia is pacing and wringing his hands. He states that another client is out to get him. Then he says, "Protect me. Select me. Reject me." Which of the following nursing diagnoses is most appropriate?

☐ **1.** *Disturbed sensory perception: Visual* related to paranoia as evidenced by thinking a client is out to get him.

☐ **2.** *Impaired verbal communication* related to severe anxiety as evidenced by clang associations.

☐ **3.** *Delayed growth and development* related to mild anxiety as evidenced by incomplete sentences.

☐ **4.** *Defensive coping* related to noncompliance as evidenced by pacing and wringing of hands.

28. When a client who exhibits feelings of inferiority is asked to attend group activities, she gets more anxious. Within 10 minutes, she begins ridiculing others in the group and receives negative attention. Which of the following statements best reflects the nurse's interpretation of the client's behavior? Select all that apply.

☐ **1.** Increased anxiety levels can cause defensive coping.

☐ **2.** Negative attention reinforces acting-out behaviors.

☐ **3.** Negative attention is better than no attention at all.

☐ **4.** Increased anxiety is a reason to exclude the client from groups.

☐ **5.** The client needs medication to control her anxiety.

29. In a family education group for those who have relatives with paranoid schizophrenia, which of the following comments indicates the need for further teaching about symptom management?

☐ **1.** "When the clients get overwhelmed, it's best if they spend some time in their room."

☐ **2.** "The more we push the clients to spend time with friends, the more their voices decrease."

☐ **3.** "Until we get the clients up and going, they seem to have no motivation to do anything."

☐ **4.** "We still have to remind the clients that we don't hear the voices they do."

30. A client is being successfully treated with clozapine (Clozaril). Which of the following statements by the client reflects a need for further teaching about managing the drug's adverse effects?

☐ **1.** "If I eat too many fruits, I'll get constipated."

☐ **2.** "I need to take the medicine with food to avoid nausea."

☐ **3.** "I have to get up slowly so I don't get dizzy."

☐ **4.** "Sometimes I have to push myself because I'm sleepy."

31. Which of the following statements indicates increased insight by the client about her newly diagnosed paranoid schizophrenia being stabilized on medications?
- ☐ **1.** "Now that the voices are gone, I can decrease my medicines."
- ☐ **2.** "I would feel better if I knew there wasn't poison in my food."
- ☐ **3.** "Since I feel better, I know I can restart school next week."
- ☐ **4.** "The voices go away when I tell them to, except if I'm really nervous."

32. A client is aware that he is experiencing auditory hallucinations as a result of his paranoid schizophrenia. At this point, which of the following is most appropriate for the nurse to do?
- ☐ **1.** "I know you hear voices, but I don't hear them."
- ☐ **2.** "Time and medicines will make the voices go away."
- ☐ **3.** "What seems to help make the voices less bothersome?"
- ☐ **4.** "The only voices I hear right now are yours and mine."

33. A client who is suspicious of others including staff is brought to the hospital wearing a wrinkled dress with stains on the front and appearing confused. Assessment also reveals a flat affect and slow movements. Which goal should the nurse identify as the initial priority when planning this client's care?
- ☐ **1.** Helping the client feel safe and accepted.
- ☐ **2.** Introducing the client to other clients.
- ☐ **3.** Giving the client information about the program.
- ☐ **4.** Providing the client with clean, comfortable clothes.

34. A suspicious client states, "I know you nurses are spraying my food with poison as you take it out of the cart." Which of the following actions would most likely be successful?
- ☐ **1.** Serving only foods that come in sealed packages.
- ☐ **2.** Asking what kind of poison the client suspects is being used.
- ☐ **3.** Giving the client canned supplements until the delusion subsides.
- ☐ **4.** Allowing the client to be the first to open the cart and get a tray.

35. The parent of a young adult client diagnosed with paranoid schizophrenia is asking questions about his son's antipsychotic medication, ziprasidone (Geodon). Which of the following statements by the father reflects a need for further teaching?
- ☐ **1.** "If he experiences restlessness or muscle stiffness, he should tell the doctor."
- ☐ **2.** "I should give him benztropine to help prevent constipation from the ziprasidone."
- ☐ **3.** "If he becomes dizzy, I'll make sure he doesn't drive."
- ☐ **4.** "The ziprasidone should help him be more motivated and less withdrawn."

The Client with Other Types of Schizophrenia and Psychotic Disorders

36. As hospital-based care has become more oriented to crisis intervention, criteria for admission to the hospital have also changed. Which client has priority for admission to an acute care facility? Select all that apply.
- ☐ **1.** Clients who live alone.
- ☐ **2.** Clients who are acutely psychotic.
- ☐ **3.** Clients who are acutely depressed.
- ☐ **4.** Clients who are dangerous to self or others.
- ☐ **5.** Clients who are not sleeping and have a lack of appetite.
- ☐ **6.** Clients who are not complying with medication regimens.

37. A 79-year-old woman is brought to the outpatient clinic by her daughter for a routine medication evaluation. The daughter reports that her mother is quite stable and has no adverse effects from the risperidone (Risperdal) she is taking. Then the daughter says, "I just think my mother could be even better if she was on a larger dosage. My son takes 1 mg of Risperdal every day and my mother is only on 0.5 mg." What is the most helpful response by the nurse?
- ☐ **1.** "Maybe your son is sicker than your mother is."
- ☐ **2.** "We could increase your mother's dosage if you want."
- ☐ **3.** "Older clients generally need only one-third to one-half the dose of younger people."
- ☐ **4.** "I'm not seeing any symptoms of illness in your mother. Let's wait until the next visit."

38. At an outpatient visit 3 months after discharge from the hospital, a client says he has stopped his olanzapine (Zyprexa) even though it controls his symptoms of schizophrenia better than other medications. "I have gained 20 lb already. I can't stand any more." Which response by the nurse is most appropriate?

- ☐ 1. "I don't think you look fat, why do you think so?"
- ☐ 2. "I can help you with a diet and exercise plan to keep your weight down."
- ☐ 3. "You can be switched to another medicine."
- ☐ 4. "Your weight gain will level off if you stay on the medication 3 more months."

39. A client diagnosed with schizophrenia is being switched to risperidone long-acting injection (Risperdal Consta). He is told that he will remain on his oral dose of risperidone (Risperdal) daily for approximately 1 month. The client says, "I didn't have to take pills when I was on fluphenazine decanoate (Prolixin Decanoate) shots in the past." Which of the following responses by the nurse is most accurate?

- ☐ 1. "Taking fluphenazine orally and by injection would not be as effective as the injection alone."
- ☐ 2. "Risperdal Consta is less potent than Prolixin Decanoate."
- ☐ 3. "The doctor didn't believe you would take both the pills and Prolixin Decanoate."
- ☐ 4. "Risperdal Consta initially takes a little longer to reach the ideal blood level."

40. One of the important aspects of the client's rights is the right to treatment in the least restrictive environment. The nurse observes this principle when making which decisions? Select all that apply.

- ☐ 1. Referring a client to a group home or supervised apartment living.
- ☐ 2. Releasing client information to a primary care physician or a relative.
- ☐ 3. Placing a client in seclusion or restraints.
- ☐ 4. Respecting the client's right to accept or refuse treatment.
- ☐ 5. Placing a committed client in a daily outpatient group or a weekly self-help group.

41. A client has been perceiving her roommate's stuffed animal as her own dog at home. The nurse determines that this misperception of reality (illusion) is improving when the client makes which of the following statements?

- ☐ 1. "Jan's stuffed dog looks somewhat like my dog, Trixie."
- ☐ 2. "Jan's dog and my dog could be twins."
- ☐ 3. "I wish Jan hadn't had my dog stuffed."
- ☐ 4. "I guess Jan needs a dog as much as I do."

42. When asked about her stresses before admission, an anxious client stares blankly at the nurse and mutters unintelligibly. Which of the following descriptions of the client's behaviors should the nurse document in the client's chart?

- ☐ 1. "Client cannot answer any questions asked at this time."
- ☐ 2. "Client is uncooperative during admission procedure, refusing to answer any questions."
- ☐ 3. "Client responded to questions with a blank look and incomprehensible mumble."
- ☐ 4. "Client stared at wall when asked questions and was disoriented and incoherent."

43. The nurse identifies a nursing diagnosis of *Dressing or grooming self-care deficit* related to apathy, as evidenced by an inability to shower and dress herself for a female client diagnosed with schizophrenia. Which of the following outcomes should the nurse expect as most therapeutic for the client to achieve by the end of 4 days?

- ☐ 1. Verbalize the need to shower and dress herself.
- ☐ 2. Recognize the need to shower and dress herself.
- ☐ 3. Explain reasons for showering and dressing herself.
- ☐ 4. Perform showering and dressing for herself.

44. A client diagnosed with schizophrenia is brought to the hospital from a group home where he became agitated, threw a chair at another client, and has been refusing medication for 8 weeks. The client exhibits a flat affect, is not caring for his hygiene, and has become increasingly withdrawn and asocial. The physician orders treatment with risperidone (Risperdal) to improve the client's negative and positive symptoms of schizophrenia. When evaluating the drug's effectiveness on the client's negative symptoms, the nurse should expect improvement in which of the following?

- ☐ 1. Apathy, affect, social isolation.
- ☐ 2. Agitation, delusions, hallucinations.
- ☐ 3. Hostility, ideas of reference, tangential speech.
- ☐ 4. Aggression, bizarre behavior, illusions.

45. A 77-year-old client is brought to the emergency department by her son. The client is complaining of a severe headache and lack of sleep because, "I'm so worried about everything." Her son says that she has heart failure and chronic schizophrenia. "In addition to all of her heart medicines, she is on aripiprazole (Abilify), which was increased to 30 mg by her family doctor 3 days ago." In addition to documenting all of the client's medications and exact dosages, the nurse should particularly investigate which of the following? Select all that apply.

- ☐ 1. The qualifications of the client's family doctor.
- ☐ 2. The client's symptoms of schizophrenia.
- ☐ 3. The dose of aripiprazole.
- ☐ 4. The client's symptoms of heart failure.
- ☐ 5. The client's relationship with her son.

46. A client with schizophrenia comes to the outpatient mental health clinic 5 days after being discharged from the hospital. The client was given a 1-week supply of clozapine (Clozaril). The client tells the nurse that she has too much saliva and frequently needs to spit. The nurse interprets the client's statement as indicating which of the following?
- ☐ 1. Delusion, requiring further assessment.
- ☐ 2. Unusual reaction to clozapine.
- ☐ 3. Expected adverse effect of clozapine.
- ☐ 4. Unresolved symptom of schizophrenia.

47. The client with an Axis I diagnosis of schizophrenia, undifferentiated type, is acutely psychotic and exhibits religious delusions and hallucinations, loose associations, and concrete thinking. When the nurse offers the client her medication, the client states, "I don't need that. God will heal me." Which of the following responses by the nurse is most appropriate at this time?
- ☐ 1. "God helps those who help themselves."
- ☐ 2. "God wants you to take your medicine."
- ☐ 3. "God is important in your life, but the medicine will help you too."
- ☐ 4. "This medicine will help clear your thoughts and decrease anxiety."

48. The nurse hands the medication cup to a client who is psychotic and exhibiting concrete thinking, and tells the client to take his medicine. The client takes the cup, holds it in his hand, and stares at it. Which of the following should the nurse do next?
- ☐ 1. Tell the client to put the medicine in his mouth and swallow it with some water.
- ☐ 2. Instruct the client to sit in the dayroom and wait for the nurse to assist him.
- ☐ 3. Ask another staff member to stay with the client until he takes the medication.
- ☐ 4. Say nothing and wait for the client to put the medication in his mouth and swallow it.

49. A client is admitted to the unit with a diagnosis of Axis I delusional disorder, persecutory type. The nurse includes the nursing diagnosis *Defensive coping* secondary to suspiciousness as evidenced by the statement, "My wife and coworker are conspiring against me," in the client's plan of care. Which statement about the client should be an expected outcome for this nursing diagnosis?
- ☐ 1. Demonstrate an absence of hostile behavior.
- ☐ 2. Express own needs using assertive communication.
- ☐ 3. Use adaptive coping strategies appropriately.
- ☐ 4. Accurately interpret the behaviors of his wife and coworker.

50. Which action by the nurse is likely to increase the anxiety and suspiciousness of a client who is delusional?
- ☐ 1. Informing the client of schedule changes.
- ☐ 2. Whispering with others where the client can observe.
- ☐ 3. Telling the client gently that the nurse does not share the client's view.
- ☐ 4. Inviting the client to join in leisure activities.

51. A client with undifferentiated schizophrenia tells the nurse that he doesn't go out much because he doesn't have anywhere to go and he doesn't know anyone in the apartment where he's staying. Which of the following actions is most beneficial for the client at this time?
- ☐ 1. Encouraging him to call his family to visit more often.
- ☐ 2. Making an appointment for the client to see the nurse daily for 2 weeks.
- ☐ 3. Thinking about the need for rehospitalization for the client.
- ☐ 4. Arranging for the client to attend day treatment at the clinic.

52. A client with chronic undifferentiated schizophrenia has positive and negative symptoms of schizophrenia but does not meet the criteria for paranoid, disorganized, or catatonic schizophrenia. Based on the interpretation of this information, the nurse should expect the client to exhibit which of the following as the most likely symptoms?
- ☐ 1. Auditory hallucinations and asocial behaviors.
- ☐ 2. Preoccupation with persecutory delusions and hallucinations.
- ☐ 3. Grossly disorganized behaviors and speech.
- ☐ 4. Immobility and waxy flexibility.

53. The plan of care for an outpatient client with chronic undifferentiated schizophrenia (CUS) includes risperidone (Risperdal) therapy. The nurse prepares to administer this drug based on the understanding of which of the following?
- ☐ 1. The positive symptoms of CUS are usually more prominent than the negative symptoms.
- ☐ 2. Agranulocytosis is less of a risk with risperidone therapy.
- ☐ 3. Negative symptoms are more prominent than positive symptoms in CUS.
- ☐ 4. Risperidone is less expensive than traditional antipsychotics.

54. A client diagnosed with undifferentiated schizophrenia is being discharged on aripiprazole (Abilify) 5 mg every night. When developing the teaching plan about the most common adverse effects, which of the following should the nurse include? Select all that apply.
- ☐ 1. Headaches that will subside in a few weeks.
- ☐ 2. Transient mild anxiety.
- ☐ 3. Insomnia.
- ☐ 4. Torticollis.
- ☐ 5. Pill rolling movements.

55. A newly admitted client with an acute exacerbation of psychotic symptoms of chronic undifferentiated schizophrenia is having trouble deciding whether to live in a group home or a supervised apartment. When caring for this client, which of the following activities is most appropriate for the nurse to ask the client to do initially?
- ☐ 1. List the pros and cons of each housing option.
- ☐ 2. Choose between apple and orange juice for breakfast.
- ☐ 3. Identify why the client cannot live in an unsupervised apartment.
- ☐ 4. Decide which staff member the client would like to have today.

56. An outpatient client who has been receiving haloperidol (Haldol) for 2 days develops muscular rigidity, altered consciousness, a temperature of 103° F (39.4° C), and trouble breathing on day 3. The nurse interprets these findings as indicating which of the following?
- ☐ 1. Neuroleptic malignant syndrome.
- ☐ 2. Tardive dyskinesia.
- ☐ 3. Extrapyramidal adverse effects.
- ☐ 4. Drug-induced parkinsonism.

57. A client with chronic undifferentiated schizophrenia reports to the nurse that he does very little all day except sleep and eat. Which of the following interventions is most appropriate for this client?
- ☐ 1. Having three meals per day brought in to increase the amount of time the client spends out of bed.
- ☐ 2. Asking a relative to call the client at least 10 times a day to decrease the sleeping.
- ☐ 3. Helping the client set up a daily activity schedule to include setting a wake-up alarm.
- ☐ 4. Arranging for the client to move to a group home with structured activities.

58. The nurse notes that a client sitting in a chair has not gotten up in 1 hour. The client does not respond to verbal directions, and her arm has been extended over the armrest for 30 minutes. Which of the following should the nurse do next?
- ☐ 1. Assist the client out of the chair to lead her back to bed.
- ☐ 2. Give p.r.n.-ordered doses of haloperidol (Haldol) and lorazepam (Ativan).
- ☐ 3. Ask the client to describe what is being experienced right now.
- ☐ 4. Sit quietly with the client until she begins to respond.

59. What is the most appropriate long-term goal for an outpatient client with chronic undifferentiated schizophrenia who has been withdrawn from friends and family for 3 weeks?
- ☐ 1. Calling his mother once a day.
- ☐ 2. Attending day therapy three times a week.
- ☐ 3. Allowing two friends to visit every day.
- ☐ 4. Remaining out of bed for 10 hours a day.

60. For the client with catatonic behaviors, which of the following should the nurse use to determine that the medication administered p.r.n. has been most effective in the long term?
- ☐ 1. The client can move all extremities occasionally.
- ☐ 2. The client walks with the nurse to her room.
- ☐ 3. The client responds to verbal directions to eat.
- ☐ 4. The client initiates simple activities without directions.

61. The mother of a client with chronic undifferentiated schizophrenia calls the nurse in the outpatient clinic to report that her daughter has not answered the phone in 10 days. "She was doing so well for months. I don't know what's wrong. I'm worried." Which of the following responses by the nurse is most appropriate?
- ☐ 1. "Maybe she's just mad at you. Did you have an argument?"
- ☐ 2. "She may have stopped taking her medications. I'll check on her."
- ☐ 3. "Don't worry about this. It happens sometimes."
- ☐ 4. "Go over to her apartment and see what's going on."

62. During a home visit, the nurse discovers that the client is less verbal, less active, less responsive to directions, severely anxious, and more stuporous. The nurse interprets these findings to indicate that the client needs which intervention?
- ☐ 1. A sleep aid.
- ☐ 2. A clinic appointment.
- ☐ 3. An increase in medication.
- ☐ 4. Hospitalization.

63. A client diagnosed with disorganized schizophrenia has been well maintained on olanzapine (Zyprexa) for 1 year. Two days ago, the client was found in the backyard without any clothes on and unable to communicate well because of loose associations. His mother died 2 weeks ago. Which intervention should the nurse anticipate will be included in the client's plan of care first?
- ☐ 1. Addition of a short course of haloperidol (Haldol).
- ☐ 2. A significant increase in the dose of olanzapine.
- ☐ 3. Grief counseling.
- ☐ 4. A switch to risperidone (Risperdal) instead of olanzapine.

64. A client admitted with a diagnosis of schizoaffective disorder, manic phase, who is currently taking fluoxetine (Prozac), valproic acid (Depakote), and olanzapine (Zyprexa) as ordered has had an increase in manic symptoms in the past week. The psychiatrist orders a valproic acid blood level to be drawn stat. The nurse understands the rationale for this order as which of the following?
☐ 1. All clients taking valproic acid need periodic valproic acid levels drawn.
☐ 2. Fluoxetine can decrease the effectiveness of the valproic acid.
☐ 3. A decrease in the level of valproic acid could explain the increase in manic symptoms.
☐ 4. The valproic acid level is needed before a short course of lorazepam (Ativan) for agitation is ordered.

65. A 22-year-old client is being admitted with a diagnosis of brief psychotic disorder. Two weeks ago, his girlfriend broke off their engagement and canceled the wedding. Given the *Diagnostic and Statistical Manual of Mental Disorders,* 4th edition, text revised, criteria for this disorder, the nurse should expect to find which data during the interview with the client?
☐ 1. Current treatment for pneumonia.
☐ 2. Regular use of alcohol or marijuana.
☐ 3. Evidence of delusions or hallucinations.
☐ 4. A history of chronic depression.

66. A successful real estate agent brought to the clinic after being arrested for harassing and stalking his ex-wife denies any other symptoms or problems except anger about being arrested. The ex-wife reports to the police, "He is fine except for this irrational belief that we will remarry." Which of the following should the nurse expect to include in this client's plan of care?
☐ 1. An order for olanzapine (Zyprexa) 10 mg daily.
☐ 2. A joint session with the client and his ex-wife.
☐ 3. An order for fluoxetine (Prozac) 20 mg every morning.
☐ 4. Referral to an outpatient therapist.

Clients and Families Affected by Chronic Mental Illnesses

67. When working with clients who are experiencing chronic mental illnesses, which of the following should the nurse expect to be generally the least necessary for this client population?
☐ 1. Community-based treatment programs.
☐ 2. Psychosocial rehabilitation.
☐ 3. Employment opportunities.
☐ 4. Custodial care in long-term hospitals.

68. The nurse is offered a position as a psychiatric nurse in a psychosocial rehabilitation program for chronically mentally ill clients. Which of the following strategies should the nurse expect to be least beneficial for the client population?
☐ 1. Teaching independent living skills.
☐ 2. Assisting clients with living arrangements.
☐ 3. Helping clients in insight-oriented therapy.
☐ 4. Linking clients with community resources.

69. A nurse working at an outpatient mental health center primarily with chronically mentally ill clients receives a telephone call from the mother of a client who lives at home. She reports that the client has not been taking her medication and now is refusing to go to the sheltered workshop where she has worked for the past year. What should the nurse do first?
☐ 1. Call the director of the workshop for information about the client.
☐ 2. Reserve an inpatient bed in preparation for the client's admission.
☐ 3. Ask to speak to the client directly on the phone.
☐ 4. Make an appointment for the client to see the doctor.

70. The nurse invites a new client's parents to attend the psychoeducational program for families of the chronically mentally ill. The program is most likely to help the family with which of the following issues?
☐ 1. Feeling guilty about the client's illness.
☐ 2. Developing a support network with other families.
☐ 3. Managing financial concerns and problems.
☐ 4. Recognizing the client's weaknesses.

71. A nurse is teaching the families of clients with chronic mental illnesses about causes of relapse and rehospitalization. What should the nurse include as the primary cause?
☐ 1. Loss of family support.
☐ 2. Noncompliance with medications.
☐ 3. Sudden changes in medications.
☐ 4. Nonattendance at treatment programs.

72. The director of a workshop program tells the nurse that the client with schizophrenia had done well for 6 months until last week, when a new person started at the workshop. This new person worked faster than the client did and took his place as leader of the group. Based on this information, which of the following interventions is most appropriate?
- ☐ 1. Make a home visit and tell the client that if he does not return to the workshop, he will lose his place there.
- ☐ 2. Ask the director to assign the client to another work group when he returns to the workshop.
- ☐ 3. Make an appointment to meet the client at the mental health center and ask him about the situation.
- ☐ 4. Arrange for the placement of the client in a skill-training program.

73. A 25-year-old client diagnosed with chronic schizophrenia states, "I stopped my medications a week ago. I was just tired of not being able to drink with my friends. Besides, I feel fine without them." Which of the following responses by the nurse is most appropriate?
- ☐ 1. "It's important for you to go back on your medicines."
- ☐ 2. "I hear how difficult it must be to live with the changes caused by your illness."
- ☐ 3. "You will have to talk to your doctor about stopping your medications."
- ☐ 4. "Your buddies will understand that you can't drink anymore."

74. A 23-year-old client diagnosed with schizophrenia cheerfully announces, "My mom and I are so excited that I'm pregnant. She's willing to help us take care of the baby too." Which of the following reasons should cause the nurse to be concerned about this situation?
- ☐ 1. The client did not say that the father of the baby was excited about this.
- ☐ 2. The mother is not likely to provide enough help for what the client needs.
- ☐ 3. Symptom management will be difficult in early pregnancy without medications.
- ☐ 4. The client will have difficulty financially supporting the baby.

75. Mental health professionals are concerned about the care of chronically ill clients who have aging parents. The primary reason for this concern is associated with which of the following?
- ☐ 1. Clients will have to face grieving issues when one or both parents die.
- ☐ 2. Parents experience much guilt about abandoning their child.
- ☐ 3. Clients will lose a source of emotional support.
- ☐ 4. Parents are commonly providing financial support and/or housing.

76. The discovery of the biochemical hypothesis for the cause of schizophrenia has helped families of ill clients in many ways. Which new information should the nurse understand to be most significant when planning care for a client with schizophrenia and his family?
- ☐ 1. Family dysfunction, if it exists, is viewed as an effect rather than a cause of the disorder.
- ☐ 2. Professionals are more likely to view families as allies than as villains.
- ☐ 3. Families are less likely to participate in "families of schizophrenics" studies.
- ☐ 4. Families are less likely to be involved in providing care to their ill relatives.

77. As a result of the effects of managed care, hospitalization is commonly reserved for emergency care. Which of the following situations should the nurse recognize as having the least priority for admission?
- ☐ 1. Potential for self-harm.
- ☐ 2. Potential for harm to others.
- ☐ 3. Grave disability (cannot care for self).
- ☐ 4. Decline in functioning at work.

78. Given the decrease in length of hospital stay for the chronically mentally ill, the nurse recognizes the increased need for emphasizing discharge planning. For the client who is being discharged before complete stabilization of symptoms, the nurse should anticipate that he would require which of the following?
- ☐ 1. More medical consultations after discharge.
- ☐ 2. Monthly outpatient visits.
- ☐ 3. Many coordinated services.
- ☐ 4. A caring and supportive family.

79. Clients with chronic mental illnesses need to develop trust in their care providers and gain education about their illness and its treatment. What is another critical need for these clients?
- ☐ 1. Family support.
- ☐ 2. Advocacy for improved mental health statutes.
- ☐ 3. Diligent monitoring for medication compliance.
- ☐ 4. Support groups.

80. When developing a teaching plan for the community about managed care models and their effect on clients with chronic mental illnesses, which of the following factors should the nurse include as critical for this population? Select all that apply.
- ☐ 1. Restriction in the range and quantity of services.
- ☐ 2. Hospitalization reserved for emergency services.
- ☐ 3. Nonshifting of allocated funding to outpatient services.
- ☐ 4. Loss of the principle of "least restrictive alternative for care."
- ☐ 5. Development of enough group homes.

81. When developing a community-based service program for clients with chronic mental illnesses, which of the following is the least important?
- ☐ **1.** Partial programs.
- ☐ **2.** Psychiatric home care.
- ☐ **3.** Residential services.
- ☐ **4.** Long-term hospitals.

82. Crisis intervention plays a major role in the management of care for clients with chronic mental illnesses. Although the safety of the client and others is always a priority, these clients typically need crisis intervention in which of the following situations? Select all that apply.
- ☐ **1.** Inability to keep outpatient appointments.
- ☐ **2.** Signs of relapse and decompensation.
- ☐ **3.** Threat of eviction from housing.
- ☐ **4.** Unpaid bills and lack of food.
- ☐ **5.** Occasionally missing a dose of medication.

83. The most common reason given by mentally ill clients for noncompliance with medications is their uncomfortable adverse effects. When teaching the families, what need should the nurse identify as the greatest?
- ☐ **1.** Alternative ways to manage the adverse effects.
- ☐ **2.** Home visits to set up a week's supply of medications.
- ☐ **3.** Family monitoring of the administration of medication.
- ☐ **4.** Outpatient monitoring of medication compliance.

84. The stigma related to having a mental illness, especially a chronic illness, persists despite improvements in the management of illnesses and an increase in public education. Which of the following views most perpetuates the stigma?
- ☐ **1.** Mental illness is hereditary.
- ☐ **2.** Mental illnesses have biochemical bases.
- ☐ **3.** Clients cannot prevent mental illness if they want to do so.
- ☐ **4.** Clients can recover from mental illness if they have willpower.

The Client with Cognitive Disorders

85. In planning for the discharge of a client with a cognitive disorder, it is important to assess the client's caregiver support system. Which aspects are the most crucial to assess? Select all that apply.
- ☐ **1.** Availability of resources for caregiver support.
- ☐ **2.** Ability to provide the level of care and supervision needed by the client.
- ☐ **3.** Willingness to transport the client to medical and psychiatric services.
- ☐ **4.** Interest in engaging the cognitively disordered family member in reminiscence and games.
- ☐ **5.** Willingness to install door alarms and make other safety changes.
- ☐ **6.** Understanding the client's abilities and limitations.

86. The son of an elderly client who has cognitive impairments approaches the nurse and says, "I'm so upset. The physician says I have 4 days to decide on where my dad is going to live." The nurse responds to the son's concerns, gives him a list of types of living arrangements, and discusses the needs, abilities, and limitations of the client. The nurse should intervene further if the son makes which comment?
- ☐ **1.** "Boy, I have a lot to think about before I see the social worker tomorrow."
- ☐ **2.** "I think I can handle most of Dad's needs with the help of some home health care."
- ☐ **3.** "I'm so afraid of making the wrong decision, but I can move him later if I need to."
- ☐ **4.** "I want the social worker to make this decision so Dad won't blame me."

87. Transfer data for a client brought by ambulance to the hospital's psychiatric unit from a nursing home indicate that the client has become increasingly confused and disoriented. The client's behavior is found to be the result of cerebral arteriosclerosis. Which of the following behaviors of the nursing staff should positively influence the client's behavior? Select all that apply.
- ☐ **1.** Limiting the client's choices.
- ☐ **2.** Accepting the client as he is.
- ☐ **3.** Allowing the client to do as he wishes.
- ☐ **4.** Acting nonchalantly.
- ☐ **5.** Explaining to the client what he needs to do step-by-step.

88. A nurse is planning care for an elderly client with cognitive impairment who is still living at home. Which action should the nurse identify as a priority for safety in planning care for this client?
- ☐ **1.** Having two people accompany the client whenever the client is up and about.
- ☐ **2.** Ensuring the removal of objects in the client's path that may cause him to trip.
- ☐ **3.** Putting the client's favorite belongings in a safe place so that he will not lose them.
- ☐ **4.** Giving the client his medications in liquid form to make certain that he swallows them.

89. The nurse manager of a psychiatric unit notices that one of the nurses commonly avoids a 75-year-old client's company. Which of the following factors should the nurse manager identify as being the most likely cause of this nurse's discomfort with older clients?
- ☐ **1.** Fears and conflicts about aging.
- ☐ **2.** Dislike of physical contact with older people.
- ☐ **3.** A desire to be surrounded by beauty and youth.
- ☐ **4.** Recent experiences with her mother's elderly friends.

90. The nurse observes a client in a group who is reminiscing about his past. Which effect should the nurse expect reminiscing to have on the client's functioning in the hospital?

☐ 1. Increase the client's confusion and disorientation.

☐ 2. Cause the client to become sad.

☐ 3. Decrease the client's feelings of isolation and loneliness.

☐ 4. Keep the client from participating in therapeutic activities.

The Client with Delirium

91. A 69-year-old client is admitted and diagnosed with delirium. Later in the day, he tries to get out of the locked unit. He yells, "Unlock this door. I've got to go see my doctor. I just can't miss my monthly Friday appointment." Which of the following responses by the nurse is most appropriate?

☐ 1. "Please come away from the door. I'll show you your room."

☐ 2. "It's Tuesday and you are in the hospital. I'm Anne, a nurse."

☐ 3. "The door is locked to keep you from getting lost."

☐ 4. "I want you to come eat your lunch before you go the doctor."

92. An 83-year-old woman is admitted to the unit after being examined in the emergency department (ED) and diagnosed with delirium. After the admission interviews with the client and her grandson, the nurse explains that there will be more laboratory tests and X-rays done that day. The grandson says, "She has already been stuck several times and had a brain scan or something. Just give her some medicine and let her rest." Which response by the nurse is appropriate? Select all that apply.

☐ 1. "I agree she needs to rest, but there is no one specific medicine for your grandmother's condition."

☐ 2. "The doctor will look at the results of those tests in the ED and decide what other tests are needed."

☐ 3. "Delirium commonly results from underlying medical causes that we need to identify and correct."

☐ 4. "Tell me about your grandmother's behaviors and maybe I could figure out what medicine she needs."

☐ 5. "I'll ask the doctor to postpone more tests until tomorrow."

93. The nurse is attempting to draw blood from a woman with a diagnosis of delirium who was admitted last evening. The client yells out, "Stop; leave me alone. What are you trying to do to me? What's happening to me?" Which response by the nurse is most appropriate?

☐ 1. "The tests of your blood will help us figure out what is happening to you."

☐ 2. "Please hold still so I don't have to stick you a second time."

☐ 3. "After I get your blood, I'll get some medicine to help you calm down."

☐ 4. "I'll tell you everything after I get your blood tests to the laboratory."

94. A client with uremia, admitted to a medical unit, is suddenly experiencing sleep disturbances, an inability to focus, poor recent memory, altered perceptions, and disorientation to time and place. The psychiatric liaison nurse conducts an evaluation of the client. Based on an analysis of the findings, the psychiatric liaison nurse suspects which of the following?

☐ 1. Bipolar disorder.

☐ 2. Dementia.

☐ 3. General anxiety disorder.

☐ 4. Delirium.

95. When caring for the client diagnosed with delirium, which condition is the most important for the nurse to investigate?

☐ 1. Cancer of any kind.

☐ 2. Impaired hearing.

☐ 3. Prescription drug intoxication.

☐ 4. Heart failure.

96. In addition to developing over a period of hours or days, the nurse should assess delirium as distinguishable by which of the following characteristics?

☐ 1. Disturbances in cognition and consciousness that fluctuate during the day.

☐ 2. The failure to identify objects despite intact sensory functions.

☐ 3. Significant impairment in social or occupational functioning over time.

☐ 4. Memory impairment to the degree of being called amnesia.

97. Which of the following is most critical when caring for a client who is experiencing delirium?

☐ 1. Controlling behavioral symptoms with low-dose psychotropics.

☐ 2. Identifying the underlying causative condition or illness.

☐ 3. Manipulating the environment to increase orientation.

☐ 4. Decreasing or discontinuing all previously prescribed medications.

98. Which of the following should the nurse identify as a realistic short-term goal to be accomplished in 2 to 3 days for a client with delirium?
☐ **1.** Explain the experience of having delirium.
☐ **2.** Resume a normal sleep-wake cycle.
☐ **3.** Regain orientation to time and place.
☐ **4.** Establish normal bowel and bladder function.

99. Which of the following should the nurse expect to include as a priority in the plan of care for a client with delirium based on the nurse's understanding about the disturbances in orientation associated with this disorder?
☐ **1.** Identifying self and making sure that the nurse has the client's attention.
☐ **2.** Eliminating the client's napping in the daytime as much as possible.
☐ **3.** Engaging the client in reminiscing with relatives or visitors.
☐ **4.** Avoiding arguing with a suspicious client about his perceptions of reality.

100. A client has been in the critical care unit for 3 days following a severe myocardial infarction. Although he is medically stable, he has begun to have fluctuating episodes of consciousness, illogical thinking, and anxiety. He is picking at the air to "catch these baby angels flying around my head." While waiting for medical and psychiatric consults, the nurse must intervene with the client's needs. Which of the following needs have the highest priority? Select all that apply.
☐ **1.** Decreasing as much "foreign" stimuli as possible.
☐ **2.** Avoiding challenging the client's perceptions about "baby angels."
☐ **3.** Orienting the client about his medical condition.
☐ **4.** Gently presenting reality as needed.
☐ **5.** Assisting the client with deep-breathing and relaxation techniques.
☐ **6.** Calling the client's family to report his onset of dementia.

The Client with Dementia

101. A client with dementia who prefers to stay in his room has been brought to the dayroom. After 10 minutes, the client becomes agitated and retreats to his room again. The nurse decides to assess the conditions in the dayroom. Which is the most likely occurrence that is disturbing to this client?
☐ **1.** There is only one other client in the dayroom; the rest are in a group session in another room.
☐ **2.** There are 3 staff members and 1 physician in the nurse's station working on charting.
☐ **3.** A relaxation tape is playing in one corner of the room, and a television airing a special on crime is playing in the opposite corner.
☐ **4.** A housekeeping staff member is washing off the countertops in the kitchen, which is on the far side of the dayroom.

102. Nursing staff are trying to provide for the safety of an elderly female client with moderate dementia. She is wandering at night and has trouble keeping her balance. She has fallen twice but has had no resulting injuries. Which intervention is most appropriate?
☐ **1.** Move the client to a room near the nurse's station and install a bed alarm.
☐ **2.** Have the client sleep in a reclining chair across from the nurse's station.
☐ **3.** Help the client to bed and raise all four bedrails.
☐ **4.** Ask a family member to stay with the client at night.

103. During a home visit to an elderly client with mild dementia, the client's daughter reports that she has one major problem with her mother. She says, "She sleeps most of the day and is up most of the night. I can't get a decent night's sleep anymore." Which suggestions should the nurse make to the daughter? Select all that apply.
☐ **1.** Ask the client's physician for a strong sleep medicine.
☐ **2.** Establish a set routine for rising, hygiene, meals, short rest periods, and bedtime.
☐ **3.** Engage the client in simple, brief exercises or a short walk when she gets drowsy during the day.
☐ **4.** Promote relaxation before bedtime with a warm bath or relaxing music.
☐ **5.** Have the daughter encourage the use of caffeinated beverages during the day to keep her mother awake.

104. A client is experiencing agnosia as a result of vascular dementia. She is staring at dinner and utensils without trying to eat. Which intervention should the nurse attempt first?
☐ **1.** Pick up the fork and feed the client slowly.
☐ **2.** Say, "It's time for you to start eating your dinner."
☐ **3.** Hand the fork to the client and say, "Use this fork to eat your green beans."
☐ **4.** Save the client's dinner until her family comes in to feed her.

105. A client with early dementia exhibits disturbances in her mental awareness and orientation to reality. The nurse should expect to assess a loss of ability in which of the following other areas?
☐ **1.** Speech.
☐ **2.** Judgment.
☐ **3.** Endurance.
☐ **4.** Balance.

106. The client with dementia states to the nurse, "I know you. You're Margaret, the girl who lives down the street from me." Which of the following responses by the nurse is most therapeutic?
- ☐ **1.** "Mrs. Jones, I'm Rachel, a nurse here at the hospital."
- ☐ **2.** "Now Mrs. Jones, you know who I am."
- ☐ **3.** "Mrs. Jones, I told you already, I'm Rachel and I don't live down the street."
- ☐ **4.** "I think you forgot that I'm Rachel, Mrs. Jones."

107. When assessing a client with dementia, which of the following behaviors should the nurse interpret as a manifestation of disinhibition?
- ☐ **1.** Wandering and getting lost.
- ☐ **2.** Auditory and/or visual hallucinations.
- ☐ **3.** Decreased interest in bathing and hygiene.
- ☐ **4.** Inappropriate language and sexual behaviors.

108. The term motor apraxia relates to a decline in motor patterns essential for complex motor tasks. However, the client with severe dementia may be able to perform which of the following actions?
- ☐ **1.** Balance a checkbook accurately.
- ☐ **2.** Brush the teeth when handed a toothbrush.
- ☐ **3.** Use confabulation when telling a story.
- ☐ **4.** Find misplaced car keys.

109. When communicating with the client who is experiencing dementia and exhibiting decreased attention and increased confusion, which of the following interventions should the nurse employ as the first step?
- ☐ **1.** Using gentle touch to convey empathy.
- ☐ **2.** Rephrasing questions the client doesn't understand.
- ☐ **3.** Eliminating distracting stimuli such as turning off the television.
- ☐ **4.** Asking the client to go for a walk while talking.

110. While educating the daughter of a client with dementia about the illness, the daughter complains to the nurse that her mother distorts things. The nurse understands that the daughter needs further teaching about dementia when she makes which statement?
- ☐ **1.** "I tell her reality, such as, 'That noise is the wind in the trees.'"
- ☐ **2.** "I understand the misperceptions are part of the disease."
- ☐ **3.** "I turn off the radio when we're in another room."
- ☐ **4.** "I tell her she is wrong and then I tell her what's right."

The Client with Alzheimer's Disease

111. The client in the early stage of Alzheimer's disease and his adult son attend an appointment at the community mental health center. While conversing with the nurse, the son states, "I'm tired of hearing about how things were 30 years ago. Why does Dad always talk about the past?" Which response by the nurse is the most appropriate?
- ☐ **1.** "Your dad lost his short-term memory, but he still has his long-term memory."
- ☐ **2.** "You need to be more accepting of your dad's behavior."
- ☐ **3.** "I want you to understand your dad's level of anxiety."
- ☐ **4.** "Telling your dad that you are tired of hearing about the past will help him stop."

112. The nurse discusses the possibility of a client's attending day treatment for clients with early Alzheimer's disease. Which of the following is the best rationale for encouraging day treatment?
- ☐ **1.** The client would have more structure to his day.
- ☐ **2.** Staff are excellent in the treatment they offer clients.
- ☐ **3.** The client would benefit from increased social interaction.
- ☐ **4.** The family would have more time to engage in their daily activities.

113. When describing Alzheimer's disease to a group of nursing students, which of the following should the nurse identify as the characteristic found in Alzheimer's disease that distinguishes it from other dementias?
- ☐ **1.** Hypoxic destruction of brain cells.
- ☐ **2.** Hyperkinesis causing choreiform movements.
- ☐ **3.** Neurofibrillary tangles and plaques.
- ☐ **4.** An infectious particle called a prion.

114. When developing the plan of care for a client with Alzheimer's disease who is experiencing moderate impairment, which of the following types of care should the nurse expect to include?
- ☐ **1.** Prompting and guiding activities of daily living.
- ☐ **2.** Managing a medication schedule.
- ☐ **3.** Constant supervision and total care.
- ☐ **4.** Supervision of risky activities such as shaving.

115. Families of clients with Alzheimer's disease report that they have the most difficulty in managing their relatives' aggression and wandering. Which of the following suggestions is least important for the nurse to suggest to help manage wandering?
- ☐ **1.** A Medical Alert bracelet.
- ☐ **2.** Motion and sound detectors.
- ☐ **3.** Door alarms.
- ☐ **4.** Antidepressant medications.

116. Which of the following is a priority to include in the plan of care for a client with Alzheimer's disease who is experiencing difficulty processing and completing complex tasks?
☐ 1. Repeating the directions until the client follows them.
☐ 2. Asking the client to do one step of the task at a time.
☐ 3. Demonstrating for the client how to do the task.
☐ 4. Maintaining routine and structure for the client.

117. The client with Alzheimer's disease may have delusions about being harmed by staff and others. When the client expresses fear of being killed by staff, which of the following responses is most appropriate?
☐ 1. "What makes you think we want to kill you?"
☐ 2. "We like you too much to want to kill you."
☐ 3. "You are in the hospital. We are nurses trying to help you."
☐ 4. "Oh, don't be so silly. No one wants to kill you here."

118. When helping the families of clients with Alzheimer's disease cope with vulgar or sexual behaviors, which of the following suggestions is most helpful?
☐ 1. Ignore the behaviors, but try to identify the underlying need for the behaviors.
☐ 2. Give feedback on the inappropriateness of the behaviors.
☐ 3. Employ anger management strategies.
☐ 4. Administer the prescribed risperidone (Risperdal).

119. The nurse determines that the son of a client with Alzheimer's disease needs further education about the disease when he makes which of the following statements?
☐ 1. "I didn't realize the deterioration would be so incapacitating."
☐ 2. "The Alzheimer's support group has so much good information."
☐ 3. "I get tired of the same old stories, but I know it's important for Dad."
☐ 4. "I woke up this morning expecting that my old Dad would be back."

120. The husband of a client with Alzheimer's disease that was diagnosed 6 years ago approaches the nurse and says, "I'm so excited that my wife is starting to use donepezil (Aricept) for her illness." The nurse needs to inform the husband of which of the following facts about this drug?
☐ 1. Improvements are usually seen in the early stages.
☐ 2. The adverse effects of the drug are numerous.
☐ 3. The client will attain a functional level of that of 6 years ago.
☐ 4. Effectiveness in the terminal phase of the illness is scientifically proven.

121. The physician orders risperidone (Risperdal) for a client with Alzheimer's disease. The nurse anticipates administering this medication to help decrease which of the following behaviors?
☐ 1. Sleep disturbances.
☐ 2. Concomitant depression.
☐ 3. Agitation and assaultiveness.
☐ 4. Confusion and withdrawal.

122. Which of the following agents would the nurse expect to administer, if ordered, for an anxious elderly client with Alzheimer's disease?
☐ 1. Lorazepam (Ativan).
☐ 2. Diazepam (Valium).
☐ 3. Chlordiazepoxide (Librium).
☐ 4. Venlafaxine (Effexor).

123. When providing family education for those who have a relative with Alzheimer's disease about minimizing stress, which of the following suggestions is most relevant?
☐ 1. Allow the client to go to bed four to five times during the day.
☐ 2. Test the cognitive functioning of the client several times a day.
☐ 3. Provide reality orientation even if the memory loss is severe.
☐ 4. Maintain consistency in environment, routine, and caregivers.

Correct Answers and Rationales

The letter in parentheses after each rationale identifies the client need addressed in the item, including management of care (M), safety and infection control (S), health promotion and maintenance (H), psychosocial adaptation (P), basic care and comfort (C), pharmacological and parenteral therapies (D), reduction of risk potential (R), and physiological adaptation (A).

The Client with Paranoid Schizophrenia

1. 4. It is critical for the nurse to ensure the safety of others by knowing who the client might think needs elimination. Asking the client to explain what she means or discuss her concerns at the group session are possible interventions for later in the client's hospital stay. Wearing appropriate clothing while hospitalized is generally a unit expectation for all clients. (P)

2. 2. Knowing the client's interests is the best place to begin to help the client resocialize. Knowing with whom the client wishes to socialize, what transportation she has, or how much spending money she has may be relevant questions, but should be asked after the question concerning what activities the client enjoyed in the past. (P)

3. **1.** It is appropriate to talk alone with this client about her feelings. A suspicious client is unlikely to agree to talk about feelings in a group. It is a violation of the client's privacy to reveal a client's problems to group members. The other clients in the group have no reason to apologize, and the nurse should not ask them to do so. (P)

4. **2.** Schizoaffective disorder is commonly treated with a combination of antipsychotic and mood stabilizing medications. Risperdal alone will not manage the mood symptoms even in large doses. The severity of the mood symptoms is not a factor in selecting treatments. The mood swings are upsetting to the client and need to be treated whether or not there are suicidal thoughts. (P)

5. **2.** The nurse's nonverbal behavior, moving away from the window as the client requests, indicates agreement with the client's false ideas. The client's behavior is likely to be reinforced if the nurse takes steps to agree with the false ideas he holds. (P)

6. **2.** The nursing diagnosis *Disturbed thought processes* related to increased anxiety, as evidenced by delusional thinking, most accurately reflects this client's problem with paranoid delusions. *Disturbed sensory perception: Visual* would be appropriate if the client is hallucinating. *Impaired verbal communication* would be appropriate if the client demonstrates less coherent speech. *Social isolation* would be appropriate if the client refuses to come out of his room. (P)

7. **2, 3, 4, 6.** Assessing the client's risk for harm to self and others is important because she could direct her anger at her ex-husband or turn it on herself. It is important to know more about her current situation and her immediate and priority needs. Obtaining information from the ex-husband's case manager and the police would help clarify the risk of harm to the client. Problems leading to the divorce are less important than the situation following the divorce. The nurse is responsible for assessing the client before requesting a psychiatric consult. (P)

8. **1.** When a client becomes restless during a conversation with the nurse, the first course of action is to reduce the client's anxiety, commonly by walking with the client. Then the nurse can help the client recognize and acknowledge her feelings by sharing observations with her. Changing the subject of the conversation or leaving the client after pointing out that she doesn't appear to want to talk is inappropriate because this does not help the client to recognize and acknowledge her feelings. Additionally, it does not encourage the client to express her anxiety. (P)

9. **4.** The client exhibits aggression against his perceived adversary when he names another client as his adversary. The staff will need to watch him carefully for signs of impending violent behavior that may injure others. Crying about a divorce would be appropriate, not pathologic,

behavior demonstrating grief over a loss. A petition to delay bedtime would be a positive, direct action aimed at a bothersome situation. Although declining to attend group therapy needs follow-up, there may be any number of unknown reasons for this action. (P)

10. **2.** The drug of choice for a client experiencing extrapyramidal adverse effects from haloperidol is benztropine mesylate because of its anticholinergic properties. Lorazepam is an antianxiety agent. Paroxetine is an antidepressant. Olanzapine is an antipsychotic agent. (D)

11. **2.** Clients with paranoid schizophrenia experience alterations in thought resulting in introspection, confusion, and distraction from external reality. Simple tasks that require concentration and effort, including activities involving self-care, may be difficult for the client, especially during the acute phase of the illness. However, the mother should not need to do everything for her daughter. Rather, the mother should encourage the daughter to do things for herself with guidance. Visits from friends should be discussed with the client, and the client should be encouraged to visit with friends to minimize the risk of social isolation. Although relapse typically occurs with medication noncompliance, vulnerability to stress, a low threshold for stress, the number of stresses, and the client's lack of adaptive coping behaviors contribute to relapse. (P)

12. **1.** The nurse recognizes the mother's feelings of being overwhelmed with the issues concerning the management of her daughter at home as caregiver role strain. Anxiety, fear, and sleep disturbances all contribute to caregiver role strain. The nurse should help the mother elicit the support of other family members or friends, continue with psychoeducation, and help the family connect with the Alliance for the Mentally Ill for support, reassurance, and education. (P)

13. **1.** The client is voicing paranoid delusions of being followed and monitored. Presence of delusions is described in the area of thought content in the mental status examination. The speech section would typically include documentation of disturbances in speech or pressured speech. In the insight section, the nurse would document information reflecting a lack of insight—for example, statements such as "I don't have a problem." In the judgment section, the nurse would document information reflecting a lack of judgment—for example, poor choices such as buying a gun for self protection. (P)

14. **2.** For the client with paranoid schizophrenia, 2 days on medication is too short a time for improvement to be seen. Therefore, the nurse evaluates the client's wife as needing education or knowledge about paranoid schizophrenia, the course of the illness, and medications. Expecting an absence of delusions by the end of the client's 2nd day of hospitalization is unrealistic. Rather, the nurse would reasonably expect delusions to decrease, disappearing by 5 to 9 days of hospitalization. The wife's inquiry is not reasonable because not enough time has elapsed to evaluate the effectiveness of treatment. An increase in the client's medication would be unreasonable because not enough time has elapsed to evaluate the effectiveness of the medication. Generally, a time frame of 5 to 7 days is needed before the effectiveness of medications can be determined. (D)

15. 1. The client is describing an auditory hallucination that is most likely related to unresolved guilt about a perceived sin. *Social isolation* would be supported by evidence indicating that the client refuses to come out of her room. *Disturbed thought processes* would be evidenced, for example, by the client's saying that someone in her life is trying to punish her. Loose associations are reflections of racing thoughts, not problems with verbal communication. (P)

16. 4. Benztropine commonly causes the adverse effect of blurred vision. Quetiapine, an atypical antipsychotic, and buspirone, an antianxiety agent, are not likely to produce blurred vision. Although haloperidol, a high-potency antipsychotic, may cause blurred vision, this adverse effect is more common with benztropine. (D)

17. 4. The client is exhibiting suspiciousness of and a lack of trust in the staff, not aggression. Seeking out staff indicates the development of trust and decreased suspiciousness. Although completing activities of daily living and participating in recreation with other clients are important, the major problem presented is related to the client's isolation and perception of being harmed—not, for example, showering, hygiene, or other clients. (P)

18. 3. The client is exhibiting negative symptoms of schizophrenia. Olanzapine, an atypical antipsychotic, is likely to be effective with negative symptoms. Haloperidol, a high-potency antipsychotic agent, and chlorpromazine, a low-potency antipsychotic agent, are effective with the positive symptoms of schizophrenia, such as delusions and hallucinations, but have very little effect on negative symptoms. Trihexyphenidyl is an antiparkinsonian agent, not an antipsychotic agent. (D)

19. 2. Chlorpromazine is a low-potency antipsychotic that is likely to cause sun-sensitive skin. Therefore the client needs instructions about using sunscreen with a sun protection factor of 25 or higher. Typically, chlorpromazine is not associated with an increased risk of seizures. Although constipation is a common adverse effect of this drug, it can be managed with diet, fluids, and exercise. The drug does not need to be discontinued. Chlorpromazine is associated with postural hypotension, not hypertension. Additionally, if postural hypotension occurs, safety measures, such as changing positions slowly and dangling the feet before arising, not stopping the drug, are instituted. (D)

20. 1. The nurse needs to present the reality of the situation. By explaining that the men are groundskeepers and probably talking about work, the nurse is reinforcing reality to counter the client's illusion (misinterpretation of reality). Additionally, this response voices doubt in the client's paranoid interpretation. Telling the client not to take things personally is flippant and judgmental. Telling the client to not pay attention to the men fails to address the client's misinterpretations and misperceptions. Closing the drapes so that the client doesn't see the men ignores the client's misperceptions and misinterpretation. (P)

21. 4. Clozapine is associated with agranulocytosis. Therefore, the nurse must instruct the client about the need for weekly blood tests to monitor for this adverse effect. Akathisia and drug-induced parkinsonism are associated with high-potency antipsychotics. These effects are not common with this atypical antipsychotic agent. Constipation and sedation may occur with this drug. (D)

22. 2. Before intervening with the client experiencing hallucinations, the nurse must validate what the client is experiencing. Asking the client what he hears right now accomplishes this. Asking about seeing someone near the client would be appropriate to validate visual hallucinations. Asking the client about what is going on may be helpful. However, the question is too general to validate that the client is experiencing auditory hallucinations. Asking the client if he wants to go to the recreation room might be appropriate after the nurse has validated what the client is experiencing. (P)

23. 3. The client may act on command hallucinations and harm himself or others. Therefore, the staff need to know when the client is hearing such commands, to ensure safety first. Telling the client that the voices are real but that the nurse doesn't hear them would be an appropriate response later in the client's hospitalization when the client's safety is no longer an issue because antipsychotics are beginning to take effect. Telling the client that the hallucinations are part of the illness or that medications will help control the voices would be appropriate once the client has developed some insight into the symptoms of the illness. (S)

24. 2. The newer antipsychotics block dopamine and serotonin receptors. They do not block GABA acid and norepinephrine receptors. Antidepressants more commonly affect norepinephrine receptors and levels. (D)

25. 3. Tactile hallucinations are more common in alcohol withdrawal than in schizophrenia. Therefore, the nurse should explain that these hallucinations are the result of withdrawal from alcohol. Because the client stopped drinking 4 days ago, the client is not intoxicated. Risperidone has little effect on symptoms of alcohol withdrawal. It is prescribed for symptoms of schizophrenia. Alcohol and risperidone have an additive effect, not one of causing hallucinations. (P)

26. **1, 3, 4, 5.** Documentation provided in option 2 is the most factual and without conclusions or assumptions. Stating that the client was noncompliant with medications is not the only cause of decreased sleep and activities of daily living or increased delusions and hallucinations. Also, the client did not say that his parents wanted to harm him directly. Stating that the client's relationship with his parents is strained is an assumption, even if he did indeed state that they wanted him dead. The client does not state a wish to be dead or harm others, although further assessment would be necessary. Documenting that his parents may be abusing him makes an assumption, although the nurse should further assess for this possibility. (M)

27. **2.** The client is visibly upset and anxious, as demonstrated by his behaviors. In addition, the client's statement reflects clang associations, phrases that rhyme. Panic level anxiety can disturb thought processes, resulting in severely impaired communication such as clang associations. Thinking that a client is out to get him is a delusion but reflects less anxiety and impairment. Incomplete sentences are unrelated to growth and development issues. Data, such as pacing and wringing of the hands, and the client's statements do not indicate noncompliance. (P)

28. **1, 2, 3.** Ridiculing others is a defensive coping strategy in response to the client's feelings of increased anxiety. Negative attention does reinforce inappropriate behaviors. For many clients, negative attention is better than no attention. The client's increased level of anxiety is something that can be dealt with in the group. It is not a reason for excluding the client. There are not sufficient data to indicate a need for medication; behavioral approaches to anxiety management will be more effective. (P)

29. **2.** Pushing a suspicious client into social situations is likely to increase anxiety, which increases, not decreases, the hallucinations. The statement about spending some time alone if the client is overwhelmed indicates awareness and understanding of how to intervene when the client is exposed to stress. The statement about lack of motivation indicates awareness and understanding of avolition. The statement about reminding the client that the family doesn't hear the voices indicates awareness and understanding of the client's hallucinations. (P)

30. **1.** Clozapine is the one atypical antipsychotic associated with severe anticholinergic adverse effects such as constipation. Consuming fruits would not be the cause of the client's constipation. The client should take clozapine with food to avoid nausea. Getting up slowly indicates that the client understands that postural hypotension may occur with clozapine. The statement about sleepiness indicates that the client understands that sedation may occur with this drug. (D)

31. **4.** The statement about the voices occurring if the client is nervous reflects awareness that stress and anxiety can increase the positive symptoms of schizophrenia. Decreasing the medications because the voices are gone reveals a lack of awareness about the need for the medications to control the client's symptoms. Stating that there is still poison in her food demonstrates a lack of insight into the client's delusions. Restarting school in a week reflects an unrealistic expectation for a client who is newly diagnosed and being stabilized on medications. (P)

32. **3.** Because the client is aware that he is experiencing auditory hallucinations, he has some insight into his current problem. Therefore, the nurse should help the client take an active role in trying to control the hallucinations. Telling the client that the nurse doesn't hear voices even though the client does is appropriate to help the client gain insight and awareness of the problem. Although time and medications will make the voices go away, the focus is on helping the client to develop coping strategies to control the hallucinations. Telling the client that the nurse hears only the client's and the nurse's voices is appropriate when the client lacks insight and awareness of the problem. (P)

33. **1.** The initial priority for this client is to help her overcome suspiciousness of others, including staff, and thereby feel safe and accepted. Introducing the client to others, giving the client information about the program, and providing clean clothes are important, but these are of lower priority than helping the client feel safe and accepted. (P)

34. **4.** Allowing the client to be the first to open the cart and take a tray presents the client with the reality that the nurses are not touching the food and tray, thereby dispelling the delusion. Serving foods in sealed packages is unrealistic because most hospital food does not arrive this way. Additionally, if this were possible, sealing the packages would further reinforce the client's delusion. Asking the client about the type of poison or giving the client canned supplements confirms the reality of the client's suspicions, reinforcing the delusion. (P)

35. **2.** Constipation caused by medication is best managed by diet, fluids, and exercise. Benztropine (Cogentin) can increase constipation. However, it may be prescribed for restlessness and stiffness. Restlessness and stiffness should be reported to the physician. Drowsiness and dizziness are adverse effects of ziprasidone. Clients should not drive if they are experiencing dizziness. Ziprasidone does help improve the negative symptoms of schizophrenia such as avolition. (D)

The Client with Other Types of Schizophrenia and Psychotic Disorders

36. **2, 4.** Safety, including protection of the client and others, are the priorities for admission. Acute psychosis commonly involves issues of safety. Living alone is not a sufficient reason to be admitted to a health care facility. Depression, insomnia, lack of appetite, and noncompliance are important issues but not sufficient for admission unless combined with one of the other criteria. (M)

37. **3.** Elderly clients are typically on lower dosages of antipsychotic medications due to the metabolic changes of aging. Comparing dosages is not relevant. Each client is unique in metabolizing medications. Changing medication dosages is based on an assessment of illness symptoms and the adverse effect profile, not on family preferences. Urging the daughter to wait discounts her concerns and gives no rationale for waiting. (P)

38. **2.** Helping the client control his weight is the most appropriate approach. The nurse's contradiction of the client's complaint is inappropriate. Most atypical antipsychotics cause weight gain and are not a solution to the weight gain. There is little evidence that weight gain from taking olanzapine decreases with time. (D)

39. **4.** Achieving a therapeutic blood level is a slower process with risperidone long-acting injection. Oral fluphenazine (Prolixin) does not decrease the effectiveness of the intramuscular version and might increase the incidence of adverse effects. There is no evidence that the potency of the two medications is significantly different. Blaming the client for noncompliance with these two medications is inappropriate. (D)

40. **1, 3, 5.** Group homes, apartment programs, seclusion, restraints, day treatment programs, and self-help groups all involve degrees of restriction and supervision. Releasing information about the client is governed by rules of confidentiality and the Health Insurance Portability and Accountability Act of 1996. Accepting or refusing treatment is governed by laws related to informed consent. (M)

41. **1.** Recognition by the client that there is a difference between the stuffed animal and her live dog indicates that the client perceives the reality of the situation. Stating that the stuffed animal and the client's dog could be twins reflects the client's continued misperception of reality, thinking that the stuffed animal and her dog are one and the same. Stating that she wishes her dog hadn't been stuffed reflects her continued misperception of reality. Stating that the roommate needs a dog as much as she does is unrelated to the client's perception or misperception of reality. (P)

42. **3.** The nurse must be objective in documenting the client's behavior, recording exactly what the client did or did not say or do in a particular situation. Recording that the client could not answer any questions, was uncooperative and refused to answer questions, or was disoriented and incoherent is not described and is a subjective interpretation on the nurse's part. (P)

43. **4.** By the end of 4 days, the client should be able to perform showering and dressing for herself. The client with schizophrenia commonly appears to be apathetic and lack initiative. Therefore, demonstrating the ability to complete the tasks indicates improvement. Although the client may be able to recognize, verbalize, or explain the need to shower and dress herself, she may be unable to do so because of the ambivalence associated with schizophrenia that impedes the client's ability to initiate and complete self-care. Therefore, evidence of improvement would be lacking. (P)

44. **1.** When determining the effectiveness of risperidone, the nurse would expect improvement in the client's negative symptoms of apathy, flat affect, and social withdrawal. Delusions, hallucinations, illusions, and ideas of reference are positive symptoms of schizophrenia. Agitation, hostility, and aggression are the result of the positive symptoms. (D)

45. **2, 3, 4.** The client's symptoms are likely to be adverse effects of aripiprazole, especially at the reported dose. The normal adult dose is 5 to 10 mg. The elderly client commonly needs a lower dose compared with other adults. The anxiety and sleep disturbance could be symptoms of schizophrenia or medication adverse effects. A holistic approach would include assessing the client's heart failure. Questioning the qualifications of the family doctor is unproductive. There are no indications of problems in the client's relationship with her son. (D)

46. **3.** Sialorrhea, excessive salivation, is commonly associated with clozapine therapy. The client can use a washcloth to wipe the saliva instead of spitting. It is an expected adverse effect of the drug, not a delusion, an unusual reaction, or an unresolved symptom of schizophrenia. (D)

47. **3.** Stating that God is important in the client's life recognizes the client's cognitive and perceptual disturbances and level of anxiety and acknowledges the client's message in a respectful and neutral manner, while adding that the medicine also will help, clearly and directly states the need for medication. Stating, "God helps those who help themselves" challenges the client. Stating, "God wants you to take your medicine" is deceitful. Stating, "Medicine will help clear your thinking and decrease anxiety" would be helpful to the client later when she is less acutely psychotic and anxious. (P)

48. 1. The nurse instructs the client clearly and directly to put the medication in his mouth and then to swallow it with some water. Clear, step-by-step directions assist the client to process what the nurse is saying. Telling the client to sit in the dayroom and wait, asking another staff member to stay with the client, or saying nothing is not helpful. (D)

49. 4. Based on the nursing diagnosis of *Defensive coping* secondary to suspiciousness, the client's ability to accurately interpret the behaviors of his wife and coworker would be the expected outcome. The underlying problem is the client's suspiciousness. Therefore, improvement in this behavior would be the focus of the outcome. Although demonstrating an absence of hostile behavior, developing the ability to express one's own needs assertively, and using adaptive coping strategies are desirable, the focus of the outcome needs to address the client's underlying problem, which is interpreting the behaviors of others. (P)

50. 2. Whispering and laughing with another person where the client can see or observe the nurse but not hear the conversation increases the client's anxiety and suspiciousness. Therefore, this action should be avoided. Informing the client of schedule changes, telling the client gently that the nurse does not share the client's interpretation of an event, and inviting the client to participate in leisure activities help the client to decrease anxiety and suspiciousness and to focus on actual or realistic events. (P)

51. 4. Because the client can live in an apartment setting, further development of independent functioning and the skills to gain as much independence as he is capable of need to be fostered, including getting out and developing new friendships. Arranging for participation in day treatment is most beneficial at this time. Family visits and daily nursing visits do not encourage the client to do this. Making an appointment for 2 weeks later puts the client's needs off. Lack of social relationships is not a sufficient reason for rehospitalization. (P)

52. 1. Hallucinations and asocial behaviors are typical symptoms of undifferentiated schizophrenia. Preoccupation with persecutory delusions and hallucinations are associated with paranoid schizophrenia. Grossly disorganized behaviors and speech are associated with disorganized schizophrenia. Immobility and waxy flexibility are associated with catatonic schizophrenia. (P)

53. 2. With CUS, negative symptoms are more prominent. Therefore, risperidone is given to help control negative symptoms. Any positive symptoms of CUS initially could be treated with a high-potency antipsychotic agent such as haloperidol (Haldol). Agranulocytosis is commonly associated with clozapine (Clozaril). Because it is a newer drug, risperidone usually is more expensive than traditional antipsychotics. (D)

54. 1, 2, 3. Transient headaches, anxiety, and insomnia are the most common adverse effects of aripiprazole. Torticollis and pill rolling are more common with the older antipsychotics. (D)

55. 2. The client is in an acute psychotic state and cannot process complex decisions or explain complex situations. Therefore, the nurse would focus on decision making involving simple choices. Listing the pros and cons of each housing option and identifying why the client cannot live in an unsupervised apartment involve complex decision-making skills. Deciding which staff member to have today is a difficult and threatening decision for a client who is psychotic. (P)

56. 1. The client is exhibiting hallmark signs and symptoms of life-threatening neuroleptic malignant syndrome induced by the haloperidol. Tardive dyskinesia usually occurs later in treatment, typically months to years later. Extrapyramidal adverse effects (dystonia, akathisia) and drug-induced parkinsonism, although common, are not life-threatening. (R)

57. 3. The client with chronic undifferentiated schizophrenia needs more structure every day to improve functioning. Therefore, helping the client to set up a daily activity schedule is most appropriate. However, a group home is not necessary. The client is already eating. Having meals brought in would increase the client's dependence, not his activity level. Asking a relative to call the client 10 times per day is unrealistic given the typical daily responsibilities of a healthy relative. (P)

58. 2. The client is exhibiting catatonic behavior, an acutely serious result of severe anxiety and psychosis. In this situation, the nurse needs to administer the p.r.n.-ordered doses of haloperidol and lorazepam; they can be given together safely. Assisting the client out of the chair to go back to bed or sitting quietly until the client responds ignores the seriousness of the client's condition. It is unlikely that the client can describe what is being experienced. (P)

59. 2. Attending day therapy three times per week is a long-term goal that will show the most progress in overcoming withdrawal. The client's calling his mother is a first step in getting out of a severe withdrawal. Allowing two friends to visit every day would be appropriate if the client is successful with calling his mother once a day. Insufficient information is presented in the scenario to indicate that excessive sleep is a problem. (P)

60. 4. Although all the actions indicate improvement, the ability to initiate simple activities without directions indicates the most improvement in the catatonic behaviors. Moving all extremities occasionally, walking with the nurse to the client's room, and responding to verbal directions to eat represent single steps toward the client initiating her own actions. (D)

61. **2.** Noncompliance with medications is common in the client with chronic undifferentiated schizophrenia. The nurse has the responsibility to assess this situation. Asking the mother if they've argued or if the client is mad at the mother or telling the mother to go over to the apartment and see what's going on places the blame and responsibility on the mother and therefore is inappropriate. Telling the mother not to worry ignores the seriousness of the client's symptoms. (P)

62. **4.** The client is exhibiting symptoms of becoming catatonic and unable to care for himself, and needs hospitalization. A sleep aid is not sufficient to treat this client. The client's worsening condition dictates action without waiting for a clinic appointment. An increase in medication may be indicated, but hospitalization is required first for safety. (P)

63. **1.** The client recently lost his mother, causing the client to experience increased stress. This increase in stress can decrease the effectiveness of medications. Therefore, a short course of a fast-acting medication, such as haloperidol, would be added to the client's drug therapy regimen. An increase in olanzapine is not likely to relieve the immediate symptoms quickly. Grief counseling would not be effective until the client's other symptoms are controlled. Changing to a new medication is premature. This would be done only if the client failed to respond to the addition of haloperidol to his drug regimen. (D)

64. **3.** Valproic acid is commonly used to treat manic symptoms. Therefore, a decrease in the valproic acid level could explain the increase in manic symptoms. Periodic determinations of the valproic acid level are necessary to determine the effectiveness of the drug. However, the stat nature of the specimen to be drawn indicates an immediate problem. Fluoxetine is not known to decrease the effectiveness of valproic acid. The valproic acid level is not needed before beginning a short course of therapy with lorazepam. (D)

65. **3.** According to the criteria of the *Diagnostic and Statistical Manual of Mental Disorders,* 4th edition, text revised, a diagnosis of brief psychotic disorder is made when the client exhibits delusions, hallucinations, and disorganized speech or behaviors in the absence of a mood disorder, substance-induced disorder, or general medical condition. (P)

66. **4.** Follow-up counseling is appropriate because of the client's anger and inappropriate behaviors. The goal is to help the client deal with the end of his marriage. A joint session might have been useful before the divorce and arrest, but not after. The client is exhibiting no signs or symptoms of schizophrenia or psychosis, so olanzapine is not indicated. The client is not exhibiting signs of depression, so fluoxetine is not indicated. (P)

Clients and Families Affected by Chronic Mental Illnesses

67. **4.** During necessary periods of hospitalization, active treatment, rather than custodial care, is needed. Among the more common needs of the chronically mentally ill are community-based treatment programs, psychosocial rehabilitation programs, and employment opportunities. (P)

68. **3.** Insight-oriented therapy is less beneficial for this client population. The nurse's role in a psychosocial rehabilitation program involves teaching the client to live independently by using interpersonal skills and community resources. (P)

69. **3.** The first thing that the nurse should do is to speak with the client on the phone and question her about perceptions or reasons that are interfering with her going to the sheltered workshop. This conveys that the nurse is interested and willing to help the client. The nurse should call the director of the workshop for information only if the nurse receives the client's permission. Making preparations for the client's admission is inappropriate and would not be done until the client's needs have been assessed and it is determined that the client requires hospitalization. Making an appointment with the doctor is inappropriate until the nurse has assessed the client's needs. (P)

70. **2.** Psychoeducational groups for families primarily help them to develop a support network. They provide education about the biochemical etiology of psychiatric disease to reduce, not increase family guilt. Financial problems may or may not be addressed. The focus should be on client strengths, not weaknesses. (P)

71. **2.** Noncompliance with medications is documented as the primary cause of relapse. Although loss of family support, sudden changes in medications, and nonattendance at treatment programs may contribute to relapse, these factors are not as significant as medication noncompliance as causes of relapse. (P)

72. **3.** The most therapeutic action at this time is for the nurse to make an appointment with the client at the mental health center to explore his feelings and behavior. Doing so acknowledges the client's importance and makes him a partner in resolving the problem. The nurse needs to determine what is going on in the situation first, and then plan accordingly. Threatening the client with loss of the position, asking for a new assignment for the client, or arranging for the placement of the client in a skill-training program is inappropriate and premature. (P)

73. **2.** By acknowledging the difficulties of living with the illness, the nurse conveys empathy for the client's feelings and opens up the lines of communication. Although it is important for the client to maintain compliance with medication therapy, telling the client that it is important to start taking them again or to talk with the doctor about stopping the medications ignores the underlying feelings of the client's initial statements. Stating that the client's buddies will understand may or may not be true. Additionally, this statement ignores the underlying feelings. (P)

74. **3.** Because antipsychotic agents cross the placental barrier and can be teratogenic, they are to be avoided during pregnancy, especially during the first trimester. Later in the pregnancy, low doses of medications may be given if necessary. Although the degree of excitement by the father, the mother's ability to provide help, and the client's financial situation may or may not be of concern, the priority in this situation is the safety of the fetus and risks associated with the need for antipsychotic therapy. (P)

75. **4.** Although all of the options are commonly true, the primary reason for concern is that parents commonly provide financial support and housing for their chronically mentally ill children. The most critical needs after loss of the parents are the lack of financial support and housing, which are hard to replace. (P)

76. **2.** Families are more likely to be seen as allies in the care of clients because they are no longer viewed as causing the illness. Although family dysfunction is viewed as an effect of rather than a cause of the disorder, the most significant aspect is that families are now viewed as allies by health care professionals. Families may or may not be less likely to participate in studies or to be involved in caring for the ill relatives. (P)

77. **4.** Although a decline in functioning is important, this situation would have the least priority when compared with other situations that put the client or others in danger of direct or indirect harm. (S)

78. **3.** Many coordinated services is needed, including medication management, more frequent outpatient visits, day treatment, or some combination of these, to decrease the risk of relapse, which is common among chronically ill clients. Medical consultations (if needed) would be included in the coordinated services provided. Chronically mentally ill clients who are discharged early, before becoming truly stable, typically require more than monthly outpatient visits because of the high risk of relapse. A caring and supportive family is ideal for all clients but not always available. (P)

79. **3.** Noncompliance with medications is the most common cause of relapse and rehospitalization for chronically mentally ill persons. Preventing relapse is a daily goal. Support groups are not always appropriate for chronically ill clients. Family support is desirable but is less likely to be available for these clients. Advocacy is a long-term goal. (P)

80. **1, 3.** Without a sufficient range and quantity of services, care is inadequate and hospitalization rates increase. Nonshifting of allocated funding to outpatient services has increased the problem with the range and quantity of services. Reserving hospitalization for emergency services was a practice before managed care. The principle of "least restrictive alternative" is still as relevant as it was before managed care. There are not enough group homes available. (P)

81. **4.** For a community-based program, the need for long-term hospitalization is least needed if the other services, such as partial programs, psychiatric home care, and residential services, are available and accessible. (M)

82. **2, 3, 4.** Although all of the situations require immediate attention, the inability to keep outpatient appointments is less critical than signs of relapse and decompensation, threat of eviction, and unpaid bills and lack of food. Occasionally missing a dose of medication usually will not precipitate a crisis for a client. (P)

83. **1.** Ways to decrease or manage adverse effects without additional medications is crucial. Although home visits, family monitoring, and outpatient monitoring may help, if the adverse effects are not controlled, the client is less likely to take the drug, which would interfere with its effectiveness. (D)

84. **4.** Many Americans still believe that recovery from mental illness is a matter of willpower—for example, "pull yourself up by your bootstraps" or "just get over it." This belief persists despite awareness that mental illness is hereditary and has a biochemical basis. Mental illness can be prevented only if there is early intervention. Clients cannot prevent it just by the desire to do so. (P)

The Client with Cognitive Disorders

85. **1, 2, 3, 5, 6.** It is important for a caregiver to have support for herself as well as be able to provide adequate safety, supervision, and medical care to the client. The caregiver must also have realistic expectations of the client, given his abilities and limitations. Reminiscing and engaging the client in games is desirable but not crucial to care. (M)

86. **4.** Expecting the social worker to make the decision indicates that the son is avoiding participating in decisions about his father. The other responses convey that the son understands the importance of a careful decision, the availability of resources, and the ability to make new plans if needed. (M)

87. **1, 2, 5.** Confused clients need fewer choices, acceptance as a person, and step-by-step directions. Allowing the client to do as he wishes can lead to substandard care and the risk of harm. Acting nonchalantly conveys a lack of caring. (P)

88. **2.** When caring for a client with cognitive impairment, the priority is to ensure that all objects in the client's path are removed to prevent the client from falling. Additional measures, such as having two people accompany the client when he ambulates, placing his favorite things in safekeeping, and giving medications in a liquid form to be sure he swallows them, are less crucial and available. (S)

89. **1.** The most common reason for the nurse's discomfort with elderly clients is that she has not examined her own fears and conflicts about aging. Until nurses resolve their fears, it is unlikely that they will feel comfortable with elderly clients. A dislike of physical contact with older people, a desire to be surrounded by beauty and youth, and recent experiences with a parent's elderly friends are possible explanations, but not common or likely. (P)

90. **3.** Reminiscing can help reduce depression in an elderly client and lessens feelings of isolation and loneliness. Reminiscing encourages a focus on positive memories and accomplishments as well as shared memories with other clients. An increase in confusion and disorientation is most likely the result of other cognitive and situational factors, such as loss of short-term memory, not reminiscing. The client will not likely become sad because reminiscing helps the client connect with positive memories. Keeping the client from participating in therapeutic activities is less likely with reminiscing. (P)

The Client with Delirium

91. **2.** Loss of orientation, especially for time and place, is common in delirium. The nurse should orient the client by telling him the time, date, place, and who the client is with. Taking the client to his room and telling him why the door is locked does not address his disorientation. Telling the client to eat before going to the doctor reinforces his disorientation. (P)

92. **1, 2, 3.** The client does need rest and it is true that there is no specific medicine for delirium, but it is crucial to identify and treat the underlying causes of delirium. Other tests will be based on the results of already completed tests. Although some medications may be prescribed to help the client with her behaviors, this is not the primary basis for medication orders. Because the underlying medical causes of delirium could be fatal, treatment must be initiated as soon as possible. It is not the nurse's role to determine medications for this client. Postponing tests until the next day is inappropriate. (P)

93. **1.** Explaining why blood is being taken responds to the client's concerns or fears about what is happening to her. Threatening more pain or promising to explain later ignores or postpones meeting the client's need for information. The client's statements do not reflect loss of self control requiring medication intervention. (P)

94. **4.** Based on the assessment findings, delirium is the most likely cause of the sudden onset of symptoms. Uremia is a common cause of delirium resulting from the buildup of toxins in the body. Disorientation and memory deficits are not commonly seen in bipolar or general anxiety disorder. Grandiosity and hyperactivity are more common in bipolar disorder. Dementia has a slow but progressive onset, not a sudden onset as described. (A)

95. **3.** Polypharmacy is much more common in the elderly. Drug interactions increase the incidence of intoxication from prescribed medications, especially with combinations of analgesics, digoxin, diuretics, and anticholinergics. With drug intoxication, the onset of the delirium typically is quick. Although cancer, impaired hearing, and heart failure could lead to delirium in the elderly, the onset would be more gradual. (R)

96. **1.** Fluctuating symptoms are characteristic of delirium. The failure to identify objects despite intact sensory functions, significant impairment in social or occupational functioning over time, and memory impairment to the degree of being called amnesia all indicate dementia. (A)

97. **2.** The most critical aspect when caring for the client with delirium is to institute measures to correct the underlying causative condition or illness. Controlling behavioral symptoms with low-dose psychotropics, manipulating the environment, and decreasing or discontinuing all medications may be dangerous to the client's health. (R)

98. **3.** In approximately 2 to 3 days, the client should be able to regain orientation and thus become oriented to time and place. Being able to explain the experience of having delirium is something that the client is expected to achieve later in the course of the illness, but ultimately before discharge. Resuming a normal sleep-wake cycle and establishing normal bowel and bladder function probably will take longer, depending on how long it takes to resolve the underlying condition. (P)

99. **1.** Identifying oneself and making sure that the nurse has the client's attention addresses the difficulties with focusing, orientation, and maintaining attention. Eliminating daytime napping is unrealistic until the cause of the delirium is determined and the client's ability to focus and maintain attention improves. Engaging the client in reminiscing and avoiding arguing are also unrealistic at this time. (P)

100. **1, 2, 4, 5.** The abnormal stimuli of the critical care unit can aggravate the symptoms of delirium. Arguing with hallucinations is inappropriate. When a client has illogical thinking, gently presenting reality is appropriate as is reducing his anxiety level. Disorientation is not described. Dementia is not the likely cause of the client's symptoms. The client is experiencing delirium, not dementia. (P)

The Client with Dementia

101. **3.** The tape and television are competing, even conflicting, stimuli. Crime events portrayed on television could be misperceived as a real threat to the client. A low number of clients and the presence of a few staff members quietly working are less intense stimuli for the client and not likely to be disturbing. (M)

102. **1.** Using a bed alarm enables the staff to respond immediately if the client tries to get out of bed. Sleeping in a chair at the nurse's station interferes with the client's restful sleep and privacy. Using all four bedrails is considered a restraint and unsafe practice. It is not appropriate to expect a family member to stay all night with the client. (S)

103. **2, 3, 4.** A set routine and brief exercises help decrease daytime sleeping. Decreasing caffeine and fluids and promoting relaxation at bedtime promote nighttime sleeping. A strong sleep medicine for an elderly client is contraindicated due to changes in metabolism, increased adverse effects, and the risk of falls. Using caffeinated beverages may stimulate metabolism but can also have long-lasting adverse effects and may prevent sleep at bedtime. (M)

104. **3.** Agnosia is the lack of recognition of objects and their purpose. The nurse should inform the client about the fork and what to do with it. Feeding the client does not address the agnosia or give the client specific directions. It should only be attempted if identifying the fork and explaining what to do with it is ineffective. Waiting for the family to care for the client is not appropriate unless identifying the fork and explaining or feeding the client are not successful. (M)

105. **2.** Clients with chronic cognitive disorders experience defects in memory orientation and intellectual functions, such as judgment and discrimination. Loss of other abilities, such as speech, endurance, and balance, is less typical. (P)

106. **1.** Because of the client's short-term memory impairment, the nurse gently corrects the client by stating her name and who she is. This approach decreases anxiety, embarrassment, and shame and maintains the client's self-esteem. Telling the client that she knows who the nurse is or that she forgot can elicit feelings of embarrassment and shame. Saying, "I told you already" sounds condescending, as if blaming the client for not remembering. (P)

107. **4.** Loss of judgment decreases the ability to control impulses and behaviors in social situations. Therefore, the client typically exhibits inappropriate language and sexual behaviors. Wandering and getting lost involve cognitive changes, not disinhibition. Hallucinations are sensory perceptual disturbances. Decreased interest in activities of daily living is related to apathy and cognitive changes. (P)

108. **2.** Highly conditioned motor skills, such as brushing the teeth, may be retained by the client who has dementia and motor apraxia. Balancing a checkbook involves calculations, a complex skill that is lost with severe dementia. Confabulation is fabrication of details to fill a memory gap. This is more common when the client is aware of a memory problem, not when dementia is severe. Finding keys is a memory factor, not a motor function. (P)

109. **3.** Competing and excessive stimuli lead to sensory overload and confusion. Therefore, the nurse should first eliminate any distracting stimuli. After this is accomplished, then using touch and rephrasing questions are appropriate. Going for a walk while talking has little benefit on attention and confusion. (P)

110. **4.** Telling the client that she is wrong and then telling her what is right is argumentative and challenging. Arguing with or challenging distortions is least effective because it increases defensiveness. Telling the client about reality indicates awareness of the issues and is appropriate. Acknowledging that misperceptions are part of the disease indicates an understanding of the disease and an awareness of the issues. Turning off the radio helps to limit environmental stimuli and indicates an awareness of the issues. (P)

The Client with Alzheimer's Disease

111. **1.** The son's statements regarding his father's recalling past events is typical for family members of clients in the early stage of Alzheimer's disease, when recent memory is impaired. Telling the son to be more accepting is critical and not an attempt to educate. Understanding the client's level of anxiety is unrelated to the memory loss of Alzheimer's disease. The client cannot stop reminiscing at will. (P)

112. **3.** The best rationale for day treatment for the client with Alzheimer's disease is the enhancement of social interactions. More daily structure, excellent staff, and allowing caregivers more time for themselves are all positive aspects, but they are less focused on the client's needs. (P)

113. **3.** Neurofibrillary tangles and plaques are found in postmortem examinations of Alzheimer's disease clients, distinguishing it from other dementias. Hypoxic destruction of brain cells is associated with multi-infarct dementia. Hyperkinesis causing choreiform movements is associated with Huntington's disease. Evidence of an infectious particle called a prion is associated with Creutzfeldt-Jakob disease. (P)

114. **1.** Considerable assistance is associated with moderate impairment when the client cannot make decisions but can follow directions. Managing medications is needed even in mild impairment. Constant care is needed in the terminal phase, when the client cannot follow directions. Supervision of shaving is appropriate with mild impairment—that is, when the client still has motor function but lacks judgment about safety issues. (P)

115. **4.** Antidepressant medications have little impact on wandering. A Medical Alert bracelet helps in identifying the client should he wander. Motion and sound detectors and door alarms can alert family members to the possibility of the client's leaving the area. (P)

116. **2.** Because the client is experiencing difficulty processing and completing complex tasks, the priority is to provide the client with only one step at a time, thereby breaking the task up into simple steps, ones that the client can process. Repeating the directions until the client follows them or demonstrating how to do the task is still too overwhelming to the client because of the multiple steps involved. Although maintaining structure and routine is important, it is unrelated to task completion. (P)

117. **3.** The nurse needs to present reality without arguing with the delusions. Therefore, stating that the client is in the hospital and the nurses are trying to help is most appropriate. The client doesn't recognize the delusion or why it exists. Telling the client that the staff likes him too much to want to kill him is inappropriate because the client believes the delusions and doesn't know that they are false beliefs. It also restates the word, kill, which may reinforce the client's delusions. Telling the client not to be silly is condescending and disparaging and therefore inappropriate. (P)

118. **1.** The vulgar or sexual behaviors are commonly expressions of anger or more sensual needs that can be addressed directly. Therefore, the families should be encouraged to ignore the behaviors but attempt to identify their purpose. Then the purpose can be addressed, possibly leading to a decrease in the behaviors. Because of impaired cognitive function, the client is not likely to be able to process the inappropriateness of the behaviors if given feedback. Likewise, anger management strategies would be ineffective because the client would probably be unable to process the inappropriateness of the behaviors. Risperidone (Risperdal) may decrease agitation, but it does not improve social behaviors. (P)

119. **4.** The statement about expecting that the old Dad would be back conveys a lack of acceptance of the irreversible nature of the disease. The statement about not realizing that the deterioration would be so incapacitating is based in reality. The statement about the Alzheimer's group is based in reality and demonstrates the son's involvement with managing the disease. Stating that reminiscing is important reflects a realistic interpretation on the son's part. (P)

120. **1.** When compared with other similar medications, donepezil (Aricept) has fewer adverse effects. Donepezil is effective primarily in the early stages of the disease. The drug helps to slow the progression of the disease if started in the early stages. After the client has been diagnosed for 6 years, improvement to the level seen 6 years ago is highly unlikely. Data are not available to support the drug's effectiveness for clients in the terminal phase of the disease. (D)

121. **3.** Antipsychotics are most effective with agitation and assaultiveness. Antipsychotics have little effect on sleep disturbances, concomitant depression, or confusion and withdrawal. (D)

122. **1.** Lorazepam is the antianxiety drug of choice for the elderly client because it is one of the safest agents. Diazepam and chlordiazepoxide have an extended half-life and active metabolites. The elderly client is less able to break down and excrete these medicines. Venlafaxine is an antidepressant and is not used to treat anxiety. (D)

123. **4.** Change increases stress. Therefore, the most important and relevant suggestion is to maintain consistency in the client's environment, routine, and caregivers. Although rest periods are important, going to bed interferes with the sleep-wake cycle. Rest in a recliner chair is more useful. Testing cognitive functioning and reality orientation are not likely to be successful and may increase stress if memory loss is severe. (P)

Personality Disorders, Substance-Related Disorders, and Anxiety-Related Disorders

- The Client with a Personality Disorder
- The Client with an Alcohol-Related Disorder
- The Client with Disorders Related to Other Addictive Substances
- The Client with an Anxiety-Related Disorder
- The Client with a Somatoform Disorder
- Correct Answers and Rationales

The Client with a Personality Disorder

1. A client with borderline personality disorder has self-inflicted cuts on her arms. The nurse is assessing the client for the risk of suicide. What should the nurse ask the client first?
- [ ] 1. About medications she has taken recently.
- [ ] 2. If she is taking antidepressants.
- [ ] 3. If she has a suicide plan.
- [ ] 4. Why she cut herself.

2. When developing the plan of care for a client with a personality disorder, the nurse expects to assist the client primarily with which of the following?
- [ ] 1. Specific dysfunctional behaviors.
- [ ] 2. Psychopharmacologic compliance.
- [ ] 3. Examination of developmental conflicts.
- [ ] 4. Manipulation of the environment.

3. A client with paranoid personality disorder is hospitalized for physically threatening his wife because he suspects her of having an affair with a coworker. Which of the following approaches should the nurse employ with this client?
- [ ] 1. Authoritarian.
- [ ] 2. Parental.
- [ ] 3. Matter-of-fact.
- [ ] 4. Controlling.

4. When planning care for a client with schizotypal personality disorder, which of the following helps the client become involved with others?
- [ ] 1. Participating solely in group activities.
- [ ] 2. Being involved with primarily one-to-one activities.
- [ ] 3. Leading a sing-along in the afternoon.
- [ ] 4. Attending an activity with the nurse.

5. A client is complaining to other clients about not being allowed by staff to keep food in her room. Which of the following interventions is most appropriate?
- [ ] 1. Ignoring the client's behavior.
- [ ] 2. Setting limits on the behavior.
- [ ] 3. Reprimanding the client.
- [ ] 4. Allowing the snack to be kept in her room.

6. A client with an Axis II diagnosis of antisocial personality disorder has a potential for violence and aggressive behavior. Which of the following client outcomes to be accomplished in the short term is most appropriate for the nurse to include in the plan of care?
- [ ] 1. Use humor when expressing anger.
- [ ] 2. Discuss feelings of anger with staff.
- [ ] 3. Ask the nurse for medication when upset.
- [ ] 4. Use indirect behaviors to express anger.

7. A client with an Axis II diagnosis of antisocial personality disorder has been stealing equipment from his place of employment. He states, "It's not a big deal. My boss can afford a few missing pieces. He doesn't like me." The nurse interprets the client's behavior as indicative of problems in which of the following stages of growth and development defined by Erikson?
- [ ] 1. Trust versus mistrust.
- [ ] 2. Autonomy versus shame and doubt.
- [ ] 3. Initiative versus guilt.
- [ ] 4. Industry versus inferiority.

8. Which of the following approaches should the nurse expect to include in the plan of care for a client with antisocial personality disorder who has a history of stealing and jail time?
- [ ] 1. Helping the client develop a conscience.
- [ ] 2. Teaching the client consequences of her actions.
- [ ] 3. Assisting the client with understanding right from wrong.
- [ ] 4. Using strategies to help the client become passive.

9. A 28-year-old client with an Axis I diagnosis of major depression and an Axis II diagnosis of dependent personality disorder has been living at home with very supportive parents. The client is thinking about independent living on the recommendation of the treatment team. The client states to the nurse, "I don't know if I can make it in an apartment without my parents." Which of the following responses by the nurse is most therapeutic?

☐ **1.** "You're a 28-year-old adult now, not a child who needs to be cared for."
☐ **2.** "Your parents won't be around forever. After all, they are getting older."
☐ **3.** "Your parents need a break, and you need a break from them."
☐ **4.** "Your parents have been supportive and will continue to be even if you live apart."

10. The client with major depression and dependent personality disorder has made the decision to live independently in an apartment. The nurse and the client meet with his parents to discuss his decision. Which statement by the nurse is most helpful to foster the client's independence?

☐ **1.** "You'll still be able to see your son and help him as much as you want."
☐ **2.** "All of you will gain from his independent living; he needs our support."
☐ **3.** "You'll need to help monitor his medication and clinic appointments."
☐ **4.** "You'll live nearby and be able to help with meals and laundry."

11. A client who had been living with her family after her boyfriend of 4 weeks told her to leave is admitted to the subacute unit complaining of feeling empty and lonely, being unable to sleep, and hardly eating for the past week. Her arms are scarred from frequent self-mutilation. The nurse interprets these findings as indicating which of the following personality disorders?

☐ **1.** Antisocial personality disorder.
☐ **2.** Avoidant personality disorder.
☐ **3.** Borderline personality disorder.
☐ **4.** Compulsive personality disorder.

12. The client approaches various staff with numerous requests and needs to the point of disrupting the staff's work with other clients. The nurse meets with the staff to decide on a consistent, therapeutic approach for this client. Which of the following approaches should the nurse expect to institute?

☐ **1.** Telling the client to stay in his room until staff approach him.
☐ **2.** Limiting the client to the dayroom and dining area.
☐ **3.** Giving the client a list of permissible requests.
☐ **4.** Having the client address needs to the staff person assigned.

13. The client with borderline personality disorder tells the nurse, "You're the best nurse here. I can talk to you and you listen. You're the only one here that can help me." Which of the following responses by the nurse is most therapeutic?

☐ **1.** "Thank you, you're a good person."
☐ **2.** "All of the nurses here provide good care."
☐ **3.** "Other clients have told me that too."
☐ **4.** "Mary and Sam are good nurses too."

14. The client with borderline personality disorder is admitted to the unit after having attempted to cut her wrists with a pair of scissors. The client has several scars on both arms from self-mutilation and suicide gestures. A staff member states to the nurse, "It's just attention that she wants, she's not going to kill herself." Which of the following responses by the nurse is most appropriate?

☐ **1.** "She's here now and we have to do our best."
☐ **2.** "She needs to be here until she can control her behavior."
☐ **3.** "I'm ashamed of you; you know better than to say that."
☐ **4.** "Any attempt at self-harm is serious, and safety is a priority."

15. The nurse assesses a client to be at risk for self-mutilation and implements a safety contract with the client. Which of the following client behaviors would indicate that the contract is working?

☐ **1.** The client withdraws to his room when feeling overwhelmed.
☐ **2.** The client notifies staff when anxiety is increasing.
☐ **3.** The client suppresses his feelings when angry.
☐ **4.** The client displaces his feelings onto the physician.

16. The client with borderline personality disorder who is to be discharged soon threatens to "do something" to herself if discharged. Which of the following actions by the nurse is most important?

☐ **1.** Request an immediate extension for the client.
☐ **2.** Ignore the client's statement because it's a sign of manipulation.
☐ **3.** Ask a family member to stay with the client at home temporarily.
☐ **4.** Discuss the meaning of the client's statement with her.

17. A 19-year-old client is admitted to a psychiatric unit with an Axis I diagnosis of alcohol abuse and an Axis II diagnosis of personality disorder not otherwise specified. The client's mother states, "He's always in trouble, just like when he was a boy. Now he's just a bigger prankster and out of control." In view of the client's history, which of the following is most important initially?

☐ **1.** Letting the client know the staff has the authority to subdue him if he gets unruly.

☐ **2.** Keeping the client isolated from other clients until he is better known by the staff.

☐ **3.** Emphasizing to the client that he will have to pay for any damage he causes.

☐ **4.** Closely observing the client's behavior to establish a baseline pattern of functioning.

18. The client tells the nurse at the outpatient clinic that she doesn't need to attend groups because she's "not a regular like these other people here." Which of the following responses by the nurse is best?

☐ **1.** "Because you're not a regular client, sit in the hall when the others are in group."

☐ **2.** "Your family wants you to attend, and they will be very disappointed if you don't."

☐ **3.** "I'll have to mark you absent from the clinic today and speak to the doctor about it."

☐ **4.** "You say you're not a regular here, but you're experiencing what others are experiencing."

19. After a client with an antisocial personality disorder belches loudly, a staff member asks the client, "Do you wonder why people find you repulsive?" This comment most likely would elicit which of the following client reactions?

☐ **1.** Defensiveness.

☐ **2.** Remorsefulness.

☐ **3.** Shame.

☐ **4.** Embarrassment.

20. The client who has a history of using angry outbursts when frustrated begins to curse at the nurse during an appointment after being informed that she will have to wait to have her medication refilled. Which of the following responses by the nurse is most appropriate?

☐ **1.** "You're being very childish."

☐ **2.** "I'm sorry if you can't wait."

☐ **3.** "I will not continue to talk with you if you curse."

☐ **4.** "Come back tomorrow and your medication will be ready."

21. Which of the following behaviors indicates to the nurse that the client with avoidant personality disorder is improving?

☐ **1.** Interacting with two other clients.

☐ **2.** Listening to music with headphones.

☐ **3.** Sitting at a table and painting.

☐ **4.** Talking on the telephone.

22. One evening the client takes the nurse aside and whispers, "Don't tell anybody, but I'm going to call in a bomb threat to this hospital tonight." Which of the following actions is the priority?

☐ **1.** Warning the client that his telephone privileges will be taken away if he abuses them.

☐ **2.** Offering to disregard the client's plan if he does not go through with it.

☐ **3.** Notifying the proper authorities after saying nothing until the client has actually completed the call.

☐ **4.** Explaining to the client that this information will have to be shared immediately with the staff and the physician.

23. When teaching a nursing assistant new to the unit about the principles for the care of a client with a personality disorder, which of the following should the nurse include as the most important basic principle?

☐ **1.** The clients are accepted although their behavior may not be.

☐ **2.** Clients need limits on their behavior.

☐ **3.** The staff members are the primary ones left to care about these clients.

☐ **4.** The staff should use minimal humor when working with these clients.

24. The nurse is talking with a client who has been diagnosed with antisocial personality disorder about how to socialize during activities without being seductive. The nurse should focus the discussion on which of the following areas?

☐ **1.** Explaining the negative reactions of others toward his behavior.

☐ **2.** Suggesting he apologize to others for his behavior.

☐ **3.** Asking him to explain the reasons for his seductive behavior.

☐ **4.** Discussing his relationship with his mother.

25. The client with an Axis II diagnosis of narcissistic personality disorder tells the nurse he can get an executive position with the best company around anytime he wants. The history reveals that the client, whose highest level of education completed is high school, has held only a series of short-term part-time jobs for the past 2 years. The nurse interprets the client's statement to be an example of which of the following?
☐ **1.** Grandiose delusion.
☐ **2.** Blatant lie.
☐ **3.** Grandiose self-importance.
☐ **4.** Sense of entitlement.

26. Which of the following approaches is most appropriate to use with the client who has a narcissistic personality disorder when discrepancies exist between what the client states and what actually exists?
☐ **1.** Limit setting.
☐ **2.** Supportive confrontation.
☐ **3.** Consistency.
☐ **4.** Rationalization.

27. The client with a histrionic personality disorder is melodramatic and responds to others and situations in an exaggerated manner. The nurse should recommend which of the following activities for this client?
☐ **1.** Party planning.
☐ **2.** Music group.
☐ **3.** Cooking class.
☐ **4.** Role-playing.

28. When developing the plan of care for a client with an Axis I diagnosis of major depression and an Axis II diagnosis of borderline personality disorder, the nurse should most likely anticipate an order for which of the following medications?
☐ **1.** A selective serotonin reuptake inhibitor.
☐ **2.** A benzodiazepine.
☐ **3.** A mood stabilizer.
☐ **4.** An antipsychotic.

The Client with an Alcohol-Related Disorder

29. A client known to abuse alcohol is admitted to the emergency department with a temperature of 99° F (37.2° C), pulse of 110 bpm, respirations of 26, and blood pressure of 150/92 mm Hg. The client is belligerent with slurred speech. His blood alcohol level is 400 mg/dl. What should the nurse do first?
☐ **1.** Start an I.V. infusion.
☐ **2.** Restrain the client.
☐ **3.** Place the client in a quiet room.
☐ **4.** Administer naloxone (Narcan).

30. A client has been admitted to the emergency department with alcohol withdrawal delirium. The nurse is assessing the client for signs of withdrawal. At 9 a.m. on 10/25, the nurse notes that the client is confused. His vital signs are T = 99° F, P = 60, R = 10, and BP = 118/70. The nurse compares these findings to the nurses' progress notes from admission 24 hours ago (shown below). What should the nurse do first?
☐ **1.** Contact the physician.
☐ **2.** Increase the rate of the I.V. infusion.
☐ **3.** Attempt to arouse the client.
☐ **4.** Administer magnesium sulfate.

PROGRESS NOTES

Date	Time	Progress Notes
10/24/07	09:00 pm	T = 99° F; P = 110; R = 18; BP = 140/90; Client has I.V. D₅W keep open rate started; Valium administered as ordered. Client oriented × 3.
10/25/07	01:00 am	T = 99.2° F; P = 90; R = 14; BP = 130/80; Client resting.
10/25/07	05:00 am	T = 99° F; P = 70; R = 14; BP = 126/80; Client oriented × 3.

31. An intoxicated client is admitted to the hospital for alcohol withdrawal. Which of the following should the nurse do to help the client become sober?
☐ **1.** Give the client black coffee to drink.
☐ **2.** Walk the client around the unit.
☐ **3.** Have the client take a cold shower.
☐ **4.** Provide the client with a quiet room to sleep in.

32. The client is admitted to the hospital for alcohol detoxification. Which of the following interventions should the nurse use? Select all that apply.
☐ **1.** Taking vital signs.
☐ **2.** Monitoring intake and output.
☐ **3.** Placing the client in restraints as a safety measure.
☐ **4.** Reinforcing reality if the client is disoriented or hallucinating.
☐ **5.** Explaining to the client that the symptoms of withdrawal are temporary.

33. A client is entering the chemical dependency unit for treatment of alcohol dependency. Which of the client's possessions should the nurse place in a locked area?
☐ **1.** Toothpaste.
☐ **2.** Dental floss.
☐ **3.** Shaving cream.
☐ **4.** Antiseptic mouthwash.

34. When obtaining the history from a client entering rehabilitation for alcohol dependency, the nurse questions the client about the amount of alcohol he consumes daily. The client responds, "I just have a few drinks with the guys after work." The nurse interprets this statement as the client's using which of the following as a defense?
- ☐ **1.** Projection.
- ☐ **2.** Minimization.
- ☐ **3.** Denial.
- ☐ **4.** Rationalization.

35. While admitting a client to the alcohol treatment program, the nurse asks the client how long she's been drinking, how much she's been drinking, and when she had her last drink. The client replies that she has been drinking about a liter of vodka a day for the past week and her last drink was about an hour ago. This information helps the nurse to determine which of the following?
- ☐ **1.** The severity of the disease.
- ☐ **2.** The severity of withdrawal symptoms.
- ☐ **3.** The possibility of alcoholic hallucinosis.
- ☐ **4.** The occurrence of delirium tremens.

36. The client is feeling better as the symptoms of alcohol withdrawal abate. She refuses information about alcohol rehabilitation and states, "I don't have a problem. I'll never drink like that again. I learned my lesson this time. I guess I'll just have to switch to beer or wine." Which of the following is most effective in decreasing the client's denial?
- ☐ **1.** Discussing how alcohol has gotten her into trouble.
- ☐ **2.** Explaining the effects of drinking on her family.
- ☐ **3.** Urging her to attend Alcoholics Anonymous meetings.
- ☐ **4.** Telling her about the physiologic damage that can result.

37. A client who is experiencing alcohol withdrawal exhibits tremors, diaphoresis, and hyperactivity. Blood pressure is 190/87 mm Hg and pulse is 92 bpm. Which of the following medications should the nurse expect to administer?
- ☐ **1.** Haloperidol (Haldol).
- ☐ **2.** Lorazepam (Ativan).
- ☐ **3.** Benztropine (Cogentin).
- ☐ **4.** Naloxone (Narcan).

38. Which of the following assessments provides the best information about the client's physiologic response and the effectiveness of the medication prescribed specifically for alcohol withdrawal?
- ☐ **1.** Nutritional status.
- ☐ **2.** Evidence of tremors.
- ☐ **3.** Vital signs.
- ☐ **4.** Sleep pattern.

39. A client who had been drinking heavily over the weekend could not remember specific events of where he had been or what he had done. The nurse interprets this information as indicating that the client experienced which of the following conditions?
- ☐ **1.** Blackout.
- ☐ **2.** Hangover.
- ☐ **3.** Tolerance.
- ☐ **4.** Delirium tremens.

40. A client is entering the alcohol treatment program for the fourth time in 5 years. Which of the following statements by the nurse is be most helpful to the client?
- ☐ **1.** "I hope you are serious about maintaining your sobriety this time."
- ☐ **2.** "I'm Maria, a nurse here. I don't know you from past attempts but you'll get it right this time."
- ☐ **3.** "I know someone who was successful after the fifth program."
- ☐ **4.** "I'm Maria, a nurse in the program. The staff and I will help you through the program."

41. The wife of a client with alcohol dependency tells the nurse, "I'm tired of making excuses for him to his boss and coworkers when he can't make it into work. I believe him every time he says he's going to quit." The nurse recognizes the wife's statement as indicating which of the following behaviors?
- ☐ **1.** Helpfulness.
- ☐ **2.** Self-defeat.
- ☐ **3.** Enabling.
- ☐ **4.** Masochism.

42. Which of the following statements by the nurse participating in a group confrontation of a coworker is most helpful in reducing the coworker's denial about alcohol being a problem?
- ☐ **1.** "Your behavior is unprofessional."
- ☐ **2.** "As a nurse you should have sought help earlier."
- ☐ **3.** "Nurses are the worst when it comes to asking for help."
- ☐ **4.** "You have alcohol on your breath."

43. The husband of a nurse who is being confronted by a group about her problem with alcohol asks the nurse acting as the group leader what he should say to his wife during the meeting. The nurse leader directs the husband to use which of the following statements to facilitate his wife's entrance into treatment?
- ☐ **1.** "The children and I want you to get help."
- ☐ **2.** "If your parents were alive, they would be extremely disappointed in you."
- ☐ **3.** "Either you get help or the kids and I will move out of the house."
- ☐ **4.** "You need to enter treatment now or be a drunk if that's what you want."

44. A nurse working in an alcohol rehabilitation program is teaching staff how to give clients constructive feedback. Which of the following statements given as an example illustrates that the staff member understands the nurse's teaching regarding the use of constructive feedback?

☐ **1.** "I think you're a real con artist."
☐ **2.** "You're dominating the conversation."
☐ **3.** "You interrupted Terry twice in 4 minutes."
☐ **4.** "You don't give anyone a chance to finish talking."

45. A client ashamedly tells the nurse that he hit his wife while intoxicated and asks the nurse if his wife will ever forgive him. Which of the following replies by the nurse is best in this situation?

☐ **1.** "Perhaps you could ask her and find out."
☐ **2.** "That's something you can explore in family therapy."
☐ **3.** "It would depend on how much she really cares for you."
☐ **4.** "You seem to have some feelings about hitting your wife."

46. While meeting with the nurse, a client's wife states, "I don't know what else to do to make him stop drinking." The nurse should anticipate initiating a referral for the wife to which of the following organizations?

☐ **1.** Alateen.
☐ **2.** Al-Anon.
☐ **3.** Employee assistance program.
☐ **4.** Alcoholics Anonymous.

47. Which of the following nursing actions is contraindicated for the client who is experiencing severe symptoms of alcohol withdrawal?

☐ **1.** Helping the client walk.
☐ **2.** Monitoring intake and output.
☐ **3.** Assessing vital signs.
☐ **4.** Using short, concrete statements.

48. Which of the following client statements indicates to the nurse that the client needs further teaching about disulfiram (Antabuse)?

☐ **1.** "I can drink one or two beers and not get sick while on Antabuse."
☐ **2.** "I can take Antabuse at bedtime if it makes me sleepy."
☐ **3.** "A metallic or garlic taste in my mouth is normal when starting on Antabuse."
☐ **4.** "I'll read the labels on cough syrup and mouthwash for possible alcohol content."

49. While receiving disulfiram (Antabuse) therapy, the client becomes nauseated and vomits severely. Which of the following questions should the nurse ask first?

☐ **1.** "How long have you been taking Antabuse?"
☐ **2.** "Do you feel like you have the flu?"
☐ **3.** "How much alcohol did you drink today?"
☐ **4.** "Have you eaten any foods cooked in wine?"

50. A coworker, new to the chemical dependency unit, questions the use of thiamine for all clients being treated for an alcohol problem. The nurse responds based on the understanding that thiamine is used for which of the following reasons?

☐ **1.** It prevents the development of Wernicke's encephalopathy.
☐ **2.** It decreases clients' withdrawal symptoms.
☐ **3.** It aids clients in regaining their strength sooner.
☐ **4.** It promotes elimination of alcohol from the body faster.

51. Which of the following client statements indicates an understanding of the signs of alcohol relapse?

☐ **1.** "I know I can stay dry if my wife keeps alcohol out of the house."
☐ **2.** "Stopping Alcoholics Anonymous (AA) and not expressing feelings can lead to relapse."
☐ **3.** "I'll have my sponsor at AA keep the list of symptoms for me."
☐ **4.** "If someone tells me I'm about to relapse, I'll be sure to do something about it."

52. The client sees no connection between her liver disorder and her alcohol intake. She believes that she drinks very little and that her family is making something out of nothing. The nurse interprets these behaviors as indicative of the client's use of which of the following defense mechanisms?

☐ **1.** Denial.
☐ **2.** Displacement.
☐ **3.** Rationalization.
☐ **4.** Reaction formation.

53. A client with alcohol dependency is prescribed a B-complex vitamin. The client states, "Why do I need a vitamin? My appetite is just fine." Which of the following responses by the nurse is most appropriate?

☐ **1.** "Your doctor wants you to take it for at least 4 months."
☐ **2.** "You've been drinking alcohol and eating very little."
☐ **3.** "The vitamin is a nutritional supplement important to your health."
☐ **4.** "The amount of vitamins in the alcohol you drink is very low."

54. The client with alcohol dependency suffers from numbness, itching, and pain in her extremities. Which of the following should the nurse suspect?

☐ **1.** Neuralgia.
☐ **2.** Bell's palsy.
☐ **3.** Neurasthenia.
☐ **4.** Peripheral neuritis.

55. Which of the following foods should the nurse eliminate from the diet of a client in alcohol withdrawal?
☐ **1.** Milk.
☐ **2.** Regular coffee.
☐ **3.** Orange juice.
☐ **4.** Eggs.

56. A client with alcohol dependency has peripheral neuropathy. Which of the following areas is most important to include in the client's teaching plan?
☐ **1.** Washing and drying the feet daily.
☐ **2.** Massaging the feet with lotion.
☐ **3.** Trimming the toenails carefully.
☐ **4.** Avoiding use of an electric blanket.

57. A client who is brought to the emergency department by ambulance begins to thrash about on the stretcher, slapping the sheets and yelling, "Go away, bugs, go away!" Assessment reveals disorientation, a blood pressure of 189/75 mm Hg, and a pulse of 86 bpm. The friend who accompanied the client to the hospital states, "He was drinking a lot when I saw him 4 days ago and asked me for money to get more liquor, but I didn't have any cash to give him." Based on an analysis of these findings, the nurse suspects that the client is experiencing:
☐ **1.** Stupor.
☐ **2.** Mild alcohol withdrawal.
☐ **3.** Impaired consciousness.
☐ **4.** Delirium.

58. When a client experiencing alcohol withdrawal thrashes in bed and yells, "Go away, bugs, go away," the nurse should expect to classify this behavior as reflective of which of the following nursing diagnoses?
☐ **1.** *Disturbed sensory perception: Visual.*
☐ **2.** *Disturbed thought processes.*
☐ **3.** *Risk for injury.*
☐ **4.** *Ineffective coping.*

59. The nurse is teaching unlicensed staff about caring for the client with alcohol dependency. Which of the following statements by the staff indicates the need for additional teaching?
☐ **1.** "Alcohol dependency affects the entire family."
☐ **2.** "The client is a weak individual and could stop if he desires."
☐ **3.** "Alcohol is a problem when it interferes with the client's daily life."
☐ **4.** "The client who can't stop drinking even though he wants to is alcohol dependent."

60. Which of the following measures should the nurse include in the plan of care for a client with alcohol withdrawal delirium?
☐ **1.** Using restraints continuously.
☐ **2.** Touching the client before saying anything.
☐ **3.** Remaining with the client when she is confused or disoriented.
☐ **4.** Informing the client about alcohol treatment programs.

61. Which of the following is an accurate response when a client asks the nurse about requirements to become a member of Alcoholics Anonymous (AA)?
☐ **1.** "You must be sober for at least a month before joining."
☐ **2.** "AA is open to anyone who wants sobriety."
☐ **3.** "The members will interview you and decide if you can join the group."
☐ **4.** "AA requires daily attendance at meetings."

62. A client is to be discharged from an alcohol rehabilitation program. Which of the following should the nurse emphasize in the discharge plan as a priority?
☐ **1.** Supportive friends.
☐ **2.** A list of goals.
☐ **3.** Family forgiveness.
☐ **4.** Follow-up care.

63. The client is to be discharged from the hospital after a safe, medically supervised withdrawal from alcohol. Which of the following outcomes indicate client readiness for an outpatient alcohol treatment program? Select all that apply.
☐ **1.** The client states the need to cut down on his alcohol intake.
☐ **2.** The client verbalizes the damaging effects of alcohol on his body.
☐ **3.** The client plans to attend Alcoholics Anonymous meetings.
☐ **4.** The client takes naltrexone (ReVia) daily.
☐ **5.** The client says he is indestructible.

64. A client is being admitted to the unit with a dual diagnosis. The nurse should expect that the client's diagnoses would include which of the following?
☐ **1.** Schizophrenia and dependent personality disorder.
☐ **2.** Bipolar disorder and suicide attempt.
☐ **3.** Major depression and alcohol abuse.
☐ **4.** Chronic paranoid schizophrenia and borderline personality disorder.

65. While caring for a client who has a dual diagnosis of bipolar disorder and alcohol dependency, which of the following areas is the priority for daily assessment?
☐ **1.** Sleep pattern.
☐ **2.** Mental status.
☐ **3.** Eating habits.
☐ **4.** Self-care ability.

66. A client diagnosed with schizophrenia and alcohol abuse decides to drink alcohol with his buddies. The nurse interprets this behavior, recognizing which of the following as an underlying dynamic of the client's alcohol use?
- ☐ **1.** The decision to use alcohol results in a feeling of autonomy and power.
- ☐ **2.** The decision to drink increases the client's guilt and shame.
- ☐ **3.** The client abused alcohol before developing a mental illness.
- ☐ **4.** The client is compelled to drink because of cognitive difficulties.

The Client with Disorders Related to Other Addictive Substances

67. The friend of a client brought to the emergency department states, "I guess she had some bad junk (heroin) today." The client is drowsy and verbally nonresponsive. Which of the following assessment findings is of immediate concern to the nurse?
- ☐ **1.** Respiratory rate of 9 breaths/minute.
- ☐ **2.** Urinary retention.
- ☐ **3.** Hypotension.
- ☐ **4.** Reduced pupil size.

68. A client is brought to the emergency department by a friend who states, "He's been using a lot of heroin until he ran out of money about 2 days ago." The nurse judges the client to be in opioid withdrawal if he exhibits which of the following? Select all that apply.
- ☐ **1.** Rhinorrhea.
- ☐ **2.** Diaphoresis.
- ☐ **3.** Piloerection.
- ☐ **4.** Synesthesia.
- ☐ **5.** Formication.

69. The nurse prepares to administer which of the following medications to a client with heroin overdose?
- ☐ **1.** Haloperidol (Haldol).
- ☐ **2.** Naloxone (Narcan).
- ☐ **3.** Lorazepam (Ativan).
- ☐ **4.** Oxazepam (Serax).

70. Which of the following should the nurse expect to assess for a client who is exhibiting late signs of heroin withdrawal?
- ☐ **1.** Vomiting and diarrhea.
- ☐ **2.** Yawning and diaphoresis.
- ☐ **3.** Lacrimation and rhinorrhea.
- ☐ **4.** Restlessness and irritability.

71. After administering naloxone (Narcan), an opioid antagonist, the nurse should monitor the client carefully for which of the following?
- ☐ **1.** Cerebral edema.
- ☐ **2.** Kidney failure.
- ☐ **3.** Seizure activity.
- ☐ **4.** Respiratory depression.

72. When teaching a client who is to receive methadone therapy for opioid addiction, the nurse should instruct the client that methadone is useful primarily for which of the following reasons?
- ☐ **1.** It is not an addictive substance.
- ☐ **2.** A maintenance dose is taken twice a day.
- ☐ **3.** The client will no longer be addicted to opioids.
- ☐ **4.** The client may work and live normally.

73. A client states to the nurse, "I'm not going to any more Narcotics Anonymous meetings. I felt out of place there." Which of the following responses by the nurse is best?
- ☐ **1.** "Try attending a meeting at a different location; you may feel more comfortable there."
- ☐ **2.** "Maybe it just wasn't a good day for you. Everybody has bad days now and then."
- ☐ **3.** "Perhaps you weren't paying close enough attention to what they were saying."
- ☐ **4.** "Sometimes the meetings can seem like a waste of time, but you need to attend to stay clean."

74. Which of the following should the nurse use as the best measure to determine a client's progress in rehabilitation?
- ☐ **1.** The kinds of friends he makes.
- ☐ **2.** The number of drug-free days he has.
- ☐ **3.** The way he gets along with his parents.
- ☐ **4.** The amount of responsibility his job entails.

75. Which of the following should lead the nurse to suspect that a client is addicted to heroin?
- ☐ **1.** Hilarity.
- ☐ **2.** Aggression.
- ☐ **3.** Labile mood.
- ☐ **4.** Hypoactivity.

76. A client brought by ambulance to the emergency department after taking an overdose of barbiturates is comatose. The nurse should be especially alert for which of the following?
- ☐ **1.** Kidney failure.
- ☐ **2.** Cerebrovascular accident.
- ☐ **3.** Status epilepticus.
- ☐ **4.** Respiratory failure.

77. The client's friend reports that the client has been taking about eight "reds" (800 mg of secobarbital [Seconal]) daily, besides drinking more alcohol than usual. The client's friend asks anxiously, "Do you think she will live?" Which of the following responses by the nurse is *most* appropriate?
- ☐ **1.** "We can only wait and see. It's too soon to tell."
- ☐ **2.** "Do you know her well? She's so young."
- ☐ **3.** "She is very ill and may not live. Some don't pull through."
- ☐ **4.** "Her condition is serious. You sound very worried about her."

78. Before his hospitalization, a client needed increasingly larger doses of barbiturates to achieve the same euphoric effect he initially realized from their use. From this information, the nurse develops a plan of care that takes into account that the client is most likely suffering from which of the following?
- [ ] **1.** Tolerance.
- [ ] **2.** Addiction.
- [ ] **3.** Abuse.
- [ ] **4.** Dependence.

79. Which of the following statements by the nurse is most appropriate when addressing a client with a barbiturate overdose who awakens in a confused state and exhibits stable vital signs?
- [ ] **1.** "I'm here to help you beat your drug habit. But it's you who will need to work hard."
- [ ] **2.** "It's time to get straight and stay clean and put an end to your torture."
- [ ] **3.** "I'm glad you pulled through; it was touch and go with you for a while."
- [ ] **4.** "You're in the hospital because of a drug problem; I'm one of the nurses who will help you."

80. During an interaction with the nurse, the client states that her "life has gone down the tubes" since her divorce 6 months ago. Afterwards, she lost her job and apartment and then she "took those pills to sleep and not wake up." From these data, the nurse should identify which of the following nursing diagnoses as the priority?
- [ ] **1.** *Situational low self-esteem* related to losses.
- [ ] **2.** *Risk for self-directed violence* related to suicide attempt.
- [ ] **3.** *Ineffective coping* related to hopelessness.
- [ ] **4.** *Powerlessness* related to helplessness.

81. The nurse identifies a nursing diagnosis of *Situational low self-esteem* for a client who has experienced the loss of her husband through divorce, the loss of her job and apartment, and the development of drug dependency. Which of the following outcomes is most appropriate initially?
- [ ] **1.** The client will discuss her feelings related to her losses.
- [ ] **2.** The client will identify two positive qualities.
- [ ] **3.** The client will explore her strengths.
- [ ] **4.** The client will prioritize problems.

82. The nurse notices that a client recovering from a barbiturate overdose spends most of his time with other young adults who have substance-related problems. This group of clients is a dominant force on the unit, keeping the non–drug users entertained with stories of their "highs." Which of the following methods is best to use when dealing with this problem?
- [ ] **1.** Providing additional recreation.
- [ ] **2.** Breaking up drug-oriented discussions.
- [ ] **3.** Speaking with the clients individually about their behavior.
- [ ] **4.** Discussing the behavior at the daily community meeting.

83. A client recovering from a drug overdose is interacting with the nurse and recounting her exploits at numerous rave parties she's attended. Which of the following actions is most therapeutic?
- [ ] **1.** Allowing the client to continue with her stories.
- [ ] **2.** Telling the client you've heard the stories before.
- [ ] **3.** Questioning the client further about her exploits.
- [ ] **4.** Directing the conversation to realistic concerns.

84. The nurse is speaking to a sixth grade class about drugs. A student states, "I know someone who smokes marijuana and he says it's safe." Which of the following responses by the nurse is most appropriate?
- [ ] **1.** "Marijuana isn't safe and it is illegal."
- [ ] **2.** "Do you really believe him?"
- [ ] **3.** "That drug causes more damage to your body than regular cigarettes."
- [ ] **4.** "Marijuana usage can lead to using other chemicals."

85. When developing a teaching plan for a group of middle school children about the drug 3,4-methylenedioxymethamphetamine (Ecstasy), what information should the nurse expect to include? Select all that apply.
- [ ] **1.** Using Ecstasy is similar to using speed.
- [ ] **2.** Ecstasy is used at "raves."
- [ ] **3.** Candylike pacifiers are used for teeth grinding.
- [ ] **4.** It can cause death.
- [ ] **5.** It reduces self-consciousness.

86. A client tells the nurse that he "sees sounds and hears colors" when he uses lysergic acid diethylamide. The nurse interprets this information as indicating that the client has experienced which of the following?
- [ ] **1.** Impaired judgment.
- [ ] **2.** Synesthesia.
- [ ] **3.** Flashback.
- [ ] **4.** Panic.

87. Which of the following actions is most appropriate for the nurse to do for a client who is experiencing a "bad trip" from lysergic acid diethylamide use and is frightened and paranoid?
- ☐ **1.** Staying with the client to talk her down.
- ☐ **2.** Placing the client in seclusion.
- ☐ **3.** Leaving the client alone until the "bad trip" subsides.
- ☐ **4.** Telling another caregiver to check on the client periodically.

88. A client who is a chronic user of cocaine reports that he feels like he has bugs crawling under his skin. His arms are red from scratching. The nurse interprets these findings as possibly indicating which of the following?
- ☐ **1.** Illusion.
- ☐ **2.** Formication.
- ☐ **3.** Confusion.
- ☐ **4.** Flashback.

89. A client walks into the clinic and tells the nurse she has run out of money for crack, has crashed, and wants something to help her feel better. Which of the following is most important for the nurse to assess?
- ☐ **1.** Suspiciousness.
- ☐ **2.** Loss of appetite.
- ☐ **3.** Drug craving.
- ☐ **4.** Suicidal ideation.

90. A client in the emergency department is diagnosed with amphetamine psychosis. The nurse should prepare to administer which of the following medications?
- ☐ **1.** Haloperidol (Haldol).
- ☐ **2.** Lorazepam (Ativan).
- ☐ **3.** Diazepam (Valium).
- ☐ **4.** Chlordiazepoxide (Librium).

91. A client has been taking increased amounts of alprazolam (Xanax) for about 6 months for anxiety. To safely withdraw the client from this drug, the nurse anticipates which of the following to be ordered?
- ☐ **1.** Immediate discontinuation of the alprazolam.
- ☐ **2.** A slow decrease in dose and frequency of the drug.
- ☐ **3.** Administration of alprazolam on an as-needed basis.
- ☐ **4.** Tapering off of the drug over a 24-hour period.

92. The client is fidgeting and has trouble sitting still. He has difficulty concentrating and is tangential. Which of the following interventions should help decrease this client's level of anxiety? Select all that apply.
- ☐ **1.** Refocusing attention.
- ☐ **2.** Allowing ventilation.
- ☐ **3.** Suggesting a time-out.
- ☐ **4.** Giving intramuscular medication.
- ☐ **5.** Assisting with problem solving.

93. When caring for a client who has overdosed on phencyclidine (PCP), the nurse should be especially cautious about which of the following client behaviors?
- ☐ **1.** Visual hallucinations.
- ☐ **2.** Violent behavior.
- ☐ **3.** Bizarre behavior.
- ☐ **4.** Loud screaming.

94. Which of the following liquids would the nurse administer to a client who is intoxicated on phencyclidine (PCP) to hasten excretion of the chemical?
- ☐ **1.** Water.
- ☐ **2.** Milk.
- ☐ **3.** Cranberry juice.
- ☐ **4.** Grape juice.

95. When assessing a client with possible alcohol poisoning, the nurse should investigate the client's use of which of the following substances while drinking alcohol?
- ☐ **1.** Marijuana.
- ☐ **2.** Lysergic acid diethylamide.
- ☐ **3.** Peyote.
- ☐ **4.** Psilocybin.

96. A client with a cocaine dependency is irritable, anxious, highly sensitive to stimuli, and over-reactive to clients and staff on the unit. Which of the following actions is most therapeutic for this client?
- ☐ **1.** Secluding and restraining the client as needed.
- ☐ **2.** Telling the client to stay in his room until he can control himself.
- ☐ **3.** Providing the client with frequent "time-outs."
- ☐ **4.** Confronting the client about his behaviors.

97. A client with symptoms of amphetamine psychosis that are improving is anxious and still experiencing some delusions. When developing the client's plan of care, which of the following measures should the nurse include?
- ☐ **1.** Assign the client to a group about the physiologic effects of drugs.
- ☐ **2.** Advise the client to watch television.
- ☐ **3.** Wait for the client to approach the nurse.
- ☐ **4.** Invite the client to play a game of ping-pong with the nurse.

98. For the client who has difficulty falling asleep at night because of withdrawal symptoms from alcohol, which are abating, which of the following nursing interventions is best?
- ☐ **1.** Inviting the client to play a board game with the nurse.
- ☐ **2.** Allowing the client to sit in the community room until she feels sleepy.
- ☐ **3.** Advising the client to sleep on the sofa in the dayroom.
- ☐ **4.** Teaching the client relaxation exercises to use before bedtime.

The Client with an Anxiety-Related Disorder

99. A client is taking diazepam (Valium) for generalized anxiety disorder. Which instruction should the nurse give to this client? Select all that apply.
- ☐ 1. To consult with his health care provider before he stops taking the drug.
- ☐ 2. To avoid eating cheese and other tyramine-rich foods.
- ☐ 3. To take the medication on an empty stomach.
- ☐ 4. Not to use alcohol while taking the drug.
- ☐ 5. To stop taking the drug if he experiences swelling of the lips and face and difficulty breathing.

100. An adult client with anxiety disorder becomes anxious when she touches fruits and vegetables. What should the nurse do?
- ☐ 1. Instruct the woman to avoid touching these foods.
- ☐ 2. Ask the woman why she becomes anxious in these situations.
- ☐ 3. Assist the woman to make a plan for her family to do the food shopping and preparation.
- ☐ 4. Teach the woman to use cognitive behavioral approaches to manage her anxiety.

101. A client who is pacing and wringing his hands states, "I just need to walk" when questioned by the nurse about what he is feeling. Which of the following responses by the nurse is most therapeutic?
- ☐ 1. "You need to sit down and relax."
- ☐ 2. "Are you feeling anxious?"
- ☐ 3. "Is something bothering you?"
- ☐ 4. "You must be experiencing a problem now."

102. A client is brought to the emergency department by his brother. The client is perspiring profusely, breathing rapidly, and complaining of dizziness and palpitations. Problems of a cardiovascular nature are ruled out, and the client's diagnosis is tentatively listed as a panic attack. After the symptoms pass, the client states, "I thought I was going to die." Which of the following responses by the nurse is best?
- ☐ 1. "It was very frightening for you."
- ☐ 2. "We would not have let you die."
- ☐ 3. "I would have felt the same way."
- ☐ 4. "But you're okay now."

103. A client commonly jumps when spoken to and complains of feeling uneasy. She says, "It's as though something bad is going to happen." Which of the following actions is most beneficial to the client?
- ☐ 1. Leaving her alone.
- ☐ 2. Demonstrating technical competency.
- ☐ 3. Conveying optimistic verbalizations.
- ☐ 4. Reducing environmental stimulation.

104. Which of the following points should the nurse include when teaching a client about panic disorder?
- ☐ 1. Staying in the house will eliminate panic attacks.
- ☐ 2. Medication should be taken when symptoms start.
- ☐ 3. Symptoms of a panic attack are time limited and will abate.
- ☐ 4. Maintaining self-control will decrease symptoms of panic.

105. A client with panic disorder is taking alprazolam (Xanax) 1 mg P.O. three times daily. The nurse understands that this medication is effective in blocking the symptoms of panic because of its specific action on which of the following neurotransmitters?
- ☐ 1. Gamma-aminobutyrate.
- ☐ 2. Serotonin.
- ☐ 3. Dopamine.
- ☐ 4. Norepinephrine.

106. While a client is taking alprazolam (Xanax), which of the following should the nurse instruct the client to avoid?
- ☐ 1. Chocolate.
- ☐ 2. Cheese.
- ☐ 3. Alcohol.
- ☐ 4. Shellfish.

107. Which of the following statements by a client who has been taking buspirone (BuSpar) as prescribed for 2 days indicates the need for further teaching?
- ☐ 1. "This medication will help my tight, aching muscles."
- ☐ 2. "I may not feel better for 7 to 10 days."
- ☐ 3. "The drug does not cause physical dependence."
- ☐ 4. "I can take the medication with food."

108. A week ago, a tornado destroyed the client's home and seriously injured her husband. The client has been walking around the hospital in a daze without any outward display of emotions. She tells the nurse that she feels like she's going crazy. Which of the following actions should the nurse use initially?
- ☐ 1. Explain the effects of stress on the mind and body.
- ☐ 2. Reassure the client that her feelings are typical reactions to serious trauma.
- ☐ 3. Reassure the client that her symptoms are temporary.
- ☐ 4. Acknowledge the unfairness of the client's situation.

109. After being discharged from the hospital with acute stress disorder, a client is referred to the outpatient clinic for follow-up. Which of the following is most important for the client to use for continued alleviation of anxiety?
- ☐ 1. Recognizing when she is feeling anxious.
- ☐ 2. Understanding reasons for her anxiety.
- ☐ 3. Using adaptive and palliative methods to reduce anxiety.
- ☐ 4. Describing the situations preceding her feelings of anxiety.

110. A client with acute stress disorder states to the nurse, "I keep having horrible nightmares about the car accident that killed my daughter. I shouldn't have taken her with me to the store." Which of the following responses by the nurse is most therapeutic?
- ☐ **1.** "Don't keep torturing yourself with such horrible thoughts."
- ☐ **2.** "Stop blaming yourself. It's only hurting you."
- ☐ **3.** "Let's talk about something that is a bit more pleasant."
- ☐ **4.** "The accident just happened and could not have been predicted."

111. The client, a veteran of the Vietnam war who has posttraumatic stress disorder, tells the nurse about the horror and mass destruction of war. He states, "I killed all of those people for nothing." Which of the following responses by the nurse is most appropriate?
- ☐ **1.** "You did what you had to do at that time."
- ☐ **2.** "Maybe you didn't kill as many people as you think."
- ☐ **3.** "How many people did you kill?"
- ☐ **4.** "War is a terrible thing."

112. A client with acute stress disorder has avoided feelings of anger toward her rapist and cannot verbally express them. The nurse suggests which of the following activities to assist the client with expressing her feelings?
- ☐ **1.** Working on a puzzle.
- ☐ **2.** Writing in a journal.
- ☐ **3.** Meditating.
- ☐ **4.** Listening to music.

113. When developing the plan of care for a client with acute stress disorder who lost her sister in a boating accident, which of the following should the nurse expect to initiate?
- ☐ **1.** Helping the client to evaluate her sister's behavior.
- ☐ **2.** Telling the client to avoid details of the accident.
- ☐ **3.** Facilitating progressive review of the accident and its consequences.
- ☐ **4.** Postponing discussion of the accident until the client brings it up.

114. A client with posttraumatic stress disorder needs to find new housing and wants to wait for a month before setting another appointment to see the nurse. The nurse interprets this action as which of the following?
- ☐ **1.** A method of avoidance.
- ☐ **2.** A detriment to progress.
- ☐ **3.** The end of treatment.
- ☐ **4.** A necessary occurrence.

115. The nurse should teach a client with an anxiety disorder who is taking a benzodiazepine about using which of the following in combination with his medication?
- ☐ **1.** Antacids.
- ☐ **2.** Acetaminophen (Tylenol).
- ☐ **3.** Vitamins.
- ☐ **4.** Aspirin.

116. Which of the following client statements would indicate the need for additional teaching about benzodiazepines?
- ☐ **1.** "I can't drink alcohol while taking diazepam (Valium)."
- ☐ **2.** "I can stop taking the drug anytime I want."
- ☐ **3.** "Valium can make me drowsy, so I shouldn't drive for a while."
- ☐ **4.** "Valium will help my tight muscles feel better."

117. A client with agoraphobia without panic disorder asks the nurse to advise her on which type of treatment is best for her illness. Which of the following should the nurse suggest?
- ☐ **1.** Insight therapy.
- ☐ **2.** Group therapy.
- ☐ **3.** Behavior therapy.
- ☐ **4.** Psychoanalysis.

118. The client with a fear of eating in public places or in front of other people has finished eating lunch in the dining area in the nurse's presence. Which of the following statements by the nurse should reinforce the client's positive action?
- ☐ **1.** "It wasn't so hard, now was it?"
- ☐ **2.** "At supper, I hope to see you eat with a group of people."
- ☐ **3.** "You must have been hungry today."
- ☐ **4.** "It's a sign of progress to eat in the dining area."

119. The client with agoraphobia refuses to walk down the hall to the group room. Which of the following responses by the nurse is most appropriate?
- ☐ **1.** "I know you can do it."
- ☐ **2.** "Try holding onto the wall as you walk."
- ☐ **3.** "You can miss group this one time."
- ☐ **4.** "I'll walk with you."

120. A client with obsessive-compulsive disorder arrives late for an appointment with the nurse at the outpatient clinic. During the interview, he fidgets restlessly, has trouble remembering what topic is being discussed, and says he thinks he is going crazy. Which of the following statements by the nurse best deals with the client's feelings of "going crazy?"
- ☐ **1.** "What do you mean when you say you think you're going crazy?"
- ☐ **2.** "Most people feel that way occasionally."
- ☐ **3.** "I don't know enough about you to judge."
- ☐ **4.** "You sound perfectly sane to me."

121. A client with obsessive-compulsive disorder reveals that he was late for his appointment "because of my dumb habit. I have to take off my socks and put them back on 41 times! I can't stop until I do it just right." The nurse interprets the client's behavior as most likely representing an effort to obtain which of the following?
- ☐ 1. Relief from anxiety.
- ☐ 2. Control of his thoughts.
- ☐ 3. Attention from others.
- ☐ 4. Safe expression of hostility.

122. A client with obsessive-compulsive disorder, who was admitted early yesterday morning, must make his bed 22 times before he can have breakfast. Because of his behavior, the client missed having breakfast yesterday with the other clients. Which of the following actions should the nurse institute to help the client be on time for breakfast?
- ☐ 1. Tell the client to make his bed one time only.
- ☐ 2. Wake the client an hour earlier to perform his ritual.
- ☐ 3. Insist that the client stop his activity when it's time for breakfast.
- ☐ 4. Advise the client to have breakfast first before making his bed.

123. The nurse notices that a client with obsessive-compulsive disorder must get up and move to another area when someone sits next to her. Which of the following actions by the nurse is most therapeutic?
- ☐ 1. Ignoring the client's behavior.
- ☐ 2. Questioning the client about her ritual.
- ☐ 3. Conveying awareness of the need for the ritual.
- ☐ 4. Telling the other clients to follow the client when she moves.

124. The client with obsessive-compulsive disorder is taking clomipramine (Anafranil) for his disorder. The nurse should expect the client to exhibit side effects similar to those of which of the following medications?
- ☐ 1. Fluoxetine (Prozac).
- ☐ 2. Sertraline (Zoloft).
- ☐ 3. Imipramine (Tofranil).
- ☐ 4. Fluvoxamine (Luvox).

The Client with a Somatoform Disorder

125. At 10 a.m., a client with an Axis I diagnosis of pain disorder demands that the nurse call the physician for more pain medication because she's still in pain after the 9 a.m. analgesic. Which of the following should the nurse do next?
- ☐ 1. Call the physician as the client requests.
- ☐ 2. Suggest the client lie down because she has to wait for the next dosage.
- ☐ 3. Tell the client that the physician will be in later to talk to her about it.
- ☐ 4. Inform the client that the nurse cannot give her additional medication at this time.

126. The nursing assistant tells the nurse that the client is not in the dining room for lunch. The nurse should direct the nursing assistant to do which of the following?
- ☐ 1. Take the client a lunch tray and let him eat in his room.
- ☐ 2. Tell the client he'll need to wait until supper to eat if he misses lunch.
- ☐ 3. Invite the client to lunch and accompany him to the dining room.
- ☐ 4. Inform the client that he has 10 minutes to get to the dining room for lunch.

127. The client with conversion disorder has a paralyzed arm. A staff member states, "I would just tell the client her arm is paralyzed because she had an affair and neglected her baby's care to the point where the baby had to be hospitalized for dehydration." Which of the following responses by the nurse is best?
- ☐ 1. "Ignore the client's behaviors and treat her with respect."
- ☐ 2. "Pushing insight will increase the client's anxiety and the need for physical symptoms."
- ☐ 3. "Pushing awareness will be helpful and further the client's recovery."
- ☐ 4. "We'll meet with the client and confront her with her behavior."

128. The physician refers a client with somatization disorder to the outpatient clinic because of problems with nausea. The client's past symptoms involved back pain, chest pain, and problems with urination. The client tells the nurse that the nausea began when his wife asked him for a divorce. Which of the following is most appropriate?
- ☐ 1. Asking the client to describe his problem with nausea.
- ☐ 2. Directing the client to describe his feelings about his impending divorce.
- ☐ 3. Allowing the client to talk about the physicians he has seen and the medications he has taken.
- ☐ 4. Informing the client about a different medication for his nausea.

129. A client with pain disorder is talking with the nurse about fishing when he suddenly reverts to talking about the pain in his arm. Which of the following should the nurse do next?
- ☐ 1. Allow the client to talk about his pain.
- ☐ 2. Ask the client if he needs more pain medication.
- ☐ 3. Get up and leave the client.
- ☐ 4. Redirect the interaction back to fishing.

130. Which of the following statements indicates to the nurse that the client is progressing toward recovery from a somatoform disorder?

☐ 1. "It's okay if I feel nauseous when I'm worried about my divorce."

☐ 2. "My stomach pain will go away once I get properly diagnosed."

☐ 3. "My headache feels better when I time my medication dose."

☐ 4. "I need to find a doctor who understands what my pain is like."

Correct Answers and Rationales

The letter in parentheses after each rationale identifies the client need addressed in the item, including management of care (M), safety and infection control (S), health promotion and maintenance (H), psychosocial adaptation (P), basic care and comfort (C), pharmacological and parenteral therapies (D), reduction of risk potential (R), and physiological adaptation (A).

The Client with a Personality Disorder

1. 3. The client is at risk for suicide and the nurse should determine how serious the client is, including if she has a plan and the means to implement the plan. While medication history may be important, the nurse should first attempt to determine suicide risk. Asking the client why she cut herself will likely cause the client to respond with insufficient information to determine suicide risk. (R)

2. 1. The nurse should plan to assist the client who has a personality disorder primarily with specific dysfunctional behaviors that are distressing to the client or others. The client with a personality disorder has lifelong, inflexible, and dysfunctional patterns of relating and behaving. The client commonly does not view his behavior as distressful to himself. The client becomes distressed because of others' reactions and behaviors toward him, which cause the client emotional pain and discomfort. Psychopharmacologic compliance is not a primary need because medication does not cure a personality disorder. Medication is prescribed if the client has a severe symptom that interferes with functioning, such as severe anxiety or depression, or if the client has an Axis I disorder. Examination of developmental conflicts usually is not helpful because of the ingrained dysfunctional ways of thinking and behaving. It is more useful to help the client with changing dysfunctional behaviors. Although milieu management is a component of care, the client usually is proficient in manipulation of the environment to meet his needs. (P)

3. 3. For this client, the nurse needs to use a calm, matter-of-fact approach to create a nonthreatening and secure environment because the client is experiencing problems with suspiciousness and trust. Use of "I" statements and responses would be therapeutic to reduce the client's suspiciousness and increase his trust in the staff and the environment. An authoritarian approach is nontherapeutic and inappropriate because the client may perceive this approach as an attack, subsequently responding with anger and threatening behavior. A parental or controlling approach may be perceived as authoritarian, and the client may become defensive and angry. (P)

4. 4. Attending an activity with the nurse assists the client to become involved with others slowly. The client with a schizotypal personality disorder needs support, kindness, and gentle suggestion to improve social skills and interpersonal relationships. The client commonly has problems in thinking, perceiving, and communicating and appears similar to clients with schizophrenia except that psychotic episodes are infrequent and less severe. Participation solely in group activities or leading a sing-along would be too overwhelming for the client, subsequently increasing the client's anxiety and withdrawal. Engaging primarily in one-to-one activities would not be helpful because of the client's difficulty with social skills and interpersonal relationships. However, activities with the nurse could be used to establish trust. Then the client could proceed to activities with others. (P)

5. 2. The nurse needs to set limits on the client's manipulative behavior to help the client control dysfunctional behavior. The manipulative client bends rules to have her needs met without regard for rules or the needs or rights of others. A consistent approach by the staff is necessary to decrease manipulation. Ignoring the client's behavior reinforces or promotes the continuation of the client's manipulative behavior. Reprimanding the client may be perceived as a threat, resulting in aggressive behavior. Allowing the client to keep a snack in her room reinforces the dysfunctional behavior. (P)

6. 2. The nurse assists the client with identifying and putting feelings into words during one-to-one interactions. This helps the client express her feelings in a nonthreatening setting and avoid directing anger toward other clients. A client with an antisocial personality disorder needs to understand how others feel and react to her behaviors and why they react the way they do. The client also needs to understand the consequences of her behaviors. Using humor or indirect behaviors to express anger is a passive–aggressive method that will not help the client learn how to express her anger appropriately. Asking the nurse for medication when upset is a way to avoid dealing with feelings and is not helpful. However, medication may be necessary if talking and engaging in a physical activity have not been effective in lowering anxiety or if the client is about to lose control of her behavior. (P)

7. **3.** The client with an antisocial personality disorder is manifesting behavior indicative of problems in Erikson's stage of initiative versus guilt. Typical behaviors of a client with an antisocial personality disorder are engaging in illegal activities, violating the rights of others, lack of guilt or remorse, recklessness, impulsiveness, aggressive behavior, and irresponsibility in work and with finances. A lack of guilt or remorse for offenses, such as stealing, is typically present, as if the client does not have a conscience. Behaviors indicating problems in the stage of trust versus mistrust include suspiciousness, projection of blame and feelings, and withdrawal. Behaviors indicating problems in the stage of autonomy versus shame and doubt include self-doubt and self-consciousness, dependency on others for approval, and denial of problems. Behaviors indicating problems in the stage of industry versus inferiority include poor work history, inadequate problem-solving skills, and manipulation of others. (H)

8. **2.** The nurse should teach the client consequences of her actions to help the client understand that if she steals she will get into legal trouble and be put in jail. So, if she wants to avoid jail, she needs to not steal. Helping the client to develop a conscience or to understand right from wrong is impossible. However, the client needs to be taught that her actions do lead to consequences. Using strategies to help the client become passive is not helpful, is nontherapeutic, and does not help the client to understand the consequences of her actions. (P)

9. **4.** Some characteristics of a client with a dependent personality are an inability to make daily decisions without advice and reassurance and the preoccupation with fear of being alone to care for oneself. The client needs others to be responsible for important areas of his life. The nurse should respond, "Your parents have been supportive of you and will continue to be supportive even if you live apart," to gently challenge the client's fears and suggest that they may be unwarranted. Stating, "You're a 28-year-old adult now, not a child who needs to be cared for," or "Your parents need a break, and you need a break from them," is reprimanding and would diminish the client's self-worth. Stating, "Your parents won't be around forever; after all they are getting older," may be true, but it is an insensitive response that may increase the client's anxiety. (P)

10. **2.** Stating, "All of you will gain from his independent living; he needs our support," encourages the client's independent behaviors and fosters autonomous functioning for the entire family. The other statements minimize the son's independence and decrease his self-esteem. (P)

11. **3.** This client's signs and symptoms indicate borderline personality disorder, characterized by impulsiveness, self-mutilating behavior, unstable and intense personal relationships, identity disturbances, chronic feelings of emptiness, frantic avoidance of abandonment, and problems with anger. Antisocial personality disorder is characterized by lack of guilt or remorse, engaging in illegal activities, impulsiveness, recklessness, irresponsibility at work, aggressive behavior, and violation of the rights of others. The client with avoidant personality disorder demonstrates social withdrawal, hypersensitivity to criticism, and reluctance to engage in new activities. The client with compulsive personality disorder is characterized by a preoccupation with details and rules to the exclusion of other life activities, perfectionism, and rigidity. (P)

12. **4.** For the client with attention-seeking behaviors, the nurse would institute a behavioral contract with the client to help decrease dysfunctional behaviors and promote self-sufficiency. Having the client approach only his assigned staff person sets limits on his attention-seeking behavior. Telling the client to stay in his room until staff approach him, limiting the client to a certain area, or giving the client a list of permissible requests is punitive and does nothing to help the client gain control over the dysfunctional behavior. (M)

13. **2.** The most therapeutic response is, "All of the nurses here provide good care." This statement corrects the client's unrealistic and exaggerated perception. "Splitting," defined as the inability to integrate good and bad aspects of an individual and the self, is a hallmark behavior of a client with borderline personality disorder. The client sees himself and others as all good or all bad. Components of "splitting" include behaviors that idealize and devalue others. It is a defense that allows the client to avoid pain and feelings associated with past abuse or a current situation involving the threat of rejection or abandonment. The other statements promote the client's idealistic view and do nothing to help correct the client's distortion. (P)

14. **4.** The client with borderline personality disorder is usually in a crisis situation when hospitalized for self-mutilation and suicidal ideation or behavior. The statement, "Any attempt at self-harm is serious and safety is a priority," is the best response because the misperception that self-mutilation is used to gain attention can result in death of the client. The client can accidentally commit suicide. Any form of self-harm is an indication that the client needs treatment. The statement, "She's here now and we have to do our best," is not helpful and does not educate the staff member about the client's needs. The statement, "She needs to be here until she can control her behavior," may be true but does not provide information about the client's priority needs. The statement, "I'm ashamed of you; you know better than to say that," is punitive, diminishes self-worth, and may not be a correct assumption of the staff member's knowledge. (M)

15. **2.** For the client who is at risk for self-mutilation, the nurse develops a contract to assist the client with assuming responsibility for his behavior and to help the client develop adaptive methods of coping with feelings. Self-mutilation is usually an expression of intense anxiety, anger, helplessness, or guilt or a means to block psychological pain by inducing physical pain. A typical contract helpful to the client would have the client notify staff when anxiety is increasing. Withdrawing to his room when feeling overwhelmed, suppressing feelings when angry, or displacing feelings onto the physician is not an adaptive method to help the client deal with his feelings and could still result in self-mutilation. (S)

16. 4. Any suicidal statement must be assessed by the nurse. The nurse should discuss the client's statement with her to determine its meaning in terms of suicide, overwhelming feelings of anxiety, abandonment, or other need that the client cannot express appropriately. It is not uncommon for a client with borderline personality disorder to make threatening comments before discharge. Extending the hospital stay is inappropriate because it would encourage dependency and manipulation. Ignoring the client's statement on the assumption that it is a sign of manipulation is an error in judgment. Asking a family member to stay with the client temporarily at home is not appropriate and places the responsibility for the client on the family instead of the client. (P)

17. 4. The best initial course of action when admitting a client is to observe him to establish baseline information. This assessment provides valuable information about the client's behavior and forms the basis for the plan of care. Telling the client that the staff has authority to subdue him if he gets unruly or that he will have to pay for any damage he causes is threatening and may incite or provoke trouble. Isolating a client is not recommended unless there is a very good reason for it, such as a very active, combative client who is dangerous to himself and others. (P)

18. 4. The best response is, "You say you're not a regular here, but you're experiencing what others are experiencing." This statement helps the client to identify factors that precipitate denial by helping her to confront that which inhibits compliance. Denial is used to help a client feel better and more secure when a situation provokes a high level of anxiety and is threatening to the client. The statement, "Because you're not a regular client, sit in the hall when the others are in group," agrees with and promotes denial in the client and interferes with treatment. The statement, "Your family wants you to attend and they will be disappointed if you don't," causes the client to feel guilty and decreases her self-esteem. The statement, "I'll have to mark you absent from the clinic today and speak to the doctor about it," is punitive and threatening to the client, subsequently decreasing her self-esteem. (P)

19. 1. When the staff member asks the client if he wonders why others find him repulsive, the client is likely to feel defensive because the question is belittling. The natural tendency is to counterattack the threat to the client's self-image. Because the client with an antisocial personality disorder is egocentric and unconcerned about his effect on others, he is unlikely to feel ashamed, remorseful, or embarrassed. (P)

20. 3. Stating, "I will not continue to talk with you if you curse," sets limits on the client's behavior and points out the negative effects of her behavior. Therefore, this response is most appropriate and therapeutic. The statement, "You're being very childish," reprimands the client, possibly causing the anger to escalate. The statement, "I'm sorry if you can't wait," fails to provide feedback to the client about her behavior. The statement, "Come back tomorrow and your medication will be ready," ignores the client's behavior, failing to provide feedback to the client about the behavior. It also shows poor nursing judgment because the client may need her medication before tomorrow or may not return to the clinic the following day. (P)

21. 1. The client with avoidant personality disorder is showing signs of improvement when interacting with two other clients. A client with avoidant personality disorder is timid, socially uncomfortable, withdrawn, and hypersensitive to criticism. Social contact with others decreases isolation and withdrawal. Listening to music with headphones, sitting at a table and painting, and talking on the telephone are solitary activities and therefore do not indicate improvement, which is evidenced by social contact. (P)

22. 4. The priority is to explain to the client that this information has to be shared immediately with the staff and the physician because of its serious nature. Safety of all is crucial regardless of whether the client follows through on his plan. It is possible that the client is asking to be stopped and that he is indirectly pleading for help in a dysfunctional manner. Bargaining with the client, such as warning him that his telephone privileges will be taken away if he abuses them or offering to disregard his plan if he does not go through with it, is inappropriate. Saying nothing to anyone until the client has actually completed the call and then notifying the proper authorities represents serious negligence on the part of the nurse. (S)

23. 1. The most basic and important idea to convey to a client is that, as a person, he or she is accepted, although his or her behavior may not be. Empathy is conveyed for emotional pain regardless of the client's behavior. Although some clients need limits placed on their behavior, not all clients require limit setting. That the staff members are the primary ones left to care about these clients is not necessarily true, nor is it true that the staff should use very little humor with these clients. Clients who are rigid and perfectionists and who have a restricted affect may need help with displaying humor. (M)

24. 1. The nurse should explain the negative reactions of others toward the client's behaviors to make him aware of the impact of his seductive behaviors on others. Suggesting that the client apologize to others for his behavior is futile because the client cannot feel remorse for wrongdoing. Asking him to explain reasons for his seductive behavior is not helpful because this client is skillful at using projection and rationalization. Discussing his relationship with his mother is not helpful because the focus should be oriented to the present situation and managing his behavior at the present time. (P)

25. **3.** The nurse judges the client's statement to be an example of grandiose self-importance, which is not a lie but an overvaluing of oneself. The grandiosity of a client with a narcissistic personality disorder is not a delusion because it usually is based somewhat in reality. However, it can be distorted, embellished, or convoluted to meet the client's need of self-importance. Sense of entitlement is a symptom of the narcissistic client but refers to deserving to be favored or given special treatment. (P)

26. **2.** The nurse would specifically use supportive confrontation with the client to point out discrepancies between what the client states and what actually exists to increase responsibility for self. Limit setting and consistency also may be used. However, limit setting helps the client control unacceptable behavior and consistency helps reduce the frequency of negative behaviors; they do not point out discrepancies. Rationalization is typically used by the client, not the nurse, to blame others, make excuses, and provide alibis for self-centered behaviors. (P)

27. **4.** The nurse should use role-playing to teach the client appropriate responses to others in various situations. This client dramatizes events, draws attention to self, and is unaware of and does not deal with feelings. The nurse works to help the client clarify true feelings and learn to express them appropriately. Party planning, music group, and cooking class are therapeutic activities, but will not help the client specifically learn how to respond appropriately to others. (P)

28. **1.** The client with major depression and borderline personality disorder would probably be taking a selective serotonin reuptake inhibitor to improve depression and reduce feelings of anger and impulsiveness. A benzodiazepine (antianxiety agent) may be used cautiously for anxiety and restlessness. A mood stabilizer would be used for the client with rapid mood swings. An antipsychotic would be used only temporarily and in low doses for the client with borderline personality disorder who is experiencing transient psychotic symptoms. (D)

The Client with an Alcohol-Related Disorder

29. **1.** The client is experiencing an overdose of alcohol as indicated by his blood alcohol level. The nurse should establish an intravenous line and administer fluids. The physician may order magnesium sulfate to reduce the risk of seizures. The client should not be restrained because that will agitate the client further. The nurse should observe the client at this point; quiet rooms are used while the client is withdrawing from the alcohol (alcohol withdrawal delirium). Naloxone (Narcan) is used for an opioid overdose. (S)

30. **1.** The nurse should first contact the physician. The client's vital signs and level of consciousness are deteriorating, indicating complications of withdrawal, which can be life-threatening. Increasing the rate of the infusion may cause fluid overload and has not been ordered by the physician. Arousing the client will not address the underlying problems. Magnesium sulfate is used to treat seizures precipitated by alcohol withdrawal, but the client is not demonstrating signs of actual or impending seizures. (S)

31. **4.** The nurse should provide the client with a quiet room to sleep in. Alcohol is destroyed and oxidized in the body at a slow, steady rate. The rate of alcohol metabolism is not influenced by drinking black coffee, walking around the unit, or taking a cold shower. Therefore, it is best to have the client sleep off the effects of the alcohol. (P)

32. **1, 2, 4, 5.** For the client experiencing symptoms of alcohol withdrawal, the nurse monitors vital signs and intake and output, reinforces reality for the client who is confused, disoriented, or hallucinating, explains that the symptoms of withdrawal are temporary, reduces stimulation, and stays with the client if he is confused or agitated. The nurse administers medications to prevent the progression of symptoms, such as seizures and delirium tremens, and to ensure the client's safety. Restraints are not used as a precautionary measure. Restraints are used only as a least restrictive measure to protect the client and others when the client is a danger to himself or others. (P)

33. **4.** Antiseptic mouthwash commonly contains alcohol and should be kept in a locked area unless labeling clearly indicates that the product does not contain alcohol. A client with an intense craving for alcohol may drink mouthwash that contains alcohol. Personal care items, such as toothpaste, dental floss, and shaving cream, do not contain alcohol, and the client would be allowed to keep them in the room. (S)

34. **2.** The client with alcohol dependency is using minimization when he states that he just has a few drinks with the guys after work. Minimization, projection, denial, and rationalization are defenses that are part of the "stinkin' thinkin'" that permits the client with an alcohol problem to continue drinking. Projection involves blaming someone else for one's difficulties. An example is, "My wife keeps getting on my case about nothing. She drives me crazy." Denial involves an unconscious refusal to admit an unacceptable idea or behavior. An example is, "I can stop drinking anytime I want. I don't have a problem." Rationalization is an attempt to make or prove that one's feelings or behaviors are justifiable. An example is, "If my boss wasn't so hard on me, I wouldn't be so stressed out. I just need a few drinks to relax." (P)

35. **2.** The client's response helps the nurse determine the severity of withdrawal symptoms because the length and extent of drinking alcohol has an effect on the severity of symptoms the client experiences during withdrawal. Decreased use of alcohol can also result in withdrawal symptoms in the client who has developed a high tolerance to alcohol and is physically dependent. The severity of the disease, the possibility of hallucinations, and the occurrence of delirium tremens are not determined by the information given. The Axis I diagnosis of alcohol dependency is just that—it is not classified as mild, moderate, or severe. Alcoholic hallucinosis is a state of auditory hallucinations that develops about 48 hours after the client has stopped drinking. The client hears voices or noises within the context of a clear sensorium, meaning that the auditory hallucination is the only symptom the client experiences. Severe withdrawal symptoms that are not managed medically can progress to delirium tremens or a severe abstinence syndrome. Delirium tremens occurs about 3 to 5 days after the client's last drink and is characterized by confusion, agitation, severe psychomotor activity, hallucinations, sleeplessness, tachycardia, elevated blood pressure, elevated temperature, and possibly seizures. (R)

36. **1.** The most effective way to help decrease the client's denial is to point out how alcohol has gotten the client into trouble, using specific, concrete data based on fact, not opinion. Explaining the effects of drinking on family, urging the client to attend Alcoholics Anonymous meetings, and telling her about the physiologic damage that can result are important components of the treatment process but are not as effective in decreasing denial as discussing how alcohol has affected her life. (P)

37. **2.** The nurse would most likely administer a benzodiazepine, such as lorazepam, to the client who is experiencing symptoms of alcohol withdrawal. The benzodiazepine substitutes for the alcohol to suppress withdrawal symptoms. The client experiences symptoms of withdrawal because of the "rebound phenomenon" when sedation of the central nervous system (CNS) from alcohol begins to decrease. Haloperidol (Haldol) is an antipsychotic and is not indicated for alcohol withdrawal symptoms. Benztropine is used to treat extrapyramidal symptoms associated with antipsychotic therapy. Naloxone is used in opioid overdose to reverse the CNS depression caused by the opioid. (D)

38. **3.** Monitoring vital signs provides the best information about the client's overall physiologic status during alcohol withdrawal and the physiologic response to the medication used. Vital signs reflect the degree of central nervous system irritability and indicate the effectiveness of the medication in easing withdrawal symptoms. Although assessment of nutritional status and sleep pattern and assessment for evidence of tremors are important, they provide only indirect information about single aspects of the client's physiologic status. (R)

39. **1.** A client is suffering from a blackout when he cannot recall what he did while under the influence of alcohol. A hangover refers to symptoms experienced the day after a bout of heavy drinking. Common symptoms include headaches and gastrointestinal distress, typically after heavy alcohol consumption. Tolerance refers to the need to increase the amount of the substance or to ingest the substance more often to achieve the same effects. Delirium tremens refers to severe alcohol withdrawal or abstinence syndrome with confusion, psychomotor agitation, sleeplessness, hallucinations, and elevated vital signs. (A)

40. **4.** Stating, "I'm Maria, a nurse in the program; the staff and I will help you," is a nonjudgmental, caring approach that promotes trust and a therapeutic relationship. The statement, "I hope you are serious about maintaining your sobriety this time," blames the client, subsequently decreasing the client's self-worth. Saying, "You'll get it right this time" is threatening to the client, possibly leading to decreased self-worth by reinforcing the client's past failures at maintaining sobriety. The statement, "I know someone who was successful after the fifth program," is impersonal and irrelevant to the client's situation. (P)

41. **3.** The wife of the man with alcohol dependency is exhibiting enabling behavior when she makes excuses for her husband's absenteeism. Enabling behavior is not helpful to the client but rescues him from adverse consequences in relation to his employment. Self-defeating behavior would be evidenced by putting oneself in a position that will lead to failure. Masochistic behavior would be evidenced by the need to experience emotional or physical pain to become sexually aroused. (P)

42. **4.** To be most helpful, the nurse should calmly and objectively present facts by saying, "You have alcohol on your breath," to help the coworker overcome denial and resistance. This statement also helps to reinforce the coworker's awareness of the problem. The other statements blame the coworker and may reinforce denial. Blaming, nagging, and yelling diminish self-esteem in the individual with a substance abuse problem who has low frustration tolerance. (P)

43. **3.** The nurse leader should direct the husband to say, "Either you get help or the kids and I will move out of the house." This statement facilitates entrance into treatment because it is a direct statement of what the consequences are if the alcohol abuse continues. The statement, "The children and I want you to get help," is not effective. Most likely, the husband has already made a similar statement before the confrontation session. Saying, "If your parents were alive, they would be extremely disappointed in you," or "You need to enter treatment now or be a drunk if that's what you want," shames the wife and further decreases her self-esteem. (P)

44. **3.** The statement, "You interrupted Terry twice in 4 minutes," indicates an understanding of the use of constructive feedback by describing specifically what was seen and heard in an objective manner. The other statements are judgmental and blame the client without specifying what the objectionable behavior is. (P)

45. **4.** The client is feeling remorse about hitting his wife. It is best to make a comment that will help him focus on his feelings and express them. Reflecting what the client has said is a good technique to accomplish these goals. Suggesting the client ask his wife or explore the issue in family therapy is inappropriate because it gives advice and ignores the client's underlying feelings. Saying, "It would depend on how much she really cares for you," is inappropriate because it ignores the client's feelings and reinforces the negative aspects, such as the shamefulness, of the behavior. (P)

46. **2.** Al-Anon is a self-help group for spouses and significant others that provides education and support and helps participants learn to lead their own life without feeling responsible for the individual with an alcohol problem. Alateen provides support for teenaged children of a person with an alcohol problem. Employee assistance programs help employees recover from alcohol or drug dependence while retaining their positions or jobs. Alcoholics Anonymous provides support for the individual with alcohol problems to attain and maintain sobriety. (M)

47. **1.** Having the client who is experiencing severe symptoms of alcohol withdrawal walk is contraindicated because increased activity and stimulation may confuse the client and promote hallucinations. The client may also sustain an injury if he has a seizure as part of the alcohol withdrawal process. The nurse should monitor intake and output to ensure fluid and electrolyte balance and hydration. The nurse should assess vital signs to assess the physiologic status of the client and the response to medications. The nurse should use short, concrete statements to decrease confusion and ambiguity. (R)

48. **1.** Any amount of alcohol consumed while taking disulfiram (Antabuse) can cause an alcohol-disulfiram reaction. The reaction experienced is in proportion to the amount of alcohol ingested. The alcohol-disulfiram reaction can begin 5 to 10 minutes after alcohol is ingested. Symptoms can be mild, as in flushing, throbbing in the head and neck, nausea, and diaphoresis. Other symptoms include vomiting, respiratory difficulty, hypotension, vertigo, syncope, and confusion. Severe reactions involve respiratory depression, convulsions, coma, and even death. Disulfiram can be taken at bedtime if the client feels sleepy from the medication. Some clients experience a metallic or garlic taste when initiating disulfiram treatment. Anything containing alcohol, such as cough medicine, aftershave lotion, and mouthwash, can cause a reaction. Therefore, the client needs to check the labels of these items for their alcohol content. (D)

49. **3.** The first question should be to ask the client how much alcohol she has had today because nausea with severe vomiting is a sign of an alcohol-disulfiram (Antabuse) reaction. Asking the client whether she feels like she has flu symptoms is important after inquiring about alcohol intake. Foods cooked in an alcoholic beverage, such as wine, could also cause a reaction, but the reaction would be less severe because the alcohol dissipates with cooking. Asking how long the client has been taking Antabuse would be least important at this time. (D)

50. **1.** Thiamine specifically prevents the development of Wernicke's encephalopathy, a reversible amnestic disorder caused by a diet deficient in thiamine secondary to poor nutritional intake that commonly accompanies chronic alcoholism. It is characterized by nystagmus, ataxia, and mental status changes. Because the client would rather drink alcohol than eat, the client is depleted of vitamins and nutrients. Alcohol also is an irritant that causes a "malabsorption syndrome" in which vitamins and nutrients are not absorbed properly in the gastrointestinal tract. Thiamine is not associated with decreasing withdrawal symptoms, helping clients regain their strength, or promoting elimination of alcohol from the body. (D)

51. **2.** The statement, "Stopping Alcoholics Anonymous and not expressing feelings can lead to relapse," indicates the client's understanding of signs of relapse. The client is responsible for sobriety and must understand the signs of relapse. Other antecedents to relapse include severe craving, being around users, and severe emotional crises. The other statements place the responsibility for the client's sobriety on someone else. (R)

52. **1.** The client is using denial, an unconscious defense mechanism, when she refuses to acknowledge that she has a problem with alcohol. This is further evidenced by the client's inability to connect the liver disorder with alcohol ingestion. Displacement involves transfer of a feeling to someone else or to an object. Rationalization involves an attempt to make or prove that one's feeling or behavior is justifiable. Reaction formation is a conscious behavior that is the exact opposite of an unconscious feeling. (P)

53. **3.** Stating that the vitamin is a nutritional supplement important to the client's health is the best response. The client is nutritionally depleted, and the B-complex vitamins produce a calming effect on the irritated central nervous system and prevent anemia, peripheral neuropathy, and Wernicke's encephalopathy. Although the statements about drinking alcohol and eating very little and that there is a low amount of vitamins in the alcohol consumed may be true, they fail to address the client's concerns directly and fail to provide the necessary information, as does telling the client that the doctor wants the client to take the vitamin for 4 months. (D)

54. **4.** The client is most likely experiencing peripheral neuritis secondary to chronic alcohol consumption. Typical symptoms of peripheral neuritis include numbness, itching, and pain in the extremities and a predisposition to footdrop. Neuralgia refers to severe pain along the course of a nerve. Bell's palsy is a type of facial paralysis involving the seventh cranial nerve. Neurasthenia refers to motor and mental fatigue. (R)

55. **2.** Regular coffee contains caffeine, which acts as a psychomotor stimulant and leads to feelings of anxiety and agitation. Serving coffee to the client may add to tremors and wakefulness. Milk, orange juice, and eggs are part of a well-balanced, high-protein diet needed by the client in alcohol withdrawal, who is nutritionally depleted. (R)

56. **4.** The nurse should teach the client with peripheral neuropathy to avoid using an electric blanket because the client is likely to have decreased sensitivity in the extremities owing to the damaging effects of alcohol on the nerve endings. It is particularly important to guard against burns because the client may not be able to discern the appropriate degree of heat on the feet. Daily washing and drying, massaging with lotion, and trimming the toenails are appropriate foot care measures for any client. (R)

57. **4.** Based on the assessment findings, the nurse should suspect that the client is experiencing delirium, specifically delirium tremens, severe symptoms of alcohol withdrawal. Delirium tremens is characterized by disorientation, confusion, hallucinations, agitation, and elevated vital signs. Stupor refers to a level of consciousness in which a client responds only to repeated verbal stimuli and painful tactile stimuli. Mild alcohol withdrawal is characterized by mild tremors, nausea, nervousness, diaphoresis, rapid heartbeat, and increased blood pressure. Impaired consciousness is characterized by drowsiness, lethargy, loss of recent memory, and slowed thought processes. (A)

58. **1.** The client is demonstrating visual hallucinations, one of the defining characteristics of *Disturbed sensory perception: Visual.* Although *Disturbed thought processes, Risk for injury,* and *Ineffective coping* may occur in the client experiencing alcohol withdrawal, they are not reflected in the client's statement about bugs. *Disturbed thought processes* refers to the state when the client experiences a disruption in cognitive operations and activities as evidenced by memory problems, hypovigilance or hypervigilance, distractibility, or egocentricity. *Risk for injury* is a result of an environmental condition that interacts with a client's adaptive and defensive resources. *Ineffective coping* refers to a client's impairment of adaptive behavior and problem-solving ability in meeting life's demands and roles. (P)

59. **2.** The statement, "The client is a weak individual and could stop if he desires," is false and indicates a lack of understanding regarding alcohol dependency. The *Diagnostic and Statistical Manual of Mental Disorders,* 4th edition, text revised, criteria for substance dependency includes the inability to stop using even when wanting to do so. The client cannot stop or control the amount used when dependent on a substance. Alcohol dependency affects individuals from every culture and socioeconomic background and has nothing to do with being a "weak" individual. The devastating effects of alcohol dependency are felt by every member of the family and not just the individual with the alcohol problem. Family members need education about the physical, physiologic, and psychological effects of alcohol and referrals to self-help groups for support. They have felt and lived with the devastating effects of the disease. A simple and commonly held view of alcoholism is that alcohol is a problem when it interferes with life or disrupts family, work, or social relationships. (M)

60. **3.** The client with alcohol withdrawal delirium should not be left unattended when confused, disoriented, or hallucinating. Injury or unintentional suicide is a possibility when the client attempts to get away from hallucinations. Restraints are used only when the client loses control and is a danger to herself or others, to protect the client from injury or harm. Touching the client before saying anything is an additional stimulus that would most likely add to the client's agitation. Informing the client about the alcohol treatment program while the client is delirious is inappropriate and shows poor nursing judgment. The client should be given information about alcohol treatment when the withdrawal symptoms are lessening and the client can comprehend the information. (S)

61. **2.** AA, a self-help program based on 12 steps, is open to anyone whose goal is sobriety. The first step requires that the individual admit that he is powerless over alcohol and needs help. Members are in various stages of recovery, and the individual does not have to be sober for at least a month before joining. Potential members are not interviewed. The individual decides how many meetings to attend each week. AA does not require attendance at meetings daily, but some individuals choose to do so, especially at the beginning of recovery. (P)

62. **4.** Follow-up care is essential to prevent relapse. Recovery has just begun when the treatment program ends. The first few months after program completion can be difficult and dangerous for the chemically dependent client. The nurse is responsible for discharge plans that include arrangements for counseling, self-help group meetings, and other forms of aftercare. Supportive friends, a list of goals, and family forgiveness may be important and helpful to the client, but follow-up care is essential. (M)

63. **2, 3, 4.** The client who plans to attend Alcoholics Anonymous meetings, verbalizes the damaging effects of alcohol on his body, and takes naltrexone daily may be ready for alcohol rehabilitation. Other key outcomes include admitting that a problem with alcohol exists and realizing the negative effects of alcohol on his life. Stating that he needs to cut down on his alcohol intake and that he is indestructible are signs of denial of an alcohol problem. (P)

64. **3.** The term dual diagnosis refers to the presence of at least one psychiatric disorder and a substance abuse or dependency problem. The psychiatric disorder can be a mental illness or a personality disorder (or both). Therefore, major depression and alcohol abuse is a dual diagnosis. (P)

65. **2.** The nurse should assess the client's mental status daily to note changes that could occur from exacerbation of the mental illness or withdrawal from alcohol. Changes in mental status is important for treatment issues such as medication and participation in groups. Assessment of mental status takes priority because mental status affects the client's ability to sleep, eat, and care for himself. Flexibility is necessary on the part of nurses and staff members who are working with a heterogeneous client population. (M)

66. **1.** The client's decision to drink alcohol results in a feeling of autonomy and a temporary increase in self-esteem. The client feels better, problems are avoided, and he is in temporary control of himself. Guilt or shame may result later because the client is aware that he should not use alcohol because of his mental illness. The combination of a mental illness and substance abuse results in increased recidivism and treatment complications. It may not be true that the client abused alcohol before developing a mental illness or that the client is compelled to drink because of cognitive difficulties. The client may be predisposed to developing a substance abuse problem and a mental illness because of heredity and biologic factors. The largest group of dual diagnosis clients have separate etiologies for their mental illness and substance abuse problem. The client who is not experiencing acute symptoms of his mental illness is probably not impaired cognitively but can decide whether he wants to drink alcohol. (P)

The Client with Disorders Related to Other Addictive Substances

67. **1.** A respiratory rate of less than 12 breaths/minute is cause for concern because of central nervous system depression. Respiratory depression and arrest is the primary cause of death among clients who abuse opioids. Peripheral nervous system effects associated with opioid abuse include urinary retention, hypotension, reduced pupil size, constipation, and decreased gastric, biliary, and pancreatic secretions. Pinpoint pupils are a sign of opioid overdose. However, respiratory depression is the immediate concern. (R)

68. **1, 2, 3.** Symptoms of opioid withdrawal include yawning, rhinorrhea, sweating, chills, piloerection (goose bumps), tremors, restlessness, irritability, leg spasms, bone pain, diarrhea, and vomiting. Symptoms of withdrawal occur within 36 to 72 hours of usage and subside within a week. Withdrawal from heroin is seldom fatal and usually does not necessitate medical intervention. Synesthesia (a blending of senses) is associated with lysergic acid diethylamide use, and formication (feeling of bugs crawling beneath the skin) is associated with cocaine use. (P)

69. **2.** Heroin is an opioid. Naloxone, an opioid antagonist, is used to treat suspected opioid overdose. Naloxone blocks the neuroreceptors affected by opioids. Usually, the client responds in a few minutes to an intravenous injection of the drug. Respirations improve, but the nurse must monitor the client carefully to determine whether additional naloxone is needed. Haloperidol is an antipsychotic, and lorazepam and oxazepam are antianxiety agents; they would further depress the central nervous system. (D)

70. **1.** Vomiting and diarrhea are usually late signs of heroin withdrawal, along with muscle spasm, fever, nausea, repetitive sneezing, abdominal cramps, and backache. Early signs of heroin withdrawal include yawning, tearing (lacrimation), rhinorrhea, and sweating. Intermediate signs of heroin withdrawal are flushing, piloerection, tachycardia, tremor, restlessness, and irritability. (R)

71. **4.** After administering naloxone, the nurse should monitor the client's respiratory status carefully because the drug is short-acting and respiratory depression may recur after its effects wear off. Cerebral edema, kidney failure, and seizure activity are not directly related to opioid overdose or naloxone therapy. (D)

72. **4.** The client takes methadone primarily to be able to work, live normally, and function productively without the mental and physical deterioration caused by opioid addiction. Methadone lessens physiologic dependence on opioids and is used to prevent withdrawal symptoms. Methadone, a substance similar to morphine, is an addictive substance; the client is still considered addicted to opioids. Because methadone has a long half-life of 15 to 30 hours, it can be taken once a day on an outpatient basis. (P)

73. **1.** Suggesting that the client try attending a meeting at a different location is a supportive, positive response and encourages the client to continue participating in treatment. Saying, "Maybe it just wasn't a good day for you," or "Perhaps you weren't paying close enough attention," places blame on the client and is not helpful. The statement, "Sometimes the meetings can seem like a waste of time, but you need to attend to stay clean," diminishes the importance of the self-help group and offers little support to the client. (P)

74. **2.** The best measure to determine a client's progress in rehabilitation is the number of drug-free days he has. The longer the client abstains, the better the prognosis is. Although the kinds of friends the client makes, the way he gets along with his parents, and the degree of responsibility his job requires could influence his decision to stay clean, the number of drug-free days is the best indicator of progress. (P)

75. **4.** The client who is addicted to heroin is most likely to exhibit hypoactivity. Initially, the client feels euphoric. This is followed by drowsiness, hypoactivity, anorexia, and a decreased sex drive. Hilarity, aggression, and a labile mood usually are not associated with heroin addiction. (P)

76. **4.** Because barbiturates are central nervous system depressants, the nurse should be especially alert for the possibility of respiratory failure. Respiratory failure is the most likely cause of death from barbiturate overdose. Kidney failure, cerebrovascular accident, and status epilepticus are not associated with barbiturate overdose. (R)

77. **4.** When a friend asks whether a seriously ill client will live, it is best for the nurse to respond by explaining the seriousness of the client's condition and acknowledging the friend's concern. This type of comment does not offer false hope. Telling the friend to wait and see and that it is too soon to tell is a stereotypical statement that offers no support to the friend. Asking the friend to describe his or her relationship with the client ignores the friend's concern and does not focus on the problem. Simply saying that the client is very ill and may not live and that some don't pull through is harsh and not supportive. (P)

78. 1. Tolerance for a drug occurs when a client requires increasingly larger doses to obtain the desired effect. Therefore, the plan of care would address the client's state of tolerance. The term addiction refers to psychological and physiologic symptoms indicating that an individual cannot control his or her use of psychoactive substances. This term has been replaced with the term dependence. Abuse refers to the excessive use of a substance that differs from societal norms. Drug dependence occurs when the client must take a usual or increasing amount of the drug to prevent the onset of abstinence symptoms, cannot keep drug intake under control, and continues to use even though physical, social, and emotional processes are compromised. (A)

79. 4. For a client who is confused when awakening after taking a large dose of barbiturates, the nurse should speak in concrete terms using simple statements in a calm, nonjudgmental, gentle manner to assist the client with cognitive-perceptual impairment, enhance understanding, and decrease anxiety. The other statements contain abstract information and some slang terms that may further confuse the client and thus increase the client's anxiety. (P)

80. 2. The priority nursing diagnosis would be *Risk for self-directed violence* related to suicide attempt. Although the client may be experiencing a self-esteem disturbance, ineffective coping, or feelings of powerlessness, the priority here is the client's safety. (P)

81. 1. The most appropriate initial outcome for the client is to discuss thoughts and feelings related to her losses. The nurse should help the client identify and verbalize her feelings so that she can externalize her thoughts and emotions and begin to deal with them. This prevents the client from internalizing feelings, which leads to depression and self-harm. The ability to identify two positive qualities, explore strengths, and prioritize problems would be appropriate after the client has explored her thoughts and feelings, gained awareness of the issues, and then can participate in the treatment plan. (P)

82. 4. The best method to deal with the problem is to discuss observations with clients at the daily community meeting because the problem involves all of the clients and this provides them with the opportunity to offer their views. Peer pressure is valuable in confronting self-defeating and destructive behaviors. Providing additional recreation avoids or ignores the problem and is damaging to all clients because it decreases trust in the nurse. Breaking up drug-oriented discussions would not be sufficient to stop the behavior. Speaking with the clients individually about their behavior is not as effective as dealing with the problem openly and directly with everyone. (P)

83. 4. The nurse directs the conversation to realistic concerns or issues to decrease denial and focus on rebuilding a substance-free life. Allowing the client to continue with the stories or questioning the client further about her exploits reinforces the denial. Telling the client you've heard the stories before is nondirective. Additionally, these actions do nothing to help the client focus on rebuilding a substance-free life. (P)

84. 3. The statement that marijuana causes more damage to your body than regular cigarettes is a direct, correct, educational response to the student's statement that does not decrease the student's or the friend's self-worth. Marijuana causes harmful pulmonary effects, weakens heart contractions, causes immunosuppression, and reduces serum testosterone and sperm count. Telling the student that marijuana is unsafe and illegal, or that using marijuana leads to using other chemicals, does not provide the student with factual information to answer the student's question. Asking whether the student really believes the friend challenges the student and may lead to defensive behavior. (P)

85. 1, 2, 3, 4, 5. Ecstasy is chemically related to methamphetamine (speed) and is used at "raves" (all-night dance parties) to enhance dancing, closeness to others, affection, and the ability to communicate. Euphoria, heightened sexuality, disinhibition, and diminished self-consciousness can occur. Adverse effects include tachycardia, elevated blood pressure, anorexia, dry mouth, and teeth grinding. Pacifiers, including candy-shaped pacifiers and lollipops, are used to ease the discomfort associated with teeth grinding and jaw clenching. Hyperthermia, dehydration, renal failure, and death can occur. (P)

86. 2. Synesthesia is the blending of senses, a phenomenon caused by lysergic acid diethylamide. The client can taste colors, see sounds, or smell rainbows. Impaired judgment is exhibited by a client who thinks he can fly. A flashback—the cognitive, emotional, and physical reexperiencing of a traumatic event—can instill panic in a client because he experiences a sense of "going crazy" or paranoia. Acute panic occurs when the client is on a "bad trip" and becomes extremely frightened. (P)

87. 1. When the client experiences a "bad trip" and is frightened and paranoid, the nurse should stay with the client and talk her down. The nurse supports the client through the experience, ensures her safety, and orients her to where she is. The nurse should tell the client that she is experiencing the effects of lysergic acid diethylamide, she is safe, and the effects of the drug will end. Placing the client in seclusion or leaving the client alone until the "bad trip" subsides is poor judgment and irresponsible on the part of the nurse, possibly leading to increased anxiety, panic, and injury. Telling another caregiver to check on the client periodically demonstrates poor management of the client's care and is also unfair to the caregiver. (S)

88. **2.** The feeling of bugs crawling under the skin, termed *formication,* is associated with cocaine use. An illusion is misinterpretation of sensory input such as walking past a tree and thinking it's a ghost. Confusion is a state of being bewildered or unclear. A flashback is a cognitive, emotional, and physical reexperiencing of a traumatic event. (P)

89. **4.** The nurse assesses the client for feelings of depression and suicidal ideation. After experiencing an instantaneous high from crack, a crash immediately follows and the client has an intense craving for more crack. A crash commonly leads to a cocaine-induced depression when additional crack is unavailable. At times, the depression is so severe that users attempt suicide. Although suspiciousness, loss of appetite, and drug craving are also associated with cocaine use, they are less of a priority than suicidal ideation. (P)

90. **1.** The nurse should prepare to administer an antipsychotic medication, such as haloperidol, to a client experiencing amphetamine psychosis to decrease agitation and psychotic symptoms, including delusions, hallucinations, and cognitive impairment. Lorazepam and diazepam, which are benzodiazepines, and chlordiazepoxide are antianxiety agents that have no effect on the client's symptoms of psychosis. (D)

91. **2.** The client is physically dependent on alprazolam. Therefore, the client is slowly tapered off of the benzodiazepine by decreasing the dose and frequency over several days. Doing so helps to minimize withdrawal symptoms (similar to those of alcohol withdrawal) while safely withdrawing the client from the medication. Benzodiazepines should never be stopped abruptly because of withdrawal symptoms, especially convulsions and tachycardia. Administering alprazolam on an as-needed basis would not help the client withdraw from the medication. (R)

92. **1, 2, 5.** The client is exhibiting symptoms of moderate anxiety. At this level of anxiety, the nurse should help the client to decrease anxiety by allowing ventilation, crying, exercise, and relaxation techniques. The nurse would further assist the client by refocusing his attention, relating behaviors and feelings to anxiety, and then assisting with problem solving. Oral medication may be needed if the client's anxiety is prolonged or does not decrease with the nurse's interventions. Suggesting a time-out and giving intramuscular medication are possible interventions for a client whose anxiety level is severe. (P)

93. **2.** The nurse must be especially cautious when providing care to a client who has taken PCP because of unpredictable, violent behavior. The client can appear to be in a calm state or even in a coma, then become violent, and then return to a calm or comatose state. Visual hallucinations, bizarre behavior, and loud screaming are associated with PCP-intoxicated clients. However, the unpredictable, violent behavior presents a major issue of safety for clients and staff. (S)

94. **3.** An acid environment aids in the excretion of phencyclidine (PCP). Therefore, the nurse should give the client with PCP intoxication cranberry juice to acidify the urine to a pH of 5.5 and accelerate excretion. (R)

95. **1.** Smoking marijuana while using alcohol can lead to alcohol poisoning because marijuana masks the nausea and vomiting associated with excessive alcohol consumption. Marijuana contains tetrahydrocannabinol (THC), which is responsible for suppressing nausea. With dangerous levels of alcohol in the body, respiratory depression, coma, and death can occur. Lysergic acid diethylamide, peyote, and psilocybin do not contain THC. (P)

96. **3.** Providing frequent "time-outs" when the client is highly anxious, sensitive, irritable, and over-reactive is needed to calm the client and reduce the possibility of escalating behaviors and violence. Secluding and restraining the client is not appropriate and would only be used if the client was threatening others and other alternative actions had been unsuccessful. Telling the client to stay in his room until he can control himself is unrealistic and futile because the client cannot eliminate behaviors induced by chemicals. Confronting the client about his behaviors would most likely lead to aggression and possibly violent behavior. (S)

97. **4.** The nurse should invite the client who is anxious to participate in an activity that involves gross motor movements. Doing so helps to direct energy toward a therapeutic activity. Appropriate activities include walking, riding a stationary bicycle, or playing volleyball. Assigning the client to an educational group is not helpful because the anxious client would be unable to sit in a group setting and concentrate on what was occurring in the group. Watching television may be too stimulating for the client, possibly increasing anxiety. Additionally, the client may be too anxious to sit and focus. Waiting for the client to approach the nurse is not helpful or appropriate. The nurse is responsible for initiating contact with the client. (P)

98. **4.** The best action by the nurse to help a client who has difficulty falling asleep would be to teach the client relaxation exercises to use before bedtime to reduce anxiety and promote relaxation. This activity will also be useful for the client when out of the hospital. Inviting the client to play a board game is inappropriate because this activity can be competitive and thus stimulate the client. Allowing the client to sit in the community room until she feels sleepy is inappropriate because it does nothing to help the client relax; nor does advising the client to sleep on the sofa in the dayroom, which may be against unit policy. (C)

The Client with an Anxiety-Related Disorder

99. **1, 4, 5.** The nurse should instruct the client who is taking diazepam to take the medication as prescribed; stopping the medication suddenly can cause withdrawal symptoms. This medication is used for a short term only. The drug dose can be potentiated by alcohol and the client should not drink alcoholic beverages while taking this drug. Swelling of the lips and face and difficulty breathing are signs and symptoms of an allergic reaction. The client should stop taking the drug and seek medical assistance immediately. The client does not need to avoid eating foods containing tyramine; tyramine interacts with monoamine oxidase inhibitors, not Valium. The client can take the medication with food. (H)

100. **4.** Cognitive behavioral therapy is effective in treating anxiety disorders. The nurse can assist the client in identifying the onset of the fears that cause the anxiety and develop strategies to modify the behavior associated with the fears. Avoiding touching foods, asking about reasons for the anxiety, and providing ways to work around touching the foods do not deal with the anxiety and are not interventions that will help this client. (P)

101. **2.** Asking, "Are you feeling anxious?" helps the client to specifically label the feeling as anxiety so that he can begin to understand and manage it. Some clients need assistance with identifying what they are feeling so they can recognize what is happening to them. Stating, "You need to sit down and relax," is not appropriate because the client needs to continue his pacing to feel better. Asking if something is bothering the client or saying that he must be experiencing a problem is vague and does not help the client identify his feelings as anxiety. (P)

102. **1.** The nurse responds with the statement, "It was very frightening for you," to express empathy, thus acknowledging the client's discomfort and accepting his feelings. The nurse conveys respect and validates the client's self-worth. The other statements do not focus on the client's underlying feelings, convey active listening, or promote trust. (P)

103. **4.** Reducing the client's environmental stimulation helps to reduce anxiety. For the client who is already anxious, noise and activity further increase anxiety. Leaving the client alone is not therapeutic because the nurse's presence provides comfort, safety, and support. Making optimistic statements ignores the client's feelings and offers little help when she feels uneasy. Although demonstrating technical competence is helpful to the anxious client, environmental stimulation must be reduced to reduce the client's anxiety. (P)

104. **3.** It is important for the nurse to teach the client that the symptoms of a panic attack are time limited and will abate. This helps decrease the client's fear about what is occurring. Clients benefit from learning about their illness, what symptoms to expect, and the helpful use of medication. A simple biologic explanation of the disorder can convince clients to take their medication. Telling the client to stay in the house to eliminate panic attacks is not correct or helpful. Panic attacks can occur "out of the blue," and clients with panic disorder can become agoraphobic because of fear of having a panic attack where help is not available or escape is impossible. Medication should be taken on a scheduled basis to block the symptoms of panic before they start. Taking medication when symptoms start is not helpful. Telling the client to maintain self-control to decrease symptoms of panic is false information because the brain and biochemicals may account for its development. Therefore, the client cannot control when a panic attack will occur. (P)

105. **1.** Alprazolam, a benzodiazepine used on a short-term or temporary basis to treat symptoms of anxiety, increases gamma-aminobutyrate, a major inhibitory neurotransmitter. Because gamma-aminobutyric acid is increased and the reticular activating system is depressed, incoming stimuli are muted and the effects of anxiety are blocked. Alprazolam does not directly target serotonin, dopamine, or norepinephrine. (D)

106. **3.** Using alcohol or any central nervous system depressant while taking a benzodiazepine, such as alprazolam, is contraindicated because of additive depressant effects. Ingestion of chocolate, cheese, or shellfish is not problematic. (D)

107. **1.** Buspirone, a nonbenzodiazepine anxiolytic, is particularly effective in treating the cognitive symptoms of anxiety, such as worry, apprehension, difficulty with concentration, and irritability. BuSpar is not effective for the somatic symptoms of anxiety (muscle tension). Therapeutic effects may be experienced in 7 to 10 days, with full effects not occurring for 3 to 4 weeks. This drug is not known to cause physical or psychological dependence. It can be taken with food or small meals to reduce gastrointestinal upset. (D)

108. **2.** The nurse initially reassures the client that her feelings and behaviors are typical reactions to serious trauma to help decrease anxiety and maintain self-esteem. Explaining the effects of stress on the body may be helpful later. Telling the client that her symptoms are temporary is less helpful. Acknowledging the unfairness of the client's situation does not address the client's needs at this time. (P)

109. **3.** The client with anxiety may be able to learn to recognize when she is feeling anxious, understand the reasons for her anxiety, and be able to describe situations that preceded her feelings of anxiety. However, she is likely to continue to experience symptoms unless she has also learned to use adaptive and palliative methods to reduce anxiety. (P)

110. **4.** Saying, "The accident just happened and could not have been predicted," provides the client with an objective perception of the event instead of the client's perceived role. This type of statement reflects active listening and helps to reduce feelings of blame and guilt. Saying, "Don't keep torturing yourself," or "Stop blaming yourself," is inappropriate because it tells the client what to do, subsequently delaying the therapeutic process. The statement, "Let's talk about something that is a bit more pleasant," ignores the client's feelings and changes the subject. The client needs to verbalize feelings and decrease feelings of isolation. (P)

111. **1.** The nurse states, "You did what you had to do at that time," to help the client evaluate past behavior in the context of the trauma. Clients commonly feel guilty about past behaviors when viewing them in the context of current values. The other statements are inappropriate because they do not help the client to evaluate past behavior in the context of the trauma. (P)

112. **2.** Writing in a journal can help the client safely express feelings, particularly anger, when the client cannot verbalize them. Safely externalizing anger by writing in a journal helps the client to maintain control over her feelings. (P)

113. **3.** The nurse should facilitate progressive review of the accident and its consequences to help the client integrate feelings and memories and to begin the grieving process. Helping the client to evaluate her sister's behavior, telling the client to avoid details of the accident, or postponing the discussion of the accident until the client brings it up is not therapeutic and does not facilitate the development of trust in the nurse. Such actions do not facilitate review of the accident, which is necessary to help the client integrate feelings and memories and begin the grieving process. (P)

114. **4.** The nurse judges the client's request for an interruption in treatment as a necessary occurrence. A "time-out" is common and necessary to enable the client to focus on pressing problems and solutions. It is not necessarily a method of avoidance, a detriment to progress, or the end of treatment. A problem like housing can be very stressful and require all of the client's energy and attention, with none left for the emotional stress of treatment. (P)

115. **1.** Combining a benzodiazepine with an antacid impairs the absorption rate of the benzodiazepine. Acetaminophen, vitamins, and aspirin are safe to take with a benzodiazepine because no major drug interactions occur. (D)

116. **2.** Valium, like any benzodiazepine, cannot be stopped abruptly. The client must be slowly tapered off of the medication to decrease withdrawal symptoms, which would be similar to withdrawal from alcohol. Alcohol in combination with a benzodiazepine produces an increased central nervous system depressant effect and therefore should be avoided. Valium can cause drowsiness, and the client should be warned about driving until tolerance develops. Valium has muscle relaxant properties and will help tight, tense muscles feel better. (D)

117. **3.** The nurse should suggest behavior therapy, which is most successful for clients with phobias. Systematic desensitization, flooding, exposure, and self-exposure treatments are most therapeutic for clients with phobias. Self-exposure treatment is being increasingly used to avoid frequent therapy sessions. Insight therapy, exploration of the dynamics of the client's personality, is not helpful because the process of anxiety underlies the disorder. Group therapy or psychoanalysis, which deals with repressed, intrapsychic conflicts, is not helpful for the client with phobias because it does not help to manage the underlying anxiety or disorder. (P)

118. **4.** Saying, "It's a sign of progress to eat in the dining area," conveys positive reinforcement and gives the client hope and confidence, thus reinforcing the adaptive behavior. Stating, "It wasn't so hard, now was it," decreases the client's self-worth and minimizes his accomplishment. Stating, "At supper, I hope to see you eat with a group of people," will overwhelm the client and increase anxiety. Stating, "You must have been hungry today," ignores the client's positive behavior and shows the nurse's lack of understanding of the dynamics of the disorder. (P)

119. **4.** The nurse should walk with the client to activate adaptive coping for the client experiencing high anxiety and decreased motivation and energy. Stating, "I know you can do it," "Try holding on to the wall," or "You can miss group this one time," maintains the client's avoidance, thus reinforcing the client's behavior, and does not help the client begin to cope with the problem. (P)

120. **1.** When the client says he thinks he is "going crazy," it is best for the nurse to ask him what "crazy" means to him. The nurse must have a clear idea of what the client means by his words and actions. Using an open-ended question facilitates client description to help the nurse assess his meaning. The other statements minimize and dismiss the client's concern and do not give him the opportunity to openly discuss his feelings, possibly leading to increased anxiety. (P)

121. **1.** A client who is exhibiting compulsive behavior is attempting to control his anxiety. The compulsive behavior is performed to relieve discomfort and to bind or neutralize anxiety. The client must perform the ritual to avoid an extreme increase in tension or anxiety even though the client is aware that the actions are absurd. The repetitive behavior is not an attempt to control thoughts; the obsession or thinking component cannot be controlled. It is not an attention-seeking mechanism or an attempt to express hostility. (P)

122. **2.** The nurse should wake the client an hour earlier to perform his ritual so that he can be on time for breakfast with the other clients. The nurse provides the client with time needed to perform rituals because the client needs to keep his anxiety in check. The nurse should never take away a ritual, because panic will ensue. The nurse should work with the client later to slowly set limits on the frequency of the action. (D)

123. **3.** The nurse conveys empathy and awareness of the client's need to perform the ritual to show acceptance and understanding to the client, thereby promoting trust. Ignoring the behavior, questioning the client about her ritual, or telling the other clients to follow her when she moves is not therapeutic or appropriate. (P)

124. **3.** Clomipramine is used to treat obsessive-compulsive disorder and is related to the tricyclic antidepressants (TCAs). Side effects of Anafranil would be similar to those of the TCA imipramine. Fluoxetine, sertraline, and fluvoxamine are selective serotonin reuptake inhibitors and have minimal side effects. (D)

The Client with a Somatoform Disorder

125. **4.** The nurse sets limits by informing the client in a matter-of-fact manner that the nurse cannot give her additional pain medication at this time. Then the nurse invites the client to participate in a card game to decrease rumination about pain by directing the client's attention to an activity. By telling the client the nurse will call the physician as requested, the nurse is manipulated to do what the client demands. Suggesting that the client lie down because she has to wait for the next dosage or telling the client that the physician will be in later ignores the client and her needs and is not helpful in decreasing rumination about her pain. (P)

126. **3.** The nurse instructs the nursing assistant to invite the client to lunch and accompany him to the dining room to decrease manipulation, secondary gain, dependency, and reinforcement of negative behavior while maintaining the client's self-worth. Taking the client a lunch tray and allowing him to eat in his room reinforces negative behaviors and secondary gain. Telling the client he'll need to wait until supper to eat if he misses lunch or informing the client that he has 10 minutes to get to the dining room challenges the client and may increase feelings of anger and the need for physical complaints. (M)

127. **2.** Pushing insight or awareness into conflicts or problems increases anxiety and the need for physical symptoms to handle or take care of the anxiety. Awareness or insight must be developed slowly as the client's need for symptoms diminishes. Saying, "Ignore the client's behavior and treat her with respect," is not helpful to the staff member or the client. This statement fails to educate the staff member about the client's disorder and simply dismisses the needs of both. It is not true that pushing awareness will be helpful and further the client's recovery; this is the opposite of what is needed. Meeting with the client to confront her behavior is not therapeutic and will greatly increase the client's anxiety and the need for the conversion symptoms. (M)

128. **2.** The nurse helps the client to focus on his feelings about his impending divorce to decrease the client's anxiety and decrease his focus on physical ailments. The client with a somatoform disorder typically has problems with identifying, describing, and dealing with feelings. Internalizing feelings leads to increased anxiety and the need for protective mechanisms. Asking the client to describe his problem with nausea, allowing the client to talk about the many physicians he has seen and the medications he has taken, and informing the client about a different medication for nausea are counterproductive toward recovery because they reinforce the focus on the symptoms. (P)

129. **4.** The nurse should redirect the interaction back to fishing or another focus whenever the client begins to ruminate about physical symptoms or impairment. Doing so helps the client talk about topics that are more therapeutic and beneficial to recovery. Allowing the client to talk about his pain or asking if he needs additional pain medication is not therapeutic because it reinforces the client's need for the symptom. Getting up and leaving the client is not appropriate unless the nurse has set limits previously by saying, "I will get up and leave if you continue to talk about your pain." (P)

130. **1.** The client who states, "It's okay if I feel nauseous when I'm worried about my divorce," recognizes the connection between his nausea and the divorce and is developing insight and awareness into his problem. The nurse should then be able to assist the client with developing adaptive coping strategies. The other statements indicate a lack of insight into his disorder and lack of progress toward recovery. The client is still searching for the "right" diagnosis, medication, and doctor. (P)

Crisis, Violence, and Disorders in Children and Adolescents

The Client in Crisis

1. An anxious teenage girl is brought to the interviewing room of a crisis shelter, sobbing and saying that she thinks she is pregnant but does not know what to do. Which of the following nursing interventions is most appropriate at this time?
- ☐ 1. Ask the client about the type of things that she had thought of doing.
- ☐ 2. Give the client some ideas about what to expect to happen next.
- ☐ 3. Recommend a pregnancy test after acknowledging the client's distress.
- ☐ 4. Question the client about her feelings and possible parental reactions.

2. A potentially pregnant 14-year-old client says that she and her boyfriend have engaged in "mostly heavy petting and necking." Which of the following responses by the nurse is best initially?
- ☐ 1. "You mean you have had sexual intercourse?"
- ☐ 2. "Describe what you mean by heavy petting and necking."
- ☐ 3. "I think we need to talk about what's involved in sexual intercourse."
- ☐ 4. "All you have been doing with your boyfriend is heavy petting and necking?"

3. A 40-year-old client who is quite anxious says that she would "rather die than be pregnant." Which of the following responses by the nurse is most helpful?
- ☐ 1. "Try not to worry until after the pregnancy test."
- ☐ 2. "You know, pregnancy is a normal event."
- ☐ 3. "You're only 40 years old and not too old to have a baby."
- ☐ 4. "I see you're upset. Take some deep breaths to relax a little."

4. After the results of a pregnancy test for a 15-year-old client are found to be negative, the nurse teaches her about sexual intercourse and contraception. At the end of the teaching session, the client states, "No more fooling around for me!" Which of the following replies by the nurse is most appropriate?
- ☐ 1. "Just in case, why don't you try the pills for a while?"
- ☐ 2. "The last person who said that ended up having a baby."
- ☐ 3. "It's your decision, but if you change your mind, we're here to help you."
- ☐ 4. "Aren't you being a little bit overconfident about it, as attractive as you are?"

5. On a crisis shelter hotline, the nurse talks to two 11-year-old boys who think a friend sniffs glue. They say his breath sometimes smells like glue and he acts drunk. They say they are afraid to tell their parents about the friend. When formulating a reply, the nurse should consider which of the following?
- ☐ 1. The boys probably fear punishment.
- ☐ 2. Sniffing glue is illegal.
- ☐ 3. The boys' observations could be wrong.
- ☐ 4. Glue-sniffing is a minor form of substance abuse.

6. While teaching a group of volunteers for a crisis hotline, a volunteer asks, "What if I'm not sure why someone is calling?" Which of the following statements by the nurse is most helpful?
- ☐ 1. "Ask the caller to tell you why he or she is calling you today."
- ☐ 2. "Tell the caller to make an appointment at the walk-in crisis clinic."
- ☐ 3. "Instruct the caller to go to the nearest emergency room."
- ☐ 4. "Tell the caller to let you speak to anyone else in the house."

7. After teaching a group of students who are volunteering for a local crisis hotline, the nurse judges that further education about crisis and intervention is needed when a student states which of the following?

☐ **1.** "Callers to a crisis line use this service when they're overwhelmed and exhausted."

☐ **2.** "People use crisis hotlines when they're in the most pain and nothing is working for them."

☐ **3.** "Most people in crisis will be calling the line once every day for at least a year."

☐ **4.** "One benefit is that a person will know how to handle stressful situations better in the future."

8. Three months after the death of her husband in an automobile accident, a client is admitted to the hospital after attempting to overdose on her antidepressant. She states, "I can't live without him. It's no use. I just want to die." Which of the following nursing diagnoses is the priority in the client's plan of care?

☐ **1.** *Complicated grieving* related to husband's death as evidenced by a suicide attempt.

☐ **2.** *Powerlessness* related to husband's death as evidenced by statement of "It's no use."

☐ **3.** *Hopelessness* related to husband's death as evidenced by the client's statement of inability to live without the husband.

☐ **4.** *Risk for self-directed violence* related to husband's death as evidenced by the client's wish to die.

9. A true crisis state, involving a period of severe disorganization, is difficult to endure emotionally and physically. The nurse recognizes that a client will only be able to tolerate being in crisis for which of the following lengths of time?

☐ **1.** 1 to 2 weeks.

☐ **2.** 4 to 6 weeks.

☐ **3.** 12 to 14 weeks.

☐ **4.** 24 to 26 weeks.

10. The nurse incorporates the underlying premise of crisis intervention, about providing "the right kind of help at the right time," to achieve which of the following goals initially?

☐ **1.** Regaining emotional security and equilibrium.

☐ **2.** Resolution of underlying emotional problems.

☐ **3.** Development of insight and personal growth.

☐ **4.** Formulation of more effective support systems.

11. The nurse understands that with the right help at the right time, a client can successfully resolve a crisis and function better than before the crisis, based primarily on which of the following factors?

☐ **1.** Relinquishment of dysfunctional coping.

☐ **2.** Reestablishment of lost support systems.

☐ **3.** Acquisition of new coping skills.

☐ **4.** Gain of crisis prevention knowledge.

12. A client is being discharged after 3 days of hospitalization for a suicide attempt that followed the receipt of a divorce notice. Which of the following, if verbalized by the client, indicates to the nurse that the client is ready for discharge?

☐ **1.** A readiness for discharge.

☐ **2.** Names and phone numbers of two divorce lawyers.

☐ **3.** A list of support persons and community resources.

☐ **4.** Emotional stability.

13. A distraught father is waiting for his son to come out of surgery. He accidentally backed the car into his son, causing multiple fractures and a serious head injury. Which of the following statements by the father should alert the nurse to the need for a psychiatric consultation?

☐ **1.** "My son will be fine, but I may be charged with reckless driving."

☐ **2.** "His mother is going to kill me when she finds out about this."

☐ **3.** "I just didn't see him run behind the car."

☐ **4.** "If he dies, there will be nothing for me to do but join him."

14. A grandson who calls the crisis center expressing concern about his grandmother who lost her husband a month ago states, "She has been in bed for a week and is not eating or showering. She told me that she did not want to kill herself, but it's not like her to do nothing for herself. She won't even talk to me when I visit her." The nurse encourages the grandson to bring his grandmother to the center for evaluation based on which of the following reasons?

☐ **1.** The behaviors may reflect passive suicidal thoughts.

☐ **2.** The behaviors reflect altered role performance.

☐ **3.** Seeing the grandson and grandmother together will be helpful.

☐ **4.** Refusing to talk to the grandson alone indicates a major problem.

15. A 16-year-old client who is being seen by the crisis nurse after making several superficial cuts on her wrist complains that all her friends are siding with her ex-boyfriend and won't talk to her anymore. She says she knows that the relationship is over, but "If I can't have him, no one else will." Which of the following nursing diagnoses is most important?

☐ **1.** *Situational low self-esteem* related to rejection by friends as evidenced by friends not talking to her.

☐ **2.** *Risk for other-directed violence* related to break-up of the relationship as evidenced by the statement, "If I can't have him, no one else will."

☐ **3.** *Risk for suicide* related to loss of the relationship as evidenced by client's acting-out behaviors.

☐ **4.** *Risk prone health behavior* related to rejection by the boyfriend as evidenced by self-mutilation.

16. A client who comes to the crisis center in a very distressed state tells the nurse, "I just can't get over being fired last week. I've asked for help. I've talked to friends. I've tried everything to get through this, but nothing is working. Help me!" Which of the following should the nurse anticipate using as the initial crisis intervention strategy?

☐ **1.** Referral for counseling.
☐ **2.** Support system assessment.
☐ **3.** Emotion management.
☐ **4.** Unemployment assistance.

17. A major role in crisis intervention is getting a client's significant others involved in helping with the immediate crisis as soon as possible. The nurse should determine that the support persons are prepared to help when they verbalize which of the following?

☐ **1.** The name and phone number of the client's physician.
☐ **2.** Emergency resources and when to use them.
☐ **3.** The coping strategies they are using.
☐ **4.** Long-term solutions they plan to tell the client to use.

18. During the interview, a newly widowed client reveals the wish "to join my husband in Heaven." After the nurse asks the client to sign a no harm contract, which of the following statements is most appropriate to say next?

☐ **1.** "Tell me what feelings you have been experiencing."
☐ **2.** "Has your husband's estate been settled yet?"
☐ **3.** "What was the cause of your husband's death?"
☐ **4.** "Do you have children who are willing to help you?"

The Client with Problems Expressing Anger

19. A female client in an anger management group states, "My doctor tells me I need to get mad more often and not let people tell me what to do. Maybe she thinks I should be more aggressive." What information should the nurse incorporate in the response to this client as most important?

☐ **1.** Denial of anger and lack of assertiveness can be as serious as aggressiveness.
☐ **2.** Assertive behavior in women is not culturally acceptable.
☐ **3.** The client has most likely misinterpreted what the physician said.
☐ **4.** The client is trying to gain acceptance by the group.

20. Based on a client's history of violence toward others and her inability to cope with anger, which of the following should the nurse use as the most important indicator of goal achievement before discharge?

☐ **1.** Acknowledgment of her angry feelings.
☐ **2.** Ability to describe situations that provoke angry feelings.
☐ **3.** Development of a list of how she has handled her anger in the past.
☐ **4.** Verbalization of her feelings in an appropriate manner.

21. In developing a plan of care for an angry client, the staff decides to take an educational approach. Which of the following steps is the least helpful?

☐ **1.** Assisting the client to recognize anger.
☐ **2.** Identifying those with whom the client is angry.
☐ **3.** Identifying alternative ways to express anger.
☐ **4.** Practicing how to express anger.

22. A client is admitted to the hospital because of threatening, aggressive behavior toward his family. In the first group meeting after the client is admitted, another client sits near the nurse and says loudly, "I'm sitting here because I'm afraid of Ted. He's so big, and I heard him talk about hitting people." Which of the following responses by the nurse is the most therapeutic?

☐ **1.** "Everyone is here for different problems. You know you don't have to worry."
☐ **2.** "Ted is new to the group. Let's go around and introduce ourselves to him."
☐ **3.** "You don't know Ted yet. Once you get to know him, I'm sure you won't be afraid."
☐ **4.** "It's frightening to have new people on the unit. We're here to talk about things like being afraid."

23. A client is admitted to the psychiatric hospital for evaluation after numerous incidents of threatening others, angry outbursts, and two episodes of hitting a coworker at the grocery store where he works. The client is very anxious and tells the nurse who admits him, "I didn't mean to hit him. He made me so mad that I just couldn't help it. I hope I don't hit anyone here." Which of the following is the most important initial action to take to ensure a safe environment?

☐ **1.** Letting other clients know that he has a history of hitting others so that they will not provoke him.
☐ **2.** Putting him in a private room and limiting his time out of the room to when staff can be with him.
☐ **3.** Telling him that hitting others is unacceptable behavior and asking him to tell a staff member when he begins feeling angry.
☐ **4.** Obtaining an order for a medication to be administered to decrease his anxiety and threatening behavior.

24. A client loses control and throws two chairs toward another client. What should the nurse do next?
- ☐ **1.** Ask the client to go to the quiet area and talk about the behavior.
- ☐ **2.** Administer an oral tranquilizer and prepare for a show of determination.
- ☐ **3.** Process the incident with the client and discuss alternative behaviors.
- ☐ **4.** Use restraints and administer an intramuscular tranquilizer.

25. The nurse judges that a client is ready to be released from seclusion and restraints when the client demonstrates which of the following behaviors?
- ☐ **1.** Is adequately sedated.
- ☐ **2.** Struggles less against the restraints.
- ☐ **3.** Stops swearing and yelling.
- ☐ **4.** Shows signs of self-control.

26. The treatment team recommends that a client take an assertiveness training class offered in the hospital. Which of the following behaviors indicates that the client is becoming more assertive?
- ☐ **1.** Begins to arrive late for unit activities. When asked why he's late, he says, "Because I feel like it!"
- ☐ **2.** Asks the nurse to call his employer about his insurance.
- ☐ **3.** Asks his roommate to put away his dirty clothes after telling him that this bothers him.
- ☐ **4.** Follows the nurse's advice of asking his doctor about being passive-aggressive.

27. Which of the following physiologic responses should the nurse expect as unlikely to occur when a client is angry?
- ☐ **1.** Increased respiratory rate.
- ☐ **2.** Decreased blood pressure.
- ☐ **3.** Increased muscle tension.
- ☐ **4.** Decreased peristalsis.

28. Which of the following responses to anger from others should the nurse expect as most common in clients?
- ☐ **1.** Increased self-esteem.
- ☐ **2.** Feelings of invulnerability.
- ☐ **3.** Fear of harm.
- ☐ **4.** Powerlessness.

29. When planning the care of a client experiencing aggression, the nurse incorporates the principle of "least restrictive alternative," meaning that less restrictive interventions must be tried before more restrictive measures are employed. Which of the following measures should the nurse consider to be the most restrictive?
- ☐ **1.** Tension reduction strategies.
- ☐ **2.** Haloperidol (Haldol) given orally.
- ☐ **3.** Voluntary seclusion or time-out.
- ☐ **4.** Haloperidol given intramuscularly.

30. As an angry client becomes more agitated while talking about his problems, the nurse decides to ask for staff assistance in taking control of the situation when the client demonstrates which of the following behaviors?
- ☐ **1.** Swearing about his wife's behaviors when discussing marital problems.
- ☐ **2.** Picking up a pool cue stick and telling the nurse to get out of his way.
- ☐ **3.** Making a fist and pounding loudly on the table.
- ☐ **4.** Coming out of his room instead of staying in time-out.

31. A client who is agitated but not currently psychotic is willing to take a medication ordered p.r.n. If all of the following medications were ordered for the client, which should the nurse expect to administer?
- ☐ **1.** Oral lorazepam (Ativan).
- ☐ **2.** Oral benztropine (Cogentin).
- ☐ **3.** Intramuscular (I.M.) haloperidol (Haldol).
- ☐ **4.** I.M. fluphenazine decanoate (Prolixin Decanoate).

32. When a client is about to lose control, the extra staff who come to help commonly stay at a distance from the client unless asked to move closer by the nurse who is talking to the client. Which of the following best explains the primary rationale for staying at a distance initially?
- ☐ **1.** The client is more likely to act out if there is an audience, even additional staff.
- ☐ **2.** The nurse talking to the client makes the decisions about other staff actions.
- ☐ **3.** The client is likely to perceive others as being closer than they are and feel threatened.
- ☐ **4.** When the extra staff is visible, the client is less likely to regain self-control.

33. Psychiatric staff are usually required to participate in an aggression management program annually. Evaluation of such a program would be based primarily on which of the following indicators?
- ☐ **1.** Fewer client injuries during restraint procedures.
- ☐ **2.** A reduction of complaints by clients' relatives.
- ☐ **3.** Fewer staff injuries during restraint procedures.
- ☐ **4.** A reduction in the total number of restraint procedures.

34. When preparing to use seclusion as an alternative to restraint for a client who has not yet lost control, the nurse expects to use a room with limited furniture and no access to dangerous articles. What should the nurse also consider as critical for the safety of the client?
- ☐ **1.** A security window in the door or a room camera.
- ☐ **2.** Lights that can be dimmed from outside the room.
- ☐ **3.** A staff member to stay in the room with the client.
- ☐ **4.** A doctor's order for the seclusion before it is initiated.

35. The nurse is required initially to restrain all four of a client's extremities. For which of the following reasons should the nurse anticipate the need to add a full-length restraint blanket?

☐ 1. The client complains that restraints are tight and uncomfortable.

☐ 2. The staff want extra protection for themselves.

☐ 3. The client is at risk for injury from fighting the restraints.

☐ 4. Staff assessment reveals that the client will feel more secure under the blanket.

36. Which of the following is the top priority for the client who is placed in restraints?

☐ 1. Monitoring the client every 15 minutes.

☐ 2. Assisting with nutrition and elimination.

☐ 3. Performing range-of-motion exercise for each limb, one at a time.

☐ 4. Changing the client's position every 2 hours.

37. According to hospital protocol, after a client is restrained, the staff meet and discuss the restraint situation. In addition to sharing feelings and offering support, what should the nurse identify as the long-term goal?

☐ 1. Providing feedback to each other on how procedures were handled.

☐ 2. Comparing the perceptions of the various staff members.

☐ 3. Deciding when to release the client from restraints.

☐ 4. Improving the staff's use of restraint procedures.

38. Despite education and role-play practice of restraint procedures, a staff member is injured during an actual restraint. When helping the uninjured staff deal with the incident, the nurse should anticipate addressing which of the following about the injured member?

☐ 1. The emotional responses may be similar to those of other crime victims.

☐ 2. The member is likely to resign after experiencing such an injury.

☐ 3. Legal action against the client will take time and energy.

☐ 4. The member must debrief with the assaultive client before returning.

The Client with Family Abuse or Violence

39. A married female client has been referred to the mental health center because she is depressed. The nurse notices bruises on her upper arms and asks about them. After denying any problems, the client starts to cry and says, "He didn't really mean to hurt me, but I hate for the kids to see this. I'm so worried about them." Which of the following is the most crucial information for the nurse to determine?

☐ 1. The type and extent of abuse occurring in the family.

☐ 2. The potential of immediate danger to the client and her children.

☐ 3. The resources available to the client.

☐ 4. Whether the client wants to be separated from her husband.

40. A client with suspected abuse describes her husband as a good man who works hard and provides well for his family. She does not work outside the home and states that she is proud to be a wife and mother just like her own mother. The nurse interprets the family pattern described by the client as best illustrating which of the following as characteristic of abusive families?

☐ 1. Tight, impermeable boundaries.

☐ 2. Unbalanced power ratio.

☐ 3. Role stereotyping.

☐ 4. Dysfunctional feeling tone.

41. When planning the care for a client who is being abused, which of the following measures is most important to include?

☐ 1. Being compassionate and empathetic.

☐ 2. Teaching the client about abuse and the cycle of violence.

☐ 3. Explaining to the client her personal and legal rights.

☐ 4. Helping the client develop a safety plan.

42. A nurse is assessing a client who is being abused. The nurse should assess the client for which characteristic? Select all that apply.

☐ 1. Assertiveness.

☐ 2. Self-blame.

☐ 3. Alcohol abuse.

☐ 4. Suicidal thoughts.

☐ 5. Guilt.

43. The father of a U.S. Marine who was killed 2 days ago in Iraq is admitted after a serious suicide attempt. He is medically stable and has signed a no harm contract. During a talk with the nurse, he says, "Terrorism and war are holding me and the whole world hostage. It's so unfair. I'd rather be dead than live alone in constant fear." Which of the following nursing interventions is the most crucial in the next few days? Select all that apply.

☐ 1. Discussing effective ways to express justifiable anger.

☐ 2. Teaching stress management and relaxation techniques.

☐ 3. Identifying community groups for relatives of military personnel.

☐ 4. Recommending an antiwar advocacy group.

☐ 5. Strategizing about ways to increase a personal sense of security.

44. During the third session with the nurse, a client who is being abused states, "I don't know what to do anymore. He doesn't want me to go anywhere while he's at work, not even to visit my friends." Which nursing diagnosis should the nurse formulate regarding this information?

☐ 1. *Risk for other-directed violence* related to an abusive husband, as evidenced by the victim's statement of being battered.

☐ 2. *Situational low self-esteem* related to victimization, as evidenced by not being able to leave the house.

☐ 3. *Powerlessness* related to an abusive husband, as evidenced by the inability to make decisions.

☐ 4. *Ineffective coping* related to victimization, as evidenced by crying.

45. After months of counseling, a client abused by her husband tells the nurse that she has decided to stop treatment. There has been no abuse during this time, and she feels better able to cope with the needs of her husband and children. In discussing this decision with the client, it is most important for the nurse to do which of the following?

☐ 1. Tell the client that this is a bad decision that she will regret in the future.

☐ 2. Find out more about the client's rationale for her decision to stop treatment.

☐ 3. Warn the client that abuse commonly stops when one partner is in treatment, only to begin again later.

☐ 4. Remind the client of her duty to protect her children by continuing treatment.

46. A third-grade child is referred to the mental health clinic by the school nurse because he is fearful, anxious, and socially isolated. After meeting with the client, the nurse talks with his mother, who says, "It's that school nurse again. She's done nothing but try to make trouble for our family since my son started school. And now you're in on it." Which of the following responses by the nurse is most helpful in developing a relationship with this family?

☐ 1. "The school nurse is concerned about your son and is only doing her job."

☐ 2. "We see a number of children who go to your son's school. He isn't the only one."

☐ 3. "You sound pretty angry with the school nurse. Tell me what has happened."

☐ 4. "Let me tell you why your son was referred, and then you can tell me about your concerns."

47. The mother of a school-aged child tells the school nurse that for most of the past year her husband was unemployed and she worked a second job to help. Twice during the year, she slapped her son repeatedly when he refused to obey. She says it has not happened again and that the family is "back to normal." After assessing the family, the nurse decides that the child is no longer at risk for abuse. Which of the following observations best supports such a decision?

☐ 1. The parents have a caring and supportive relationship.

☐ 2. The child has not talked about violence during his visits to the nurse.

☐ 3. The infrequent episodes were limited to a time of intense family stress.

☐ 4. The parents have a defensive attitude toward the school nurse.

48. When assessing a client who was the victim of a crime, the nurse understands that crimes, whether they cause physical injury or not, involve a sense of emotional violation and a loss of trust in others. Which of the following should the nurse identify as another developmental stage that is typically affected by crime?

☐ 1. Autonomy versus shame and doubt.

☐ 2. Identity versus role diffusion.

☐ 3. Generativity versus stagnation.

☐ 4. Integrity versus despair.

49. When caring for a client who was a victim of a crime, the nurse is aware that recovery from any crime can be a long and difficult process depending on the meaning it has for the client. Which of the following should the nurse identify as a victim's ultimate goal in reconstructing his or her life?

☐ 1. Getting through the shock and confusion.

☐ 2. Carrying out home and work routines.

☐ 3. Resolving grief over any losses.

☐ 4. Regaining a sense of security and safety.

50. A client tells the nurse that she has been raped but has not reported it to the police. After determining whether the client was injured, whether it is still possible to collect evidence, and whether to file a report, the nurse's next priority is to offer which of the following to the client?

☐ **1.** Legal assistance.
☐ **2.** Crisis intervention.
☐ **3.** A rape support group.
☐ **4.** Medication for disturbed sleep.

51. In working with a rape victim, which of the following is most important?

☐ **1.** Continuing to encourage the client to report the rape to the legal authorities.
☐ **2.** Recommending that the client resume sexual relations with her partner as soon as possible.
☐ **3.** Periodically reminding the client that she did not deserve and did not cause the rape.
☐ **4.** Telling the client that the rapist will eventually be caught, put on trial, and jailed.

52. In the process of dealing with the intense feelings about being raped, victims commonly verbalize that they were afraid they would be killed during the rape and wish that they had been. The nurse should decide that further counseling is needed if the client voices which of the following?

☐ **1.** "I didn't fight him, but I guess I did the right thing because I'm alive."
☐ **2.** "Suicide would be an easy escape from all this pain, but I couldn't do it to myself."
☐ **3.** "I wish they gave the death penalty to all rapists and other sexual predators."
☐ **4.** "I get so angry at times that I have to have a couple of drinks before I sleep."

53. One of the myths about sexual abuse of young children is that it usually involves physically violent acts. Which of the following behaviors is more likely to be used by the abusers?

☐ **1.** Tying the child down.
☐ **2.** Bribery with money.
☐ **3.** Coercion as a result of the trusting relationship.
☐ **4.** Asking for the child's consent for sex.

54. A preadolescent child is suspected of being sexually abused because he demonstrates the self-destructive behaviors of self-mutilation and attempted suicide. Which common behavior should the nurse also expect to assess?

☐ **1.** Inability to play.
☐ **2.** Truancy and running away.
☐ **3.** Head banging.
☐ **4.** Overcontrol of anger.

55. Adolescents and adults who were sexually abused as children commonly mutilate themselves. The nurse interprets this behavior as which of the following?

☐ **1.** The need to make themselves less sexually attractive.
☐ **2.** An alternative to bingeing and purging.
☐ **3.** Use of physical pain to avoid dealing with emotional pain.
☐ **4.** An alternative to getting high on drugs.

56. A young child who has been sexually abused has difficulty putting feelings into words. Which of the following should the nurse employ with the child?

☐ **1.** Engaging in play therapy.
☐ **2.** Role-playing.
☐ **3.** Giving the child's drawings to the abuser.
☐ **4.** Reporting the abuse to a prosecutor.

57. When working with a group of adult survivors of childhood sexual abuse, dealing with anger and rage is a major focus. Which strategy should the nurse expect to be successful? Select all that apply.

☐ **1.** Directly confronting the abuser.
☐ **2.** Using a foam bat while symbolically confronting the abuser.
☐ **3.** Keeping a journal of memories and feelings.
☐ **4.** Writing letters to the abusers that are not sent.
☐ **5.** Writing letters to the adults who did not protect them that are not sent.

58. After a client reveals a history of childhood sexual abuse, the nurse needs to immediately ask which of the following questions?

☐ **1.** "What other forms of abuse did you experience?"
☐ **2.** "How long did the abuse go on?"
☐ **3.** "Was there a time when you did not remember the abuse?"
☐ **4.** "Does your abuser still have contact with young children?"

59. A client with a history of self-mutilation and substance abuse begins talking about memories of torture and ritual abuse that ended 15 years ago. She describes that her parents locked her in a closet whenever they were gone, starved and beat her, sexually abused her and mutilated her genitals, and gave her drugs to keep her sedated. To her knowledge, no others were or are being abused by the parents. Which of the following is most crucial for recovery from such torture and abuse? Select all that apply.

☐ **1.** Dealing with ambivalent feelings toward her parents.
☐ **2.** Planning a confrontation with her parents.
☐ **3.** Determining alternatives to self-destructive behaviors.
☐ **4.** Filing criminal charges against her parents.
☐ **5.** Developing safe ways to deal with her rage and guilt.

60. A client who was sexually abused as a child decides to stop participating in counseling. The nurse will evaluate this as appropriate if the client states which of the following?

☐ 1. "It is all out in the open now, and I can be done with it."
☐ 2. "It is too hard to deal with all this pain all the time."
☐ 3. "I'm functioning okay now, but I know problems will come up again."
☐ 4. "Everyone tells me how much better I'm doing and I believe them."

61. A woman who was raped in her home was brought to the emergency department by her husband. After being interviewed by the police, the husband talks to the nurse. "I don't know why she didn't keep the doors locked like I told her. I can't believe she has had sex with another man now." What is the most appropriate response by the nurse?

☐ 1. "Let's talk about how you feel. Maybe it would help to talk to other men who have been through this."
☐ 2. "Maybe the doors were locked, but the man broke in anyway."
☐ 3. "Your wife needs your support right now, not your criticism."
☐ 4. "It was not consensual sex. Let's see if your wife was physically injured."

62. A young woman has been stalked and then beaten by an ex-boyfriend. Treatment of her injuries is complete and she is ready for discharge. What is a crucial step before discharge to ensure the woman's safety and security? Select all that apply.

☐ 1. Determine the current location of the ex-boyfriend.
☐ 2. Ask if she plans to see the ex-boyfriend again.
☐ 3. Give the information on resources and a safety plan.
☐ 4. Ensure that she has a safe place to stay after discharge.
☐ 5. Obtain consent to send her emergency department records to her family physician.

63. A young man makes an appointment to see the psychiatric nurse at the Employee Assistance Program of a large corporation. He complains that his female boss is making him very uncomfortable. He reports that she wants to date him, sends him provocative e-mails, and makes seductive remarks on his voice mail at home. The nurse informs him about Occupational Safety and Health Association services and Corporate Workplace Violence Guidelines. He agrees to work with Corporate Security on the issue. What should the nurse do next?

☐ 1. Refer the client to his boss's supervisor to file a report.
☐ 2. Suggest the client contact Human Resources to request a job transfer.
☐ 3. Ask the client about his reactions to this situation.
☐ 4. Report the incident to the client's coworkers who are at risk for similar harassment.

64. A 75-year-old woman was brought to the crisis center by her husband. The husband reports that his wife has been in shock and anxious since her purse was stolen outside of their home. The woman blames herself for being robbed, is worried about her stolen wallet and credit cards, and is afraid to go home. What intervention is appropriate at this time? Select all that apply.

☐ 1. Request an order for lorazepam (Ativan) to decrease her anxiety.
☐ 2. Encourage her to talk about the robbery and her feelings.
☐ 3. Discuss what changes at home would help her feel safe.
☐ 4. Investigate if she has physical injuries from the robbery.
☐ 5. Ask her what she thinks she could have done to prevent the robbery.

65. A 35-year-old has been killed as a result of a terrorist attack. What should the nurse advise the friends and relatives of the victim to do during the early stages of the recovery process? Select all that apply.

☐ 1. Keep in contact with other family and friends.
☐ 2. Attend memorial or religious services.
☐ 3. Use relaxation techniques and physical activities.
☐ 4. Speak out publicly about the impact of the loss.
☐ 5. Attend community meetings with others who have lost loved ones.

The Client with Anorexia Nervosa

66. A hospitalized adolescent diagnosed with anorexia nervosa refuses to comply with her daily before-breakfast weigh-in. She states that she just drank a glass of water, which she feels will unfairly increase her weight. What is the nurse's best response to the client?

☐ 1. "You are here to gain weight so that will work in your favor."
☐ 2. "Don't drink or eat for two hours and then I'll weigh you."
☐ 3. "You must weigh in every day at this time. Please step on the scale."
☐ 4. "If you don't get on the scale, I will be forced to call your doctor."

67. The nurse discovers that an adolescent client with anorexia nervosa is taking diet pills rather than complying with the diet. What should the nurse do first?

☐ 1. Explain to the client how diet pills can jeopardize health.
☐ 2. Listen to the client about fears of losing control of eating while being treated.
☐ 3. Talk with the client about how weight loss and emaciation worry the health care providers.
☐ 4. Inquire about the client's family's worries concerning the client's physical and emotional health.

68. When teaching a group of adolescents about anorexia nervosa, the nurse should describe this disorder as being characterized by which of the following?

☐ 1. Excessive fear of becoming obese, near-normal weight, and a self-critical body image.

☐ 2. Obsession with the weight of others, chronic dieting, and an altered body image.

☐ 3. Extreme concern about dieting, calorie-counting, and an unrealistic body image.

☐ 4. Intense fear of becoming obese, emaciation, and a disturbed body image.

69. When developing a teaching plan for a high school health class about anorexia nervosa, which of the following should the nurse include as the primary group affected by this disease?

☐ 1. Women, age at onset between 12 and 20 years.

☐ 2. Men, onset during the college years.

☐ 3. Women, onset typically after 30 years.

☐ 4. Men, onset after 20 years.

70. When assessing a client with anorexia nervosa, the nurse should expect to find which of the following?

☐ 1. Hyperthermia, oliguria, and bradycardia.

☐ 2. Lanugo, hypothermia, and hypotension.

☐ 3. Constipation, dysmenorrhea, and hypertension.

☐ 4. Diarrhea, dry skin, and menorrhagia.

71. The parents of a newly diagnosed 15-year-old with anorexia nervosa are meeting with the nurse during the admission process. Which of the following remarks by the parents should the nurse interpret as typical for a client with anorexia nervosa?

☐ 1. "We've given her everything and look how she repays us!"

☐ 2. "She's had behavior problems for the past year both at home and at school."

☐ 3. "She's been a model child. We've never had any problems with her."

☐ 4. "We have five children, all normal kids with some problems at times."

72. Which of the following nursing diagnoses should the nurse formulate as the priority for a client who is admitted to the mental health unit with a diagnosis of anorexia nervosa and who is 5 feet 4 inches tall and weighs only 82 lb?

☐ 1. *Situational low self-esteem* related to feelings of inadequacy and loss of control.

☐ 2. *Disturbed body image* related to self-view of being overweight.

☐ 3. *Interrupted family processes* related to overprotectiveness and avoidance of conflict.

☐ 4. *Imbalanced nutrition: Less than body requirements* related to severe restriction of intake.

The Client with Bulimia

73. A young adult female client and her roommate go the emergency department due to gastrointestinal problems. The client reveals that she attends college and works at a coffee shop each evening. A diet history indicates that the client has unhealthy eating habits, commonly eating large amounts of carbohydrates and junk food with few fruits and vegetables. "Her stomach is upset a lot," the roommate says. She further reports that the client is "in the bathroom all the time." Which of the following should the nurse refer the client to?

☐ 1. A mental health clinic and physician.

☐ 2. A weight loss program.

☐ 3. An overeating support group.

☐ 4. The client's family physician.

74. A nurse is working with a client with bulimia. What is a goal of nursing care? Select all that apply.

☐ 1. The client will maintain normal weight.

☐ 2. The client will comply with medication therapy.

☐ 3. The client will achieve a positive self-concept.

☐ 4. The client will acknowledge the disorder.

☐ 5. The client will never have the desire to purge again.

75. A nurse works with a client diagnosed with bulimia. What is an appropriate long-term client goal for this client?

☐ 1. Eating meals at home without bingeing or purging.

☐ 2. Being able to eat out without bingeing or purging.

☐ 3. Managing stresses in life without bingeing or purging.

☐ 4. Being able to attend college in another state without bingeing or purging.

76. While coaching a youth soccer team, the nurse has observed one of the teammates bingeing and purging on multiple occasions. The nurse asks the girl's mother to stay after practice and talk privately. Which of the following ways is best for the nurse to begin the conversation?

☐ 1. "Thank you for letting your daughter play on the team. She's a very good player and is also pleasant and easy to coach."

☐ 2. "I have some very bad news for you. Your daughter has a serious problem that is diagnosed as an eating disorder."

☐ 3. "I am a nurse. I have seen your daughter doing things that are considered to be part of an eating disorder."

☐ 4. "Let me get right to the point. Your daughter is very sick and needs to see a mental health therapist right away."

77. A client newly diagnosed with bulimia is attending the nurse-led group at the mental health center. She tells the group that she came only because her husband said he would divorce her if she didn't get help. Which of the following responses by the nurse is most appropriate?

- ☐ **1.** "You sound angry with your husband. Is that correct?"
- ☐ **2.** "You will find that you like coming to group. These people are a lot of fun."
- ☐ **3.** "Tell me more about why you are here and how you feel about that."
- ☐ **4.** "Tell me something about what has caused you to be bulimic."

78. A client diagnosed with bulimia tells the nurse that she only eats excessively when she is upset with her best friend and then vomits so she won't gain a lot of weight. Which of the following nursing diagnoses is most appropriate for this client?

- ☐ **1.** *Disabled family coping.*
- ☐ **2.** *Ineffective coping.*
- ☐ **3.** *Imbalanced nutrition: More than body requirements.*
- ☐ **4.** *Anxiety.*

79. During the initial interview, a client with a compulsive eating disorder remarks, "I can't stand myself and the way I look." Which of the following statements by the nurse is most therapeutic?

- ☐ **1.** "Everyone who has the same problem feels like you do."
- ☐ **2.** "I don't think you look bad at all."
- ☐ **3.** "Don't worry, you'll soon be back in shape."
- ☐ **4.** "Tell me more about your feelings."

80. When discussing eating disorders with a group of adolescents, the nurse incorporates information that persons living within the culture of the United States commonly experience difficulty with weight control because they unconsciously equate food with which of the following?

- ☐ **1.** Love and affection.
- ☐ **2.** Power and control.
- ☐ **3.** Status and prestige.
- ☐ **4.** Survival and growth.

Children and Adolescents with Behavior Problems

81. The school nurse assesses a 10-year-old girl who excessively cleans and categorizes. Her parents report that she has always been orderly, but since her brother died of cancer 6 months ago, her cleaning and categorizing have escalated. In school, she reads instead of playing with other children. These behaviors are now interfering with homework and leisure activities. To bolster her self-esteem, what should the nurse encourage the child to do?

- ☐ **1.** Be a library helper.
- ☐ **2.** Organize a party for the class.
- ☐ **3.** Be in charge of a group project with four peers.
- ☐ **4.** Be captain of the kickball team.

82. A 13-year-old junior high school student has come to the school nurse, stating that her father has physically abused her for 3 years. Initially, she accepted it, thinking it was because he had been laid off, but the abuse continued after he got a job 4 months ago. She fears that her mother will not believe her and her father will reject her if they discover she has revealed the abuse. What is the nurse's best initial action?

- ☐ **1.** Inform the mother in a face-to-face meeting without the girl present.
- ☐ **2.** Call the father, confront him, and then call the police to have him arrested.
- ☐ **3.** Meet with both parents together. Include the daughter in the meeting so she can speak for herself.
- ☐ **4.** Report the alleged abuse to Child Protective Services that day, and then provide for the child's safety.

83. A 15-year-old is a heavy user of marijuana and alcohol. When the nurse confronts the client about his drug and alcohol use, he admits previous heavy use in order to feel more comfortable around peers and achieve social acceptance. He says he has been trying to stay clean since his parents found out and had him seek treatment. When the nurse develops a plan of care with the client, what should be the highest priority to help him maintain sobriety?

- ☐ **1.** Peer recognition that does not involve substance use.
- ☐ **2.** Support and guidance from his parents.
- ☐ **3.** A strict no-drug policy at his high school.
- ☐ **4.** The threat of legal charges if caught drinking or smoking marijuana.

84. A 17-year-old is admitted to a psychiatric day treatment program due to severe lower back pain since her mother's death 3 years ago. Medical examinations have not discovered a physical cause for her pain. She cares for her four younger siblings after school and on weekends because of her father's long work hours. Which predischarge statement indicates that treatment for her condition has been successful?
- ☐ 1. "I understand now why my father spends so much time away from home."
- ☐ 2. "My back pain is worse on weekends with more chores and homework."
- ☐ 3. "I don't want to talk about my family. It's my back that is hurting."
- ☐ 4. "I just need more rest and relaxation and then my back will feel fine."

85. A 2-year-old child is brought into the physician's office by her parents who are concerned by her behavior. They state that she resists their affection, self-stimulates, and does not respond to other children and adults. Based on the analysis of these behaviors, which of the following should the nurse suspect?
- ☐ 1. Tourette syndrome.
- ☐ 2. Schizophrenia.
- ☐ 3. Attention deficit hyperactivity disorder.
- ☐ 4. Autism.

86. When developing the plan of care for a child diagnosed with attention deficit hyperactivity disorder (ADHD), the nurse would expect to include treatment most commonly with a combination of which of the following?
- ☐ 1. Antianxiety medications, such as buspirone (BuSpar), and home schooling.
- ☐ 2. Antidepressant medications, such as imipramine (Tofranil), and family therapy.
- ☐ 3. Anticonvulsant medications, such as carbamazepine (Tegretol), and monthly blood levels.
- ☐ 4. Psychostimulant medications, such as methylphenidate (Ritalin), and behavior modification.

87. The mental health nurse meets with the mother of a child diagnosed with attention deficit hyperactivity disorder. The mother states, "I feel so guilty that he has this disease, like I did something wrong. I feel like I need to be with him constantly in order for him to get better. But still sometimes I feel like I'm going to lose control and hurt him." Which of the following is most appropriate to suggest to the mother?
- ☐ 1. Arranging for respite care to watch her child and give herself a regular break.
- ☐ 2. Taking a job to allow herself to feel some success because her child won't ever improve.
- ☐ 3. Arranging to have coffee with friends daily as a way to begin a support group.
- ☐ 4. Considering foster care if she feels that she can't handle her child's problems.

88. The nurse is with the parents of a 16-year-old boy who recently attempted suicide. The nurse cautions the parents to be especially alert for which of the following in their son?
- ☐ 1. Expression of a desire to date.
- ☐ 2. Decision to try out for an extracurricular activity.
- ☐ 3. Giving away valued personal items.
- ☐ 4. Desire to spend more time with friends.

89. The parents of a 15-year-old girl bring their daughter for admission to the mental health center. She was recently expelled from school for repeated behavior problems and truancy. She was also arrested for vandalism and prostitution in the past week. Based on an analysis of these findings, the nurse should suspect which of the following as the most likely medical diagnosis?
- ☐ 1. Attention deficit hyperactivity disorder.
- ☐ 2. Conduct disorder.
- ☐ 3. Oppositional defiant disorder.
- ☐ 4. Tourette syndrome.

90. The nurse at the mental health clinic is meeting a new client who is a 7-year-old boy with Tourette syndrome. Which of the following should the nurse expect to assess?
- ☐ 1. Multiple motor and verbal tics.
- ☐ 2. Primarily motor tics.
- ☐ 3. Isolated verbal tics.
- ☐ 4. Alternating simple and complex motor tics.

91. When comparing the signs and symptoms of depression found in children with those found in adults, which of the following should the nurse expect?
- ☐ 1. Adults commonly display sad behaviors, while children have more somatic complaints and possible acting-out behaviors.
- ☐ 2. Adults have more problems performing in the work setting than children have in performing in the school setting.
- ☐ 3. Adults typically will not be able to function at work and at home but children continue to succeed in school activities while depressed.
- ☐ 4. Adults usually have few major problems functioning with depression, while children usually cannot function at school or with tasks at home.

92. Assessment of suicidal risk in children and adolescents requires the nurse to know which of the following?
- [ ] **1.** Children rarely commit suicide unless one of their parents has already committed suicide, especially in the past year.
- [ ] **2.** The risk of suicide increases during adolescence, with those who have recently suffered a loss, abuse, or family discord being most at risk.
- [ ] **3.** Children do have a suicidal risk that coincides with some significant event such as a recent gun purchase in the family.
- [ ] **4.** Adolescents typically don't choose suicide unless they live in certain geographical regions of the United States, including the western states.

93. When counseling a 5-year-old girl who recently suffered the loss of her mother, the nurse understands that which of the following statements reflects the typical understanding about death at this age?
- [ ] **1.** "My mommy died last week, but I'm going to see her again."
- [ ] **2.** "My daddy said mommy went to heaven and I'm glad Jesus took her there."
- [ ] **3.** "My dog died and now we got another one."
- [ ] **4.** "I think Mommy went to heaven and I'll get to see her someday when I die."

94. A child with Asperger's disorder is being referred to the mental health clinic along with his parents. To provide the best care for this family, the nurse remembers that this disorder differs from autism in which of the following areas?
- [ ] **1.** Asperger's disorder, commonly diagnosed earlier than autism, is associated with fewer major problems in interpersonal interactions.
- [ ] **2.** In Asperger's disorder, behavior commonly is similar to that of other children with autism but without the problems with school.
- [ ] **3.** Asperger's disorder is recognized later than autism, and interpersonal interaction problems typically become more apparent when the child begins school.
- [ ] **4.** There are significant problems with language development, as with autism, but there are no delays or difficulties with motor development.

95. A staff nurse on the mental health unit tells the nurse manager that kids with conduct disorders might as well be jailed because they all end up as adults with antisocial personality disorder anyway. What is the best reply by the nurse manager?
- [ ] **1.** "You really sound burned out. Do you have a vacation coming up soon?"
- [ ] **2.** "These children are more likely to have problems with depression and anxiety disorder as adults."
- [ ] **3.** "You sound really frustrated. Let's talk about the meaning of their behavior."
- [ ] **4.** "My experience hasn't been that negative. Let's see what the other staff members think; maybe I'm wrong."

96. The mother of a 14-year-old girl who is diagnosed with oppositional defiant disorder tells the nurse that she has read extensively on this disorder and does not believe the diagnosis is correct for her daughter. Which of the following responses by the nurse is most appropriate?
- [ ] **1.** "It sounds like you are very interested in your daughter. Let's focus on what is best for her."
- [ ] **2.** "Tell me what you have found in your reading that is leading you to that conclusion."
- [ ] **3.** "Your doctor has had many years of education and experience so you can believe he's right."
- [ ] **4.** "That doesn't matter now because we just need to help her get better."

97. A 12-year-old girl has been diagnosed with oppositional defiant disorder. She is observed by the nurse on the unit kissing two of the male clients. Given the client's developmental level and diagnosis, the nurse decides to intervene with the client in which of the following ways? Select all that apply.
- [ ] **1.** Discussing with the client when and where it is acceptable to kiss boys.
- [ ] **2.** Reinforcing that kissing and touching other clients is not allowed.
- [ ] **3.** Telling the client that her behavior will be reported to her psychiatrist.
- [ ] **4.** Restricting the client to her room to work on an assignment about anger.
- [ ] **5.** Showing the client a video about human reproduction.

98. At the admission interview, the father of a 4-year-old boy with attention deficit hyperactivity disorder (ADHD) says to the mental health nurse, "I know that my wife or I must have caused this disease." Which of the following is the nurse's best response?

☐ 1. "ADHD is more common within families, but there is no evidence that problems with parenting cause this disorder."

☐ 2. "What do you think you might have done that could have led to causing this disorder to develop in your son?"

☐ 3. "Many parents feel this way, but I doubt there is anything that you did that caused ADHD to develop in your child."

☐ 4. "Let's not focus on the cause but rather on what needs to be done to help your son get better. I know that you and your wife are very interested in helping him to improve his behavior."

99. A member of a nurse-led group for depressed adolescents tells the group that she is not coming back because she is taking medication and no longer needs to talk about her problems. Which of the following responses by the nurse is most appropriate?

☐ 1. "I'm glad that you are taking your medication, but how can we know that you will continue to take it? After all, you haven't been on it for very long and you might decide to stop taking it."

☐ 2. "I think that it is important to let everyone respond to what you said, so let's go around the group and let everyone give their thoughts about what you have decided."

☐ 3. "The purpose of the group is to provide each of you with a place to discuss the problems of being a teenager with depression with others who also are experiencing a similar situation."

☐ 4. "You don't have to stay in the group if you don't want to, but if you choose to leave, then you won't be able to change your mind later and return to the group."

100. When assessing a 17-year-old male client with depression for suicide risk, which of the following questions is best?

☐ 1. "What movies about death have you watched lately?"

☐ 2. "Can you tell me what you think about suicide?"

☐ 3. "Has anyone in your family ever committed suicide?"

☐ 4. "Are you thinking about killing yourself?"

101. A teacher is talking to the school nurse about a child in her classroom who has a tic disorder. She mentions that the boy frequently trips other children although no one has ever been hurt. She further states that she ignores him when that happens because it is part of his disorder. Which of the following is the best response by the nurse?

☐ 1. "Tripping other children is not a tic, so you can respond to that as you would in any other child."

☐ 2. "I can't believe that you actually allow him to get away with that!"

☐ 3. "I think that is the best choice unless some parents of the other children start to complain about it."

☐ 4. "If no one else is getting hurt then it seems harmless and might prevent the development of a worse behavior."

102. Which of the following medications should the nurse anticipate administering as a treatment for tic disorders, including Tourette disorder?

☐ 1. Chlorpromazine (Thorazine).

☐ 2. Imipramine (Tofranil).

☐ 3. Lithium.

☐ 4. Clonidine (Catapres).

103. The nurse leading a group for parents of children diagnosed with oppositional defiant disorder plans on including which of the following recommendations for discipline?

☐ 1. Avoid limiting the child's use of the television and computer for punishment.

☐ 2. Be consistent with discipline while assisting with ways for the child to more positively express anger and frustration.

☐ 3. Use primarily positive reinforcement for good behavior while ignoring any demonstrated bad behavior.

☐ 4. Use time-out as the primary means of punishment for the child regardless of what the child has done.

104. Which of the following children should the nurse identify as being more at risk for an episode of major depression?

☐ 1. Michael, a 16-year-old, who has been struggling in school, making only Cs and Ds.

☐ 2. Lauren, a 13-year-old, who was upset over not being chosen as a cheerleader.

☐ 3. Cody, a 10-year-old, who has never liked school and basically has few friends.

☐ 4. Gretchen, a 14-year-old, who recently moved to a new school after her parents' divorce.

105. A 15-year-old girl is sent to the school nurse with complaints of dizziness and nausea. While assessing the girl, who denies any health problems, the nurse smells alcohol on her breath. Which of the following responses by the nurse is most appropriate?
- ☐ 1. "Don't tell me that you have been drinking alcohol before you came to school this morning!"
- ☐ 2. "Why don't you tell me the real reason that you are feeling sick this morning?"
- ☐ 3. "Tell me everything that you have had to eat and drink yesterday and today."
- ☐ 4. "I know that high school is stressful, but drinking alcohol is not the best way to handle it."

106. Parents of a 7-year-old child newly diagnosed with attention deficit hyperactivity disorder (ADHD) ask the nurse whether their son will always have to take medication for this condition. Which of the following responses is most appropriate?
- ☐ 1. "Yes, almost everyone with this disorder has to continue taking medication forever."
- ☐ 2. "Up to 50% of individuals need to continue to take medications as adults."
- ☐ 3. "Most people with this disorder do not need to continue taking medications as adults."
- ☐ 4. "There is just a small percentage of adults with ADHD who can manage without medications."

107. A 9-year-old client with attention deficit hyperactivity disorder tells the nurse, "No one in my class likes me because they think I'm stupid. They're right, I am stupid!" The nurse identifies which of the following nursing diagnoses as relevant for this client?
- ☐ 1. *Situational low self-esteem* related to client's perception of how other's view him.
- ☐ 2. *Ineffective coping* related to an inability to be objective about peers.
- ☐ 3. *Interrupted family processes (disabling)* related to the family's difficulty in coping with the child.
- ☐ 4. *Anxiety* related to dislike of the client by his peers.

108. Which of the following should the nurse expect to include in the teaching plan for the parents of a child who is receiving methylphenidate (Ritalin)?
- ☐ 1. Giving the medication at the same time every evening.
- ☐ 2. Having the child take two doses at the same time if the last dose was missed.
- ☐ 3. Giving the single-dose form of the medication early in the day.
- ☐ 4. Allowing concurrent use of any over-the-counter medications with this drug.

109. A 6-year-old female is brought to the school nurse for refusal to sit in class. She denies feeling sick but insists that her mother be called so she can go home. She is pacing and chewing on a fingernail. This has occurred daily since school began 4 weeks ago. She tells the nurse that she is afraid something bad is going to happen to her mother. Which of the following should the nurse suspect?
- ☐ 1. Obsessive-compulsive disorder.
- ☐ 2. Major depression.
- ☐ 3. Attention deficit hyperactivity disorder.
- ☐ 4. Separation anxiety disorder.

110. A 7-year-old client is diagnosed with conduct disorder. After admission, the nurse identifies his problematic behaviors as cruelty to animals, stealing, truancy, aggression with peers, lying, and explosive angry outbursts resulting in destruction of property. The nurse is now talking with the client about his behavioral contract, which should include which crucial components? Select all that apply.
- ☐ 1. Taking prescribed medications.
- ☐ 2. Acceptable methods for expressing anger.
- ☐ 3. Consequences for unacceptable behaviors.
- ☐ 4. Rules for interacting with staff and other clients.
- ☐ 5. Personal possessions allowed on the unit.

111. Which of the following children should the nurse assess as demonstrating behaviors that need further evaluation?
- ☐ 1. Joey, age 2, who refuses to be toilet-trained and talks to himself.
- ☐ 2. Adrienne, age 6, who sucks her thumb when tired and has never spent the night with a friend.
- ☐ 3. Curt, age 10, who frequently tells his mother that he is going to run away whenever they argue.
- ☐ 4. Stephen, age 2, who is indifferent to other children and adults and is mute.

The Child or Adolescent Who Has Suffered Sexual Abuse

112. A 9-year-old girl reveals to the nurse that her uncle, a young adult who began babysitting her last month, has been touching her "privates" and fondling her breasts. The nurse should intervene based on what fact about perpetrators of sexual abuse? Select all that apply.
- ☐ 1. Perpetrators choose children in order to be in control because of difficulty with equal, same-age sexual relationships.
- ☐ 2. Perpetrators choose children, especially relatives, to introduce them to sex in a gentle manner.
- ☐ 3. Perpetrators tell the child sexual behavior is normal and initially persuade, rather than threaten the child to maintain the "secret."
- ☐ 4. Perpetrators may reverse roles and expect the child they abuse to love and nurture them.
- ☐ 5. Perpetrators are upset about being caught, but readily admit their abuse when confronted.

113. A mother of a 4-year-old preschool child is 6 months pregnant. The 4-year-old is curious about the changes in the mother's body. The child alternately displays anxiety and jealousy, and either acts out or is withdrawn. She asks her mother to quit work. At school, the child does not want to talk to her male preschool teacher or be alone with him. The nurse should counsel the mother that her daughter may be:
- ☐ 1. Having trouble adjusting to the pregnancy and impending birth of a sibling.
- ☐ 2. Demonstrating signs of possible sexual abuse.
- ☐ 3. Responding appropriately to the pregnancy for her developmental age.
- ☐ 4. Demonstrating signs of attention deficit hyperactivity disorder.

114. A 12-year-old boy is admitted due to depression and post-trauma response. Child Protective Services reports that the boy's father is now in jail for molesting him from ages 6 to 9. Given the typical reactions of incest victims, the nurse should expect which behavior? Select all that apply.
- ☐ 1. Sexualized play.
- ☐ 2. Aggression.
- ☐ 3. Isolation at home.
- ☐ 4. Running away.
- ☐ 5. Truancy.

115. A 16-year-old female was raped by an acquaintance. After the emergency department staff examine her and collect evidence, the client says, "I don't want him to do that to anyone else, but I don't know if I want to prosecute him." Which response by the nurse is most appropriate?
- ☐ 1. "As long as we have all the evidence collected, you might as well prosecute."
- ☐ 2. "Prosecuting him is the best way of making sure he doesn't do it again."
- ☐ 3. "Unless you can handle going through a trial, I'd suggest thinking twice about it."
- ☐ 4. "You can make that decision after you talk with our sexual assault advocate."

116. A 19-year-old male calls the psychiatric hotline and says he was raped about 3 months ago by 3 gang members. He reports that he can't sleep because of nightmares about it. He also says, "I'm suspicious of everyone, afraid to go out of my apartment except for work, and I've lost 20 lb." He denies having suicidal or homicidal thoughts. Which response by the nurse is most appropriate?
- ☐ 1. "Come to the hospital to be admitted."
- ☐ 2. "Give yourself a few more months to recover."
- ☐ 3. "I can give you the phone number for a sexual assault advocate."
- ☐ 4. "I think it would help to ask your family physician for a sleeping medicine."

Correct Answers and Rationales

The letter in parentheses after each rationale identifies the client need addressed in the item, including management of care (M), safety and infection control (S), health promotion and maintenance (H), psychosocial adaptation (P), basic care and comfort (C), pharmacological and parenteral therapies (D), reduction of risk potential (R), and physiological adaptation (A).

The Client in Crisis

1. 3. Before any interventions can occur, knowing whether the client is pregnant is crucial in formulating a plan of care. Asking the client about what things she had thought about doing, giving the client some ideas about what to expect next, and questioning the client about her feelings and possible parental reactions would be appropriate after it is determined that the client is pregnant. (P)

2. 2. Because of the client's potential pregnancy, the nurse needs to determine exactly what the client means by the terms "heavy petting and necking" by asking the client to describe what she has been doing in sexual encounters with her boyfriend. Asking the client if she means sexual intercourse or telling the client that they need to talk about sexual intercourse makes an assumption that may or may not be appropriate. The nurse needs to determine exactly what the client means by the terms used. Repeating the client's statement does not elicit the necessary information to interpret the client's statement. Additionally, this type of response assumes an understanding of what the client has said. (P)

3. 4. Because people in an emotional crisis find it difficult to focus their thinking, the goal is to return the client to noncrisis functioning. Pointing out and decreasing the client's level of anxiety is the first step in attaining this goal. Telling an obviously distressed person not to worry is ineffective because it ignores the client's distress and concerns. Although pregnancy is a normal event, and 40 years of age may not be too old for a pregnancy, these responses also ignore the client's distress and feelings. (P)

4. 3. The client's statement indicates that she needs no more help. Therefore, the nurse needs to inform the client that the door is open for her return. Suggesting that the client try pills for a while imposes the nurse's view on the client without allowing the client to make the decision. The statement that the last person who said that ended up with a baby is condescending, ridiculing, and somewhat threatening. Telling the client that she is overconfident is inappropriate because it is condescending and somewhat threatening. (P)

5. 1. Telephoning the crisis shelter indicates that the boys are alarmed but are reluctant to talk with their parents. The boys may fear that their parents will assume that they have been sniffing glue and punish them. The nurse should focus on helping the boys talk with their parents. Although sniffing glue is dangerous and potentially lethal, it is not illegal. To prove that the observations are incorrect requires an intervention beginning with the boys' parents. Sniffing glue is included in the *Diagnostic and Statistical Manual of Mental Disorders,* 4th edition, text revised, as inhalant abuse. It is not a minor form of substance abuse. (P)

6. 1. The crisis worker needs to use active focusing techniques to determine the crisis-precipitating event or the immediate problem. Asking the caller, "Why are you calling today?" or "What is the immediate problem?" will assist the caller to focus on the specific need or event. Telling the client to make an appointment is inappropriate because the problem might be life-threatening. Telling the caller to go to the nearest emergency room is precipitous and may be unnecessary. Asking to speak to someone else in the home may be futile because the caller might be alone. This action also ignores the caller and his or her feelings. (P)

7. 3. The concern that someone may call the crisis hotline every day for a year indicates that further understanding about crisis and crisis intervention is needed. A crisis situation is time-limited, typically resolving in 4 to 6 weeks if handled effectively. If a person calls the line daily for a year, that person has not been properly dealt with or is probably in a highly disorganized state requiring an alternative intervention. The nurse needs to further review and clarify the material presented. Callers are typically in pain, overwhelmed, and exhausted when they call. A crisis can help an individual cope better in the future if he learns to handle the situation. (P)

8. 4. *Risk for self-directed violence* is the priority nursing diagnosis for a client who has attempted or verbalizes the intent to harm herself. Although the client is depressed, feeling hopeless and powerless, and is grieving, these are not the priority concern at this time. (P)

9. 2. Generally, 4 to 6 weeks is viewed as the length of time a client can tolerate the severe level of disturbance of a true crisis. In the first week or two, the client usually is still trying to use normal coping skills and support systems. After 6 weeks of continuous crisis, a client is probably becoming so physically and emotionally drained that he has sought or has been brought by others for medical or psychiatric care. (P)

10. 1. The initial goal in crisis intervention is helping the client regain emotional security and equilibrium. Resolution of the underlying emotional problems, development of insight and personal growth, and formulation of more effective support systems are goals to address as the crisis subsides. (P)

11. 3. Learning new coping skills is the major factor necessary for higher functioning. Better coping is likely to lead to regaining support systems, giving up dysfunctional coping, and awareness of how to prevent future crises. (P)

12. 3. The risk of suicide can persist for 2 to 3 months even after a crisis has abated. Therefore, it is important for the client to be able to verbalize information about appropriate support persons and community resources and to have this information readily available. Although the client may state that she is ready to be discharged, this is not the most reliable indicator. A divorce lawyer may not be appropriate at this point. At 3 days after a suicide attempt, emotional stability is not likely. (P)

13. 4. The statement about joining the son if he dies indicates potential for self-harm and subsequent suicide, always a risk during crisis. Although the father may be charged with reckless driving, this is not an indication for a psychiatric consultation. Although the son's mother may be extremely upset and angry about the event, this statement is more likely an overstatement, not a real risk. The statement about not seeing the son run behind the car illustrates the father's attempts at trying to process the situation. (P)

14. 1. Passive suicidal thoughts, such as a wish to die or giving up on self-care, can be as much of a risk as active suicidal ideation (the idea of killing one's self directly), especially for older clients because they commonly lack the means, energy, and motivation for an active suicide attempt. Seeing the grandson and grandmother together may help later. Not talking to the grandson and experiencing altered role performance may be real issues, but these are not as critical as the risk of indirect (passive) suicide. (P)

15. 2. The threat toward the ex-boyfriend is the most immediate concern now, as the client turns her anger toward him instead of herself. Although *Situational low self-esteem, Risk for suicide,* and *Risk prone health behavior* are accurate, these nursing diagnoses are less of a concern at this time. (P)

16. 3. Letting the client express his feelings (emotion management) is essential before trying to problem solve about the situation or deciding what kind of referral is appropriate. A referral for counseling, assessment of the client's support system, and unemployment assistance may be appropriate after the client's anxiety is reduced. (P)

17. 2. During a crisis, support persons demonstrate preparedness to help the client by verbalizing the emergency resources available and knowing when to use them. Follow-up medical care may be helpful as the crisis subsides. The coping strategies used by the support persons may or may not be relevant to the client's needs and situation. Long-term solutions and advice may or may not be appropriate. The focus needs to be on the client's immediate needs and situation. (P)

18. 1. The nurse needs to focus on the client and address her feelings. Talking about her feelings helps to decrease the risk of self-harm. Doing so takes precedence over questions about the husband's estate, the cause of death, and her children's support. (P)

The Client with Problems Expressing Anger

19. 3. It is unlikely that the physician would imply that the client should be more aggressive. Denial of anger with passive, unassertive behavior and the aggressive expression of anger are dysfunctional behavior patterns. Gender-based stereotypes are not conducive to mental health, and deeming assertive behavior in women as culturally unacceptable interferes with the goal of developing assertiveness skills. Group acceptance should not be based on whether a client is demonstrating assertive or aggressive behavior. (P)

20. 4. Verbalizing feelings, especially feelings of anger, in an appropriate manner is an adaptive method of coping that reduces the chance that the client will act out these feelings toward others. The client's ability to verbalize her feelings indicates a change in behavior, a crucial indicator of goal achievement. Although acknowledging feelings of anger and describing situations that precipitate angry feelings are important in helping the client reach her goal, they are not appropriate indicators that she has changed her behavior. Asking the client to list how she has handled anger in the past is helpful if the nurse discusses coping methods with the client. However, based on this client's history, this would not be helpful because the nurse and client are already aware of the client's aggression toward others. (P)

21. 2. Identifying people with whom the client is angry is less important to the overall plan because this action focuses on other individuals instead of focusing on the client's responsibility for his behavior. Helping the client to recognize anger, identify alternative ways to express anger, and practice the expression of anger are all steps in the process of teaching the client to recognize and respond appropriately to anger. (P)

22. 4. The nurse needs to acknowledge the client's feelings. In doing so, the nurse helps the group accept a new member. Focusing on "everyone" and telling the client not to worry ignores the client's fears. Having the other group members introduce themselves places the focus on the other clients in the group and does not address the client's fears. Implying that getting to know someone will reduce the fear is false reassurance. (P)

23. 3. The nurse must clearly address behavioral expectations, such as telling the client that hitting is unacceptable and also provide alternatives for the client, such as letting staff members know when he begins to feel angry. Making others responsible for the client's behavior or isolating the client in his room is inappropriate because it does not include the client in managing his behavior. Although medication may be helpful, this action does not give the client responsibility for his behavior and is not warranted at this time. (P)

24. 4. The client is in the crisis phase of the assault cycle. Therefore, the nurse must act immediately, using restraints and an intramuscular tranquilizer to prevent injury to others or further property damage. It is too late to ask the client to go to a quiet area to talk because the client's behavior is past the triggering phase. Giving the client an oral tranquilizer and preparing for a show of determination are nursing interventions used in the escalation phase. Processing the incident with the client and discussing alternative behaviors are interventions used in the postcrisis phase. (P)

25. 4. The client is ready to be released from restraints when he shows signs of self-control, decreased anxiety and agitation, reality orientation, mood stabilization, increased attention span, and judgment. Adequate sedation, struggling less against restraints, and not swearing and yelling are not adequate signs of being calm and in control. (P)

26. 3. By requesting that the roommate respect his rights (asking the roommate to put the dirty clothes on the floor away after telling him that this bothers him), the client is asserting himself. Arriving late is commonly passive resistance and thus not an indicator that the client is becoming assertive. Asking the nurse to call is dependent behavior. Although asking the doctor is more assertive, the client is relying on the nurse's direction to do so. (P)

27. 2. Blood pressure, as well as respiratory rate and muscle tension, increase during anger because of the autonomic nervous system response to epinephrine secretion. Peristalsis also decreases. (A)

28. 3. Fear of harm is a common response to anger in clients who lack coping skills and assertiveness. Decreased self-esteem is common because most clients are aware that they have difficulty in responding to anger effectively. Although anger may provide an initial feeling of strength and invulnerability, this is rarely a sustained response. Powerlessness more commonly leads to anger, rather than resulting from it. (P)

29. **4.** When given intramuscularly, haloperidol is considered most restrictive because it is intrusive and a client usually does not receive the drug voluntarily. Oral haloperidol is considered less restrictive because the client usually accepts the pill voluntarily. Tension reduction strategies and voluntary seclusion are considered less restrictive because they are not intrusive and the client usually consents to their use. (P)

30. **2.** Asking the staff for assistance is appropriate when the client demonstrates behaviors that involve the direct threat of violence. Holding a stick and telling the nurse to move is the most direct threat of violence. Swearing and pounding on a table may be disturbing, but these actions are less of a threat. Coming out of his room may indicate noncompliance with directions. However, further assessment is needed to determine whether this behavior was a direct threat of violence. (P)

31. **1.** An orally administered drug is considered less restrictive than one administered intramuscularly. Lorazepam, a benzodiazepine, is administered for its antianxiety and sedative properties. Benztropine is an antiextrapyramidal side effects medication. Haloperidol and fluphenazine decanoate are antipsychotic agents and would not be administered because the client is not psychotic. (D)

32. **3.** The client who is about to lose control is experiencing a high degree of anxiety or agitation, which alters the client's ability to perceive reality. Initially, the client may feel threatened by the presence of others. A client who is out of control is not thinking about having an audience. Although the nurse with the client who is about to lose control is generally the one giving directions, this is not a rationale for staying at a distance. When seeing extra staff, the client may or may not be able to gain self-control. (P)

33. **4.** The primary goal of aggression management is to prevent violence. This goal is evidenced by a reduction in the total number of restraint procedures used or needed. Although fewer client and staff injuries are important, these goals are secondary to prevention. Reduction in the number of complaints by clients' relatives is affected by more variables than just restraint procedures. (P)

34. **1.** When using seclusion, the safety of the client is paramount. Therefore, staff must be able to see the client in seclusion at all times, such as through a security window in the door or with a room camera. Although outside access for dimming the lights to decrease stimuli may be appropriate, it is not critical for the client's safety. Having one staff member stay in a room alone with a potentially violent client is unsafe. A doctor's order for seclusion can be obtained before or after it is initiated. (P)

35. **3.** A full-length restraint blanket is added when the client is at risk for injury from fighting the restraints. The increased degree of restriction is justified only when the risk of client injury increases. Feeling more secure is not a sufficient cause for using a more restrictive measure. Client complaints that restraints are tight and uncomfortable require the nurse to assess the situation and adjust the restraints if necessary to ensure adequate circulation. Four-way restraints already provide adequate protection for the staff. (P)

36. **1.** Safety of the client and staff is the utmost priority. Therefore, the client must be monitored closely and frequently, such as every 15 minutes, to ensure that the client is safe and free from injury. Assisting with nutrition and elimination, performing range-of-motion exercises on each limb, and changing the client's position every 2 hours are important after the safety of the client and staff is ensured by close, frequent monitoring. (P)

37. **4.** The long-term goal of the debriefing after restraining a client is to improve aggression management procedures so that prevention of aggression improves and the frequency of restraint use decreases. Providing feedback and comparing perceptions are single aspects that would eventually lead to the ultimate goal of improving aggression management procedures. When a client can be released from restraints is not immediately predictable. (P)

38. **1.** Being injured by a client can result in emotional responses similar to those of other crime victims. A resignation after being injured is relatively rare. Legal action against the client is sometimes discussed but rarely initiated. Debriefing with the client may be inappropriate or unnecessary to resolve the situation. (P)

The Client with Family Abuse or Violence

39. **2.** The safety of the client and her children is the most immediate concern. If there is immediate danger, action must be taken to protect them. The other options can be discussed after the client's safety is assured. (P)

40. **3.** The traditional and rigid gender roles described by the client are examples of role stereotyping. Impermeable boundaries, unbalanced power ratio, and dysfunctional feeling tone are also common in abusive families. (P)

41. **4.** The client's safety, including the need to stay alive, is crucial. Therefore, helping the client develop a safety plan is most important to include in the plan of care to ensure the client's safety. Being empathetic, teaching about abuse, and explaining the person's rights are also important after safety is ensured. (P)

42. **2, 3, 4, 5.** The victim of abuse is usually compliant with the spouse and feels guilt, shame, and some responsibility for the battering. Self-blame, substance abuse, and suicidal thoughts and attempts are possible dysfunctional coping methods used by abuse victims. The victim of abuse is not likely to demonstrate assertiveness. (P)

43. **1, 2, 3, 5.** Dealing with anger, stress, and anxiety, identifying resources and support groups, and increasing a sense of safety and security are appropriate interventions at this time. However, recommending an antiwar advocacy group may or may not be appropriate, even much later in the client's recovery. (P)

44. **3.** Based on the client's statements, such as "I don't know what to do anymore," the data here best support the nursing diagnosis of *Powerlessness* related to an abusive husband, as evidenced by inability to make decisions. A nursing diagnosis of *Risk for other-directed violence* would be appropriate if the client had talked about being beaten up the previous night. A nursing diagnosis of *Situational low self-esteem* would be appropriate if the client verbalized feelings of embarrassment in leaving the house and worthlessness. A nursing diagnosis of *Ineffective coping* would be appropriate if the client was crying or talked about crying herself to sleep at night. (P)

45. **2.** The nurse needs more information about the client's decision before deciding what intervention is most appropriate. Judgmental responses could make it difficult for the client to return for treatment should she want to do so. Telling the client that this is a bad decision that she will regret is inappropriate because the nurse is making an assumption. Warning the client that abuse commonly stops when one partner is involved in treatment may be true for some clients. However, until the nurse determines the basis for the client's decision, this type of response is an assumption and therefore inappropriate. Reminding the client about her duty to protect the children would be appropriate if the client had talked about episodes of current abuse by her partner and the fear that her children might be hurt by him. (P)

46. **3.** The mother's feelings are the priority here. Addressing the mother's feelings and asking for her view of the situation is most important in building a relationship with the family. Ignoring the mother's feelings will hinder the relationship. Defending the school nurse and the school puts the client's mother on the defensive and stifles communication. (P)

47. **1.** A caring, supportive relationship among family members is a characteristic of healthy families. Therefore, evidence of such a relationship would provide data to support the decision that the child is no longer at risk for abuse. Children frequently conceal information about the abuse they are enduring. Therefore, not talking about violence during visits to the nurse would not support the nurse's decision. Episodes of abuse, even if infrequent and occurring only during times of stress, indicate family coping problems if the parents do not have a caring and supportive relationship. A strong defensive reaction by parents to appropriate concern expressed by a teacher or other professional and episodes of abuse, even if infrequent, indicates family coping problems. (P)

48. **1.** Autonomy involves the sense of control over oneself and one's life. This area is affected by any crime. The others stages listed are less affected. (P)

49. **4.** Ultimately, a victim of a crime needs to move from being a victim to being a survivor. A reasonable sense of safety and security is key to this transition. Getting through the shock and confusion, carrying out home and work routines, and resolving grief over any losses represent steps along the way to becoming a survivor. (P)

50. **2.** The experience of rape is a crisis. Crisis intervention services, especially with a rape crisis nurse, are essential to help the client begin dealing with the aftermath of a rape. Legal assistance may be recommended if the client decides to report the rape and only after crisis intervention services have been provided. A rape support group can be helpful later in the recovery process. Medications for sleep disturbance, especially benzodiazepines, should be avoided if possible. Benzodiazepines are potentially addictive and can be used in suicide attempts, especially when consumed with alcohol. (P)

51. **3.** Guilt and self-blame are common feelings that need to be addressed directly and frequently. The client needs to be reminded periodically that she did not deserve and did not cause the rape. Continually encouraging the client to report the rape pressures the client and is not helpful. In most cases, resuming sexual relations is a difficult process that is not likely to occur quickly. It is not necessarily true that the rapist will be caught, tried, and jailed. Most rapists are not caught or convicted. (P)

52. **4.** Use of alcohol reflects unhealthy coping mechanisms. A client's report of needing alcohol to calm down needs to be addressed. Survival is the most important goal during a rape. The client's acknowledging this indicates that she is aware that she made the right choice. Although suicidal thoughts are common, the statement that suicide is an easy escape but the client would be unable to do it indicates low risk. Fantasies of revenge, such as giving the death penalty to all rapists, are natural reactions and are a problem only if the client intends to carry them out directly. (P)

53. **3.** Coercion is the most common strategy used because the child commonly trusts the abuser. Tying the child down usually is not necessary. Typically the abusive person can control the child by his or her size and weight alone. Bribery usually is not necessary because the child wants love and affection from the abusive person, not money. Young children are not capable of giving consent for sex before they develop an adult concept of what sex is. (P)

54. **2.** Truancy and running away are common symptoms for young children and adolescents. The stress of the abuse interferes with school success, leading to the avoidance of school. Running away is an effort to escape the abuse and/or lack of support at home. Rather than an inability to play or a lack of play, play is likely to be aggressive with sexual overtones. Children tend to act out anger rather than control it. Head banging is a behavior typically seen with very young children who are abused. (P)

55. **3.** Dealing with the physical pain associated with mutilation is viewed as easier than dealing with the intense anger and emotional pain. The client fears an aggressive outburst when anger and emotional pain increase. Self-mutilation seems easier and safer. Additionally, self-mutilation may occur if the client feels unreal or numb or is dissociating. Here, the mutilation proves to the client that he or she is alive and capable of feeling. The client may want to be less sexually attractive, but this aspect usually is not related to self-mutilation. Bingeing and purging is commonly done in addition to, not instead of, self-mutilation. Although a few clients report an occasional high with self-mutilation, usually the experience is just relief from anger and rage. (P)

56. **1.** The dolls and toys in a play therapy room are useful props to help the child remember situations and reexperience the feelings, acting out the experience with the toys rather than putting the feelings into words. Role-playing without props commonly is more difficult for a child. Although drawing itself can be therapeutic, having the abuser see the pictures is usually threatening for the child. Reporting abuse to authorities is mandatory, but doesn't help the child express feelings. (P)

57. **2, 3, 4, 5.** Using a foam bat while symbolically confronting the abuser, keeping a journal of memories and feelings, and writing letters about the abuse but not sending them are appropriate strategies because they allow anger to be expressed safely. Directly confronting the abuser is likely to result in further harm because the abusers commonly deny the abuse, rationalize about it, or blame the victim. (P)

58. **4.** The safety of other children is a primary concern. It is critical to know whether other children are at risk for being sexually abused by the same perpetrator. Asking about other forms of abuse, how long the abuse went on, and if the victim did not remember the abuse are important questions after the safety of other children is determined. (P)

59. **1, 3, 5.** Survivors of torture and ritual abuse typically have intense feelings, including mixed emotions about the abusers, anger, rage, and guilt. With self-destructive behavior, they need ways to handle these urges, such as dealing with ambivalent feelings, determining alternatives to self-destructive behaviors, and developing safe ways to deal with rage and guilt. Confrontation with the abusers is not necessarily appropriate. Filing criminal charges is not likely due to the statute of limitations. (P)

60. **3.** The statement about functioning OK now but being aware that problems will come up again indicates insight into problems and the desire for sporadic counseling as new problems arise. Disclosing and feeling done with the work is common in early therapy because of the initial emotional release. It does not reflect the ability to work through problems resulting from the abuse. Stating that it is too hard to deal with all this pain suggests a lack of progress and a wish to escape the pain (perhaps by suicide). Client self-evaluation is more important than relying on the perceptions of others. (P)

61. **1.** The nurse should respond to the husband's needs and concerns and should offer support. Protecting or defending the wife against his criticism ignores the husband's needs. (P)

62. **1, 2, 3, 4.** The crucial interventions involve safety and support. Asking for consent is a Health Information Portability and Accountability Act issue, not a safety issue, and is not essential to the discharge process. (P)

63. **3.** It is important to know the client's reactions in order to plan appropriate interventions. Until the client's reactions are known, it is premature to suggest a job transfer, file a report to his boss's supervisor, or alert his coworkers. (P)

64. **2, 3, 4.** After the impact of a crime, the client's most important needs are for physical safety and emotional security. There is no indication that the client has a severe level of anxiety; therefore, lorazepam is not indicated. Asking her how she could have prevented the robbery implies that she could be at fault. (P)

65. **1, 2, 3, 5.** Receiving support from family, friends, other survivors, and community services is generally helpful after such events. Relaxation and participation in activities help manage stress reactions. Speaking out publicly may or may not be helpful later in the recovery process, but may actually hinder recovery in the early stages. (P)

The Client with Anorexia Nervosa

66. 3. In responding to the client, the nurse must be nonjudgmental and matter of fact. Telling her that weight gain is in her favor ignores the client's extreme fear of gaining weight. Putting off the weigh in for 2 hours allows the client to manipulate the nurse and interferes with the need to weigh the client at the same time each day. Threatening to call the doctor is not likely to build rapport or a working relationship with the client. (P)

67. 2. A client with anorexia nervosa commonly has an extreme fear of not being able to control weight. The nurse should address this fear. Explaining the dangers of diet pills or discussing health care provider or family concerns focuses on the effect of the client's weight loss on other people rather than the client. Unless the client is motivated to stop, the client will likely not be successful. (P)

68. 4. An intense fear of becoming obese, emaciation, and a disturbed body image all are considered to be characteristic of anorexia nervosa. Near-normal weight is not associated with anorexia. The weight of others is not a primary factor. Concern about dieting is not strong enough language to describe the control of food intake in the individual with anorexia nervosa. (P)

69. 1. Anorexia nervosa occurs most commonly in girls and women, with the age at onset between 12 and 20 years. It begins less commonly after 30 years. Although anorexia occurs in men, the prevalence rate is less than 5% to 10% of all cases of anorexia. (P)

70. 2. Lanugo, hypothermia, and hypotension are consistent with anorexia nervosa. Primarily what is found is a decrease or slowing down of bodily functions as starvation occurs. The only function that is increased is urination, and that is to rid the body of extra waste products. Bradycardia, constipation, and amenorrhea also are associated with anorexia. (A)

71. 3. Parents commonly describe their child as a model child who is a high achiever and compliant. These adolescents are typically well liked by teachers and peers. It is not typical for behavior problems to be reported. The description about having given the child everything and being repaid is more likely to describe an adolescent who is exhibiting behavior problems. (P)

72. 4. The client is in a state of starvation as evidenced by her body weight compared with height. The priority nursing diagnosis is *Imbalanced nutrition: Less than body requirements* because the client is in danger of dying or suffering damage to her body as a result of starvation. *Situational low self-esteem, Disturbed body image,* and *Interrupted family processes* are important and relevant, but the priority is the client's state of starvation and need for refeeding. (P)

The Client with Bulimia

73. 1. The large carbohydrate intake and significant time in the bathroom are characteristics of bulimia. To address the problem, the client must obtain an evaluation of her physical and psychological status. Suggesting going to a weight loss program or overeating support group frames the problem as strictly a weight issue and ignores the psychological etiology of the problem. Seeing the family physician does not address the psychological aspect of the client's illness, and the client must make the appointment herself. (P)

74. 1, 2, 3, 4. Because of the large number of calories ingested in a binge and the fact that a purge does not eliminate all calories consumed, the client with bulimia is of more normal weight, but still must have a goal of maintaining that weight. Research has shown that selective serotonin reuptake inhibitors are effective in treating bulimia, and the client is usually amenable to taking the medication. The client with an eating disorder (bulimia and anorexia) has negative self-concepts that fuel her disordered eating, and attaining a positive self-concept is an appropriate goal. The nurse should work with the client with bulimia to help her recognize her eating as disordered. That recognition can make the client more amenable to treatment. It is not realistic to establish a goal that the client with bulimia will never have the desire to purge again. (P)

75. 3. A successful outcome for a bulimic client is to avoid using the eating disorder as a coping measure when dealing with stress. Being able to attend college in another state, eat at home, and eat out without bingeing and purging are important goals, but do not address the primary problem of stress management and its connection to eating. (P)

76. 3. By telling the mother that the coach is a nurse and relaying the behaviors observed, the nurse gives the mother a chance to recognize the expertise of the coach and introduces the possibility of an eating disorder. Thanking the mother and complimenting the player does not begin to approach the topic. Telling the mother that the nurse has some very bad news is negative and dramatic. Additionally, although the observed behaviors suggest an eating disorder, it would be inappropriate for the nurse to medically diagnose the daughter. Although the daughter may indeed be very sick and need to see a therapist, the nurse should relate the information in a matter-of-fact, unemotional way. (P)

77. 3. Encouraging the client to talk about why she is here and her feelings may reveal more information about what led her to come to the group and what led to her diagnosis. It also provides the nurse with valuable information needed to develop an appropriate plan of care. The comment that the client sounds angry presumes what the client is feeling and focuses the talk on her husband. The focus should be on the client, not the husband. Telling the client that she will like coming to group imposes the nurse's view onto the client. The statement also focuses on having fun in the group instead of stressing the therapeutic value. Having the client tell the nurse something about the cause of her bulimia ignores the client's original statement. In addition, it requires the client to have insight into the cause of her disease, which may not be possible at this point. Also, it may be too early in the relationship to discuss this disorder. (P)

78. 2. Because the client eats excessively whenever she is upset, the best nursing diagnosis is *Ineffective coping*. There are no data on the family to support *Disabled family coping*. The client's bingeing and purging behavior occurs in response to her difficulty with coping. If the client were only overeating and not purging, then *Imbalanced nutrition: More than body requirements* would be an appropriate diagnosis. The client does not report nervousness and tension that would lead to a nursing diagnosis of *Anxiety*. (P)

79. 4. The nurse needs to explore more about the client's feelings to assess what underlies the eating disorder. The nurse also needs to evaluate the client's suicide risk. The other statements are not therapeutic because they minimize the client's feelings. (P)

80. 1. In the United States, food has been equated with love and affection. Parties and family celebrations usually include food. When someone is upset, food is commonly offered as comfort. People rarely share food with enemies. Power and control, status and prestige, and survival and growth may at times be associated with food, but these do not have the universality of association that love and affection both have. (C)

Children and Adolescents with Behavior Problems

81. 1. This child is demonstrating signs of anxiety and withdrawal. Being a library helper enables the client to use an interest (reading) when interacting with others and gaining pride in helping others. Most interaction will be one-to-one and with adults, which is likely to be more comfortable for her in her state of anxiety. Organizing a class party, a group project with her peers, and a kickball team involve multiple peer interactions, which are likely to be difficult for her at this time. Also, there is no mention of the child liking sports, so kickball would not be an appropriate activity. (P)

82. 4. All suspected child abuse must be reported, but this child's age and ability to describe the abuse make this allegation particularly strong. Because parental reaction to her allegation is not predictable, the nurse must ensure the child's safety. The nurse should not discuss the situation with the client or the parents. The nurse must refer this case to Child Protective Services. (P)

83. 1. Peer acceptance and recognition is a very powerful force in the lives of adolescents, leading to positive or negative behavior depending on the child's peers. While the influence of parents remains strong, peer acceptance combined with the adolescent's desire for independence can lead to disobeying the parents. The sanctions provided at school and in the community by law enforcement will support those teens that have other support in their lives, but are generally not sufficient to prevent substance use in adolescents lacking support at home and with peers. (P)

84. 2. This statement indicates insight into possible emotional causes for her pain. After insight is achieved, the client can make behavior changes to effectively cope with her anxiety-related disorder. Saying that she understands why her father is away so often demonstrates insight into her father's actions rather than her own. Wanting to discuss her pain and not her family indicates denial of any connection between her pain and her stress, which perpetuates her current situation. While rest may help her back, the client's statement does not address psychological issues related to the back pain. (P)

85. 4. Problems with interpersonal relationships, such as resisting affection and refusing to respond to others, and repetitive or self-stimulating behaviors suggest autism. Because the parents did not report any tics, Tourette syndrome is not suggested. Because the parents did not report any psychotic behaviors, such as hallucinations or delusions, schizophrenia can be ruled out. Attention deficit hyperactivity disorder is commonly portrayed as incessant activity with difficulty completing tasks. (P)

86. 4. ADHD is typically managed by psychostimulant medications, such as methylphenidate and pemoline (Cylert), along with behavior modification. Antianxiety medications, such as buspirone, are not appropriate for treating ADHD. Home schooling commonly is not a possibility because both parents work outside the home. Antidepressants, such as imipramine, are not recommended for use in children. Family therapy may be a part of the treatment. Anticonvulsant medications, such as carbamazepine, are not appropriate for ADHD. Also, carbamazepine levels are obtained weekly early during therapy to avoid toxicity and ascertain therapeutic levels. (P)

87. 1. Suggesting that the mother arrange for respite care so that she can have a regular break would help to alleviate some of the stress that she feels when she is with her child constantly. The mother also could use family and friends to provide some care, thereby helping with giving her a break. The child may improve, so suggesting that the mother take a job to provide a feeling of success would be inappropriate. Having coffee daily with friends may provide some opportunities for socialization. However, friends may not be able to provide the verbal support that the mother needs. Rather, attending a support group of other parents with children with attention deficit hyperactivity disorder might be helpful. Placing the child in foster care is an extreme measure that may damage the therapeutic relationship with the nurse and dramatically and negatively affect the relationship between the mother and child. (P)

88. 3. Giving away personal items has consistently been shown to be an indicator of suicide plans in a depressed and suicidal individual. Expression of a desire to date, trying out for an extracurricular activity, or the desire to spend more time with friends indicates a return of interest in normal adolescent activities. (P)

89. 2. Most likely, the client is diagnosed with conduct disorder. Conduct disorder is characterized by severe problems with behavior, authority, and the law. The individual with a conduct disorder is not concerned with the rights of others, as demonstrated by vandalism and prostitution. With attention deficit hyperactivity disorder, the client would demonstrate constant activity and problems with attention. In oppositional defiant disorder, problems with authority may result in behavior problems, but the core of the disorder is defiance to authority not including legal problems, such as vandalism and prostitution. Tourette syndrome is a tic disorder. However, tics were not described with this individual. (P)

90. 1. Tourette syndrome is characterized by motor and verbal tics. The disorder begins with simple tics, such as finger twitching, and may progress to a complex tic involving movement of the entire arm. There also may be difficulties with obsessions and compulsions. (P)

91. 1. Children are not as likely as adults to display sad behaviors but instead frequently have somatic complaints and acting-out behaviors. Both adults and children can have problems with performance. (P)

92. 2. Adolescents are more likely than children to attempt or commit suicide. Loss, abuse, and family discord remain significant risk factors. There is no evidence to support that children rarely commit suicide. Additionally, evidence fails to support the belief that children who have lost a parent to suicide will attempt it themselves. Significant events, such as a recent firearm purchase, have not been linked to suicide attempts in children. No geographical region in the United States is free from adolescent suicide. (P)

93. 1. Five-year-old children view death as reversible, so talking about seeing her mother again is a normal statement for a child of this age. A child this age would not usually state that she was glad Jesus took her mom but instead might be afraid that Jesus would also take her or her dad. The idea of replacing her mother with a new one, as hinted in the statement that they got another dog after the dog died, has not been supported by studies of grieving children. Stating that mommy went to heaven and that the child will see her someday when the child dies is reflective of more advanced abstract thinking than a 5-year-old would demonstrate. (H)

94. 3. Asperger's disorder is recognized later than autism, and the interpersonal problems worsen with school attendance. These children usually have restricted and repetitive patterns of behavior. School problems exist as a result of the interaction difficulties and behavior differences. Motor development may be delayed, but language commonly progresses normally. (P)

95. 3. The nurse manager needs to focus on the frustration that the nurse is expressing. Additionally, the nurse manager needs to correct any misinformation or misinterpretation that the staff nurse has. Saying that the nurse sounds burned out and asking about a vacation does not focus on the nurse's frustration or address the inaccuracy of the nurse's statement. There is no evidence to suggest that children with conduct disorder have more than the average adult's risk of depression or anxiety. Therefore, this response is inaccurate and inappropriate. Anecdotal information from personal experience does not supply the nurse with accurate, reliable information. (M)

96. 2. The nurse needs to find out what exactly the mother knows and has read. Reviewing what the mother has found in her reading that is leading her to doubt the diagnosis will help direct the nurse's teaching and clarify any misperceptions or misinformation that the mother may have. The physician may indeed have many years of education and experience, and the focus should be on the daughter, but the nurse needs to address the mother's concerns at this time. (P)

97. 1, 2. Discussing relationship issues related to the opposite sex with an early adolescent beginning at or near pubescence is appropriate. Kissing and touching other clients is discouraged and this needs reinforcement because she is likely to defy rules. Staying in her room with an assignment and seeing a video on reproduction may be appropriate approaches later on, but do not help the client learn appropriate sexual and social behaviors outside of the hospital. Calling her psychiatrist is not necessary because it is not an emergency. (P)

98. **1.** Stating that attention deficit hyperactivity disorder occurs more commonly in families takes the opportunity for teaching while also helping the father realize that he and his wife are not to blame. Parents, who are commonly blamed by society for their child's behavior, need help with education. Questioning the father on what he thinks he may have done implies that the parents played some role in this disorder, possibly contributing to the father's guilt. Telling the father that many parents feel this way and that the nurse does not think the parents are at fault is premature at this point. Telling the father that he should focus on what needs to be done, rather than what caused the disorder, minimizes the father's concerns and feelings. (P)

99. **3.** Focusing on the purpose of the group is the best response. Adolescents are greatly influenced by their peers. Medication alone is not typically the most successful treatment strategy. Questioning whether the client will continue the medication is negative and is not the reason for her to stay in the group. Asking the rest of the group to respond may or may not give the nurse support for the teenager remaining in the group. Groups commonly have rules regarding movement of members in and out of the group, but this does not address the reasons for the client to remain in the group. (P)

100. **4.** Asking whether the client is thinking about killing himself is the most direct and therefore the best way to assess suicidal risk. Knowing whether the client has watched movies on suicide and death, what the client thinks about suicide, and whether other family members have committed suicide will not tell the nurse whether the client is thinking about committing suicide right now. (P)

101. **1.** The teacher needs to be informed that this behavior is inappropriate. Therefore, educating the teacher and encouraging her to respond to misbehavior consistently is correct. Telling the teacher that the nurse can't believe the teacher lets the child get away with the behavior is demeaning and condescending. Allowing the child to continue the misbehavior is counterproductive to discipline and could create other problems. (P)

102. **4.** Drugs such as clonidine, haloperidol (Haldol), and pimozide (Orap) are currently being used for treatment of tic disorders. Risperidone (Risperdal) has also been used in clinical trials, with good results. Chlorpromazine is an antipsychotic, imipramine is an antidepressant, and lithium is used to manage mania and bipolar disorder. (D)

103. **2.** Consistent discipline and alternative methods of anger management are two important tools for parents who have a child with oppositional defiant disorder. Consistent discipline sets limits for the child. Helping the child learn more appropriate ways to manage anger assists the child in living within societal expectations. Avoiding restriction of television and computer time for punishment or using time-out as the primary means of punishment has not been suggested as an appropriate management method. Typically, using many strategies is more effective. Ignoring bad behavior could be dangerous and does not reinforce to the child that limits on behavior exist in society. (P)

104. **4.** Children who experience serious losses, especially multiple losses, such as old friends or a parent, are more at risk for depression. Girls also are at greater risk than boys during the adolescent years. (H)

105. **3.** Asking the client to report everything that she has had to eat and drink yesterday and today is the least judgmental approach and also provides helpful information. Confronting the client about drinking alcohol or asking the client to admit the real reason for feeling sick can put the girl on the defensive and block further communication. The nurse should avoid putting the client on the defensive to facilitate communication that may eventually enable the nurse to get the truth and identify interventions. (P)

106. **2.** Studies show that usually one-third to one-half of people diagnosed with ADHD do not need medication as adults. (P)

107. **1.** The client is stating that he is stupid like his classmates believe. Attention deficit hyperactivity disorder commonly causes problems in school, which can lead to problems with self-esteem. *Ineffective coping* would be manifested by the client's hitting a peer who laughs at him. *Interrupted family processes* would be evidenced by the parents' not being able to help their son cope or by their own inability to cope with their son and his disorder. *Anxiety* would be associated with the client's reporting tense or nervous feelings. (P)

108. **3.** The single-dose form of methylphenidate should be taken 10 to 14 hours before bedtime to prevent problems with insomnia, which can occur when the daily or last dose of the medication is taken within 6 hours (for multiple dosing) or 10 to 14 hours (for single dosing) before bedtime. It is recommended that a missed dose be taken as soon as possible; the dose is skipped if it is not remembered until the next dose is due. Any other medication, including over-the-counter medications, should be discussed with the health care provider before use to eliminate the risk of a possible drug interaction. (D)

109. **4.** The child's refusal to sit in class, insistence on calling her mother when she isn't ill, fear that something bad is going to happen to her mother, and physical appearance of anxiety best fit separation anxiety disorder. Children with separation anxiety disorder display these types of behaviors for a month or longer. Obsessive-compulsive disorder would be manifested by ritualistic, repetitive behaviors that are excessive and interfere with normal activities. Major depression in children is evidenced by sadness or acting-out behaviors. Attention deficit hyperactivity disorder is manifested by failure to complete tasks, an inability to pay attention during class, and easy distractibility. (P)

110. **1, 2, 3, 4.** The crucial elements of a behavioral contract include compliance with the medication regimen if medication is prescribed, appropriate anger management, consequences for unacceptable behaviors, and rules for interactions with others. Personal possessions may be limited by unit rules, but are not part of an individualized behavioral contract. (P)

111. **4.** Indifference to other people and mutism may be indicators of autism and would require further investigation. A 2-year-old who talks to himself and refuses to cooperate with toilet training is displaying behaviors typical for this age. Occasional thumb sucking and not having spent the night with a friend would be normal at age 6. Threats to run away when angry is considered within the range of normal behaviors for a 10-year-old child. (H)

The Child or Adolescent Who Has Suffered Sexual Abuse

112. **1, 3, 4.** Perpetrators prey on those who are younger and weaker who they can control mentally and physically. Their isolation, low self-esteem, and poor social skills mean that they commonly need love and belonging from their victims. The introduction of children to sex is inappropriate because of their age and level of maturity, no matter what the supposed motive is. When caught, perpetrators more commonly blame the victim and might use the claim to be introducing sex gently as an excuse for their actions. (P)

113. **2.** The change in the child's behavior at preschool and at home signals a potential problem, such as sexual abuse, and would require further follow up. Her previous combination of interest and jealousy is common for older siblings before the birth of a sibling. The alternating withdrawal and aggression are not normal for this developmental level. There is not sufficient hyperactivity, impulsivity, and distractibility to warrant a diagnosis of attention deficit hyperactivity disorder at this young age. (P)

114. **1, 2, 4, 5.** Children typically act out their feelings (such as depression and anger) in response to incest. Sexualized play, aggression, running away, and truancy are typical acting-out behaviors. Isolation at home is not common for incest victims who are preadolescents. (P)

115. **4.** Prosecution is the client's decision, not the nurse's, and should be carefully processed. It is inappropriate for the nurse to offer advice or opinions. (P)

116. **3.** The symptoms reported by the client indicate the need for counseling. Coming to the hospital would be recommended if he might be dangerous to himself or others. Telling the client that he needs more time to recover does not address his current concerns. Recovery can take months or years and requires professional assistance. A sleep aid without counseling is unlikely to be effective. (P)

Stress, Coping, and Therapeutic Communication

- The Client Managing Stress
- The Client Coping with Chronic Illness
- Therapeutic Communication
- Correct Answers and Rationales

The Client Managing Stress

1. The nurse cares for a middle-aged client with a below-the-knee amputation. What statement indicates the need for further assessment of the client's body image?
- ☐ 1. "When I get my prosthesis, I want to learn to walk so I can participate in walk-a-thons."
- ☐ 2. "I hope to get skilled enough at using my prosthesis to help others like me adjust."
- ☐ 3. "Whenever I start to feel sorry for myself, I remember that my buddy died in that accident."
- ☐ 4. "I hope I can handle having a prosthesis, but I'm really wondering what my wife will think."

2. A client demonstrates moderate anxiety regarding a pending medical procedure. What actions should the nurse perform to minimize the client's anxiety about the procedure?
- ☐ 1. Assuring the client that pain is not associated with the procedure.
- ☐ 2. Providing a brief explanation and then doing the procedure quickly.
- ☐ 3. Giving a demonstration of what is to be done.
- ☐ 4. Indicating to the client that it is normal to feel anxious and fearful before such a procedure.

3. A 75-year-old client is newly diagnosed with diabetes. The nurse is instructing him about blood glucose testing. After the session, the client states, "I can't be expected to remember all this stuff." The nurse should recognize this response as most likely related to which of the following?
- ☐ 1. Moderate to severe anxiety.
- ☐ 2. Disinterest in the illness.
- ☐ 3. Early-onset dementia.
- ☐ 4. Normal reaction to learning a new skill.

4. A client in a general hospital is to undergo surgery in 2 days. He is experiencing moderate anxiety about the procedure and its outcome. What anxiety reduction plans should the nurse implement?
- ☐ 1. Tell the client to distract himself with games and television.
- ☐ 2. Reassure the client that he will come through surgery without incident.
- ☐ 3. Explain the surgical procedure to the client and what happens before and after surgery.
- ☐ 4. Ask the surgeon to refer the client to a psychiatrist who can work with the client to diminish his anxiety.

5. After teaching a group of nursing students about the neurochemical changes that help facilitate rapid behavioral responses to dangerous situations, which of the following, if stated by the group as important for facilitating rapid responses, indicates effective teaching?
- ☐ 1. Increase in release of endogenous opiates.
- ☐ 2. Increase in noradrenergic and dopaminergic system activity.
- ☐ 3. Decrease in peripheral sympathetic system activity.
- ☐ 4. Decrease in glucocorticoid levels.

6. Anxiety occurs in degrees, from a level that stimulates productive problem solving to a level that is severely debilitating. At a mild, productive level of anxiety, the nurse should expect to see which of the following as a cognitive characteristic of mild anxiety?
- ☐ 1. Slight muscle tension.
- ☐ 2. Occasional irritability.
- ☐ 3. Accurate perceptions.
- ☐ 4. Loss of contact with reality.

7. As a client's level of anxiety increases to a debilitating degree, the nurse should expect which of the following as a psychomotor behavior indicating a panic level of anxiety?
- ☐ 1. Suicide attempts or violence.
- ☐ 2. Desperation and rage.
- ☐ 3. Disorganized reasoning.
- ☐ 4. Loss of contact with reality.

8. Nursing interventions with an anxious client change as the anxiety level increases. At a low level of anxiety, the primary focus of interventions is on which of the following?
- ☐ 1. Taking control of the situation for the client.
- ☐ 2. Learning and problem solving.
- ☐ 3. Reducing stimuli and pressure.
- ☐ 4. Using tension reduction activities.

9. When coping becomes dysfunctional enough to require the client to be admitted to the hospital, the nurse should expect the client to demonstrate which of the following?
- ☐ 1. Objective and rational problem solving.
- ☐ 2. Tension reduction activities and then problem solving.
- ☐ 3. Anger management strategies with no problem solving.
- ☐ 4. Minimal functioning with new problems developing.

10. In addition to teaching assertiveness and problem-solving skills when helping the client cope effectively with stress and anxiety, which of the following should the nurse also expect to address?
- ☐ 1. Suppressing anger.
- ☐ 2. Balancing a checkbook.
- ☐ 3. Following step-by-step directions.
- ☐ 4. Using conflict resolution skills.

11. Which of the following client statements indicates to the nurse that the client has coped effectively with a relationship problem?
- ☐ 1. "My wife will be happy to know that I can spend less time at work now."
- ☐ 2. "My wife and I are talking about our likes and dislikes in activities."
- ☐ 3. "I can understand how my wife and I see things differently."
- ☐ 4. "We are really listening to each other about our different view on issues."

12. In an ongoing assessment, the nurse should identify the client's thoughts and feelings about a situation in addition to which of the following?
- ☐ 1. Whether the client's behavior is appropriate in the context of the current situation.
- ☐ 2. Whether the client is motivated to decrease dysfunctional behaviors.
- ☐ 3. Which of the client's problems have the highest priority.
- ☐ 4. Which of the client's behaviors necessitates a no harm contract.

13. When developing appropriate short-term goals with clients who are inpatients, which of the following is most realistic?
- ☐ 1. The client will demonstrate a positive self-image.
- ☐ 2. The client will describe plans for how to get back into school.
- ☐ 3. The client will write a list of strengths and needs.
- ☐ 4. The client will practice assertiveness skills in confronting his mother.

14. A nurse is counseling a client with cancer who is experiencing anxiety. Which goal will provide the best long-term client outcome?
- ☐ 1. Follow up with psychiatrists.
- ☐ 2. Understand medication effects and adverse effects.
- ☐ 3. Take medication as prescribed.
- ☐ 4. Solve problems without help from others.

15. When integrating the concepts underlying the cognitive-behavioral model into a client's plan of care, the nurse should expect to focus on which of the following areas?
- ☐ 1. Substitution of rational beliefs for self-defeating thinking and behaving.
- ☐ 2. Insight into unconscious conflicts and processes.
- ☐ 3. Analysis of fears and barriers to growth.
- ☐ 4. Reduction of bodily tensions and stress management.

16. Which of the following client statements indicates that he has gained insight into his use of the defense mechanism of displacement?
- ☐ 1. "I can't think about the weekend right now. I've got to study for the exam."
- ☐ 2. "I know I'm not good in sports, but I feel good about my grades."
- ☐ 3. "Now when I'm mad at my wife, I talk to her instead of taking it out on the kids."
- ☐ 4. "For years I couldn't remember being molested; now I know I have to face it."

17. According to Erikson's developmental model, which of the following interventions is helpful for a client experiencing a problem with identity versus role confusion?
- ☐ 1. Asking for a list of goals related to family and career.
- ☐ 2. Discussing productive ways to achieve societal responsibilities.
- ☐ 3. Discussing appropriate versus inappropriate social behaviors.
- ☐ 4. Asking for a list of benefits and risks for committing in a relationship.

18. When the client is involuntarily committed to a hospital because he is assessed as being dangerous to himself or others, which of the following rights is lost?
- [ ] **1.** The right to refuse medications and treatments.
- [ ] **2.** The right to send and receive uncensored mail.
- [ ] **3.** Freedom from seclusion and restraints.
- [ ] **4.** The right to leave the hospital against medical advice.

19. In which of the following situations can a client's confidentiality be breached legally?
- [ ] **1.** To answer a request from a client's spouse about the client's medication.
- [ ] **2.** In a student nurse's clinical paper about a client.
- [ ] **3.** When a client near discharge is threatening to harm an ex-partner.
- [ ] **4.** When a client's employer requests the client's diagnosis to initiate medical claims.

20. A client is admitted after the police found he had been sleeping in his car for 3 nights. The client says, "My wife kicked me out and is divorcing me. It wasn't my fault I was fired from work. My wife and boss are plotting against me because I am smarter than they are." He then pounds the table and says, "I'm not staying here, and you can't stop me." Which of the following are the most crucial and immediate issues to include in the client's plan of care? Select all that apply.
- [ ] **1.** Collateral information from his wife and boss.
- [ ] **2.** Anxiety and anger management.
- [ ] **3.** Appropriate housing.
- [ ] **4.** Divorce counseling.
- [ ] **5.** Assault and escape precautions.
- [ ] **6.** Suspiciousness and grandiosity issues.

21. Which of the following is a crucial goal of therapeutic communication when helping the client deal with personal issues and painful feelings?
- [ ] **1.** Communicating empathy through gentle touch.
- [ ] **2.** Conveying client respect and acceptance even if not all of the client's behaviors are tolerated.
- [ ] **3.** Mutual sharing of information, spontaneity, emotions, and intimacy.
- [ ] **4.** Guaranteeing total confidentiality and anonymity for the client.

22. A client who has not left the bus station for 3 days is brought to the mental health facility by a police officer because she has been bothering other people. She denies this, holds tightly to her purse, and refuses to talk to anyone except to say, "You have no right to keep me here. I have money, and I can take care of myself." The police officer thinks she needs psychiatric evaluation. Evaluation reveals that the client stopped taking her psychotropic medication, but she agrees to start taking her medication again. The charge nurse informs the other staff members that the physician is discharging the client because involuntary commitment is not indicated. Another nurse states, "How can her physician be so cruel? She should stay in the hospital instead of being discharged." Which response is best for the nurse to make to her peer?
- [ ] **1.** "I agree with you. She does have symptoms of mental illness."
- [ ] **2.** "Although she may have a mental illness, she is not gravely disabled or dangerous to herself or others now."
- [ ] **3.** "The client wants to leave, so the physician is not going to put her through the commitment process."
- [ ] **4.** "The client has a home to go to and family to support her. She doesn't need to be here."

23. Which question or statement indicates that the nurse and client are involved in the planning stage of the nursing process?
- [ ] **1.** "It sounds as if you are feeling abandoned by your family."
- [ ] **2.** "How important is it for you to change this behavior?"
- [ ] **3.** "Tell me what you want to say to your husband this evening."
- [ ] **4.** "Which of these two options do you want to try first?"

24. Which of the following questions or statements should the nurse use to encourage client evaluation?
- [ ] **1.** "I can hear that it's still hard for you to talk about this."
- [ ] **2.** "So what does this all mean to you now?"
- [ ] **3.** "What did you do differently with your coworker this time?"
- [ ] **4.** "What will it take to carry out your new plans?"

25. With shorter lengths of stay becoming the norm, which statement is a more practical view of the stages of the nurse-client relationship, originally proposed by H. Peplau?

☐ **1.** Different phases of the relationship involve emphasizing different processes and goals related to client needs.

☐ **2.** Building trust is the most that can be accomplished during the relationship.

☐ **3.** What can be achieved during the relationship is problem identification and referrals.

☐ **4.** Teaching new skills becomes the most important aspect of the relationship phases.

26. Even when the client understands problems and is motivated to change, the client may have fears about failing. Which of the following interventions is most likely to facilitate change?

☐ **1.** Reality testing about the need for change.

☐ **2.** Asking the client about fears that need to be overcome.

☐ **3.** Teaching new communication skills.

☐ **4.** Practicing new behaviors with the nurse.

The Client Coping with Chronic Illness

27. Which client should the nurse identify as needing the most assistance in accepting being ill?

☐ **1.** An 8-year-old boy who alternately cries for his mother and is angry with the nurse about being hospitalized after a bike accident.

☐ **2.** A 32-year-old woman diagnosed with depression related to lupus erythematosus who discusses her medication's adverse effects with the nurse.

☐ **3.** A 45-year-old man who just suffered a severe myocardial infarction and talks to the nurse about concerns regarding resuming sexual relations with his wife.

☐ **4.** A 60-year-old woman diagnosed with chronic obstructive pulmonary disease who refuses to wear an oxygen mask even though poor oxygenation makes her confused.

28. An 18-year-old client is recently diagnosed with leukemia. What is the most appropriate short-term goal for the nurse and client to establish?

☐ **1.** Accepting his death as imminent.

☐ **2.** Expressing his angry feelings to the nurse.

☐ **3.** Decreasing interaction with peers to conserve energy.

☐ **4.** Gaining an intellectual understanding of the illness.

29. The nurse has been asked to develop a medication education program for clients with chronic mental illness in the rehabilitation program. When developing the course outline, which of the following topics is most important to include?

☐ **1.** A categorization of many psychotropic drugs.

☐ **2.** Interventions for common side effects of psychotropic drugs.

☐ **3.** The role of medication in the treatment of acute illness.

☐ **4.** Effects of combining common street drugs with psychotropic medication.

30. The physician recommends that a client have a partial bowel resection and an ileostomy. Later, the client says to the nurse, "That doctor of mine surely likes to play big. I'll bet the more he can cut, the better he likes it." Which of the following replies by the nurse is most therapeutic?

☐ **1.** "I can tell you more about the surgery if you like."

☐ **2.** "What do you mean by that statement?"

☐ **3.** "Aren't you being a bit hard on him? He's trying to help you."

☐ **4.** "Does that remark have something to do with the operation he wants you to have?"

31. A client becomes increasingly morose and irritable after being told that she has cancer. She is rude to visitors and pushes nurses away when they attempt to give her medications and treatments. Which of the following should the nurse do when the client has a hostile outburst?

☐ **1.** Offer the client positive reinforcement each time she cooperates.

☐ **2.** Encourage the client to discuss her immediate concerns and feelings.

☐ **3.** Continue with the assigned tasks and duties as though nothing has happened.

☐ **4.** Encourage the client to direct her anger at staff members instead of her visitors.

32. Arrangements are made for a member of the colostomy club to meet with a client before bowel surgery. Which of the following is accomplished by having a representative from the club visit the client preoperatively?

☐ **1.** Letting the client know that he has resources in the community to help him.

☐ **2.** Providing support for the physician's plan of therapy for the client.

☐ **3.** Providing the client with support and realistic information on the colostomy.

☐ **4.** Convincing the client that he will not be disfigured and can lead a full life.

33. A client who was transferred to the medical unit from intensive care after suffering a myocardial infarction 3 days ago states, "My secretary should be here by now. I don't have time to lie around here and do nothing. I've never had time to relax, and I don't plan on starting now." Based on this initial information, which of the following nursing diagnoses should the nurse judge to be of least importance?

☐ 1. *Ineffective coping* related to serious illness, as evidenced by the statement about lying around and doing nothing.

☐ 2. *Deficient knowledge* related to cardiac rehabilitation, as evidenced by the client's statement about not planning to relax at present.

☐ 3. *Hopelessness* related to serious illness, as evidenced by the client's turning over her work to her secretary.

☐ 4. *Anxiety* related to delayed arrival of the client's secretary, as evidenced by her statement of expecting that the secretary should already have arrived.

34. The client with atrial fibrillation states to the nurse, "Please hand me the telephone. I need to check on my stocks and bonds." Which of the following responses by the nurse is most therapeutic?

☐ 1. "You will get more upset if you make that call."

☐ 2. "You have atrial fibrillations. Let's talk about what that means."

☐ 3. "You really don't care about the fact that you're sick, do you?"

☐ 4. "Do you realize you have a life-threatening condition?"

35. The nurse should determine that a client lacks understanding of her acute cardiac illness and the ability to make changes in her lifestyle by which of the following statements?

☐ 1. "I already have my airline ticket so I won't miss my meeting tomorrow."

☐ 2. "These relaxation tapes sound okay; I'll see if they help me."

☐ 3. "No more working 10 hours a day for me unless it's an emergency."

☐ 4. "I talked with my husband yesterday about working on a new budget together."

36. A 45-year-old client has been rehospitalized with a severe exacerbation of lupus that affects her central nervous system. After visiting with the client, her husband approaches the nurse. He says, "My wife is scaring me. She says she does not want to live with this illness anymore. Our kids are grown and she feels useless as a mother and a wife." Which of the following statements are the most appropriate responses to the husband? Select all that apply.

☐ 1. "I will have a talk with your wife to see if she is suicidal."

☐ 2. "You need to be strong and optimistic when you are with her."

☐ 3. "I'm glad you shared this with me. I can imagine that this is scary for you."

☐ 4. "I'm sure she will feel differently when we get this episode under control."

☐ 5. "We can talk about what you can say to her that may help."

37. The client with kidney stones refuses to eat lunch and rudely tells the nurse to get out of his room. Which of the following responses by the nurse is most appropriate?

☐ 1. "I'll leave, but you need to eat."

☐ 2. "I'll get you something for your pain."

☐ 3. "Your anger doesn't bother me. I'll be back later."

☐ 4. "You sound angry. What is upsetting you?"

38. Certain personality traits are commonly attributed to the client with ulcerative colitis. Based on this theory, which of the following traits should the nurse expect to see in a client with this disorder?

☐ 1. Self-reliance.

☐ 2. Decisiveness.

☐ 3. Perfectionism.

☐ 4. Ambitiousness.

39. One day, a client receiving dialysis directs profanities at the nurse, and then abruptly hangs his head and pleads, "Please forgive me. Something just came over me. Why do I say those things?" The nurse interprets this as which of the following?

☐ 1. Neologism.

☐ 2. Confabulation.

☐ 3. Flight of ideas.

☐ 4. Emotional lability.

Therapeutic Communication

40. A nurse is helping a client with cancer develop healthy coping skills. What behavior demonstrates the use of these skills?
- ☐ **1.** Directing anger at self instead of others.
- ☐ **2.** Calling the nurse when anxiety increases.
- ☐ **3.** Crying frequently when alone.
- ☐ **4.** Openly expressing feelings to the nurse or significant others.

41. A client is hospitalized with terminal cancer. His wife, who spends many hours by his bedside, is seen in the hall looking out the window. The nurse approaches the wife and finds her crying. The wife says, "I just don't know how I'll live without him." How should the nurse respond?
- ☐ **1.** "I know it's hard for you, but things will work out in the end."
- ☐ **2.** "We should talk about how you can best cope with your husband's death."
- ☐ **3.** "You seem sad and scared when you think about life without your husband."
- ☐ **4.** "Maybe it would be helpful for you to spend less time here at the hospital."

42. A 6-year-old client is diagnosed with attention deficit hyperactivity disorder (ADHD). When asking this client to complete a task, what techniques should the nurse use to communicate most effectively with him?
- ☐ **1.** Obtain eye contact before speaking, use simple language, and have him repeat what was said. Praise him if he completes the task.
- ☐ **2.** Fully explain to the client the actions required of him, offer verbal praise and a food reward for task completion.
- ☐ **3.** Explain to the client what he is to do, the consequences if he does not comply, and follow through with praise or consequences as appropriate.
- ☐ **4.** Demonstrate to the client what he is to do, have him imitate the nurse's actions, and give a food reward if he completes the task.

43. Following a mastectomy, a client states, "I don't want my husband to see me like this. With only one breast, I can't imagine how he can look at me." Using a facilitating response, how should the nurse respond?
- ☐ **1.** "I know how you feel. All women feel that way at first."
- ☐ **2.** "Don't let it bother you. You know he loves you."
- ☐ **3.** "You'll have time to adjust. Just be patient."
- ☐ **4.** "You seem worried. You think you won't be attractive anymore."

44. A nurse is counseling a client who is depressed. What nursing action promotes trust between the client and the nurse? Select all that apply.
- ☐ **1.** Indicating an understanding for the client's feelings as well as for their cause.
- ☐ **2.** Listening and encouraging the client to say more.
- ☐ **3.** Acknowledging that the nurse heard what the client said.
- ☐ **4.** Maintaining eye contact with the client at all times.
- ☐ **5.** Standing very close to the client.

45. A nurse is teaching a client diagnosed with diabetes to regulate his insulin dose. What is a desired outcome of the nurse's use of effective communication skills in teaching a client to regulate his insulin dose? Select all that apply.
- ☐ **1.** Increased control over the client's behavior.
- ☐ **2.** Client's understanding of expectations regarding health care procedures.
- ☐ **3.** Enhancement of the quality of care provided.
- ☐ **4.** Promotion of trust and collaboration with the client.
- ☐ **5.** Understanding of the client's concerns about regulating insulin.

46. A newly admitted young-adult male client asks the nurse to go to a movie with him when he is discharged. Which nursing response is most appropriate?
- ☐ **1.** "You don't understand the limits imposed in our relationship."
- ☐ **2.** "It seems you are having difficulties taking the step of asking a girl out."
- ☐ **3.** "You aren't showing me the respect I deserve as a professional."
- ☐ **4.** "Let's review our relationship and its purpose again."

47. A nurse has been working one-to-one with a client in an outpatient clinic who is nearing termination from the program. The nurse becomes seriously ill, is hospitalized, and is expected to be away from work for 4 to 6 weeks. What is the most appropriate way for the nurse to manage the sudden nurse-client termination?
- ☐ **1.** Ask another nurse to give the client a letter stating the reason for the termination and apologizing for the nurse's absence.
- ☐ **2.** Have another nurse work with the client until the ill nurse can return to work and complete the termination.
- ☐ **3.** No intervention is needed because the client was nearing termination. The client is strong enough to deal with the abrupt, unplanned termination.
- ☐ **4.** Wait until the nurse recovers enough to telephone the client and terminate the relationship over the phone.

48. A 17-year-old female client is at a family planning clinic for assistance in developing a birth control program. After discussing the available options, she indicates her preference for oral contraceptives and asks, "Since I'm only 17, I am worried about how these pills will affect me." What response by the nurse is most appropriate?

☐ 1. "This type of pill has been proven safe for all ages."

☐ 2. "Are you thinking that because you are young these pills will affect you differently?"

☐ 3. "Tell me about your concern about taking the pills."

☐ 4. "If the pill worries you, perhaps you'd like to consider another option."

Correct Answers and Rationales

The letter in parentheses after each rationale identifies the client need addressed in the item, including management of care (M), safety and infection control (S), health promotion and maintenance (H), psychosocial adaptation (P), basic care and comfort (C), pharmacological and parenteral therapies (D), reduction of risk potential (R), and physiological adaptation (A).

The Client Managing Stress

1. **4.** The client expressing doubts about his wife's response to his amputation as well as possible doubt on his part is still struggling with body image issues. Looking forward to participating in walk-a-thons and helping others indicate plans for the future that imply an acceptance of his amputee status. Remembering that his friend died in the accident that caused his amputation indicates that the client is aware that there was a worse end result to the accident than his amputation. (P)

2. **2.** A short explanation followed by quick completion of the procedure minimizes anxiety. The client may be fearful of pain, and assuring him that there will be no pain offers false reassurance. A demonstration may cause increased anxiety. Informing the client that his feelings are common normalizes anxiety and puts the client more at ease, but it is not the most reassuring approach. (P)

3. **1.** Anxiety, especially at higher levels, interferes with learning and memory retention. After the client's anxiety lessens, it will be easier for him to learn the steps of the blood glucose monitoring. Because the client's illness is a chronic, lifelong illness that severely changes his lifestyle, it is unlikely that he is uninterested in the illness or how to treat it. It is also unlikely that dementia would be the cause of the client's frustration and lack of memory. The client's response indicates anxiety. Client responses that would indicate lessening anxiety would be questions to the nurse or requests to repeat part of the instruction. (P)

4. **3.** An explanation of what to expect decreases anxiety about upcoming events that could be seen as traumatic by the client. Distraction, such as with games or television, only decreases anxiety temporarily and does not fulfill the client's need for information about the procedure. Reassurance about an uncomplicated outcome is not appropriate; the nurse cannot guarantee that the client will come through surgery without problems. Referring the client to a psychiatrist is not indicated for moderate, expected preoperative anxiety. (A)

5. **2.** An increase in the noradrenergic and dopaminergic system activity leads to central nervous system hyperarousal and hypervigilance. An increased release of endogenous opiates allows tolerance of fear and pain rather than increasing activity. A decrease in peripheral sympathetic system activity or glucocorticoid levels leads to a decrease in behavioral responses. (A)

6. **3.** With mild anxiety, perceptions are accurate. Slight muscle tension reflects a motor response. Occasional irritability is an emotional response. Loss of contact with reality is a cognitive characteristic of severe anxiety. (A)

7. **1.** Suicide attempts and violence are psychomotor responses to a panic level of anxiety. Desperation and rage are emotional responses. Disorganized reasoning and loss of contact with reality are cognitive responses. (A)

8. **2.** Mild anxiety motivates the client to focus on issues and resolve them. Therefore, learning and problem solving can occur at a mild level of anxiety. Taking control for the client is reserved for a near-panic level of anxiety. Severe anxiety interferes with reasoning and functioning. Therefore, reducing stimuli and pressure is crucial at a severe level. Tension reduction is appropriate at a moderate level to help the client think more clearly and engage in problem solving. (A)

9. **4.** Minimal functioning, causing new problems to develop, is a reflection of dysfunctional coping. The ability to objectively and rationally problem solve demonstrates adaptive coping. Tension reduction activities demonstrate palliative coping. However, such activities alone do not solve problems; they must be followed by problem solving. Anger management alone may prevent new problems, such as violence toward oneself or others, but it does not solve problems directly. It is considered maladaptive coping. (A)

10. 4. Because relationships inherently lead to stress and anxiety, conflict resolution skills are essential for solving relationship problems. Dealing with anger is more effective than suppressing it. Suppression is a mechanism that avoids the issue rather than solving it. Balancing a checkbook involves calculations, not coping skills. Following directions is a passive activity that reflects a lack of problem solving by the client. (P)

11. 4. The client's statement that he and his wife listen to each other reflects improved efforts at communicating about issues. The other statements provide some insight into the need for better communication. However, they are but steps along the way to coping effectively with the problem. (P)

12. 1. Assessment examines the client's thoughts, feelings, and behaviors within a context. Whether the client's behavior is appropriate for the situation is important assessment data. Setting priorities is part of making nursing diagnoses and planning; motivation to change and identifying the need for a no harm contract are part of the planning stage. (P)

13. 3. Writing a list of strengths and needs is short-term, achievable, and measurable. Achieving positive self-esteem would occur over the long term. Going to school involves complex future steps to a long-term goal. Using skills is likely to be stressful and is best attempted after the client has done a self-assessment. (P)

14. 4. The ultimate outcome is to have the client solve problems by himself, collaborating in his own care. Client follow-up with the psychiatrist, while desirable, does not ensure that the client will fully comply with treatment or medication. Knowledge of the medication's effects and adverse effects and compliance can help the client but alone will not ensure success unless the client knows how to address and solve problems without help from others. (H)

15. 1. Substituting rational beliefs is a major goal when using cognitive-behavioral models, which focus more on thinking and behaviors than feelings. Unconscious processes are the focus of psychoanalytic models. Analysis of fears and barriers to growth are the focus of developmental models. Tension and stress are targets of the stress models. (P)

16. 3. Displacement refers to a defense mechanism that involves taking feelings out on a less-threatening object or person instead of tackling the issue or problem directly. Talking to his wife directly reflects insight into the client's use of the defense mechanism and his ability to overcome it. Not thinking about the weekend is suppression. Here the client is focusing on the issue with the highest priority. Focusing on academic rather than athletic achievement is compensation, highlighting one's strengths instead of weaknesses. Not remembering the molestation is repression. (P)

17. 1. Lack of goals reflects identity problems. Societal responsibility is related to generativity issues. Social behaviors are learned in the initiative stage. Commitment in relationships is part of intimacy. (H)

18. 4. When a client is committed involuntarily, the right to leave against medical advice is forfeited. All the other rights are preserved unless there is further court action or a case of imminent danger to self or others (hitting staff, cutting self). (S)

19. 3. Legally there is a duty to warn a potential victim of a client's intent to harm. Staff can be held accountable if the client injures the ex-partner and the staff failed to warn that person. The client's permission is needed to share information with a spouse. Only client initials are used in student papers. Release of information is made directly to the client's insurance company, not to the employer. (S)

20. 2, 5. The client is showing increased anxiety and anger as well as refusing to stay in the hospital, which are immediate and crucial concerns at admission. The client is not likely to give permission to talk to his wife and boss at this point. Housing issues and divorce counseling may be relevant before discharge, but not initially. Suspiciousness and grandiosity may be relevant after the client's anxiety and anger are under control. (P)

21. 2. The nurse is required to set limits on inappropriate behavior while conveying respect and acceptance of the person. Doing so conveys to the client that he is worthy without posing any harm or embarrassment to the client. Touch is a complex issue that must be used cautiously. Touch may be misinterpreted or misperceived by a client who has been abused or who has perceptual or thought disturbances. Mutual sharing reflects a social friendship, not a therapeutic one. Total confidentiality is not desirable. For example, treatment team members and insurance companies need selected information to ensure quality services. (P)

22 2. To be committed involuntarily, a client must not only be suffering from a mental illness but must be gravely disabled (unable to care for self or likely to come to harm if discharged) or dangerous to self or others. Having a mental illness alone is not grounds for commitment. Wanting to leave the hospital is not sufficient cause for discharge if the client is dangerous to self or others or is gravely disabled. The physician would not avoid committing a client who meets the criteria to be committed. Having a supportive family or home but not wanting treatment may still result in involuntary commitment if indicated or necessary to ensure the well-being of the client or another person. (P)

23. 4. Encouraging decisions, such as asking the client to pick one of two options, is part of planning. Verbalizing the implied to clarify a message, as in the comment, "It sounds as if you are feeling abandoned by your family," is part of assessment. Asking for meaning and importance, such as, "How important is it for you to change this behavior," is related to nursing diagnosis. Rehearsing new behaviors is part of implementation. (P)

24. 3. Asking for descriptions of changes in behavior (what the client did differently) encourages evaluation. Conveying empathy, such as stating that it is still hard for the client to talk about it, encourages data collection. Asking for meaning helps with nursing diagnosis. Formulating plans is related to planning. (P)

25. 1. With the shorter lengths of stay, the processes and goals of a particular stage are chosen according to the client's current needs and abilities. Building trust (orientation stage) is a priority with psychotic and suspicious clients. It is less crucial for the client ready to work on issues. Making referrals (termination stage) is appropriate for all clients regardless of their needs. The other needs will be addressed in counseling after discharge. Teaching skills (working stage) is appropriate for clients with insight and readiness for change. They may not be appropriate for clients with severe psychosis or suspiciousness, especially if denial is present. (M)

26. 4. Practicing new behaviors builds confidence and reinforces appropriate behaviors. Reality testing, asking about fears, and teaching new communication skills are some of the many steps when trying out new behaviors. (P)

The Client Coping with Chronic Illness

27. 4. The 60-year-old woman is acting in a way that worsens her physical and mental condition because she does not want to be sick. The 8-year-old child is acting normally for someone his age who is unexpectedly hospitalized. The cooperation demonstrated by the client with lupus and the client who had a myocardial infarction indicates a level of acceptance of their illnesses and of their role as being ill. (P)

28. 2. Diagnosis of a serious illness would be a shock to anyone, but particularly a young person. Feelings of anger are normal and should be expressed. Gaining an intellectual understanding of his illness would also be necessary, but such learning will not take place if the client's feelings have not been addressed. There is no indication that the client needs to conserve energy because of his condition, nor is it clear that death is imminent. Neither situation is likely at the point of first diagnosis unless the disease is well advanced, which is not indicated here. (P)

29. 2. The psychotropic drugs used to treat chronic mental illnesses have side effects that can lead to noncompliance. Therefore, teaching the clients measures to deal with the common side effects would be most important. Teaching should be focused on the need for compliance and the specific interests of the target audience. Teaching should concentrate on the medications commonly used to treat chronic mental illness, not on many psychotropic drugs or those used in acute illness. Such topics as the role of medication in the treatment of chronic mental illness and the effects of using common street drugs with psychotropic medication should be discussed after the issue of compliance is addressed. (P)

30. 2. When the client seems to be questioning the physician's goals, it is best for the nurse to present an open statement and ask the client what he means. This technique helps the client express his feelings. Telling the client about the surgery is less therapeutic when he is upset. Chastising the client and defending the physician is likely to inhibit communication about the client's needs and feelings. Making assumptions can also interfere with communication, especially if the assumption is incorrect. (P)

31. 2. When the client has hostile outbursts, it is best for the nurse to help her express her feelings. This serves as a release valve for the client. Offering positive reinforcement for cooperation does not help the client express herself appropriately. Continuing with assigned tasks ignores the client's feelings and may lead to further escalation. Encouraging the client to direct anger to the staff is inappropriate. The client needs to express her feelings appropriately. (P)

32. 3. Preoperative visits and talks with others who have made successful adjustments to colostomies are helpful and tend to make the client less fearful of the operation and its consequences. Knowing about resources in the community will be helpful as the client approaches discharge. Supporting the physician is less important than supporting the client and giving him information. The client will have a change in body image, with disfigurement due to the creation of a colostomy. However, the client should be able to lead a full life. (P)

33. 3. *Hopelessness* is the least appropriate nursing diagnosis because the client projects an image of a person who is planning for the future and is usually in charge and productive. *Ineffective coping* is an appropriate diagnosis because the client is rushing to resume her normal activities. *Deficient knowledge* is an appropriate diagnosis because the client indicates a lack of awareness about the need for relaxation. *Anxiety* is an appropriate diagnosis because the client is demonstrating impatience and an inability to relax. (P)

34. **2.** The nurse must present reality to the client about his condition to help decrease his denial about his physical status. By stating the name of the condition and talking about what it means, the nurse provides the client with information and conveys concerns about him and a willingness to help him understand his illness. It may not be true that the client would be made more upset by the call; the news might be good. However, this statement does not provide the client with the reality of his condition. Telling the client that he really doesn't care or asking the client if he realizes that he has a life-threatening condition is belittling and may make the client defensive. (P)

35. **1.** Leaving the hospital and immediately flying to a meeting indicates poor judgment by the client and little understanding of what she needs to change regarding her lifestyle. The other statements show that the client understands some of the changes she needs to make to decrease her stress and lead a more healthy lifestyle. (P)

36. **1, 3, 5.** Suicide is a risk with chronic illnesses. The husband needs validation of his feelings and support as well as suggestions for helping his wife with her concerns. Telling him to be strong and optimistic ignores the client's needs. It is false to assume that the client will no longer be suicidal when the lupus is under control. (P)

37. **4.** The nurse's best response is one that directly expresses the nurse's observations to the client and offers the client the opportunity to talk about his feelings or concerns to decrease somatization (the need to express feelings through physical symptoms). Leaving, offering to provide pain medication, and stating that anger does not bother the nurse ignore the client's needs. (P)

38. **3.** The client with ulcerative colitis commonly has a personality trait described as obsessive-compulsive with behaviors such as perfectionism, conformity, rigidity, and obstinacy. (P)

39. **4.** This type of behavior illustrates *emotional lability*, which is a readily changeable or unstable emotional affect. *Neologism* is using a word when it can have two or more meanings, or a play on words. *Confabulation* involves replacing memory loss by fantasy to hide confusion; it is unconscious behavior. *Flight of ideas* refers to a rapid succession of verbal expressions that jump from one topic to another and are only superficially related. (P)

Therapeutic Communication

40. **4.** A client who can openly express feelings to the nurse or significant others is coping in a healthy way. A client who directs anger at himself is in danger of becoming depressed and, possibly, suicidal. If the client calls the nurse each time he is anxious, the client is not learning to use coping skills to express feelings. Crying frequently is also a sign of depression that can deepen if not addressed. (P)

41. **3.** Active listening is a helping response that communicates caring and understanding. Understanding that it's hard but assuring the wife that things will work out expresses empathy but follows it with false reassurance. Discussing coping strategies for her husband's death is premature at this stage of the wife's grieving when she has not fully considered her life after her husband dies. Urging her to spend less time at the hospital suggests that she avoid confronting her husband's dying, an action that won't assist her in coping with the loss. (P)

42. **1.** Because the client with ADHD is easily distractable, it is important to obtain eye contact before explaining the task. Simple language and having him repeat what he is told are necessary because of his age. Praise encourages the client to repeat the task in the future as well as building the client's self-esteem. A full explanation with verbal praise and a food reward is inappropriate because a food reward increases the chance that he will expect a physical reward for completing tasks. In addition, a full explanation might be too confusing for someone his age. Explaining consequences focuses on punishment, rather than praise. Although demonstration and imitation is an effective teaching method, rewarding with food fosters dependence on food reward for task completion. (P)

43. **4.** In a facilitating response, the client's feelings and their underlying cause are acknowledged. The nurse should not assume that she knows how the client feels. The nurse should also avoid offering false reassurance that the client's husband will love her and find her attractive or that everything will eventually be fine, neither of which may be true. (P)

44. **1, 2, 3.** Active listening facilitates trust. It means that the nurse acknowledges that she has heard the client and indicates in her own words an understanding of what the client says and the emotions underlying what is said. It also involves encouraging the client to say more. Constant eye contact and standing very close to a client can be unnerving and can hamper trust building. (P)

45. 2, 3, 4, 5. The nurse's effective communication helps the client know what to expect regarding treatment, which promotes trust and cooperation. Such trust and cooperation result in an enhanced quality of nursing care. Effective communication also involves listening to the client's concerns. Nurses should not aim to control the actions of their clients. (P)

46. 4. Because the client is new to the unit and may not have fully comprehended the limits of the nurse-client relationship, a review of the purpose of the nurse-client relationship is appropriate. Telling the client that he does not understand the limits of this relationship acknowledges the client's lack of understanding, but does not adequately address his lack of knowledge. Attempts to interpret the client's behavior as an indication of other difficulties might be accurate, but could upset the client. The nurse would need to validate the interpretation with the client. The nurse should not assume that the client's invitation demonstrates a lack of respect for her, rather than a potential socialization problem. (P)

47. 2. Having another nurse work with the client allows the client to make progress toward completion of the program. Having the original nurse meet with the client after the nurse's recovery acknowledges their bond and helps the client learn how to acknowledge and manage termination with a trusted caregiver. A letter is impersonal and implies that the nurse is at fault for becoming ill. Doing nothing ignores the challenges of termination altogether and abandons the client. Waiting until the nurse is well enough to telephone the client puts the burden of termination on the ill nurse at a time that the nurse may still not feel well or be ready to deal with emotional issues. Any termination done on the phone is less personal than a face-to-face meeting and should be done only if no other option is viable. (P)

48. 3. Asking the client to explain more gives her an opportunity to express her concerns. In offering reassurance that the pill is safe for all ages, the nurse fails to adequately explore the client's concern. Asking if the client thinks her age is her concern, the nurse suggests what might be the client's concern, and does not allow the client the opportunity to identify her own concerns. Although offering another option acknowledges the concern and suggests other possibilities, it does not provide an opportunity for the client to express her own views. (P)

Postreview tests

1. A client with human immunodeficiency virus (HIV) and acquired immunodeficiency syndrome confides that he is homosexual and his employer does not know his HIV status. Which response by the nurse is best?

☐ **1.** "Would you like me to help you tell them?"

☐ **2.** "The information you confide in me is confidential."

☐ **3.** "I must share this information with your family."

☐ **4.** "I must share this information with your employer."

2. The mother of a child with bronchial asthma tells the nurse that the child wants a pet. Which of the following pets should the nurse tell the mother is most appropriate?

☐ **1.** Cat.

☐ **2.** Fish.

☐ **3.** Gerbil.

☐ **4.** Canary.

3. An elderly client is being admitted to same-day surgery for cataract extraction. The client has several diamond rings. The nurse should explain to the client that:

☐ **1.** Her rings will be taped before the surgery.

☐ **2.** She will sign a valuables envelope that will be placed in a safe.

☐ **3.** The rings will be locked in the narcotics box.

☐ **4.** The nursing supervisor will hold onto the rings during the surgery.

4. When an infant resumes taking oral feedings after surgery to correct intussusception, the parents comment that the child seems to suck on the pacifier more since the surgery. The nurse explains that sucking on a pacifier:

☐ **1.** Provides an outlet for emotional tension.

☐ **2.** Indicates readiness to take solid foods.

☐ **3.** Indicates intestinal motility.

☐ **4.** Is an attempt to get attention from the parents.

5. Under which circumstance may a nurse communicate medical information without the client's consent?

☐ **1.** When certifying the client's absence from work.

☐ **2.** When requested by the client's family.

☐ **3.** When treating the client with a sexually transmitted disease.

☐ **4.** When ordered by another physician.

6. A 22-year-old client is brought to the emergency department with his fiancée after being involved in a serious motor vehicle accident. His Glasgow Coma Scale score is 7 and he demonstrates evidence of decorticate posturing. Which of the following is appropriate for obtaining permission to place a catheter for intracranial pressure (ICP) monitoring?

☐ **1.** The nurse will obtain a signed consent from the client's fiancée because he is of legal age and they are engaged to be married.

☐ **2.** The physician will get a consultation from another physician and proceed with placement of the ICP catheter until the family arrives to sign the consent.

☐ **3.** Two nurses will receive a verbal consent by telephone from the client's next of kin before inserting the catheter.

☐ **4.** The physician will document the emergency nature of the client's condition and that an ICP catheter for monitoring was placed without a consent.

7. A 68-year-old client's daughter is asking about the follow-up evaluation for her father after his pneumonectomy for primary lung cancer. The nurse's best response is which of the following?

☐ **1.** "The usual follow-up is chest X-ray and liver function tests every 3 months."

☐ **2.** "The follow-up for your father will be a chest X-ray and a computed tomography scan of the abdomen every year."

☐ **3.** "No follow-up is needed at this time."

☐ **4.** "The follow-up for your father will be a chest X-ray every 6 months."

8. The nurse is preparing to administer blood to an otherwise healthy client who requires postoperative blood replacement. The nurse is aware that the blood administration set must include a:

☐ **1.** Micron mesh filter.

☐ **2.** Nonfiltered blood administration set.

☐ **3.** Special leukocyte-poor filter.

☐ **4.** Microdrip administration set.

9. During the health history interview, which of the following strategies is the most effective for the nurse to use to help clients feel that they have an active role in their health care?
☐ **1.** Ask clients to complete a questionnaire.
☐ **2.** Provide clients with written instructions.
☐ **3.** Ask clients for their description of events and for their views concerning past medical care.
☐ **4.** Ask clients if they have any questions.

10. A client with severe major depression states, "My heart has stopped and my blood is black ash." The nurse interprets this statement to be evidence of which of the following?
☐ **1.** Hallucination.
☐ **2.** Illusion.
☐ **3.** Delusion.
☐ **4.** Paranoia.

11. When a client wants to read his chart, the nurse should:
☐ **1.** Call the doctor to obtain permission.
☐ **2.** Give the client the chart and answer questions for him.
☐ **3.** Tell the client that he can read the chart when the doctor makes rounds.
☐ **4.** Ask the client what he wants to know and answer those questions without giving him the chart.

12. A client with a fractured leg has been instructed to ambulate without weight bearing on the affected leg. The nurse evaluates that the client is ambulating correctly if she uses which of the following crutch-walking gaits?
☐ **1.** Two-point gait.
☐ **2.** Four-point gait.
☐ **3.** Three-point gait.
☐ **4.** Swing-to gait.

13. A client with major depression states, "Life isn't worth living anymore. Nothing matters." Which of the following responses by the nurse is best?
☐ **1.** "Are you thinking about killing yourself?"
☐ **2.** "Things will get better, you know."
☐ **3.** "Why do you think that way?"
☐ **4.** "You shouldn't feel that way."

14. A client with bipolar 1 disorder has been prescribed olanzapine (Zyprexa) 5 mg two times a day and lamotrigine (Lamictal) 25 mg two times a day. Which of the following adverse effects should the nurse report to the physician immediately? Select all that apply.
☐ **1.** Rash.
☐ **2.** Nausea.
☐ **3.** Sedation.
☐ **4.** Hyperthermia.
☐ **5.** Muscle rigidity.

15. A client is prescribed atropine 0.4 mg intramuscularly. The atropine vial is labeled 0.5 mg/ml. How many milliliters should the nurse plan to administer?

_____ ml

16. A multiparous client tells the nurse that she is using medroxyprogesterone (Depo-Provera) for contraception. The nurse instructs the client to increase her intake of which of the following?
☐ **1.** Folic acid.
☐ **2.** Vitamin C.
☐ **3.** Magnesium.
☐ **4.** Calcium.

17. Which of the following statements made by a pregnant woman in the first trimester are consistent with this stage of pregnancy? Select all that apply.
☐ **1.** "My husband told his friends we will have to give up the Mustang for a minivan."
☐ **2.** "Oh my, how did this happen? I don't need this now."
☐ **3.** "I can't wait to see my baby. Do you think it will have my blond hair and blue eyes?"
☐ **4.** "I used a Disney theme for decorating the room."
☐ **5.** "I wonder how it will feel to buy maternity clothes and be fat."
☐ **6.** "We went to the mall yesterday to buy a crib and dressing table."

18. The nurse is teaching a client about topical gentamicin sulfate (Garamycin). Which of the following comments by the client indicates the need for additional teaching?
☐ **1.** "I will avoid being out in the sun for long periods."
☐ **2.** "I should stop applying it once the infected area heals."
☐ **3.** "I'll call the physician if the condition worsens."
☐ **4.** "I should apply it to large open areas."

19. A client has been taking imipramine (Tofranil) for his depression for 2 days. His sister asks the nurse, "Why is he still so depressed?" Which of the following responses by the nurse is most appropriate?
☐ **1.** "Your brother is experiencing a very serious depression."
☐ **2.** "I'll be sure to convey your concern to his physician."
☐ **3.** "It takes 2 to 4 weeks for the drug to reach its full effect."
☐ **4.** "Perhaps we need to change his medication."

20. Which interventions should the nurse use to assist the client with grandiose delusions? Select all that apply.
- [ ] **1.** Accepting the client while not arguing with the delusion.
- [ ] **2.** Focusing on the feelings or meaning of the delusion.
- [ ] **3.** Focusing on events and topics based in reality.
- [ ] **4.** Confronting the client's beliefs.
- [ ] **5.** Interacting with the client only when he is based in reality.

21. A multigravid client visiting the prenatal clinic at 16 weeks' gestation exhibits facial swelling, a brownish vaginal discharge, and fundal height of 22 cm. The client's blood pressure is 160/90 mm Hg and her pulse is 80 bpm. The nurse interprets these findings as suggestive of which of the following?
- [ ] **1.** Placenta previa.
- [ ] **2.** Fetal anemia.
- [ ] **3.** Multifetal pregnancy.
- [ ] **4.** Gestational trophoblastic disease.

22. Which of the following responses is most helpful for a client who is euphoric, intrusive, and interrupts other clients engaged in conversations to the point where they get up and leave or walk away?
- [ ] **1.** "When you interrupt others, they leave the area."
- [ ] **2.** "You are being rude and uncaring."
- [ ] **3.** "You should remember to use your manners."
- [ ] **4.** "You know better than to interrupt someone."

23. The nurse coordinates with the laboratory staff to have the gentamicin trough serum level drawn. At what time should the blood be drawn in relation to the administration of the I.V. dose of gentamicin sulfate (Garamycin)?
- [ ] **1.** 2 hours before the administration of the next I.V. dose.
- [ ] **2.** 3 hours before the administration of the next I.V. dose.
- [ ] **3.** 4 hours before the administration of the next I.V. dose.
- [ ] **4.** Just before the administration of the next I.V. dose.

24. Older adults with known cardiovascular disease must balance which of the following measures for optimum health?
- [ ] **1.** Diet, exercise, and medication.
- [ ] **2.** Stress, hypertension, and pain.
- [ ] **3.** Mental health, diet, and stress.
- [ ] **4.** Social events, diet, and smoking.

25. A 4-year-old is brought to the emergency department with sudden onset of a temperature of 103° F (39.5° C), sore throat, and refusal to drink. The child will not lie down and prefers to lean forward while sitting up. Which of the following should the nurse do next?
- [ ] **1.** Give 600 mg of acetaminophen (Tylenol) rectally, as ordered.
- [ ] **2.** Inspect the child's throat for redness and swelling.
- [ ] **3.** Have an appropriate-sized tracheostomy tube readily available.
- [ ] **4.** Obtain a specimen for a throat culture.

26. Assessment of a client taking lithium reveals dry mouth, nausea, thirst, and mild hand tremor. Based on an analysis of these findings, which of the following should the nurse do next?
- [ ] **1.** Hold the lithium and obtain a stat lithium level to determine therapeutic effectiveness.
- [ ] **2.** Continue the lithium and immediately notify the physician about the assessment findings.
- [ ] **3.** Continue the lithium and reassure the client that these temporary side effects will subside.
- [ ] **4.** Hold the lithium and monitor the client for signs and symptoms of increasing toxicity.

27. A client asks the nurse how long she has to take her medicine for hypothyroidism. The nurse's response is based on the knowledge that:
- [ ] **1.** Lifelong daily medicine is necessary.
- [ ] **2.** The medication is expensive, and the dose can be reduced in a few months.
- [ ] **3.** The medication can be gradually withdrawn in 1 to 2 years.
- [ ] **4.** The medication can be discontinued after the client's thyroid-stimulating hormone level is normal.

28. Assessment of which of the following clients should lead the nurse to expect the physician to order an adjustment in lithium dosage?
- [ ] **1.** A client who continues work as a computer programmer.
- [ ] **2.** A client who attends college classes.
- [ ] **3.** A client who can now care for her children.
- [ ] **4.** A client who is beginning training for a tennis team.

29. A client admitted with a gastric ulcer has been vomiting bright red blood. His hemoglobin level is 5.11 g/dl, and his blood pressure is 100/50 mm Hg. The client and his family state that their religious beliefs do not support the use of blood products and refuse blood transfusions as a treatment for the bleeding. The nurse should expect that the next step in the treatment plan is to:
- [ ] **1.** Discontinue all measures.
- [ ] **2.** Notify the hospital attorney.
- [ ] **3.** Attempt to stabilize the client through the use of fluid replacement.
- [ ] **4.** Give enough blood to keep the client from dying.

30. The parents of a child with cystic fibrosis express concern about how the disease was transmitted to their child. The nurse should explain that:
☐ **1.** A disease carrier also has the disease.
☐ **2.** Two parents who are carriers may produce a child who has the disease.
☐ **3.** A disease carrier and an affected person will never have children with the disease.
☐ **4.** A disease carrier and an affected person will have a child with the disease.

31. A client with angina shows the nurse her nitroglycerin (Nitrostat) that she carries in a plastic bag in her pocket. The nurse instructs the client that nitroglycerin should be kept in:
☐ **1.** The refrigerator.
☐ **2.** A cool, moist place.
☐ **3.** A dark container to shield from light.
☐ **4.** A plastic bag where it is readily available.

32. The nurse caring for a client on the telemetry unit determines that the client is in sinus bradycardia by recognizing which characteristics? Select all that apply.
☐ **1.** P wave present.
☐ **2.** Ventricular rate of 50 bpm.
☐ **3.** Atrial rate of 120 bpm.
☐ **4.** PR interval ranging from 0.12 to 0.20 second.
☐ **5.** ST-segment elevation greater than 0 .01 mm.
☐ **6.** A P wave in front of every QRS complex.

33. When teaching a client with bipolar disorder, mania, who has started to take valproic acid (Depakene) about possible side effects of this medication, the nurse should include which of the following in the teaching plan?
☐ **1.** Increased urination.
☐ **2.** Slowed thinking.
☐ **3.** Sedation.
☐ **4.** Weight loss.

34. An infant is born with facial abnormalities, growth retardation, mental retardation, and vision abnormalities. These abnormalities are probably caused by maternal:
☐ **1.** Alcohol consumption.
☐ **2.** Vitamin B_6 deficiency.
☐ **3.** Vitamin A deficiency.
☐ **4.** Folic acid deficiency.

35. Nonsteroidal anti-inflammatory drugs (NSAIDs) are commonly used in the treatment of musculoskeletal conditions. It is important for the nurse to remind the client to:
☐ **1.** Take NSAIDs at least three times per day.
☐ **2.** Exercise the joints at least 1 hour after taking the medication.
☐ **3.** Take antacids 1 hour after taking NSAIDs.
☐ **4.** Take NSAIDs with food.

36. The nurse should suspect that the client taking disulfiram (Antabuse) has ingested alcohol when the client exhibits which of the following symptoms?
☐ **1.** Sore throat and muscle aches.
☐ **2.** Nausea and flushing of the face and neck.
☐ **3.** Fever and muscle soreness.
☐ **4.** Bradycardia and vertigo.

37. The nurse holds the gauze pledget against an I.M. injection site while removing the needle from the muscle. This technique helps to:
☐ **1.** Seal off the track left by the needle in the tissue.
☐ **2.** Speed the spread of the medication in the tissue.
☐ **3.** Avoid the discomfort of the needle pulling on the skin.
☐ **4.** Prevent organisms from entering the body through the skin puncture.

38. A client whose condition remains stable after a myocardial infarction gradually increases his activity. Which the following conditions should the nurse assess to determine whether the activity is appropriate for the client?
☐ **1.** Edema.
☐ **2.** Cyanosis.
☐ **3.** Dyspnea.
☐ **4.** Weight loss.

39. When a client with alcohol dependency begins to talk about not having a problem with alcohol, the nurse should use which of the following approaches?
☐ **1.** Questioning the client about how much alcohol she drinks.
☐ **2.** Confronting the client with the fact that she was intoxicated 2 days ago.
☐ **3.** Pointing out how alcohol has gotten her into trouble.
☐ **4.** Listening to what the client states and then asking her how she plans to stay sober.

40. Which of the following correctly describes Medicaid?
☐ **1.** A program designed to assist ill, low-income older adults.
☐ **2.** A federal insurance program for pregnant women.
☐ **3.** A joint federal-state program for low-income persons.
☐ **4.** A program administered by health maintenance organizations.

41. The nurse is preparing a teaching plan for a 45-year-old client recently diagnosed with type 2 diabetes mellitus. What is the first step in this process?
☐ **1.** Establish goals.
☐ **2.** Choose video materials and brochures.
☐ **3.** Assess the client's learning needs.
☐ **4.** Set priorities of learning needs.

42. A loading dose of digoxin (Lanoxin) is given to a client newly diagnosed with atrial fibrillation. The nurse begins instructing the client about the medication and the importance of monitoring his heart rate. An expected outcome of the education program will be:
☐ 1. A return demonstration of palpating the radial pulse.
☐ 2. A return demonstration of how to take the medication.
☐ 3. Verbalization of why the client has atrial fibrillation.
☐ 4. Verbalization of the need for the medication.

43. A multigravid client is scheduled for a percutaneous umbilical blood sampling procedure. The nurse instructs the client that this procedure is useful for diagnosing which of the following?
☐ 1. Twin pregnancies.
☐ 2. Fetal lung maturation.
☐ 3. Rh disease.
☐ 4. Alpha fetoprotein level.

44. Which of the following is an adverse effect of vancomycin (Vancocin) and needs to be reported promptly?
☐ 1. Vertigo.
☐ 2. Tinnitus.
☐ 3. Muscle stiffness.
☐ 4. Ataxia.

45. Which of the following statements indicates that the client with a peptic ulcer understands the dietary modifications he needs to follow at home?
☐ 1. "I should eat a bland, soft diet."
☐ 2. "It is important to eat six small meals a day."
☐ 3. "I should drink several glasses of milk a day."
☐ 4. "I should avoid alcohol and caffeine."

46. The client with a nasogastric (NG) tube begins to complain of abdominal distention. Which of the following measures should the nurse implement first?
☐ 1. Call the physician.
☐ 2. Irrigate the NG tube.
☐ 3. Check the function of the suction equipment.
☐ 4. Reposition the NG tube.

47. A male client has been diagnosed as having a low sperm count during infertility studies. After instructions by the nurse about some causes of low sperm counts, the nurse determines that the client needs further instructions when he says low sperm counts may be caused by which of the following?
☐ 1. Varicocele.
☐ 2. Frequent use of saunas.
☐ 3. Endocrine imbalances.
☐ 4. Decreased body temperature.

48. The nurse assesses a client and notes puffy eyelids, swollen ankles, and crackles at both lung bases. The nurse understands that these clinical findings are most specifically associated with fluid excess in which of the following compartments?
☐ 1. Interstitial compartment.
☐ 2. Intravascular compartment.
☐ 3. Extracellular compartment.
☐ 4. Intracellular compartment.

49. An expected physiologic response to a low potassium level is:
☐ 1. Cardiac dysrhythmias.
☐ 2. Hyperglycemia.
☐ 3. Hypertension.
☐ 4. Increased energy.

50. When teaching unlicensed assistive personnel about the importance of handwashing in preventing disease, the nurse makes which of the following statements?
☐ 1. "It is not necessary to wash your hands as long as you use gloves."
☐ 2. "Handwashing is the best method for preventing cross-contamination."
☐ 3. "Waterless commercial products are not effective for killing organisms."
☐ 4. "The hands do not serve as a source of infection."

51. The nurse is performing Leopold's maneuvers on a woman who is in her eighth month of pregnancy. The nurse is palpating the uterus as shown below. Which of the following maneuvers is the nurse performing?
☐ 1. First maneuver.
☐ 2. Second maneuver.
☐ 3. Third maneuver.
☐ 4. Fourth maneuver.

52. A client in a cardiac rehabilitation program states that he would like to make sure he is eating the right foods to ensure adequate endurance on the treadmill. Which of the following nutrients is most helpful for promoting endurance during sustained activity?
- ☐ **1.** Protein.
- ☐ **2.** Carbohydrate.
- ☐ **3.** Fat.
- ☐ **4.** Water.

53. A client's chest tube is connected to a drainage system with a water seal. The nurse notes that the fluid in the water-seal column is fluctuating with each breath that the client takes. The fluctuation means that:
- ☐ **1.** There is an obstruction in the chest tube.
- ☐ **2.** The client is developing subcutaneous emphysema.
- ☐ **3.** The chest tube system is functioning properly.
- ☐ **4.** There is a leak in the chest tube system.

54. A client with diabetes is explaining to the nurse how she will care for her feet at home. Which statement indicates that the client understands proper foot care?
- ☐ **1.** "When I injure my toe, I will plan to put iodine on it."
- ☐ **2.** "I should inspect my feet at least once a week."
- ☐ **3.** "It is okay to go barefoot in the house."
- ☐ **4.** "It is important to dry my feet carefully after my bath."

55. The nurse assesses a client with diverticulitis and suspects peritonitis when which of the following symptoms is noted?
- ☐ **1.** Hyperactive bowel sounds.
- ☐ **2.** Rigid abdominal wall.
- ☐ **3.** Explosive diarrhea.
- ☐ **4.** Excessive flatulence.

56. A nurse is assessing a client who has a potential diagnosis of pancreatitis. Which risk factors predispose the client to pancreatitis? Select all that apply.
- ☐ **1.** Excessive alcohol use.
- ☐ **2.** Gallstones.
- ☐ **3.** Abdominal trauma.
- ☐ **4.** Hypertension.
- ☐ **5.** Hyperlipidemia with excessive triglycerides.
- ☐ **6.** Hypothyroidism.

57. When performing chest percussion on a child, which of the following techniques should the nurse use?
- ☐ **1.** Firmly but gently striking the chest wall to make a popping sound.
- ☐ **2.** Gently striking the chest wall to make a slapping sound.
- ☐ **3.** Percussing over an area from the umbilicus to the clavicle.
- ☐ **4.** Placing a blanket between the nurse's hand and the child's chest.

58. The nurse walks into the room of a client who has a do not resuscitate order and finds the client without a pulse, respirations, or blood pressure. What is the most appropriate action?
- ☐ **1.** Stay in the room and notify the nursing team for assistance.
- ☐ **2.** Push the emergency alarm to call a code.
- ☐ **3.** Dial the hospital phone number for a code.
- ☐ **4.** Pull the curtain and leave the room.

59. A client is trying to lose weight at a moderate pace. If the client eliminates 1,000 calories per day from his normal intake, how many pounds would he lose in 1 week?
- ☐ **1.** 1 lb.
- ☐ **2.** 2 lb.
- ☐ **3.** 3 lb.
- ☐ **4.** 4 lb.

60. A nulligravid client calls the clinic and tells the nurse that she forgot to take her oral contraceptive this morning. Which of the following should the nurse instruct the client to do?
- ☐ **1.** Take the medication immediately.
- ☐ **2.** Restart the medication in the morning.
- ☐ **3.** Use another form of contraception for 2 weeks.
- ☐ **4.** Take two pills tonight before bedtime.

61. The nurse recognizes that a client with pain disorder is improving when the client says which of the following?
- ☐ **1.** "I need to have a good cry about all the pain I've been in and then not dwell on it."
- ☐ **2.** "I need to find another physician who can accurately diagnose my condition."
- ☐ **3.** "The pain medicine that you gave me helps me to relax."
- ☐ **4.** "I'm angry with all of the doctors I've seen who don't know what they're doing."

62. A client admitted in an acute psychotic state says that she hears terrible voices in the head and thinks her neighbor is out to get her. Which of the following is the nurse's best response?
- ☐ **1.** "What has your neighbor been doing that bothers you?"
- ☐ **2.** "How long have you been hearing these terrible voices?"
- ☐ **3.** "We won't let your neighbor visit, so you'll be safe."
- ☐ **4.** "What exactly are these terrible voices saying to you?"

63. The nurse should assess the client with severe diarrhea for which acid-base imbalance?
- ☐ **1.** Respiratory acidosis.
- ☐ **2.** Respiratory alkalosis.
- ☐ **3.** Metabolic acidosis.
- ☐ **4.** Metabolic alkalosis.

64. A nurse is assessing a client who has heart failure. Which outcome is appropriate for a client with excess fluid volume?
- [ ] **1.** A weight reduction of 10% will occur.
- [ ] **2.** Pain will be controlled effectively.
- [ ] **3.** Arterial blood gas values will be within normal limits.
- [ ] **4.** Serum osmolality will be within normal limits.

65. A 7-year-old child is admitted to the hospital with the medical diagnosis of acute rheumatic fever. Which of the following laboratory blood findings confirms that the child probably has had a streptococcal infection?
- [ ] **1.** High leukocyte count.
- [ ] **2.** Low hemoglobin count.
- [ ] **3.** Elevated antibody concentration.
- [ ] **4.** Low erythrocyte sedimentation rate.

66. A client is scheduled for hip replacement surgery and is interviewed by the nurse in the preadmission testing unit. The client states that he wishes to receive his own blood for the upcoming surgery. What is the nurse's most appropriate response?
- [ ] **1.** Document the client's request on the chart.
- [ ] **2.** Notify the hematology laboratory.
- [ ] **3.** Notify the surgeon's office.
- [ ] **4.** Call the blood bank.

67. A client needs surgery to relieve an intestinal obstruction. The nurse receives the following set of orders for the client. Which of the following orders should the nurse question before performing?
- [ ] **1.** Tap water enemas until clear.
- [ ] **2.** Out of bed as tolerated.
- [ ] **3.** Neomycin sulfate 1 g P.O. every 4 hours.
- [ ] **4.** Betadine scrub to abdomen.

68. After teaching a client about collecting a stool sample for occult testing, which client statement indicates effective teaching? Select all that apply.
- [ ] **1.** "I will avoid eating meat for 1 to 3 days before getting a stool sample."
- [ ] **2.** "I need to eat foods low in fiber a few days before collecting the sample."
- [ ] **3.** "I'll take the sample from different areas of the stool that I have passed."
- [ ] **4.** "I need to send the stool sample to the lab in a covered container right away."
- [ ] **5.** "I can continue to take all of my regular medications at home."

69. A client who is on nothing-by-mouth status is constantly asking for a drink. Which of the following is the most appropriate nursing intervention?
- [ ] **1.** Reexplain to the client why she cannot drink.
- [ ] **2.** Offer ice chips every hour to decrease thirst.
- [ ] **3.** Offer the client frequent oral hygiene care.
- [ ] **4.** Divert the client's attention by turning on the television.

70. A female client is admitted with complaints of fatigue, cold intolerance, weight gain, and muscle weakness. The initial nursing assessment reveals brittle nails, dry hair, constipation, and possible goiter. The client is most likely experiencing signs and symptoms of:
- [ ] **1.** Cushing's disease.
- [ ] **2.** Hypothyroidism.
- [ ] **3.** Hyperthyroidism.
- [ ] **4.** A pituitary tumor.

71. A mother visiting the clinic for a routine visit with her 10-year-old daughter reports that her daughter has an increase in hair growth and breast enlargement. The nurse explains to the mother and daughter that after the symptoms of puberty are noticed, menstruation typically occurs within which of the following time frames?
- [ ] **1.** 6 months.
- [ ] **2.** 12 months.
- [ ] **3.** 30 months.
- [ ] **4.** 36 months.

72. While a mother is feeding her full-term neonate 1 hour after birth, she asks the nurse, "What are these white dots in my baby's mouth? I tried to wash them out, but they're still there." After assessing the neonate's mouth, the nurse explains that these spots are which of the following?
- [ ] **1.** Koplik's spots.
- [ ] **2.** Epstein's pearls.
- [ ] **3.** Precocious teeth.
- [ ] **4.** Thrush curds.

73. The nurse should suspect esophageal atresia and tracheoesophageal fistula (TEF) in a newborn exhibiting which of the following symptoms initially? Select all that apply.
- [ ] **1.** Copious frothy mucus.
- [ ] **2.** Episodes of cyanosis.
- [ ] **3.** Several loose stools.
- [ ] **4.** Initial weight loss.
- [ ] **5.** Poor gag reflex.

74. Which of the following factors is most important for healing an infected decubitus ulcer?
- [ ] **1.** Adequate circulatory status.
- [ ] **2.** Scheduled periods of rest.
- [ ] **3.** Balanced nutritional diet.
- [ ] **4.** Fluid intake of 1,500 ml/day.

75. A client is receiving digoxin (Lanoxin). His pulse range is normally 70 to 76 bpm. After assessing the apical pulse for 1 minute and finding it to be 60 bpm, the nurse should initially:
- [ ] **1.** Call the physician for orders.
- [ ] **2.** Withhold the digoxin.
- [ ] **3.** Administer the digoxin.
- [ ] **4.** Notify the charge nurse.

76. While shopping at a local mall, the nurse hears a pregnant client yell, "Oh my! The baby's coming!" After placing the client in a supine position and trying to maintain some privacy, the nurse sees that the neonate's head is delivering. Which of the following should the nurse do first?
☐ **1.** Suction the mouth with two fingertips.
☐ **2.** Check for presence of a cord around the neck.
☐ **3.** Tell the client to bear down with force.
☐ **4.** Advise the mother that help is on the way.

77. The nurse is preparing a discharge plan for a 16-year-old who has fractured her femur and ulna. The client asks the nurse how quickly her fractures will heal so she can return to her normal activities. Which of the following responses is most appropriate for the nurse to make?
☐ **1.** "The healing of your leg will be delayed because you have had skeletal traction."
☐ **2.** "It will take your arm about 12 weeks to heal completely, but it will take your leg about 24 weeks."
☐ **3.** "Because you are young and healthy, your bones should heal in less than 12 weeks."
☐ **4.** "You will require long-term rehabilitation and should expect it to take at least 8 months for your bones to heal."

78. A client with delirium becomes very anxious and says, "I can't stop what is happening to me. Make it stop, please!" Which of the following is the nurse's most appropriate response?
☐ **1.** "I'll get you some medicine to help you relax. The more you worry, the worse it will get."
☐ **2.** "As soon as we know what's causing this, we can try to stop it. I'll get you some medicine to help you relax."
☐ **3.** "I wish I could do something to make it stop, but unfortunately I can't."
☐ **4.** "I'll sit with you until you calm down a little."

79. After teaching a primigravid client at 10 weeks' gestation about the recommendations for exercise during pregnancy, which of the following client statements indicates successful teaching?
☐ **1.** "While pregnant, I should avoid contact sports."
☐ **2.** "Even though I'm pregnant, I can learn to ski next month."
☐ **3.** "While we are on vacation next month, I can continue to scuba dive."
☐ **4.** "Sitting in a hot tub after exercise will help me to relax."

80. The nurse is caring for a client who has had a myocardial infarction involving a large section of the heart muscle. The nurse anticipates that the client is at risk for:
☐ **1.** Cardiogenic shock.
☐ **2.** Hypovolemic shock.
☐ **3.** Neurogenic shock.
☐ **4.** Metabolic shock.

81. The nurse is assessing a client who has had a myocardial infarction. The nurse notes the cardiac rhythm shown below. The nurse identifies that this rhythm is:
☐ **1.** Atrial fibrillation.
☐ **2.** Ventricular tachycardia.
☐ **3.** Premature ventricular contractions.
☐ **4.** Third-degree heart block.

82. The physician has ordered a chemotherapy drug to be administered to a client every day for the next week. The client is on an adult medical-surgical floor but the nurse assigned to the client has not been trained to handle chemotherapy agents. What is the nurse's most appropriate response?
☐ **1.** Send the client to the oncology floor for administration of the medication.
☐ **2.** Ask a nurse from the oncology floor to come to the client and administer the medication.
☐ **3.** Ask another nurse to help mix the chemotherapy agent.
☐ **4.** Ask the pharmacy to mix the chemotherapy agent and administer it.

83. Which of the following nursing diagnoses should the nurse identify as a priority after surgical repair of a cleft lip?
☐ **1.** *Acute pain.*
☐ **2.** *Risk for infection.*
☐ **3.** *Impaired physical mobility.*
☐ **4.** *Impaired parenting.*

84. Which of the following is an appropriate outcome for a client with rheumatoid arthritis?
☐ **1.** The client will manage joint pain and fatigue to perform activities of daily living.
☐ **2.** The client will maintain full range of motion in joints.
☐ **3.** The client will prevent the development of further pain and joint deformity.
☐ **4.** The client will take anti-inflammatory medications as indicated by the presence of disease symptoms.

85. A client's burn wounds are being cleaned twice a day in a hydrotherapy tub. Which of the following interventions should be included in the plan of care before a hydrotherapy treatment is initiated?
- ☐ **1.** Limit food and fluids 45 minutes before therapy to prevent nausea and vomiting.
- ☐ **2.** Increase the I.V. flow rate to offset fluids lost through the therapy.
- ☐ **3.** Apply a topical antibiotic cream to burns to prevent infection.
- ☐ **4.** Administer pain medication 30 minutes before therapy to help manage pain.

86. A health care provider has been exposed to hepatitis B through a needlestick. Which of the following drugs should the nurse anticipate administering as postexposure prophylaxis?
- ☐ **1.** Hepatitis B immune globulin.
- ☐ **2.** Interferon.
- ☐ **3.** Hepatitis B surface antigen.
- ☐ **4.** Amphotericin B.

87. When performing an otoscopic examination of the tympanic membrane of a 2-year-old child, the nurse should pull the pinna in which of the following directions?
- ☐ **1.** Down and back.
- ☐ **2.** Down and slightly forward.
- ☐ **3.** Up and back.
- ☐ **4.** Up and forward.

88. Which of the following findings should the nurse note in the client who is in the compensatory stage of shock?
- ☐ **1.** Decreased urinary output.
- ☐ **2.** Significant hypotension.
- ☐ **3.** Tachycardia.
- ☐ **4.** Mental confusion.

89. A client has been prescribed hydrochlorothiazide (HydroDIURIL) to treat heart failure. For which of the following symptoms should the nurse monitor the client?
- ☐ **1.** Urinary retention.
- ☐ **2.** Muscle weakness.
- ☐ **3.** Confusion.
- ☐ **4.** Diaphoresis.

90. The son of a client with Alzheimer's disease excitedly tells the nurse, "Mom was singing one of her favorite old songs. I think she's getting her memory back!" Which of the following responses by the nurse is most appropriate?
- ☐ **1.** "She still has long-term memory, but her short-term memory will not return."
- ☐ **2.** "I'm so happy to hear that. Maybe she is getting better."
- ☐ **3.** "Don't get your hopes up. This is only a temporary improvement."
- ☐ **4.** "I'm glad she can sing even if she can't talk to you."

91. The nurse collects a urine specimen from a client for a culture and sensitivity analysis. Which of the following is the correct care of the specimen?
- ☐ **1.** Promptly send the specimen to the laboratory.
- ☐ **2.** Send the specimen with the next pickup.
- ☐ **3.** Send the specimen the next time a nursing assistant is available.
- ☐ **4.** Store the specimen in the refrigerator until it can be sent to the laboratory.

92. A 16-year-old client is in the emergency department for treatment of minor injuries from a car accident. A crisis nurse is with her because she became hysterical and was saying, "It's my fault. My Mom is going to kill me. I don't even have a way home." Which of the following should be the nurse's initial intervention?
- ☐ **1.** Hold her hands and say, "Slow down. Take a deep breath."
- ☐ **2.** Say, "Calm down. The police can take you home."
- ☐ **3.** Put a hand on her shoulder and say, "It wasn't your fault."
- ☐ **4.** Say, "Your mother is not going to kill you. Stop worrying."

93. The nurse is developing a community health education program about sexually transmitted diseases. Which information about women who acquire gonorrhea should be included?
- ☐ **1.** Women are more reluctant than men to seek medical treatment.
- ☐ **2.** Gonorrhea is not easily transmitted to women who are menopausal.
- ☐ **3.** Women with gonorrhea are usually asymptomatic.
- ☐ **4.** Gonorrhea is usually a mild disease for women.

94. A client has his leg immobilized in a long leg cast. Which of the following assessments indicates the early beginning of circulatory impairment?
- ☐ **1.** Inability to move toes.
- ☐ **2.** Cyanosis of toes.
- ☐ **3.** Complaints of cast tightness.
- ☐ **4.** Tingling of toes.

95. While feeding a term neonate at age 2 hours, the nurse observes that the neonate has a drooping appearance on the left side of the face. The nurse notifies the physician based on the understanding that this is associated with which of the following?
- ☐ **1.** Craniotabes.
- ☐ **2.** Meningitis.
- ☐ **3.** Facial nerve damage.
- ☐ **4.** Skull fracture.

96. A client tells the nurse that she has had sexual contact with someone whom she suspects has genital herpes. Which of the following instructions should the nurse give the client in response to this information?

☐ **1.** Anticipate lesions within 25 to 30 days.

☐ **2.** Continue sexual activity unless lesions are present.

☐ **3.** Report any difficulty urinating.

☐ **4.** Drink extra fluids to prevent lesions from forming.

97. The nurse is assigned to a client with irreversible shock. The nurse realizes that the negative outcomes of irreversible shock include severe hypoperfusion to all vital organs and failure of vital functions. Therefore, the nurse will monitor the client for:

☐ **1.** Increased alertness.

☐ **2.** Circulatory collapse.

☐ **3.** Hypertension.

☐ **4.** Diuresis.

98. The nurse is caring for a client who has been diagnosed with deep vein thrombosis. When assessing the client's vital signs, the nurse notes an apical pulse of 150 bpm, a respiratory rate of 46 breaths/minute, and blood pressure of 100/60 mm Hg. The client appears anxious and restless. What should be the nurse's first course of action?

☐ **1.** Notify the physician.

☐ **2.** Administer a sedative.

☐ **3.** Try to elicit a positive Homan's sign.

☐ **4.** Increase the flow rate of intravenous fluids.

99. The charge nurse should give a new graduate nurse who made an insulin medication error which of the following advice?

☐ **1.** "Trust your judgment; don't listen to your client."

☐ **2.** "Compare the insulin doses that other clients are receiving."

☐ **3.** "Large doses must always be double-checked."

☐ **4.** "Use 'U' as an abbreviation for 'unit.'"

100. A client who has Ménière's disease is trying to cope with the chronic tinnitus that she is experiencing. Which of the following interventions is most appropriate for the nurse to suggest for coping with the tinnitus?

☐ **1.** Maintain a quiet environment.

☐ **2.** Play background music.

☐ **3.** Avoid caffeine and nicotine.

☐ **4.** Take a mild sedative.

101. A 4-year-old child who has been ill for 4 hours is admitted to the hospital with difficulty swallowing, a sore throat, and severe substernal retractions. The child's temperature is 104° F (40° C), and the apical pulse is 140 bpm. The white blood cell count is 16,000/mm³. Which of the following should the nurse identify as the immediate priority nursing diagnosis?

☐ **1.** *Anxiety* related to need for immediate and unplanned hospitalization.

☐ **2.** *Risk for injury* (airway obstruction) related to epiglottal edema.

☐ **3.** *Impaired gas exchange* related to excessive respiratory effort.

☐ **4.** *Ineffective airway clearance* related to aspiration.

102. Pulmonary function studies have been ordered for a client with emphysema. The nurse should anticipate that the test will demonstrate which of the following results?

☐ **1.** Increased residual volume, decreased forced expiratory volume, increased total lung capacity, decreased vital capacity.

☐ **2.** Increased residual volume, increased forced expiratory volume, decreased total lung capacity, decreased vital capacity.

☐ **3.** Decreased residual volume, decreased forced expiratory volume, decreased total lung capacity, increased vital capacity.

☐ **4.** Decreased residual volume, increased forced expiratory volume, increased total lung capacity, increased vital capacity.

103. The nurse caring for a client with diabetes realizes that the client has a higher risk of developing cataracts and:

☐ **1.** Background retinopathy.

☐ **2.** Proliferative retinopathy.

☐ **3.** Neuropathy.

☐ **4.** Diabetic retinopathy.

104. The nurse assesses the assigned clients for the shift. Of the following assigned clients, which client is at greatest risk for falling?

☐ **1.** A 22-year-old man with three fractured ribs and a fractured left arm.

☐ **2.** A 70-year-old woman with episodes of syncope.

☐ **3.** A 50-year-old man with angina.

☐ **4.** A 30-year-old woman with a fractured ankle.

105. Which of the following baseline laboratory data should be established before a client is started on tissue plasminogen activator or alteplase recombinant (Activase)?

☐ **1.** Potassium level.

☐ **2.** Lee-White clotting time.

☐ **3.** Hemoglobin level, hematocrit, and platelet count.

☐ **4.** Blood glucose level.

106. The nurse is developing an education plan for clients with hypertension. Which of the following long-term goals is most appropriate for the nurse to emphasize?
- ☐ 1. Develop a plan to limit stress.
- ☐ 2. Participate in a weight reduction program.
- ☐ 3. Commit to lifelong therapy.
- ☐ 4. Monitor blood pressure regularly.

107. The nurse should consider which of the following principles when developing a plan of care to manage a client's pain from cancer?
- ☐ 1. Individualize the pain medication regimen for the client.
- ☐ 2. Select medications that are least likely to lead to addiction.
- ☐ 3. Administer pain medication as soon as the client requests it.
- ☐ 4. Change pain medications periodically to avoid drug tolerance.

108. After explaining to a multigravid client at 36 weeks' gestation who is diagnosed with severe hydramnios about the possible complications of this condition, which of the following statements indicates that the client needs further instruction?
- ☐ 1. "Because I have hydramnios, I may gain weight."
- ☐ 2. "Hydramnios has been associated with gastrointestinal disorders in the fetus."
- ☐ 3. "I should continue to eat high-fiber foods and avoid constipation."
- ☐ 4. "I can continue to work at my job at the automobile factory until labor starts."

109. An obese diabetic client complains of bilateral leg aching. His physician has referred him to cardiac rehabilitation to start an exercise program. Which of the following activities is most helpful for the client?
- ☐ 1. Interval training on the stationary bicycle.
- ☐ 2. Interval training on the treadmill.
- ☐ 3. Interval training on a commercial ski machine.
- ☐ 4. Interval training on the stair climber.

110. The nurse is assigned to a client with jaundice and collects the following data: poor appetite, complaints of nausea, and two episodes of emesis in the past 2 hours. Which of the following nursing diagnoses best acknowledges the client's problems?
- ☐ 1. *Imbalanced nutrition: Less than body requirements.*
- ☐ 2. *Acute pain* related to abdominal muscle spasms.
- ☐ 3. *Adult failure to thrive.*
- ☐ 4. *Ineffective health maintenance.*

111. Which of the following interventions is recommended protocol for all clients who are at risk for pressure sore development?
- ☐ 1. Identify at-risk clients on admission to the health care facility.
- ☐ 2. Place at-risk clients on an every-2-hour turning schedule.
- ☐ 3. Automatically place clients in specialty beds.
- ☐ 4. Provide at-risk clients with a high-protein, high-carbohydrate diet.

112. A client has been prescribed digoxin (Lanoxin). Which of the following symptoms should the nurse tell the client to report as a potential indication of digoxin toxicity?
- ☐ 1. Urticaria.
- ☐ 2. Shortness of breath.
- ☐ 3. Visual disturbances.
- ☐ 4. Hypertension.

113. The nurse is instructing a client on how to care for skin that has become dry after radiation therapy. Which of the following statements by the client indicates that the client understands the teaching?
- ☐ 1. "I should take antihistamines to decrease the itching I am experiencing."
- ☐ 2. "It is safe to apply a nonperfumed lotion to my skin."
- ☐ 3. "A heating pad, set on the lowest setting, will help decrease my discomfort."
- ☐ 4. "I can apply an over-the-counter cortisone ointment to relieve the dryness."

114. The appetite-suppressing neurotransmitter that is made from tryptophan is:
- ☐ 1. Epinephrine.
- ☐ 2. Norepinephrine.
- ☐ 3. Serotonin.
- ☐ 4. Phenylalanine.

115. A neonate is experiencing respiratory distress and is using a neonatal oxygen mask. An unlicensed assistive personnel has positioned the oxygen mask as shown below. The nurse is assessing the neonate and determines that the mask:
- ☐ 1. Is appropriate for the neonate.
- ☐ 2. Is too large because it covers the neonate's eyes.
- ☐ 3. Is too small because it is obstructing the nose.
- ☐ 4. Should be covered with a soft cloth before being placed against the skin.

116. The nurse is preparing a client for a thoracentesis. How should the nurse position the client for the procedure?
- ☐ 1. Supine with the arms over the head.
- ☐ 2. Sims' position.
- ☐ 3. Prone position without a pillow.
- ☐ 4. Sitting forward with the arms supported on the bedside table.

117. The antidote for heparin is:
- ☐ 1. Vitamin K.
- ☐ 2. Warfarin (Coumadin).
- ☐ 3. Thrombin.
- ☐ 4. Protamine sulfate.

118. Which of the following actions is most appropriate when dealing with a client who is expressing anger verbally, is pacing, and is irritable?
- ☐ 1. Conveying empathy and encouraging ventilation.
- ☐ 2. Using calm, firm directions to get the client to a quiet room.
- ☐ 3. Putting the client in restraints.
- ☐ 4. Discussing alternative strategies for when the client is angry in the future.

119. A client with myasthenia gravis is seen in the emergency department for epistaxis. A priority nursing diagnosis is:
- ☐ 1. *Ineffective breathing pattern.*
- ☐ 2. *Risk for aspiration.*
- ☐ 3. *Risk for injury.*
- ☐ 4. *Feeding self-care deficit.*

120. Which of the following measures should be implemented promptly after a client's nasogastric (NG) tube has been removed?
- ☐ 1. Provide the client with oral hygiene.
- ☐ 2. Offer the client liquids to drink.
- ☐ 3. Encourage the client to cough and deep breathe.
- ☐ 4. Auscultate the client's bowel sounds.

121. The nurse prepares a warm compress to apply to a client's leg. The nurse understands that the reason for applying a heat treatment is to:
- ☐ 1. Reduce tissue metabolism.
- ☐ 2. Decrease mobility of leukocytes.
- ☐ 3. Promote circulation to the area.
- ☐ 4. Prevent swelling in the area.

122. While assisting the physician with an amniocentesis on a multigravid client at 38 weeks' gestation, the nurse observes that the fluid is very cloudy and thick. The nurse interprets this finding as indicating which of the following?
- ☐ 1. Intrauterine infection.
- ☐ 2. Fetal meconium staining.
- ☐ 3. Erythroblastosis fetalis.
- ☐ 4. Normal amniotic fluid.

123. The nurse instructs the unlicensed assistive personnel on how to collect a 24-hour urine specimen. Which of the following instructions is correct for a collection that is scheduled to start at 7 a.m. Monday and end at 7 a.m. Tuesday?
- ☐ 1. Collect and save the urine voided at 7 a.m. on Monday.
- ☐ 2. Send the first voided urine specimen on Monday to the laboratory for culture.
- ☐ 3. Collect and save the urine voided at 7 a.m. on Tuesday.
- ☐ 4. Keep each day's urine collection in separate containers.

124. Which of the following abnormal serum chemistry values is present in a client with cirrhosis who has developed ascites?
- ☐ 1. Decreased aspartate aminotransferase.
- ☐ 2. Hypoalbuminemia.
- ☐ 3. Hyperkalemia.
- ☐ 4. Decreased alanine aminotransferase.

125. An infant is brought to the clinic for a regular checkup and the diphtheria, tetanus, and acellular pertussis (DTaP) and inactivated polio vaccine (IPV) immunizations. The child is recovering from a cold and is afebrile. The child's sibling has cancer and is receiving chemotherapy. Which of the following actions is most appropriate?
- ☐ 1. Giving the DTaP and withholding the IPV.
- ☐ 2. Administering the DTaP and IPV immunizations.
- ☐ 3. Postponing both immunizations until the sibling is in remission.
- ☐ 4. Withholding both immunizations until the infant is well.

126. When creating a program to decrease the primary cause of disability and death in children, which of the following is most effective for the community health nurse to do?
- ☐ 1. Encourage state legislators to draft legislation to promote prenatal care.
- ☐ 2. Recommend that the health department make immunizations available at no cost to all children.
- ☐ 3. Teach health and safety practices to children and their parents.
- ☐ 4. Have a nurse practitioner hired for each of the schools in the community.

127. A client has had an incisional cholecystectomy. Which of the following nursing interventions has the highest priority in postoperative care for this client?
- ☐ 1. Using incentive spirometry every 2 hours while awake.
- ☐ 2. Performing leg exercises every shift.
- ☐ 3. Maintaining a weight-reduction diet.
- ☐ 4. Promoting incisional healing.

128. During a home visit, the nurse is evaluating an infant for auditory ability. Which of the following is the expected response in an infant with normal hearing?
- ☐ 1. Stoppage of body movements when sound is introduced.
- ☐ 2. Evidence of shy and withdrawn behaviors.
- ☐ 3. Saying "da-da" by age 5 months.
- ☐ 4. Absence of squealing by age 4 months.

129. A client who had a transurethral resection of the prostate (TURP) 1 day earlier has a three-way Foley catheter inserted for continuous bladder irrigation. Which of the following statements best explains why continuous irrigation is used after TURP?
- ☐ 1. To control bleeding in the bladder.
- ☐ 2. To instill antibiotics into the bladder.
- ☐ 3. To keep the catheter free from clot obstruction.
- ☐ 4. To prevent bladder distention.

130. Which of the following sounds should the nurse expect to hear when percussing a distended bladder?
- ☐ 1. Hyperresonance.
- ☐ 2. Tympany.
- ☐ 3. Dullness.
- ☐ 4. Flatness.

131. A tour bus has overturned on an exit ramp. Many passengers are injured, but there are no fatalities. While the emergency department nurse prepares for treating the injured, the nurse also calls the crisis nurse based on the understanding about which of the following?
- ☐ 1. The accident victims will be experiencing grief and mourning.
- ☐ 2. Many of the passengers may be experiencing feelings of victimization.
- ☐ 3. There is a need for someone to coordinate calls from relatives about the passengers.
- ☐ 4. Some of the passengers will need psychiatric hospitalization.

132. A postoperative nursing goal for the infant who has had surgery to correct imperforate anus is to prevent tension on the perineum. To achieve this goal, the nurse should avoid placing the neonate on the:
- ☐ 1. Abdomen, with legs pulled up under the body.
- ☐ 2. Back, with legs suspended at a 90-degree angle.
- ☐ 3. Left side, with hips elevated.
- ☐ 4. Right side, with hips elevated.

133. A child with meningococcal meningitis seen in the emergency department is to be admitted to the pediatric unit. In preparation for the child's arrival, the nurse should expect to do which of the following first?
- ☐ 1. Institute droplet precautions.
- ☐ 2. Obtain the child's vital signs.
- ☐ 3. Ask the parent about medication allergies.
- ☐ 4. Inquire about the health of siblings at home.

134. When developing the plan of care for a 14-year-old boy with a nursing diagnosis of *Deficient diversional activity* related to immobility, which of the following activities is most appropriate?
- ☐ 1. Playing a card game with a boy the same age.
- ☐ 2. Putting together a puzzle with his mother.
- ☐ 3. Playing video games with a 9-year-old.
- ☐ 4. Watching a movie with his younger brother.

135. An adolescent is being prepared for an emergency appendectomy. Which of the following should the nurse include in the teaching plan? Select all that apply.
- ☐ 1. Friends can visit whenever they want.
- ☐ 2. The scar will be small.
- ☐ 3. The teen will be back in school in 1 week.
- ☐ 4. Antibiotics will be given to prevent an infection.
- ☐ 5. A dressing will stay in place for 1 week.

136. A client receives morphine for postoperative pain. Considering the effects of morphine, which of the following assessments should the nurse include in the client's plan of care?
- ☐ 1. Take apical heart rate after each dose of morphine.
- ☐ 2. Assess urinary output every shift.
- ☐ 3. Assess mental status every shift.
- ☐ 4. Check for pedal edema every shift.

137. A client who is complaining of back and left flank pain is diagnosed with renal calculi. The client is experiencing periods of complete comfort alternating with periods of excruciating pain, accompanied by nausea and difficulty walking. Based on these data, what is the priority nursing diagnosis for this client?
- ☐ 1. *Activity intolerance.*
- ☐ 2. *Acute pain.*
- ☐ 3. *Deficient fluid volume.*
- ☐ 4. *Imbalanced nutrition: Less than body requirements.*

138. When infusing total parenteral nutrition (TPN), the nurse should assess the client for which of the following complications?
- ☐ 1. Essential amino acid deficiency.
- ☐ 2. Essential fatty acid deficiency.
- ☐ 3. Hyperglycemia.
- ☐ 4. Infection.

139. When assessing for signs of a blood transfusion reaction in a client with dark skin, the nurse should assess for which of the following?
- ☐ 1. Hypertension.
- ☐ 2. Diaphoresis.
- ☐ 3. Polyuria.
- ☐ 4. Warm skin.

140. After surgery to create a urinary diversion, the client is at risk for a urinary tract infection. The nurse should plan to incorporate which of the following interventions into the client's care?
- ☐ **1.** Clamp the urinary appliance at night.
- ☐ **2.** Empty the urinary appliance when one-third full.
- ☐ **3.** Administer prophylactic antibiotics.
- ☐ **4.** Change the urinary appliance daily.

141. When suctioning a client's tracheostomy tube, the nurse should incorporate which of the following steps into the procedure?
- ☐ **1.** Oxygenate the client before suctioning.
- ☐ **2.** Insert the suction catheter about 2 inches into the cannula.
- ☐ **3.** Use a bolus of sterile water to stimulate cough.
- ☐ **4.** Use clean gloves during the procedure.

142. When making a home visit, the nurse notices that a 14-month-old child has a severe diaper rash. Which of the following recommendations should the nurse provide to the parents?
- ☐ **1.** Continue to use the baby wipes.
- ☐ **2.** Change the diaper every 4 to 6 hours.
- ☐ **3.** Wash the buttocks using mild soap.
- ☐ **4.** Apply powder to the diaper area.

143. On entering a toddler's room, the nurse finds the mother sitting about 8 feet from the child and watching television while the toddler is screaming. Which of the following is the *most* appropriate response by the nurse?
- ☐ **1.** "What happened between you and your child?"
- ☐ **2.** "Why is your child screaming?"
- ☐ **3.** "Did something cause your child to be upset?"
- ☐ **4.** "Have you tried to calm down your child?"

144. A client has a total hip replacement. Which of the following client statements indicates a need for further teaching before discharge?
- ☐ **1.** "I will implement my exercise program as soon as I get home."
- ☐ **2.** "I will be careful not to cross my legs."
- ☐ **3.** "I will need an elevated toilet seat."
- ☐ **4.** "I can't wait to take a tub bath when I get home."

145. An adolescent tells the school nurse she thinks she has infectious mononucleosis. What common symptoms should the nurse expect the student to exhibit?
- ☐ **1.** Sore throat and malaise.
- ☐ **2.** Fatigue and weight loss.
- ☐ **3.** Coldlike symptoms and fever.
- ☐ **4.** Skin rash and abdominal pain.

146. While assessing the fundus of a multiparous client on the first postpartum day, the nurse performs hand-washing and dons clean gloves. Which of the following should the nurse do next?
- ☐ **1.** Place the nondominant hand above the symphysis pubis and the dominant hand at the umbilicus.
- ☐ **2.** Ask the client to assume a side-lying position with the knees flexed.
- ☐ **3.** Perform massage vigorously at the level of the umbilicus if the fundus feels boggy.
- ☐ **4.** Place the client on a bedpan in case the uterine palpation stimulates the client to void.

147. A nulligravid client with gestational diabetes tells the nurse that she had a reactive nonstress test 3 days ago and asks, "What does that mean?" The nurse explains that a reactive nonstress test indicates which of the following about the fetus?
- ☐ **1.** Evidence of some compromise that will require delivery soon.
- ☐ **2.** Fetal well-being at this point in the pregnancy.
- ☐ **3.** Evidence of late decelerations occurring during the test.
- ☐ **4.** No accelerations demonstrated within a 20-minute period.

148. A client has been diagnosed with right-sided heart failure. Which of the following clinical manifestations should the nurse expect to find in the client?
- ☐ **1.** Intermittent claudication.
- ☐ **2.** Dyspnea.
- ☐ **3.** Dependent edema.
- ☐ **4.** Crackles.

149. To help prevent hip flexion deformities associated with rheumatoid arthritis, the nurse should help the client assume which of the following positions in bed several times a day?
- ☐ **1.** Prone.
- ☐ **2.** Very low Fowler's.
- ☐ **3.** Modified Trendelenburg.
- ☐ **4.** Side-lying.

150. Which of the following should be the nurse's priority assessment after an epidural anesthetic has been given to a nulligravid client in active labor?
- ☐ **1.** Level of consciousness.
- ☐ **2.** Blood pressure.
- ☐ **3.** Cognitive function.
- ☐ **4.** Contraction pattern.

151. Assessment of a nulligravid client in active labor reveals the following: complaints of moderate discomfort; cervix dilated 3 cm, 0 station and completely effaced; fetal heart rate of 136 bpm. Which of the following should the nurse plan to do next?
- ☐ **1.** Assist the client with comfort measures and breathing techniques.
- ☐ **2.** Turn the client from the left side-lying position to the right side-lying position.
- ☐ **3.** Prepare the client for epidural anesthesia to relieve pain.
- ☐ **4.** Instruct the client that internal fetal monitoring is necessary.

152. The nurse monitors the serum electrolyte levels of a client who is taking digoxin (Lanoxin). Which of the following electrolyte imbalances is a common cause of digoxin toxicity?
- ☐ **1.** Hyponatremia.
- ☐ **2.** Hypomagnesemia.
- ☐ **3.** Hypocalcemia.
- ☐ **4.** Hypokalemia.

153. After abdominal surgery, a client has an order for meperidine (Demerol) I.M. 100 mg every 3 to 4 hours and acetaminophen (Tylenol) with codeine 30 mg. The client has been taking meperidine every 4 hours for the past 48 hours, but she tells the nurse that the meperidine is no longer lasting 4 hours and she needs to have it every 3 hours. Which of the following nursing actions is most appropriate?
- ☐ **1.** Realizing that the client is developing tolerance to the meperidine, the nurse administers the meperidine every 3 hours.
- ☐ **2.** The nurse urges the client to take the acetaminophen with codeine to prevent addiction to the meperidine.
- ☐ **3.** The nurse requests an order from the physician to change the dose to an equianalgesic dose of morphine.
- ☐ **4.** The nurse encourages the client to do relaxation exercises to provide distraction from the pain.

154. The nurse assesses a 7-month-old infant's growth and development. Which behavior should the nurse consider unusual?
- ☐ **1.** Drinking from a cup and spilling little of the liquid.
- ☐ **2.** Raising the chest and upper abdomen off the bed with the hands.
- ☐ **3.** Imitating sounds that the nurse makes.
- ☐ **4.** Crying loudly in protest when the mother leaves the room.

155. A 13-year-old client is dying of cancer and struggling with the emotional aspects of this. When providing care for this client, the nurse should incorporate the developmental tasks for this age. According to Erikson's developmental model, the child normally is expected to be working on which of the following psychosocial issues?
- ☐ **1.** Lifetime vocation.
- ☐ **2.** Social conscience.
- ☐ **3.** Personal values.
- ☐ **4.** Sense of competence.

156. The physician has prescribed amiodarone (Cordarone) for a client with cardiomyopathy. The nurse understands that the client's rhythm should be monitored to determine the effectiveness of the medication in controlling:
- ☐ **1.** Sinus node dysfunction.
- ☐ **2.** Heart block.
- ☐ **3.** Severe bradycardia.
- ☐ **4.** Life-threatening ventricular dysrhythmias.

157. An 18-year-old female client who is sexually active with her boyfriend visits the clinic complaining of a purulent vaginal discharge that is sometimes frothy. The nurse interprets this as suggesting which of the following?
- ☐ **1.** Sexually transmitted disease.
- ☐ **2.** Normal variations in vaginal discharge.
- ☐ **3.** Need for vaginal douching.
- ☐ **4.** Change in birth control method.

158. An elderly client has been bedridden since a cerebrovascular accident that resulted in total right-sided paralysis. The client has become increasingly confused, is occasionally incontinent of urine, and is refusing to eat. In planning the client's care, which of the following factors should the nurse consider as most critical in contributing to skin breakdown in this client?
- ☐ **1.** Nutritional status.
- ☐ **2.** Urinary incontinence.
- ☐ **3.** Episodes of confusion.
- ☐ **4.** Right-sided paralysis.

159. Assessment of a client who has just been admitted to the inpatient psychiatric unit reveals an unshaven face, noticeable body odor, visible spots on the shirt and pants, slow movements, gazing at the floor, and a flat affect. Which of the following should the nurse interpret as indicating psychomotor retardation?
- ☐ **1.** Slow movements.
- ☐ **2.** Flat affect.
- ☐ **3.** Unkempt appearance.
- ☐ **4.** Avoidance of eye contact.

160. A nurse working in the newborn nursery notices that an infant has a swelling in the scrotal area. The nurse interprets this swelling as indicative of hydrocele if which of the following occurs?
- [ ] **1.** The swollen bulge can be reduced.
- [ ] **2.** The increase in scrotal size is bilateral.
- [ ] **3.** The scrotal sac can be transilluminated.
- [ ] **4.** The bulge appears during crying.

161. When cleaning the skin around an incision and drain site, which of the following procedures should the nurse follow?
- [ ] **1.** Clean the incision and drain site separately.
- [ ] **2.** Clean from the incision to the drain site.
- [ ] **3.** Clean from the drain site to the incision.
- [ ] **4.** Clean the incision and drain site simultaneously.

162. An Hispanic mother who does not speak English and is very upset brings her child to the clinic with bleeding from the mouth. Which of the following is the most appropriate action by the nurse who does not speak Spanish?
- [ ] **1.** Call for the Spanish interpreter.
- [ ] **2.** Grab the child and take the child to the treatment room.
- [ ] **3.** Immediately apply ice to the child's mouth.
- [ ] **4.** Give the ice to the mother and demonstrate what to do.

163. The nurse is instructing an unlicensed assistive personnel on the prevention of postoperative pulmonary complications. Which of the following statements indicates that the assistant has understood the nurse's instructions?
- [ ] **1.** "I will turn the client every 4 hours."
- [ ] **2.** "I will keep the client's head elevated."
- [ ] **3.** "I should suction the client every 2 hours."
- [ ] **4.** "I will have the client take 5 to 10 deep breaths every hour."

164. Which of the following outcomes is most appropriate for a nursing diagnosis of *Ineffective tissue perfusion* related to interruption of arterial flow? Select all that apply.
- [ ] **1.** Extremities warm to touch.
- [ ] **2.** Improved respiratory status.
- [ ] **3.** Decreased muscle pain with activity.
- [ ] **4.** Participation in self-care measures.
- [ ] **5.** Lungs clear to auscultation.

165. The infusion rate of total parenteral nutrition is tapered before being discontinued. This is done to prevent which of the following complications?
- [ ] **1.** Essential fatty acid deficiency.
- [ ] **2.** Dehydration.
- [ ] **3.** Rebound hypoglycemia.
- [ ] **4.** Malnutrition.

166. While assessing the psychosocial aspects of a primigravid client at 30 weeks' gestation, the nurse should anticipate that the client will most likely have feelings of which of the following?
- [ ] **1.** Vulnerability.
- [ ] **2.** Confirmation.
- [ ] **3.** Ambivalence.
- [ ] **4.** Body image disturbance.

167. The nurse teaches a client scheduled for an I.V. pyelogram what to expect when the dye is injected. The nurse knows that the client has correctly understood what was taught when he states that he may experience which of the following sensations when the dye is injected?
- [ ] **1.** A metallic taste.
- [ ] **2.** Flushing of the face.
- [ ] **3.** Cold chills.
- [ ] **4.** Chest pain.

168. To prevent development of peripheral neuropathies associated with isoniazid administration, the nurse should teach the client to:
- [ ] **1.** Avoid excessive sun exposure.
- [ ] **2.** Follow a low-cholesterol diet.
- [ ] **3.** Obtain extra rest.
- [ ] **4.** Supplement the diet with pyridoxine (vitamin B_6).

169. A usually reliable interpreter called by the nurse to help communicate with a mother of a child who does not speak English and has brought her child in for a routine visit has yet to arrive in the clinic. The nurse has paged the interpreter several times. Which of the following should the nurse do next?
- [ ] **1.** Allow the pediatric nurse practitioner to examine the infant.
- [ ] **2.** Reschedule the infant's appointment for later in the week.
- [ ] **3.** Ask the mother to stay longer in the hope that the interpreter arrives.
- [ ] **4.** Try to page the interpreter one more time.

170. Oxygen toxicity results from oxygen concentrations greater than:
- [ ] **1.** 21%.
- [ ] **2.** 28%.
- [ ] **3.** 40%.
- [ ] **4.** 60%.

171. Before discharge from the hospital after a myocardial infarction, a client is taught to exercise by gradually increasing the distance walked. Which vital sign should the nurse teach the client to monitor to determine whether to increase or decrease the exercise level?
- [ ] **1.** Pulse rate.
- [ ] **2.** Blood pressure.
- [ ] **3.** Body temperature.
- [ ] **4.** Respiratory rate.

172. During an appointment with the nurse, a client says, "I could hate God for that flood." The nurse responds, "Oh, don't feel that way. We're making progress in these sessions." The nurse's statement demonstrates a failure to do which of the following?

- ☐ **1.** Look for meaning in what the client says.
- ☐ **2.** Explain to the client why he may think as he does.
- ☐ **3.** Add to the strength of the client's support system.
- ☐ **4.** Give the client credit for solving his own problems.

173. The nurse has just received the change of shift report on the following clients on the labor, delivery, recovery, and postpartum unit. Which of these clients should the nurse assess first?

- ☐ **1.** An 18-year-old single primigravid client, in labor for 9 hours, with cervical dilation at 6 cm, 0 station, contractions occurring every 5 minutes, and receiving epidural anesthesia.
- ☐ **2.** A 24-year-old primiparous client who delivered a 7 lb, 3 oz boy vaginally 1 hour ago, has a firm fundus and scant lochia rubra, and is attempting to breast-feed.
- ☐ **3.** A 26-year-old multigravid client, in labor for 8 hours, with cervical dilation at 8 cm, 1+ station, contractions every 3 to 4 minutes, and receiving no anesthesia.
- ☐ **4.** A 30-year-old multipara who delivered a 6 lb, 5 oz girl by cesarean section owing to fetal distress 3 hours ago, has a firm fundus and scant lochia rubra, and is receiving morphine by patient-controlled analgesia.

174. A client with type 1 diabetes mellitus is scheduled to have surgery. The client has been on nothing-by-mouth status since midnight in preparation for the surgery. In the morning before sending the client to the operating room, the nurse notices that the client's daily insulin has not been ordered. Which of the following interventions is most appropriate for the nurse at this time?

- ☐ **1.** Obtain the client's blood glucose values and evaluate the client's need for insulin.
- ☐ **2.** Contact the physician for further orders regarding insulin administration.
- ☐ **3.** Give the client's usual morning dose of insulin.
- ☐ **4.** Notify the recovery room staff to obtain an order for the insulin after surgery.

175. A client's chest tube is to be removed by the physician. Which of the following items should the nurse have ready to be placed directly over the wound when the chest tube is removed?

- ☐ **1.** Butterfly dressing.
- ☐ **2.** Montgomery strap.
- ☐ **3.** Fine mesh gauze dressing.
- ☐ **4.** Petrolatum gauze dressing.

176. While visiting a client with multiple sclerosis, the community health nurse observes that the client looks untidy and sad. The client suddenly says, "I can't even find the strength to comb my hair," and bursts into tears. Which of the following responses by the nurse is best?

- ☐ **1.** "It must be frustrating not to be able to care for yourself."
- ☐ **2.** "How many days have you been unable to comb your hair?"
- ☐ **3.** "Why hasn't your husband been helping you?"
- ☐ **4.** "Tell me more about how you're feeling."

177. A client newly diagnosed with bulimia is attending a nurse-led group at the mental health center. She tells the group that she only came because her husband said he would divorce her if she didn't get help. Which of the following responses by the nurse is most appropriate?

- ☐ **1.** "You sound angry with your husband. Is that correct?"
- ☐ **2.** "You will find that you like coming to group. These people are a lot of fun."
- ☐ **3.** "Tell me more about why you are here and how you feel about that."
- ☐ **4.** "Tell me something about what has caused you to be bulimic."

178. A client has tried without success to modify her lifestyle to lower her blood pressure. Which of the following will most likely be added to the program of continued lifestyle modification?

- ☐ **1.** Starting an antihypertensive medication.
- ☐ **2.** Beginning an exercise program.
- ☐ **3.** Quitting smoking.
- ☐ **4.** Losing weight.

179. A diabetic client has been diagnosed with hypertension and the physician has prescribed atenolol (Tenormin), a beta blocker. When performing discharge teaching, it is important for the client to recognize that the addition of Tenormin can cause:

- ☐ **1.** A decrease in the hypoglycemic effects of insulin.
- ☐ **2.** An increase in the hypoglycemic effects of insulin.
- ☐ **3.** An increase in the incidence of ketoacidosis.
- ☐ **4.** A decrease in the incidence of ketoacidosis.

180. The parent of a child who is taking an antibiotic for bilateral otitis media tells the nurse that he has stopped the medicine since his child is better, saving the rest of the medication to use the next time the child gets sick. Which of the following is the nurse's best response?

- ☐ **1.** "It is important to give the medicine as ordered."
- ☐ **2.** "How do you know your child's ears are cured?"
- ☐ **3.** "Your child needs all of the medicine so that the infection clears."
- ☐ **4.** "Stopping the medicine is not what's best for your child!"

181. The nurse is to administer 1 g of cefazolin (Ancef) in normal saline solution 50 ml over 45 minutes. The nurse should set the I.V. infusion pump to run at how many milliliters per hour?

_____ ml/hour

182. A 19-year-old client just finding out that she is approximately 8 weeks pregnant says, "I can't believe I'm pregnant. I just started college full-time!" The nurse interprets the client's statement as indicating which of the following?
☐ **1.** Ambivalence about the pregnancy.
☐ **2.** Disappointment about the pregnancy.
☐ **3.** Abortion is a likely option.
☐ **4.** Bonding may be difficult after delivery.

183. A mother visits the clinic with her 11-year-old daughter for a routine physical examination. The mother tells the nurse that her daughter is beginning to have slight breast enlargement. When teaching the mother and daughter about pubertal changes, the nurse should explain that breast enlargement is caused by the rise in which of the following?
☐ **1.** Prolactin.
☐ **2.** Estrogen.
☐ **3.** Progesterone.
☐ **4.** Testosterone.

184. The nurse monitors a client receiving mechanical ventilation for which of the following complications?
☐ **1.** Gastrointestinal hemorrhage.
☐ **2.** Immunosuppression.
☐ **3.** Increased cardiac output.
☐ **4.** Pulmonary emboli.

185. A client is going home with a prescription for nitroglycerin (Nitrostat) for his anginal symptoms. Which of the following statements accurately conveys information the client must understand to safely self-medicate?
☐ **1.** Store the nitroglycerin in the refrigerator.
☐ **2.** Take one tablet every 15 minutes.
☐ **3.** Sit down or lie down before taking the nitroglycerin.
☐ **4.** Swallow the nitroglycerin tablet.

186. Which of the following nursing interventions is most likely to be beneficial initially in helping the parents of an adolescent hospitalized for appendicitis deal with the hospitalization?
☐ **1.** Reassure the parents that their adolescent will be fine.
☐ **2.** Assess the parents' current knowledge level before providing information.
☐ **3.** Encourage the parents to participate in the client's physical care.
☐ **4.** Interact with the parents when they ask for information.

187. The nurse instructs a female client about contraceptive options. The nurse explains that the intrauterine device (IUD) is a good contraceptive option for women who:
☐ **1.** Desire short-term use of a contraceptive.
☐ **2.** Are in a monogamous relationship.
☐ **3.** Have a history of sexually transmitted diseases (STDs).
☐ **4.** Have had a history of ectopic pregnancies.

188. Before the parents of a 3-month-old child who died from sudden infant death syndrome (SIDS) leave the hospital, the nurse asks the parents what they understand about the cause of SIDS. The nurse evaluates their understanding as correct when the parents state:
☐ **1.** "The cause is unknown."
☐ **2.** "The cause is apnea."
☐ **3.** "The cause is infection."
☐ **4.** "The cause is cardiac dysrhythmias."

189. A client has been diagnosed with peripheral arterial occlusive disease. Which of the following instructions is appropriate for the nurse to give the client for promoting circulation to the extremities?
☐ **1.** Keep the extremities elevated slightly.
☐ **2.** Participate in a regular walking program.
☐ **3.** Use a heating pad to promote warmth.
☐ **4.** Massage the calf muscles if pain occurs.

190. A primigravid client at 16 weeks' gestation visits the clinic for a routine examination. The client tells the nurse that she knows someone whose baby was born with congenital toxoplasmosis. Which of the following should the nurse instruct the client to do to prevent transmission of the toxoplasmosis protozoan?
☐ **1.** Avoid contact with anyone diagnosed with this disease.
☐ **2.** Consider a course of prophylactic penicillin as prevention.
☐ **3.** Plan to be vaccinated for this condition at the next visit.
☐ **4.** Cook all meats, such as beef and pork, thoroughly.

Correct Answers and Rationales

The letter in parentheses after each rationale identifies the client need addressed in the item, including management of care (M), safety and infection control (S), health promotion and maintenance (H), psychosocial adaptation (P), basic care and comfort (C), pharmacological and parenteral therapies (D), reduction of risk potential (R), and physiological adaptation (A).

1. 2. The nurse is responsible for maintaining confidentiality of this disclosure by the client. (P)

2. **2.** Pets are discouraged when parents are trying to allergy-proof a home for a child with bronchial asthma, unless the pets are kept outside. Pets with hair or feathers are especially likely to trigger asthma attacks. A fish is a satisfactory pet for this child, but the parents should be taught to keep the fish tank clean to prevent it from harboring mold. (H)

3. **2.** Under the policy for valuables, the nurse documents the description on an envelope with the client, the client and nurse sign the envelope, and the valuables envelope is locked in the safe. The other options increase the risk of loss or damage to the client's valuables. (M)

4. **1.** Sucking provides the infant with a sense of security and comfort. It also is an outlet for releasing tension. The infant should not be discouraged from sucking on the pacifier. Fussiness after feeding may indicate that the infant's appetite is not satisfied. Sucking is not manipulative in the sense of seeking parental attention. (H)

5. **3.** Sexually transmitted diseases are communicable diseases that must be reported. The nurse is responsible for reporting these diseases to the appropriate public health agency, and to otherwise maintain the client's confidentiality. The client's family cannot request release of medical information without the client's consent. A physician's order is not a substitute for a client's consent to release medical information in the absence of a communicable disease. (M)

6. **4.** In a life-threatening emergency where time is of the essence in saving life or limb, consent is not required. This client has a Glasgow Coma Scale score of 7, which means he is comatose. The client has deteriorated to a level where he cannot be aroused, withdraws in a purposeless manner from painful stimuli, exhibits decorticate posturing, and may or may not have brain stem reflexes intact. The placement of the ICP monitor is crucial to determine cerebral blood flow and prevent herniation. The client's fiancée cannot sign his consent because, until she is his wife or has designated power of attorney, she is not considered his next of kin. The physician should insert the catheter in this emergency. He does not need to get a consultation from another physician. When consent is needed for a situation that is not a true emergency, two nurses can receive a verbal consent by telephone from the client's next of kin. (M)

7. **4.** Follow-up generally involves semiannual chest radiographs. Recurrence usually occurs locally in the lungs and may be identified on chest radiographs. Follow-up after cancer treatment is an important component of the treatment plan. Serum markers (liver function tests) have not been shown to detect recurrence of lung cancer. There are no data to support the need for an abdominal computed tomography scan. (R)

8. **1.** All blood products should be administered through a micron mesh filter. Blood is never administered without a filter. Leukocytes can be removed by using leukocyte-poor filters, and this is recommended to decrease reactions in clients, such as hemophiliacs, who require frequent transfusions. Blood is too concentrated to administer through a microdrip set. (D)

9. **3.** One of the best strategies to help clients feel in control is to ask them their view of situations, and to respond to what they say. This technique acknowledges that clients' opinions have value and relevance to the interview. It also promotes an active role for clients in the process. Use of a questionnaire or written instructions is a means of obtaining information but promotes a passive client role. Asking whether clients have questions encourages participation, but alone it does not acknowledge their views. (M)

10. **3.** A client with severe depression may experience symptoms of psychosis such as hallucinations and delusions that are typically mood congruent. The statement, "My heart has stopped and my blood is black ash," is a mood-congruent somatic delusion. A delusion is a firm, false, fixed belief that is resistant to reason or fact. A hallucination is a false sensory perception unrelated to external stimuli. An illusion is a misinterpretation of a real sensory stimulus. Paranoia refers to suspiciousness of others and their actions. (P)

11. **2.** The client should be allowed to see his chart. As a client advocate, the nurse should answer questions for the client. The nurse helps the client understand that he is a primary partner in the health team. The Bill of Rights for Patients has existed since the 1960s, and every client should be aware of this document. The doctor should not need to give permission for the client to see his chart. As a client advocate, the nurse should not make excuses to put the client off in regard to seeing his chart. (M)

12. **3.** The three-point gait, in which the client advances the crutches and the affected leg at the same time while weight is supported on the unaffected extremity, is the appropriate gait of choice. This allows for non-weight-bearing on the affected extremity. The two-point, four-point, and swing-to gaits require some weight bearing on both legs, which is contraindicated for this client. (A)

13. **1.** When the client verbalizes that life isn't worth living anymore, the nurse needs to ask the client directly about suicide by saying, "Are you thinking about killing yourself?" Asking directly does not provoke suicide but conveys concern, understanding, and the worth of the client. Commonly, the client experiences a sense of relief that someone finally hears him. It also helps the nurse plan responsible care by identifying the client who is at risk for suicide. The nurse should then evaluate the seriousness of the suicidal ideation by inquiring about the intent and plan. Stating, "Things will get better," offers hope too soon without first evaluating the intent of the suicidal ideation. Asking, "Why do you think that way?" implies a lack of understanding and knowledge on the part of the nurse. Major depression usually is endogenous and biochemically based. Therefore, the client may not know why he doesn't want to live. Saying, "You shouldn't feel that way," admonishes the client, decreases self-worth, and conveys a lack of understanding. (P)

14. **1, 4, 5.** Lamotrigine, an antiepileptic, is used as a mood stabilizer for clients with bipolar disorder and has been found to be effective for the depressive phase of bipolar disorder. Common adverse effects are dizziness, headache, sedation, tremors, nausea, vomiting, and ataxia. The development of a rash needs to be reported and evaluated by the physician because it could indicate the start of a severe systemic rash known as Stevens-Johnson syndrome, a toxic epidermal necrolysis, which would necessitate the discontinuation of lamotrigine. Hyperthermia in conjunction with muscle rigidity suggests the development of neuroleptic malignant syndrome, a life-threatening complication associated with olanzapine. (D)

15. **0.8**

$$\frac{0.4 \text{ mg}}{X} = \frac{0.5 \text{ mg}}{1 \text{ ml}}$$

$$0.4 = 0.5X$$

$$\frac{0.4}{0.5} = X$$

$$0.8 \text{ ml} = X.$$

(D)

16. **4.** The nurse should instruct the client to increase her intake of calcium because there is a slight increase in the risk of osteoporosis with this medication. Weight-bearing exercises are also advised. The drug may also impair glucose tolerance in women who are at risk for diabetes. (D)

17. **1, 2, 5.** The first trimester is when the couple works through the psychological task of accepting the pregnancy. These statements describe the client and her partner coping with the pregnancy, how it feels, and how it will impact their lives. The feelings include pleasure, excitement, and ambivalence. Wondering what the baby will look like and planning for the baby's room occur later in the pregnancy. (H)

18. **4.** The aminoglycoside antibiotic gentamicin sulfate should not be applied to large denuded areas because toxicity and systemic absorption are possible. The nurse should instruct the client to avoid excessive sun exposure because gentamicin sulfate can cause photosensitity.

The client should be instructed to apply the cream or ointment for only the length of time prescribed because a superinfection can occur from overuse. The client should contact the physician if the condition worsens after use. (D)

19. **3.** The nurse needs to inform the sister that it takes 2 to 4 weeks before a full clinical effect occurs with the drug. The nurse should let her know that her brother will gradually get better and symptoms of depression will improve. Telling the sister that her brother is experiencing a very serious depression does not give the sister important information about the medication. Additionally, this statement may cause alarm and anxiety. Conveying the sister's concern to the physician does not provide her with the necessary information about the client's medication. Telling the sister that the client's medication may need to be changed is inappropriate because a full clinical effect occurs after 2 to 4 weeks. (D)

20. **1, 2, 3.** For the client with grandiose delusions, the nurse should accept the client but not argue with the delusion to build trust and the client's self-esteem. Focusing on the underlying feeling or meaning of the delusion helps to meet the client's needs. Focusing on events and topics based in reality distracts the client from the delusional thinking. Confronting the client's delusions or beliefs can lead to agitation in the client and the need to cling to the grandiose delusion to preserve self-esteem. Interacting with the client only when he is based in reality ignores the client's needs and therapeutic nursing intervention. (P)

21. **4.** Symptoms of pregnancy-induced hypertension (PIH), such as hypertension and facial swelling, before 24 weeks' gestation and a fundal height larger than expected are suggestive of gestational trophoblastic disease or hydatidiform mole. This condition occurs when trophoblasts develop abnormally. Ultrasound can confirm the condition. Medical management includes evacuation of the mole and follow-up to detect any malignant changes. Painless vaginal bleeding suggests placenta previa. Fetal anemia is commonly caused by Rh sensitization. The client with a multifetal pregnancy may exhibit a larger fundal height than expected, but she usually does not have a brownish discharge or symptoms of PIH at this stage of gestation. (R)

22. **1.** Saying, "When you interrupt others, they leave the area," is most helpful because it serves to increase the client's awareness of how others view him by giving him specific feedback about his behavior. The other statements are punitive and authoritative, possibly threatening to the client, and likely to increase defensiveness, decrease self-worth, and increase feelings of guilt. (P)

23. **4.** To determine how low the gentamicin serum level drops between doses, the trough serum level should be drawn just before the administration of the next I.V. dose of gentamicin sulfate. (D)

24. **1.** Health-promoting strategies for clients with a history of cardiovascular disease require knowledge in three areas: diet, exercise, and medication. Pain management and management of social activities are not usually features of health promotion activities for these clients. (H)

25. **3.** The child is exhibiting signs and symptoms of possible epiglottiditis. As a result the child is at high risk for laryngospasm and airway occlusion. Therefore, the nurse should have a tracheostomy tube and setup readily available should the child experience an airway occlusion. Although acetaminophen is an antipyretic, the dosage of 600 mg to be administered rectally is too high. A typical 4-year-old weighs approximately 40 lb. The recommended dose is 125 mg. When any type of respiratory illness, and especially epiglottiditis, is suspected, putting any object, including a tongue depressor for inspection or a cotton-tipped applicator to obtain a throat culture, in the back of the mouth or throat or having the child open the mouth is inappropriate because doing so may predispose the child to laryngospasm or occlusion of the airway by a swollen epiglottis. (A)

26. **3.** The client is exhibiting temporary side effects associated with lithium therapy. Therefore, the nurse should continue the lithium and explain to the client that he is experiencing temporary side effects of lithium that will subside. Common side effects of lithium are nausea, dry mouth, diarrhea, thirst, mild hand tremor, weight gain, bloating, insomnia, and light-headedness. Immediately notifying the physician about these common side effects is not necessary. (D)

27. **1.** Thyroid replacement is a lifelong maintenance therapy. The medication is usually given as one dose in the morning. It cannot be tapered or discontinued because the client needs thyroid supplementation to maintain health. The medication cannot be discontinued after the thyroid-stimulating hormone (TSH) level is normal; the dose will be maintained at the level that normalizes the TSH concentration. (D)

28. **4.** A client who is beginning training for a tennis team would most likely require an adjustment in lithium dosage because excessive sweating can increase the serum lithium level, possibly leading to toxicity. Adjustments in lithium dosage would also be necessary when other medications have been added, when an illness with high fever occurs, and when a new diet begins. (D)

29. **3.** The most appropriate response is to continue all treatments and attempt to stabilize the client using fluid replacement without administering blood or blood products. It is imperative that the health care team respect the client's religious beliefs and wishes, even if they are not those of the health care team. Discontinuing all measures is not an option. The health care team should continue to provide the best care possible and does not need to notify the attorney. (M)

30. **2.** Cystic fibrosis is the most common inherited disease in children. It is inherited as an autosomal recessive trait, meaning that the child inherits the defective gene from both parents. The chances are one in four for each of this couple's pregnancies. (A)

31. **3.** Nitroglycerin in all dosage forms (sublingual, transdermal, or intravenous) should be shielded from light to prevent deterioration. The client should be instructed to keep the nitroglycerin in the dark container that is supplied by the pharmacy, and it should not be removed or placed in another container. (D)

32. **1, 2, 4, 6.** Sinus bradycardia has the following characteristics: P wave is normal and consistent in shape, occurring in front of every QRS complex; a ventricular and atrial rate of less than 60 bpm; and a PR interval between 0.12 to 0.20 second. An atrial rate of 120 bpm indicates tachycardia. ST-segment elevation may indicate a myocardial infarction. (R)

33. **3.** Valproic acid causes sedation as well as nausea, vomiting, and indigestion. Sedation is important because the client needs to be cautioned about driving or operating machinery that could be dangerous while feeling sedated from the medication. Depakene does not cause increased urination, slowed thinking, or weight loss. However, some clients may experience weight gain. (D)

34. **1.** These effects and others when seen after birth are known as a cluster of symptoms called fetal alcohol syndrome. Vitamin B_6 and vitamin A deficiency can affect growth and development but not with these specific effects. Folic acid deficiency contributes to neural tube defects. (A)

35. **4.** NSAIDs irritate the gastric mucosa and should be taken with food. NSAIDs are usually taken once or twice daily. Joint exercise is not related to the drug administration. Antacids may interfere with the absorption of NSAIDs. (D)

36. **2.** The client who drinks alcohol while taking disulfiram experiences sweating, flushing of the neck and face, tachycardia, hypotension, a throbbing headache, nausea and vomiting, palpitations, dyspnea, tremor, and weakness. (D)

37. **3.** Holding the gauze pledget against an I.M. injection site while removing the needle from the muscle avoids the discomfort of the needle pulling on the skin. (D)

38. **3.** Physical activity is gradually increased after a myocardial infarction while the client is still hospitalized and through a period of rehabilitation. The client is progressing too rapidly if activity significantly changes respirations, causing dyspnea, chest pain, a rapid heartbeat, or fatigue. When any of these symptoms appears, the client should reduce activity and progress more slowly. Edema suggests a circulatory problem that must be addressed but doesn't necessarily indicate overexertion. Cyanosis indicates reduced oxygen-carrying capacity of red blood cells and indicates a severe pathology. It is not appropriate to use cyanosis as an indicator for overexertion. Weight loss indicates several factors but not overexertion. (A)

39. 3. When a client talks about not having a problem with alcohol, the nurse needs to point out how alcohol has gotten the client into trouble. Concrete facts are helpful in decreasing the client's denial that alcohol is a problem. The other approaches allow the client to use defense mechanisms, such as rationalization, projection, and minimization, to explain her actions. Therefore, these approaches are not helpful. (P)

40. 3. Medicaid is state funded, with matching federal funds, and provides medical assistance for low-income persons without health insurance. The program for older adults is Medicare. (M)

41. 3. Before development and implementation of the teaching plan, it is vital to determine what the client currently knows regarding diabetes and what the client needs to know. (M)

42. 1. The goal of the education program is to instruct the client to take his pulse; therefore, the expected outcome would be the ability to give a return demonstration of how to palpate the heart rate. (R)

43. 3. Percutaneous umbilical blood sampling is a useful procedure for diagnosing Rh disease, obtaining fetal complete blood count, and karyotyping chromosomes to evaluate for genetic disorders. Ultrasound commonly is used to detect twins. A lecithin-sphingomyelin ratio is the procedure of choice to diagnose fetal lung maturation. A maternal blood test is used to determine the alpha fetoprotein level. (R)

44. 2. The client should report tinnitus because vancomycin can affect the acoustic branch of the eighth cranial nerve. Vancomycin does not affect the vestibular branch of the acoustic nerve; vertigo and ataxia would occur if the vestibular branch were involved. Muscle stiffness is not associated with vancomycin. (D)

45. 4. Caffeinated beverages and alcohol should be avoided because they stimulate gastric acid production and irritate gastric mucosa. The client should avoid foods that cause discomfort; however, there is no need to follow a soft, bland diet. Eating six small meals daily is no longer a common treatment for peptic ulcer disease. Milk in large quantities is not recommended because it actually stimulates further production of gastric acid. (R)

46. 3. When a client with a NG tube exhibits abdominal distention, the nurse should first check the suction machine. If the suction equipment is functioning properly, then the nurse should take other steps, such as repositioning the tube or checking tube patency by irrigating it. If these steps are not effective, then the physician should be called. (R)

47. 4. Increased, not decreased, body temperature resulting from occupations or infections can contribute to low sperm counts caused by decreased sperm production. Heat can destroy sperm. Varicocele, an abnormal dilation of the veins in the spermatic cord, is an associated cause of a low sperm count. The varicosity increases the temperature within the testes, inhibiting sperm production. Frequent use of saunas or hot tubs may lead to a low sperm count. The temperature of the scrotum becomes elevated, possibly inhibiting sperm production. Endocrine imbalances (thyroid problems) are associated with low sperm counts in men because of possible interference with spermatogenesis. (A)

48. 1. The clinical findings of edema are consistent with fluid excess in the interstitial compartment. The extracellular compartment consists of fluid in two locations, the interstitial (tissue) spaces and plasma (intravascular) spaces. Fluid shifts within the extracellular compartment can occur either from the plasma space to the interstitial space, or from the interstitial space to the plasma space. When fluid shifts from the plasma space into the interstitial space, usually as a result of abnormal retention of fluids in such conditions as heart failure or renal failure, edema results. The intracellular compartment consists of fluid within the cells. (A)

49. 1. Low potassium can cause an imbalance at the cellular level that leads to dysrhythmias and cardiac arrest. Hyperglycemia is caused by elevated blood sugar. Hypertension is unrelated to potassium levels. Increased energy is unrelated to potassium levels. (R)

50. 2. Handwashing with the correct technique is the best method for preventing cross-contamination. The hands serve as a source of infection. Waterless commercial products containing at least 60% alcohol are as effective at killing organisms as handwashing. (S)

51. 3. The third maneuver is used to identify the presenting part. This maneuver is used to identify the part of the fetus that lies over the inlet to the pelvis. While facing the client, the nurse places the tips of the first three fingers on the side of the woman's abdomen above the symphysis pubis and palpates deeply around the presenting part to identify its contour and size. The first maneuver involves using the tips of the fingers of both hands to palpate the uterine fundus. The second maneuver identifies the back of the fetus, and the fourth maneuver identifies the cephalic prominence. (R)

52. **2.** The stored glucose of muscle glycogen is the major fuel during sustained activity. Glucose production slows as the body begins to depend on fat stores for glucose and fatty acids. Protein is not the body's preferred energy source. Fat is a secondary source of energy. Water is not an energy source, although sufficient water is required to engage in aerobic activity without causing dehydration. (H)

53. **3.** Fluctuation of fluid with respirations in the water-seal column indicates that the system is functioning properly. If an obstruction were present in the chest tube, fluid fluctuation would be absent. Subcutaneous emphysema occurs when air pockets can be palpated beneath the client's skin around the chest tube insertion site. A leak in the system is indicated when bubbling occurs in the water-seal column. (A)

54. **4.** It is important to dry the feet carefully after a bath to prevent a fungal infection. Diabetic clients should seek medical attention when they injure their toes or feet to prevent complications. Iodine is highly toxic to the tissues. Diabetic clients should inspect their feet daily and should wear shoes that support their feet while in the house. (R)

55. **2.** Diverticular rupture causes peritonitis from the release of intestinal contents (chemicals and bacteria) into the peritoneal cavity. A rigid abdominal wall results from a diverticular cavity. The inflammatory response of the peritoneal tissue produces severe abdominal rigidity and pain, diminished intestinal motility, and retention of intestinal contents (air, fluid, and stool). Hyperactive bowel sounds, explosive diarrhea, and excessive flatulence do not indicate peritonitis. (A)

56. **1, 2, 3, 5.** Pancreatitis, a chronic or acute inflammation of the pancreas, is a potentially life-threatening condition. Excessive alcohol intake and gallstones are the greatest risk factors. Abdominal trauma can potentiate inflammation. Hyperlipidemia is a risk factor for recurrent pancreatitis. Hypertension and hypothyroidism are not associated with pancreatitis. (R)

57. **1.** The nurse should firmly yet gently strike the chest wall with the hand cupped to make a hollow popping sound. A slapping sound indicates that an incorrect technique is being used. The area over the rib cage is percussed to loosen mucus from the underlying lung passages. The child should wear a thin piece of clothing (T-shirt) over the chest area to protect the skin without diminishing the effect of the percussion. (R)

58. **1.** The nurse should call to the desk to ask for assistance. The nurse needs to notify the doctor of the client's death and the family must then be notified. A code should not be called. Nursing personnel should begin postmortem care so that the family does not walk in unannounced to find their loved one deceased and looking disarrayed. (M)

59. **2.** One pound of weight is approximately equivalent to 3,500 calories. Removing 1,000 calories per day results in a 2-lb weight loss per week (7,000 calories divided by 7 days). If a client wanted to lose 1 lb in a 7-day period, he would need to cut out 500 calories per day (3,500 calories divided by 7 days). It is unsafe to try to lose more than 2 lb per week. (H)

60. **1.** The nurse should instruct the client to take the medication immediately or as soon as she remembers that she missed the medication. There is only a slight risk that the client will become pregnant when only one pill has been missed, so there is no need to use another form of contraception. However, if the client wishes to increase the chances of not getting pregnant, a condom can be used by the male partner. The client should not omit the missed pill and then restart the medication in the morning because there is a possibility that ovulation can occur, after which intercourse could result in pregnancy. Taking two pills is not necessary and also will result in putting the client off her schedule. (D)

61. **1.** Pain disorder is a somatoform disorder involving severe pain in one or more anatomic sites causing severe distress or impaired function. The statement, "I need to have a good cry about all the pain I've been in and then not dwell on it," indicates improvement because the client has a realistic view of the physical symptoms and pain and is willing to let them go and move on. The other statements indicate the continued presence of denial, lack of insight, and the need for symptoms to manage anxiety. (P)

62. **4.** The nurse needs to collect additional information about the client's complaint of hearing voices. Assessing the content of hallucinations is essential to determine whether they are command hallucinations that the client might act on. Asking about what the neighbor has been doing or telling the client that the neighbor won't visit indirectly reinforces the delusion about the neighbor. Although determining the onset and duration of the voices is important, the nurse needs to assess the content of the hallucinations first. (P)

63. **3.** A client with severe diarrhea loses large amounts of bicarbonate, resulting in metabolic acidosis. Metabolic alkalosis does not result in this situation. Diarrhea does not affect the respiratory system. (A)

64. **4.** Serum osmolality indicates the water balance of the body. A normal plasma osmolality between 275 and 295 mOsm/kg indicates that the fluid volume excess has been resolved. A weight reduction of 10% may not necessarily return the client to a state of normal serum osmolality. Clients with excess fluid volume do not necessarily have pain or abnormal arterial blood gas values. (A)

65. 3. Exactly why rheumatic fever follows a streptococcal infection is not known, but it is theorized that an antigen-antibody response occurs to an M protein present in certain strains of streptococci. The antibodies developed by the body attack certain tissues such as in the heart and joints. Antistreptolysin O titer findings show elevated or rising antibody levels. This blood finding is the most reliable evidence of a streptococcal infection. (R)

66. 3. The nurse should call the surgeon's office so that arrangements can be made for the client to donate a unit of his blood for possible future autotransfusion. This must be done in sufficient time before surgery so that the client is not at risk for being anemic at the time of the scheduled procedure. The client's request must be scheduled through the surgeon's office because the surgeon has ultimate responsibility for the client. The nurse can document that the surgeon's office was notified of the client's request. Notifying the hematology laboratory or blood bank is not an appropriate response. (D)

67. 1. High colonic irrigation can increase the risk of perforation in a distended and inflamed colon. Tap water is hypotonic in the bowel and would draw increased fluid into the area. The other orders are part of standard preparation for intestinal surgery. (R)

68. 1, 3. When a client collects stool for occult blood, the nurse should instruct him to avoid eating meat, especially red meat, for 1 to 3 days before the sample collection because meat eliminated in the stool can lead to false-positive results. Eating foods high in fiber a few days before sample collection may be recommended because doing so improves the chances of finding occult blood if a lesion is present. The client should take stool samples from different sites of the stool for a better sample. The stool sample should be covered to protect everyone from body secretions. The specimen does not have to be sent to the laboratory immediately. Some medications, herbs, foods, and activities can lead to false results of the occult testing. For example, iron pills, turnips, and horseradish lead to false-positive results. Vitamin C leads to false-negative results. Some anti-inflammatory drugs and aspirin should be avoided due to antiplatelet properties that increase the risk of gastrointestinal bleeding. (R)

69. 3. The most appropriate intervention is to offer the client frequent mouth care to moisten the dry oral mucosa. Reexplaining why the client cannot drink may be helpful but will not relieve her thirst. Ice chips cannot be given to a client who is on nothing-by-mouth status. Diverting the client's attention does not treat her complaint. (C)

70. 2. This client is demonstrating classic symptoms of hypothyroidism. Primary hypothyroidism results from pathologic changes in the thyroid gland. In this case, the thyroid gland cannot secrete sufficient amounts of thyroid hormone, leading to a decrease in cellular metabolic activity, decreased oxygen consumption, and decreased heat production. Cushing's disease is manifested by a buffalo hump, moonface, hypertension, fatigability, and weakness, resulting from the inappropriate release of cortisol. Hyperthyroidism, or Graves' disease, is manifested by increased appetite with weight loss, increased anxiety, hand tremors, palpitations, heat intolerance, and insomnia. A pituitary tumor can have many symptoms, depending on the location. (A)

71. 3. After the symptoms of puberty, such as increased hair growth and enlargement of the breasts, are noticed, menstruation typically begins within 30 months. (H)

72. 2. Epstein's pearls are tiny, hard, white nodules found in the mouth of some neonates. They are considered normal and usually disappear without treatment. Koplik's spots, associated with measles in children, are patchy and bright red with a bluish-white speck in the middle. Precocious teeth are actual teeth that some neonates have at birth. Usually only one or two teeth are present. *Candida albicans*, or thrush, is not apparent in the mouth immediately after birth but may appear a day or two later. This infection is manifested by yellowish-white spots or lesions that resemble milk curds and bleed when attempts are made to wipe them away. (H)

73. 1, 2. The initial signs of esophageal atresia and TEF include lots of frothy mucus and unexplained episodes of cyanosis usually caused by overflow of mucus from the esophagus. Loose stools and poor gag reflex are not signs of TEF. Initial weight loss is common in newborns and not related to TEF. (R)

74. 1. Adequate circulatory status is the most important factor in the healing process of an infected decubitus ulcer. Blood flow to the area must be present to bring nutrients and prescribed antibiotics to the tissues. Rest and a balanced diet are essential to health maintenance but are not the priority for healing an infected decubitus ulcer. A fluid intake of 2,000 to 3,000 ml/day, if not contraindicated, is recommended to provide hydration to the client's tissues. (R)

75. 2. The nurse's initial response should be to withhold the digoxin . The nurse should then notify the physician if the apical pulse is 60 bpm or lower because of the risk of digoxin toxicity. The charge nurse does not need to be notified, but the nurse needs to document the notification and follow-up in the chart. (D)

76. **2.** In an emergency in which the neonate's head is already delivering, the first action by the nurse should be to check for the presence of a cord around the neonate's neck. If the cord is present, the nurse should gently remove it from around the neck. The mother should be told to breathe gently and avoid forceful bearing-down efforts, which could lead to lacerations. Although blood and bodily fluid precautions are always present in client care, this is an emergency. If possible, the nurse should put on gloves. Suctioning the mouth can be done after the nurse has checked that the cord is not around the neonate's neck. Telling the mother that help is on the way is not reassuring because emergency medical technicians may take some time to arrive. Delivery is imminent because the neonate's head is delivering. (R)

77. **2.** The ulna heals in approximately 12 weeks. The femur takes approximately 24 weeks to heal because of the size of the bone and the muscle forces exerted on the femur. Skeletal traction does not delay healing but can actually promote healing by properly aligning the fracture. (A)

78. **2.** The client needs to know that there is a cause for the delirium, that there is hope for treatment, and that medications can help decrease anxiety. Giving medications can help the anxiety, but the client also needs an explanation about the condition. Saying that the more the client worries, the worse the delirium will get is inappropriate and most likely would add to the client's anxiety. (P)

79. **1.** The client understands the instructions when she says she should avoid contact sports because they may result in injury to the client and the fetus. Learning to ski while pregnant is not recommended because injury may occur. Scuba diving should be avoided because depth pressures could cause fetal damage. Hot tubs should be avoided during the first trimester because sitting in them can result in fetal hyperthermia and fetal hypoxia. Mild exercises, such as walking, can help strengthen the muscles and prevent some discomforts such as backache. (H)

80. **1.** Cardiogenic shock is a negative outcome of a myocardial infarction that involves a significant amount of cardiac tissue. Lack of blood and oxygen leads to death of the contractile elements of the tissue, resulting in pump failure. Hypovolemic shock results from blood loss. Neurogenic shock results from loss of sympathetic tone. Metabolic acidosis is commonly caused by uncontrolled diabetes mellitus. (A)

81. **4.** Third-degree heart block occurs when atrial stimuli are blocked at the atrioventricular junction. Impulses from the atria and ventricles are conducted independently of each other. The atrial rate is 60 to 100 bpm; the ventricular rate is usually 10 to 60 bpm. (A)

82. **1.** The nurse should call the oncology unit to institute a transfer. The nurse handling chemotherapy agents should be specially trained. It is an unwise use of nursing resources to send a nurse from one unit to administer medications to a client on another unit. It is better to centralize and send the client who needs chemotherapy to one unit. Even if the pharmacy mixes the agent, the drug must be administered by a specially trained nurse. (M)

83. **2.** After surgery, the most important nursing diagnosis is *Risk for infection*. Surgery involves an incision, which places the infant at risk for infection. The infant with this type of procedure does have discomfort, which can be relieved with acetaminophen (Tylenol). *Acute pain* is an important nursing diagnosis but not the priority. The infant may be in arm restraints or have the cuff of the sleeve pinned to the diaper or pants. It is important that the infant not touch the incision line or disrupt the sutures. There is no indication for a nursing diagnosis of *Impaired parenting*. The parents would be reacting normally with a first reaction of shock. (A)

84. **1.** An appropriate outcome for the client with rheumatoid arthritis is that he will adopt self-care behaviors to manage joint pain, stiffness, and fatigue and be able to perform activities of daily living. Range-of-motion (ROM) exercises can help maintain mobility, but it may not be realistic to expect the client to maintain full ROM. Depending on the disease progression, there may be further development of pain and joint deformity, even with appropriate therapy. It is important for the client to understand the importance of taking the prescribed drug therapy even if symptoms have abated. (R)

85. **4.** Hydrotherapy wound cleaning is very painful for the client. The client should be medicated for pain about 30 minutes before the treatment in anticipation of the increased pain the client will experience. Wounds are debrided but excessive fluids are not lost during the hydrotherapy session. However, electrolyte loss can occur from open wounds during immersion, so the sessions should be limited to 20 to 30 minutes. There is no need to limit food or fluids 45 minutes before hydrotherapy unless it is an individualized need for a given client. Topical antibiotics are applied after hydrotherapy. (R)

86. **1.** Hepatitis B immune globulin is given as prophylactic therapy to individuals who have been exposed to hepatitis B. Interferon has been approved to treat hepatitis B. Hepatitis B surface antigen is a diagnostic test used to detect current infection. Amphotericin B is an antifungal. (D)

87. **1.** When examining the tympanic membrane of a child younger than age 3 years, the nurse should pull the pinna down and back. For an older child, the nurse should pull the pinna up and back to view the tympanic membrane. (R)

88. **3.** In the compensatory stage of shock, the client exhibits moderate tachycardia. If the shock continues to the progressive stage, decreased urinary output, hypotension, and mental confusion develops as a result of failure to perfuse and ineffective compensatory mechanisms. These findings are indications that the body's compensatory mechanisms are failing. (A)

89. **2.** Hydrochlorothiazide is a thiazide diuretic. Muscle weakness can be an indication of hypokalemia. Polyuria is associated with this diuretic, not urinary retention. Confusion and diaphoresis are not side effects of hydrochlorothiazide. (D)

90. **1.** The ability to remember an old song is related to long-term memory, which persists after short-term memory is lost. Therefore, the nurse should respond by providing the son with this information. Stating that the nurse is happy to hear about the change and that the client is getting better is inappropriate and inaccurate. This statement ignores the issue of long-term versus short-term memory. Telling the client not to get his hopes up because the improvement is only temporary is inappropriate. The information provided does not indicate that the client has expressive aphasia, which would be suggested by the statement that the client can't talk to the son. (P)

91. **1.** A specimen for culture and sensitivity should be sent to the laboratory promptly so that a smear can be taken before organisms start to grow in the specimen. (R)

92. **1.** The client is in a crisis and has a high anxiety level. Holding the client's hands and encouraging the client to slow down and take a deep breath conveys caring and helps decrease anxiety. Telling the client to calm down or stop worrying offers no concrete directions for accomplishing this task. It is unknown from the data who was at fault in the accident. Therefore, it is inappropriate for the nurse to state that it wasn't the client's fault. (P)

93. **3.** Many women who acquire gonorrhea are asymptomatic or experience mild symptoms that are easily ignored. They are not necessarily more reluctant than men to seek medical treatment, but they are more likely not to realize they have been affected. Gonorrhea is easily transmitted to all women and can result in serious consequences, such as pelvic inflammatory disease and infertility. (S)

94. **4.** Tingling and numbness of the toes would be the earliest indication of circulatory impairment. Inability to move the toes and cyanosis are later indicators. Complaints of cast tightness should be investigated because cast tightness can lead to circulatory impairment; it is not, however, an indicator of impairment. (R)

95. **3.** The nurse notifies the physician because a drooping of one side of the face or a "one-side cry" is asso-

ciated with facial nerve damage. Additionally, the mother's delivery record and history need to be reviewed for a possible cause. Craniotabes is a softening of the skull bones. The bones are so soft that indentation from the pressure of an examining finger can occur. Meningitis, or inflammation of the meninges, is associated with a rigid neck. Other symptoms may include lethargy, poor sucking reflexes, weak cry, seizures, and apnea. Skull fracture is not associated with a drooping facial appearance. Rather, it would be evidenced by a crack in the skull bone, possibly accompanied by leaking cerebrospinal fluid. (R)

96. **3.** The client should be encouraged to report painful urination or urinary retention. Lesions may appear 2 to 12 days after exposure. The client is capable of transmitting the infection even when asymptomatic, so a barrier contraceptive should be used. Drinking extra fluids will not stop the lesions from forming. (S)

97. **2.** Severe hypoperfusion to all vital organs results in failure of the vital functions and then circulatory collapse. Hypotension, anuria, respiratory distress, and acidosis are other symptoms associated with irreversible shock. The client in irreversible shock will not be alert. (A)

98. **1.** Pulmonary embolism is a potentially life-threatening complication of deep vein thrombosis. The client's change in mental status, tachypnea, and tachycardia indicate a possible pulmonary embolism. The nurse should promptly notify the doctor of the client's condition. Administering a sedative without further evaluation of the client's condition is not appropriate. There is no need to elicit a positive Homans' sign; the client is already diagnosed with deep vein thrombosis. Increasing the I.V. flow rate may be an appropriate action, but not without first notifying the physician. (R)

99. **3.** The nurse should always double-check a large dose of insulin before administering it. A nurse should always listen to the client; if a client who has been taking insulin for a long time suggests that the insulin dose is not right, the nurse should recheck the physician's order. Comparing insulin doses of other clients has no bearing on a particular client's dose. The nurse should not use "U" or "u"; the nurse should specify "unit" to avoid errors. (M)

100. **2.** Coping with the chronic tinnitus of Ménière's disease can be very frustrating. Providing background sound, such as music, can help camouflage the low-pitched, roaring sound of tinnitus. Maintaining a quiet environment can make the sounds of tinnitus more pronounced. Avoiding caffeine and nicotine is recommended, because this can decrease the occurrence of the tinnitus. However, avoiding these substances does not help the client with coping with tinnitus when it occurs. Taking a sedative does not affect tinnitus. (A)

101. **2.** The child's signs and symptoms in conjunction with the acute onset suggest possible croup or epiglottiditis. The priority diagnosis at this time is *Risk for injury.* The airway may become completely occluded by the epiglottis at any time. Although the child is probably experiencing fear and anxiety, and impaired gas exchange may occur with continued respiratory distress, the immediate priority is a patent airway. No evidence is provided to support aspiration and ineffective airway clearance. (A)

102. **1.** In emphysema, the client's lungs lose elasticity and only partially deflate. Air is trapped in the alveoli. As a result of these pathologic changes, the amount of air remaining in the lungs after forced expiration (residual volume) is increased and the amount of air that can be forcibly exhaled (forced expiratory volume) is decreased. Total lung capacity is increased owing to hyperinflation of the lungs. The maximum amount of air that can be exhaled after maximum inhalation (vital capacity) is decreased. (A)

103. **4.** Diabetic retinopathy involves background and proliferative retinopathy. Both forms are associated with vascular changes in the basement membrane of the arterioles and capillaries of the choroid and retina. Neuropathy is usually associated with the lower extremities. (R)

104. **2.** The 70-year-old woman with syncopal episodes is at greatest risk for falling. The nurse should assess the client's gait and balance and the syncopal episodes. The 22-year-old man with upper body fractures and the 50-year-old man with angina are not at risk for falling. The 30-year-old woman could be at risk for falling, but she is at less risk than the 70-year-old client with syncope. (M)

105. **3.** The baseline laboratory data that are established before a client is started on tissue plasminogen activator or alteplase recombinant include hematocrit, hemoglobin level, and platelet count. (R)

106. **3.** The most appropriate long-term goal for the client with hypertension is to commit to lifelong therapy. A significant problem in the long-term management of hypertension is compliance with the treatment plan. It is essential that the client understand the reasons for modifying lifestyle, taking prescribed medications, and obtaining regular health care. Limiting stress, losing weight, and monitoring blood pressure are important aspects of care for the client with hypertension; however, the treatment plan must be individualized to include aspects of care that are appropriate for each client. (H)

107. **1.** The nurse should work with the client to individualize the plan of care for managing pain. Cancer pain is best managed with a combination of medications, and each client needs to be worked with individually to find the treatment regimen that works best. Cancer pain is commonly undertreated because of fear of addiction. The client who is in pain needs the appropriate level of analgesic and needs to be reassured that he will not become addicted. Cancer pain is best treated with regularly scheduled doses of medication. Administering the medication only when the client asks for it will not lead to adequate pain control. As drug tolerance develops, the dosage of the medication can be increased. (C)

108. **4.** The client needs further instructions when she says, "I can continue to work at my job at the automobile factory until labor starts." The goal is to avoid preterm labor. Because the client is experiencing severe hydramnios, she will most likely be maintained on bed rest to increase uteroplacental circulation and reduce pressure on the cervix. Hydramnios has been associated with increased weight gain caused by increased amniotic fluid volume. Hydramnios has been associated with gastrointestinal disorders in the fetus, such as tracheoesophageal fistula with stenosis or intestinal obstruction. The client should continue to eat high-fiber foods and should avoid straining, which could lead to ruptured membranes. Stool softeners may also be ordered. The client should report any symptoms of fluid rupture or labor. (R)

109. **1.** The stationary bicycle is the most appropriate training modality because it is a non-weight-bearing exercise. Interval training involves rest and exercise. The time that the individual exercises on the stationary bicycle is increased with improved functional capacity, and the rest time is decreased. (H)

110. **1.** Nausea and anorexia, and in some situations weight loss, are symptoms experienced by clients with jaundice. Jaundice is associated with high levels of bilirubin in the blood. Causes include hepatitis, yellow fever, and alcoholism. The nursing diagnoses of *Acute pain* related to muscle spasms and *Ineffective health maintenance* are not supported by the data. *Adult failure to thrive* is a possible nursing diagnosis; however, more data is needed to support it. (A)

111. **1.** The protocol recommended by the Agency for Healthcare Research and Quality is that all clients who are at risk for pressure ulcer development be identified on admission to health care facilities so that preventive actions can be implemented by the nursing staff. These preventive actions need to be individualized to the client, so automatic placement of all at-risk clients on an every-2-hour turning schedule, a specialty bed, or a high-protein, high-carbohydrate diet is not appropriate. (R)

112. **3.** Visual disturbances are a symptom of digoxin (Lanoxin) toxicity. These disturbances can include double, blurred, or yellow vision. Cardiovascular manifestations of digoxin toxicity include bradycardia, other dysrhythmias, and pulse deficit. Gastrointestinal symptoms include anorexia, nausea, and vomiting. (D)

113. **2.** Irradiated skin can become dry and irritated, resulting in itching and discomfort. The client should be instructed to clean the skin gently and apply nonperfumed, nonirritating lotions to help relieve dryness. Taking an antihistamine does not relieve the skin dryness that is causing the itching. Heat should not be applied to the area because it can cause further irritation. Medicated ointments, especially corticosteroids, which is controversial, should not be applied to the skin without the order of the radiation therapist. (R)

114. **3.** Serotonin, a principal neurotransmitter and appetite suppressant, is produced in the brain from tryptophan. Epinephrine and norepinephrine are made from tyrosine. Phenylalanine is an amino acid found in food. (A)

115. **1.** The mask is appropriate because it covers the nose and mouth and fits snugly against the cheeks and chin. Masks that are too large may cover the eyes. Masks that are too small obstruct the nose. The mask does not need to be covered with a cloth. (M)

116. **4.** In preparation for a thoracentesis, the client should be asked to sit forward and place his arms on the bedside table for support. This position provides access to the chest wall and intercostal spaces for insertion of the needle. The supine, Sims', or prone position would not provide adequate access to the chest wall or separate the intercostal spaces sufficiently for needle insertion. (R)

117. **4.** The antidote for heparin is 1% protamine sulfate. Vitamin K is the antidote for warfarin, an oral anticoagulant. Thrombin is a topical anticoagulant. (D)

118. **1.** At this time, the client's anger is not out of control, so empathy and talking are appropriate to diffuse the anger. Using time-out is appropriate when the client's anger is escalating and the client can no longer talk about the anger rationally. Restraints are appropriate only when there is imminent risk of harm to the client or others. Future strategies are discussed after the initial incident is resolved. (P)

119. **2.** The client with myasthenia gravis may have an impaired ability to swallow. Blood draining down the back of the throat may be aspirated if swallowing is impaired. This client may have an impaired breathing pattern due to weak intercostal muscles; however, the priority is to prevent aspiration. The nursing diagnosis of *Risk for injury* is not specific enough in this situation. There are no data to support the diagnosis of *Feeding self-care deficit*. (A)

120. **1.** The nurse's first action after the removal of a NG tube is to provide the client with oral hygiene. Then it is appropriate to give the client liquids to drink if the client is no longer on nothing-by-mouth status. There is no association between removal of an NG tube and having the client cough and deep-breathe. Auscultating the client's bowel sounds should be done before removal of the NG tube. (C)

121. **3.** Heat applications cause vasodilation, which promotes circulation to the area, and increase tissue metabolism and leukocyte mobility. Heat applications do not prevent swelling; applications of cold are used to prevent swelling by causing vasoconstriction. (R)

122. **1.** Thick, cloudy amniotic fluid indicates an intrauterine infection. Typically, the client has a fever, lethargy, and malaise. Greenish-colored amniotic fluid is associated with meconium staining. A strong yellowish color is associated with erythroblastosis fetalis because of the presence of bilirubin and hemolyzed red blood cells. The normal color of amniotic fluid is clear or with a very slight yellow tint later in pregnancy. (R)

123. **3.** When finishing a 24-hour urine collection, the final voided urine is saved and added to the collection container. The first urine specimen, voided at 7 a.m. Monday, is discarded. The urine is not sent for a urine culture. It is not necessary to separate each day's collection of urine. (R)

124. **2.** Hypoalbuminemia occurs in cirrhosis because the liver cannot synthesize albumin. This causes a decrease in colloidal osmotic pressure, resulting in ascites. Hyperkalemia is not an expected electrolyte imbalance of cirrhosis. The aspartate aminotransferase and alanine aminotransferase values are increased in liver disease. (A)

125. **2.** At this time, the infant can be given the vaccines. The fact that the child's sibling is immunosuppressed because of chemotherapy is not a reason to withhold the vaccines. The fact that the child has a cold is not grounds for delaying the immunizations. However, if the child had a high fever, the immunizations would be delayed. (H)

126. **3.** The primary cause of disability and death in children is injury from accidents. Teaching safety measures to children and their parents is the best way to decrease injury and accidents. (S)

127. **1.** A major goal of postoperative care for the client who has had an incisional cholecystectomy is the prevention of respiratory complications. Because of the location of the incision, the client has a difficult time breathing deeply. Use of incentive spirometry promotes chest expansion and decreases atelectasis. Performing leg exercises each shift is not frequent enough; they should be performed hourly. Maintaining a weight reduction diet may be appropriate for the client, but it is not the highest priority in the immediate postoperative phase. Promoting wound healing is important, but respiratory complications are most common after a cholecystectomy. (R)

128. **1.** In response to hearing a noise, normally hearing infants blink or startle and stop body movements. Shy and withdrawn behaviors are characteristic of older children with hearing impairment. Squealing occurs in 90% of infants by age 4 months. Most infants can say "da-da" by age 9 months. (H)

129. **3.** Continuous irrigation, usually consisting of sterile normal saline, is used after TURP to keep blood clots from obstructing the catheter and impeding urine flow. Antibiotics may be instilled in the bladder with the use of an irrigating solution, but this is not the primary reason for using continuous irrigation in TURP. The irrigating solution may secondarily help prevent bladder distention because it keeps the catheter from becoming obstructed. (R)

130. **3.** A distended bladder produces dullness when percussed because of the presence of urine. Hyperresonance is a percussion sound that is present in hyperinflated lungs. Tympany, a loud drumlike sound, occurs over gas-filled areas such as the intestines. Flat sounds occur over very dense tissue that has no air present. (A)

131. **2.** Major accidents can induce feelings similar to those of victims of other kinds of disasters and crime. Therefore, the nurse calls the crisis nurse to assist the passengers with their feelings of victimization. Passengers may mourn the loss of a vacation, but, with no fatalities, major grief reactions are not expected. Other personnel can take calls from relatives while the crisis nurse helps the passengers. Psychiatric hospitalization is a premature assumption. (P)

132. **1.** When placed on the abdomen, a neonate pulls the legs up under the body, which puts tension on the perineum. Therefore, after surgery, the neonate should be positioned either supine with the legs suspended at a 90-degree angle or on either side with the hips elevated. (R)

133. **1.** The child with meningococcal meningitis requires droplet precautions for at least the first 24 hours after effective therapy is initiated to reduce the risk of transmission to others on the unit. After the child has been placed on droplet precautions, other actions, such as taking the child's vital signs, asking about medication allergies, and inquiring about the health of siblings at home, can be performed. (S)

134. **1.** Teenagers usually enjoy activities with peers in preference to socializing with their parents or siblings. Peer relationships help the adolescent develop self-identity. (H)

135. **2, 3.** Teens are very concerned about their body image and knowing about the size of the scar is important to them. Typically, teens return to school in 1 week. While hospitalized, friends can visit during visiting hours. Clients are usually hospitalized for an uncomplicated appendectomy for about 24 hours. Antibiotics are not routinely given to prevent an infection. The dressing is removed within a few days. (A)

136. **2.** Morphine can cause urinary retention. The nurse should assess the client for urinary hesitancy or retention, and note the urinary output. It is not necessary to take the apical heart rate after each dose of morphine. Mental status should be assessed after each dose because morphine can cause such effects as sedation, delirium, and disorientation. Assessing for pedal edema is not necessary. (D)

137. **2.** Pain is a priority for the client with renal calculi. The pain is typically described as excruciating and intermittent, occurring as the stone moves. Analgesics are a major part of therapy. *Activity intolerance* is secondary to the excruciating pain. Although the client experiences occasional nausea, there are no data to support a nursing diagnosis of *Deficient fluid volume* or *Imbalanced nutrition: Less than body requirements*. (A)

138. **4.** Infection is the greatest concern to the nurse. Infection occurs more frequently because of the number of procedures performed on clients that require this therapy and people they come in contact with in the hospital. Infection can be reduced if proper infection control techniques are used and human contact is reduced. Deficiencies and toxicities of nutrients are rare because of the use of standard protocols and orders for TPN formulas. Hyperglycemia can occur with TPN administration; however, all clients receiving TPN have their serum glucose concentration monitored frequently, and the hyperglycemia can easily be managed by adding insulin to the TPN solution. An infection is a much more serious complication. (D)

139. **2.** The nurse should assess for signs of impending shock such as diaphoresis. The client would have hypotension, dysuria, and cool skin. (D)

140. **2.** The urinary appliance should be emptied before the pouch is one-third full to prevent urinary reflux. The appliance should be attached to a leg bag at night to allow for adequate drainage. It is not appropriate to administer prophylactic antibiotics when incorporating positive self-care activities into the client's routine can prevent most urinary tract infections. The urinary appliance is not changed daily. If no leakage occurs and the client's skin remains free from irritation, the appliance can be left in place for 1 week or more. (C)

141. **1.** Preoxygenating the client before suctioning helps prevent the development of hypoxia during the procedure. The suction catheter is inserted about 5 to 6 inches into the cannula. A bolus of 3 to 5 ml of sterile normal saline solution may be inserted into the cannula before suctioning to stimulate coughing and loosen secretions. The nurse uses sterile technique when suctioning a client. (R)

142. **3.** Because the toddler has a severe diaper rash, it may be best to change all that the parents are doing. The buttocks need to be washed thoroughly with mild soap and dried well. In fact, it is helpful to leave the diaper off and expose the buttocks to the air. Baby wipes commonly contain additives and perfumes that may be irritating to the baby's sensitive skin. The diaper needs to be changed more often than every 4 to 6 hours. Otherwise, the moist diaper environment will continue to irritate the skin, causing the rash to worsen. Powder has limited absorbing ability and will most likely irritate the area more. In addition, some powders contain perfumes or are scented and can irritate the skin. (C)

143. **2.** The toddler is screaming for a reason, so it is most therapeutic to ask the mother why the child is screaming. This type of question is nonaccusatory, just seeking information. Asking the mother what happened between her and the child makes the assumption that something did happen and limits the amount of information to be gained from the question. Asking whether something caused the child to be upset makes an assumption that something happened and limits the answer to a yes or no response, cutting off communication. Asking whether the mother has tried to calm the child is accusatory and also limits the response to yes or no, thus cutting off communication. (H)

144. **4.** The client will need to avoid extremes of motion in the hip to avoid dislocation. The hip should not be flexed more than 90 degrees, internally rotated, or legs crossed. It is not possible to safely sit in the bathtub without flexing the hip beyond the recommended 90 degrees. The client can implement the prescribed exercise program at the time of discharge home. The client should take care not to stress the hip for 3 to 6 months after surgery. An elevated toilet seat will be necessary during the recovery from surgery. (R)

145. **1.** The common presenting symptoms of infectious mononucleosis vary greatly but commonly include fever, malaise, sore throat, and lymphadenopathy. Skin rash, cold symptoms, abdominal pain, and weight loss are less common symptoms. (A)

146. **1.** The nurse should place the nondominant hand above the symphysis pubis and the dominant hand at the umbilicus to palpate the fundus. This prevents uterine inversion and trauma, which can be very painful to the client. The nurse should ask the client to assume a supine, not side-lying, position with the knees flexed. The fundus can be palpated in this position and the perineal pads can be evaluated for lochia amounts. The fundus should be massaged gently if the fundus feels boggy. Vigorous massaging may fatigue the uterus and cause it to become firm and then boggy again. The nurse should ask the client to void before fundal evaluation. A full bladder can cause discomfort to the client, the uterus to be deviated to one side, and postpartum hemorrhage. (H)

147. **2.** A reactive nonstress test is a positive sign indicating that the fetus is doing well at this point in the pregnancy. For a nonstress test to be a reactive test, at least two accelerations (15 beats or more) of the fetal heart rate lasting at least 15 seconds must occur after movement. If the fetus were compromised, the nonstress test would demonstrate no accelerations in fetal heart rate; a contraction stress test would show fetal heart rate decelerations during simulated labor. Late decelerations are associated with a positive or abnormal contraction stress test. No accelerations in a 20-minute period during a nonstress test may mean that the fetus is sleeping; however, this is interpreted as a nonreactive nonstress test. (R)

148. **3.** Right-sided heart failure causes venous congestion resulting in such symptoms as peripheral (dependent) edema, splenomegaly, hepatomegaly, and neck vein distention. Intermittent claudication is associated with arterial occlusion. Dyspnea and crackles are associated with pulmonary edema, which occurs in left-sided heart failure. (A)

149. **1.** To help prevent flexion deformities, a client with rheumatoid arthritis should lie in a prone position in bed for about ½ hour several times a day. This positioning helps keep the hips and knees in an extended position and prevents joint flexion. Low Fowler's, modified Trendelenburg, and side-lying positions do not prevent hip flexion. (C)

150. **2.** Administration of an epidural anesthetic can result in a hypotensive effect on maternal blood pressure. Therefore, the priority assessment is the mother's blood pressure. Ephedrine or wedging the client to a position to keep pressure off the vena cava, such as on the left side, can be used to elevate maternal blood pressure should it drop too low. Epidural anesthesia has no effect on the level of consciousness or the client's cognitive function. Although the client's contraction pattern may decrease in frequency after administration of the anesthesia, the priority assessment is the client's blood pressure. After blood pressure is maintained, contractions can be assessed. (D)

151. **1.** The client's assessment findings indicate that the client is in the latent phase of the first stage of labor. Therefore, the nurse should plan to assist the client with comfort measures and breathing techniques to relieve discomfort. The client can move around, walk, or ambulate at this phase of labor. If the client chooses to remain in bed, a left side-lying position provides the greatest perfusion. It is too early for the client to have an epidural anesthetic. Epidural anesthesia is usually administered when the cervix is dilated 4 to 5 cm. The fetal heart rate is normal, so internal fetal monitoring is not warranted at this time. (H)

152. **4.** Hypokalemia is one of the most common causes of digoxin (Lanoxin) toxicity. It is essential that the nurse carefully monitor the potassium levels of clients taking digoxin to avoid toxicity. Low serum potassium levels can cause cardiac dysrhythmias. (D)

153. **3.** Current pain guidelines recommend the removal of meperidine from formularies and the substitution of morphine commonly administered by patient-controlled analgesia. Meperidine can be ordered for severe pain but its use is limited by the high incidence of neurotoxicity (seizures) associated with the accumulation of its metabolite, normeperidine. It is contraindicated in clients with acute pain lasting more than 2 days and in those for whom large daily doses (more than 600 mg) are needed. It would be inappropriate to urge the client to take the acetaminophen and codeine to prevent addiction. Addiction is a psychological condition in which a client is driven to take drugs for reasons that are not therapeutic. The client is in pain and her need for the morphine is therapeutic. Although the client may obtain some relief from relaxation exercises, this alone is not sufficient to provide pain relief. (D)

154. **1.** Infants at age 7 months are not capable of drinking from a cup without spilling. At age 6 months, infants can partially lift their weight on the hands, enjoy imitating sounds, and are developing separation anxiety. (H)

155. **3.** According to Erikson, a child of 13 years is normally seeking to meet the need to develop personal identity. Personal values are a component of this identity. Developing a conscience is a component of achieving initiative during the preschool years. Developing a sense of competence is a component of achieving industry in the school-age years. Developing a lifetime vocation is a component of achieving generativity in adulthood. (P)

156. **4.** Cardiomyopathy means that the myocardium is weak and irritable. Amiodarone is an antiarrhythmic and acts directly on the cardiac cell membrane. In this situation, amiodarone is used to increase the ventricular fibrillation threshold. Amiodarone is contraindicated in sinus node dysfunction, heart block, and severe bradycardia. (A)

157. **1.** A frothy, purulent vaginal discharge in a sexually active female client is typically caused by a sexually transmitted disease such as trichomonas. Other diseases, such as chlamydia, may also be present. Both the client and the boyfriend need treatment after the disease is determined. Normal variations in female vaginal discharge should be clear to white, not frothy or purulent. The client should be instructed to wear cotton underwear and avoid pantyhose, wet gym clothes, and tight-fitting garments, such as jeans, so that air can circulate. (S)

158. **4.** The most common factor in skin breakdown is immobility. Right-sided paralysis, in which the client can-not perceive the need to change position and lacks control over movement of the extremities, is the condition most likely to lead to skin breakdown. It is essential that the nurse plan to change the client's position at least every 2 hours. Nutritional status and urinary incontinence can contribute to skin breakdown, but neither is the most critical factor. Confusion does not directly influence skin breakdown. (R)

159. **1.** Psychomotor retardation refers to a general slowdown of motor activity commonly seen in a client with depression. Movements appear lethargic, energy is absent or lacking, and performance of activity is slow and difficult. A flat affect reflects a lack of emotion. An unkempt appearance reflects lack of self-care. Avoiding eye contact reflects low self-esteem or suspiciousness. (P)

160. **3.** A hydrocele, defined as fluid in the processus vaginalis, is determined when the scrotal sac can be transilluminated. A swelling in the scrotal area that can be reduced indicates an inguinal hernia. Both hydroceles and hernias can enlarge the scrotal sac, and both can be either unilateral or bilateral. A hernia typically is more obvious during crying. (A)

161. **1.** When cleaning the skin around an incision and drain, the nurse should clean the incision and drain separately to avoid contaminating either wound. This is applying the principle of working from the least contaminated area to the most contaminated area. In this case, both areas are fresh wounds and should be kept separate. (S)

162. **4.** Any injury to the mouth results in copious amounts of blood because the mouth is a highly vascular area. Because the nurse does not know the mother and does not speak Spanish, the most appropriate action is to give the mother the ice and demonstrate what she is to do. The child will be less fearful if the ice is applied by the mother. Calling for an interpreter is appropriate after caring for the immediate need of the child. Grabbing the child away will probably upset the mother more, further adding to the stress experienced by the child. (P)

163. **4.** Having the client deep-breathe hourly is the most appropriate action for the assistant to take to help prevent pulmonary complications. The client should be turned at least every 2 hours. Keeping the client's head elevated will not prevent pulmonary complications. Suctioning the client is not an assistant's responsibility, nor does it prevent pulmonary complications. (M)

164. **1, 3.** The outcomes to achieve for a nursing diagnosis of *Ineffective tissue perfusion* involve evidence of adequate blood flow to the area. The temperature of the involved extremity is an important indicator for a client with peripheral vascular disease. The temperature will indicate the degree to which the blood supply is getting to the extremity. Warmth indicates adequate blood flow. Pain is also an indicator of blood flow. Pain, such as muscle pain, suggests ischemia and lack of oxygen that results when the oxygen demand becomes greater than the supply. Thus, a decrease in muscle pain with activity would suggest improvement in blood flow to the area. Improved respiratory status and clear lungs are unrelated to ineffective tissue perfusion. Although participation in self-care measures is always helpful, this outcome is more appropriate for a nursing diagnosis of *Activity intolerance, Fatigue,* or *Self-care deficit.* (A)

165. 3. When dextrose is abruptly discontinued, rebound hypoglycemia can occur. The nurse should assess the client for symptoms of hypoglycemia. Essential fatty acid deficiency is very unlikely to occur because some of these fatty acids are stored. Preventing dehydration or malnutrition is not the reason for tapering the infusion rate; the client's hydration and nutritional status and ability to maintain adequate intake must be established before total parenteral nutrition is discontinued. (D)

166. 1. During the third trimester, particularly in the seventh month of pregnancy, the client typically exhibits feelings of vulnerability and fear that the baby will be lost. Confirmation that the fetus is real occurs during the second trimester. Ambivalence is typically seen and resolved during the first trimester. Body image disturbance commonly occurs during the second trimester because of the profound changes that occur to the body during this time. (H)

167. 2. As the dye is injected, the client may experience a feeling of warmth, flushing of the face, and a salty taste in the mouth. The client should not experience chest pain or cold chills; these would be adverse reactions warranting close monitoring of the client. (R)

168. 4. Isoniazid competes for the available vitamin B_6 in the body and leaves the client at risk for developing neuropathies related to vitamin deficiency. Supplemental vitamin B_6 is routinely prescribed to address this issue. Avoiding sun exposure is a preventive measure to lower the risk of skin cancer. Following a low-cholesterol diet lowers the individual's risk of developing atherosclerotic plaque. Rest is important in maintaining homeostasis but has no real impact on neuropathies. (D)

169. 2. The interpreter must have gotten delayed somewhere. Therefore, the nurse's best action would be to reschedule the child's appointment when the interpreter can be scheduled as well. Because the mother does not speak English, there is no point in having the pediatric nurse practitioner see the infant because history information is needed and most likely would be too difficult to obtain. Asking the mother to stay longer is rude to her. Also, doing so would probably be difficult because of the communication gap. Paging one more time is a desperate measure and inappropriate. (M)

170. 3. Oxygen concentrations greater than 40% have been found to cause oxygen toxicity in adults. (D)

171. 1. The client who is on a progressive exercise program at home after a myocardial infarction should be taught to monitor his pulse rate. The pulse rate can be expected to increase with exercise, but exercise should not be increased if the pulse rate increases more than about 25 bpm from baseline or exceeds 100 to 125 bpm. The client should also be taught to decrease exercise if chest pain or dyspnea occurs. (C)

172. 1. The nurse's response fails to identify the meaning in what the client has said. The nurse needs to explore the client's statement about hating God for that flood because the meaning of the client's statement is unclear. Also, clichés such as, "Don't feel that way," are not helpful because they ignore the client's feelings and his interpretation of the situation in which he finds himself. Explaining to the client why he may think as he does (offering a rationale) is inappropriate. The nurse's response fails to identify the meaning in what the client has said and is not supportive. There is no evidence that the client is solving his problems. (P)

173. 3. The client who should be assessed first is the multigravid client who has been in labor for 8 hours and whose cervix is 8 cm dilated at 1+ station with contractions every 3 to 4 minutes. A multigravid client typically has a shorter labor than a primigravid, and this client's station is 1+, which means that delivery of the fetus is imminent. (M)

174. 2. The nurse should contact the physician and clarify whether the client's usual insulin dose should be given before surgery. Practices vary, and it should not be assumed by the nurse that the usual insulin dose is to be given. It is not the nurse's responsibility to evaluate the client's need for insulin. It is not appropriate for the nurse to defer decision-making on this issue until after surgery. (R)

175. 4. Immediately after chest tube removal, a petrolatum gauze is placed over the wound and covered with a dry sterile dressing. This serves as an airtight seal to prevent air leakage or air movement in either direction. Bandages or straps are not applied directly over wounds. Mesh gauze allows air movement. (S)

176. 4. By asking the client to tell more about how she is feeling, the nurse is not making any assumptions about what is troubling the client. The nurse should acknowledge the client's feelings and encourage her to discuss them. Saying that this situation must be frustrating involves assumptions by the nurse about why the client is crying and is not a therapeutic response. Asking how long the client has been unable to comb her hair takes the focus off her feelings and inhibits therapeutic communication.

Inquiring why the client's husband hasn't helped insinuates that the husband is not helping enough, which is inappropriate, takes the focus off the client's feelings, and inhibits therapeutic communication. (P)

177. **3.** Encouraging the client to talk about why she is here and about her feelings may reveal more information about what led her to come to the group and what led to her diagnosis. It also provides the nurse with valuable information needed to develop an appropriate plan of care. The comment that the client sounds angry presumes what the client is feeling and asks her to talk about her husband. The focus here should be on the client, not the husband. Telling the client that she will like coming to group imposes the nurse's view onto the client. The statement stresses that the group is fun instead of giving its therapeutic value. Having the client tell the nurse something about the cause of her bulimia ignores the client's original statement. Additionally, this statement requires the client to have insight into the cause of her disease, which may not be possible at this time. Also, it may be too early in the relationship to discuss the disorder. (P)

178. **1.** Introduction of medication is most likely to be added to continue lifestyle modifications. Exercise, smoking cessation, and weight reduction are part of the first steps involved in lifestyle modification. (R)

179. **2.** There is a direct interaction between the effects of insulin and those of beta blockers. The nurse must be aware that there is a potential for increased hypoglycemic effects of insulin when a beta blocker is added to the client's medication regimen. The client's blood sugar should be monitored. Ketoacidosis occurs in hyperglycemia. Although a decrease in the incidence of ketoacidosis could occur when a beta blocker is added, the direct result is an increase in the hypoglycemic effect of insulin. (D)

180. **3.** Commonly, when a child appears better, the parents stop the medication. Unfortunately, the infection remains. Therefore, the nurse needs to explain that all of the medication is needed to clear up the infection. Explaining why the medicine should be continued is more helpful to parents than saying it needs to be given. Asking how the mother knows that her child's ears are better blames the mother and diminishes her self-esteem. Telling the mother that stopping the medication is not what is best for the child implies blame and is condescending. (D)

181. **67**

Using a proportion: The nurse should set the I.V. infusion pump at 67 ml/hour to administer 1 g of cefazolin (Ancef) in normal saline solution 50 ml over 45 minutes. (D)

182. **1.** Ambivalence is a common reaction, even when the pregnancy was planned. Manifested by conflicting feelings about the pregnancy, it usually resolves during the first trimester. There is no indication of disappointment. A statement such as, "I really don't want to be pregnant," indicates disappointment. There is no indication that the client desires an abortion, although this is an option for the client. There is no reason to suspect that bonding will be a problem after delivery, unless the client shows no signs of wanting to care for the infant after delivery. (P)

183. **2.** Increasing estrogen levels during puberty are responsible for breast development. Prolactin is a hormone necessary for milk production during pregnancy and lactation. Progesterone maintains a pregnancy after conception. Testosterone is responsible for male sexual development during puberty. (H)

184. **1.** Gastrointestinal hemorrhage occurs in about 25% of clients receiving prolonged mechanical ventilation. Other possible complications include incorrect ventilation, oxygen toxicity, fluid imbalance, decreased cardiac output, pneumothorax, infection, and atelectasis. Immunosuppression and pulmonary emboli are not direct consequences of mechanical ventilation. (A)

185. **3.** The nurse should encourage the client to sit down or lie down when he has angina. Nitroglycerin relaxes smooth muscles and dilates vascular beds; therefore, nitroglycerin causes hypotension and the client could fall, causing injury. Nitroglycerin should be stored in a dark container. It should be taken once every 5 minutes for three doses and is placed sublingually, not swallowed. (A)

186. **2.** Before giving information, it is important for the nurse to assess the learner's current level of knowledge. When dealing with parents of an ill child, the nurse considers their emotional strength and the intensity of the situation and deals with them in an accepting, nonthreatening manner. Parents may feel overwhelmed by the events, and they need time to adjust to the situation. (P)

187. **2.** The IUD is suitable for clients who desire long-term contraceptive use and are in a monogamous relationship. Because of the increased risk of infection with an IUD if an STD occurs, the device is not appropriate for women with multiple partners or a history of STDs. Previous ectopic pregnancy is also a contraindication for an IUD because the incidence of ectopic implantation is slightly higher. (H)

188. **1.** One of the main techniques used in crisis intervention in the hospital is helping parents begin to gain an intellectual understanding of SIDS. Numerous theories have been proposed, but no specific cause of SIDS has been identified. Evidence suggests that infants with SIDS have chronic hypoxia, possibly from prolonged periodic apnea. (A)

189. **2.** Clients diagnosed with peripheral arterial occlusive disease should be encouraged to participate in a regular walking program to help develop collateral circulation. They should be advised to rest if pain develops and to resume activity when pain subsides. Extremities should be kept in a dependent position to promote circulation; elevation of the extremities will decrease circulation. Heating pads should not be used by anyone with impaired circulation to avoid burns. Massaging the calf muscles will not decrease pain. Intermittent claudication subsides with rest. (R)

190. **4.** Toxoplasmosis is a protozoal infection caused by *Toxoplasma gondii*, which is transmitted through ingestion of raw or undercooked meat, through contact with infected cat feces, or across the placental barrier from the mother to the fetus. The mother should be instructed to cook all meats thoroughly, avoid touching the mucous membranes when handling raw meat, thoroughly clean all kitchen surfaces that have come in contact with raw meat, avoid uncooked eggs, and avoid contact with cat litter boxes and cat feces. The disease is not spread by contact with an infected person. Although prophylactic penicillin may be used for pregnant clients who test positive for group B streptococcus, penicillin is not used to treat toxoplasmosis. Toxoplasmosis may be treated with a combination of pyrimethamine (Daraprim) and sulfadiazine, accompanied by folic acid to reduce the toxicity of the other two drugs. However, controversy exists about whether to treat the mother. There is no vaccine for toxoplasmosis. Although a vaccine exists for rubella, this is given within 72 hours postpartum if the client is not immune. (H)

1. The unit secretary who transcribes the physicians' orders asks the nurse to interpret an order because he cannot read the writing. The nurse's best action is to:
- ☐ **1.** Interpret the order according to the client's previous medication record.
- ☐ **2.** Clarify the order with the pharmacist.
- ☐ **3.** Clarify the order by calling the physician.
- ☐ **4.** Clarify the client's medications with the client's family.

2. Propantheline bromide (Pro-Banthine) is ordered for a client who has cholecystitis. What is the primary purpose for administering this drug to clients who have cholecystitis?
- ☐ **1.** To increase bile production.
- ☐ **2.** To decrease biliary spasm.
- ☐ **3.** To treat infection.
- ☐ **4.** To relieve nausea.

3. The nurse refers the parents of a child with cystic fibrosis to the local chapter of the National Cystic Fibrosis Foundation. The Foundation has been especially beneficial for parents of children with cystic fibrosis by helping them:
- ☐ **1.** Find tutors to educate their children at home.
- ☐ **2.** Obtain genetic counseling.
- ☐ **3.** Meet with other parents of children with cystic fibrosis for mutual support.
- ☐ **4.** Obtain financial assistance to purchase medications for their children.

4. After a bronchoscopy with biopsy, the nurse assesses the client. Which of the following signs should be reported immediately to the physician?
- ☐ **1.** Green sputum.
- ☐ **2.** Dry cough.
- ☐ **3.** Hemoptysis.
- ☐ **4.** Laryngeal stridor.

5. A client complains that "the hospital food is horrible." Which of the following is the most appropriate response by the nurse?
- ☐ **1.** "The staff is doing the best they can to cook in such large quantities."
- ☐ **2.** "I'll report this to the physician."
- ☐ **3.** "Would you like to speak with the dietitian about the food and meal selection?"
- ☐ **4.** "I don't like the hospital cafeteria food either."

6. The nurse must be aware that adverse drug reactions in the elderly client may be underestimated because:
- ☐ **1.** Adverse reactions rarely have an atypical presentation.
- ☐ **2.** Cognitive impairment is an expected finding in the elderly client.
- ☐ **3.** Physical or psychological symptoms are attributed to the effects of aging.
- ☐ **4.** Excess sedation is difficult to assess in the elderly client.

7. An elderly man experiences a thrombotic cerebrovascular accident and subsequent flaccid hemiplegia of his right side. When planning his care, rehabilitation begins:
- ☐ **1.** As soon as anticoagulant therapy is started.
- ☐ **2.** When the client is admitted to the hospital.
- ☐ **3.** When the client can first work cooperatively with health care personnel.
- ☐ **4.** As directed by the physical therapist.

8. When considering quality-of-life issues for a client diagnosed with lung cancer, the nurse should be aware that:
- ☐ **1.** Lung cancer is an aggressive disease.
- ☐ **2.** Small cell lung cancer has a good prognosis if treated aggressively.
- ☐ **3.** A client diagnosed with squamous cell carcinoma can get a complete response with chemotherapy.
- ☐ **4.** The overall 5-year survival rate is 45%.

9. An unmarried pregnant teenager tells the nurse that she is undecided about having an abortion or giving the baby up for adoption. The best response for the nurse to offer is which of the following?
- ☐ **1.** "You should give the baby up so that it can have a better home and opportunities."
- ☐ **2.** "Research studies show that babies do better with their natural mothers."
- ☐ **3.** "It must be a difficult decision. What have you thought about so far?"
- ☐ **4.** "Why don't you try keeping the baby. You can always give it up for adoption later."

10. When administering blood, the nurse must check the name on the label of the blood with the name on the client's:
- ☐ **1.** Wristband.
- ☐ **2.** Wristband in the presence of another nurse.
- ☐ **3.** Medical chart.
- ☐ **4.** Medication administration record.

11. A client is admitted to the emergency department with crushing chest injuries sustained in a car accident. Which of the following signs indicates a possible pneumothorax?
- [ ] **1.** Cheyne-Stokes respirations.
- [ ] **2.** Increased fremitus.
- [ ] **3.** Diminished or absent breath sounds on the affected side.
- [ ] **4.** Decreased sensation on the affected side.

12. Which of the following statements by a client taking valproic acid (Depakene) for bipolar disorder indicates that further teaching about this medication is necessary?
- [ ] **1.** "I need to take the pills at the same time each day."
- [ ] **2.** "I can chew the pills if necessary."
- [ ] **3.** "I can take the pills with food."
- [ ] **4.** "I need to call my doctor if I start bruising easily."

13. A nurse is obtaining the history of an infant with suspected acute otitis media. What should the nurse ask the parent about?
- [ ] **1.** Position of the infant when taking a bottle.
- [ ] **2.** Covering of the infant's ears when out in the cold.
- [ ] **3.** Thorough drying of the infant's ears after a bath.
- [ ] **4.** Immunization status of the infant.

14. A client is having elective surgery under general anesthesia. Who is responsible for obtaining the informed consent?
- [ ] **1.** The nurse.
- [ ] **2.** The surgeon.
- [ ] **3.** The anesthesiologist.
- [ ] **4.** The nurse anesthetist.

15. The family of an elderly client with terminal cancer inquires about hospice services. The nurse explains that hospice care:
- [ ] **1.** Focuses only on the needs of the client.
- [ ] **2.** Can only be provided in the inpatient setting.
- [ ] **3.** Is staffed exclusively by professional health care workers.
- [ ] **4.** Focuses on supportive care for the client and family.

16. A primigravid client at 8 weeks' gestation tells the nurse that she doesn't like milk. To ensure that the client consumes an adequate intake of milk products, the nurse should instruct the client that an 8-oz glass of milk is equal to which of the following?
- [ ] **1.** 2 tablespoons of Parmesan cheese.
- [ ] **2.** ½ cup of a milkshake.
- [ ] **3.** 1½ to 2 slices of presliced American cheese.
- [ ] **4.** ½ cup of cottage cheese.

17. A primigravid client at 35 weeks' gestation is scheduled for a biophysical profile. After instructing the client about the test, which of the following, if stated by the client as one of the parameters of this test, indicates effective teaching?
- [ ] **1.** Amniotic fluid volume.
- [ ] **2.** Placement of the placenta.
- [ ] **3.** Amniotic fluid color.
- [ ] **4.** Fetal gestational age.

18. When caring for a child who has been receiving long-term steroid therapy, which of the following should the nurse expect to assess?
- [ ] **1.** Usual behavior and temperament.
- [ ] **2.** Loss of weight from baseline.
- [ ] **3.** Development of truncal obesity.
- [ ] **4.** Demonstration of a growth spurt.

19. The nurse manager has assigned a nurse as the circulating nurse for a surgical abortion. The nurse is Roman Catholic and wishes to refuse to participate in an abortion. The nurse manager of the operating room should:
- [ ] **1.** Require the nurse to do this assignment.
- [ ] **2.** Change the assignment, and record the behavior on the nurse's evaluation.
- [ ] **3.** Change the assignment without comment.
- [ ] **4.** Change the assignment to circulate, but have the nurse prepare the equipment.

20. A client is taking phenytoin (Dilantin) as an antiepileptic medication. The nurse emphasizes that the client needs:
- [ ] **1.** Increased iron.
- [ ] **2.** Increased calcium.
- [ ] **3.** Frequent dental examinations.
- [ ] **4.** Frequent eye examinations.

21. The nurse should establish baseline data on a client who is starting on long-term gentamicin sulfate (Garamycin) therapy. Which of the following is least important for assessment screening in this client?
- [ ] **1.** Visual acuity.
- [ ] **2.** Vestibular function.
- [ ] **3.** Renal function.
- [ ] **4.** Auditory function.

22. The nurse prepares to discharge a 5-year-old child from the 1-day surgery unit. The nurse leaves the room to get supplies and then, on returning, finds that the child is not breathing. The client is pulseless, and the nurse begins chest compressions. Because effective chest compressions depend on proper technique, the nurse should apply pressure:
- [ ] **1.** On the lower sternum with the heel of one hand.
- [ ] **2.** Midway on the sternum with the tips of two fingers.
- [ ] **3.** Over the apex of the heart with the heel of one hand.
- [ ] **4.** On the upper sternum with the heels of both hands.

23. When developing a nutritional plan for a child who needs to increase protein intake, which of the following foods is the nurse least likely to include?

☐ **1.** Bacon.
☐ **2.** Cooked dry beans.
☐ **3.** Peanut butter.
☐ **4.** Yogurt.

24. The nurse is auscultating S_1 and S_2 in a client. Identify the area where the nurse should hear S_1 the loudest.

25. The nurse instructs a client with coronary artery disease in the proper use of nitroglycerin (Nitrostat). At the onset of chest pain, the client should:

☐ **1.** Call 911 when three nitroglycerin tablets taken every 5 minutes are ineffective.
☐ **2.** Call 911 when five nitroglycerin tablets taken every 5 minutes are ineffective.
☐ **3.** Take three nitroglycerin tablets, 10 minutes apart, and call 911.
☐ **4.** Go to the emergency department if three nitroglycerin tablets are ineffective.

26. A diet high in which of the following food substances contributes to increases in serum cholesterol?

☐ **1.** Polyunsaturated fat.
☐ **2.** Saturated fat.
☐ **3.** Monounsaturated fat.
☐ **4.** Phospholipids.

27. During the health history, a client bluntly states, "I think I'm better off dead." The best response by the nurse is which of the following?

☐ **1.** "Has a family member ever committed suicide?"
☐ **2.** "When did these feelings begin?"
☐ **3.** "Do you have someone at home to help you?"
☐ **4.** "Are you thinking about suicide?"

28. A client is taking methotrexate (Rheumatrex) for severe rheumatoid arthritis. The nurse instructs the client that it will be necessary to monitor her:

☐ **1.** Serum glucose.
☐ **2.** Serum electrolytes.
☐ **3.** Complete blood count (CBC) with differential and platelet count.
☐ **4.** Sedimentation rate.

29. An elderly client complains to the nurse about constipation and reports that he has never been constipated before. The best response for the nurse to make is which of the following?

☐ **1.** "Constipation is an expected problem at your age."
☐ **2.** "You need to eat more fiber."
☐ **3.** "You need to drink more water."
☐ **4.** "The new onset of constipation may be a sign of a more serious problem."

30. A nurse is interviewing a client who will begin rehabilitation for alcohol dependency. Which approach by the nurse is most helpful to the client before starting the program?

☐ **1.** "You need to be very serious about this program."
☐ **2.** "You need to want to be alcohol free before we can help you."
☐ **3.** "This program requires you to do a lot of hard work."
☐ **4.** "We'll help you be successful so that you can stay alcohol free."

31. A newly diagnosed type 1 diabetic client asks the nurse, "Why do I have to take two shots of insulin? Shouldn't one shot be enough?" The best response for the nurse to make is which of the following?

☐ **1.** "A single shot of long-acting insulin would be preferable."
☐ **2.** "You might be able to change to oral medications soon."
☐ **3.** "Two shots will give you better control and decrease complications."
☐ **4.** "I'll ask the physician to change your insulin schedule."

32. The nurse understands that peak and trough serum levels from a client who is receiving gentamicin sulfate (Garamycin) are used to:

☐ **1.** Adjust the dosage to the therapeutic range.
☐ **2.** Avoid allergic reactions.
☐ **3.** Prevent side effects.
☐ **4.** Reach therapeutic levels more quickly.

33. The nurse is helping a client who has heart disease to assess his vitamin needs. The nurse is aware that recent updates to the U.S. Recommended Dietary Allowances expanded the description of nutrient needs to include Adequate Intakes, Tolerable Upper Limits, and Estimated Average Requirements. All these recommendations are called:
☐ **1.** Dietary Guidelines.
☐ **2.** Recommended Daily Allowances (RDAs).
☐ **3.** Recommended Daily Intakes.
☐ **4.** Dietary Reference Intakes (DRIs).

34. A client with a history of diabetes mellitus and chronic obstructive pulmonary disease should have which of the following immunizations?
☐ **1.** Influenza.
☐ **2.** Hepatitis A.
☐ **3.** Measles-mumps-rubella.
☐ **4.** Varicella.

35. A parent confides to the nurse that she thinks her 8-month-old infant is anxious or nervous. Which of the following suggestions by the nurse is most appropriate to help the mother lessen her anxiety about her infant?
☐ **1.** Limit holding the infant to feeding times.
☐ **2.** Talk quietly to the infant while he is awake.
☐ **3.** Play music in his room for most of the day and night.
☐ **4.** Have a close friend keep the infant for a few days.

36. The parent of a 2-week-old infant brings the child to the clinic for a checkup. The parent expresses concern about the baby's breathing because the infant breathes quickly for a while and then breathes slowly. The nurse interprets this finding as an indication of which of the following?
☐ **1.** A normal pattern in infants of this age.
☐ **2.** The need for an apnea monitor.
☐ **3.** A need for close monitoring for the mother.
☐ **4.** The need for a chest radiograph.

37. Which of the following complications is associated with a tracheostomy?
☐ **1.** Decreased cardiac output.
☐ **2.** Damage to the laryngeal nerve.
☐ **3.** Pneumothorax.
☐ **4.** Acute respiratory distress syndrome.

38. The nurse who is caring for a client with type 1 diabetes mellitus should use which of the following assessment tools to determine how well the child's insulin, diet, and exercise are balanced?
☐ **1.** Fasting serum glucose level.
☐ **2.** One-week dietary recall.
☐ **3.** Home log of blood glucose levels.
☐ **4.** Glycosylated hemoglobin level.

39. A client is receiving a unit of packed red blood cells. Before the transfusion started, the client's blood pressure was 90/50 mm Hg, pulse rate 100 bpm, respirations 20 breaths/minute, and temperature 98° F (36.7° C). Fifteen minutes after the transfusion starts, the client's blood pressure is 92/54 mm Hg, pulse 100 bpm, respirations 18 breaths/minute, and temperature is 101.4° F (38.6° C). The nurse should first:
☐ **1.** Stop the transfusion.
☐ **2.** Raise the head of the bed.
☐ **3.** Obtain an order for antibiotics.
☐ **4.** Offer the client a cool washcloth.

40. Which of the following findings in a client receiving opioid epidural analgesia would lead the nurse to notify the physician? Select all that apply.
☐ **1.** Blood pressure of 80/40 mm Hg; baseline blood pressure of 110/60 mm Hg.
☐ **2.** Respiratory rate of 14 breaths/minute; baseline respiratory rate of 18 breaths/minute.
☐ **3.** Report of crushing headache.
☐ **4.** 1.5 cc of blood aspirated from the catheter before the bolus injection.
☐ **5.** Pain rating of 3 on a scale of 1 to 10.

41. Which of the following dietary strategies best meets the nutritional needs of a client with acquired immunodeficiency syndrome (AIDS)?
☐ **1.** Tell the client to eat large meals frequently.
☐ **2.** Encourage megadoses of nutritional supplements.
☐ **3.** Instruct the client to cook foods thoroughly and adhere to safe food-handling practices.
☐ **4.** Tell the client to prepare food in advance and leave it out to eat small amounts throughout the day.

42. Before an incisional cholecystectomy is performed, the nurse instructs the client in the correct use of an incentive spirometer. Why is incentive spirometry essential after surgery in the upper abdominal area?
☐ **1.** The client will be maintained on bed rest for several days.
☐ **2.** Ambulation is restricted by the presence of drainage tubes.
☐ **3.** The operative incision is near the diaphragm.
☐ **4.** The presence of a nasogastric tube inhibits deep breathing.

43. The nurse is examining a 6-week-old African American infant. There are large spots of deep blue pigmentation across the infant's buttocks. The nurse should identify this sign as characteristic of:
☐ **1.** Vascular disease.
☐ **2.** Telangiectatic nevi.
☐ **3.** Infant milia.
☐ **4.** Mongolian spots.

44. A nulliparous client has been given a prescription for oral contraceptives. Which of the following should the nurse instruct the client to report to her health care provider immediately?
☐ **1.** Blurred vision.
☐ **2.** Nausea.
☐ **3.** Weight gain.
☐ **4.** Mild headache.

45. A client experienced a pneumothorax after the placement of a central venous pressure line. Which of the following assessments supports a medical diagnosis of pneumothorax?
☐ **1.** Sudden, sharp pain on the affected side.
☐ **2.** Tracheal deviation toward the affected side.
☐ **3.** Bradypnea and elevated blood pressure.
☐ **4.** Presence of crackles and wheezes.

46. When developing the plan of care for a client who is experiencing a flashback from the use of lysergic acid diethylamide, which of the following approaches should the nurse anticipate using?
☐ **1.** Confronting the client's misperceptions.
☐ **2.** Reassuring the client while presenting reality.
☐ **3.** Secluding the client until the flashback ends.
☐ **4.** Challenging the client's unrealistic statements.

47. The nurse should dispose of a used needle and syringe by:
☐ **1.** Cutting the needle at the hilt in a needle cutter before disposing of it in the universal precaution container in the client's room.
☐ **2.** Placing uncapped, used needles and syringes immediately in the universal precaution container in the client's room.
☐ **3.** Recapping the needle and placing the needle and syringe in the universal precaution container in the client's room.
☐ **4.** Separating the needle and syringe and placing both in the universal precaution container in the client's room.

48. An 80-year-old client is admitted with nausea and vomiting. He has a history of heart failure and is being treated with digoxin (Lanoxin). He tells the nurse he has been nauseated for a week and began vomiting 2 days ago. Laboratory values indicate that he has hypokalemia. Because of these clinical findings, the nurse should assess the client carefully for signs of which of the following conditions?
☐ **1.** Chronic renal failure.
☐ **2.** Exacerbation of heart failure.
☐ **3.** Digoxin toxicity.
☐ **4.** Metabolic acidosis.

49. The nurse instructs the client with osteoporosis that food products high in calcium include:
☐ **1.** Rice.
☐ **2.** Broccoli.
☐ **3.** Apples.
☐ **4.** Meat.

50. A woman is using progestin injections (Depo-Provera) for contraception. The nurse instructs the client to return for an appointment in:
☐ **1.** 1 month.
☐ **2.** 3 months.
☐ **3.** 4 months.
☐ **4.** 6 months.

51. A client is admitted through the emergency department with third-degree burns. The nurse assesses the client for edema, which can develop as a result of which of the following mechanisms?
☐ **1.** Increase in tissue colloidal osmotic pressure.
☐ **2.** Increase in plasma colloidal osmotic pressure.
☐ **3.** Decrease in capillary hydrostatic pressure.
☐ **4.** Decrease in interstitial fluid pressure.

52. A client exhibits increased restlessness. The results of the arterial blood gas test are as follows: pH, 7.52; partial pressure of carbon dioxide, 38 mm Hg; bicarbonate, 34 mg/L. These findings indicate which of the following acid-base imbalances?
☐ **1.** Respiratory alkalosis.
☐ **2.** Respiratory acidosis.
☐ **3.** Metabolic acidosis.
☐ **4.** Metabolic alkalosis.

53. While the nurse is caring for a multigravid client at 39 weeks' gestation in active labor whose cervix is dilated to 7 cm and completely effaced at +1 station, the client says, "I need to push!" Which of the following should the nurse do next?
☐ **1.** Turn the client to her left side.
☐ **2.** Tell her to push when she has the urge.
☐ **3.** Have her pant quickly during the contraction.
☐ **4.** Tell her to focus on an object in the room to relax.

54. Many antibiotics are nephrotoxic. When teaching a client who is taking antibiotics about signs and symptoms to report, the nurse should encourage the client to promptly report changes in urine output and appearance. Of the following descriptions of urine, which is an expected, normal description?
☐ **1.** Straw-colored.
☐ **2.** Cloudy.
☐ **3.** Smoky.
☐ **4.** Pink.

55. The school nurse is to monitor a child with suspected juvenile hypothyroidism. Which of the following should the nurse expect this child to manifest?
☐ **1.** Short attention span and weight loss.
☐ **2.** Weight loss and flushed skin.
☐ **3.** Rapid pulse and heat intolerance.
☐ **4.** Dry skin and constipation.

56. A 10-year-old diagnosed with attention deficit hyperactivity disorder (ADHD) has been switched from a stimulant to atomoxetine (Strattera) 40 mg two times a day. The nurse is instructing the client and her mother about the change in medication. Which statement indicates that the client's mother needs further education about the medication? Select all that apply.
☐ **1.** "I have to give her both doses before lunch."
☐ **2.** "I'll have to make sure she's gaining weight appropriately."
☐ **3.** "She may have nausea or dizziness for 1 or 2 months."
☐ **4.** "If she has mood swings, I should call her psychiatrist."
☐ **5.** "She can't take monoamine oxidase inhibitors while on Strattera."
☐ **6.** "If her ADHD symptoms don't improve in 2 to 3 weeks, I should stop the Strattera."

57. The nurse should anticipate which of the following medical orders for reducing a client's fluid volume excess?
☐ **1.** Low-sodium diet.
☐ **2.** Serum electrolytes daily.
☐ **3.** Monitor intake and output.
☐ **4.** Elevation of the client's feet.

58. The nurse observes a darkish blue pigment on the buttocks and back of an African American neonate. Which of the following actions is most appropriate?
☐ **1.** Ask the obstetrician to assess the child.
☐ **2.** Assess the child for other areas of cyanosis.
☐ **3.** Document this observation in the child's record.
☐ **4.** Advise the mother that laser therapy is needed.

59. During a physical examination, the nurse observes a copper bracelet on a client's wrist. The client states that she is wearing it to treat her arthritis. Because the nurse is aware of different cultural beliefs, the nurse recognizes this as a health practice:
☐ **1.** In which a protective object is believed to ward off illness.
☐ **2.** That is harmful to the client and must be discontinued.
☐ **3.** That is quackery and should not be tolerated.
☐ **4.** That is medically supported to treat arthritis and other conditions.

60. The heart rate of a newly delivered term neonate is found to be regular at 142 bpm. Which of the following should the nurse do next?
☐ **1.** Notify the neonate's pediatrician.
☐ **2.** Check for the presence of cyanosis.
☐ **3.** Assess the heart rate again in 3 hours.
☐ **4.** Document this as a normal neonatal finding.

61. The fetus of a multigravid client at 38 weeks' gestation is determined to be in a frank breech presentation. The nurse describes this presentation to the client as which of the following fetal parts coming in contact with the cervix?
☐ **1.** Buttocks.
☐ **2.** Head.
☐ **3.** Both feet.
☐ **4.** Shoulder.

62. The nurse teaches the client that the therapeutic effects of desmopressin nasal spray (DDAVP) are obtained when the client no longer has:
☐ **1.** Polydipsia.
☐ **2.** Nasal congestion.
☐ **3.** Headache.
☐ **4.** Blurred vision.

63. The nurse advises a 42-year-old client to have a screening mammogram. The client asks why this is necessary since she performs a breast self-examination (BSE) monthly. The nurse's best response is:
☐ **1.** "All women over 35 should have an annual mammogram."
☐ **2.** "A mammogram can identify breast cancer before it's detectable by BSE."
☐ **3.** "Most women don't perform BSE thoroughly enough to detect cancer."
☐ **4.** "A mammogram can detect other endocrine abnormalities as well."

64. A client is recovering from an infected abdominal wound. Which of the following foods should the nurse encourage the client to eat to support wound healing and recovery from the infection?
☐ **1.** Chicken and orange slices.
☐ **2.** Cheeseburger and french fries.
☐ **3.** Cheese omelet and bacon.
☐ **4.** Gelatin salad and tea.

65. The nurse teaches the client with iron deficiency anemia that food sources with high iron content include:
☐ **1.** Cheese.
☐ **2.** Squash.
☐ **3.** Eggs.
☐ **4.** Beef.

66. The mother of a toddler diagnosed with iron deficiency anemia asks what foods she should give her child. The nurse should evaluate the teaching as successful when the mother later reports that she feeds the toddler which of the following?

☐ **1.** Milk, carrots, and beef.
☐ **2.** Raisins, chicken, and spinach.
☐ **3.** Beef, lettuce, and juice.
☐ **4.** Eggs, cheese, and milk.

67. A toddler admitted in respiratory distress keeps pulling at the oxygen mask, trying to remove it. Which action by the nurse is most appropriate? Select all that apply.

☐ **1.** Restraining the child.
☐ **2.** Having the parent read to the child.
☐ **3.** Administering a sedative.
☐ **4.** Encouraging the parent to hold the child.
☐ **5.** Telling the child the mask will help him breathe better.
☐ **6.** Asking the parent to leave the child's bedside.

68. Four hours after a cast has been applied for a fractured ulna, the nurse assesses that the client's fingers are pale and cool and capillary refill is delayed for 4 seconds. How should the nurse interpret these findings?

☐ **1.** Nerve impairment is developing in the fingers.
☐ **2.** Arterial blood supply to the fingers is decreased.
☐ **3.** Venous stasis is occurring in the fingers.
☐ **4.** The finding is normal for this recovery period.

69. The nurse is developing a plan of care for a client who has joint stiffness due to rheumatoid arthritis. Which of the following interventions is most effective in relieving stiffness?

☐ **1.** A warm shower before performing activities of daily living.
☐ **2.** Aspirin after activity to decrease inflammation.
☐ **3.** A 10-lb weight loss to limit stress on joints.
☐ **4.** Cold compresses to joints for 30 minutes to relieve stiffness.

70. The nurse walks into the room and finds that a client who has just had surgery is diaphoretic, appears to have no respirations, and has a barely palpable pulse. The client is a full code. What is the most appropriate immediate response?

☐ **1.** Call a code.
☐ **2.** Open the airway.
☐ **3.** Start rescue breathing.
☐ **4.** Start cardiac compressions.

71. A client with obsessive-compulsive disorder washes her hands multiple times daily and is late for meals and milieu activities. Which of the following is most appropriate for the nurse to do initially?

☐ **1.** Totally eliminate the client's ritual.
☐ **2.** Allow the client to decide whether she wants to attend meals and activities.
☐ **3.** Inform the client that absence from meals and activities is not permitted.
☐ **4.** Remind the client about meal and activity times so that the ritual can be completed on time.

72. After discussing preconception needs with an Asian-American nulliparous client, which of the following client statements indicates the need for further instruction?

☐ **1.** "I should take folic acid supplements before I get pregnant."
☐ **2.** "If I become pregnant, I can continue to eat sushi twice a week."
☐ **3.** "I should continue to steam my vegetables rather than cooking them for a long time."
☐ **4.** "Eating soy products can increase my protein levels once I'm pregnant."

73. A client with osteoarthritis purchased a copper bracelet to wear. He tells the nurse that he feels better since he started wearing it. Which response by the nurse is most appropriate?

☐ **1.** Tell the client to remove the bracelet because it does not have any therapeutic value.
☐ **2.** Warn the client not to spend any more money on quackery such as bracelets.
☐ **3.** Instruct the client to remove the bracelet because the copper in it can interfere with salicylate metabolism.
☐ **4.** Acknowledge that the client feels better, but encourage the client to continue with the prescribed therapy.

74. The client is started on simvastatin (Zocor) as a component of cholesterol management. Which of the following laboratory tests needs to be monitored while on this therapy?

☐ **1.** Complete blood count.
☐ **2.** Serum glucose.
☐ **3.** Total protein.
☐ **4.** Liver function tests.

75. A man of Chinese descent is admitted to the hospital with multiple injuries after a motor vehicle accident. His pain is not under control. The client states, "If I could be with my people, I could receive acupuncture for this pain." The nurse should understand that acupuncture in the Asian culture is based on the theory that it:

☐ **1.** Purges evil spirits.
☐ **2.** Promotes tranquility.
☐ **3.** Restores the balance of energy.
☐ **4.** Blocks nerve pathways to the brain.

76. A client is taking large doses of aspirin daily to treat her rheumatoid arthritis. Which of the following side effects should the nurse instruct her to report?
- ☐ **1.** Abdominal cramps.
- ☐ **2.** Tinnitus.
- ☐ **3.** Rash.
- ☐ **4.** Hypotension.

77. A client is transferred from the coronary care unit to the step-down unit. Which of the following is not necessary in the transfer report?
- ☐ **1.** The client needs oxygen at 2 L/minute.
- ☐ **2.** The client has a do not resuscitate order.
- ☐ **3.** The client uses the bedpan.
- ☐ **4.** The client has four grandchildren.

78. The nurse is assessing fetal presentation in a multiparous client. The figure below indicates which of the following types of presentations?
- ☐ **1.** Frank breech.
- ☐ **2.** Complete breech.
- ☐ **3.** Footling breech.
- ☐ **4.** Vertex.

79. A multigravid client at 26 weeks' gestation with a history of pregnancy-induced hypertension (PIH) asks the nurse about traveling to a village in India by airplane to visit her father, who wishes to see her before she delivers. Which of the following responses by the nurse is most appropriate?
- ☐ **1.** "Air travel at this point in your pregnancy can lead to preterm labor."
- ☐ **2.** "You can travel by airplane as long as you take frequent walks during the trip."
- ☐ **3.** "You need to avoid traveling because of your history of PIH."
- ☐ **4.** "You'd be placing yourself and your fetus at risk for communicable diseases common in India."

80. To which national food assistance program should the nurse refer a low-income, pregnant client for help in obtaining food for herself and later her infant?
- ☐ **1.** Home-delivered meals.
- ☐ **2.** Congregate meals.
- ☐ **3.** Women, Infants, and Children Supplemental Food Program (WIC).
- ☐ **4.** Food bank.

81. The nurse is caring for a client who has severe burns on the head, neck, trunk, and groin areas. Which position would be most appropriate for preventing contractures?
- ☐ **1.** High Fowler's.
- ☐ **2.** Semi-Fowler's.
- ☐ **3.** Prone.
- ☐ **4.** Supine.

82. The client sustained an open fracture of the femur from an automobile accident. For which of the following types of shock should the client be assessed?
- ☐ **1.** Cardiogenic.
- ☐ **2.** Hypovolemic.
- ☐ **3.** Neurogenic.
- ☐ **4.** Anaphylactic.

83. The client has various sensory impairments associated with diabetic disease. The nurse determines that the client needs further instruction when he states which of the following?
- ☐ **1.** "I'll carefully test the temperature of my bathwater."
- ☐ **2.** "I'll avoid kitchen activities."
- ☐ **3.** "I'll avoid hot water bottles or heating pads."
- ☐ **4.** "I'll inspect my skin daily for pressure points and injury."

84. The nurse is providing discharge instructions to the client with peripheral vascular problems. Which of the following instructions should be included in the discussion with this client? Select all that apply.
- ☐ **1.** Avoiding prolonged standing and sitting.
- ☐ **2.** Limiting walking so as not to activate the "muscle pump."
- ☐ **3.** Keeping extremities elevated on pillows.
- ☐ **4.** Keeping the legs in a dependent position.
- ☐ **5.** Using a heating pad to promote vasodilation.

85. The father of an adolescent calls to talk to the nurse in the clinic about behaviors he has seen over the past 6 months in his son. The father recounts that the adolescent spends lots of time in his room, his grades are falling, and he has given away a few of his most favorite compact disks. Which of the following is the most appropriate action for the nurse?
☐ **1.** Give the father the telephone number for the local crisis hotline.
☐ **2.** Have the father take the adolescent to the nearest mental health outpatient facility now.
☐ **3.** Make a same-day appointment for the adolescent with his usual health care provider.
☐ **4.** Obtain more history information from the distraught father before making a decision.

86. A 7-year-old child is admitted to the hospital with the medical diagnosis of acute rheumatic fever. If the child develops chorea-like movements, which of the following eating utensils should the nurse suggest the parents not allow the child to use?
☐ **1.** Fork.
☐ **2.** Spoon.
☐ **3.** Plastic cup.
☐ **4.** Drinking straw.

87. Which of the following should the nurse expect in immediate postoperative care of a child after reversal of a colostomy? Select all that apply.
☐ **1.** Nasogastric (NG) tube attached to low intermittent suction.
☐ **2.** Administration of I.V. fluids.
☐ **3.** Daily measurement of abdominal girth.
☐ **4.** Calculation of intake and output every 8 hours.
☐ **5.** Assessment of vital signs every 6 hours.

88. A client's catheter is removed 4 days after a transurethral resection of the prostate (TURP). He is experiencing urinary dribbling. Which one of the following nursing interventions is appropriate in this situation?
☐ **1.** Teach the client Kegel exercises.
☐ **2.** Obtain a urine culture and sensitivity analysis to screen for a urinary infection.
☐ **3.** Encourage voiding every hour to prevent dribbling.
☐ **4.** Inform him that the dribbling will stop after a few days.

89. An adolescent primigravid client at 26 weeks' gestation who has gained 25 lb since becoming pregnant visits the prenatal clinic for a routine visit. Which of the following is the recommended amount of weight gain during the third trimester?
☐ **1.** 1 lb per week.
☐ **2.** 2 lb per week.
☐ **3.** 7 lb per month.
☐ **4.** 5 to 6 lb for the trimester.

90. The nurse is preparing to administer 0.1 mg of digoxin (Lanoxin) intravenously. Digoxin comes in a concentration of 0.5 mg/2 ml. How many milliliters should the nurse administer?
☐ **1.** 0.2 ml.
☐ **2.** 0.4 ml.
☐ **3.** 2.2 ml.
☐ **4.** 2.5 ml.

91. The mother of a 2-month-old infant with colic states, "I don't know what to do anymore. She's up in the middle of the night crying all the time." Which of the following is the nurse's best suggestion?
☐ **1.** Walk the floor with the baby at night.
☐ **2.** Take the infant for a short drive in the car.
☐ **3.** Allow the infant to cry it out in her crib.
☐ **4.** Offer cereal to fill the baby's stomach.

92. After the application of an arm cast, the client complains of pain on passive stretching of his fingers, finger swelling and tightness, and loss of function. Based on these data, the nurse anticipates that the client may be developing which of the following?
☐ **1.** Delayed bone union.
☐ **2.** Compartment syndrome.
☐ **3.** Fat embolism.
☐ **4.** Osteomyelitis.

93. Which of the following cardiac rehabilitation interventions is a priority for a client who has just had a myocardial infarction?
☐ **1.** Low-back training program.
☐ **2.** Risk modification education.
☐ **3.** Strength training program.
☐ **4.** Jogging exercise program.

94. While assessing a 4-day-old neonate delivered at 28 weeks' gestation, the nurse cannot elicit the neonate's Moro reflex, which was present 1 hour after birth. The nurse notifies the physician because this may indicate which of the following?
☐ **1.** Postnatal asphyxia.
☐ **2.** Skull fracture.
☐ **3.** Intracranial hemorrhage.
☐ **4.** Facial nerve paralysis.

95. After transurethral resection of the prostate, the nurse notices that the client's urine is bright red, has numerous clots, and is viscous. Which nursing action is most appropriate?
☐ **1.** Irrigate the catheter to remove clots.
☐ **2.** Milk the catheter tube vigorously.
☐ **3.** Increase the client's fluid intake.
☐ **4.** Assess vital signs and notify the surgeon.

96. The nurse is teaching the client about the appropriate use of lorazepam (Ativan) to manage anxiety. Which of the following statements indicates that the client understands the nurse's teaching?
☐ **1.** "I can take my medicine whenever I feel anxious."
☐ **2.** "It's okay to double my dose if I need to."
☐ **3.** "My medicine isn't for the everyday stress of life."
☐ **4.** "It's safe to have a glass of wine while taking this medicine."

97. The physician orders a maternal blood test for alpha fetoprotein for a nulligravid client at 16 weeks' gestation. When developing the teaching plan, the nurse bases the explanations on the understanding that this test is used to detect which of the following?
☐ **1.** Neural tube defects.
☐ **2.** Chromosomal anomalies.
☐ **3.** Inborn errors of metabolism.
☐ **4.** Lecithin-sphingomyelin ratio.

98. A nursing assistant recorded a client's 6 a.m. blood glucose level as 126 instead of 216. The nursing assistant did not recognize the error until 9 a.m. but reported it to the nurse right away. The nurse's correct response includes:
☐ **1.** Reassigning the nursing assistant to another client.
☐ **2.** Waiting and observing the client for symptoms of hyperglycemia.
☐ **3.** Reprimanding the nursing assistant for the error.
☐ **4.** Calling the physician and completing an incident report.

99. A client recovering from an abdominal hysterectomy complains of pain in her right calf. Which of the following additional assessments is appropriate at this time?
☐ **1.** Palpate the calf to note pain.
☐ **2.** Measure the circumference of both calves and note the difference.
☐ **3.** Have the client flex and extend her leg and note the presence of pain.
☐ **4.** Raise the right leg and lower it to detect changes in skin color.

100. The nurse is caring for an elderly client who has experienced a sensorineural hearing loss. The nurse anticipates that the client will exhibit which one of the following symptoms?
☐ **1.** Difficulty hearing high-pitched sounds.
☐ **2.** Difficulty with speaking clearly.
☐ **3.** Inability to assign meaning to sound.
☐ **4.** Vertigo when changing positions.

101. A client recently diagnosed with lung cancer tells the nurse that she has been having difficulty sleeping and is often preoccupied with thoughts about how her life has changed. She says, "I wish my life could just go on the way it was." Which of the following nursing diagnoses is most appropriate for this client?
☐ **1.** *Ineffective coping* related to cancer diagnosis.
☐ **2.** *Insomnia* related to fear of the unknown.
☐ **3.** *Grieving* related to cancer diagnosis.
☐ **4.** *Anxiety* related to the need for chemotherapy treatment.

102. The physician orders I.V. nalbuphine (Nubain) for a primigravid client in early active labor. After administering the drug, which of the following should the nurse do first?
☐ **1.** Elevate the head of the bed.
☐ **2.** Cover the client with a blanket.
☐ **3.** Pull the side rails up.
☐ **4.** Dim the lights in the room.

103. A client with emphysema has been admitted to the hospital. Which one of the following signs and symptoms is associated with his emphysema?
☐ **1.** Frequent coughing.
☐ **2.** Bronchospasms.
☐ **3.** Underweight appearance.
☐ **4.** Copious sputum.

104. A 12-year-old boy has a fractured femur and is immobilized in traction as shown in the figure below. The nurse should:
☐ **1.** Add additional weight until the foot is only 2 inches from the bed.
☐ **2.** Offer foods that are easy to eat.
☐ **3.** Place a pillow under the fractured leg to provide support.
☐ **4.** Provide opportunities for age-appropriate activities.

105. The nurse is participating in a blood pressure screening event. After three separate readings taken at least 2 minutes apart, the nurse determines that a client has a blood pressure of 160/90 mm Hg. Based on the nurse's knowledge of blood pressure screening guidelines, which of the following recommendations is appropriate at this time?
☐ 1. Have blood pressure evaluated within 1 month.
☐ 2. Begin an exercise program.
☐ 3. Examine lifestyle to decrease stress.
☐ 4. Schedule a complete physical immediately.

106. Which of the following activities is least effective in preventing sensory deprivation during a client's stay in the cardiac care unit?
☐ 1. Watching television.
☐ 2. Visiting with family.
☐ 3. Reading the newspaper.
☐ 4. Keeping the door closed to provide privacy.

107. The nurse is teaching a client who is taking dexamethasone (Decadron) for cerebral edema about early symptoms of Cushing's disease. Which of the following is a symptom of hyperadrenocorticism?
☐ 1. Hypotension.
☐ 2. Increased urinary frequency.
☐ 3. Increased muscle mass.
☐ 4. Easy bruising.

108. A client's wife arrives on the unit 6 hours after her husband's car accident, explaining that she has been out of town. She is distraught because she was not with her husband when he was admitted. What is the most appropriate initial intervention for the nurse to make?
☐ 1. Allow her to verbalize her feelings and concerns.
☐ 2. Describe her husband's medical treatment since admission.
☐ 3. Explain the nature of the injury and reassure her that her husband's condition is stable.
☐ 4. Reassure her that the important fact is that she is here now.

109. A client is scheduled to have a graded exercise test. The nurse explains to the client that the test will determine how:
☐ 1. Well he thinks under pressure.
☐ 2. Well his body reacts to controlled exercise stress.
☐ 3. Far he can walk.
☐ 4. Long he can walk.

110. A client who has asthma is taking albuterol (Ventolin) to treat bronchospasms. The nurse should anticipate that the client may experience which of the following adverse effects as a result of taking this drug? Select all that apply.
☐ 1. Lethargy.
☐ 2. Nausea.
☐ 3. Headache.
☐ 4. Nervousness.
☐ 5. Constipation.

111. A client tells the nurse that she is afraid to undergo chemotherapy because of what she has heard about the side effects. What is the nurse's best response to the client's concerns?
☐ 1. "Your health has been excellent. It's unlikely that you'll experience serious side effects."
☐ 2. "We'll give you medications to prevent the side effects, so you shouldn't be too concerned."
☐ 3. "Each person responds differently to chemotherapy treatments. We'll monitor your responses closely."
☐ 4. "It's important for you to accept this treatment. If you refuse your chemotherapy treatments, you'll die."

112. The mother of an infant with hemophilia tells the nurse that she is planning to do home teaching when the child reaches school age. She does not want her child in school because the teacher will not watch the child as well as she would. The mother's comments represent what common parental reaction to a child's chronic illness?
☐ 1. Overprotection.
☐ 2. Devotion.
☐ 3. Mistrust.
☐ 4. Insecurity.

113. A mother tells a nurse that her child has been exposed to roseola. After teaching the mother about the illness, which of the following, if stated by the mother as the most characteristic sign of roseola, indicates successful teaching?
☐ 1. Fever and sore throat.
☐ 2. Normal temperature followed by a low-grade fever.
☐ 3. High fever followed by a drop and then a rash.
☐ 4. Coldlike signs and symptoms and a rash.

114. A client with acute psychosis, not otherwise specified, has been taking haloperidol (Haldol) for 3 days. When evaluating the client's response to the medication, which of the following comments reflects the greatest improvement?
☐ 1. "I know these voices aren't really real, but I'm still scared of them."
☐ 2. "I'm feeling so restless, and I can't sit still."
☐ 3. "Boy, do I need a shower. I think it has been days since I've had one."
☐ 4. "I'll be fine if you just let me out of here today."

115. A 58-year-old homeless male is brought to the emergency department by the police after being found unconscious on the street. Following examination and evaluation of laboratory test results, a diagnosis of diabetic ketoacidosis is confirmed. Which of the following information is most crucial to document on the client's chart? Select all that apply.
- [ ] **1.** Size of pupils and reaction of pupils to light.
- [ ] **2.** Response to verbal and painful stimuli.
- [ ] **3.** Skin condition and presence of any rashes, lesions, or ulcers.
- [ ] **4.** Blood pressure.
- [ ] **5.** Length of time the client has had diabetes.
- [ ] **6.** Hourly urine output.

116. A 78-year-old client who experienced a brief delirium knows that the condition was caused by prescription medication intoxication. Which of the following statements indicates the need for further education?
- [ ] **1.** "I never realized that taking a little extra medication now and then could cause such a problem."
- [ ] **2.** "I get medicines from three different doctors and they don't all know what I'm taking."
- [ ] **3.** "I thought that the herbal medicines would help me. I never realized they would make me sick."
- [ ] **4.** "I didn't know that cold and flu medicines might not mix with my regular medicines."

117. A physician has asked for I.V. calcium to treat a client with hypocalcemia. What is the nurse's first response?
- [ ] **1.** Hand the physician calcium chloride for I.V. use.
- [ ] **2.** Check with the physician for his complete order.
- [ ] **3.** Hand the physician calcium gluconate for I.V. use.
- [ ] **4.** Hand the physician the kind of calcium available on the unit.

118. The nurse is administering an I.V. potassium chloride supplement to a client who has heart failure. When developing a plan of care for this client, which of the following should the nurse incorporate?
- [ ] **1.** Hyperkalemia will intensify the action of the client's digoxin (Lanoxin) preparation.
- [ ] **2.** The client's potassium levels will be unaffected by his potassium-sparing diuretic.
- [ ] **3.** The administration of the I.V. potassium chloride should not exceed 10 mEq/hour or a concentration of 40 mEq/L.
- [ ] **4.** Metabolic alkalosis will increase the client's serum potassium levels.

119. A client is receiving morphine sulfate by a patient-controlled analgesia (PCA) system after a left lower lobectomy about 4 hours ago. The client complains of moderately severe pain in his left thorax that worsens when he coughs. The nurse's first course of action is to:
- [ ] **1.** Reassure the client that the PCA system is working and will relieve his pain.
- [ ] **2.** Encourage the client to rest; no further assessment is needed.
- [ ] **3.** Assess the pain systematically with the hospital-approved scale.
- [ ] **4.** Encourage the client to ignore the pain and sleep because pain is expected after this type of surgery.

120. Which of the following factors can alter tissue tolerance and lead to the development of a pressure ulcer?
- [ ] **1.** The client's age.
- [ ] **2.** Exposure to moisture.
- [ ] **3.** Presence of hypertension.
- [ ] **4.** Smoking.

121. The nurse is screening clients for cancer prevention. Which of the following is the recommended screening protocol for colon cancer in asymptomatic clients who have a low-risk profile?
- [ ] **1.** Guaiac testing of stools should be performed annually after age 50 years.
- [ ] **2.** Digital rectal examinations are recommended every 5 years after age 40 years.
- [ ] **3.** Sigmoidoscopy is recommended if symptoms of colon problems are present.
- [ ] **4.** A low-fat diet should be implemented by age 50 years.

122. The nurse is evaluating the effectiveness of antipsychotic medications in a client with severe Alzheimer's disease. Which of the following changes indicates improvement resulting from medications?
- [ ] **1.** Adjustment to the structured daily routine.
- [ ] **2.** Return of the client's short-term memory.
- [ ] **3.** Decrease in verbal and physical aggression.
- [ ] **4.** Diminished resistance with activities of daily living done one step at a time.

123. After vaginal delivery of a term neonate, the nurse determines that the placenta is about to separate when which of the following occurs?
- [ ] **1.** The uterus becomes oval shaped.
- [ ] **2.** The uterus enlarges.
- [ ] **3.** A sudden gush of dark blood occurs.
- [ ] **4.** The client expends efforts pushing.

124. The nurse should complete which of the following assessments on a client who has received tissue plasminogen activator or alteplase recombinant (Activase) therapy?

☐ **1.** Neurologic signs frequently throughout the course of therapy.
☐ **2.** Excessive bleeding every hour for the first 8 hours.
☐ **3.** Blood glucose level.
☐ **4.** Arterial blood gas values.

125. During the emergency phase of burn management, the nurse should anticipate which of the following fluid and electrolyte imbalances to occur?

☐ **1.** Hypokalemia, hyponatremia.
☐ **2.** Hyperkalemia, increased hematocrit.
☐ **3.** Decreased hematocrit, hypernatremia.
☐ **4.** Hypocalcemia, increased hematocrit.

126. A 6-year-old child is to have a cardiac catheterization and asks the nurse if it will hurt. Which of the following statements provides the nurse with the best guide for responding to the child's question?

☐ **1.** "The medication used to numb the insertion site will sting."
☐ **2.** "A momentary sharp pain usually occurs when the catheter enters the heart."
☐ **3.** "Most 6-year-olds feel some discomfort during the procedure."
☐ **4.** "It's a painless procedure, although a tingling sensation may be felt in the extremities."

127. A 10-year-old with a history of recent respiratory infection comes to the clinic and reports swelling around the eyes in the morning and dark urine. Which of the following should the nurse ask first?

☐ **1.** "Has the child had a rash and fever?"
☐ **2.** "Has the child had a sore throat?"
☐ **3.** "Does the child have any allergies?"
☐ **4.** "Does the child drink lots of liquids?"

128. After a nasogastric (NG) tube has been inserted, the nurse can most accurately determine that the tube is in the proper place if which of the following can be demonstrated?

☐ **1.** The client is no longer gagging or coughing.
☐ **2.** The pH of the aspirated fluid is measured.
☐ **3.** Thirty milliliters of normal saline can be injected without difficulty.
☐ **4.** A whooshing sound is auscultated when 10 ml of air is inserted.

129. A client at 40+ weeks' gestation visits the emergency department because she thinks she is in labor. Which of the following is the best indication that the client is in true labor?

☐ **1.** Fetal descent into the pelvic inlet.
☐ **2.** Cervical dilation and effacement.
☐ **3.** Painful contractions every 3 to 5 minutes.
☐ **4.** Leaking amniotic fluid clear in color.

130. Which of the following should be considered the highest priority during the first 24 hours postoperatively for the client who had a total laryngectomy due to cancer of the larynx?

☐ **1.** Provide adequate nourishment.
☐ **2.** Prevent skin breakdown.
☐ **3.** Maintain proper bowel elimination.
☐ **4.** Maintain a patent airway.

131. It has been 5 months since a client lost his wife and child in a car-train accident. The nurse should determine that the client needs continuing counseling if he makes which of the following statements?

☐ **1.** "I'm sleeping, eating, and working pretty well, but I still get so sad at times."
☐ **2.** "I miss them so much, but I can tell I'm getting better day by day."
☐ **3.** "I wish I didn't have to sleep. I hate the nightmares about what the car looked like."
☐ **4.** "I never thought I'd get over this, but I'm working with my congressman for train crossing safety."

132. A client is hearing voices that are telling her to kill herself. She is demanding a knife to use on her wrists. Which of the following is most appropriate at this time?

☐ **1.** Put the client in restraints after giving an I.M. dose of p.r.n. medication.
☐ **2.** Ask the client to talk about her anger and what is causing it.
☐ **3.** Give oral p.r.n. doses of haloperidol (Haldol) and lorazepam (Ativan) as ordered.
☐ **4.** Search the client's room for potential weapons after locking the unit kitchen.

133. The nurse should adjust a client's heparin dose according to a prescribed anticoagulation order based on maintaining which laboratory value at what therapeutic level for anticoagulant therapy?

☐ **1.** Partial thromboplastin time, 1.5 to 2.5 times the normal control.
☐ **2.** Prothrombin time, 1.5 to 2.5 times the normal control.
☐ **3.** International Normalized Ratio, 2 to 3 seconds.
☐ **4.** Thrombin clotting time, 10 to 15 seconds.

134. Which of the following measures is contraindicated when the nurse assists a child who has leukemia with oral hygiene?

☐ **1.** Applying petroleum jelly to the lips.
☐ **2.** Cleaning the teeth with a toothbrush.
☐ **3.** Swabbing the mouth with moistened cotton swabs.
☐ **4.** Rinsing the mouth with a nonirritating mouthwash.

135. The nurse realizes that a medication error has been made and a client has received the wrong medication. What should be the nurse's first action when realizing an error has been made?
- ☐ **1.** Assess the client's condition.
- ☐ **2.** Notify the physician of the error.
- ☐ **3.** Complete an incident report.
- ☐ **4.** Report the error to the unit manager.

136. The nurse has been assigned to a client who has had diabetes for 10 years. The nurse gives the client's usual dose of Humulin Regular insulin at 7 a.m. At 10:30 a.m., the client complains of light-headedness and sweating. The nurse suspects that the client is experiencing:
- ☐ **1.** Metabolic acidosis.
- ☐ **2.** Hyperglycemia.
- ☐ **3.** Hypoglycemia.
- ☐ **4.** Ketoacidosis.

137. A 6-year-old boy is being treated in the emergency department for injuries inflicted by his stepfather. The client's mother says, "This never happened before. Jim got fired today. He got drunk and came home in a tirade. I'm so sorry that Jason got hurt, but I don't think it will ever happen again." Which of the following responses is most appropriate initially?
- ☐ **1.** "I'm sorry too, but I agree it probably won't happen again."
- ☐ **2.** "I'm not as forgiving as you are. I think you need to file charges on Jim."
- ☐ **3.** "This is child abuse and I have to file a report with Child Protective Services."
- ☐ **4.** "I want to know more about your situation. Let's sit and talk."

138. The nurse administers a tap water enema to a client. While the solution is being infused, the client begins to complain of abdominal cramping. What should be the nurse's first response to the client's complaint?
- ☐ **1.** Clamp the tubing and carefully withdraw the tube.
- ☐ **2.** Temporarily stop the infusion and have the client take deep breaths.
- ☐ **3.** Raise the height of the enema container.
- ☐ **4.** Rub the client's abdomen gently until the cramps subside.

139. In preparing for insertion of a peripheral I.V. catheter, the nurse must select an appropriate site. Which of the following areas should the nurse try first if an appropriate vein is found?
- ☐ **1.** Back of the hand.
- ☐ **2.** Inner aspect of the elbow.
- ☐ **3.** Inner aspect of the forearm.
- ☐ **4.** Outer aspect of the forearm.

140. The nurse administers lactulose (Duphalac) to a client with cirrhosis. What is the expected outcome from the administration of the lactulose?
- ☐ **1.** Stimulation of peristalsis of the bowel.
- ☐ **2.** Reduced peripheral edema and ascites.
- ☐ **3.** Reduced serum ammonia levels.
- ☐ **4.** Prevention of hemorrhage.

141. A 12-month-old child is seen in the neighborhood clinic for a regular checkup. The child's mother states that the child is caught up with immunizations. The nurse interprets this statement as indicating that the toddler has already received which of the following?
- ☐ **1.** Diphtheria, tetanus and acellular pertussis (DTaP) #1 and 2; hepatitis B (HepB) #1 and 2; inactivated poliovirus (IPV) #1 and 2.
- ☐ **2.** DTaP #1, 2, and 3; HepB #1, 2, and 3; IPV #1 and 2.
- ☐ **3.** DTaP #1 and 2; HepB #1, 2, and 3; oral polio vaccine (OPV) #1 and 2.
- ☐ **4.** DTaP #1, 2, and 3; *Haemophilus* b #1 and 2; OPV #1 and 2.

142. When conducting a health promotion class with a group of women, the nurse should include which of the following strategies to help reduce the risk of developing osteoarthritis?
- ☐ **1.** Follow a high-protein diet.
- ☐ **2.** Exercise at least three times per week.
- ☐ **3.** Prevent obesity.
- ☐ **4.** Take a multivitamin supplement daily.

143. A deficiency of which of the following vitamins is thought to be the first step in the formation of plaque and oxidative changes?
- ☐ **1.** Vitamin C.
- ☐ **2.** Vitamin A.
- ☐ **3.** Vitamin E.
- ☐ **4.** Vitamin B_6.

144. A neonate circumcised with a Plastibell 1 hour ago is brought to his mother for feeding. The nurse instructs the mother to do which of the following?
- ☐ **1.** Read a pamphlet about circumcision care.
- ☐ **2.** Remove the petroleum jelly gauze in 24 hours.
- ☐ **3.** Tell the nurse when the neonate voids.
- ☐ **4.** Place petroleum jelly over the site every 2 hours.

145. A client has been diagnosed with early alcoholic cirrhosis. The client should be taught that incorporating which of the following behaviors into his lifestyle could potentially reverse the pathologic changes occurring in the liver?
- ☐ **1.** Avoid overexertion and fatigue.
- ☐ **2.** Avoid drinking alcohol.
- ☐ **3.** Eliminate smoking.
- ☐ **4.** Eat a high-carbohydrate, low-fat diet.

146. A child is to receive dexamethasone (Decadron) intravenously at the ordered dosage of 7.6 mg. The drug concentration in the vial is 4 mg/ml. Which of the following amounts should the nurse administer?
- ☐ **1.** 0.05 ml.
- ☐ **2.** 0.72 ml.
- ☐ **3.** 1.9 ml.
- ☐ **4.** 3.8 ml.

147. A 40-year-old primigravid client with AB-positive blood visits the outpatient clinic for an amniocentesis at 16 weeks' gestation. The nurse determines that the most likely reason for the client's amniocentesis is to determine if the fetus has which of the following?
- ☐ **1.** Cri du chat syndrome.
- ☐ **2.** ABO incompatibility.
- ☐ **3.** Erythroblastosis fetalis.
- ☐ **4.** Down syndrome.

148. The nurse is assessing a client who has benign prostatic hypertrophy (BPH). Which symptom is the client most likely to exhibit?
- ☐ **1.** Impotence.
- ☐ **2.** Flank pain.
- ☐ **3.** Difficulty starting the urinary stream.
- ☐ **4.** Hematuria.

149. Which of the following is the most helpful strategy to use for anger management when dealing with a verbally aggressive client?
- ☐ **1.** Role-playing assertive statements with the nurse.
- ☐ **2.** Watching a videotape about assertiveness.
- ☐ **3.** Describing feelings that occur after aggressive outbursts.
- ☐ **4.** Discussing situations that appear to be threatening.

150. Which of the following actions should the nurse anticipate using when caring for a term neonate diagnosed with transient tachypnea at 2 hours after birth?
- ☐ **1.** Monitoring the neonate's color and cry every 4 hours.
- ☐ **2.** Feeding the neonate with a bottle every 3 hours.
- ☐ **3.** Obtaining extracorporeal membrane oxygenation equipment.
- ☐ **4.** Providing warm, humidified oxygen in a warm environment.

151. A client is to receive sulfisoxazole (Gantrisin) 1.5 g every 6 hours orally. The Gantrisin comes in an elixir of 300 mg in 2 ml. How many milliliters should the nurse give?

_____ ml

152. The skin tone of a client of Vietnamese descent with dark skin who has early signs of iron deficiency anemia appears:
- ☐ **1.** Reddish-brown.
- ☐ **2.** Yellowish-brown.
- ☐ **3.** Black-brown.
- ☐ **4.** Whitish-brown.

153. Which of the following laboratory findings is present in nephrotic syndrome?
- ☐ **1.** Decreased total serum protein.
- ☐ **2.** Hypercalcemia.
- ☐ **3.** Hyperglycemia.   *read careful*
- ☐ **4.** Decreased hematocrit.

154. While caring for several preterm infants in the special care nursery, which of the following actions is most important for preventing nosocomial infections in these neonates?
- ☐ **1.** Using sterile supplies for all treatments.
- ☐ **2.** Performing thorough handwashing before giving infant care.
- ☐ **3.** Donning cover gowns for nurses and visitors to the unit.
- ☐ **4.** Wearing a mask, and changing it frequently when giving care.

155. Which of the following types of restraints is best for the nurse to use for a child in the immediate postoperative period after cleft palate repair?
- ☐ **1.** Safety jacket.
- ☐ **2.** Elbow restraints.
- ☐ **3.** Wrist restraints.
- ☐ **4.** Body restraints.

156. When preparing to present a community program about women who are victims of physical abuse, which of the following should the nurse stress about the incidence of battering?
- ☐ **1.** Death from battering is rare.
- ☐ **2.** Battering is a major cause of injury to women.
- ☐ **3.** Lower socioeconomic groups are primarily affected.
- ☐ **4.** Battering rarely involves pregnant women.

157. A client undergoes a nephrectomy. In the immediate postoperative period, which nursing intervention has the highest priority?
- ☐ **1.** Monitoring blood pressure.
- ☐ **2.** Encouraging the use of the incentive spirometer.
- ☐ **3.** Assessing urine output hourly.
- ☐ **4.** Checking the flank dressing for urine drainage.

158. A nulliparous client tells the nurse that during her last pelvic examination the physician said that her uterus was in a severe retroverted position. The nurse determines that the client may experience which of the following?
☐ **1.** Frequent vaginal infections.
☐ **2.** Pain from endometriosis.
☐ **3.** Severe menstrual cramping.
☐ **4.** Difficulty conceiving a child.

159. A mother tells the nurse that she wants her 4-year-old to stop sucking her thumb. When developing the teaching plan, which of the following should the nurse suggest?
☐ **1.** Apply a special medicine that tastes terrible on the thumb.
☐ **2.** Get the child to agree to stop the thumb sucking.
☐ **3.** Remind the child every time the mother sees the thumb in her mouth.
☐ **4.** Put the child in time-out every time the mother observes thumb sucking.

160. A client in severe respiratory distress is admitted to the hospital. When assessing the client, the nurse should:
☐ **1.** Conduct a complete health history.
☐ **2.** Complete a comprehensive physical examination.
☐ **3.** Delay assessment until client's respiratory distress is resolved.
☐ **4.** Focus assessment on the respiratory system and distress.

161. A client has had a total hip replacement. Which of the following signs most likely indicates that the hip has dislocated?
☐ **1.** Abduction of the affected leg.
☐ **2.** Loosening of the prosthesis.
☐ **3.** External rotation of the affected leg.
☐ **4.** Shortening of the affected leg.

162. A client with paranoid schizophrenia is withdrawn and suspicious of others and projects blame. The client's behavior reflects problems in which of the following stages of development as identified by Erikson?
☐ **1.** Trust versus mistrust.
☐ **2.** Autonomy versus shame and doubt.
☐ **3.** Initiative versus guilt.
☐ **4.** Intimacy versus isolation.

163. During the initial interview, a client with a compulsive eating disorder remarks, "I can't stand myself and the way I look." Which of the following statements by the nurse is most therapeutic?
☐ **1.** "Everyone who has the same problem feels like you do."
☐ **2.** "I don't think you look bad at all."
☐ **3.** "Don't worry. You'll soon be back in shape."
☐ **4.** "Tell me more about your feelings."

164. A client with a new ileal conduit asks the nurse when he needs to wear his appliance. Which of the following responses by the nurse is correct?
☐ **1.** "You need to wear your appliance all the time."
☐ **2.** "You need to wear your appliance after you irrigate."
☐ **3.** "It is only necessary to wear your appliance at night."
☐ **4.** "The appliance must be worn after your meals."

165. A child who is admitted after having suffered trauma has also been exposed to varicella. Which of the following should the nurse institute for infection control?
☐ **1.** Airborne precautions.
☐ **2.** Droplet precautions.
☐ **3.** Contact precautions.
☐ **4.** Indirect contact precautions.

166. Which of the following expected outcomes is appropriate for a client with multiple myeloma?
☐ **1.** Achieve effective management of bone pain.
☐ **2.** Recover from the disease with minimal disabilities.
☐ **3.** Decrease episodes of nausea and vomiting.
☐ **4.** Monitor for signs of hyperkalemia.

167. A client with major depression is completing his morning care independently. When the nurse approaches the client with his medication, he tells the nurse that he is a failure as a husband and a father and is worthless. His wife told the nurse previously that the client is a good provider and a wonderful father and husband. Which of the following responses by the nurse is most appropriate?
☐ **1.** "You were able to shower and dress without help this morning."
☐ **2.** "Your wife told me that you are a good husband and father."
☐ **3.** "You don't have any reason why you should feel that way."
☐ **4.** "This medication will help your thinking."

168. The nurse uses Montgomery straps primarily to achieve which of the following client outcomes?
☐ **1.** The client is free from falls.
☐ **2.** The client is free from bruises.
☐ **3.** The client is free from skin breakdown.
☐ **4.** The client is free from wandering.

169. After an episode of severe pain, a client says to the nurse, "The pain really frightened me. I thought I was going to die." Which statement is the most appropriate response from the nurse?
☐ **1.** "I understand that pain can be a frightening experience."
☐ **2.** "Why were you frightened? You have had pain before."
☐ **3.** "There's no need to be frightened of pain."
☐ **4.** "Pain can't cause you to die. Try to relax."

170. A child returns to the pediatric unit after a bowel resection. Which of the following actions has the highest priority?
- ☐ **1.** Administer I.V. fluids.
- ☐ **2.** Keep the child on nothing-by-mouth status.
- ☐ **3.** Monitor vital signs frequently.
- ☐ **4.** Assess the child's pain level.

171. During a health history, a 59-year-old male client is being evaluated for possible type 2 diabetes mellitus. Which of the following client statements supports the diagnosis of type 2 diabetes?
- ☐ **1.** "I have some shortness of breath when I exercise."
- ☐ **2.** "No matter how much I drink, I'm still thirsty all the time."
- ☐ **3.** "I wake up early in the morning and can't return to sleep."
- ☐ **4.** "In the past couple of weeks, I've been having a lot of trouble urinating."

172. A common nursing diagnosis for a client who has hypothyroidism and is complaining of fatigue, muscular weakness, and muscle cramping is:
- ☐ **1.** *Activity intolerance.*
- ☐ **2.** *Anxiety.*
- ☐ **3.** *Hopelessness.*
- ☐ **4.** *Ineffective coping.*

173. A client is diagnosed with metastatic bone cancer. Because of this diagnosis, which of the following abnormal laboratory values should the nurse expect to see?
- ☐ **1.** Hypocalcemia.
- ☐ **2.** Elevated serum alkaline phosphatase.
- ☐ **3.** Elevated aspartate transaminase.
- ☐ **4.** Hypokalemia.

174. A 25-year-old man has been diagnosed with hypertrophic cardiomyopathy. The nurse plans to assess the client for:
- ☐ **1.** Angina.
- ☐ **2.** Fatigue and shortness of breath.
- ☐ **3.** Abdominal pain.
- ☐ **4.** Hypertension.

175. The nurse should advise the mother of a toddler suspected of having pinworms to do the cellophane tape test at which of the following times?
- ☐ **1.** Before bathing.
- ☐ **2.** After a bowel movement.
- ☐ **3.** While the child is asleep.
- ☐ **4.** After a meal.

176. Which of the following conditions occurring in a mother's pregnancy provides a clue that the newborn might have a gastrointestinal tract anomaly?
- ☐ **1.** Meconium in the amniotic fluid.
- ☐ **2.** Low implantation of the placenta.
- ☐ **3.** Increased amount of amniotic fluid.
- ☐ **4.** Toxemia in the last trimester.

177. As part of the treatment plan, a client is prescribed steroids to treat ulcerative colitis. The nurse should assess the client for which of the following common complications related to steroid therapy?
- ☐ **1.** Peptic ulcer.
- ☐ **2.** Hypoglycemia.
- ☐ **3.** Tachycardia.
- ☐ **4.** Renal failure.

178. A client's abdominal incision eviscerates. The nurse's priority action on detecting the evisceration is to:
- ☐ **1.** Take the client's vital signs and call the physician.
- ☐ **2.** Lower the client's head and elevate the feet.
- ☐ **3.** Cover the incision with a dressing moistened with sterile normal saline solution.
- ☐ **4.** Start an emergency infusion of I.V. fluids.

179. What is the priority nursing intervention for a client who is admitted to the emergency department with burns over an estimated 27% of the body surface area?
- ☐ **1.** Insert a large-caliber I.V. line.
- ☐ **2.** Administer morphine intramuscularly.
- ☐ **3.** Establish an airway.
- ☐ **4.** Administer tetanus toxoid.

180. Which of the following clients should the nurse expect to place on one-to-one suicide precautions?
- ☐ **1.** A client who is withdrawn and anorectic.
- ☐ **2.** A client who refuses to sign a no harm contract.
- ☐ **3.** A client who is visibly crying.
- ☐ **4.** A client who refuses his medication.

181. To prepare a client who has a fractured femur for ambulation, the nurse teaches her how to do quadriceps setting exercises. Which of the following client instructions is most accurate?
- ☐ **1.** "Contract and relax your buttocks."
- ☐ **2.** "Try to lift your legs up when I press against your feet."
- ☐ **3.** "Press the back of your knee against the bed."
- ☐ **4.** "Flex and extend your toes."

182. A client with an ileostomy calls the nurse to report that she is experiencing abdominal cramps, vomiting, and watery discharge from her ileostomy. What is the nurse's best response?
- ☐ **1.** Tell the client to take 30 ml of milk of magnesia.
- ☐ **2.** Encourage the client to increase her fluid intake.
- ☐ **3.** Have the client measure her abdominal girth.
- ☐ **4.** Notify the physician immediately.

183. Which of the following signs and symptoms indicates that a client with human immunodeficiency virus (HIV) infection has developed acquired immunodeficiency syndrome (AIDS)?
- ☐ **1.** Severe fatigue at night.
- ☐ **2.** Pain on standing and walking.
- ☐ **3.** Weight loss of 10 lb over 3 months.
- ☐ **4.** Herpes simplex ulcer persisting for 2 months.

184. The nurse has been teaching a client with genital herpes how to care for the lesions. Which of the following statements by the client indicates that she needs additional instruction?
- ☐ 1. "I'll use a sitz bath to decrease the inflammation of the sores."
- ☐ 2. "I'll wear occlusive underwear to prevent transmission of the virus."
- ☐ 3. "I can use a hair dryer to dry the lesions as long as I use a cool setting."
- ☐ 4. "It's important that I drink plenty of fluids."

185. A client has just received the first I.M. injection of 30 mg of risperidone (Risperdal Consta). The client states, "At least I won't have to take the Risperdal pills anymore." How should the nurse respond?
- ☐ 1. "You're correct and understand your medication."
- ☐ 2. "You'll only need to take one pill per day."
- ☐ 3. "You'll need to continue taking oral Risperdal for 3 weeks."
- ☐ 4. "You'll need to take your usual dose as a supplement."

186. The client has been taking famotidine (Pepcid) at home. The nurse prepares a teaching plan for the client indicating that the medication acts primarily to achieve which of the following?
- ☐ 1. Inhibit gastric acid secretions.
- ☐ 2. Neutralize acid in the stomach.
- ☐ 3. Shorten the time required for digestion in the stomach.
- ☐ 4. Improve the mixing of foods and gastric secretions.

187. Which of the following dietary changes should the nurse emphasize to a client with fibrocystic breast disease?
- ☐ 1. Increase sodium consumption.
- ☐ 2. Use only bottled water.
- ☐ 3. Decrease consumption of caffeine.
- ☐ 4. Decrease calcium intake.

188. A very obese client wants to lose weight and attends an introductory class on how to eat properly. The nurse provides him with a brochure that contains information, updated every 5 years, that guides healthy eating. This brochure is called:
- ☐ 1. The Dietary Guidelines for Hearty Eating.
- ☐ 2. The Dietary Guidelines for Americans.
- ☐ 3. The Guidelines and Goals for Americans.
- ☐ 4. Food for Lifestyle.

189. A client with an Axis I diagnosis of bipolar disorder, mania, states to the nurse, "I'm the Prince of Wales and you will be my Queen Anna. Get ready for our wedding." Which of the following replies by the nurse is most appropriate?
- ☐ 1. "Sorry, but I'm already happily married and won't be getting ready for a wedding."
- ☐ 2. "No, you know better, we aren't going to be married. There will be no wedding."
- ☐ 3. "You are Sam Smith, a client here in the hospital, and I'm Marjorie, a nurse here on the unit."
- ☐ 4. "You aren't a prince and I can't be your queen. We aren't going to be married."

190. A client with a new colostomy tells the nurse she thinks she is ready to learn how to care for it. Which of the following interventions would most likely be effective in preparing the client to look at the colostomy?
- ☐ 1. Tell her how quickly other clients have adjusted to caring for their colostomies.
- ☐ 2. Encourage her to handle the colostomy appliance.
- ☐ 3. Ask a female member of the local ostomy club to visit her.
- ☐ 4. Show the client pictures that illustrate how a colostomy looks and functions.

Correct Answers and Rationales

The letter in parentheses after each rationale identifies the client need addressed in the item, including management of care (M), safety and infection control (S), health promotion and maintenance (H), psychosocial adaptation (P), basic care and comfort (C), pharmacological and parenteral therapies (D), reduction of risk potential (R), and physiological adaptation (A).

1. 3. Illegible writing is one of the most common reasons for medication errors. The physician should be called to clarify the order. The previous medication record should not be used as a substitute for the exact order written by the physician. The pharmacist or the client's family cannot interpret an order written by a physician. (M)

2. 2. Propantheline bromide is an anticholinergic used to decrease biliary spasm. Decreasing biliary spasm helps to reduce pain in cholecystitis. Propantheline does not increase bile production or have an antiemetic effect, and it is not effective in treating infection. (D)

3. 3. An important function of the National Cystic Fibrosis Foundation is to put parents of children with cystic fibrosis in touch with each other. Other parents can commonly offer support and help. In some instances, the Foundation gives parents financial assistance for equipment required for home care of their child with cystic fibrosis (but not for medications). The Foundation does not obtain tutors for children or provide genetic counseling for parents. (M)

4. 4. Laryngeal stridor is characteristic of respiratory distress from inflammation and swelling after bronchoscopy. It must be reported immediately. Green sputum indicates infection and would occur 3 to 5 days after bronchoscopy. A mild cough or hemoptysis is typical after bronchoscopy. If a tissue biopsy specimen was obtained, sputum may be blood-streaked for several days. (R)

5. 3. Strategies for meeting client satisfaction include involving hospital department personnel to improve service. Saying, "The staff is doing the best they can," or, "I will report this to the physician," does not offer a practical resolution to the client's complaint. Expressing a personal dislike for the food negates the client's complaint and does not offer a solution. (M)

6. 3. The elderly client commonly has vague or atypical responses to medications and diseases that are erroneously attributed to aging. A new cognitive change needs to be investigated and is not an expected change with aging. Changes in a client's behavior should be investigated to see whether there is a relation to excessive sedation. The nurse can interview the family members to obtain information. (H)

7. 2. Rehabilitation for a client who has sustained a cerebrovascular accident begins at the time he is admitted to the hospital. The first goal of rehabilitation should be to help prevent deformities. This goal is achieved through such techniques as positioning the client properly in bed, changing his position frequently, and supporting all parts of his body in proper alignment. Passive range-of-motion exercises may also be started, unless contraindicated. (M)

8. 1. Lung cancer is a very aggressive disease. Small cell lung cancer is commonly metastatic at the time of diagnosis. The client with non-small-cell lung cancer may have a longer survival time, but lung cancer continues to be an aggressive disease that disseminates rapidly. The overall 5-year survival rate for all types of lung cancer is 14%. (A)

9. 3. The nurse's response should suggest exploration of the difficult decision-making process the client must go through. The client should be encouraged to verbalize the various options in order to make the choice that is right for her. Telling the client that she should give the baby up so it can have a better home or that research shows babies do better with their birth mothers is judgmental and does not place the control of the decision with the client. Suggesting that the client try keeping the baby at first minimizes the situation and also does not put the control of the decision with the client. (P)

10. 2. Two nurses must verify the name and label of the blood with the client's wristband. (D)

11. 3. Accumulation of air in the pleural cavity after a crushing chest injury may be assessed by unilateral diminished or absent breath sounds. Cheyne-Stokes respirations with periods of apnea commonly precede death. They indicate heart failure or brain death. Fremitus is increased with lung consolidation and decreased with pleural effusion or pneumothorax. Pain occurs at the injury site and increases with inspiration. (A)

12. 2. Chewing the pill or capsule form of valproic acid can cause mouth and throat irritation and is contraindicated. Taking the pills at the same time each day is important to maintain therapeutic effectiveness of the drug. Taking the pills with food is appropriate if the client is experiencing gastrointestinal upset. Valproic acid may cause clotting problems; therefore, bruising should be reported. (D)

13. 1. A significant association between feeding position and otitis media exists. Children fed in a supine position have a high incidence of otitis media because of the reflux of milk into the eustachian tubes during feedings. Keeping the infant's ears covered when out in the cold or thoroughly drying the ears after a bath has not been identified as a contributing factor to an infant's development of ear infections. Although the infant's immunization status is always important to ascertain, other factors, such as the position of the infant when taking a bottle, have more impact. (R)

14. 2. It is the role of the surgeon or the person performing the procedure to obtain the informed consent. This consists of informing the client about the procedure, the risks of treatment, the side effects, other types of treatments available, and the effects without the procedure. (M)

15. 4. Hospice care focuses on supportive care for the client and family. Care for the family may continue throughout the bereavement period. Hospice care involves care of the client at home as well as in an inpatient setting. Although professional care is provided in hospice, family members, volunteers, and unlicensed nursing personnel also participate in the care of the client. (C)

16. **3.** An 8 oz glass of milk is equivalent to $1\frac{1}{2}$ to 2 slices of presliced American cheese. Two tablespoons of Parmesan cheese or $\frac{1}{2}$ cup of milkshake is equivalent to 4 oz of milk, and $\frac{1}{2}$ cup of cottage cheese is equivalent to 2 oz of milk. (H)

17. **1.** The biophysical profile typically measures five parameters to assess the fetus: fetal breathing, movement, and tone; amniotic fluid volume; and fetal heart reactivity. The test uses a scale of 0 to 2 for each parameter with a maximum score of 10. (A)

18. **3.** One of the side effects of steroid therapy is fat deposition on the trunk and face, producing classic Cushingoid signs. Therefore, the nurse should expect to find truncal obesity. Steroids also can cause altered moods or mood swings. Typically, long-term steroid use results in weight gain. Steroids may inhibit the action of growth hormone. Therefore, a growth spurt is not likely. (D)

19. **3.** The nurse should not be required to participate in an abortion if it contradicts the nurse's religious beliefs. The behavior should not be reflected negatively on the nurses' evaluation. Preparing equipment and supplies for the case may be viewed as the same as circulating for the case. The nurse has a right not to participate in an abortion unless it is an absolute emergency and no one else is available to care for the client. (M)

20. **3.** Phenytoin causes hyperplasia of the gums, and the client needs frequent dental examinations and meticulous oral hygiene. Phenytoin therapy may contribute to a folic acid deficiency, but it is not related to iron or calcium metabolism. A need for frequent eye examinations is not related to the side effects of phenytoin. (D)

21. **1.** Visual acuity is not affected by long-term gentamicin sulfate therapy. The nurse should establish baseline data for vestibular, renal, and auditory function because gentamicin sulfate is ototoxic and causes renal toxicity. (D)

22. **1.** The chest is compressed with the heel of one hand positioned on the lower sternum, two fingerbreadths above the sternal notch. Fingertips are used to compress the sternum in infants, and the heels of both hands are used in adult cardiopulmonary resuscitation. (S)

23. **1.** Bacon is high in fat and therefore a poor choice for protein. Yogurt, dry beans, and peanut butter all contain protein in amounts that make them good sources of protein for the child. (C)

24. S_1 is loudest at the mitral area. (H)

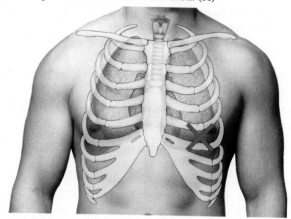

25. **1.** Nitroglycerin (Nitrostat) tablets should be taken 5 minutes apart for three doses; if this is ineffective, 911 should be called to obtain an ambulance to take the client to the emergency department. The client should not drive or have a family member drive the client to the hospital. (D)

26. **2.** Saturated fats raise blood cholesterol. Polyunsaturated fats maintain blood cholesterol. Monounsaturated fats may help to maintain or lower blood cholesterol. Phospholipids do not have an effect on cholesterol but act as emulsifiers, keeping fats dispersed in water. (H)

27. **4.** The client who voices death wishes must be asked directly about thoughts of suicide and specific suicide plans. The other questions are important history questions but are not crucial to address the follow-up needed when the client verbalizes a death wish. (P)

28. **3.** This client should be monitored for blood dyscrasias, evidenced by decreased platelet count and white blood cell count with changes in the CBC differential. (D)

29. **4.** The new onset of constipation may be a sign of a tumor from colon cancer. Constipation is not an expected change of aging. Increased fiber and fluid intake is helpful with constipation, but in this case the client needs to be seen by a health care provider to rule out colon cancer. (R)

30. **4.** Saying, "We'll help you be successful so that you can stay alcohol-free," conveys interest in the client as a worthwhile individual who needs help and treatment. This statement also helps to build trust and enhances self-esteem. The other statements confront the client and may result in the client's feeling belittled, judged, and rejected. (P)

31. **3.** Research has shown that at least two injections daily provide improved blood glucose control and decreased incidence of target end-organ damage. Type 1 diabetes requires insulin replacement and cannot be managed with oral medications alone. It would be inappropriate to ask the physician to change the insulin schedule. (D)

32. **1.** Peak and trough serum levels are used to adjust the dosage within a therapeutic range. (D)

33. **4.** DRIs are sets of nutrient intake values suggested for the dietary intake of healthy people in the United States and Canada. The DRIs were developed to establish levels of nutrient intake required to prevent chronic disease. The DRIs are meant to replace U.S. RDAs, which represented the minimum amount required to prevent symptoms of deficiency. The DRIs do not include recommended daily intake. Dietary Guidelines describe food choices that promote good health. (H)

34. **1.** The client with diabetes and a chronic respiratory condition is most at risk for influenza and should receive the vaccine yearly. Diabetes and chronic respiratory conditions do not increase the risk of hepatitis A. An adult client is not as likely to need the measles-mumps-rubella or varicella immunizations, but titers can be checked if the client has not had childhood immunizations or the disease. (R)

35. **2.** Infants are sensitive to stress in their caretakers. The best way to handle an anxious infant is to talk quietly to him, thereby soothing the infant. Limiting holding of the infant to feeding periods interferes with meeting the infant's needs for close contact, possibly compromising his ability to develop trust. Playing music in the room for most of the day and night will make it difficult for the infant to differentiate days from nights. Having a friend take the infant for several days will not necessarily take care of the problem because when the infant returns to the mother the same behaviors will recur unless the mother makes some changes. (P)

36. **1.** The infant is exhibiting periodic breathing, which is normal in infants of this age. The infant typically alternates short periods of rapid, louder respirations with periods of slower, quieter respirations. (H)

37. **2.** Tracheostomy tubes are associated with several potential complications, including laryngeal nerve damage, bleeding, and infection. Tracheostomy tubes do not cause decreased cardiac output, pneumothorax, or acute respiratory distress syndrome. (A)

38. **4.** A glycosylated hemoglobin level gives the nurse data about the average blood glucose concentration over 2 to 3 months, providing a picture of the client's overall glucose control. A fasting serum glucose level gives a picture of the child's recent glucose level, not the overall effectiveness of the child's therapeutic regimen. A 1-week diet recall is not always accurate. Although a home log would provide some information about the child's overall control and compliance, the log may not have all of the glucose levels recorded. (R)

39. **1.** The nurse's first action should be to clamp off the transfusion because the client is having a transfusion reaction. It is most important that the client not receive any more blood. Other measures may be appropriate after the blood has been stopped. The nurse should raise the head of the bed if the client becomes short of breath. There is no need for antibiotic therapy for a blood transfusion related to a temperature spike. The nurse can provide a cool washcloth for a headache or fever; however, this is not a priority. (D)

40. **1, 3, 4.** A drop in blood pressure to 80/40 mm Hg is significant and should be reported to the physician. Hypotension and vasodilation may occur as a result of sympathetic nerve blockage along with the pain nerve blockage. A report of a crushing headache suggests that the epidural catheter may be dislodged and in the subarachnoid space rather than the epidural space. The physician also should be notified anytime more than 1 ml of fluid or blood is aspirated from the catheter before a bolus injection. A respiratory rate of 14 breaths/minute, although somewhat decreased from baseline, is within acceptable parameters. However, if the rate drops to 10 breaths/minute or less, the physician should be notified. A pain rating of 3 out of 10 suggests that pain is being relieved with the epidural analgesia. (D)

41. **3.** A client with AIDS is immunocompromised, and food safety is an important concern. Food-borne illnesses and infections can be devastating to the client with AIDS. Large, frequent meals are not necessary. Megadoses of vitamins can result in toxicities that may aggravate the client's clinical condition. Leaving food out encourages growth of microorganisms. (S)

42. **3.** The incisions made for upper abdominal surgeries, such as cholecystectomies, are near the diaphragm and make deep breathing painful. Incentive spirometry, which encourages deep breathing, is essential to prevent atelectasis after surgery. The client is not maintained on bed rest for several days. The client is encouraged to ambulate by the first postoperative day, even with drainage tubes in place. Nasogastric tubes do not inhibit deep breathing and coughing. (A)

43. **4.** This finding describes Mongolian spots, which are common in newborns of African, Asian, or Latin descent. Telangiectatic nevi, or "stork bites," are pink lesions commonly found on the back of the neck. Milia are small white papules over the nose and cheek that indicate blocked sebaceous glands. (H)

44. 1. Blurred vision is a serious adverse effect of oral contraceptives, possibly because of severe hypertension as a result of the medication. If the client experiences blurred vision, she needs to contact her health care provider immediately. Nausea, weight gain, and mild headache are common and possibly bothersome side effects and should be noted. However, they do not need to be reported immediately unless they are severe, prolonged, or accompanied by other symptoms. (D)

45. 1. Signs and symptoms of a pneumothorax include sudden, sharp pain with breathing or coughing on the affected side, tachypnea, dyspnea, diminished or absent breath sounds on the affected side, tachycardia, anxiety, and restlessness. Tracheal deviation away from the affected side indicates a tension pneumothorax, which is a medical emergency. (A)

46. 2. When a client is experiencing a flashback, the nurse should stay with the client, offer reassurance, and present reality in a nonthreatening manner to minimize the client's anxiety and agitation. The client needs to be told that she is experiencing an effect from lysergic acid diethylamide and that she is safe and the flashback will end. Confronting the client's misperceptions or challenging her unrealistic statements could increase her anxiety and agitation, possibly leading to aggressive behavior. Secluding the client until the flashback ends usually is not necessary or appropriate unless the client threatens or demonstrates aggression toward herself or others. (P)

47. 2. The nurse should dispose of any used needle and syringe by immediately placing uncapped, used needles and syringes in the universal precaution container. (D)

48. 3. Nausea and vomiting, along with hypokalemia, are likely indicators of digoxin toxicity. Hypokalemia is a common cause of digoxin toxicity; therefore, serum potassium levels should be carefully monitored if the client is taking digoxin. The earliest clinical signs of digoxin toxicity are anorexia, nausea, and vomiting. Bradycardia, other dysrhythmias, and visual disturbances are also common signs. Chronic renal failure usually causes hyperkalemia. With persistent vomiting, the client is more likely to develop metabolic alkalosis than metabolic acidosis. (D)

49. 2. Food sources high in calcium include steamed broccoli, dairy products, and fortified cereals. Rice, apples, and meat are not calcium-rich sources. Menopausal women need 1,500 mg of calcium daily. (R)

50. 2. At the time a client receives a Depo-Provera injection, a follow-up appointment should be made for 3 months later. The nurse should emphasize the need to adhere to the medication schedule to prevent an unplanned pregnancy. One of the most common reasons for failure of this contraceptive is lack of adherence to the appointment schedule for injections every 3 months. (D)

51. 1. In major burns, there is a significant initial shift of fluid out of the plasma space into the interstitial spaces. This is the result of increased capillary permeability. Because of the increased permeability of capillary walls, water, sodium, and plasma protein escape into the tissues, increasing the tissue colloidal osmotic pressure and causing edema. Plasma colloidal pressure is decreased as a result of protein loss. A decrease in capillary hydrostatic pressure does not result in edema; an increase does. As fluid escapes into the tissues, it creates an increase in interstitial fluid pressure, not a decrease. (A)

52. 4. The pH of 7.52 indicates that the body is in a state of alkalosis. The partial pressure of carbon dioxide value is normal and the bicarbonate value is elevated. The increased bicarbonate value indicates that the acid-base imbalance is metabolic alkalosis. Restlessness can be a clinical finding in metabolic alkalosis. (A)

53. 3. Panting will alleviate the client's urge to push. The client risks edema or tearing of the cervix if pushing begins before complete cervical dilation (10 cm) is achieved. Although turning the client to her left side improves uteroplacental blood flow, it will have no effect on diminishing the client's urge to push. Although focusing on an object in the room may help the client to relax, it will have no effect on diminishing the client's urge to push due to the pressure of a fetus at +1 station. (H)

54. 1. The client who is taking potentially nephrotoxic antibiotics does not need to report straw-colored urine because this is normal. The client needs to report if the urine is cloudy, smoky, or pink; early signs of nephrotoxicity are manifested by changes in urine color. (D)

55. 4. Clinical manifestations of juvenile hypothyroidism include dry skin, constipation, sparse hair, and sleepiness. Short attention span, weight loss, moist flushed skin, rapid pulse, and heat intolerance suggest hyperthyroidism. (A)

56. 1, 6. Atomoxetine is a selective norepinephrine reuptake inhibitor antidepressant, not a stimulant. Therefore, a two-times-a-day dosing schedule is appropriate, with a dose given in the morning and late afternoon. It may take more than 2 to 3 weeks to see the full effects of this medication. Nausea and dizziness are transient side effects. Monoamine oxidase inhibitors are contraindicated with atomoxetine. (D)

57. 1. In clients with excess fluid volume, sodium restriction may be necessary to promote fluid loss. Monitoring electrolytes daily may be appropriate but will not reduce the excess fluid. Maintaining a record of the client's intake and output is also an independent nursing intervention. Elevating the client's feet helps promote venous return and fluid reabsorption but in itself will not reduce the volume of excess fluid. The nurse can elevate the client's feet without a medical order. (R)

58. **3.** The bluish pigment on the buttocks and back of an African American infant is a common finding and should be documented as Mongolian spots in the child's record. These spots typically fade by the time the child is 5 or 6 years. Additional assessment by the physician is not indicated. Laser therapy is not used. Rather, laser therapy is useful for port wine stains, which are dark purple and disfiguring. (H)

59. **1.** The client might wear objects as a protection against specific medical disorders. Typically these practices bring no harm to the client and should not be discouraged. The client should continue to be encouraged to follow the medical guidance of her health care provider. If the practice is not harming the client, it is inappropriate to label it quackery and demand that the client discontinue it. There is no medical evidence to support the wearing of a copper bracelet. (H)

60. **4.** Normally, a neonate's heart rate should be between 120 and 160 bpm shortly after birth. The nurse should document this as a normal neonatal finding. The physician does not need to be notified. Assessing for cyanosis is a routine assessment at birth, but with the neonate's heart rate at 142 bpm, cyanosis should be minimal and typically located in the hands and feet. Heart rate assessments are performed routinely according to facility protocol. For example, the heart rate is assessed soon after birth, every 15 minutes for 1 hour, every 30 minutes for 1 hour, and then every 4 hours. (H)

61. **1.** In a frank breech, the buttocks alone are at the cervix, while the knees are extended to rest on the chest. In a cephalic presentation, the head is the fetal body part first coming in contact with the cervix. Both feet at the cervix is termed double footling breech. In a shoulder presentation, one of the shoulders (actually the acromion process) presents to the cervix. Typically, the fetus is lying horizontally (transverse lie). (H)

62. **1.** The therapeutic effects of desmopressin nasal spray are relief from polydipsia and control of polyuria and nocturia in the client with diabetes insipidus. Side effects include nasal congestion and headache. Blurred vision is not related to desmopressin. (D)

63. **2.** A mammogram can detect a lesion the size of a pinhead, and a lump is about 2 cm before it can be detected by a BSE. The American Cancer Society guidelines recommend a mammogram yearly after age 40. A mammogram will not detect other endocrine abnormalities. (H)

64. **1.** Protein and vitamin C are particularly important in promoting wound healing and recovery from infection. A diet high in carbohydrates is also essential. Because the client with an infection commonly does not feel like eating, it is important that what he is encouraged to eat should be nutritious. Chicken and orange slices would help meet the client's protein and vitamin needs. A meal of cheeseburger and fries or cheese omelet and bacon is high in fat and low in vitamins. Gelatin salad and tea contain minimal nutrients. (C)

65. **4.** Beef, liver, iron-fortified cereals, and spinach are iron-rich foods. Cheese, squash, and eggs are not significant sources of iron. (R)

66. **2.** Good sources of dietary iron include red meats, poultry, green leafy vegetables, and dried fruits such as raisins. Milk products are poor sources of iron. Carrots are high in vitamin A. (R)

67. **2, 4.** Children in respiratory distress need to be kept as quiet as possible to decrease respiratory and heart rates. Toddlers need a parent with them for security. The best way to quiet toddlers is to read to or hold them. Restraints increase heart and respiratory rates. A sedative will mask the signs of further respiratory distress. Although telling toddlers that a mask will help with breathing, they cannot understand the rationale and thus fully comprehend its importance. Asking the parents to leave the bedside will most likely result in greater upset, further contributing to respiratory distress. (C)

68. **2.** The pallor and cool temperature of the fingers and the decreased return time for capillary refill indicate decreased arterial blood supply to the fingers. These findings are not normal for any time in the recovery process. Nerve impairment includes numbness, tingling, and impaired movement of the fingers. Signs of venous stasis include edema and reddening of the fingers, not pallor and cool temperature. (A)

69. **1.** Warm showers, baths, or hand soaks can help relieve joint stiffness and allow the client to more comfortably perform activities of daily living. Aspirin or other anti-inflammatory drugs should be taken before activity to help decrease inflammation and reduce joint pain and inflammation. Although weight loss may decrease stress on joints, pain and stiffness will continue to be a problem. Cold compresses are most effective for relieving joint pain, whereas moist heat is useful for decreasing pain and stiffness. When cold compresses are applied, their use should be limited to 10 to 15 minutes at a time to decrease the risk of tissue damage. (C)

70. **2.** The most appropriate immediate response is to open the airway. The nurse then should look, listen, and feel for respirations. Noting none, the nurse calls a code and attempts ventilations with a bag mask or mask with a one-way valve until the full code team responds. Using standard precautions with the mask protects the nurse from exposure to possible client microorganisms. (A)

71. **4.** The nurse should remind the client about meal and activity times so that the ritual can be completed beforehand and not interfere with meals and activities. The client must be allowed to complete her ritual because it keeps anxiety in check. Totally eliminating the client's ritual will increase her anxiety and the need for the handwashing. Allowing the client to decide whether she wants to attend meals and activities is not appropriate or in the client's best interest because she must perform the ritual to assuage anxiety. Informing the client that absence from meals and activities is not permitted scolds the client, increasing her anxiety and her need for the ritual. (P)

72. 2. The client needs further instructions when she says, "If I become pregnant, I can continue to eat sushi twice a week." Raw fish, including tuna, should be avoided while the client is pregnant because of the risk of contamination with mercury and other potential teratogens. Folic acid supplements taken before the client gets pregnant and during pregnancy can help reduce the risk of neural tube defects. Steaming vegetables reduces the risk that vitamins will be lost in the cooking water. Soy products can increase the client's protein levels. (H)

73. 4. The nurse should acknowledge that the client feels better, but should also remind the client to continue his drug therapy and other self-care activities of rest, exercise, joint protection, and adequate nutrition. Wearing the bracelet is not harmful, and the nurse should not instruct the client to remove it or label it quackery. Copper bracelets do not interfere with salicylate metabolism. (P)

74. 4. Liver function tests, including aspartate transaminase (AST) should be monitored before therapy, 6 to 12 weeks after initiation of therapy or after dose elevation, and then every 6 months. If AST levels increase to three times normal, therapy should be discontinued. Simvastatin does not influence serum glucose, complete blood count, or total protein. Serum cholesterol and triglyceride levels should be evaluated before initiating therapy, after 4 to 6 weeks of therapy, and periodically thereafter. (H)

75. 3. Acupuncture, like acumassage and acupressure, is performed in certain Asian cultures to restore the energy balance within the body. Pressure, massage, and fine needles are applied to energy pathways to help restore the body's balance. Acupuncture is not based on a belief in purging evil spirits. Although pain relief through acupuncture can promote tranquility, acupuncture is performed to restore energy balance. In the Western world, many researchers think that the gate-control theory of pain may explain the success of acupuncture, acumassage, and acupressure. (C)

76. 2. Tinnitus or ringing in the ears is a sign of aspirin toxicity and should be reported. Clients should be instructed to take aspirin as prescribed and to avoid overdosage. Gastrointestinal symptoms associated with aspirin include nausea, heartburn, and epigastric discomfort caused by gastric irritation. Abdominal cramps, rash, and hypotension are not related to aspirin therapy. (D)

77. 4. The nurse does not need to know that the client has four grandchildren in the transfer report because this is not information needed to help with the client's continuity of care. (M)

78. 3. Although breech presentations are rare, footling breech occurs when there is an extension of the fetal knees and one or both feet protrude through the pelvis. In frank breech, there is flexion of the fetal thighs and extension of the knees. The feet rest at the sides of the fetal head. In complete breech, there is flexion of the fetal thighs and knees; the fetus appears to be squatting. Vertex position occurs in 95% of deliveries; in such cases, the head is engaged in the pelvis. (H)

79. 3. Traveling is not advised because of the client's history of PIH. The client may be in jeopardy if complications occur and medical care is not available. In some cases, insurance companies will not cover costs of medical care in foreign countries. Air travel is not associated with preterm labor, although some airlines advise clients who are at 28 weeks' gestation or beyond not to travel by air. Any travel that causes fatigue should be avoided. Additionally, any pregnant client should get frequent exercise while traveling to avoid venous stasis from prolonged sitting. The client is not at greater risk for communicable diseases. The priority is the client's history of PIH, which, if it occurs, could lead to complications. (R)

80. 3. WIC is the best option. Home-delivered and congregate meals are for adults older than age 60 years. The food bank does not ensure adequate intake of the appropriate nutrients during pregnancy. (M)

81. 4. A supine position in extension is the position most likely to prevent contractures. Clients who have experienced burns will find a flexed position most comfortable. However, flexion promotes the development of contractures. The high Fowler's and semi-Fowler's positions create hip flexion. The prone position is contraindicated because of head and neck burns. In clients with head and neck burns, pillows should not be used under the head or neck because it promotes neck flexion contractures. (R)

82. 2. A fractured femur, especially an open fracture, can cause much soft tissue damage and lead to significant blood loss. Hypovolemic shock can develop. Cardiogenic shock occurs when cardiac output is decreased as a result of ineffective pumping. Neurogenic shock occurs as a result of an impaired autonomic nervous system function. Anaphylactic shock is the result of an allergic reaction. (A)

83. 2. Safety concerns are essential for a client with sensory impairment. Water temperature should be tested carefully, hot water bottles should be avoided, and the skin should be inspected regularly. Independence and self-care are also important; the client should not be instructed to avoid kitchen activities out of fear of injury. (S)

84. **1, 3.** Elevating the extremities counteracts the forces of gravity and promotes venous return and reduces venous stasis. Walking is encouraged to activate the muscle pump and promote collateral circulation. Prolonged sitting and standing leads to venous stasis and should be avoided. Although heat promotes vasodilation, use of a heating pad is to be avoided to reduce the risk of thermal injury secondary to diminished sensation. (R)

85. **3.** These behaviors suggest that the adolescent is thinking of suicide. Because of these behaviors, it is imperative for the adolescent to see his health care professional as soon as possible to determine whether he has suicidal thoughts. After the nurse makes the appointment, then obtaining more information would be appropriate. Giving the father the telephone number for the local crisis hotline is appropriate after the appointment is made, to ensure that the father has additional support should the adolescent's behavior escalate and an emergency arises. Taking the adolescent to the nearest mental health outpatient facility now is not warranted unless the adolescent's behavior escalates. (P)

86. **1.** For a child with chorea-like movements, safety is of prime importance. Feeding the child may be difficult. Forks should be avoided because of the danger of injury to the mouth and face with the tines. (S)

87. **1, 2, 4.** After bowel surgery, an NG tube attached to low intermittent suction is used to remove gastric fluids. The amount of fluid from the NG tube suction is important because it contributes to the child's overall fluid and electrolyte balance. I.V. fluids are used to maintain hydration, and intake and output is measured to determine hydration status. Postoperative vital signs are assessed more frequently than every 6 hours. Bowel sounds will be auscultated to determine when they return. Measuring abdominal girth is not necessary following colostomy reversal. (A)

88. **1.** After TURP, sphincter tone is poor, resulting in dribbling or incontinence. Kegel exercises can increase sphincter tone and decrease dribbling. Voiding every hour will not prevent dribbling or improve sphincter tone. It may take up to 12 months for urinary continence to be regained. (R)

89. **1.** The pattern of weight gain is commonly more important than the amount. Clients should be advised to gain a total of 25 to 35 lb if they are of average weight when becoming pregnant. The recommended pattern is 1 lb per month in the first trimester, then 1 lb per week in the second and third trimesters. A sudden increase in weight gain is associated with pregnancy-induced hypertension, whereas a sudden weight loss may indicate an illness. (H)

90. **2.** The nurse should administer 0.4 ml to administer 0.1 mg of digoxin I.V. if it comes in a concentration of 0.5 mg/2 ml, or 0.25 mg/ml. (D)

91. **2.** Numerous things have been tried by mothers with babies crying with colic. However, research has identified that the motion of a car is soothing to a baby with colic, commonly quieting the infant. The more the infant cries, the more air is swallowed, adding to the colic pain. Cereal should not be offered until the infant is age 4 to 6 months because of the increased risk of food allergies. Additionally, cereal has not been found to help with colic. (H)

92. **2.** Compartment syndrome, caused by compression of blood vessels and nerves, can lead to irreversible muscle and nerve damage if not detected early. Common signs of compartment syndrome in the arm include pain unrelieved by analgesics, pain on passive extension of fingers, loss of function, numbness and tingling, pallor, coolness of the extremity, and decreased or absent peripheral pulse. Delayed bone union does not cause symptoms of neurovascular impairment. Fat embolism is characterized primarily by confusion and respiratory symptoms. Osteomyelitis is a bone infection and is manifested by signs and symptoms of inflammation and infection. (R)

93. **2.** Cardiac rehabilitation includes client and family education and individualized activity counseling. Generally, the educational programs focus on presenting all of the risk factors associated with coronary artery disease. Low-back training is associated with a back injury recovery program. A strength training or jogging exercise program is not appropriate immediately after a cardiac event. (C)

94. **3.** When the nurse cannot elicit the Moro reflex of a 4-day-old preterm infant and the Moro reflex was present at birth, intracranial hemorrhage or cerebral edema should be suspected. Other symptoms include lethargy, bulging fontanels, and seizure activity. Confirmation can be made by ultrasound. Postnatal asphyxia is suggested by respiratory distress, grunting, nasal flaring, and cyanosis. A skull fracture can be confirmed by radiography. However, it is unlikely to occur in a preterm neonate. Rather, it is more common in the large-for-gestational-age neonate. Facial nerve paralysis is indicated when there is no movement on one side of the face. This condition is more common in the large-for-gestational-age neonate. (R)

95. **4.** Blood clots are normal after transurethral resection of the prostate, but bright red urine can indicate a hemorrhage. The nurse should assess the client's vital signs and notify the surgeon. Irrigation of the catheter may help remove clots, but it does not decrease bleeding. Milking a urinary catheter or increasing fluid intake is not effective for controlling bleeding or decreasing clots. (R)

96. **3.** The statement, "My medicine is not for the everyday stress of life," indicates an accurate understanding of the nurse's teaching about the use of lorazepam. Antianxiety agents like the benzodiazepines are used to treat anxiety that is unmanageable by other means and beyond the client's ability to cope. For the drug to be effective, it must be taken as prescribed. Lorazepam can cause physical and psychological dependence. Tolerance can occur, and doubling the dose of lorazepam may increase the risk of tolerance. Lorazepam is a central nervous system depressant. When it is taken in combination with alcohol, the depressant effect increases, posing a danger to the client. (D)

97. **1.** A blood test for alpha fetoprotein is recommended at 15 to 20 weeks' gestation to screen for neural tube defects such as spina bifida. Chorionic villi sampling is used to detect chromosomal anomalies. Amniotic fluid amino acid determination is used to detect inborn errors of metabolism such as phenylketonuria. An amniocentesis is used to determine the lecithin-sphingomyelin ratio for fetal lung maturity, indicated by a ratio of 2:1, or chromosomal abnormalities. (R)

98. **4.** The error should be reported to the physician promptly for orders. The nurse should complete an incident report because an unusual occurrence happened during the client's care. The nurse should observe the client for symptoms of hyperglycemia but first must call the physician and complete an incident report. The nursing assistant does not need to be reassigned for this error. The nurse does not need to reprimand the nursing assistant for the error because the nursing assistant already knows an error was made. (M)

99. **2.** After abdominal pelvic surgery, the client is especially prone to thrombophlebitis. Measuring calf circumference can help detect edema in the affected leg. The calf should not be rubbed or palpated because a clot could be loosened and travel to the lungs as a pulmonary embolism. Homans' sign, which is calf pain on dorsiflexion of the foot when the leg is raised, is sometimes associated with thrombophlebitis. Having the client flex and extend the leg does not provide useful assessment data; the leg will not change color when raised and lowered. (R)

100. **1.** The client with sensorineural hearing loss has difficulty hearing high-pitched sounds. Aging and ototoxicity are two causes of sensorineural hearing loss. The client's ability to speak is not affected. The client who cannot assign meaning to sound has central hearing loss. Vertigo is commonly an indication of an inner ear problem. (A)

101. **3.** *Grieving* best describes the client as she grieves for the changes occurring in her life since her cancer diagnosis. The other nursing diagnoses may be appropriate, but *Grieving* is the most applicable diagnosis for this client. (P)

102. **3.** Nalbuphine is an analgesic that is used for clients in labor. It has a sedative effect and can slow the respiratory rate. After administering the drug, the nurse should first put the side rails up to prevent injury to the client and then assess her vital signs. Then the nurse can lower the head of the bed slightly to allow the client to sleep, cover the client with a blanket, and dim the lights. (D)

103. **3.** The client with emphysema is commonly underweight in appearance. It is theorized that weight loss is caused by the increased energy required to support the work of breathing. Frequent coughing, bronchospasms, and copious sputum are clinical manifestations of chronic bronchitis. (A)

104. **4.** The traction is set up correctly. Additional weights are not needed. A well-balanced diet with fiber should be offered. A pillow under the leg would negate the effects of the traction. Because the adolescent is positioned this way for an extended period, the nurse can help by finding activities that interest the client. (C)

105. **1.** The client with a systolic blood pressure of 160 to 179 mm Hg should be evaluated by a health care professional within 1 month of the screening. The client with a diastolic blood pressure of 90 to 99 mm Hg should be rechecked within 2 months. Exercise and stress reduction may be desirable activities, but it is first necessary to evaluate the cause of elevated blood pressure. In the absence of other symptoms, it is not necessary to have the client evaluated immediately. (H)

106. **4.** Keeping the client's door closed is likely to contribute to feelings of isolation and sensory deprivation. Such activities as watching television, visiting with a relative, and reading a newspaper help prevent sensory deprivation and yet do not require physical effort. (P)

107. **4.** The client taking dexamethasone needs to know the early signs of Cushing's disease, which include easy bruising, moonface, buffalo hump, and osteoporosis. Loss of collagen makes the skin weaker and thinner; therefore, the client bruises more easily. The nurse should instruct the client to report any of these signs to the physician. Hypertension is a symptom of Cushing's disease, and muscle mass is decreased. Increased urinary frequency is not a symptom of Cushing's disease. (D)

108. **1.** Verbalizing feelings and concerns helps decrease anxiety and allows the family member to move on to understanding the current situation. Describing events or explaining equipment is appropriate when the person is not distraught and is ready to learn. Reassuring the family member does not allow verbalization of feelings and discounts the person's feelings. (P)

109. **2.** Graded exercise testing is a diagnostic and prognostic tool used to determine the physiologic responses to controlled exercise stress. Information gained from a graded exercise test can achieve diagnostic, functional, and therapeutic objectives for the client. Graded exercise tests involve the use of a treadmill, stationary bicycle, or arm ergometry. Thinking under pressure, distance walked, and duration of walking are not the purpose of a graded exercise test. (R)

110. **2, 3, 4.** Albuterol is a beta-adrenergic agonist. Possible adverse effects include nausea, headache, and nervousness as well as insomnia and vomiting. Constipation is not associated with this drug. The client will not become lethargic; instead, he may experience restlessness. (D)

111. **3.** It is normal for the client who is beginning chemotherapy to be anxious and fearful about possible side effects. It is important that the nurse listen to the client's concerns, correct any misconceptions, and explain the supportive care that will be provided during the chemotherapy treatments. The client needs to understand that individuals do respond differently to the treatments, and her experience may be very different from those of other people she knows. A previously excellent health record does not necessarily ensure that the client will not experience side effects. Medications may lessen but not prevent the side effects, so client concerns should not be dismissed. Telling the client that she will die if she refuses treatment does nothing to allay her fears and concerns. (P)

112. **1.** Overprotection is a typical parental reaction to chronic illness in a child. Characteristics include sacrifice of self and family for the child, failure to recognize the child's capabilities and sense of responsibility, placement of overly stringent restrictions on play and peer friendship, and a lack of confidence in other peoples' capabilities. (P)

113. **3.** Children with roseola have a high fever for 3 days, which drops suddenly. Then a nonpruritic rash appears, typically lasting for 1 to 2 days. High fever followed by a rash is a characteristic sign. Associated symptoms include cold symptoms, cough, and lymphadenopathy. (A)

114. **1.** Knowing that the voices are not real is a reflection that the haloperidol is effective in decreasing psychosis. Restlessness may be a side effect of haloperidol, not an indication of improvement. Awareness of need for activities of daily living is an indicator of improvement.

However, recognizing that the voices are not real demonstrates a greater awareness of the client's disorder than the need for hygiene does. Wanting discharge reflects denial of illness. (D)

115. **1, 2, 3, 4, 6.** Diabetic ketoacidosis is a potentially life-threatening problem. The state of unconsciousness requires very astute monitoring of the neurologic condition. Frequent assessments of neurologic status (including the client's ability to respond to stimuli), blood pressure, and urinary output need to be documented. Assessment of skin condition for the presence of lesions, bruises, ulcers, or bumps is documented to assess for possible injuries, such as falls associated with head injury or internal injuries. Although it would be helpful to know how long the client has had diabetes, this information is not essential to document. (A)

116. **2.** The elderly client commonly has multiple physicians. The client needs to inform every doctor about all the medications being prescribed by all of them. (D)

117. **2.** The nurse should first check with the physician for the complete order of calcium because calcium chloride has a concentration of 13.6 mEq of calcium per gram and calcium gluconate has 4.65 mEq of calcium per gram. The nurse can always offer the doctor the type of calcium available after the conversion in calcium has been made; otherwise, the error could be fatal. (D)

118. **3.** When administering I.V. potassium chloride, the administration should not exceed 10 mEq/hour or a concentration of 40 mEq/L via a peripheral line. These limits are extremely important to prevent the development of hyperkalemia and the possibility of cardiac dysrhythmias. In some situations, with dangerously low serum potassium levels, the client may need cardiac monitoring and more than 10 mEq of potassium per hour. Potassium-sparing diuretics may lead to hyperkalemia because they affect the kidney's ability to excrete excess potassium. Metabolic alkalosis can cause potassium to shift into the cells, thus decreasing the client's serum potassium levels. Hypokalemia can lead to digoxin toxicity. (D)

119. **3.** Systematic pain assessment is necessary for adequate pain management in the postoperative client. Guidelines from the Agency for Healthcare Research and Quality recommend that facilities adopt a pain assessment scale to facilitate pain management. Even though the client is receiving morphine sulfate by PCA, assessment is needed if he is experiencing pain. Encouraging the client to rest or to ignore pain without further assessment is not a sufficient intervention. (C)

120. **2.** Exposure to moisture can lead to maceration and the development of pressure ulcers. It is important for the client's skin to be kept clean and dry with prompt attention to cleanliness after incidents of incontinence. The client's age and the presence of hypertension are not factors leading to pressure ulcers. Smoking affects the oxygen status of the client but does not directly lead to the development of pressure ulcers. (R)

121. **1.** The screening protocol recommended by the American Cancer Society for early detection of cancer in asymptomatic people includes: Beginning at age 50, men and women should have fecal occult blood testing every year or flexible sigmoidoscopy every 5 years or colonoscopy every 10 years. A diet low in fat and high in fruit and fiber is not a screening protocol but is good dietary advice for all clients. (H)

122. **3.** A low dose of an antipsychotic can decrease aggression. Adjustment to the structured daily routine and diminished resistance with activities of daily living are improvements related to the nursing care given, not the medications. No medications currently given to treat Alzheimer's disease return short-term memory. (D)

123. **3.** A sudden gush of dark blood, a lengthening of the umbilical cord, a smaller uterus, and changing of the uterus to a round or spherical shape are impending signs of placental separation. Pushing effort from the client is not a reliable indicator for impending placental separation, nor is it necessary for placental expulsion. (H)

124. **1.** The nurse needs to assess neurologic status throughout the therapy. Altered sensorium or neurologic changes may indicate intracranial bleeding for the client who has received tissue plasminogen activator or alteplase. The nurse should carefully check for bleeding every 15 minutes during the first hour of therapy, every 15 to 30 minutes during the next 9 hours, and at least every 4 hours during the duration of therapy. Bleeding may occur from sites of invasive procedures or from body orifices. The blood glucose level does not need to be evaluated. Arterial blood gas values relate to acid base status and oxygenation and are avoided due to the invasiveness of arterial puncture at this time. (D)

125. **2.** In the emergency phase of burn management, hyperkalemia develops as a result of the destruction of red blood cells. The hematocrit is increased in response to the plasma loss that has occurred and the resulting hemoconcentration. Initially, hyponatremia may occur as sodium shifts into the interstitial spaces. (A)

126. **1.** The nurse should explain that the child will feel a stinging when the numbing medicine is inserted into the area around the introduction site of the catheter. There may also be a feeling of pressure when the catheter is introduced. Because the child will be sedated and will feel little during the procedure, telling the child that a momentary sharp pain is felt on entering the heart is inappropriate. A tingling sensation in the extremities is not felt. (R)

127. **2.** In conjunction with the child's history of recent respiratory infection and report of dark urine, swelling around the eyes should lead the nurse to suspect acute glomerulonephritis. Therefore, the nurse should ask about a recent sore throat because a child with glomerulonephritis typically would have had a sore throat in the past 10 days. Drinking lots of liquids is unrelated to the periorbital edema. (A)

128. **2.** Measuring the pH of the aspirated gastric fluid is the most accurate determination of the placement of the NG tube. A pH lower than 4 indicates that the tube is in the stomach. Whether or not the client is gagging or coughing is not an accurate way to determine if the tube is placed correctly. No fluids should be inserted into the tube until the placement has been determined. Inserting air into the tube and listening for the resulting whoosh can be used, but this is not as accurate as pH measurement. (R)

129. **2.** True labor is present when cervical dilation and effacement occur. Fetal descent into the pelvic inlet is an indication that labor will begin soon. However, for a nulligravid client, this may take 1 to 2 weeks. Painful contractions every 3 to 5 minutes may be Braxton Hicks contractions. Contractions that disappear when the client lies down are a sign of false labor. Although leaking amniotic fluid should be reported, it is not a sign of true labor. (H)

130. **4.** During the first 24 hours after a total laryngectomy, maintaining a patent airway is a priority goal. After a total laryngectomy, the client will have a tracheostomy with increased secretions and will require suctioning and tracheostomy care. Providing adequate nutrition, preventing skin breakdown, and maintaining proper bowel elimination will be appropriate as the client recovers, but maintaining a patent airway is the initial priority goal. (R)

131. **3.** Not sleeping to avoid nightmares reflects inadequate grief resolution. The client is not letting go or resolving the vivid memories of the trauma as expected. Statements that the client gets sad at times but can function in daily activities or that the client still misses his family but acknowledges improvement indicate that the client is recovering and continued counseling is not necessary. Working for train crossing safety indicates motivation to help others escape what he has experienced. This action also denotes a goal for the future, indicating recovery. (P)

132. **3.** Haloperidol and lorazepam together decrease hallucinations and agitation, thus decreasing the risk of self-harm. Putting the client in restraints is premature because danger is not imminent. Asking the client to talk about her anger is inappropriate because the client is beyond rational conversation. A room search is appropriate only after the crisis with the client is handled. (D)

133. **1.** The nurse should adjust the heparin dose to maintain the client's partial thromboplastin time between 1.5 and 2.5 times the normal control. The prothrombin time and International Normalized Ratio are used to maintain therapeutic levels of warfarin (Coumadin), oral anticoagulation therapy. The thrombin clotting time is used to confirm disseminated intravascular coagulation. (D)

134. **2.** The oral mucous membranes are easily damaged and are commonly ulcerated in the client with leukemia. It is better to provide oral hygiene without using a toothbrush, which can easily damage sensitive oral mucosa. Applying petroleum jelly to the lips, swabbing the mouth with moistened cotton swabs, and rinsing the mouth with a nonirritating mouthwash are appropriate oral care measures for a child with leukemia. (C)

135. **1.** The nurse's first response to the error is to assess the client for any untoward reactions as a result of the error. Notifying the physician and unit manager of the error as well as completing an incident report are all appropriate later actions, but the first action is to assess the client. (M)

136. **3.** The peak action of Regular insulin is approximately 2 to 3 hours after administration. The client is having typical hypoglycemic symptoms. Acidosis results from uncontrolled diabetes mellitus, with hyperpnea (Kussmaul respirations) as the outstanding symptom. The hallmark symptoms of hyperglycemia are increased thirst, fruity breath, and glycosuria. The signs and symptoms of diabetic ketoacidosis include Kussmaul respirations, fruity breath, tachycardia, abdominal pain, nausea, vomiting, headache, thirst, dry skin, and dehydration. (D)

137. **4.** The nurse needs to obtain more information before plans are developed. Therefore, asking to know more about the situation is most appropriate. The nurse has no way of predicting whether abuse will occur again. Therefore, it is inappropriate for the nurse to agree with the mother, stating that the abuse probably will not happen again. Filing charges and a Child Protective Services report may be needed, but more information is needed first. These actions would not be done without the mother's understanding why. (P)

138. **2.** If the client begins to experience abdominal cramping during administration of the enema fluid, the nurse's first action is to temporarily stop the infusion and have the client take a few deep breaths. After the cramping subsides, the nurse can continue with the enema solution. If the cramping does not subside, the nurse should clamp the tubing and remove it. Raising the height of the container will increase the flow of fluid and cause the cramping to increase. Rubbing the abdomen while infusing the enema fluid will not stop the cramping. (C)

139. **1.** When inserting an I.V. catheter needle, the nurse initially uses veins low on the hand or arm if available, unless contraindicated. Should the I.V. fluid infiltrate or the vein become irritated at this insertion site, veins higher on the arm are still available for use. After a vein higher up on the arm has been damaged, veins below it cannot be used. (D)

140. **3.** Lactulose is used to treat hepatic encephalopathy by reducing serum ammonia levels. It is not used to stimulate bowel peristalsis, even though diarrhea can be a side effect of the drug. Lactulose does not have any effect on edema, ascites, or hemorrhage. (D)

141. **2.** A 12-month-old whose immunizations are current has received three diphtheria, tetanus, and acellular pertussis; three hepatitis B; and two inactivated poliovirus immunizations. Oral polio vaccine is not used routinely. *Haemophilus* b is administered at 2, 4, and 6 months, and a booster is given at 12 to 15 months. (H)

142. **3.** Obesity is a risk factor for osteoarthritis because it places increased stress on the joints. A high-protein diet, regular exercise, and vitamin supplements do not reduce a client's risk of developing osteoarthritis. (H)

143. **3.** Vitamin E is a powerful antioxidant that helps to prevent oxidation of the cell membrane. Vitamins C, A, and B_6 are helpful in the prevention of heart disease, but vitamin E plays a more important role. (H)

144. **3.** The nurse should instruct the mother to report the first voiding after the circumcision because edema could cause a urinary obstruction. Although reading a pamphlet about circumcision care may be helpful, it may not be appropriate for all mothers. Some mothers could have difficulty reading or understanding the information. Petroleum jelly gauze is used with Gomco clamp circumcisions, not Plastibell. Petroleum jelly should not be used with Plastibell circumcision methods, because the bell prevents further bleeding. (H)

145. **2.** Alcoholic cirrhosis is associated with excessive alcohol intake. In the early stages, the liver develops fatty changes. If alcohol intake stops, the fatty changes can be reversed. Avoiding overexertion is important in the client with cirrhosis, but it does not reverse the disease. Stopping smoking is a positive, healthy lifestyle change, but it does not have an impact on cirrhosis. A diet high in carbohydrates and low in fat is also recommended for the client with cirrhosis, but the diet does not reverse the pathologic changes that have occurred in the liver. (R)

146. **3.** Using the ratio-proportion method, the equations are as follows:

$$4 \text{ mg}/1 \text{ ml} = 7.6 \text{ mg}/X \text{ ml}$$

$$4X = 7.6$$

$$X = 7.6/4 = 1.9 \text{ ml.}$$

(D)

147. **4.** Because of the client's age, the amniocentesis is most likely being done to evaluate for Down syndrome (trisomy 21). Women older than 35 years are at higher risk for having a child with Down syndrome. Cri du chat syndrome is a genetic disorder involving a short arm on chromosome 5. This disorder is not associated with mothers who are older than 35 years. The client is AB-positive, so the amniocentesis is not being done for ABO incompatibility, in which the mother is type O and the fetus is type A, B, or AB. The amniocentesis is not being done to detect erythroblastosis fetalis because the mother is Rh-positive. (R)

148. **3.** The symptoms of BPH are related to obstruction as a result of an enlarged prostate. Difficulty in starting the urinary stream is a common symptom, along with dribbling, hesitancy, and urinary retention. Impotence does not result from BPH. Flank pain is most commonly related to pyelonephritis. Hematuria occurs in urinary tract infections, renal calculi, and bladder cancer, to name some of the most common causes. (A)

149. **1.** Having the client role-play assertive statements assists the client in learning how to use assertiveness and practicing appropriate behaviors in a safe environment. Watching a videotape on assertiveness or discussing situations that appear threatening is a step toward actually using assertive techniques. Describing feelings that occur after an angry outburst motivates the client to make changes in behavior. (P)

150. **4.** Symptoms of transient tachypnea include respirations as high as 150 breaths/minute, retractions, flaring, and cyanosis. Treatment is supportive and includes provision of warm, humidified oxygen in a warm environment. The nurse should continuously monitor the neonate's respirations, color, and behaviors to allow for early detection and prompt intervention should problems arise. Feedings are given by gavage rather than bottle to decrease respiratory stress. Obtaining extracorporeal membrane oxygenation equipment is not necessary but may be used for the neonate diagnosed with meconium aspiration syndrome. (A)

151. **10**

First, convert 1.5 g to 1,500 mg. Then set up a proportion:

$$1,500 \text{ mg}/X \text{ ml} = 300 \text{ mg}/2 \text{ ml}$$

$$X = 10 \text{ ml.}$$

(D)

152. **2.** One of the early signs of iron deficiency anemia in a client of Vietnamese descent with dark skin is yellowish-brown skin tones. The nurse can assess for petechiae or jaundice, which may be observed in the conjunctiva or buccal mucosa. (A)

153. **1.** A decreased total serum protein occurs as extensive amounts of protein are excreted from the body through the urine. Clients may develop hypocalcemia. Hyperglycemia is not a finding related to nephrotic syndrome. A decreased hematocrit is not a finding related to nephrotic syndrome. (A)

154. **2.** The number one cause of nosocomial infections in hospital units is not washing the hands. Nosocomial infections can be significantly reduced by thorough handwashing before caring for each infant. Sterile supplies are not necessary for all treatments. Cover gowns and masks, although helpful in reducing the risk of exposure to blood and body fluids, do not decrease the risk of nosocomial infection. (S)

155. **2.** Recommended restraints for a child who has had palate surgery is elbow restraints. They minimize the limitation placed on the child but still prevent the child from injuring the repair with fingers and hands. A safety jacket or wrist or body restraints restrict the child unnecessarily. (S)

156. **2.** Battering is a major cause of injury to women. Although battering occurs in all socioeconomic groups, it may appear to be more common in members of lower socioeconomic groups because they are more likely to use emergency department services. Pregnant women are frequent victims of battering. Death from battering is not rare. (P)

157. **3.** After a nephrectomy, a specific aspect of immediate postoperative management includes monitoring urine output at least hourly. Monitoring blood pressure and encouraging the use of incentive spirometry are other important considerations, but because of the surgical disruption of the urinary system, urine output is a priority. Measurement of urine output should also include an estimation of the amount of urine drainage on the flank dressing. (R)

158. **4.** Severe retroversion or anteversion may lead to infertility or difficulty conceiving a child because these positions can block the deposition or migration of sperm. The normal position of the uterus is tipped slightly forward. Frequent vaginal infections commonly are associated with diabetes or human immunodeficiency virus infection, not abnormal uterine positions. Pain from endometriosis (abnormal myometrial growth outside the uterus) is not associated with abnormal uterine positions. Severe menstrual cramping or dysmenorrhea (primary) is caused by increased prostaglandin production, not abnormal uterine positions. Secondary dysmenorrhea is associated with pelvic inflammatory disease or endometriosis. (H)

159. **2.** A 4-year-old is old enough to be able to cooperate and stop the behavior. Therefore, the first step is to obtain the child's cooperation. When this has occurred, then the mother makes sure it is okay to remind the child when the behavior is viewed. The mother also should be encouraged to praise the child when she sees her not engaging in the behavior. (H)

160. **4.** During an episode of acute respiratory distress, it is important that the nurse focus the assessment on the client's respiratory system and distress to quickly address the client's problem. Conducting a complete health history and a comprehensive physical examination can be deferred until the client's condition is stabilized. It is not appropriate to delay all assessments until the respiratory distress is resolved because the nurse must have data to guide treatment. (A)

161. **4.** The most likely indication of a dislocated hip is a shortening of the affected leg. Other indications of dislocation include increasing pain, loss of function to the extremity, and deformity. Abduction of the leg after total hip replacement is a desirable position to prevent dislocation. Loosening of the prosthesis does not necessarily indicate that the hip has dislocated. External rotation of the hip can occur without the hip's being dislocated. However, a neutral position of rotation is the desired position. (A)

162. **1.** The client who is withdrawn, is suspicious, and projects blame is exhibiting problems in trust versus mistrust. Shame and doubt would be reflected as low self-esteem and suspiciousness. Guilt would be reflected in self-blame for all problems. Isolation would be reflected in a lack of long-term relationships. (P)

163. **4.** The nurse needs to explore more about the client's feelings to assess what underlies the eating disorder. The nurse also needs to evaluate the client's suicide risk. The other statements are not therapeutic because they minimize the client's feelings. (P)

164. **1.** An ileal conduit is a urinary diversion that requires the client to wear an appliance, or pouch, at all times because urine drains continuously. Ileal conduits are not irrigated. The urinary drainage is affected by fluid intake, not meals. (A)

165. **1.** Children with varicella or suspected varicella should be treated under airborne precautions in addition to standard precautions. Varicella is transmitted by airborne nuclei. Droplet precautions are indicated for conditions, such as pertussis, meningococcal pneumonia, and rubella. Contact precautions are indicated for conditions, such as draining major abscesses, acute viral conjunctivitis, and *Clostridium difficile* gastroenteritis. Indirect contact is not a method of controlling infection. Rather it is a mode of transmission involving contamination via some intermediate object, such as an instrument, needle, or dressing, or by hands that are not washed or gloves that are not changed between clients. (S)

166. **1.** In multiple myeloma, neoplastic plasma cells invade the bone marrow and begin to destroy the bone. As a result of this skeletal destruction, pain can be significant. There is no cure for multiple myeloma. Nausea and vomiting are not characteristics of the disease, although the client may experience anorexia. The client should be monitored for signs of hypercalcemia resulting from bone destruction, not for hyperkalemia. (A)

167. **1.** Stating, "You were able to shower and dress without any help this morning," points out a visible, realistic accomplishment and strength to the client with self-deprecatory statements, thereby helping to increase the client's self-worth. The statements, "Your wife told me that you are a good husband and father," and, "You don't have any reason why you should feel this way," are not helpful because logical statements are ineffective in changing the thinking of a client who is depressed. The client may agree with what the nurse states but be just as depressed because intellectual understanding does not help the severely depressed client. The statement, "This medication will help your thinking," although true, does not recognize the client's accomplishment and will have no positive effect on his self-esteem. (P)

168. **3.** The nurse uses Montgomery straps primarily to avoid the removal of long-term abdominal dressing tape and ultimate skin breakdown. (C)

169. **1.** The nurse's most appropriate response is to acknowledge and validate the client's concerns. Questioning the client's fears is not a therapeutic response and can make the client feel defensive. False reassurance that the client should not be afraid disregards the client's fears and does not promote further communication between the client and nurse. Dismissing the client's feelings and telling the client to relax does not encourage sharing of feelings. (P)

170. **3.** In a child with abdominal surgery, it is important to check vital signs frequently to assess for internal bleeding. Administering I.V. fluids, assessing pain, and keeping the child on nothing-by-mouth status are all important, but monitoring vital signs frequently is the priority. (R)

171. **2.** Polydipsia, or increased thirst, is a classic clinical manifestation of diabetes. The excessive loss of fluids is the result of the osmotic diuresis that occurs with glycosuria. It is unlikely that shortness of breath, early awakening, or trouble urinating is related to diabetes mellitus. (A)

172. **1.** *Activity intolerance* is a common nursing diagnosis for clients with hypothyroidism. Cellular metabolism and oxygen consumption are decreased. *Anxiety* is a symptom of hyperthyroidism, and *Hopelessness* is associated with depression; they are not supported by the data given here. *Ineffective coping* could be relevant at some point, but not based on the facts given. (A)

173. **2.** The client's serum alkaline phosphatase, which is produced by osteoblasts in the bone, is elevated in bone cancer. Hypercalcemia may occur in bone cancer. An elevated aspartate transaminase is present in liver disease. Potassium levels are not affected in bone cancer. (A)

174. **2.** Cardiomyopathy is a broad term that includes three major forms: dilated, hypertrophic, and restrictive cardiomyopathies. The underlying etiology of hypertrophic cardiomyopathy is unknown; it is typically observed in young men but is not limited to them. Common symptoms are fatigue, low tolerance to activity related to the low ejection fraction, and shortness of breath. Angina may be observed if coronary artery disease is present. Abdominal pain and hypertension are not common. (A)

175. **3.** Pinworms come out of the rectum during the nighttime and early morning hours. Therefore, the best time to apply the tape to get results is while the child is asleep. (A)

176. **3.** Maternal hydramnios occurs when the fetus has a congenital obstruction of the gastrointestinal tract, such as in the presence of a tracheoesophageal fistula. The fetus normally swallows amniotic fluid and absorbs the fluid from the gastrointestinal tract. Excretion then occurs through the kidneys and placenta. Most fluid absorption occurs in the colon. Absorption cannot occur when the fetus has a gastrointestinal obstruction. Meconium in the amniotic fluid, low implantation of the placenta, and toxemia could occur but are more specifically associated with fetal hypoxia. (H)

177. **1.** A common complication of steroid therapy is gastric irritation and peptic ulcers. Hyperglycemia is a potential complication. Tachycardia and renal failure are not associated with steroid therapy. (D)

178. **3.** When an incision eviscerates, it is a medical emergency. The nurse's first response is to apply a sterile dressing that has been moistened with sterile normal saline solution. The client should also be placed in semi-Fowler's position to release any tension on the abdominal area. Vital signs should be taken, and an I.V. line may be started for emergency treatment; however, the first action is to protect the wound and abdominal contents. (R)

179. **3.** Establishing a patent airway is the priority intervention. Prophylactic intubation is initiated if heat has been inhaled or if the neck, head, or face is involved. Swelling of the upper airways can progress to obstruction. Fluid replacement can best be achieved using a large-caliber peripheral I.V. catheter, and morphine sulfate is appropriate for analgesia in a burn client. Although these are priorities, they are secondary to establishing a patent airway. Administering tetanus toxoid is a secondary priority. (R)

180. **2.** The client who refuses to sign a no harm contract is an immediate and serious threat for suicide. Therefore, the nurse should place this client on one-to-one suicide precautions to protect the client from self-harm. Although a client who is withdrawn and anorectic or visibly crying may have symptoms of depression, these symptoms alone do not warrant one-to-one suicide precautions. Refusal of medication indicates a lack of insight by the client into his illness and lack of participation in treatment, but it is not an immediate suicide threat. However, the nurse must be alert for the cheeking and hoarding of medication as a possible means for self-harm. (P)

181. **3.** Quadriceps setting exercises help the immobilized client keep the quadriceps muscles strong and ready for resuming ambulation. Pressing the back of the knee against the bed promotes tightening of the quadriceps muscle. (R)

182. **4.** The physician should be notified immediately because the client's symptoms indicate that an intestinal obstruction may have developed. Taking milk of magnesia or any laxatives with a suspected obstruction can worsen the client's condition. Increasing oral fluids while the client is vomiting will not be effective. Measuring the abdominal girth is not an essential activity at this time. (A)

183. **4.** A diagnosis of AIDS cannot be made until the HIV-infected person meets case criteria established by the Centers for Disease Control and Prevention. The immune system becomes compromised. The CD4 T-cell count drops below 200 cells and develops one of the opportunistic diseases, such as *Pneumocystis carinii* pneumonia, candidiasis, cytomegalovirus, or herpes simplex. (A)

184. **2.** The client should wear loose, cotton underwear to promote cleanliness and dryness in the genital area. Sitz baths can promote cleanliness and decrease inflammation in the area. A hair dryer, set on a cool setting, can be used to carefully dry the lesions in the perineal area. Drinking plenty of fluids is advised to decrease dysuria, which accompanies genital herpes. (C)

185. **3.** Risperdal Consta, an atypical antipsychotic, is the I.M., long-acting form of risperidone (Risperdal). Risperdal Consta is given every 2 weeks, typically in a dose of 30 mg. The client must continue oral Risperdal for 3 weeks after treatment with Risperdal Consta begins. After 3 weeks, oral Risperdal is discontinued. (D)

186. **1.** Famotidine is useful for treating and preventing ulcers and managing gastroesophageal reflux disease. It functions by inhibiting the action of histamine at the H-2 receptor site located in the gastric parietal cells, thus inhibiting gastric acid secretion. (D)

187. **3.** Methylxanthines, a chemical found in coffee, tea, cola, and chocolate, contribute to fibrocystic breast disease in many women. Although the response has not been universal, decreasing caffeine intake has been very beneficial for many women in helping treat fibrocystic breast disease. In the absence of other health conditions, a woman is not advised to increase sodium or decrease calcium. A woman is not advised to use bottled water. (H)

188. **2.** The Dietary Guidelines for Americans discusses healthy nutritional guidelines. Dietary Reference Intakes include protein, vitamins, and mineral needs but do not address energy and health guidelines. (H)

189. **3.** The nurse needs to clarify reality in response to the client's grandiose delusions. The statement, "You are Sam Smith, a client here in the hospital, and I'm Marjorie, a nurse here on the unit," clarifies the client's identity and status and that of the nurse. The other statements do not help to clarify the identity of the client and nurse and do not address the reality of the situation, thereby correcting the client's grandiose delusions. The statement, "You know better; we are not going to be married," is blaming. (P)

190. **4.** When the client demonstrates a readiness to look at and learn about the colostomy, providing literature that shows the client how the colostomy looks and functions is a helpful teaching tool. Telling the client how others have adjusted to caring for their colostomy does not focus on the client's feelings as an individual. Handling colostomy appliances will be important before the client learns to care for the colostomy, but it is not essential to preparing the client to look at the stoma. Having a member of the local ostomy club visit can be beneficial, but it will probably be more effective after the client has looked at the colostomy and has some knowledge of how it functions. (P)

1. A primigravid client at 10 weeks' gestation tells the nurse that she eats fruits and vegetables but isn't fond of them. After teaching the client about possible serving sizes, the nurse determines that the teaching has been successful when the client states that one serving of fruit is equivalent to which of the following?

☐ **1.** One-fourth of a cantaloupe.
☐ **2.** 3 oz of vegetable juice cocktail.
☐ **3.** Three tomatoes.
☐ **4.** One raw apricot.

2. A nurse performs care on the client's Hickman catheter according to hospital policy. The client develops an infection and is considering litigation. The nurse's practice is:

☐ **1.** Malpractice.
☐ **2.** *Respondeat superior.*
☐ **3.** Negligent.
☐ **4.** Tort.

3. A Hispanic client is admitted to the surgical unit from the emergency department for an appendectomy. The nurse conducts the preoperative preparations and determines that the client has difficulty understanding English. The surgeon needs to obtain the client's informed consent. The best course for obtaining the client's informed consent is to:

☐ **1.** Have the client call a family member to act as interpreter.
☐ **2.** Have the client sign the Spanish surgical consent form.
☐ **3.** Call the Spanish interpreter to translate the surgeon's explanation of the procedure, risks, and alternatives to obtain the client's consent and to answer the client's questions.
☐ **4.** Notify the surgical charge nurse of the situation.

4. A client who has glaucoma has been prescribed timolol (Timoptic) eyedrops. Which of the following instructions should the nurse give the client about the administration of the eyedrops?

☐ **1.** Instill the eyedrops whenever the eyes feel irritated.
☐ **2.** The medication may cause some transient eye discomfort.
☐ **3.** Keep the medication refrigerated between doses.
☐ **4.** The need to use the eyedrops will be reevaluated after 1 month.

5. A 6-year-old child is admitted to the hospital for heart surgery to repair tetralogy of Fallot. The child asks the nurse if the cardiac catheterization will hurt. Which of the following statements offers the nurse the best guide for responding to the child's question?

☐ **1.** The medication used to numb the insertion site will sting.
☐ **2.** Momentary sharp pain usually occurs when the catheter enters the heart.
☐ **3.** It is usual for a 6-year-old to feel discomfort during the procedure.
☐ **4.** It is a painless procedure, although a tingling sensation may be felt in the extremities.

6. The nurse is assessing a 55-year-old client with chronic obstructive pulmonary disease. The client weighs 200 lb and is 6 feet tall. Using the diagram below, the nurse should record in the health history that the client's chest is:

☐ **1.** Barrel-shaped.
☐ **2.** Muscular.
☐ **3.** Normal for the client's age, height, and weight.
☐ **4.** Showing the effects of long-term use of bronchodilators.

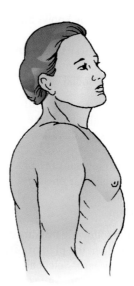

7. A diabetic primigravid client at 38 weeks' gestation asks the nurse why she had a fetal acoustic stimulation during her last nonstress test. Which of the following should the nurse include as the rationale for this test?
☐ 1. To listen to the fetal heart rate. ✓
☐ 2. To startle and awaken the fetus.
☐ 3. To stimulate mild contractions.
☐ 4. To confirm amniotic fluid amount.

8. The mother of an older infant reports stopping the prescribed iron supplements after 2 weeks of treatment. Which of the following responses by the nurse is most appropriate?
☐ 1. "Bring the child in so that we can retest him."
☐ 2. "You need to continue the iron for several more weeks."
☐ 3. "Let's start a diet that is high in iron."
☐ 4. "No more medication is needed at this time."

9. A Jewish client requests an orthodox diet while she is hospitalized. The nurse should refer this request to the:
☐ 1. Dietitian.
☐ 2. Physician.
☐ 3. Unit case manager.
☐ 4. Rabbi in pastoral care.

10. A mother reports to the nurse that she cannot afford the antibiotic azithromycin (Zithromax), which was ordered by the physician for her toddler's otitis media. The nurse's best response is to:
☐ 1. Instruct the mother on the importance of the medication.
☐ 2. Ask the mother if she knows anyone who could loan her the money.
☐ 3. Confer with the physician about whether a less expensive drug cold be ordered.   → advocate
☐ 4. Consult with the social worker.

11. The doctor has prescribed nitroglycerin to a client with angina. The client also has closed-angle glaucoma. The nurse contacts the physician to discuss the potential for:
☐ 1. Decreased intraocular pressure.
☐ 2. Increased intraocular pressure.
☐ 3. Hypotension.
☐ 4. Hypertension.

12. Which of the following nursing diagnoses is most appropriate to include in the plan of care for a client with peripheral vascular disease? Select all that apply.
☐ 1. *Imbalanced nutrition: More than body requirements* related to sedentary activity level.
☐ 2. *Acute pain* related to imbalance between oxygen demand and oxygen supply.
☐ 3. *Activity intolerance* related to pain.
☐ 4. *Deficient fluid volume* related to decreased fluid intake.
☐ 5. *Ineffective tissue perfusion (peripheral)* related to compromised circulation.

13. A client states she thinks she is experiencing premenstrual syndrome (PMS). The nurse instructs the client that common symptoms are:
☐ 1. Menstrual cycle irregularity with increased menstrual flow.
☐ 2. Mood swings immediately after menses.
☐ 3. Tension and fatigue before menses and through the second day of the menstrual cycle.
☐ 4. Midcycle spotting and abdominal pain at the time of ovulation.

14. For which of the following should the nurse closely assess a client who is reversing from halothane (Fluothane) general anesthesia and receiving clindamycin (Cleocin)?
☐ 1. Tachycardia.
☐ 2. Respiratory depression.
☐ 3. Hypotension.
☐ 4. Renal failure.

15. An adolescent with type 1 diabetes mellitus is hospitalized for appendicitis. He is weak and nauseated with poor skin turgor. The nurse notes a fruity odor to the client's breath. The client uses Lispro insulin. His last meal was lunch, 2 hours ago. Place the following nursing actions in the order in which the nurse should perform them.

Ketoacidosis.

| 1. Obtain a fingerstick test for blood glucose. |
| 2. Start an I.V. infusion with normal saline solution. |
| 3. Administer Lispro. |
| 4. Notify the physician. |

| 2 |
| 1 |
| 4 |
| 3 |

16. A nulliparous client visiting the clinic tells the nurse that she stopped taking oral contraceptives 6 months ago but doesn't think she is ovulating. Which of the following should the nurse anticipate that the physician would order if the client is anovulatory?
☐ 1. Dienestrol (Ortho Dienestrol).
☐ 2. Clomiphene citrate (Clomid).   – stimulates ovulation
☐ 3. Medroxyprogesterone (Depo-Provera).
☐ 4. Norgestrel (Ovrette).

17. A client who has been recently diagnosed with acquired immunodeficiency syndrome (AIDS) inquires about hospice services. The nurse explains that hospice care is appropriate:
- ☐ **1.** For clients with an inevitable death within weeks to months.
- ☐ **2.** For all clients with AIDS at any stage.
- ☐ **3.** Only for clients with cancer.
- ☐ **4.** When the client is ready to discuss his prognosis.

18. While assessing a neonate at age 24 hours, the nurse observes several irregularly shaped, red, flat patches on the back of the neonate's neck. The nurse interprets this finding as which of the following?
- ☐ **①** Stork bite.
- ☐ **2.** Port wine stain.
- ☐ **3.** Newborn rash.
- ☐ **4.** Café au lait spot.

19. A Mexican mother brings her 2-month-old son to the emergency department with a high fever and possible sepsis. A lumbar puncture is ordered, but the mother will not sign the consent until the father arrives to give permission. The nurse is aware that:
- ☐ **1.** This needs to be reported to the social worker.
- ☐ **2.** This needs to be reported to Child Protective Services.
- ☐ **③** The Mexican man is considered the family head and makes the major decisions.
- ☐ **4.** This behavior is unusual for Mexican cultural norms.

20. A client with Alzheimer's disease is started on a low dose of lorazepam (Ativan) because of agitation and a sleep disturbance. While monitoring the client for possible adverse effects, the nurse should expect to find which of the following as the most common?
- ☐ **1.** Confusion and nighttime agitation. *Akuthesia*
- ☐ **2.** Extrapyramidal side effects. → *cant move*
- ☐ **3.** Vomiting and profuse sweating.
- ☐ **④** Anticholinergic side effects.

21. A postmenopausal client with an intact uterus asks the nurse why her hormone medicine has two drugs, estrogen and progesterone. Which of the following statements by the nurse provides the client with accurate information?
- ☐ **1.** "The progesterone will help prevent cervical cancer." ✓
- ☐ **2.** "The progesterone will help prevent breast cancer."
- ☐ **3.** "The progesterone will help prevent liver disease."
- ☐ **④** "The progesterone will help prevent endometrial cancer."

22. The nurse should turn the client on bed rest every 2 hours to prevent the development of pressure ulcers. In addition, the nurse should:
- ☐ **1.** Have the client walk at least twice a day.
- ☐ **2.** Insert an indwelling urinary catheter.
- ☐ **③** Monitor serum albumin. → *nutrition needed for heal.*
- ☐ **4.** Monitor the white blood cell count.

23. A client has been hospitalized with heart failure. He is receiving digoxin (Lanoxin) and furosemide (Lasix) intravenously. He tells the nurse that he hears a continuous ringing in his ears and that he has never had this problem before. What is the appropriate action for the nurse to take at this time?
- ☐ **1.** Obtain a digoxin level to check for toxicity.
- ☐ **2.** Note the observation in the chart and plan to reassess in 2 hours.
- ☐ **③** Ask the client if he has been taking aspirin in addition to his other medications.
- ☐ **④** Discontinue the furosemide and notify the physician.

24. Which of the following instructions about thermal injury should be given to a client with peripheral vascular disease? Select all that apply.
- ☐ **1.** "Warm the fingers or toes by using an electric heating pad."
- ☑ **2.** "Avoid sunburn during the summer." ✓
- ☑ **3.** "Wear extra socks in the winter." ✓
- ☑ **4.** "Choose loose, soft, cotton socks." ✓
- ☐ **5.** "Use an electric blanket when you are sleeping." ✓

25. A client receives an I.V. dose of gentamicin sulfate (Garamycin). How long after the completion of the dose should the peak serum concentration level be measured?
- ☐ **1.** 10 minutes.
- ☐ **2.** 20 minutes.
- ☑ **3.** 30 minutes.
- ☐ **4.** 40 minutes.

26. A client with hydrocephalus complains of a headache in the morning on arising, but it disappears later in the day. The nurse is aware that intracranial pressure (ICP) is highest in the:
- ☐ **①** Early morning.
- ☐ **2.** Late afternoon.
- ☐ **3.** Evening.
- ☐ **4.** Middle of the night.

27. A primigravid client visits the clinic for a routine examination at 35 weeks' gestation. The client's blood pressure is near the baseline of 120/74 mm Hg with no proteinuria or evidence of facial edema. The client asks the nurse, "What should I take if I get an occasional headache after looking at my computer at work all day?" The nurse instructs the client that she can occasionally take which of the following?
☐ **1.** Acetaminophen (Tylenol).
☐ **2.** Aspirin.
☐ **3.** Ibuprofen (Advil).
☐ **4.** Naproxen (Aleve).

28. A 19-year-old client has undergone an examination and had evidence collected after being raped. Her father is overheard yelling at his daughter, "You're going to tell me who did this to you. What's his name?" Which of the following is the nurse's most immediate action?
☐ **1.** "Please come with me, sir. I need some important information."
☐ **2.** "Stop yelling. You're being inappropriate."
☐ **3.** "Please be quiet. You're not helping your daughter this way."
☐ **4.** "If you don't stop yelling, I'll have to call Security."

29. Which of the following groups is more likely to develop severe hypertension?
☐ **1.** Asian.
☐ **2.** African American.
☐ **3.** European.
☐ **4.** American Indian.

30. During a neonate's assessment shortly after birth, the nurse observes a large pad of fat at the back of the neck, widely set eyes, simian hand creases, and epicanthal folds. Which of the following actions is most appropriate?
☐ **1.** Notify the physician immediately.
☐ **2.** Ask the mother to consent to genetic studies.
☐ **3.** Explain these deviations to the newborn's mother.
☐ **4.** Document these findings as minor deviations.

31. A client with severe arthritis has been receiving maintenance therapy of prednisone (Deltasone) 10 mg/day for the past 6 weeks. The nurse should instruct the client to immediately report symptoms of:
☐ **1.** Respiratory infection.
☐ **2.** Joint pain.
☐ **3.** Constipation.
☐ **4.** Joint swelling.

32. A 90-year-old client discloses that he has two guns at home. The nurse asks him whether he has any grandchildren who come to visit or other school-age visitors because the most common risk factor for school-age children associated with injury or death from firearms is:
☐ **1.** An argument with a stranger.
☐ **2.** Firearm access.
☐ **3.** Substance use.
☐ **4.** Peer pressure.

33. A 7-year-old child is admitted to the hospital with the medical diagnosis of acute rheumatic fever. During the acute phase of the illness, it is least desirable to interest the child in which of the following diversional activities?
☐ **1.** Reading a book to the father.
☐ **2.** Playing with a doll with the nurse.
☐ **3.** Watching the television with a sibling.
☐ **4.** Playing checkers with a roommate.

34. A woman is taking oral contraceptives. The nurse teaches the client to report which of the following danger signs?
☐ **1.** Breakthrough bleeding.
☐ **2.** Severe calf pain.
☐ **3.** Mild headache.
☐ **4.** Weight gain of 3 lb.

35. Which of the following is most essential for the hospitalized client with a new tracheostomy?
☐ **1.** Decrease secretions.
☐ **2.** Provide client teaching regarding tracheostomy care.
☐ **3.** Relieve anxiety related to the tracheostomy.
☐ **4.** Maintain a patent airway.

36. Immediately after the client receives an injection of bupivacaine (Marcaine), he becomes restless and nervous and reports a feeling of impending doom. Which of the following actions by the nurse is appropriate at this time?
☐ **1.** Ask the client to talk more about what he is feeling.
☐ **2.** Reassure the client that it is normal to feel restless before a procedure.
☐ **3.** Assess the client's vital signs.
☐ **4.** Administer epinephrine.

37. A menopausal woman is taking hormone replacement therapy. The nurse teaches the client that a warning sign for endometrial cancer that needs to be reported is:
☐ **1.** Hot flashes.
☐ **2.** Irregular vaginal bleeding.
☐ **3.** Urinary urgency.
☐ **4.** Dyspareunia.

38. When teaching a group of students in health class about cystic fibrosis, which of the following should the school nurse use when explaining how this disorder is transmitted?
☐ **1.** Both parents have the recessive gene.
☐ **2.** The gene is carried on the X chromosome.
☐ **3.** The disease is restricted to males, implicating the Y chromosome.
☐ **4.** It usually happens by chance; neither parent has the gene.

39. The client complains of a severe vulvar pruritus and a yellow-green, malodorous vaginal discharge. The nurse recognizes that the symptoms suggest:
- ☐ **1.** Gonorrhea.
- ☐ **2.** Syphilis.
- ☐ **3.** Chlamydia.
- ☐ **4.** Trichomoniasis.

40. To evaluate the effectiveness of the client's use of an incentive spirometer, the nurse should understand that this device is used primarily to accomplish which of the following objectives?
- ☐ **1.** Stimulate circulation.
- ☐ **2.** Prepare the client for ambulation.
- ☐ **3.** Strengthen abdominal muscles.
- ☐ **4.** Increase respiratory effectiveness.

41. A client was talking with her husband by telephone, and then she began swearing at him. The nurse interrupts the call and offers to talk with the client. She says, "I can't talk about that bastard right now. I just need to destroy something." At this point, which of the following should the nurse do next?
- ☐ **1.** Tell her to write her feelings in her journal.
- ☐ **2.** Urge her to talk with the nurse now.
- ☐ **3.** Ask her to calm down or she will be restrained.
- ☐ **4.** Offer her a phone book to "destroy" while staying with her.

42. The nurse is caring for a multigravid client in active labor when the nurse detects variable fetal heart rate decelerations on the electronic monitor. The nurse interprets this as the compression of which of the following structures?
- ☐ **1.** Head.
- ☐ **2.** Chest.
- ☐ **3.** Umbilical cord.
- ☐ **4.** Placenta.

43. Which of the following assessment findings should lead the nurse to suspect that a client who had a cesarean delivery 8 hours earlier is developing disseminated intravascular coagulation (DIC)? Select all that apply.
- ☐ **1.** Petechiae on the arm where the blood pressure was taken.
- ☐ **2.** Heart rate of 126 bpm.
- ☐ **3.** Abdominal incision dressing with bright red drainage.
- ☐ **4.** Platelet count of 80,000/mm^3.
- ☐ **5.** Urine output of 350 ml in the past 8 hours.
- ☐ **6.** Temperature of 98.4° F (36.9° C).

44. Two days after placement of a pleural chest tube, the tube is accidentally pulled out of the chest wall. The nurse should first:
- ☐ **1.** Immerse the tube in sterile water.
- ☐ **2.** Apply an occlusive dressing such as petroleum jelly gauze.
- ☐ **3.** Instruct the client to cough to expand the lung.
- ☐ **4.** Auscultate the lung to determine whether it collapsed.

45. A client is admitted to the hospital with a diagnosis of a pulmonary embolism. Which of the following problems should the nurse address first?
- ☐ **1.** Nonproductive cough.
- ☐ **2.** Activity intolerance.
- ☐ **3.** Ineffective breathing pattern.
- ☐ **4.** Impaired gas exchange.

46. Which of the following is characteristic of cardiogenic shock?
- ☐ **1.** Hypovolemia.
- ☐ **2.** Increased cardiac output.
- ☐ **3.** Decreased myocardial contractility.
- ☐ **4.** Infarction.

47. The nurse is reviewing the laboratory results of a client with hypothyroidism. An expected finding is:
- ☐ **1.** Decreased thyroxine (T_4) and increased thyroid-stimulating hormone (TSH) levels.
- ☐ **2.** Decreased TSH and increased T_4 levels.
- ☐ **3.** Decreased creatine phosphokinase levels.
- ☐ **4.** Absence of antithyroid antibodies.

48. The mother of a 7-month-old child born 6 weeks early asks the nurse what play activities and toys is appropriate for her child. Which of the following should the nurse suggest?
- ☐ **1.** Picture books.
- ☐ **2.** Peek-a-boo.
- ☐ **3.** Rattle.
- ☐ **4.** Colored blocks.

49. Which of the following is the most accurate method of determining the extent of a client's fluid loss?
- ☐ **1.** Measuring intake and output.
- ☐ **2.** Assessing vital signs.
- ☐ **3.** Weighing the client.
- ☐ **4.** Assessing skin turgor.

50. The nurse is counseling a client regarding treatment of the client's newly diagnosed depression. The nurse emphasizes that full benefit from antidepressant therapy usually takes how long?
- ☐ **1.** 1 week.
- ☐ **2.** 2 to 4 weeks.
- ☐ **3.** 5 to 7 weeks.
- ☐ **4.** 8 weeks.

51. A 70-year-old, previously well client asks the nurse, "I notice I have tremors. Is this just normal for my age?" The best response for the nurse to make is which of the following?
- ☐ 1. "I wouldn't be worried because this is common with aging."
- ☐ 2. "You should report this to the physician because it may indicate a problem."
- ☐ 3. "You should drink orange juice when this occurs."
- ☐ 4. "You should have your blood pressure checked when this occurs."

52. A school-age child diagnosed with attention deficit hyperactivity disorder is prescribed methylphenidate (Ritalin). Assessment of which of the following should alert the school nurse to the possibility that the child is experiencing a common side effect of the drug?
- ☐ 1. Loss of appetite.
- ☐ 2. Vomiting.
- ☐ 3. Photosensitivity.
- ☐ 4. Weight gain.

53. A client complains of a dull headache and dizziness and has an increased pulse rate. The results of arterial blood gas analysis are as follows: pH, 7.26; partial pressure of carbon dioxide, 50 mm Hg; and bicarbonate, 24 mEq/L. These findings indicate which of the following acid-base imbalances?
- ☐ 1. Respiratory alkalosis.
- ☐ 2. Respiratory acidosis.
- ☐ 3. Metabolic acidosis.
- ☐ 4. Metabolic alkalosis.

54. Which of the following interventions is appropriate for a client with metabolic alkalosis?
- ☐ 1. Monitor serum potassium levels.
- ☐ 2. Maintain the client on bed rest.
- ☐ 3. Have the client inhale carbon dioxide using a paper bag.
- ☐ 4. Administer sodium bicarbonate as ordered.

55. Which of the following demonstrates that the client needs further instruction after being taught about ciprofloxacin (Cipro)?   *Drink w off*
- ☐ 1. "I must drink 1,000 to 1,500 ml of water a day."
- ☐ 2. "I shouldn't take an antacid before taking the Cipro."
- ☐ 3. "I should let the doctor know if I start vomiting from the Cipro."
- ☐ 4. "I may get light-headed from the Cipro."

56. When developing the plan of care for a client with Alzheimer's disease, which of the following activities is least beneficial to the client?
- ☐ 1. Reminiscence group.
- ☐ 2. Walking.
- ☐ 3. Pet therapy.
- ☐ 4. Stress management.

57. The nurse should instruct the parents of a school-age child with hemophilia to implement which of the following when the child develops bleeding into a joint? Select all that apply.
- ☐ 1. Having the child rest. ✓
- ☐ 2. Applying heat to the joint area.
- ☐ 3. Beginning factor VIII therapy. *w*
- ☐ 4. Starting physical therapy.
- ☐ 5. Applying a topical antifibrinolytic. *x*

58. Which of the following nursing diagnoses should the nurse implement as part of the long-term care for a child with hemophilia?
- ☐ 1. *Deficient knowledge.*
- ☐ 2. *Risk for injury.*
- ☐ 3. *Situational low self-esteem.*
- ☐ 4. *Acute pain.*

59. When preparing a 3-year-old child to have blood specimens drawn for laboratory testing, which of the following should the nurse do?
- ☐ 1. Explain the procedure in advance.
- ☐ 2. Explain why the blood needs to be drawn.
- ☐ 3. Use distraction techniques during the procedure.
- ☐ 4. Provide verbal explanations about what will occur.

60. The client has been prescribed lisinopril (Prinivil) to treat hypertension. Which of the following electrolyte imbalances may occur?
- ☐ 1. Hyponatremia.
- ☐ 2. Hypocalcemia.
- ☐ 3. Hyperkalemia.   *Ace takes out K + watch K*
- ☐ 4. Hypermagnesemia.

61. A client with a chronic mental illness who does not always take her medications is separated from her husband and receives Supplemental Security Income. She lives with her mother and older sister and manages her own medication. The client's mother is in poor health and receives Social Security benefits. The client's sister works outside the home, and the client's father is dead. Which of the following issues should the nurse need to address first?
- ☐ 1. Family.
- ☐ 2. Marital.
- ☐ 3. Financial.
- ☐ 4. Medication.

62. A client is receiving total parenteral nutrition (TPN). The nurse notices that the bag of TPN solution has been infusing for 24 hours but has 300 ml of solution left. What is the most appropriate action for the nurse to take?
- ☐ 1. Continue the infusion until the remaining 300 ml is infused.
- ☐ 2. Change the filter on the tubing and continue with the infusion.
- ☐ 3. Notify the physician and obtain orders to alter the flow rate of the solution.
- ☐ 4. Discontinue the current solution, change the tubing, and hang a new bag of TPN solution.

no longer than 24 hrs

63. A client with a history of cardiac problems complains of severe chest pain. What should be nurse's first response?
- ☐ **1.** Notify the physician.
- ☐ **2.** Administer an analgesic to control the pain.
- ☐ **3.** Assess the client's pain.
- ☐ **4.** Start oxygen at 2 L/minute via nasal cannula.

64. Which of the following characteristics should the nurse include in the teaching plan for a multiparous client after delivering a neonate diagnosed with trisomy 13?
- ☐ **1.** Webbed neck.
- ☐ **2.** Small testes.
- ☐ **3.** Congenital heart defects.
- ☐ **4.** Polydactyly.

65. A client is being treated for acute low back pain. Which of these clinical manifestations must be reported to the physician immediately?
- ☐ **1.** Diffuse, aching sensation in the L4 to L5 area.
- ☐ **2.** New onset of footdrop.
- ☐ **3.** Pain in the lower back when the leg is lifted.
- ☐ **4.** Pain in the lower back that radiates to the hip.

66. A client with type 1 diabetes mellitus asks the nurse whether he can take ginseng at home. The nurse's best response to the client is which of the following?
- ☐ **1.** "No, ginseng isn't good for people."
- ☐ **2.** "No, taking ginseng will increase the risk of hypoglycemia."
- ☐ **3.** "Yes, ginseng is good for you and will help your memory."
- ☐ **4.** "I'm not certain."

67. The nurse teaches the client with cirrhosis that the expected effect of lactulose (Cephulac) is:
- ☐ **1.** One regular bowel movement a day.
- ☐ **2.** Two to three soft stools per day.
- ☐ **3.** Four to five loose stools per day.
- ☐ **4.** Five to six loose stools per day.

68. The nurse is evaluating the laboratory results of a client who was recently admitted to the hospital. Which one of the following results indicates the presence of inflammation?
- ☐ **1.** Decreased sedimentation rate.
- ☐ **2.** Thrombocytopenia.
- ☐ **3.** Leukocytosis.
- ☐ **4.** Erythrocytosis.

69. The nurse is assessing teenaged girls at a well child clinic. The nurse should describe the girl shown below as having:
- ☐ **1.** Normal posture.
- ☐ **2.** Kyphosis.
- ☐ **3.** Scoliosis.
- ☐ **4.** Lordosis.

70. A client complains of pain in his casted left arm that is unrelieved by pain medication. The nurse assesses the arm and notes that the fingers are swollen and difficult to separate. Which action is most appropriate for the nurse to take at this time?
- ☐ **1.** Administer morphine 2 mg intravenously.
- ☐ **2.** Apply an ice bag to the fingers to relieve pain.
- ☐ **3.** Elevate the arm on two pillows and reassess in 30 minutes.
- ☐ **4.** Call the physician to report swelling and pain.

71. A primiparous client develops uterine atony and postpartum hemorrhage 1 hour after a vaginal delivery. The physician has ordered I.M. prostaglandin-F_{2a}. After administration of the medication, the nurse should observe the client for which of the following?
- ☐ **1.** Tachycardia.
- ☐ **2.** Hypotension.
- ☐ **3.** Constipation.
- ☐ **4.** Abdominal distention.

72. While caring for a mother and her 1-day-old neonate delivered vaginally at 30 weeks' gestation, the nurse explains about the neonate's need for gavage feeding at this time instead of the mother's plan for bottle feeding. Which of the following should the nurse include as the rationale for this?

☐ **1.** The neonate has difficulty coordinating sucking, swallowing, and breathing.

☐ **2.** A high-calorie formula, presently needed at this time, is more easily delivered via gavage.

☐ **3.** Gavage feedings can minimize the neonate's increased risk of developing hypoglycemia.

☐ **4.** This type of feeding, easily given in the Isolette, decreases the neonate's risk of cold stress.

73. The nurse is evaluating the client's ability to manage the fatigue associated with her rheumatoid arthritis. Which statement by the client indicates she understands how to manage her fatigue?

☐ **1.** "I sleep for 8 to 10 hours every night so that I'll have the energy to care for my children during the day."

☐ **2.** "I schedule afternoon rest periods for myself in addition to sleeping 10 hours every night."

☐ **3.** "I spend one weekend day a week resting in bed while my husband cares for the children."

☐ **4.** "I get up early in the morning and get all my household chores completed before my children wake up."

74. The school nurse is caring for a child with hemophilia who is actively bleeding from the leg. Which of the following should the nurse apply?

☐ **1.** Direct pressure, checking every few minutes to see if the bleeding has stopped.

☐ **2.** Ice to the injured leg area several times a day.

☐ **3.** Direct pressure to the injured area continuously for 10 minutes.

☐ **4.** Ice bag with elevation of the leg twice a day.

75. Which of the following is least likely a danger associated with pancytopenia?

☐ **1.** Anemia.

☐ **2.** Bleeding.

☐ **3.** Infection.

☐ **4.** Hypothyroidism.

76. A client suspected of being a victim of abuse returns to the emergency department and, sobbing, tells the nurse, "I guess you really know that my husband beats me and that's why I have bruises all over my body. I don't know what to do. I'm afraid he'll kill me one of these times." Which of the following responses best demonstrates that the nurse recognizes the client's needs at this time?

☐ **1.** "The fear that your husband will kill you is unfounded."

☐ **2.** "We can begin by discussing various options open to you."

☐ **3.** "You can legally leave your husband because he has no right to hurt you."

☐ **4.** "We can begin by listing ways to avoid making your husband angry with you."

77. A client has just returned from surgery for a gastrectomy. The nurse should position the client in which position?

☐ **1.** Prone.

☐ **2.** Supine.

☐ **3.** Low Fowler's.

☐ **4.** Right or left Sims'.

78. A child with heart disease starts on oral digoxin (Lanoxin). When preparing to administer the medication, which of the following should the nurse do first?

☐ **1.** Check the last serum electrolyte results for the child.

☐ **2.** Verify the dosage with a licensed practical nurse who is working that day.

☐ **3.** Ask the mother if she is willing to administer the medication.

☐ **4.** Teach the mother how to measure the child's heart rate.

79. The nurse is caring for a client who has suffered deep partial-thickness and full-thickness burns. During the emergent (resuscitative) phase of burn management, the nurse would anticipate a fluid shift from the:

☐ **1.** Intracellular to extracellular compartment.

☐ **2.** Extracellular to intravascular compartment.

☐ **3.** Interstitial to the intracellular compartment.

☐ **4.** Intravascular to the interstitial compartment.

80. The nurse is evaluating the effectiveness of fluid resuscitation during the emergency period of burn management. Which of the following indicates that adequate fluid replacement has been achieved in the client?

☐ **1.** An increase in body weight.

☐ **2.** Fluid intake less than urinary output.

☐ **3.** Urine output greater than 35 ml/hour.

☐ **4.** Blood pressure of 90/60 mm Hg.

81. A client who comes to the emergency department with multiple bruises on her face and arms, a black eye, and a broken nose says that these injuries occurred when she fell down the stairs. The nurse suspects that the client may have been physically assaulted. Which of the following should the nurse do next?

☐ 1. Ask the client specifically about the possibility of physical abuse.

☐ 2. Tell the client that it is difficult to believe that such injuries resulted from a fall.

☐ 3. Ask the client what she did to make someone beat her so badly.

☐ 4. Discuss with the client what she can do to deescalate the situation next time.

82. What is the primary outcome for the care of a client who is in shock?

☐ 1. Achieve adequate tissue perfusion.

☐ 2. Preserve renal function.

☐ 3. Prevent hypostatic pneumonia.

☐ 4. Maintain adequate vascular tone.

83. A 2-year-old child is brought into the physician's office by his parents who are concerned by his behavior. They describe how the child resists their affection, twirls around frequently, and refuses to respond to other children and adults. Based on the analysis of these behaviors, which of the following should the nurse suspect?

☐ 1. Tourette syndrome.

☐ 2. Schizophrenia.

☐ 3. Attention deficit hyperactivity disorder.

☐ 4. Autism.

84. The parent of a young child diagnosed with low-dose lead exposure asks about long-term effects. Which of the following should the nurse mention as possible long-term effects to this mother? Select all that apply.

☐ 1. Seizures.

☐ 2. Depression.

☐ 3. Hyperactivity.

☐ 4. Aggression.

☐ 5. Impulsiveness.

85. Which of the following is appropriate to include in an incident report?

☐ 1. An interpretation of the likely cause of the incident.

☐ 2. What the nurse saw and did.

☐ 3. The client's statement about the incident that occurred.

☐ 4. The extenuating circumstances involved in the situation.

86. To reduce urethral irritation, where should the nurse tape the female client's Foley catheter?

☐ 1. Inner thigh.

☐ 2. Groin area.

☐ 3. Lower abdomen.

☐ 4. Lower thigh.

87. The physician has determined that a primigravid client in active labor requires a cesarean delivery because of cephalopelvic disproportion. After the delivery of a male neonate, for which of the following should the nurse assess first?

☐ 1. Nasopharyngeal secretions.

☐ 2. High-pitched cry.

☐ 3. Skull fracture.

☐ 4. Decreased muscle tone.

88. The nurse understands that most accidental scalding of young children occur:

☐ 1. On the back of the body.

☐ 2. On the front of the body.

☐ 3. In a circular or glove pattern.

☐ 4. On the buttocks.

89. A 17-year-old client visits the clinic at 36 weeks' gestation. The client's blood pressure is 130/90 mm Hg. On previous visits, her blood pressure ranged from 100 to 110 mm Hg systolic, 70 to 80 mm Hg diastolic. Further assessment reveals slight edema of her hands and 1+ proteinuria. The nurse anticipates that the physician will most likely order which of the following?

☐ 1. I.V. magnesium sulfate.

☐ 2. Labetalol (Normodyne).

☐ 3. Bed rest with bathroom privileges.

☐ 4. Hourly blood pressure checks.

90. The nurse observes that an area in the mouth of a child with leukemia is bleeding. Which of the following items should the nurse use because it is most effective for promoting homeostasis over the lesion?

☐ 1. Karaya gum.

☐ 2. A cotton ball imbedded with petroleum jelly.

☐ 3. A nonsticking gauze sponge.

☐ 4. A dry tea bag.

91. Which of the following interventions is appropriate for the nurse to include in a plan for the prevention of pressure ulcers?

☐ 1. Daily skin cleaning with soap and hot water.

☐ 2. Gentle massage of bony prominences every shift.

☐ 3. Encouraging the client to sit up as much as possible.

☐ 4. Systematic skin assessment at least once per shift.

92. Which of the following acid-base imbalances should the nurse anticipate developing in the client with a nasogastric tube inserted?

☐ 1. Respiratory alkalosis.

☐ 2. Respiratory acidosis.

☐ 3. Metabolic alkalosis.

☐ 4. Metabolic acidosis.

93. A client at 36 weeks' gestation tells the nurse, "I've been having a lot of backaches lately." After giving instructions about how to decrease the backaches, the nurse determines that the client needs further instruction when she says which of the following?
- ☐ 1. "I should walk with my pelvis tilted backward."
- ☐ 2. "I may need to put a board under my mattress."
- ☐ 3. "I should squat and not bend to pick up objects."
- ☐ 4. "I should wear flat or low-heeled shoes."

94. Which of the following is usually the initial clinical manifestation of gonorrhea in men?
- ☐ 1. Impotence.
- ☐ 2. Scrotal pain.
- ☐ 3. Penile lesion.
- ☐ 4. Urethral discharge.

95. A client's blood pressure was elevated at 160/90 mm Hg when the physician ordered "clonidine (Catapres) 1 mg by mouth now." The nurse sent the order to pharmacy at 7:10 a.m., but the medication still has not arrived at 8 a.m. The most appropriate responses of the nurse include all but which of the following?
- ☐ 1. Check all appropriate places on the unit to which the drug could have been delivered.
- ☐ 2. Check the client's blood pressure.
- ☐ 3. Call the pharmacy.
- ☐ 4. Go to the pharmacy to obtain the drug.

96. The client with major depression states, "I'm too tired to get out of bed to go to group. I just want to rest." Which of the following is the nurse's best response?
- ☐ 1. "Perhaps you'll feel better later on."
- ☐ 2. "I'll let you rest for as long as you need."
- ☐ 3. "Attending group is an important part of your treatment plan."
- ☐ 4. "You've been in bed long enough and need to get up."

97. After teaching the mother of a 7-month-old diagnosed with bronchiolitis, the nurse determines that the teaching has been effective when the mother states which of the following as a sign to report immediately?
- ☐ 1. Seven wet diapers a day.
- ☐ 2. Temperature of 100° F (37.8° C) for 2 days.
- ☐ 3. Clear nasal discharge for longer than 2 days.
- ☐ 4. Longer periods of sleep than usual.

98. Which of the following clients would benefit from the application of warm moist heat?
- ☐ 1. A client with appendicitis.
- ☐ 2. A client with a recently sprained joint.
- ☐ 3. A client with a suspected malignancy.
- ☐ 4. A client with low back pain.

99. A 65-year-old client is newly diagnosed with pernicious anemia. The nurse emphasizes to the client the need to increase vitamin B_{12} intake by:
- ☐ 1. Increasing dietary intake of vitamin B_{12}.
- ☐ 2. Taking an oral vitamin B_{12} replacement.
- ☐ 3. Taking vitamin B_{12} injections or nasal spray replacement.
- ☐ 4. Chelation therapy.   *– removing metals.*

100. The nurse is caring for a client with an acute exacerbation of Crohn's disease. The nurse has received an order to add 20 mEq of potassium chloride to a 1,000-ml bottle of I.V. fluid. The nurse has a 30-ml, multiple-dose vial of potassium chloride. The label reads 2 mEq/ml. How many milliliters should the nurse add to the I.V. fluid?

_____ ml

101. A client with major depression and suicidal ideation is suddenly calmer and more energetic. Which of the following conclusions should the nurse reach?
- ☐ 1. The client is improving.
- ☐ 2. The client's medication dosage is too high.
- ☐ 3. The client is overstimulated.
- ☐ 4. The client is imminently suicidal.

102. A multigravid client at 38 weeks' gestation is scheduled to undergo a contraction stress test. Which of the following should the nurse include in the explanation as the purpose of this test?
- ☐ 1. Evaluation of fetal lung maturity.
- ☐ 2. Determination of the fetal biophysical profile.
- ☐ 3. Assessment of fetal ability to tolerate labor.
- ☐ 4. Determination of fetal response during movements.

103. The nurse is caring for a client who has been diagnosed with atypical pneumonia. When conducting a client assessment, which of the following symptoms should the nurse anticipate observing?
- ☐ 1. High fever.
- ☐ 2. Tachypnea.
- ☐ 3. Dry cough.
- ☐ 4. Severe chills.

104. The nurse is teaching a client with emphysema how to do pursed-lip breathing. What is the primary reason to use pursed-lip breathing?
- ☐ 1. To increase oxygenation.
- ☐ 2. To prolong exhalation.
- ☐ 3. To prevent respiratory infection.
- ☐ 4. To decrease shortness of breath.

105. The advantage of using automated medication dispensing equipment includes which of the following?
- ☐ 1. It facilitates the change-of-shift count of narcotics.
- ☐ 2. It keeps a record of narcotic usage.
- ☐ 3. It allows nurses unmonitored access to narcotics.
- ☐ 4. It cancels the charges for narcotics.

106. A 21-year-old male client is transported by ambulance to the emergency department after a serious automobile accident. He complains of severe pain in his right chest where he struck the steering wheel. He also has a compound fracture of his right tibia and fibula and multiple lacerations and contusions. The primary goal at this point is to:
- ☐ **1.** Reduce the client's anxiety.
- ☐ **2.** Maintain adequate oxygenation.
- ☐ **3.** Decrease chest pain.
- ☐ **4.** Maintain adequate circulating volume.

107. While assessing a primiparous client 8 hours after delivery, the nurse inspects the episiotomy site, finding it edematous and slightly reddened. Which of the following interpretations by the nurse is most appropriate?
- ☐ **1.** The client needs application of an ice pack.
- ☐ **2.** The episiotomy site is probably infected.
- ☐ **3.** A hematoma will likely develop.
- ☐ **4.** The client has had a repair of a vaginal laceration.

108. When administering an I.M. injection, the nurse uses the Z-track technique when the medication:
- ☐ **1.** Takes a long time to absorb.
- ☐ **2.** Takes effect very quickly.
- ☐ **3.** Is irritating to tissues.
- ☐ **4.** Is viscous in consistency.

109. A client with an Axis I diagnosis of bipolar disorder, mania, is monopolizing the use of the telephone by making several calls each day, interfering with the ability of other clients to use the telephone. Which of the following actions is most appropriate?
- ☐ **1.** Instructing the other clients to be patient.
- ☐ **2.** Limiting the amount of calls the client can make each day.
- ☐ **3.** Reminding the client that others need to use the telephone.
- ☐ **4.** Taking away the client's telephone privileges.

110. When preparing a 20-month-old with a foreign body in the nasal passage for removal of the foreign body by the health care provider, which of the following is most appropriate?
- ☐ **1.** Jacket restraint.
- ☐ **2.** Elbow restraint.
- ☐ **3.** Use of father to hold.
- ☐ **4.** Papoose board.

111. The nurse auscultates the lungs of a client who has been diagnosed with lung cancer and notes wheezing over one lung. The nurse understands that the most likely cause of this clinical finding is:
- ☐ **1.** The presence of exudate in the airways.
- ☐ **2.** The result of the client's history of smoking.
- ☐ **3.** An indication of pleural effusion.
- ☐ **4.** Obstruction of the airway by a tumor.

112. The nurse is teaching a client who is taking insulin about the signs of diabetic ketoacidosis, which include:
- ☐ **1.** Kussmaul's respirations.
- ☐ **2.** Excessive hunger.
- ☐ **3.** Dry, flaky skin.
- ☐ **4.** High blood pressure.

113. A nurse at the outpatient clinic receives a lithium level report of l.0 mEq/L for a client who has been taking lithium for 2 months. The nurse should interpret this level to indicate which of the following?
- ☐ **1.** An error in reporting.
- ☐ **2.** Too low to be therapeutic.
- ☐ **3.** Too high, indicating toxicity.
- ☐ **4.** Within the therapeutic range.

114. A 16-year-old Hispanic client at 10 weeks' gestation has been diagnosed with mild iron deficiency anemia. The client tells the nurse that she doesn't like to eat much meat. Which of the following foods should the nurse suggest to provide the client with the greatest amount of iron in her diet?
- ☐ **1.** 1 cup of lentils.
- ☐ **2.** 1 cup of sunflower seeds.
- ☐ **3.** 1½ oz of hard cheese.
- ☐ **4.** 2 poached eggs.

115. A client has been receiving radiation therapy for 3 weeks to treat his cancer. He is complaining of fatigue. Which of the following should be considered while the nurse plans interventions to help the client cope with the fatigue?
- ☐ **1.** Fatigue is a temporary problem that requires no active intervention.
- ☐ **2.** The client should be closely examined to determine the cause of fatigue.
- ☐ **3.** Fatigue indicates that the client's cancer is not under control.
- ☐ **4.** The client should be encouraged to maintain activity to combat the fatigue.

116. Which of the following nutrients provides the base for the Food Guide Pyramid?
- ☐ **1.** Fat.
- ☐ **2.** Protein.
- ☐ **3.** Carbohydrate.
- ☐ **4.** Table sugar.

117. When educating unlicensed assistants on how to prevent the development of pressure ulcers, the nurse should emphasize that most tissue injuries related to shearing can be prevented by implementing which of the following activities?
- ☐ **1.** Close adherence to a turning schedule.
- ☐ **2.** Keeping the skin clean and dry.
- ☐ **3.** Proper positioning and moving of the client.
- ☐ **4.** Use of skin lubricants.

118. When using crutches, the client should be instructed to bear weight primarily on the:
- [ ] 1. Axillae.
- [ ] 2. Elbows.
- [ ] 3. Upper arms.
- [ ] (4.) Hands.

119. Which of the following nursing diagnoses is a priority for the family whose child is dying of leukemia?
- [ ] 1. *Disabled family coping.*
- [ ] 2. *Impaired parenting.*
- [ ] 3. *Fear.*
- [ ] 4. *Grieving.*

120. Which of the following should the nurse do first for a toddler just admitted with croup?
- [ ] 1. Monitor vital signs.
- [ ] (2.) Assess respiratory status.
- [ ] 3. Ensure adequate fluid intake.
- [ ] 4. Place a tracheostomy set at the bedside.

121. Before the nurse administers I.V. replacement of 5% dextrose in water with potassium chloride, what nursing intervention must be completed first?
- [ ] 1. Adding potassium chloride to the bag at the bedside.
- [ ] 2. Evaluating laboratory results for electrolytes.
- [ ] 3. Priming tubing using sterile technique.
- [ ] 4. Checking the rate for I.V. push administration.

122. Homocysteine may be cleared from the blood with the help of which of the following vitamins?
- [ ] 1. Vitamin C.
- [ ] 2. Vitamin E.
- [ ] 3. Vitamin K.
- [ ] (4.) Vitamin B_6.

123. Which of the following signs and symptoms is an early indication that a client has developed hypocalcemia?
- [ ] (1.) Tingling in the fingers. → tingling.
- [ ] 2. Depressed reflexes.
- [ ] 3. Ventricular dysrhythmias.
- [ ] 4. Memory changes.

124. The nurse is auscultating the lung sounds of a client with long-standing emphysema. Which of the following abnormal lung sounds should the nurse anticipate hearing?
- [ ] 1. Fine crackles.
- [ ] (2.) Diminished breath sounds. → over inflated
- [ ] 3. Stridor.
- [ ] 4. Pleural friction rub.

125. A client with a paranoid personality disorder sees some clients laughing during a group activity and asks the nurse, "Why are they laughing at me? I bet they're making fun of me." Which of the following responses by the nurse is most appropriate?
- [ ] 1. "You shouldn't let yourself get so upset."
- [ ] 2. "Don't worry about them. They don't mean any harm."
- [ ] 3. "Look. They seem to be having fun."
- [ ] 4. "They're laughing at a joke John told. They aren't laughing at you." *older than 1 yr*

126. Mebendazole (Vermox) is prescribed for an 8-year-old child with pinworms. The child has an 18-month-old brother and a 4-year-old sister. The nurse should expect to treat which of the following family members with this drug?
- [ ] 1. Both of the child's siblings.
- [ ] 2. The child's parents and brother.
- [ ] 3. Everyone who lives in the household.
- [ ] (4.) The parents and sister.

127. When planning a presentation on the topic of osteoporosis to a group of middle-aged women, which of the following should the nurse expect to include?
- [ ] 1. An early symptom of osteoporosis is the dowager's hump.
- [ ] 2. African American and Latina women are at greater risk.
- [ ] 3. Loss of height is an early symptom of the disease.
- [ ] 4. Conventional radiographs are usually used to confirm the disease.

128. Which of the following statements best explains why the nurse should evaluate gastric residual before administering the client's next enteral feeding?
- [ ] 1. To determine how well nutrients are being absorbed.
- [ ] 2. To determine if the client is receiving enough feeding.
- [ ] (3.) To prevent overdistention of the stomach.
- [ ] 4. To prevent mixing undigested formula with partially digested formula.

129. Which of the following serologic tests should the nurse have on the chart before a client is started on tissue plasminogen activator or alteplase recombinant (Activase)?
- [ ] (1.) Partial thromboplastin time.
- [ ] 2. Potassium level.
- [ ] 3. Lee-White clotting time.
- [ ] 4. Fibrin split product.

130. When planning the care for a client diagnosed with hepatitis A, which of the following nursing interventions should the nurse expect to include? Select all that apply.
- [ ] 1. Implementing an exercise program.
- [ ] 2. Providing relief from nausea and vomiting. ✓
- [ ] 3. Administering pain medication. ✓
- [ ] 4. Encouraging multiple small meals daily. ✓
- [ ] 5. Planning frequent rest periods. ✓

131. An older adult man has been referred by his physician to participate in the cardiac rehabilitation program. The client is a diabetic and has complaints of bilateral leg discomfort with walking. The nurse should use a stationary bicycle and intermittent training because of the client's:
- [ ] 1. Diabetic neuropathy.
- [ ] 2. Muscle atrophy.
- [ ] 3. Raynaud's disease.
- [ ] 4. Transient ischemic attacks.

132. The client with borderline personality disorder spends much time around the nurse's station, making numerous minor requests. The nurse interprets these behaviors as indicating which of the following?
- [ ] 1. Fears of abandonment and attention seeking.
- [ ] 2. Enjoyment of bothering the staff.
- [ ] 3. Boredom suggesting the need for something to do.
- [ ] 4. Lack of desire for involvement in milieu activities.

133. A client has soft wrist restraints to prevent her from pulling out her nasogastric tube. Which of the following nursing interventions should be implemented while the restraints are on the client?
- [ ] 1. Instruct the client not to move while the restraints are in place.
- [ ] 2. Remove the restraints every 4 hours to provide skin care.
- [ ] 3. Secure the restraints to side rails of the bed.
- [ ] 4. Check on the client every 30 minutes while the restraints are on.

134. A client with alcohol dependence states, "I feel so bad because of what I've done to my wife and kids. I'm just no good." Which of the following responses by the nurse is most appropriate?
- [ ] 1. "You'll need to make up for a lot of things."
- [ ] 2. "They will need to forgive your shortcomings."
- [ ] 3. "Alcohol dependence is a disease that can be treated."
- [ ] 4. "Alcoholism is painful for everyone involved."

135. After teaching the parents of a toddler about appropriate snack foods for their child, the nurse judges that the instructions about not giving the child raisins for snacks are effective when the father states which of following?
- [ ] 1. "Raisins are low in nutritional value."
- [ ] 2. "Raisins can increase tooth decay."
- [ ] 3. "Raisins are easy to choke on."
- [ ] 4. "Raisins are hard to digest entirely."

136. A client has been diagnosed with atrial fibrillation. The physician ordered warfarin (Coumadin) to be taken on a daily basis. The nurse instructs the client to avoid using which of the following over-the-counter medications while taking warfarin?
- [ ] 1. Aspirin.
- [ ] 2. Diphenhydramine (Benadryl).
- [ ] 3. Digoxin (Lanoxin).
- [ ] 4. Pseudoephedrine (Sudafed).

137. The nurse should inform a client taking carba- — *seizure* mazepine (Tegretol) that it can affect other medications in which of the following ways?
- [ ] 1. It decreases the effects of oral anticoagulants.
- [ ] 2. It decreases the serum concentration of verapamil (Calan).
- [ ] 3. It increases the serum concentration of other anticonvulsants.
- [ ] 4. It increases the effects of oral contraceptives.

138. A client has been diagnosed with viral hepatitis. Which of the following expected outcomes is most appropriate for the client?
- [ ] 1. Achieve control of abdominal pains.
- [ ] 2. Increase activity levels gradually.
- [ ] 3. Be able to breathe without difficulty.
- [ ] 4. Experience relief from edema.

139. Which of the following activities by the mother offers the most support to the child during the first few days after surgery to repair a cleft lip?
- [ ] 1. Holding and cuddling the child.
- [ ] 2. Helping the child play with some toys.
- [ ] 3. Reading some of the child's favorite stories.
- [ ] 4. Staying at the bedside and holding the child's hand.

140. Which of the following is the public health nurse's best strategy to reduce the number of children involved in automobile accidents who were not wearing seat belts?
- [ ] 1. Contact the local state representative to discuss new legislation about child seat belts.
- [ ] 2. Attend a school board meeting to advocate for classes teaching children seat belt safety.
- [ ] 3. Call the town mayor's office with this information so that the mayor can discuss it with the media.
- [ ] 4. Start a letter-writing campaign to the school superintendent about seat belt importance.

141. A basic principle of any rehabilitation program, including a cardiac rehabilitation program, is that rehabilitation begins:
- ☐ 1. On discharge from the hospital.
- ☐ 2. On discharge from the cardiac care unit.
- ☐ 3. On admission to the hospital.
- ☐ 4. 4 weeks after the onset of illness.

142. A child is admitted to the emergency department with dyspnea related to bronchospasms. The nurse should place the client in which of the following positions?
- ☐ 1. High Fowler's.
- ☐ 2. Side-lying.
- ☐ 3. Prone.
- ☐ 4. Supine.

143. The nurse is preparing to administer I.M. morphine sulfate to a client who is in pain. On checking the physician's order, the nurse notes that the order states, "morphine sulfate 60 mg I.M. every 4 hours as needed for pain." The nurse understands that a usual dose of morphine is 10 to 15 mg. What is the most appropriate action for the nurse to take?
- ☐ 1. Administer the medication as ordered.
- ☐ 2. Reduce the ordered dosage to 20 mg and give that.
- ☐ 3. Contact the physician to verify the order.
- ☐ 4. Ask another nurse to review the order.

144. The nurse is preparing a client for paracentesis. Which of the following activities should the nurse complete in preparation for this test?
- ☐ 1. Have the client void before the procedure. *perform*
- ☐ 2. Prepare the client's abdomen with Betadine solution.
- ☐ 3. Position the client supine.
- ☐ 4. Put the client on nothing-by-mouth (NPO) status 4 hours before the procedure.

145. A nurse working in a community health center suspects that a 20-month-old is being abused. Which of the following behaviors should lead the nurse to suspect this?
- ☐ 1. Absence of crying during the examination.
- ☐ 2. Clinging to the parent during the examination.
- ☐ 3. Playing with toys on the examination room floor.
- ☐ 4. Talking easily with the nurse.

146. Which of the following should the nurse plan to include when teaching the client and family about a substance abuse problem?
- ☐ 1. The role of the family in perpetuating the problem.
- ☐ 2. The family's responsibility for the client.
- ☐ 3. The physical, physiologic, and psychological effects of substances.
- ☐ 4. The reasons that could have led the client to use the substance.

147. A client who has had a laparoscopic cholecystectomy receives discharge instructions from the nurse. Which statement indicates that the client has understood the instructions?
- ☐ 1. "I need to maintain a low-fat diet for the next 6 months."
- ☐ 2. "I can remove the dressing from my incision tomorrow and take a shower."
- ☐ 3. "I can anticipate some nausea for several days after surgery."
- ☐ 4. "I can return to work in 4 to 6 weeks."

148. The nurse should recognize that Mexican American culture most highly values:
- ☐ 1. Children.
- ☐ 2. Materialism.
- ☐ 3. Firstborn sons.
- ☐ 4. The elderly.

149. A client comes into the emergency department complaining of extreme fatigue. He is malnourished, and laboratory tests reveal that he is severely anemic. Based on an understanding of how vitamin and mineral deficiencies are associated with anemia, the nurse asks the client about his intake of food high in which of the following nutrients?
- ☐ 1. Vitamins A, E, and C.
- ☐ 2. Vitamins B_6 and B_{12}, folate, iron, and copper.
- ☐ 3. Thiamin, riboflavin, and niacin.
- ☐ 4. Vitamins A and B.

150. The nurse is assessing a neonate born to a diabetic mother. Which of the following findings should the nurse expect to see in the infant?
- ☐ 1. Hypertonia.
- ☐ 2. Hyperactivity.
- ☐ 3. Large size.
- ☐ 4. Scaly skin.

151. A client who had transurethral resection of the prostate complains of dribbling urine after his Foley catheter is removed on the second postoperative day. The nurse notes that the client had 200 ml of urine output in the last 8 hours with a 1,000 ml intake. Which of the following interventions is a priority for the nurse at this time?
- ☐ 1. Apply a condom catheter.
- ☐ 2. Assess for bladder distention.
- ☐ 3. Obtain a urine specimen for culture.
- ☐ 4. Teach the client Kegel exercises.

152. A client has atrial fibrillation. The nurse should monitor the client for:
- ☐ 1. Cardiac arrest.
- ☐ 2. Cerebrovascular accident. *Clots*
- ☐ 3. Heart block.
- ☐ 4. Ventricular fibrillation.

153. A child diagnosed with tinea is being treated with griseofulvin (Grifulvin V). Which of the following instructions should the nurse give to the parents?
- ☐ **1.** Give the medication before a meal.
- ☐ **2.** Have the child avoid intense sunlight.
- ☐ **3.** Give the medication for 10 days.
- ☐ **4.** Encourage increased fluid intake.

154. The nurse is teaching a client who had a myocardial infarction about her diet. What percentage of calories should come from fat?
- ☐ **1.** 10%.
- ☐ **2.** 20%.
- ☐ **3.** 30%.
- ☐ **4.** 40%.

155. After going through the necessary procedures for collecting physical evidence after a rape, a client is crying and talking about what happened to her. Which of the following actions is most appropriate?
- ☐ **1.** Advising the client to try to forget about what happened.
- ☐ **2.** Recommending that the client be thankful for the fact that she's alive.
- ☐ **3.** Questioning the client about what she could have done to deter the attack.
- ☐ **4.** Listening to the client's descriptions about what occurred.

156. A client undergoes cystoscopy with bladder biopsy. After the procedure, which assessment is most appropriate for the nurse to make?
- ☐ **1.** Assess the patency of the Foley catheter.
- ☐ **2.** Assess urine for excessive bleeding.
- ☐ **3.** Percuss the bladder for distention.
- ☐ **4.** Obtain a urine specimen for culture.

157. When a client of Mexican American descent tells the nurse that she treated her infection by drinking milk, the nurse interprets the client's remark as:
- ☐ **1.** Confusion from fever.
- ☐ **2.** Use of the hot disease concept.
- ☐ **3.** Use of milk as a laxative.
- ☐ **4.** The need for a dietitian to assist her with meal planning.

158. A female client with paranoid schizophrenia has been hearing negative voices and "getting special messages from various sources." Which of the following interventions is most appropriate for the client's symptoms?
- ☐ **1.** Asking her to make simple decisions.
- ☐ **2.** Being matter-of-fact with her.
- ☐ **3.** Monitoring her reactions to television programs.
- ☐ **4.** Reinforcing appropriate dress and hygiene.

159. A 20-year-old client who reports vaginal itching and a thick, white, cheese-like vaginal discharge beginning 2 days ago tells the nurse that she has been taking oral contraceptives for 2 months. The nurse determines that the client is most likely exhibiting signs of which of the following?
- ☐ **1.** *Trichomonas vaginalis.*
- ☐ **2.** Candidiasis.
- ☐ **3.** *Herpes genitalis.*
- ☐ **4.** Gonorrhea.

160. The nurse is talking with an outpatient client who was diagnosed with bulimia 3 months ago. The nurse decides that the client needs more education about the illness if she makes which of the following comments? Select all that apply.
- ☐ **1.** "I know that this illness is chronic and intermittent. I'll always have to control it."
- ☐ **2.** "If I start severely restricting my eating, I may be building up to a bingeing episode."
- ☐ **3.** "When I'm not bingeing and purging, I can skip that Eating Disorder support group."
- ☐ **4.** "I've made a real effort to be more social and involved in activities."
- ☐ **5.** "My depression is gone so I don't need my antidepressant any longer."

161. The nurse judges that the parents of a newborn with imperforate anus know what a low defect is when they say that the rectum:
- ☐ **1.** Is below the abdominal rectus muscle.
- ☐ **2.** Is above the abdominal rectus muscle.
- ☐ **3.** Has descended through the puborectalis muscle.
- ☐ **4.** Has ascended through the puborectalis muscle.

162. A 75-year-old man is receiving meperidine (Demerol) after surgery. For which of the following side effects of meperidine should the nurse carefully evaluate the client?
- ☐ **1.** Respiratory depression.
- ☐ **2.** Dysrhythmias.
- ☐ **3.** Constipation.
- ☐ **4.** Seizures.

163. A client with iron deficiency anemia is taking iron supplements. The nurse emphasizes to the client that the drug will have increased absorption if taken with:
- ☐ **1.** Milk.
- ☐ **2.** Orange juice.
- ☐ **3.** Food.
- ☐ **4.** Beta-carotene.

164. When obtaining the nursing history of a client who has diabetes mellitus, the nurse should identify which of the following as a potential early symptom of renal insufficiency?

- ☐ **1.** Polyuria.
- ☐ **2.** Dysuria.
- ☐ **3.** Hematuria.
- ☐ **4.** Oliguria. → later.

165. A client is planning to be treated for infertility with the zygote intrafallopian transfer (ZIFT) method. Which of the following should the nurse include when teaching the client about this type of treatment method?

- ☐ **1.** Fertilization takes place outside of the body.
- ☐ **2.** ZIFT is helpful for clients with bilateral blocked fallopian tubes.
- ☐ **3.** Ova and sperm are needed for instillation into the fallopian tube.
- ☐ **4.** Fertilized ova are instilled into the vagina to enter the uterus.

166. When assessing for oxygenation in a client with dark skin, the nurse should examine the client's:

- ☐ **1.** Skin.
- ☐ **2.** Buccal mucosa.
- ☐ **3.** Nape of the neck.
- ☐ **4.** Forehead.

167. Which of the following rehabilitative measures should the nurse teach the client to perform after chest surgery to prevent shoulder ankylosis?

- ☐ **1.** Turn from side to side.
- ☐ **2.** Raise and lower the head.
- ☐ **3.** Raise the arm on the affected side over the head.
- ☐ **4.** Flex and extend the elbow on the affected side.

168. A client with a tracheostomy tube coughs and dislodges the tracheostomy tube. The nurse's first action should be to:

- ☐ **1.** Call for emergency assistance.
- ☐ **2.** Attempt reinsertion of tracheostomy tube.
- ☐ **3.** Position the client in semi-Fowler's position with the neck hyperextended.
- ☐ **4.** Insert the obturator into the stoma to reestablish the airway.

169. An infant is to return to the clinic for a regular check-up and receive immunizations. In preparation for this next visit, which of the following should the nurse suggest to the parents?

- ☐ **1.** "Be prepared for the infant to be very fussy."
- ☐ **2.** "Give the infant acetaminophen (Tylenol) before coming."
- ☐ **3.** "Plan to keep the infant out of day care for that day."
- ☐ **4.** "Bring someone else to the appointment to support you."

170. A first-time mother is concerned that her 6-month-old infant is not gaining enough weight. The best response for the nurse to make is which of the following?

- ☐ **1.** "Birth weight doubles by 6 months of age."
- ☐ **2.** "Birth weight doubles by 3 months of age."
- ☐ **3.** "The baby will eat what he needs."
- ☐ **4.** "You need to make sure the baby finishes each bottle."

171. In accurately assessing a client who reports a back injury, it is critical for the nurse to question the client concerning which of the following?

- ☐ **1.** Family history of back problems.
- ☐ **2.** Previous hospitalizations.
- ☐ **3.** Personal history of illness.
- ☐ **4.** Mechanism of injury.

172. The nurse realizes that an antihypertensive medication functions to:

- ☐ **1.** Lower the individual's blood pressure.
- ☐ **2.** Alter cardiac output.
- ☐ **3.** Alter cardiac output or peripheral vascular resistance.
- ☐ **4.** Alter peripheral vascular resistance.

173. The nurse is examining a client with possible early rheumatoid arthritis. Which of the following symptoms should the nurse observe?

- ☐ **1.** Nausea.
- ☐ **2.** Joint swelling.
- ☐ **3.** Fatigue. early
- ☐ **4.** Limitation of movement.

174. The nurse instructs the client in mixing and administering regular and NPH insulin. Which of the following statements indicates that the client needs additional instruction?

- ☐ **1.** "I draw up the regular insulin first."
- ☐ **2.** "I shake the bottle of NPH insulin before drawing it up."
- ☐ **3.** "I store the insulin in a cool place."
- ☐ **4.** "I insert the needle at a 90-degree angle."

175. The mother of a child with newly diagnosed Duchenne's muscular dystrophy asks how her child developed the disease. The nurse formulates a response incorporating which of the following statements about its transmission?

- ☐ **1.** It is an autosomal recessive genetic disorder.
- ☐ **2.** It is a genetic disorder carried by males and transmitted to male children.
- ☐ **3.** It is a disorder primarily transmitted by males in the family.
- ☐ **4.** It is a disorder usually carried by females and transmitted to male children.

176. Which of the following should the nurse identify as a priority nursing diagnosis for an infant with intussusception?
☐ **1.** *Deficient fluid volume.*
☐ **2.** *Diarrhea.*
☐ **3.** *Impaired skin integrity.*
☐ **4.** *Acute pain.* colick ab pain

177. The physician orders I.V. cefazolin (Kefzol) 1 g for a client. In preparing to administer the Kefzol, the nurse notes that the client is allergic to penicillin. Based on this information, what is an appropriate action for the nurse to take?
☐ **1.** Continue to prepare to administer the Kefzol as ordered.
☐ **2.** Notify the physician of the client's allergy to penicillin.
☐ **3.** Administer the Kefzol, staying at the client's bedside during the infusion.
☐ **4.** Call the pharmacist to verify that the Kefzol should be administered as ordered.

178. A client is prescribed buspirone (BuSpar) 5 mg two times a day. Which of the following statements indicates that the client has understood the nurse's teaching about this drug? Select all that apply.
☐ **1.** "This medicine will make me sleepy."
☐ **2.** "BuSpar will relax my muscles."
☐ **3.** "My anxiety will be completely gone by tomorrow."
☐ **4.** "BuSpar will help me not to worry so much."
☐ **5.** "I'll be able to focus better."

179. When a client has a tearing of tissue with irregular wound edges, the nurse should document this as a:
☐ **1.** Contusion.
☐ **2.** Abrasion.
☐ **3.** Laceration.
☐ **4.** Colonization.

180. A client with schizophrenia is responding well to risperidone (Risperdal) and is no longer psychotic. After teaching the client about managing his illness, which of the following statements reflects a need for further education?
☐ **1.** "I just don't know if I can afford to keep taking medicines every day."
☐ **2.** "When my thoughts start racing, I know I need to relax more."
☐ **3.** "I can name the side effects of Risperdal, but I'm not having any."
☐ **4.** "I don't listen to my mom's religious beliefs about not using medicines."

181. A 3-year-old has been admitted with diarrhea. He has mild dehydration (less than 5%). The nurse is reviewing the laboratory report of the stool specimen, as indicated in the chart below.

LABORATORY RESULTS	
Test	**Result**
WBC	Mildly elevated
RBC	Few
Bacteria	Positive for *Escherichia coli*
Ova and parasites	Negative

Based on the laboratory report, what should the nurse do first?
☐ **1.** Start an I.V. infusion.
☐ **2.** Institute enteric precautions.
☐ **3.** Instruct the family to wash all family bed linens in hot water.
☐ **4.** Clean and protect the anal area.

182. Which of the following symptoms should the nurse expect to find as an early symptom of chronic heart failure?
☐ **1.** Fatigue. early = Ahzve.
☐ **2.** Pedal edema.
☐ **3.** Nocturia.
☐ **4.** Irregular pulse.

183. The nurse instructs the client with gastroesophageal reflux disease (GERD) regarding dietary measures. The recommended dietary changes for the client with GERD include:
☐ **1.** Eliminating spicy foods.
☐ **2.** Avoiding chocolate and coffee.
☐ **3.** Eliminating cucumbers and other foods with seeds.
☐ **4.** Avoiding steamed foods.

184. Signs and symptoms of which of the following is a priority when caring for a newly delivered term neonate diagnosed as small for gestational age?
☐ **1.** Iron deficiency anemia.
☐ **2.** Birth asphyxia. ABC S
☐ **3.** Persistent pulmonary hypertension.
☐ **4.** Hyperglycemia.

185. At what rate (in drops per minute) should a nurse start an I.V. infusion if the order is for 1 g of vancomycin (Vancocin) to be given in 180 ml of dextrose 5% in water over 60 minutes? The tubing delivers 15 drops/ml.

_____ drops/minute

186. A mother of a child with food allergies expresses concern that her child's 2-month-old sibling may also have food allergies. When discussing feeding techniques for the infant, the nurse should suggest that the mother:

☐ **1.** Give only rice cereal to the child.
☐ **2.** Use only apple juice as a supplementary fluid.
☐ **3.** Introduce new foods to the infant one at a time.
☐ **4.** Discontinue formula feedings when the infant begins to eat baby food.

187. The nurse enters a client's room and finds the client crying. Which of the following is the nurse's most appropriate response?

☐ **1.** "It's okay to cry."
☐ **2.** "Is there someone I can call for you?"
☐ **3.** "Tell me what you are feeling."
☐ **4.** "Do you want to talk about it?"

188. A 23-year-old client is experiencing premenstrual syndrome (PMS) symptoms. Which of the following dietary choices is appropriate for relieving PMS symptoms?

☐ **1.** Decreasing sodium and increasing calcium.
☐ **2.** Limiting fat to 9 g/day.
☐ **3.** Increasing vitamins A and C.
☐ **4.** Increasing proteins and decreasing carbohydrates.

189. A client with a fractured tibia has a long leg plaster cast. The cast is still damp, and the client complains that it feels hot to him. What should be the nurse's response?

☐ **1.** Notify the physician because this is an indication that the cast is applying pressure to soft tissue.
☐ **2.** Explain to the client that this feeling is a normal part of the drying process for plaster casts.
☐ **3.** Elevate the casted leg on two pillows.
☐ **4.** Administer prescribed pain medication to decrease discomfort.

190. A 28-year-old woman is learning about breast self-examination. The nurse teaches the woman that the best time of each month to examine her breasts is during the:

☐ **1.** Week before menstruation occurs.
☐ **2.** Week that menstruation occurs.
☐ **3.** First week after menstruation.
☐ **4.** Week that ovulation occurs.

fibrocysis - week befor menstruu

Correct Answers and Rationales

The letter in parentheses after each rationale identifies the client need addressed in the item, including management of care (M), safety and infection control (S), health promotion and maintenance (H), psychosocial adaptation (P), basic care and comfort (C), pharmacological and parenteral therapies (D), reduction of risk potential (R), and physiological adaptation (A).

1. 1. One serving of fruit is equivalent to one-fourth of a cantaloupe. The client needs 6 oz of a vegetable juice cocktail, two tomatoes, or two raw apricots to meet one fruit serving. (C)

2. 2. *Respondeat superior* is Latin for "The master is responsible for the acts of his servants." The nurse, as an employee of the hospital, acted according to the established policy of the hospital. Because the nurse followed hospital policy, it is unlikely that this incident involved malpractice, negligence, or tort law. (M)

3. 3. The surgeon is required to give the client explanations and have questions answered. The nurse has no way of assessing the client's understanding without the interpreter. The client should sign the Spanish consent form only after receiving an explanation of the procedure, its risks, and alternatives. A family member cannot be relied on to translate the surgeon's instructions. The nurse is commonly asked to witness the explanation and to obtain the client's signature on the informed consent form. Informed consent is the provision of information concerning the procedure and its risks, not obtaining the client's signature on the form. The surgical charge nurse does not need to be notified. (M)

4. 2. Timolol can cause some eye discomfort when administered. It is important for the client to continue to take the drug. Glaucoma eyedrops should be administered as prescribed, not whenever the client desires. The client with glaucoma needs to take eye medication on an ongoing basis to control the disorder and prevent vision damage. There is no need to refrigerate the drug. (D)

5. 1. The nurse's best response when a child asks if cardiac catheterization is painful is to explain that the child will feel a little stinging when the numbing medicine is inserted into the area around the introduction site of the catheter. There may also be a feeling of pressure when the catheter is introduced. The child's trust in the nurse will be quickly lost if the nurse is untruthful. The child is usually sedated and feels little during the procedure. (R)

6. 1. This client has a barrel chest. The anterior-posterior diameter of the chest is larger than the transverse diameter, as is characteristic of the client with chronic obstructive pulmonary disease. Although the client may be muscular, the barrel chest is not associated with the client's age, height, or weight. Use of bronchodilators will not change the shape of the client's chest. (A)

7. 2. Fetal acoustic stimulation involves the use of an instrument that emits sound levels of approximately 80 dB at a frequency of 80 Hz. The sharp sound startles and awakens the fetus and is used with nonstress testing as a method to evaluate fetal well-being. A fetoscope or Doppler stethoscope is used to listen to the fetal heart rate. Nipple stimulation or intravenous oxytocin is used to stimulate contractions. Ultrasound testing is used to determine amniotic fluid volume. (R)

8. 2. Typically, iron supplements are needed for at least 1 month. By the end of this time, there should be a significant rise in the hemoglobin and hematocrit. Therefore the mother needs to continue the iron supplements for several more weeks. Testing the child after only 2 weeks of treatment may not be beneficial. A significant rise in hemoglobin and hematocrit usually requires approximately 1 month of therapy. An iron-rich diet should have been started when the diagnosis was made and continued for at least the duration of iron supplement therapy. (D)

9. 1. The dietary department should meet with the client to ensure that the foods are available and prepared according to her religious beliefs. On admission, the client should be asked whether there are special dietary needs. The dietary department should be notified of these special needs, and a dietary representative should meet with the client and family when possible. The physician should be consulted if a requested food is contrary to a prescribed diet restriction. The unit case manager does not need to be contacted regarding a dietary request. The rabbi is not involved in dietary requests. (M)

10. 3. The nurse must act as an advocate for the client when the client cannot afford treatment. It is possible to substitute a less expensive antibiotic. Correct procedure includes contacting the physician to explain the mother's economic situation and request a substitution. For example, amoxicillin (Amoxil) is more economical than azithromycin. (M)

11. 2. Nitroglycerin causes vasodilation, which results in increased intraocular pressure. The vasodilatory effects of the medication can trigger an attack, causing pain and loss of vision. Hypotension is a common side effect of nitroglycerin, which dilates the blood vessels but is not a concern in the client with glaucoma. (D)

12. 2, 3, 5. In the client with peripheral vascular disease, blood flow to the extremities is decreased. As a result, peripheral tissue perfusion is altered. This altered blood flow also leads to pain because the oxygen demand exceeds the oxygen supply. In addition, the client commonly has difficulty with activity because of this pain. Nutrition and fluid volume typically are not problems related to peripheral vascular disease. (A)

13. 3. The timing of symptoms is important to the diagnosis of PMS. The client should keep a 3-month log of symptoms and menses. With PMS, the symptoms begin 3 to 7 days before menses and resolve 1 to 2 days after the menstrual cycle has started. Menstrual cycle irregularity and mood swings after menses are not related to PMS, and other causes should be investigated. Midcycle spotting and pain are related to ovulation. (H)

14. 2. The client who has received general anesthesia with halothane or other neuromuscular blocking agents must be carefully monitored when given clindamycin. A serious interaction is enhanced neuromuscular blockage, skeletal muscle weakness, or respiratory depression if this combination is used during or immediately after surgery. Concurrent use should be avoided. The combined effect of the medications places the client at increased risk and the nurse should assess the client closely for respiratory depression or paralysis. The nurse will be monitoring the client's heart rate, blood pressure, and urinary output, but not specifically because of potential drug interactions and adverse effects of clindamycin. (D)

15.

2. Start an I.V. infusion with normal saline solution.
1. Obtain a fingerstick test for blood glucose.
4. Notify the physician.
3. Administer Lispro.

The client is experiencing ketoacidosis. The first action is to initiate I.V. fluids to prevent further dehydration. Next, the nurse should obtain serum glucose values to report to the physician, who will then order the appropriate dose of insulin. (A)

16. **2.** When ovulation is suppressed for 6 to 8 months after oral contraceptive use, the physician may prescribe clomiphene citrate to stimulate ovulation. Clomiphene acts to give the hypothalamus the signal to increase secretion of follicle-stimulating hormone and luteinizing hormone, thereby stimulating ovulation. Dienestrol is an estrogen applied topically to treat atrophic vaginitis and kraurosis vulvae in postmenopausal women. Medroxyprogesterone is a progesterone derivative that prevents maturation of the follicle and ovulation. Norgestrel is a progesterone-only contraceptive that is believed to alter the cervical mucus, possibly suppress ovulation, and interfere with implantation in the uterus. (D)

17. **1.** Hospice programs are appropriate programs for clients with any type of terminal illness when death is imminent within weeks up to 6 months. Clients may discuss their prognosis of a terminal illness before it progresses to the terminal stage when a referral to hospice care is indicated. (M)

18. **1.** Several irregularly shaped red patches, common skin variations in neonates, are termed stork bites. They eventually fade away as the neonate grows older. Port wine stains are disfiguring darkish red or purplish skin discolorations on the scalp and face that may need laser therapy for removal. Newborn rash is typically generalized over the body, not localized to one body area, and is commonly raised. Café au lait spots are brown and typically found anywhere on the body. More than six spots or spots larger than 1.5 cm are associated with neurofibromatosis, a genetic condition of neural tissue. (H)

19. **3.** In the traditional Mexican household, the man is the head of the family and makes the major decisions. Efforts should be made to reach the father as soon as possible to acquire his permission. Contacting the social worker does not reflect the nurse's need to understand a client's cultural values and how they affect medical care decisions. This is not a situation of suspected child abuse. (M)

20. **1.** In the cognitively impaired client, benzodiazepines, such as lorazepam, can increase confusion and nighttime agitation. Extrapyramidal side effects are more common with antipsychotics. Vomiting and sweating are signs of benzodiazepine withdrawal. Anticholinergic side effects are more likely with antipsychotics and tricyclic antidepressants. (D)

21. **4.** A woman with a uterus who takes unopposed estrogen has an increased risk of endometrial cancer. The addition of progesterone prevents the formation of endometrial hyperplasia. (D)

22. **3.** The nurse should monitor the client's serum albumin. A decreased serum albumin indicates malnutrition and is considered a risk factor in the development of pressure ulcers. Other risk factors include immobility, incontinence, and decreased sensation. Having the client walk and inserting an indwelling catheter require a physician's order. The white blood cell count is monitored if an infection is present. (A)

23. **4.** The nurse should recognize the ringing in the ears, or tinnitus, as a sign of ototoxicity probably caused by the furosemide. The appropriate action is for the nurse to stop the furosemide and notify the physician. If the drug is stopped soon enough, permanent hearing loss can be avoided and the tinnitus should subside. The nurse should note the observation in the chart but should not delay action. Tinnitus is not a symptom of digoxin (Lanoxin) toxicity. Aspirin can cause tinnitus, but the nurse should first investigate the obvious cause of tinnitus, which in this case is the furosemide. (D)

24. **2, 3, 4.** The client should recognize the signs of potential thermal dangers to prevent skin breakdown. He should be instructed to wear clean, loose, soft cotton socks so that the feet are comfortable, air can circulate, and moisture is absorbed. In the winter or if the client complains of cold feet, the client should be encouraged to wear an extra pair of socks and a larger shoe size. Getting a sunburn during the summer puts the client at risk for tissue injury and skin breakdown. Using a heating pad to warm the feet or using an electric blanket places the client at risk for injury and should be avoided. (R)

25. **3.** The peak serum dose of an antibiotic is drawn 30 minutes after the completion of the I.V. dose of the antibiotic. (D)

26. **1.** ICP is highest in the early morning. If the client has a headache on arising, this should be reported to the physician. The client with hydrocephalus may be experiencing signs of increased ICP that need to be treated. (A)

27. **1.** The nurse should instruct the client that symptoms from an occasional headache due to eye strain or continuous work at a computer can be relieved by acetaminophen. Although this drug causes prostaglandin inhibition, this effect is rapidly reversed and cleared with no apparent harmful effects in pregnancy. If the headaches become more frequent or severe, the client should be instructed to contact her health care provider immediately. Aspirin should be avoided during pregnancy because it inhibits prostaglandin synthesis. It also decreases uterine contractility and may delay the onset of labor or prolong pregnancy and labor. Aspirin decreases platelet aggregation, possibly increasing the risk of bleeding. Ibuprofen and naproxen can lead to premature closure of the fetal ductus arteriosus and decreased amniotic fluid with prolonged use. They may also prolong pregnancy or labor because of their antiprostaglandin effects. (D)

28. **1.** With this level of anger in a crisis, the father needs simple but firm directions to leave the room, calm down, and then to talk. Doing so relieves the daughter of any pressure from her father. Telling the father to stop yelling or be quiet provides no concrete directions to the father and may embarrass him in front of his daughter. Telling the father that if he doesn't stop yelling, the nurse will call Security is a threat, possibly leading to an escalation of the situation. (P)

29. **2.** Epidemiologic and experimental research studies indicate that African Americans are more likely to develop severe hypertension. (H)

30. **1.** A large pad of fat at the back of the neck, widely set eyes, a simian crease in the hands, and epicanthal folds are typically associated with Down syndrome. The nurse should notify the physician immediately. The physician should obtain consent for genetic studies and is responsible for explaining these deviations to the parents. However, the nurse may need to provide additional teaching to the mother and to answer any questions that may arise. (H)

31. **1.** Clients receiving chronic steroid therapy can become immunosuppressed and are prone to infections. Signs of infection can also be masked with prednisone. Signs and symptoms of infection should be reported immediately. Joint pain, constipation, and joint swelling are not related to the adverse effects of steroid therapy. (D)

32. **2.** Injury and death from firearms is a major public health problem in the United States. One reason that this is such an epidemic is that children, grandchildren, and neighbor children have easy access to firearms. (S)

33. **4.** School-age children enjoy board games and are commonly intense about following rules. Their play can become emotional. Adequate rest is of utmost importance during the acute stage of rheumatic fever. Therefore, playing a game with another child probably would be too strenuous. Such diversional activities as reading a book, playing with a doll, and watching television would be more satisfactory. (H)

34. **2.** Women who take oral contraceptives are at increased risk for thromboembolic conditions. Severe calf pain needs to be investigated as a potential sign of deep vein thrombosis. Breakthrough bleeding, mild headache, or weight gain may be common benign side effects that accompany oral contraceptive use. Clients may be monitored for these side effects without a change in treatment. (D)

35. **4.** The priority for a client with a new tracheostomy is to maintain a patent airway. A new tracheostomy commonly causes bleeding and excess secretions, and the client may require frequent suctioning to maintain a patent airway. (R)

36. **3.** The nurse should assess the client's vital signs because he is most likely having a reaction to the bupivacaine. If the client's vital signs are abnormal, immediate intervention may be necessary. Although the nurse may ask the client to continue to describe how he is feeling, this is not likely to be a psychosocial reaction. Simple reassurance is inappropriate in most clinical situations and can be dangerous if physiologic causes of restlessness are overlooked. The nurse should not administer epinephrine until vital signs have been assessed. (D)

37. **2.** Endometrial cancer has very few warning signals; irregular bleeding may be the only sign. Any irregular bleeding in a menopausal woman should be investigated, and an endometrial biopsy may be ordered. Hot flashes result from the decreased estrogen levels that accompany menopause. Urinary urgency should be monitored and treated as a separate problem. Dyspareunia is the occurrence of pain in the labial, vaginal, or pelvic areas during or after sexual intercourse. It may be caused by inadequate vaginal lubrication in the menopausal woman. (D)

38. **1.** Cystic fibrosis is an autosomal recessive genetic disorder. This means that both parents have the gene. There is a one in four chance with each pregnancy from such parents that the child will have cystic fibrosis. (A)

39. **4.** Trichomoniasis is caused by a protozoan. Although the client may not have symptoms, the classic symptom of trichomoniasis is a malodorous, yellow-green discharge. Gonorrhea, syphilis, and chlamydia do not commonly manifest as a vaginal discharge. (A)

40. **4.** Incentive spirometry promotes lung expansion and increases respiratory function. When used properly, an incentive spirometer causes sustained maximal inspiration and increased cardiac output. (R)

41. **4.** At this level of aggression, the client needs an appropriate physical outlet for the anger. She is beyond writing in a journal. Urging the client to talk to the nurse now or making threats, such as telling her that she will be restrained, is inappropriate and could lead to an escalation of her anger. (P)

42. **3.** Variable decelerations are associated with compression of the umbilical cord. The nurse should alter the client's position and increase the I.V. fluid rate. Fetal head compression is associated with early decelerations. Severe compression of the fetal chest, such as during the process of vaginal delivery, may result in transient bradycardia. Compression or damage to the placenta, typically from abruptio placentae, results in severe, late decelerations. (R)

43. **1, 2, 3, 4.** DIC is diagnosed based on clinical symptoms and laboratory findings. Excessive and unusual bruising or bleeding over areas of tissue trauma, such as I.V. insertion or incision sites or application of a blood pressure cuff, is observed. Tachycardia and diaphoresis also may be noted. Laboratory results reveal low platelet, fibrinogen, proaccelerin, antihemophiliac factor, and prothrombin levels. Bleeding time is normal and partial thromboplastin time is increased. A urine output of 350 ml in 8 hours indicates adequate renal function. Temperature is not an indication of DIC. (A)

44. **2.** If the chest tube is accidentally pulled out (a rare occurrence), a petroleum jelly gauze and sterile 4-× 4-inch dressing should be applied over the chest wall insertion site immediately. The dressing should be covered with adhesive tape and be occlusive, and the surgeon should be notified. The lungs can be auscultated and vital signs can be taken after the dressing is in place and the surgeon has been called. (R)

45. **4.** Emboli obstruct blood flow, leading to a decreased perfusion of the lung tissue. Because of the decreased perfusion, a ventilation-perfusion mismatch occurs, causing hypoxemia to develop. Arterial blood gas analysis typically will indicate hypoxemia and hypocapnia. A priority objective in the treatment of pulmonary emboli is maintaining adequate oxygenation. A nonproductive cough and activity intolerance do not indicate impaired gas exchange. The client does not demonstrate an ineffective breathing pattern; rather, the problem of impaired gas exchange is caused by the inability of blood to flow through the lung tissue. (A)

46. **3.** Cardiogenic shock occurs when myocardial contractility decreases and cardiac output greatly decreases. The circulating blood volume is within normal limits or increased. Infarction is not always the cause of cardiogenic shock. (A)

47. **1.** The nurse should expect to find decreased levels of thyroxine and triiodothyronine and increased thyroid-stimulating hormone. Other indicators of hypothyroidism are the presence of antithyroid antibodies and elevation of the creatine phosphokinase (CPK-MM) level. Hypothyroidism has a metabolic effect on skeletal muscle. Muscle injury results, causing the CPK-MM to spill out of the damaged cells and into the bloodstream. (A)

48. **3.** Although chronologically the infant is 7 months old, because of being born 6 weeks early, the child is only 5½ months old developmentally. Appropriate activities for a 5- to 5½-month-old infant include placing a rattle or ball in the infant's hand. Picture books are an appropriate choice for an infant older than 9 months. Playing peek-a-boo is appropriate for a 9- to 12-month-old infant. Colored blocks are appropriate for a toddler approximately age 15 to 18 months. (H)

49. **3.** Accurate daily weight measurement provides the best measure of a client's fluid status: 1 kg (2.2 lb) is equal to 1,000 ml of fluid. To be accurate, weight should be obtained at the same time every day, with the same scale, and with minimal clothing on. (A)

50. **2.** Full benefit from an antidepressant medication usually takes about 2 to 4 weeks on an adequate dose. (D)

51. **2.** Fine tremors are the first symptom reported in 70% of clients with Parkinson's disease. A new onset of tremors needs to be investigated by the physician. Tremors are not an expected change with aging. (R)

52. **1.** Loss of appetite is one of the more common adverse effects associated with methylphenidate. Although nausea is associated with this drug, vomiting is not. Photosensitivity is not associated with this drug. Because of decreased appetite, the client will not gain more weight. (D)

53. **2.** The pH of 7.26 indicates that the body is in a state of acidosis. The elevated partial pressure of carbon dioxide value accompanied by a normal bicarbonate value indicates that the acid-base imbalance is respiratory acidosis. The additional clinical findings of a headache, dizziness, and increased pulse rate, resulting from the elevated partial pressure of carbon dioxide, further supports this diagnosis. (A)

54. **1.** With a client in metabolic alkalosis, the nurse should monitor for hypokalemia. Metabolic alkalosis can cause potassium to shift into the cells, resulting in a decrease of serum potassium. In metabolic alkalosis, the body tries to compensate by conserving carbon dioxide, so there is no need to have the client inhale carbon dioxide, as would be the case if hyperventilation were occurring. There is already a base bicarbonate excess with this condition, so the nurse should not administer sodium bicarbonate. Unless symptoms dictate, the client does not need to be placed on bed rest. (A)

55. **1.** To reduce the risk of crystalluria, the client should drink 2,000 to 3,000 ml of water a day, not 1,000 to 1,500 ml. The client should not take an antacid before taking Cipro. An antacid decreases the absorption of the Cipro. The client should let the doctor know if vomiting occurs from the medication. The client may get lightheaded from the Cipro. If so, the client should not drive a motor vehicle and should contact the physician. (D)

56. **4.** Stress management is not beneficial to the client with Alzheimer's disease because of cognitive impairment, confusion, and short-term memory loss. Reminiscence group, walking, and pet therapy is beneficial. (P)

57. **1, 3.** When a child with hemophilia develops bleeding into a joint, the parents should have the child rest and begin factor VIII therapy. If therapy is started immediately, usually other interventions such as ice are not necessary. Heat causes vasodilation and promotes bleeding. Starting factor VIII immediately helps prevent chronic joint disease. Starting physical therapy further traumatizes the joint, possibly increasing the bleeding. Applying a topical agent does not control internal bleeding. (R)

58. **2.** The priority long-term nursing diagnosis for this child is *Risk for injury*. This is always a concern for the child with hemophilia. As with all chronic illnesses, there is a potential for self-esteem problems, but no data are presented to support this diagnosis. The parents should have a good understanding of the disease process and realize the importance of obtaining regular health care for their child. *Acute pain* is an appropriate nursing diagnosis for the child who has bleeding into a joint, but this is a transient situation. (R)

59. **3.** A 3-year-old child responds best to distraction during a procedure because of the typical level of cognitive development of a 3-year-old and the fear of painful events. Preparation for the procedure should be done immediately beforehand, so that the child will not become too frightened. A 3-year-old is not concerned about the why of the procedure but about whether the procedure will hurt. This child is too young for verbal explanations alone because of the limited verbal abilities at this age and the fear of a painful event. (H)

60. **3.** Lisinopril is an angiotensin-converting enzyme (ACE) inhibitor. Hyperkalemia can be a side effect of ACE inhibitors. Because of this side effect, ACE inhibitors should not be administered with potassium-sparing diuretics. (D)

61. **4.** Medication noncompliance is a primary cause of exacerbation in chronic mental illnesses. Of the issues listed, medications should be addressed first. Other issues, such as family, marriage, and finances can be addressed as client stabilization is maintained. (P)

62. **4.** I.V. fluids should not be infused for longer than 24 hours because of the risk of bacterial growth in the solution. The appropriate action for the nurse to take is to discontinue the current TPN solution, change the tubing, and hang a new bag of solution. Changing the filter does not decrease the risk of contamination. Notifying the physician for a change in flow rate is not an acceptable solution. (D)

63. **3.** The nurse's first response is to further assess the client's pain. After a thorough assessment, additional appropriate actions may be to notify the physician, administer an analgesic, and administer oxygen. (C)

64. **4.** Trisomy 13 (Patau's syndrome) is an autosomal disorder. Characteristics include cleft lip and palate, polydactyly, malformed ears, and mental retardation. These neonates typically die during infancy. A webbed neck is associated with Turner's syndrome (45 total chromosomes). Small testes and absence of sperm are associated with Klinefelter's syndrome (47 chromosomes). Congenital heart defects are associated with trisomy 21 (Down syndrome) and trisomy 18 (Edwards' syndrome). (A)

65. **2.** Neurologic symptoms, such as footdrop, or bowel or bladder changes should be reported to the physician immediately. When musculoskeletal strain causes back pain, these symptoms may take 4 to 6 weeks to resolve. As an accompanying symptom of acute low back pain, the client may have a diffuse, aching sensation in the L4 to L5 area, pain in the lower back when the leg is lifted, or pain that radiates to the hip. (R)

66. **2.** Taking ginseng when on insulin is not encouraged because ginseng increases the risk of hypoglycemia. Ginseng can be therapeutic in certain situations. If the nurse does not know about the interaction, she should ask the pharmacist. (D)

67. **2.** The expected effect of lactulose is for the client to have two to three soft stools a day to help reduce the pH and serum ammonia levels, which will prevent hepatic encephalopathy. (D)

68. **3.** Leukocytosis, an increased white blood cell count, indicates the presence of inflammation, infection, or a leukemia process. In inflammation and infection, the client's sedimentation rate is increased. Thrombocytopenia, a platelet deficiency, occurs in the client with leukemia, immunocompromise, aplastic anemia, or other conditions. Erythrocytosis, an elevation of the red blood cell count, occurs in polycythemia vera. (A)

69. **4.** This girl has an exaggeration of the lumbar spine, swayback, or lordosis. Kyphosis is an increased convexity or roundness of the curve of the thoracic spine. Scoliosis is a lateral curvature of the spine. (H)

70. **4.** The most appropriate action is to report the swelling, loss of mobility, and unrelieved pain to the physician. These symptoms are indicators of neurovascular impairment. Administering opioids will not eliminate the cause of the problem, which is unrelieved pressure on nerves and blood supply. If prompt action (cutting the cast) is not taken to relieve the pressure, permanent muscular and neurologic injury may result. Applying the ice bag would have been appropriate earlier to decrease or prevent swelling, but applying it at this time could actually lead to further decreased circulation. The arm should be elevated, but the nurse cannot wait 30 minutes to reassess the client without risking permanent damage. (R)

71. 1. Prostaglandin F_{2a} promotes uterine contractions, thereby minimizing uterine atony and subsequent hemorrhage. Possible side effects include nausea, tachycardia, hypertension, and diarrhea. Abdominal distention is not associated with the use of prostaglandin F_{2a}. **(D)**

72. 1. Before 32 weeks' gestation, most neonates have difficulty coordinating sucking and swallowing reflexes along with breathing. Increased respiratory distress may occur with bottle feeding. Bottle feedings can be given after the neonate shows sucking and swallowing behaviors. High-calorie formulas can be given by bottle or by gavage feeding. Although frequent feeding prevents hypoglycemia, the feeding does not have to be given via a gavage tube. Although these neonates can be stressed by cold, they can be kept warm with blankets while being bottle-fed or fed while in the warm isolette environment. **(H)**

73. 2. Regularly scheduled rest periods during the day along with 8 to 10 hours of sleep at night helps relieve the fatigue, pain, and stiffness associated with rheumatoid arthritis. Even with mild rheumatoid arthritis, the client may find it difficult to perform activities of daily living without some rest periods. Spending 1 day a week in bed to relieve fatigue does not adequately manage the disease. The client must recognize the need for rest before feeling exhausted because overexertion can cause exacerbations. In addition, prolonged periods of inactivity can increase joint stiffness and pain. Getting up early to do household chores before the children are awake does not allow for adequate rest. **(C)**

74. 3. For the child with hemophilia who is actively bleeding, the nurse should apply direct pressure to the injured area for 10 minutes continuously along with elevating the leg. The continuous application of direct pressure aids in stopping the bleeding. Elevating the leg reduces blood flow to the area, thereby minimizing the extent of blood loss. Although ice will cause local vasoconstriction and slow the bleeding, applying continuous direct pressure is essential. **(A)**

75. 4. Hypothyroidism is not associated with pancytopenia. Various anemias are associated with pancytopenia owing to the reduction in all cellular elements of the blood. Bleeding and clotting difficulties can be associated with pancytopenia. Infection is a common danger associated with pancytopenia. **(A)**

76. 2. The client's return to the emergency department and her statement about not knowing what to do about being abused by her husband indicate that the client is asking for help. The nurse's best course of action is to explain the various options available to her. This helps the client make decisions based on appropriate knowledge. Research reveals that women are more likely to be killed by partners than by strangers. Although the client can legally leave her husband, this answer provides the client with no safety options. Listing ways to avoid making the husband angry ignores the dynamics of abuse and blames the victim. **(P)**

77. 3. The nurse places a postoperative client who has had abdominal surgery in low Fowler's position. This position relaxes abdominal muscles and promotes maximum respiratory and cardiovascular function. **(R)**

78. 1. It is most important to know the child's serum potassium level when administering digoxin. Digoxin increases contractility of the heart and increases renal perfusion, resulting in a diuretic effect with increased loss of potassium and sodium. Hypokalemia increases the risk of digoxin toxicity. Verifying the dosage is specified by facility policy and varies among facilities. Although the child may take the medication better from the mother than from the nurse, asking the mother to give the medication is not necessary. In addition, this would be done after the nurse has checked the electrolyte levels. Teaching the parent how to measure the child's heart rate can be done at any time, not necessarily when preparing to give digoxin. **(D)**

79. 4. During the emergent phase of burn management, there is a massive shift of fluid from the blood vessels (intravascular compartment) into the tissues (interstitial compartment). The result of this shift is hypovolemic shock and edema formation. The fluid shift, which occurs between the intravascular and interstitial extracellular compartments, is caused by increased capillary permeability that allows water, sodium, and protein to shift to the tissues. As the emergent period ends and capillary permeability returns to normal, the fluid in the interstitial compartment will return to the intravascular compartment. **(A)**

80. 3. A urine output of 30 to 50 ml/hour indicates adequate fluid replacement in the client with burns. An increase in body weight may indicate fluid retention. A urine output greater than fluid intake does not represent a fluid balance. Depending on the client, blood pressure of 90/60 mm Hg could indicate the presence of a hypovolemic state; by itself, it does not indicate adequate fluid replacement. **(A)**

81. 1. Many clients who experience abuse are hesitant to talk about it and need help to do so. The nurse should ask the client directly about abuse when it is suspected, using a sensitive, empathetic, and compassionate approach. In this way, the client can feel comfortable revealing information about the abuse. Telling the client that it's difficult to believe her injuries resulted from a fall is not helpful because it is blameful and puts the client on the defensive. Asking the client what she did to make someone hit her or discussing what she can do the next time blames and alienates the client. (P)

82. **1.** A primary outcome for the care of the client in shock is to achieve adequate tissue perfusion, thus avoiding multiple organ dysfunction. The lungs are susceptible to injury, especially acute respiratory distress syndrome. Vasoconstriction occurs as a compensatory mechanism until the client enters the irreversible stage of shock. (R)

83. **4.** Problems with interpersonal relationships, such as resisting affection and refusing to respond to others, and repetitive behaviors, such as twirling around frequently, suggest autism. Because the parents did not report tics, Tourette syndrome is not suggested. No psychotic behaviors, such as hallucinations or delusions, were reported, so schizophrenia can be ruled out. Attention deficit hyperactivity disorder is commonly portrayed as incessant activity with difficulty completing tasks. (P)

84. **3, 4, 5.** The neurologic system can be affected and cause long-term consequences in a young child exposed to lead. Common behavioral effects include hyperactivity, impulsivity, and aggression. Seizures may occur in a child with high-dose lead exposure. Depression is not usually associated with lead exposure. (A)

85. **2.** The incident report includes only what the nurse saw and did—the objective data. The nurse does not try to interpret the likely cause of the incident, include statements from the client about the incident, or comment on extenuating circumstances. (M)

86. **1.** To reduce urethral irritation and allow drainage, the nurse should tape the Foley catheter to a female client's inner thigh. Taping the catheter also prevents excessive traction against the bladder neck. Taping the catheter to the groin or lower abdomen would not allow for proper drainage and would cause urethral discomfort. Taping the catheter to the lower thigh would pull on the catheter and cause urethral irritation. (R)

87. **1.** A neonate delivered by cesarean delivery has not had the benefit of the chest-squeezing action of a vaginal delivery, which helps remove some of the nasopharyngeal secretions. The nurse should place the neonate under the radiant warmer and suction the mouth and nares with a bulb syringe to remove nasopharyngeal secretions. A high-pitched cry is associated with neurologic involvement or neonatal drug withdrawal and is unrelated to cesarean delivery. Skull fractures may occur with difficult vaginal deliveries and are not typically seen with cesarean deliveries. Decreased muscle tone is associated with oversedation, neurologic impairment, or use of general anesthesia. (H)

88. **2.** Accidental scaldings are usually splash-related and occur on the front of the body. Any burns on the back of the body or in a well-defined circular or glove pattern may indicate physical abuse. Immersion burns on the buttocks are also suspicious injuries. (H)

89. **3.** A client exhibiting mild preeclampsia is initially treated with activity restriction. Bed rest, or lying on the left side, decreases pressure on the vena cava and improves circulatory blood flow. Restriction of visitors and a quiet environment are also necessary. I.V. magnesium sulfate, a central nervous system depressant, is usually ordered for the client with severe preeclampsia. Labetalol is used for the client with severe preeclampsia. Frequent monitoring of the client's blood pressure is important. However, hourly blood pressure checks are more routinely ordered for the client with severe preeclampsia. Additionally, the client needs to rest, and checking her blood pressure hourly could interfere with her ability to rest. (R)

90. **4.** A dry tea bag placed on the bleeding area can be effective to control bleeding from lesions on the oral mucosa. The tannic acid in the tea apparently helps control bleeding. (R)

91. **4.** The best treatment for a pressure ulcer is prevention. If a client has been determined to be at risk for developing a pressure ulcer, a systematic skin assessment should be conducted at least once per shift. Other preventive measures include daily gentle cleaning of the skin and avoiding harsh soaps and hot water, which are damaging to the skin. Massage of bony prominences is not done because it can increase damage to the underlying tissue. The client should be encouraged to change position at least every 2 hours to avoid pressure on any one area for a prolonged period. (R)

92. **3.** Nasogastric suctioning removes gastric acid from the gastrointestinal tract, thus creating a base bicarbonate excess and a state of metabolic alkalosis. The respiratory system is not affected by the presence of a nasogastric tube. Metabolic acidosis is not created when gastric acid is removed. (A)

93. **1.** The client needs further instructions when she says, "I should walk with my pelvis tilted backward." Walking in this position puts greater strain on the back. The client should walk with her pelvis tilted forward. Pelvic tilt exercises can also help the client with backaches. Putting a board under the mattress makes the mattress firmer and provides more support. Squatting and not bending to pick up objects helps decrease back strain. Squatting involves the use of the large thigh muscles rather than those of the back. Flat or low-heeled shoes provide better balance and greater support and can help decrease backaches. (R)

94. **4.** Urethritis is usually the initial clinical manifestation of gonorrhea in men. The symptoms include a profuse, purulent discharge and dysuria. Complications are uncommon, but they include prostatitis and sterility. Impotence, scrotal pain, and penile lesions are not associated with gonorrhea. (S)

95. **4.** Although the nurse needs to obtain and administer the medication as soon as possible, it is inappropriate for the nurse to go to the pharmacy and request the drug without first calling the pharmacy and checking to see whether the medication was delivered. The drug may have been delivered to several appropriate spots on the unit, such as the client's drug bin, the transport system, or the delivery box. The nurse should assess the client's blood pressure to determine the immediacy of the condition for which the medication was ordered. (S)

96. **3.** The client with major depression suffers from lack of energy and withdrawal. The nurse should emphasize the importance of group involvement for the client to gain support from others and to see that others have similar problems and concerns. Attendance at group sessions and activities decreases social isolation and destructive rumination. The other statements are not therapeutic and interfere with increasing the client's involvement with others. (P)

97. **4.** An infant's sleeping longer than usual can indicate that the child is expending too much energy to breathe and is tiring, suggesting that the child's condition is getting worse. This should be reported to the physician. Fewer than seven wet diapers a day indicates that the child is not drinking enough. A temperature of 100° F (37.8° C) for longer than 2 days should be reported. Clear nasal drainage is normal. However, yellow nasal drainage lasting longer than 24 hours should be reported. (R)

98. **4.** Direct application of warm moist heat would benefit a client with low back pain because the heat relaxes muscle spasms. Heat should not be applied to a client who has appendicitis because it can lead to rupture of the appendix and peritonitis. Ice is applied to recently sprained joints to help decrease edema. Applying heat to the area of a suspected malignancy can increase blood flow to the tumor and promote nourishment of the cancer cells. (C)

99. **3.** The client with pernicious anemia will require lifelong supplementation of vitamin B_{12}, available through injection or nasal spray administration. It must be given in these forms to ensure absorption. Oral vitamin B_{12} would not be absorbed because the client lacks the intrinsic factor in the stomach necessary for absorption. Chelation therapy is used to extract metals at toxic levels such as in lead poisoning. (D)

100. **10.**

To administer 20 mEq of potassium chloride, the nurse needs to administer 10 ml. The following formula is used to calculate the correct dosage:

$$20 \text{ mEq}/X \text{ ml} = 2 \text{ mEq}/1 \text{ ml}$$

$$X = 10 \text{ ml}.$$

(D)

101. **4.** When a client with major depression and suicidal ideation displays a sudden elevation in mood, seems calmer, has more energy, and is more peaceful, the nurse should judge these behaviors as an indication that a suicide attempt is imminent. These symptoms may indicate relief from ambivalent thoughts about suicide and that the client has an immediate plan for killing himself. (P)

102. **3.** The purpose of a contraction stress test is to determine fetal response during labor. If late decelerations are noted with the contractions, the test is considered positive or abnormal. Fetal lung maturity is evaluated through amniocentesis to obtain the lecithin-sphingomyelin ratio. The nonstress test is part of the biophysical profile. Determining fetal response during movements is evaluated as part of the nonstress test. (R)

103. **3.** Atypical pneumonia is characterized by a gradual onset of symptoms, such as dry cough, headache, sore throat, fatigue, nausea, and vomiting. Typical pneumonia is characterized by tachypnea, fever, chills, and productive cough with purulent sputum. (A)

104. **2.** The primary reason for instructing the client with emphysema about how to pursed-lip breathe is to prolong exhalation. Prolonging exhalation helps to prevent bronchiolar collapse and the trapping of air. It does not directly prevent respiratory infection. Because pursed-lip breathing affects the expiratory phase of the respiratory cycle, it does not affect oxygenation. It may decrease shortness of breath, but this is not the primary reason for the technique. (R)

105. **2.** The primary purpose of the automated dispensing machine for nurses is to keep an up-to-date record of the narcotic usage and count. The automated dispensing machine has eliminated the need for change-of-shift counts for narcotics. It does not include unmonitored access by nurses to narcotics, which would not be considered an advantage. The pharmacy has direct information about the narcotics being used on the client at what intervals and by whom, and it automatically records the charges of narcotics used. Not recording the charges would not be an advantage. (M)

106. **2.** Blunt chest trauma can lead to respiratory failure. Maintenance of adequate oxygenation is the priority for the client. Decreasing the client's anxiety is related to maintaining effective respirations and oxygenation. Although pain is distressing to the client and can increase anxiety and decrease respiratory effectiveness, pain control is secondary to maintaining oxygenation, as is maintaining adequate circulatory volume. (A)

107. **1.** An episiotomy that is edematous and slightly reddened 8 hours after delivery is normal. Therefore, the nurse should offer the client an ice pack to provide some relief from the perineal pain for the first 24 hours. An infection is present if greenish, purulent drainage is observed from the site. The edema and discoloration of the episiotomy at this time after delivery are normal and do not indicate that a hematoma is likely to develop. A laceration when repaired should appear intact with edges well-approximated, clean, and dry. (H)

108. **3.** The Z-track technique is used with medications that are irritating to tissues. It allows the medication to be trapped in the muscle and prevents it from leaking back through the tissues. (C)

109. **2.** The nurse should limit the amount of telephone calls the client can make. Setting limits for a client with bipolar disorder, mania, helps to control the hyperactive client who has excessive goal-directed activity, especially when it interferes with the rights of other clients. Instructing the other clients to be patient is neither fair to them nor helpful to the hyperactive client in managing behavior. Reminding the client that others need to use the telephone will probably be futile because the client with mania is experiencing cognitive impairment and needs to be active. Taking away the client's telephone privileges is not the best action because the client has a right to use the telephone. The nurse is responsible for helping the client manage behavior by setting constructive limits. (P)

110. **4.** Because a toddler is strong and moves frequently, the child needs to be restrained during the removal procedure by a total body restraint. To protect the child, the papoose board is best because the arms, legs, chest, and head can be fully restrained. A jacket restraint would immobilize only the child's upper body. Elbow restraints would immobilize only the child's arms. The father should be available to provide comfort before and after the procedure, but not to hold the child down during the procedure. (S)

111. **4.** Wheezing over one lung in the presence of lung cancer is most likely caused by obstruction of the airway by a tumor. Exudate would be more likely to cause crackles. The client's history of smoking would not cause unilateral wheezing. Pleural effusion would produce diminished or absent breath sounds. (A)

112. **1.** The client with diabetic ketoacidosis exhibits Kussmaul respiration, as well as flushed skin, dry mouth, urinary frequency, glucosine, and ketonuria. Excessive hunger and high blood pressure are not associated with diabetic ketoacidosis. (R)

113. **4.** For the client who has been receiving lithium therapy for the past 2 months, a maintenance serum lithium level of 0.6 to 1.2 mEq/L is considered therapeutic. A lithium level greater than 1.2 mEq/L suggests toxicity. (D)

114. **2.** One cup of sunflower seeds contains 15 mg of iron. During pregnancy, 30 mg of iron is recommended daily. One cup of lentils provides the equivalent of 6.9 mg of iron. One and one-half ounces of hard cheese provides the equivalent of the amount of calcium in 1 cup of milk. Two poached eggs provides only 2 mg of iron. (H)

115. **4.** The plan of care to treat fatigue associated with radiation therapy should include encouraging the client to remain active and to plan scheduled rest periods as necessary before activity. Engaging in activities, such as walking, has been shown to decrease the cycle of fatigue, anxiety, and depression that can occur during treatment. Fatigue is a very common side effect of radiation therapy that typically begins during the third or fourth week of treatment and persists until after treatment ends. The presence of fatigue does not mean that the cancer is not responding to treatment or that the client has developed another health problem. (R)

116. **3.** Carbohydrate is the base of the diet; it is found in grains, fruits, vegetables, and milk. Carbohydrate provides the base because it is the primary fuel for energy in the human body. Protein is near the top of the food pyramid, above carbohydrates and fruits and vegetables, indicating it should be used moderately. Fats and sweets are at the very top of the pyramid, indicating that they should be used sparingly. (H)

117. **3.** Shearing forces occur because of improper movement and positioning, which causes the underlying tissues and capillary blood supply to be pulled and disrupted. This leads to tissue trauma and the potential beginning of skin breakdown. To prevent shearing, clients should be moved with the use of lift sheets and other devices, thus preventing dragging of the skin across the mattress and linens. Clients should also be positioned and supported to prevent pulling or tension of the skin across bony prominences. Turning clients, if not done properly, can cause shearing injuries. Keeping the skin clean, dry, and lubricated is an important aspect of care, but care must be used to decrease the amount of pulling forces exerted on the tissues. (R)

118. **4.** The proper use of crutches requires supporting the body weight primarily on the hands. Improper use of crutches can cause nerve damage from excess pressure on the axillary nerve. (R)

119. **4.** Because this family is waiting for the child to die, the most appropriate nursing diagnosis is *Grieving*. Families grieve at the time of diagnosis as well as during the illness, as the child is dying, and after death has occurred. This is a normal process and does not indicate *Disabled family coping*, *Impaired parenting*, or *Fear*. (P)

120. **2.** For the child with croup, assessing the child's respiratory status is the priority. It is especially important to assess airway patency because laryngeal spasms can occur suddenly. After the nurse has assessed the toddler's respiratory status, having a tracheostomy set at the bedside would be the next priority. Monitoring vital signs is important, as is ensuring adequate fluid intake to keep secretions loose, but assessing respiratory status is key. (A)

121. **2.** I.V. solutions are ordered based upon the fluid and electrolyte status of the client, so laboratory results should be monitored first. Safety recommendations are for standard premixed solutions. If solutions are not premixed, additives are completed by the pharmacy, not at the bedside. Potassium chloride is never given by I.V. push because this could be fatal. Administration guidelines require no more than 10 mEq of potassium chloride be infused per hour on a general medical-surgical unit. An infusion device or pump is required for safe administration. (D)

122. **4.** Research indicates that vitamin B_6, vitamin B_{12}, and folate may help to clear homocysteine from the blood. Elevated homocysteine correlates with a high incidence of heart and artery disease. (H)

123. **1.** Neuromuscular irritability is usually the first indication that a client has developed a low serum calcium level. Numbness and tingling around the mouth as well as in the extremities is an early sign of neuromuscular irritability. Depressed reflexes, decreased memory, and ventricular dysrhythmias are indications of hypercalcemia. (A)

124. **2.** In emphysema, the anteroposterior diameter of the chest wall is increased. As a result, the client's breath sounds may be diminished. Fine crackles are present when there is fluid in the lungs. Stridor occurs as a result of a partially obstructed larynx or trachea; stridor can be heard without auscultation. A pleural friction rub is present when pleural surfaces are inflamed and rub together. (A)

125. **4.** The client with paranoid personality disorder interprets the actions of others as personal threats and feels vulnerable. He questions and is overly sensitive to others'

motives. Saying, "They're laughing at a joke John told. They aren't laughing at you," is a simple explanation of others' behavior, which helps to decrease the client's suspiciousness and promote trust. The other statements do not help the client to realistically interpret situations and the behavior of others and are not helpful in reducing the client's suspicions or mistrust. (P)

126. **4.** Mebendazole is prescribed for household members older than 2 years. Although the child's 18-month-old brother would not receive the drug, his 4-year-old sister and parents would. (D)

127. **3.** Loss of height and back pain are early indications of the disease that are caused by collapse of the vertebrae. Later signs include the dowager's hump and loss of the waistline. The dowager's hump is a later sign of osteoporosis that occurs when the vertebrae can no longer support the upper body in an upright position. Fair-skinned, small-boned, white and Asian women are at greater risk for osteoporosis. Conventional radiographs are little help because more than 30% of the bone mass must be lost before the disease is detected. High-density bone scans can detect the disease earlier. (R)

128. **3.** The primary reason for evaluating gastric residual is to determine whether gastric emptying has been delayed and the stomach is becoming overdistended from the feeding. With delayed gastric emptying, the possibility of aspiration of the feeding into the lungs is increased. It is not possible to determine how well the client's body is absorbing nutrients or whether the client is receiving enough feeding by checking the gastric residual. It is not necessary to keep partially digested formula separate from undigested formula. (R)

129. **1.** The baseline values of the client's partial thromboplastin time, bleeding time, and prothrombin time should be obtained. Potassium levels do not indicate a client's coagulation time. The Lee-White clotting time or baseline fibrin split product does not need to be established before starting tissue plasminogen activator or alteplase. (R)

130. **2, 4, 5.** Clients with hepatitis A commonly experience fatigue and altered nutrition due to anorexia and nausea. Because of the severe fatigue associated with hepatitis, clients are encouraged to rest and restrict activity during the active phase of the disease. It is important that frequent rest periods be planned throughout the day. Clients may experience nausea and vomiting; thus, providing relief is important. Small, frequent meals help clients manage the anorexia associated with hepatitis. An exercise program is not appropriate due to the need for rest. Clients with hepatitis do not experience pain. All medications administered to clients with hepatitis need to be evaluated for their potential for hepatotoxicity. (A)

131. 1. A common complication of diabetes is diabetic neuropathy. Diabetic neuropathy results from the metabolic and vascular factors related to hyperglycemia. Damage leads to sensory deficits and peripheral pain. Muscle atrophy can result from disuse, but it is not a direct consequence of diabetes. Raynaud's disease is associated with vasospasms in the hands and feet. Transient ischemic attacks involve the cerebrum. (R)

132. 1. Clients with borderline personality disorder have fears of abandonment and seek attention. Clients are dependent and fear being alone; this stems from disapproval, feelings of being abandoned, and not having needs met earlier in their life. The nurse intervenes by reducing attention-seeking behaviors and abandonment fears to help with intense feelings and emotions. (P)

133. 4. The application of restraints places the client in a vulnerable, confined position. The nurse should check on the client every 30 minutes while she is restrained to make sure that her needs are being met and she is safe. The client should be able to move while the restraints are in place. The restraints should be removed every 2 hours to provide skin care and exercise the extremities. Restraints should not be secured to the side rails; they should be secured to the movable bed frame so that when the bed is adjusted the restraints will not be pulled too tightly. (S)

134. 3. The most appropriate response is, "Alcohol dependence is a disease that can be treated" because it conveys hope. It also emphasizes that the client has a treatable illness, which is helpful in reducing denial and guilt and encouraging the client to seek and comply with treatment. The other statements are judgmental and guilt-producing, possibly leading to denial and furthering the need for alcohol. (P)

135. 2. Raisins are high in nutritional value but are sticky and have a high sugar content. The raisin can stick to the teeth and act like high-sugar foods in promoting tooth decay. Although anything can be aspirated, round, hard, smooth foods are more easily aspirated than raisins, which are soft and chewy. Raisins need to be chewed thoroughly for maximum nutritional value. (H)

136. 1. Aspirin is an antiplatelet medication. The use of aspirin is contraindicated while taking warfarin because it will potentiate the drug's effects. Diphenhydramine and pseudoephedrine do not affect blood coagulation. Digoxin is not an over-the-counter medication; it requires a physician's order. (D)

137. 1. The nurse should inform the client that carbamazepine can decrease the effects of oral anticoagulants. Tegretol can increase the serum concentration of verapamil and can decrease the serum concentration of other anticonvulsants and the effects of oral contraceptives. (D)

138. 2. Viral hepatitis causes fatigue. It is important for the client to rest to allow the liver to recover. Activity levels are resumed gradually as the client begins to recover. Abdominal pain is not a common manifestation of hepatitis. The client typically does not have difficulty breathing or experience edema. (A)

139. 1. The mother should be encouraged to hold and cuddle her child to provide needed emotional support. Such activities as helping the child play with toys, reading stories, and staying with the child would not be contraindicated but do not offer as much emotional support as holding and cuddling. (P)

140. 2. The best strategy to affect child seat belt safety is to attend the school board meeting and advocate for educational programming. The programming could be simple and done quickly. This action also targets the best audience. (H)

141. 3. A basic principle of rehabilitation, including cardiac rehabilitation, is that rehabilitation begins on hospital admission. Early rehabilitation is essential to promote maximum functional ability as the client recovers from an illness. Delaying rehabilitation activities is associated with poorer client outcomes. (C)

142. 1. The goal of the intervention is to decrease the child's work of breathing by decreasing pressure on the diaphragm and increase chest expansion by increasing the pull of gravity on the diaphragm. Placing the client in high Fowler's position accomplishes this. Side-lying positions make it more difficult to expand the side of the lung closest to the bed. The prone or supine position does not decrease the work of breathing unless the head of the bed is raised. (A)

143. 3. The most appropriate action is to contact the physician to verify that the order is correct. Although 60 mg of morphine is a significant dose, the amount of morphine administered to a client can vary widely, especially if a client has been taking morphine for an extended period and has developed a tolerance to the medication. The safest approach is for the nurse to verify orders that do not appear to fall within the norm. Administering the medication without verification is unsafe. The nurse cannot decide to reduce the amount of a prescribed medication without an order. Asking another nurse to review the order is not inappropriate; however, checking with the physician to verify the order should be done. (D)

144. 1. Before paracentesis, the client is asked to void. This is done to collapse the bladder and decrease the risk of accidental bladder perforation. The abdomen is not prepared with Betadine. The client is placed in a Fowler's position. The client does not need to be put on NPO status before the procedure. (R)

145. **1.** Children who are being abused may demonstrate behaviors such as withdrawal, apparent fear of parents, and lack of an appropriate reaction, such as crying, and attempting to get away when faced with a frightening event (an examination or procedure). (P)

146. **3.** The nurse should include teaching the client and family about the physical, physiologic, and psychological effects of substances to educate them about the potential injury, illness, and disability that can result from substance use. Teaching about the role of the family in perpetuating the problem, the family's responsibility for the client, or the reasons that could have led the client to use the substance is inappropriate and based on an erroneous assumption. Including these topics blames the family for the problem and attempts to rationalize the use of the substance. (P)

147. **2.** Postoperative care after a laparoscopic cholecystectomy includes removal of the dressing from the incisional site the day after surgery and allowing the client to bathe or shower. The client can resume a normal diet but may wish to follow a low-fat diet for a few weeks after surgery. Nausea is not expected to last for several days after surgery. The client usually can return to work within 1 week. (R)

148. **1.** Children are highly valued and are closely protected by godparents. The tradition of the family is all-encompassing, and the health care provider gains trust and improved compliance rates by including the family in teaching and health care matters. (P)

149. **4.** Many vitamin and mineral deficiencies can result in anemia. All of these vitamins and minerals need to be assessed, preferably through a nutrition assessment. Deficiencies of vitamins A, B_6, and C result in a small cell, microcytic anemia. Folate and vitamin B_{12} deficiencies result in large cell, macrocytic anemia. Iron, copper, and vitamin E deficiencies can also result in anemia. (A)

150. **3.** Women with diabetes mellitus generally have neonates who are large but physically immature. Other common findings in these infants are hypoglycemia, hypocalcemia, hyperbilirubinemia, polycythemia, renal thrombosis, and congestive anomalies. The neonates do not exhibit hypertonia, hyperactivity, or scaly skin. (H)

151. **2.** The imbalance between the client's intake and output indicates that the client may be retaining urine since the removal of his Foley catheter. The nurse's first action is to validate this assumption by assessing for bladder distention. Applying a condom catheter will not relieve urinary retention; condom catheters are meant to be used for incontinence. A urine specimen for a culture is obtained if a urinary infection is suspected, but this is not a priority at this point. Kegel exercises are helpful in controlling urinary dribbling but do not treat retention. (R)

152. **2.** Because of the poor emptying of blood from the atrial chambers, there is an increased risk for clot formation around the valves. The clots become dislodged and travel through the circulatory system. As a result, cerebrovascular accident is a common complication of atrial fibrillation. (A)

153. **2.** Griseofulvin is associated with photosensitivity reactions. Therefore, the nurse should instruct the parents to have the child avoid intense sunlight. Griseofulvin is best absorbed when administered after a high-fat meal. Treatment with griseofulvin typically lasts for at least 1 month. There are no indications that increased fluid intake affects absorption. (D)

154. **3.** Based on the National Cholesterol Education Program Expert Panel of Detention, Evaluation and Treatment of High Blood Cholesterol in Adults, 30% of the diet should come from fat. (H)

155. **4.** The nurse should actively listen to the client's descriptions and details about being raped and allow her to talk about the trauma. This allows the client to vent, decreases feelings of isolation, and guides the nurse to potential areas that could be problematic for the client. The nurse is a safe person to confide in, thus helping to decrease the client's apprehension about disclosing intimate details and feelings. Advising the client to try to forget about what happened, recommending that she be thankful for being alive, or questioning her about what she could have done to deter the attack is contraindicated for the victim of violence. These responses blame the victim and tend to increase her guilt, as if somehow she is to blame or would have been capable of preventing the rape. (P)

156. **2.** After cystoscopy with biopsy, the nurse would assess for excessive hematuria, which might indicate hemorrhage caused by the biopsy. Catheters are not routinely inserted after cystoscopy. The nurse would not assess for bladder distention unless the client was having difficulty voiding. Urine cultures are not routinely ordered after cystoscopy. (R)

157. **2.** The nurse interprets the client's statement as use of the hot disease concept in the Mexican American culture, where the belief of a hot and cold balance of the body exists. A hot disease such as an infection is treated with the opposite, a cold food such as milk. The nurse should focus on the cultural differences and be sensitive to the cultural diversity. (H)

158. **3.** A client who is "getting special messages" (ideas of reference) commonly misinterprets content presented on television as containing messages for the client. Therefore, it is important for the nurse to monitor the client's reactions to television programs. (P)

159. **2.** A thick, white, cottage cheese-like vaginal discharge along with vaginal itching is most likely candidiasis. This condition is associated with oral contraceptive use, diabetes, and systemic antibiotic therapy because the normal vaginal flora is altered. Candidiasis is treated with miconazole (Monistat). *Trichomonas vaginalis* typically is characterized by a greenish discharge. *Herpes genitalis* is associated with blisters and pain. Although women may not experience symptoms related to gonorrhea, the most common symptom is a purulent vaginal discharge. (H)

160. **3, 5.** Not attending the support group consistently and not taking the antidepressant may lead to a relapse and the client needs this information. Bulimia is chronic and intermittent and involves cycles of bingeing, purging, and restrictive eating. Increased socialization and activities promote healthy relationships. (P)

161. **3.** In a low anorectal anomaly, the rectum has descended normally through the puborectalis muscle. In an intermediate anomaly, the rectum is at or below the level of the puborectalis muscle; in a high anomaly, the rectum ends above the puborectalis muscle. (A)

162. **1.** It is especially important for the nurse to carefully assess the elderly client for respiratory depression after administering a dose of meperidine. It may be necessary to reduce the dosage to prevent respiratory depression. Dysrhythmias, constipation, and seizures are all potential adverse effects of meperidine, but respiratory depression is most significant in the elderly. (D)

163. **2.** Ascorbic acid (vitamin C) increases iron absorption. Taking iron with a food rich in ascorbic acid, such as orange juice, increases absorption. Milk delays iron absorption. It is best to give iron on an empty stomach to increase absorption. Beta-carotene does not affect iron absorption. (D)

164. **1.** In early renal insufficiency, the kidneys lose the ability to concentrate urine, resulting in polyuria. Oliguria occurs later. Dysuria and hematuria are not associated with renal insufficiency. (A)

165. **1.** The ZIFT method requires that fertilization take place outside the body. After fertilization has occurred, the fertilized eggs are transferred by laparoscopy to the open end of the fallopian tube. At least one tube must be patent for this procedure to succeed, so it is not beneficial if the client has bilateral blocked fallopian tubes. Ova and sperm are instilled in the fallopian tube for fertilization when the gamete intrafallopian transfer method is used. With in vitro fertilization, a fertilized ovum is instilled into the vagina to enter the uterus for implantation. (H)

166. **2.** The nurse should examine the buccal mucosa, along with the conjunctiva and sclera, nailbeds, palms, soles, lips, and tongue to assess for oxygenation in a client with dark skin. (R)

167. **3.** A client who has undergone chest surgery should be taught to raise the arm on the affected side over the head to help prevent shoulder ankylosis. This exercise helps restore normal shoulder movement, prevents stiffening of the shoulder joint, and improves muscle tone and power. (R)

168. **2.** The nurse's first action should be to attempt to replace the tracheostomy tube immediately so that the client's airway is reestablished. Although the nurse may also call for assistance, there should be no delay before attempting reinsertion of the tube. The client is placed in a supine position with the neck hyperextended to facilitate reentry of the tube. The obturator is inserted into the replacement tracheostomy tube to guide insertion and is then removed to allow passage of air through the tube. (R)

169. **2.** Many parents are advised to administer acetaminophen before the child receives immunizations to minimize local and systemic reactions. Typically, infants should not be very fussy after receiving immunizations. There is no reason to keep the infant out of day care that day; the child is not contagious. Although it may be helpful to the parents to have someone with them at the appointment, advising them to give the infant acetaminophen is more important. (H)

170. **1.** A general growth parameter is that the birth weight doubles in 6 months and triples in a year. Telling the mother that the baby will eat what he needs is not appropriate. The nurse needs to investigate whether the baby's weight is within the normal parameters of infant weight gain. A bottle-fed baby should not be forced to complete the bottle because this may contribute to obesity. (H)

171. **4.** The mechanism of injury is always the most critical information to obtain from a client with a musculoskeletal injury. In the event of a back injury, the mechanism of injury provides the greatest clue as to the extent of injury and the proper treatment plan. The other questions are important but will not give the critical information needed related to this specific complaint and injury. (A)

172. **3.** Mechanisms for regulating blood pressure involve cardiac output and peripheral vascular resistance. Therefore, the way to modify the client's blood pressure is to prescribe medications that alter one of these two variables. Alteration of the blood pressure is the result of the antihypertensive medication, but this answer does not explain the mechanism of action. (D)

173. **3.** Typical early signs of rheumatoid arthritis are nonspecific and not necessarily related to specific arthritic joint complaints. Common early symptoms include fatigue, anorexia, weight loss, and generalized feelings of stiffness. Joint swelling and limitation of movement usually occur as joint involvement becomes more specific. Nausea is not typically associated with the disease process but can be related to medications prescribed to treat rheumatoid arthritis. (A)

174. **2.** NPH insulin should be rolled between the palms to mix it before drawing it up; shaking it will introduce air bubbles into the solution, which can cause inaccurate dosing. (D)

175. **4.** The gene for Duchenne's muscular dystrophy is carried by women and transmitted to their male children. It involves an X-linked inheritance pattern. About one-third of new cases involve mutations. (A)

176. **4.** Because of colic-like abdominal pain, *Acute pain* is the priority nursing diagnosis. There are no data to indicate a skin problem or dehydration. Diarrhea or constipation may precede the appearance of currant-jelly stools. (A)

177. **2.** The nurse should notify the physician that the client is allergic to penicillin before giving the Kefzol. Cephalosporins are contraindicated in clients who are allergic to penicillin. Clients who are allergic to penicillin may have a cross-allergy to cephalosporins. (D)

178. **4, 5.** Buspirone is not a benzodiazepine but acts as a serotonin agonist. Serotonin is the neurotransmitter implicated in depression. BuSpar reduces symptoms of worry, apprehension, difficulty with concentration, and irritability. It is not sedating, does not cause a high, takes 1 to 6 weeks to be effective, does not cause muscle relaxation, and does not produce dependence, withdrawal, or tolerance. Full therapeutic benefit takes 3 to 6 weeks. (D)

179. **3.** The nurse should document a tearing of tissue with irregular wound edges as a laceration. A contusion or a bruise is a closed wound caused by a blunt object resulting in bleeding in underlying tissue. An abrasion is a superficial wound from a rubbing or a scraping of the surface of the skin such as from a fall. Colonization is a wound containing microorganisms. (S)

180. **1.** The major cause of relapse is noncompliance. If the client states that he's not sure he can afford to keep taking his medicines, it is a warning sign to the nurse that the client may be at risk for noncompliance. Therefore, the nurse needs to stress the need for compliance to prevent relapse. If money is a problem, a referral to a social worker may be necessary. (P)

181. **2.** The stool specimen indicates that the child has *Escherichia coli* in his stool. The nurse should institute enteric precautions, and all who come in contact with this child should observe good hand washing and gown technique to prevent the spread of infection. Restoring fluid balance is a goal of therapy, but because the dehydration is mild, oral rehydration will be the first choice for replacing fluids. The nurse should also clean and protect the anal area from irritation from diarrhea, but on an ongoing basis, not as the priority for care. It is not necessary for the family to wash all of their bed linens because only those in contact with the child are contaminated. (S)

182. **1.** Fatigue is commonly the earliest symptom of chronic heart failure; it is caused by decreased cardiac output and tissue oxygenation. Pedal edema and nocturia are symptoms of heart failure, but they occur later in the course of the condition. An irregular pulse can be a complication of heart failure, but it is not necessarily an early indication of the condition. (A)

183. **2.** Chocolate, tea, cola, and caffeine lower esophageal sphincter pressure, thereby increasing reflux. Clients do not need to eliminate spicy foods unless such foods bother them. Foods with seeds are restricted in diverticulosis. Steamed foods are encouraged to retain vitamins and decrease fat intake. (A)

184. **2.** The nurse should assess for signs and symptoms of birth asphyxia as a priority. Birth asphyxia is a common problem for small-for-gestational-age neonates because they have undeveloped chest muscles and a risk of meconium aspiration syndrome due to anoxia during labor. Iron deficiency anemia is not a typical problem for the small-for-gestational-age neonate. However, the neonate may have polycythemia due to anoxia during intrauterine life. Persistent pulmonary hypertension is a problem for preterm neonates, not small-for-gestational-age neonates. Hypoglycemia is a problem for small-for-gestational-age neonates. (R)

185. **45**

The nurse should administer 45 ml/minute. The formula is to divide 180 ml by 60 minutes, which yields 3 ml/minute; 3 ml/minute × 15 drops = 45 drops/minute. (D)

186. **3.** When introducing solid foods to infants, only one new food should be added at a time; if an allergic reaction occurs, the food allergen can be easily identified. In the absence of evidence of allergy, all foods are appropriate except mixed foods, which should be avoided to facilitate allergen identification. Infant formula is a major source of nutrition for the first year and should not be eliminated when solids are introduced. Rice cereal is usually recommended as the starter cereal, but other cereals, such as oatmeal, are also recommended. (S)

187. **3.** The most appropriate response for the nurse is to use an open-ended question that permits the client to voice feelings and concerns. The client does not need anyone's permission to cry. Asking if there is someone the nurse can call implies that the nurse is not willing to listen to the client. A closed question allows the client to say, "No," which interferes with the nurse's appropriate interventions. (P)

188. **1.** Studies have shown that decreasing sodium and increasing calcium improve such PMS symptoms as fluid retention, breast tenderness, and mood changes. (A)

189. **2.** The nurse should explain that the feeling of heat is a normal part of the process for a plaster cast. The sensation is not an indication that the cast is applying pressure to soft tissue. Keeping the cast exposed to room air helps facilitate drying and dissipate the heat. Elevating the casted leg is an appropriate action, but it does nothing to decrease heat. Administering pain medication also does not relieve the feeling of heat. (R)

190. **3.** It is recommended that a woman examine the breasts during the first week after menstruation. During this period, the breasts are least likely to be tender or swollen because the secretion of estrogen, which prepares the uterus for implantation, is at its lowest level. (H)

1. A primigravid client at 26 weeks' gestation asks the nurse what causes heartburn during pregnancy. The nurse should explain to the client that heartburn during pregnancy is usually caused by which of the following?

☐ **1.** Increased peristaltic action during pregnancy.

☐ **2.** Displacement of the stomach by the diaphragm.

☐ **3.** Decreased secretion of hydrochloric acid.

☐ **4.** Backflow of stomach contents into the esophagus.

2. A client at a follow-up appointment after having a miscarriage 2 weeks previously yells at the nurse, "How could God do this to me? I've never done anything wrong." Which of the following responses by the nurse would be most appropriate at this time?

☐ **1.** "God can handle your anger. It's okay."

☐ **2.** "I know you are angry. It's so hard to lose your baby."

☐ **3.** "It isn't God's fault. It was an accident."

☐ **4.** "You're a strong person. You will get through this."

3. A client with cancer has been advised by the physician that he should have chemotherapy. The client is concerned about chemotherapy and wants to take herbal treatments instead. The nurse's best response to the client is which of the following?

☐ **1.** "You are making a mistake and placing your life in jeopardy."

☐ **2.** "Herbal treatments are not approved by the Food and Drug Administration (FDA)."

☐ **3.** "Herbal treatments have not been researched with cancer."

☐ **4.** "Tell me about your concerns with chemotherapy."

4. A 4-year-old child is admitted for a cardiac catheterization. Which of the following is most important to include as the nurse teaches this child about the cardiac catheterization?

☐ **1.** A plastic model of the heart.

☐ **2.** A catheter that will be inserted into the artery.

☐ **3.** The parents.

☐ **4.** Other children undergoing a catheterization.

5. A client has a reddened area over a bony prominence. The nurse finds a nursing assistant massaging this area. The nurse should:

☐ **1.** Reinforce the nursing assistant's use of this intervention over the bony prominence.

☐ **2.** Explain to the nursing assistant that massage is effective because it improves blood flow to the area.

☐ **3.** Inform the nursing assistant that massage is even more effective when combined with the use of lotion.

☐ **4.** Instruct the nursing assistant that massage is contraindicated because it decreases blood flow to the area.

6. A worried mother confides in the nurse that she wants to change physicians because her infant is not getting better. The best response by the nurse is which of the following?

☐ **1.** "This doctor has been on our staff for 20 years."

☐ **2.** "I know you are worried, but the doctor has an excellent reputation."

☐ **3.** "You always have an option to change. Tell me about your concerns."

☐ **4.** "I take my own children to this doctor."

7. A breast-feeding mother with known food sensitivities is asking the nurse at the infant's well checkup what foods she should avoid in her diet. The nurse should advise her to avoid which foods? Select all that apply.

☐ **1.** Fish.

☐ **2.** Soy.

☐ **3.** Peanuts.

☐ **4.** Beef.

☐ **5.** Lamb.

8. A recently widowed, elderly male client is receiving chemotherapy. He tells the nurse that he does not like to cook for himself. A community resource for this client is:

☐ **1.** Hospice Association.

☐ **2.** Visiting Nurses' Association (VNA).

☐ **3.** Meals on Wheels.

☐ **4.** American Association of Retired Persons (AARP).

9. The nurse assists the physician in inserting a temporary pacemaker into the client. The nurse knows that it will be critical to document:

☐ **1.** The client's cardiovascular status.
☐ **2.** The client's emotional state.
☐ **3.** The type of sedation used.
☐ **4.** Pacemaker rate, type, and settings.

10. The nurse judges that the parent of a 9-month-old infant in a hip spica cast understands how to feed the child when the parent states which of the following?

☐ **1.** "I can lay my child flat and feed that way."
☐ **2.** "I'll raise my child's head up and leave the hips and legs on a pillow."
☐ **3.** "I can borrow a special feeding table to use."
☐ **4.** "It will take two of us, one to hold and one to feed."

11. The nurse is assessing a client who has had a myocardial infarction. The nurse notes the cardiac rhythm shown below. The nurse identifies this rhythm as:

☐ **1.** Atrial fibrillation.
☐ **2.** Atrial tachycardia.
☐ **3.** Premature ventricular contractions.
☐ **4.** Ventricular tachycardia.

12. The nursing staff has finished restraining a client. In addition to determining whether anyone was injured, the staff is mandated to evaluate the incident to obtain which of the following ultimate outcomes?

☐ **1.** Coordinate documentation of the incident.
☐ **2.** Resolve negative feelings and attitudes.
☐ **3.** Improve the use of restraint procedures.
☐ **4.** Calm down before returning to the other clients.

13. The nurse is caring for a client who has experienced severe multiple trauma. The client's arterial blood gases reveal low arterial oxygen levels that are not responsive to high concentrations of oxygen. The nurse is aware that this finding is a major indicator of the development of which of the following conditions?

☐ **1.** Hospital-acquired pneumonia.
☐ **2.** Hypovolemic shock.
☐ **3.** Acute respiratory distress syndrome (ARDS).
☐ **4.** Asthma.

14. A client asks the nurse why he was asked to complete an advance directive when he entered the hospital. The nurse's best response is which of the following?

☐ **1.** "This will provide a substitute for informed discussion with the physician."
☐ **2.** "It is a legal requirement for all clients entering a hospital to be offered the chance to make an advance directive."
☐ **3.** "The physician will make the best decisions for you in an emergency."
☐ **4.** "Are you worried that extraordinary means will be taken if you are dying?"

15. When witnessing the client's signature on a consent for a procedure, the nurse verifies that the consent was obtained in an appropriate manner. Which of the following is an unrealistic expectation for the nurse to verify?

☐ **1.** That there was adequate disclosure of information.
☐ **2.** That there was sufficient comprehension of information.
☐ **3.** That there was voluntary consent on the client's part.
☐ **4.** That the client has full awareness of the rehabilitation process.

16. An elderly client is diagnosed with temporal arteritis. The medication of choice is:

☐ **1.** Prednisone (Deltasone).
☐ **2.** Naproxen (Naprosyn).
☐ **3.** Aspirin.
☐ **4.** Azathioprine (Imuran).

17. A pregnant woman at 22 weeks' gestation is diagnosed with gonorrhea. The physician orders doxycycline (Vibramycin). The first action of the nurse should be to:

☐ **1.** Instruct the client about the effects of the drug.
☐ **2.** Make sure the record notes that the baby must receive eyedrops when born.
☐ **3.** Have the physician add a single dose of ceftriaxone (Rocephin).
☐ **4.** Discuss with the physician the need to change the order.

18. After a client undergoes a contraction stress test that is negative, which of the following should the nurse assess next?

☐ **1.** Evidence of ruptured membranes.
☐ **2.** Viability status of the fetus.
☐ **3.** Indications that contractions have ceased.
☐ **4.** Fetal heart rate variability.

19. An infant is at risk for an ileus after surgery to correct intussusception. Which observation should the nurse not include in an assessment for this complication?

☐ **1.** Measurement of urine specific gravity.
☐ **2.** Assessment of bowel sounds.
☐ **3.** Characteristics of the first stool.
☐ **4.** Measurement of gastric output.

20. A client with asthma asks the nurse if she should use her salmeterol (Serevent) inhaler when she exercises and experiences wheezing and shortness of breath. The nurse's best response is which of the following?

☐ **1.** "Yes, use the inhaler immediately for these symptoms."
☐ **2.** "No, this drug is a maintenance drug, not a rescue inhaler."
☐ **3.** "Use the inhaler 5 minutes before you exercise to prevent the wheezing."
☐ **4.** "This inhaler is for allergic rhinitis, not asthma."

21. Which of the following clinical manifestations should the nurse expect to find when assessing a child with the diagnosis of nephrotic syndrome? Select all that apply.

☐ **1.** Normal blood pressure.
☐ **2.** Generalized edema.
☐ **3.** Normal serum lipid levels.
☐ **4.** No red blood cells in the urine.
☐ **5.** Elevated streptococcal antibody titers.

22. A nurse is assessing a client who is receiving clozapine (Clozaril). The nurse reviews the chart below.

VITAL SIGNS

Date Time	06/12/07 8 am	06/12/07 12 noon
Temperature	98° F	98° F
Pulse	140	148
Respirations	22	24
Blood pressure	120/80	122/84

What should the nurse do next?

☐ **1.** Give the clozapine, and tell the client to lie down.
☐ **2.** Withhold the clozapine, and tell the client to go to an exercise group.
☐ **3.** Administer the clozapine, and notify the physician.
☐ **4.** Withhold the clozapine, and notify the physician.

23. A nurse is assessing a client with a history of myocardial infarction who is in the surgical unit following a gastric resection. The client complains of chest pains. The nurse obtains the electrocardiogram (ECG) below.

What should the nurse do first?

☐ **1.** Administer oxygen.
☐ **2.** Inspect the client's incision.
☐ **3.** Call the rapid response team.
☐ **4.** Reposition the ECG electrodes.

24. The nurse is watching two siblings, ages 7 and 9 years, verbally arguing over a toy. The nurse has counseled the parent before about how to handle this situation. The nurse should judge that the teaching has been effective when the parent does which of the following?

☐ **1.** Tells the siblings to stop arguing and shake hands.
☐ **2.** Ignores the arguing and continues what she is doing.
☐ **3.** Tells the children they will be punished when they go home.
☐ **4.** Says they will not go out to lunch now since they have argued.

25. A 64-year-old man is admitted with palpitations, hyperventilation, a choking sensation, and tightness in the chest. The nurse analyzes the results of arterial blood gas studies. Which of the following metabolic factors will be depleted?

☐ **1.** Sodium.
☐ **2.** Oxygen.
☐ **3.** Potassium.
☐ **4.** Carbon dioxide.

26. A client is diagnosed with genital herpes, (herpes simplex virus type 2, or HSV-2). The nurse should instruct the client that:

☐ **1.** Using occlusive ointments may decrease the pain from the lesions.
☐ **2.** Reducing stressful life events may decrease the incidence of herpetic outbreaks.
☐ **3.** There are no effective drug therapies to manage herpes symptoms.
☐ **4.** Herpes is transmitted to partners only when lesions are weeping.

27. The client is having ototoxic effects of the vestibular branch of the acoustic nerve. Which clinical manifestation would not be associated with this problem?
- [ ] **1.** Vertigo.
- [ ] **2.** Tinnitus.
- [ ] **3.** Nausea and vomiting with motion.
- [ ] **4.** Ataxia.

28. A young male client comes to the clinic with a bite he received in a fight. He has a bite mark on his forearm and the skin is broken. His last tetanus shot was about 8 years ago. What should the recommended treatment include?
- [ ] **1.** Administration of 0.5 ml of tetanus toxoid I.M.
- [ ] **2.** Application of a corticosteroid cream.
- [ ] **3.** Closure of the wound with sutures.
- [ ] **4.** Withholding medication to see if signs of infection develop.

29. A client 6 weeks postpartum is asking the nurse about taking progesterone (Depo-Provera) for birth control. Prior to discussing options, what should the nurse determine? Select all that apply.
- [ ] **1.** If the client has a sexually transmitted disease.
- [ ] **2.** How willing her husband is to have her take the drug.
- [ ] **3.** If the woman is experiencing postpartum depression.
- [ ] **4.** That the woman is not currently pregnant.
- [ ] **5.** If the woman is breast-feeding.

30. In the care and treatment of a client with heart failure, the nurse should expect the client to be taking which of the following types of drugs?
- [ ] **1.** Selective serotonin reuptake inhibitors (SSRIs).
- [ ] **2.** Nonsteroidal anti-inflammatory drugs (NSAIDs).
- [ ] **3.** Angiotensin-converting enzyme (ACE) inhibitors.
- [ ] **4.** Steroids.

31. A mother who is visibly upset tells the nurse she wants to take her child home because the child is dying. Which of the following would be the nurse's best response?
- [ ] **1.** "I know how you feel, but the medication will make your child feel better."
- [ ] **2.** "I can't let you do this without calling your physician first."
- [ ] **3.** "Can you tell me why you want to take your child home now?"
- [ ] **4.** "I can imagine how hard this is for you, but it's not what's best for the child."

32. Clients with chronic obstructive pulmonary disease may be bedridden at home and get little exercise. Which of the following is a normal physiologic reaction to prolonged periods of bed rest and inactivity?
- [ ] **1.** Increased sodium retention.
- [ ] **2.** Increased calcium excretion.
- [ ] **3.** Increased insulin use.
- [ ] **4.** Increased red blood cell production.

33. Which of the following parameters should indicate to the nurse that a 5-month-old weighing 15 pounds and being treated for dehydration has a normal urine output?
- [ ] **1.** 1 to 2 ml/kg/hour.
- [ ] **2.** 3 to 5 ml/kg/hour.
- [ ] **3.** 6 to 8 ml/kg/hour.
- [ ] **4.** 10 to 12 ml/kg/hour.

34. A 24-year-old client has been diagnosed with acute osteomyelitis in the left leg. He complains of acute pain in the leg that intensifies when he moves it. The client has a temperature of 101° F (38.3° C) and a reddened, warm area in the midcalf region over the shaft of the tibia. Based on this information, which of the following nursing diagnoses would be most appropriate for this client?
- [ ] **1.** *Grieving* related to possible left lower leg amputation.
- [ ] **2.** *Activity intolerance* related to severe left leg pain.
- [ ] **3.** *Disturbed body image* related to left leg swelling and inflammation.
- [ ] **4.** *Deficient fluid volume* related to elevated temperature of 101° F (38.3° C).

35. A client has undergone a vasectomy. The nurse instructs the client that he can begin having unprotected intercourse:
- [ ] **1.** When desired because sterilization is immediate.
- [ ] **2.** As soon as scrotal edema and tenderness resolve.
- [ ] **3.** When the sperm count reflects sterilization.
- [ ] **4.** After 6 to 10 ejaculations.

36. Long-term administration of gentamicin sulfate (Garamycin) to a client has been discontinued. The client should be instructed to have which of the following assessments?
- [ ] **1.** Hemoglobin level in 2 weeks.
- [ ] **2.** White blood cell count in 2 weeks.
- [ ] **3.** Vestibular check in 3 to 4 weeks.
- [ ] **4.** Serum potassium level in 1 week.

37. When assessing an infant diagnosed with bacterial meningitis, which findings should the nurse most likely expect? Select all that apply.
- [ ] **1.** Fever.
- [ ] **2.** Vomiting.
- [ ] **3.** Diarrhea.
- [ ] **4.** Poor feeding.
- [ ] **5.** Abdominal pain.

38. Which of the following nursing interventions would best accomplish the goal of preventing atelectasis and pneumonia in a postoperative client?
- [ ] **1.** Administer oxygen therapy as needed to maintain adequate oxygenation.
- [ ] **2.** Offer pain medication before having the client deep-breathe and use incentive spirometry.
- [ ] **3.** Encourage the client to cough, deep-breathe, and turn in bed once every 4 hours.
- [ ] **4.** Force fluids to 2,000 ml every 24 hours.

39. A 7-year-old child is admitted to the hospital with acute rheumatic fever. When discussing long-term care for the child with the parents, the nurse should teach them that a necessary part of this care is:
☐ **1.** Physical therapy.
☐ **2.** Antibiotic therapy.
☐ **3.** Psychological therapy.
☐ **4.** Anti-inflammatory therapy.

40. The nurse is assessing the perineal changes of a woman in the second stage of labor. The figure below represents which of the following perineal changes?
☐ **1.** Anterior-posterior slit.
☐ **2.** Oval opening.
☐ **3.** Circular shape.
☐ **4.** Crowning.

41. A client is admitted to the hospital with a diagnosis of suspected pulmonary embolism. Physician orders include the following: oxygen 2 to 4 L/minute per nasal cannula, oximetry at all times, and I.V. administration of 5% dextrose in water at 100 ml/hour. The client complains of increasing dyspnea and has a respiratory rate of 32 breaths/minute. What is the nurse's first response to this situation?
☐ **1.** Increase the oxygen flow rate from 2 to 4 L/minute.
☐ **2.** Call the physician immediately.
☐ **3.** Provide reassurance to the client.
☐ **4.** Obtain a sample for arterial blood gas analysis.

42. The mother of a 10-month-old child calls the nurse because her child has cold symptoms. The mother asks how she can clear the infant's nose. Which of the following would be the nurse's best recommendation?
☐ **1.** Use a cool air vaporizer with plain water.
☐ **2.** Use saline nose drops and then a bulb syringe.
☐ **3.** Blow into the child's mouth to clear the infant's nose.
☐ **4.** Administer a nonprescription vasoconstrictive nose spray.

43. A nurse is assessing a client with metastatic lung cancer. The nurse should assess the client for which condition?
☐ **1.** Diarrhea.
☐ **2.** Constipation.
☐ **3.** Hoarseness.
☐ **4.** Weight gain.

44. A client is at risk for development of metabolic alkalosis because of persistent vomiting. Which of the following symptoms is indicative of metabolic alkalosis?
☐ **1.** Irritability.
☐ **2.** Hyperventilation.
☐ **3.** Diarrhea.
☐ **4.** Edema.

45. Which of the following should first alert the nurse that a child is hemorrhaging after a tonsillectomy?
☐ **1.** Mouth breathing.
☐ **2.** Frequent swallowing.
☐ **3.** Requests for a drink.
☐ **4.** Increased pulse rate.

46. A nurse is caring for a client who is having an allergic reaction to a blood transfusion. In what order should the nurse provide care for this client?

1. Stop the transfusion.

2. Send the blood bag and blood slip to the blood bank.

3. Keep the vein open with normal saline solution.

4. Administer an antihistamine as directed.

47. The nurse is to administer chloramphenicol (Chloromycetin) 50 mg I.V. in 100 ml of dextrose 5% in water over 30 minutes. The infusion set administers 10 gtt/ml. At what flow rate (in drops per minute) should the nurse set the infusion?

_____ gtt/ml

48. A client's belief in her "special mission from God" can be referred to as a religious delusion of grandeur. The nurse incorporates this delusion into the client's plan of care based on the understanding that the primary purpose of such a delusion is to provide which of the following?
- ☐ **1.** Sexual outlet.
- ☐ **2.** Comfort.
- ☐ **3.** Safety.
- ☐ **4.** Self-esteem.

49. A client who has been vomiting for 2 days has a nasogastric tube inserted. The nurse notes that over the past 10 hours the tube has drained 2 L of fluid. The nurse should plan to implement treatment that will prevent which of the following electrolyte imbalances?
- ☐ **1.** Hypermagnesemia.
- ☐ **2.** Hypernatremia.
- ☐ **3.** Hypokalemia.
- ☐ **4.** Hypocalcemia.

50. During the clinical breast examination, which of the following is a normal finding?
- ☐ **1.** Pronounced unilateral venous pattern.
- ☐ **2.** Peau d'orange breast tissue.
- ☐ **3.** Long-term, bilateral nipple inversion.
- ☐ **4.** Breast tissue that is darker than the areolae.

51. A child with sickle cell crisis is being discharged. As part of discharge teaching to prevent further crisis, the nurse advises the parent to do which of the following?
- ☐ **1.** Encourage the child to drink lots of liquids.
- ☐ **2.** Take the child's temperature every morning.
- ☐ **3.** Weigh the child every day.
- ☐ **4.** Offer the child a high-protein diet.

52. While assessing a neonate 30 minutes after birth, the nurse observes that the child has a short neck covered with webbing. The nurse notifies the pediatrician based on the interpretation that this usually indicates which of the following?
- ☐ **1.** Genetic deviations.
- ☐ **2.** Cleft palate.
- ☐ **3.** Potter's syndrome.
- ☐ **4.** Neural tube defects.

53. In a client with severe diarrhea, the nurse should conclude that the client was experiencing hypokalemia if which of the following signs were observed?
- ☐ **1.** Muscle spasms.
- ☐ **2.** Thirst.
- ☐ **3.** Arrhythmia.
- ☐ **4.** Confusion.

54. The nurse identifies clinical manifestations of a superimposed infection when a client who has been taking an antibiotic returns to the medical clinic. Which of the following findings can be excluded when assessing for a superinfection?
- ☐ **1.** Black, hairy tongue.
- ☐ **2.** Pruritus.
- ☐ **3.** Glossitis.
- ☐ **4.** Anal itching.

55. Which of the following is the most reliable indicator of the existence and intensity of acute pain?
- ☐ **1.** The client's vital signs.
- ☐ **2.** The client's self-report of pain.
- ☐ **3.** The nurse's assessment of the client.
- ☐ **4.** The severity of the condition causing the pain.

56. The nurse advises a mother with a 2-year-old child to avoid encouraging excessive milk consumption (more than 3.5 cups per day) by the infant because excess milk consumption can lead to:
- ☐ **1.** Vitamin C deficiency.
- ☐ **2.** Iron deficiency.
- ☐ **3.** Biotin deficiency.
- ☐ **4.** Folate deficiency.

57. The nurse is caring for a client with a fracture of a long bone. Which of the following assessments would be the earliest symptom of a fat embolism?
- ☐ **1.** Respiratory distress.
- ☐ **2.** Confusion.
- ☐ **3.** Petechiae.
- ☐ **4.** Fever.

58. A client tells the nurse, "Everybody smiles at me because they know that I was chosen by God for this mission." The nurse interprets this statement as which of the following?
- ☐ **1.** Idea of reference.
- ☐ **2.** Thought insertion.
- ☐ **3.** Visual hallucination.
- ☐ **4.** Neologism.

59. The mother of a newborn is voicing concerns about her baby's ability to hear. Which of the following should the nurse include in the discussion?
- ☐ **1.** Newborns cannot hear well until they are at least 6 weeks old.
- ☐ **2.** The mother's concern is unfounded because hearing problems are rare in newborns.
- ☐ **3.** The majority of states now mandate that newborns undergo a screening test for hearing.
- ☐ **4.** The mother can test the baby's hearing by clapping her hands 24 inches from the infant's head.

60. The physician decides to change a client's current dose of I.M. meperidine hydrochloride (Demerol) to an oral dosage. The current I.M. dosage is 75 mg every 4 hours as needed. What dosage of oral meperidine will be required to provide an equivalent analgesic dose?
- ☐ **1.** 25 to 50 mg every 4 hours.
- ☐ **2.** 75 to 100 mg every 4 hours.
- ☐ **3.** 125 to 140 mg every 4 hours.
- ☐ **4.** 150 to 300 mg every 4 hours.

61. The parent asks the nurse about the major causes of brain injury in children. Which of the following should the nurse expect to include in the response as the major causes? Select all that apply.
- ☐ **1.** Falls.
- ☐ **2.** Motor vehicle accidents.
- ☐ **3.** Bicycle accidents.
- ☐ **4.** Child abuse.
- ☐ **5.** Tumors.

62. Which of the following nursing measures is most useful in preventing the development of osteoporosis in a client who is immobilized?
- ☐ **1.** Beginning weight-bearing activities as soon as possible.
- ☐ **2.** Increasing the client's calcium intake in the diet.
- ☐ **3.** Performing passive range-of-motion (ROM) exercises four times a day.
- ☐ **4.** Teaching the client to perform isometric exercises.

63. The mother of a toddler asks the nurse what she should do with her toddler when he has a temper tantrum. Which of the following suggestions would be most appropriate?
- ☐ **1.** Move the toddler to a time-out chair.
- ☐ **2.** Try to talk the toddler out of the tantrum.
- ☐ **3.** Leave the toddler alone during the tantrum as long as he is safe.
- ☐ **4.** Punish the toddler for having a temper tantrum.

64. The nurse who is stuck by a used needle but has not completed the hepatitis B immunization should receive:
- ☐ **1.** Both active and passive immunization.
- ☐ **2.** Active immunization.
- ☐ **3.** Passive immunization.
- ☐ **4.** Immunization only after a blood titer has been drawn.

65. Which of the following nursing interventions is appropriate for preventing pressure ulcers?
- ☐ **1.** Clean the skin daily using mild soap and hot water.
- ☐ **2.** Perform a systematic skin assessment at least once a day.
- ☐ **3.** Massage bony prominences gently every shift.
- ☐ **4.** Encourage the client to sit in a chair as much as possible.

66. The nurse is evaluating the pin insertion site of a client's skeletal traction. Which of the following signs and symptoms indicate a complication?
- ☐ **1.** Presence of crusts around the pin insertion site.
- ☐ **2.** Serous drainage on the dressing.
- ☐ **3.** Pin moves slightly at insertion site.
- ☐ **4.** Client does not feel pain at insertion site.

67. On the night before a 58-year-old wife and mother is to have a lobectomy for lung cancer, she remarks to the nurse, "I am so scared of this cancer. I should have quit smoking years ago. Now I've brought all this fear and sadness on myself and now my family." What would be the nurse's best response to the client?
- ☐ **1.** "It's normal to be scared. I would be, too. We'll help you through it."
- ☐ **2.** "Do you feel guilty because you smoked?"
- ☐ **3.** "Don't be so hard on yourself. You don't know if your smoking caused the cancer."
- ☐ **4.** "It's okay to be scared. What is it about cancer that you're afraid of?"

68. The nurse is caring for an elderly client who has hip pain related to rheumatoid arthritis. The nurse knows that the client is practicing appropriate self-care activities when the client chooses to sit in which of the following chairs?
- ☐ **1.** Recliner chair with arms to support wrists and hands.
- ☐ **2.** Couch with soft cushions to support thighs.
- ☐ **3.** Straight-back chair with elevated seat.
- ☐ **4.** Curved-back rocking chair.

69. The nurse is with the parents of a 16-year-old boy who recently attempted suicide. The nurse cautions the parents to be especially alert for which of the following in their son?
- ☐ **1.** Expression of a desire to date.
- ☐ **2.** Decision to try out for an extracurricular activity.
- ☐ **3.** The giving away of valued personal items.
- ☐ **4.** Desire to spend more time with his friends.

70. Which of the following responses would be most appropriate for the nurse when comforting a primiparous client whose critically ill neonate delivered at 25 weeks dies while the mother is present?
- ☐ **1.** "This is probably for the best because his organs were so immature."
- ☐ **2.** "You should try to get pregnant again soon to get over this loss."
- ☐ **3.** "You can stay with your baby as long as you want and say anything you want."
- ☐ **4.** "If you want me to, I can call the chaplain to stay with you."

71. A nurse is caring for a toddler who is assessed as having hypertonicity, delayed fine motor skills, and poor control of coordinated motion. This is indicative of what cerebral palsy (CP) classification? Select all that apply.
- [ ] **1.** Abnormal involuntary movements.
- [ ] **2.** Wormlike writhing movements.
- [ ] **3.** Poor coordination.
- [ ] **4.** Gross motor skills impairment.
- [ ] **5.** Hypertonicity.

72. A 32-year-old woman recently diagnosed with Hodgkin's disease is admitted to the hospital outpatient clinic for staging by undergoing a bone marrow aspiration and biopsy. The nurse assesses the client's nutrition status. Which of the following blood examinations would be most helpful in determining whether the client's diet lacks protein?
- [ ] **1.** Red blood cell count.
- [ ] **2.** Direct and indirect bilirubin levels.
- [ ] **3.** Reticulocyte count.
- [ ] **4.** Albumin level.

73. The nurse teaches a client taking desmopressin (DDAVP) nasal spray about how to manage treatment. The nurse determines that the client needs additional instruction when he makes which of the following comments?
- [ ] **1.** "I should check for sores in my nose while taking this medication."
- [ ] **2.** "I should use the same nostril each time I take the medicine."
- [ ] **3.** "I should report nasal congestion."
- [ ] **4.** "I should report any signs of respiratory infection."

74. The nurse has an order to administer ampicillin (Omnipen) 250 mg I.M. After reconstituting the ampicillin with sterile water for injection, the solution available is 500 mg/ml. How many milliliters should the nurse administer?

_____ ml

75. The nurse assesses a client and notes that he has a weak, irregular pulse, as well as soft, flabby muscles. These findings are indicative of which electrolyte imbalance?
- [ ] **1.** Hypercalcemia.
- [ ] **2.** Hypernatremia.
- [ ] **3.** Hypokalemia.
- [ ] **4.** Hypomagnesemia.

76. A primiparous client at 48 hours postpartum is to be given medroxyprogesterone acetate (Depo-Provera) before discharge. Which of the following should the nurse include in the teaching plan before administering this medication?
- [ ] **1.** There is an increased risk of ovarian cancer with use of this drug.
- [ ] **2.** Amenorrhea is common during the first 6 months.
- [ ] **3.** Heavy menstrual bleeding may occur.
- [ ] **4.** The client may experience periods of increased energy.

77. The nurse establishes the goal of preventing the development of a stress ulcer in a burn client. Which of the following interventions would most likely contribute to the achievement of this goal?
- [ ] **1.** Implementing relaxation exercises.
- [ ] **2.** Administering a sedative as needed.
- [ ] **3.** Providing a soft, bland diet.
- [ ] **4.** Administering famotidine (Pepcid) as ordered.

78. The parents of a child with acquired immunodeficiency syndrome (AIDS) ask the nurse how to look for signs and symptoms of infection. The nurse responds that they need to be especially alert for which of the following?
- [ ] **1.** Erythema around the infected area.
- [ ] **2.** Rectal temperature higher than 100.5° F (38° C).
- [ ] **3.** Tenderness of the infected area.
- [ ] **4.** Warmth of the infected area.

79. The nurse is teaching a group of unlicensed personnel new to psychiatry about providing care to clients with depression. To care effectively for these clients, the nurse should emphasize that caregivers demonstrate which of the following behaviors?
- [ ] **1.** Cheerful demeanor.
- [ ] **2.** Empathetic concern.
- [ ] **3.** Serious, business-like affect.
- [ ] **4.** Humorous light-heartedness.

80. When fluids by mouth are appropriate for the infant after surgery to correct intussusception, the nurse most likely would initiate feeding with:
- [ ] **1.** Cereal-thickened formula.
- [ ] **2.** Full-strength formula.
- [ ] **3.** Half-strength formula.
- [ ] **4.** Oral electrolyte solution.

81. A client is taking paroxetine (Paxil) 20 mg P.O. every morning. The nurse should monitor the client for which of the following adverse effects?
- [ ] **1.** Hypertensive crisis.
- [ ] **2.** Sexual problems.
- [ ] **3.** Sleep disturbance.
- [ ] **4.** Orthostatic hypotension.

82. The Dietary Approaches to Stop Hypertension diet includes ensuring the adequate intake of very specific nutrients. These specific nutrients include:
- [ ] **1.** Magnesium, potassium, vitamin C, and calcium.
- [ ] **2.** Vitamins B_6, B_{12}, E, and A.
- [ ] **3.** Iron, zinc, vitamin D, and vitamin K.
- [ ] **4.** Biotin, protein, riboflavin, and pantothenic acid.

83. Which of the following neurologic changes indicates that the client is in the progressive stage of shock?
- ☐ **1.** Restlessness.
- ☐ **2.** Confusion.
- ☐ **3.** Incoherent speech.
- ☐ **4.** Unconsciousness.

84. A child diagnosed with osteomyelitis will be discharged on I.V. nafcillin (Unipen). After teaching the parents about adverse effects that are important to report, which effects as stated by the parents indicate that they understand the teaching? Select all that apply.
- ☐ **1.** Sore mouth.
- ☐ **2.** Pain with urination.
- ☐ **3.** Headache.
- ☐ **4.** Stomach upset.
- ☐ **5.** Fever.

85. The code team and crash cart arrive in the room of a client who has had a cardiac arrest. What is the first piece of monitoring equipment applied to the client by the code team members?
- ☐ **1.** Electrocardiogram (ECG) electrodes.
- ☐ **2.** Pulse oximeter.
- ☐ **3.** Blood pressure cuff.
- ☐ **4.** Doppler for pulse check.

86. The nurse is talking to a group of parents about drug abuse among adolescents. One parent says he has heard that you can tell which drug a person is using by how the eyes look. The parent asks how you could tell a person was taking heroin. Which of the following should the nurse use to describe the eyes of a person using heroin?
- ☐ **1.** Whites red and bloodshot.
- ☐ **2.** Pupils small and constricted.
- ☐ **3.** Pupils large and dilated.
- ☐ **4.** Drooping eyelids.

87. When performing routine health evaluations in school-age children, which of the following would alert the school nurse to pediculosis capitis (head lice)?
- ☐ **1.** Spotty baldness.
- ☐ **2.** Wheals with scalp blistering.
- ☐ **3.** Frequent scalp scratching.
- ☐ **4.** Dry, scaly patches on the skin.

88. Which of the following best indicates that a client's peristaltic activity is returning to normal after surgery?
- ☐ **1.** The client passes flatus.
- ☐ **2.** The client says that she is hungry.
- ☐ **3.** Bowel sounds are hypoactive on auscultation.
- ☐ **4.** Peristalsis can be felt on abdominal palpation.

89. A client appears flushed and has shallow respirations. The arterial blood gas report shows the following: pH, 7.24; partial pressure of arterial carbon dioxide ($Paco_2$), 49 mm Hg; bicarbonate (HCO_3^-), 24 mEq/L. These findings are indicative of which of the following acid-base imbalances?
- ☐ **1.** Metabolic acidosis.
- ☐ **2.** Metabolic alkalosis.
- ☐ **3.** Respiratory acidosis.
- ☐ **4.** Respiratory alkalosis.

90. Which of the following measures is most important for pain management for a client after a lobectomy?
- ☐ **1.** Reposition the client immediately after administering pain medication.
- ☐ **2.** Reassess the client after administering pain medication.
- ☐ **3.** Reassure the client after administering pain medication.
- ☐ **4.** Readjust the pain medication dosage as needed.

91. The nurse is evaluating a female client's understanding of how to prevent sexually transmitted diseases (STDs). Which of the following statements indicates that the client understands how to protect herself?
- ☐ **1.** "I will be sure my partner uses a condom."
- ☐ **2.** "I need to be sure to take my birth control pills."
- ☐ **3.** "I will always douche after sexual intercourse."
- ☐ **4.** "I will be sure to take antibiotics to prevent an STD."

92. While assessing a multigravid client at 10 weeks' gestation, the nurse notes a purplish color to the vagina and cervix. The nurse documents this finding as which of the following?
- ☐ **1.** Goodell's sign.
- ☐ **2.** Chadwick's sign.
- ☐ **3.** Hegar's sign.
- ☐ **4.** Melasma.

93. A client with bipolar disorder, mania, has flight of ideas and grandiosity and becomes easily agitated. To prevent harmful behaviors, which of the following should the nurse do initially?
- ☐ **1.** Encourage the client to stay in his room.
- ☐ **2.** Seclude the client at the first sign of agitation.
- ☐ **3.** Tell the client to seek out staff when feeling agitated.
- ☐ **4.** Instruct the client to ask for medication when agitated.

94. The nurse is preparing written information for a client. Which of the following represents a sound approach to providing information?
- ☐ **1.** Use charts to help convey information.
- ☐ **2.** Prepare information at an eighth-grade reading level.
- ☐ **3.** Use short words.
- ☐ **4.** Print the material in a medium-sized type.

95. Which of the following signs or symptoms would the nurse expect to assess in a child newly diagnosed with hyperthyroidism? Select all that apply.
- ☐ **1.** Weight gain.
- ☐ **2.** Dry skin.
- ☐ **3.** Constipation.
- ☐ **4.** Rapid pulse.
- ☐ **5.** Heat intolerance.

96. A nurse is evaluating the proper use of crutches by a client who has fractured her right leg. Which statement by the client indicates that she is using the correct technique?
- ☐ **1.** "I move my left leg forward first as I swing forward on my crutches."
- ☐ **2.** "I need to increase my arm strength because my arms tingle after I use my crutches."
- ☐ **3.** "I padded the tops of my crutches so that I can lean more comfortably on my crutches."
- ☐ **4.** "I feel pressure on the palms of my hands when I am walking with my crutches."

97. Which of the following factors is a priority when evaluating discharge plans for a 68-year-old man after a lower left lobectomy for lung cancer?
- ☐ **1.** The distance the client lives from the hospital.
- ☐ **2.** Support available for assisting the client at home.
- ☐ **3.** The client's ability to do home blood pressure monitoring.
- ☐ **4.** The client's knowledge of the causes of lung cancer.

98. A primiparous client planning to breast-feed her term neonate delivered vaginally asks, "When will my 'real' milk come in?" The nurse explains to the client that after delivery breasts begin to fill with milk within which of the following periods?
- ☐ **1.** 12 hours.
- ☐ **2.** 24 hours.
- ☐ **3.** 2 to 4 days.
- ☐ **4.** 7 days.

99. The nurse is caring for an elderly, debilitated client who has been bedridden for an extended period. Which of the following is the predominant clinical finding indicating that the client has developed pneumonia?
- ☐ **1.** Fever and chills.
- ☐ **2.** Productive cough.
- ☐ **3.** Confusion.
- ☐ **4.** Pleuritic chest pain.

100. A child with rheumatic fever has polyarthritis and chorea. An echocardiogram shows swelling of the cardiac tissue. Which of the following should the nurse include in the child's plan of care?
- ☐ **1.** Explaining that the chorea will disappear over time.
- ☐ **2.** Performing neurologic checks every 4 hours until the chorea subsides.
- ☐ **3.** Promoting ambulation by administering aspirin every 4 hours.
- ☐ **4.** Keeping the child in a slightly cool environment.

101. A 19-year-old unmarried college student who is visiting the clinic and is found to be approximately 8 weeks pregnant asks, "If I have an abortion in the next 2 or 3 weeks, how will it be done?" The nurse instructs the client that at this gestational age an abortion is usually performed by which of the following techniques?
- ☐ **1.** Dilatation and curettage.
- ☐ **2.** Menstrual extraction.
- ☐ **3.** Dilatation and vacuum extraction.
- ☐ **4.** Saline induction.

102. The nurse is performing a respiratory assessment on a client who has a pleural effusion. Which of the following assessment data should the nurse anticipate finding to support this diagnosis?
- ☐ **1.** Decreased chest movement on the affected side.
- ☐ **2.** Normal bronchial breath sounds.
- ☐ **3.** Hyperresonance on percussion.
- ☐ **4.** Fever.

103. A nurse is caring for a child with intussusception. Which of the following is an expected client outcome related to the nursing diagnosis *Acute pain* related to cramping, which might be made for this child?
- ☐ **1.** The child exhibits no manifestations of discomfort.
- ☐ **2.** The child is very still.
- ☐ **3.** The child has a normal bowel movement.
- ☐ **4.** The child has not vomited in 3 hours.

104. Gentamicin sulfate (Garamycin) 25 mg I.M. has been ordered every 6 hours. Garamycin 40 mg/ml is available. The nurse should administer how many milliliters?

_____ ml

105. Assessment of a 36-year-old woman complaining of malaise and dysuria reveals a temperature of 100° F (37.4° C) and painful blisters on the outside of her vagina. The client tells the nurse she had intercourse with a new partner 5 days ago. Which of the following should the nurse suspect as most likely?
- ☐ **1.** Human immunodeficiency virus (HIV) infection.
- ☐ **2.** *Chlamydia trachomatis* infection.
- ☐ **3.** Syphilis.
- ☐ **4.** Herpes genitalis.

106. A child with leukemia fails to respond to therapy. Which of the following statements offers the nurse the best guide in making plans to assist the parents in dealing with their child's imminent death?

☐ **1.** Knowing that the prognosis is poor helps prepare relatives for the death of children.

☐ **2.** Relatives are especially grieved when a child does well at first but then declines rapidly.

☐ **3.** Trust in health personnel is most often destroyed by a death that is considered untimely.

☐ **4.** It is more difficult for relatives to accept the death of a 10-year-old than the death of a younger child whose family membership has been short.

107. The nurse is caring for a child receiving a blood transfusion. The child becomes flushed and is wheezing. What should the nurse do first?

☐ **1.** Notify the physician.

☐ **2.** Administer oxygen.

☐ **3.** Switch the transfusion to normal saline solution.

☐ **4.** Take the child's vital signs.

108. A client who states that he is allergic to penicillin has an order to receive cefazolin (Ancef). The nurse's initial response is to:

☐ **1.** Ask the client if he has taken cefazolin before.

☐ **2.** Consult with the physician or a clinical pharmacist.

☐ **3.** Administer cefazolin immediately.

☐ **4.** Observe the client closely for urticaria.

109. A client with chronic renal failure tells the nurse that her skin feels dry and is constantly itching. Based on these data, which of the following is an appropriate nursing diagnosis?

☐ **1.** *Ineffective health maintenance* related to poor hygiene.

☐ **2.** *Chronic pain* related to skin irritation.

☐ **3.** *Risk for impaired skin integrity* related to severe pruritus.

☐ **4.** *Ineffective coping* related to manifestations of chronic illness.

110. When preparing the teaching plan for a client and his family about lithium therapy, the nurse should expect to include teaching about which of the following?

☐ **1.** Maintaining an adequate sodium intake.

☐ **2.** Discontinuing sodium in the diet.

☐ **3.** Buying foods labeled "low in sodium."

☐ **4.** Increasing sodium in the diet.

111. A client who is undergoing radiation therapy develops mucositis. Which of the following interventions should be included in the client's plan of care?

☐ **1.** Increase mouth care to twice per shift.

☐ **2.** Provide the client with hot tea to drink.

☐ **3.** Promote regular flossing of teeth.

☐ **4.** Use half-strength hydrogen peroxide on mouth ulcers.

112. A parent calls the Poison Control Center because her 3-year-old has eaten 10 to 12 chewable acetaminophen tablets. What should the nurse instruct the parent to do?

☐ **1.** Give the child a large glass of milk.

☐ **2.** Give the child water with syrup of ipecac.

☐ **3.** Take the child to the emergency department.

☐ **4.** Monitor the child's respirations for 24 hours.

113. While waiting for the physician, the parent of a preschool-age child tells the nurse that the child is hyperactive and something needs to be done. Which of the following responses by the nurse would be most appropriate initially?

☐ **1.** "What makes you think your child is hyperactive?"

☐ **2.** "What do you think needs to be done ?"

☐ **3.** "How does your child behave normally?"

☐ **4.** "Why not wait and see what the doctor says?"

114. When preparing for the discharge of a newborn after surgery to correct tracheoesophageal fistula (TEF), the nurse teaches the parents about the need for long-term health care because their child has a high probability of developing which of the following?

☐ **1.** Recurrent mild diarrhea with dehydration.

☐ **2.** Esophageal stricture.

☐ **3.** Speech problems.

☐ **4.** Ulcers.

115. A young man with Hodgkin's disease has been readmitted to the hospital because of his aggressive disease that is unresponsive to multiple therapies. Death appears imminent. One goal for this client is to:

☐ **1.** Reduce feelings of isolation.

☐ **2.** Reduce fear of pain.

☐ **3.** Reduce fear of more aggressive therapies.

☐ **4.** Reduce feelings of social inadequacy.

116. A client is admitted in early active labor at 39 weeks' gestation with intact membranes. When assessing the fetal heart rate, the nurse locates the heart sounds above the client's umbilicus at midline. The nurse should suspect that the fetus is lying in which of the following positions?

☐ **1.** Cephalic.

☐ **2.** Frank breech.

☐ **3.** Face.

☐ **4.** Transverse.

117. The nurse is caring for a client who has been diagnosed with pernicious anemia. Which of the following statements by the client indicates an understanding of the treatment of pernicious anemia?

☐ **1.** "I will need to increase my dietary intake of foods that are high in vitamin B_{12}."

☐ **2.** "I will receive my first injection of vitamin B_{12} tomorrow, and I will return for a follow-up injection in 1 month."

☐ **3.** "I understand that the oral form of vitamin B_{12} is preferred because it is safer and less expensive than the injection form."

☐ **4.** "I will need to take vitamin B_{12} replacements for the rest of my life."

118. A client's 12:00 noon blood glucose concentration was inaccurately documented as 310 instead of 130. This error was not noticed until 1:00 p.m. The nurse administered the sliding scale insulin for a blood glucose of 310 instead of 130. What should the nurse do first?

☐ **1.** Notify the physician.

☐ **2.** Assess for hypoglycemia.

☐ **3.** Consult with the clinical pharmacist.

☐ **4.** Call the charge nurse.

119. An older infant who has been injured in an automobile accident has to wear a splint on the injured leg. The mother reports that the infant has become mobile even while wearing the splint. The nurse should advise the mother to do which of the following?

☐ **1.** Notify the physician immediately to adjust the treatment plan.

☐ **2.** Confine the infant to one room in the apartment.

☐ **3.** Keep the infant in the splint at night, removing it during the day.

☐ **4.** Remove any unsafe items from the area in which the infant is mobile.

120. While preparing a client for surgery, the nurse assesses for psychosocial problems that may cause preoperative anxiety. Which of the following is believed to be the most distressing fear a preoperative client is likely to experience?

☐ **1.** Fear of the unknown.

☐ **2.** Fear of changes in body image.

☐ **3.** Fear of the effects of anesthesia.

☐ **4.** Fear of being in pain.

121. A 56-year-old woman is admitted for a modified radical mastectomy. The client appears anxious and asks many questions. The nurse's best course of action is to:

☐ **1.** Tell the client as much as she wants to know and is able to understand.

☐ **2.** Delay discussing the client's questions with her until the convalescent phase of her care.

☐ **3.** Delay discussing the client's questions with her until her apprehension subsides.

☐ **4.** Explain to the client that she should discuss her questions with her physician.

122. The nurse asks the client to sign a consent form before undergoing surgery. The client indicates that he was not told about the risks of the surgical procedure. Which of the following statements by the nurse is most appropriate?

☐ **1.** "What are your concerns? I can answer any questions that you have."

☐ **2.** "You can go ahead and sign the form. I will be sure to tell the surgeon you have questions."

☐ **3.** "It is important that your questions are answered before you consent to the procedure. I will contact the surgeon."

☐ **4.** "Actually, the risks associated with this procedure are minimal. The surgeon has performed this surgery many times."

123. The nurse is assessing fetal position in a 32-year-old woman in her eighth month of pregnancy. From the figure below, the fetal position can be described as:

☐ **1.** Left occipital transverse.

☐ **2.** Left occipital anterior.

☐ **3.** Right occipital transverse.

☐ **4.** Right occipital anterior.

124. The father of an infant states that the physician told him that his child has a urinary tract infection. The father calls the clinic to ask about the signs and symptoms that he should watch out for in the future to indicate a recurrence. Which of the following should the nurse tell the father?

☐ **1.** Increased urine output and clear urine.

☐ **2.** Loss of appetite and fussiness.

☐ **3.** Feeding problems and jaundice.

☐ **4.** Fever and dysuria.

125. After teaching a mother about the neonate's positive Babinski's reflex, the nurse determines that the mother understands the instructions when she says that a positive Babinski's reflex indicates:
☐ 1. Possible partial paralysis.
☐ 2. Possible lower limb defect.
☐ 3. Immature central nervous system.
☐ 4. Possible injury to nerves that innervate the legs.

126. The nurse should instruct a client who is taking dexamethasone (Decadron) and furosemide (Lasix) to observe for signs and symptoms of hypokalemia, which include:
☐ 1. Excitability.
☐ 2. Muscle weakness.
☐ 3. Diarrhea.
☐ 4. Increased thirst.

127. A client with a suspected diagnosis of lung cancer has a bronchoscopy with biopsy. Which of the following interventions would be appropriate after the procedure?
☐ 1. Encourage the client to gargle with oral lidocaine to decrease throat irritation.
☐ 2. Monitor the client for signs of pneumothorax.
☐ 3. Administer pain medication as needed to relieve mediastinal discomfort.
☐ 4. Advise the client not to talk until the gag reflex returns.

128. A nurse is preparing to administer 500 ml of an I.V. solution to a child over 12 hours via tubing that delivers microdrips at 60 gtt/ml. At what rate should the nurse infuse the solution?

_____ gtt/minute

129. Which of the following techniques is correct when administering a subcutaneous injection?
☐ 1. Use a 1-inch needle for injection.
☐ 2. Insert the needle at a 45-degree angle to the skin.
☐ 3. Spread the skin tightly at the injection site.
☐ 4. Draw 0.2 ml of air into the syringe before administration.

130. Which of the following is a priority nursing diagnosis for the client presenting with pelvic inflammatory disease?
☐ 1. *Imbalanced nutrition: Less than body requirements.*
☐ 2. *Bathing/hygiene self-care deficit.*
☐ 3. *Acute pain.*
☐ 4. *Impaired skin integrity.*

131. After talking with the mother of a child, the nurse determines that the child has a difficult temperament. Which of the following should the nurse expect to include when developing this child's plan of care?
☐ 1. Allow the child to determine when feeding should occur.
☐ 2. Ensure that the child is fed even though crying does not occur.
☐ 3. Provide structured feeding times and bedtimes.
☐ 4. Instruct the mother to take extra safety precautions around the house.

132. Which of the following steps is appropriate for the nurse to include when giving a client a tube feeding?
☐ 1. Warm the feeding solution before administration.
☐ 2. Place the client in a left side-lying position.
☐ 3. Aspirate residual gastric contents before the feeding and discard.
☐ 4. Verify position of the tube before beginning feeding.

133. A multiparous client 48 hours postpartum who is breast-feeding tells the nurse, "I'm having a lot of cramping. This didn't happen when I nursed my first baby." Which of the following would be the nurse's best response?
☐ 1. "I will notify your doctor. It's possible there are some placental fragments remaining."
☐ 2. "I need to check your lochial flow. You may have a clot that is being dislodged."
☐ 3. "You must have gotten a heavy dose of oxytocin (Pitocin). It should wear off soon."
☐ 4. "The cramping is normal and is caused by your baby's sucking, which stimulates the release of oxytocin."

134. The mother of a child with moderate diarrhea calls the clinic to find out how to manage her child's illness. Which of the following should the nurse suggest?
☐ 1. Begin clear liquids for 24 hours.
☐ 2. Feed the child bananas, rice, applesauce, and toast.
☐ 3. Offer foods that are low in fat.
☐ 4. Continue the child's regular diet.

135. The nurse is performing routine tracheostomy care. Which of the following steps would be appropriate for the nurse to include in the performance of the procedure?
☐ 1. Remove the inner cannula every 2 hours for cleaning.
☐ 2. Secure the tracheostomy ties with a square knot.
☐ 3. Use cut gauze under the neck plate to protect the skin.
☐ 4. Suction the inner cannula on completion of the procedure.

136. What is the nurse's most appropriate response when finding a sealed container of I.V. 50% dextrose in a catch-all bin on the unit?
- ☐ **1.** Leave it where found and notify risk management.
- ☐ **2.** Send it to the pharmacy.
- ☐ **3.** File an incident report.
- ☐ **4.** Discard it in a sharps container.

137. To reduce the risk of pressure ulcer formation, which of the following activities should the nurse teach the client who is wheelchair-bound as a result of a spinal cord injury?
- ☐ **1.** Bathe daily.
- ☐ **2.** Eat a high-carbohydrate diet.
- ☐ **3.** Shift your weight every 15 minutes.
- ☐ **4.** Move from the bed to the wheelchair every 2 hours.

138. A client in the second stage of labor has had no anesthesia or analgesia. Anatomically, which of the following would be the most effective position for the client to begin pushing?
- ☐ **1.** Squatting with the body curved in a C shape.
- ☐ **2.** Side-lying while keeping the head elevated.
- ☐ **3.** In the knee-chest position while keeping the head down.
- ☐ **4.** Squatting with the back arched.

139. A client with antisocial personality disorder tells the nurse, "I punched the guy out because he deserved it and then the cops arrested me." Which of the following responses would be most helpful to the client?
- ☐ **1.** "It's wrong to punch others."
- ☐ **2.** "If you punch people out, you'll get into trouble."
- ☐ **3.** "I wouldn't do that again if I were you."
- ☐ **4.** "Don't ever do that again; you're an adult."

140. The nurse is teaching unlicensed personnel about the care of clients with self-mutilation. Which of the following, if stated by the unlicensed personnel about self-mutilation, demonstrates that the teaching has been effective?
- ☐ **1.** "It is a means of getting what the person wants."
- ☐ **2.** "It is a nonserious event that can be ignored."
- ☐ **3.** "It is a way to express anger and rage."
- ☐ **4.** "It is a form of manipulation."

141. The nurse has obtained the nursing history of a client diagnosed with hepatitis C. What would be considered a potential risk factor for acquiring hepatitis C?
- ☐ **1.** Drinking contaminated water.
- ☐ **2.** Traveling to India.
- ☐ **3.** Having a tattoo.
- ☐ **4.** Eating shellfish.

142. A client is experiencing symptoms of early alcohol withdrawal. His blood pressure is 150/85 mm Hg and his pulse is 98 bpm. The nurse should expect to administer which of the following medications?
- ☐ **1.** Lorazepam (Ativan).
- ☐ **2.** Naltrexone (ReVia).
- ☐ **3.** Methadone (Dolophine)
- ☐ **4.** Imipramine (Tofranil).

143. Which of the following diet instructions are appropriate when teaching a client in the early stages of cirrhosis about her nutritional needs? Select all that apply.
- ☐ **1.** "Limit your caloric intake so that you don't become overweight."
- ☐ **2.** "An adequate intake of protein is important to your health."
- ☐ **3.** "I encourage you to eat small, frequent meals."
- ☐ **4.** "Restrict your fluid intake to 1,000 ml/day."
- ☐ **5.** "Limit your alcohol intake to one glass of wine daily."

144. After a child returns from the postanesthesia care unit after surgery, which of the following should the nurse assess first?
- ☐ **1.** The I.V. fluid access site.
- ☐ **2.** The child's level of pain.
- ☐ **3.** The surgical site dressing.
- ☐ **4.** The functioning of the nasogastric tube.

145. A critical nursing intervention to protect a client who has received tissue plasminogen activator (t-PA) or alteplase recombinant (Activase) therapy includes:
- ☐ **1.** Using the radial artery to obtain blood gas samples.
- ☐ **2.** Maintaining arterial pressure for 10 seconds.
- ☐ **3.** Administering I.M. injections.
- ☐ **4.** Encouraging physical activity.

146. Two clients have been following low-sodium diets for several weeks. One of the clients states that his blood pressure has not changed and asks the nurse why not. The nurse should base the response on the fact that the percentage of the population that are able to lower their blood pressure through a sodium-restricted diet is only which of the following?
- ☐ **1.** 10%.
- ☐ **2.** 25%.
- ☐ **3.** 50%.
- ☐ **4.** 70%.

147. A client is admitted with acute pancreatitis. Which laboratory value is indicative of pancreatitis?
- ☐ **1.** Decreased urine amylase level.
- ☐ **2.** Increased calcium level.
- ☐ **3.** Decreased glucose level.
- ☐ **4.** Increased serum amylase and lipase levels.

148. For the client with a substance abuse problem, which of the following would be most helpful to aid the client in dealing with feelings and concerns related to alcohol and drugs?
☐ **1.** Individual therapy.
☐ **2.** Group sessions.
☐ **3.** Solitary activities.
☐ **4.** Recreation.

149. Which of the following assessment findings should the nurse expect to observe in a client with cystitis?
☐ **1.** Flank pain.
☐ **2.** Oliguria.
☐ **3.** Nausea and vomiting.
☐ **4.** Foul-smelling urine.

150. A client with acute stress disorder is telling the nurse about the tornado that leveled his house and killed his wife and baby while he was out of town on business. He states, "If only I'd been at home, I could have saved them." Which of the following responses would be most appropriate?
☐ **1.** "Don't blame yourself; you'll only feel worse."
☐ **2.** "It's not your fault; so stop feeling so guilty."
☐ **3.** "You might not have been at home."
☐ **4.** "You couldn't have prevented the tornado; it just happened."

151. On the first postpartum day, the nurse is caring for a primiparous client who has recently emigrated from Japan to the United States and speaks only a little English. The nurse observes that the client has been bottle-feeding her neonate on occasion, but most of the neonatal care is being performed by the client's mother-in-law. Which of the following actions would be most appropriate?
☐ **1.** Notify the social worker because bonding may be affected.
☐ **2.** Document the unusual maternal behavior in the client's chart.
☐ **3.** Determine whether this is a cultural practice for the client and her family.
☐ **4.** Obtain an order to make a home visit after the client's discharge.

152. A client is scheduled for a creatinine clearance test. Which one of the following preparations is appropriate for the nurse to make?
☐ **1.** Instruct the client about the need to collect urine for 24 hours.
☐ **2.** Prepare to insert an indwelling urethral catheter.
☐ **3.** Provide the client with a sterile urine collection container.
☐ **4.** Instruct the client to force fluids to 3,000 ml/day.

153. When the nurse is assessing a client's cultural adaptation, which of the following statements is *least* sensitive to the client's needs?
☐ **1.** "What are some of your favorite foods?"
☐ **2.** "Describe any health problems in your past."
☐ **3.** "Please tell me how you would like to be addressed."
☐ **4.** "Your eyes look dark; is this normal for you?"

154. After several months of taking olanzapine (Zyprexa), the client reports that he is no longer hearing voices of any kind. Which of the following would confirm that the client is developing insight into his illness?
☐ **1.** "That Zyprexa is the best medicine I have ever had."
☐ **2.** "I didn't realize how sick I could get from a chemical brain imbalance."
☐ **3.** "My mom is proud of me for staying on my medicines."
☐ **4.** "I think I may be able to get a little part-time job soon."

155. A client who is a computer operator has developed carpal tunnel syndrome. The nurse explains to the client that carpal tunnel syndrome is caused by which of the following pathophysiologic conditions?
☐ **1.** Decreased circulation to the brachial nerve.
☐ **2.** Muscle atrophy resulting from disuse.
☐ **3.** Median nerve compression.
☐ **4.** Progressive flexion contracture of the wrist.

156. In addition to milk and eggs, which of the following foods is commonly implicated in allergic reactions?
☐ **1.** Peanuts.
☐ **2.** Soy.
☐ **3.** Fish.
☐ **4.** Orange juice.

157. A client who is recovering from transurethral resection of the prostate (TURP) experiences urinary incontinence. He tells the nurse that he has decreased his fluid intake because of the incontinence. What would be the nurse's best response to the client?
☐ **1.** "Yes, limiting your fluids can decrease your incontinence."
☐ **2.** "Limiting your fluids will cause kidney stones."
☐ **3.** "Drink eight glasses of water a day and urinate every 2 hours."
☐ **4.** "If your incontinence continues, we will reinsert your catheter."

158. An infant has surgery to correct a tracheoesophageal fistula. The most appropriate nursing diagnosis for the nurse to identify after surgery is:
☐ **1.** *Risk for infection.*
☐ **2.** *Acute pain.*
☐ **3.** *Constipation.*
☐ **4.** *Impaired physical mobility.*

159. The nurse teaches girls age 10 to 12 about self-care during menses. The nurse emphasizes that a risk factor for toxic shock syndrome (TSS) is:
- ☐ **1.** Changing tampons every 3 hours.
- ☐ **2.** Avoiding use of deodorized tampons.
- ☐ **3.** Alternating tampons with sanitary pads.
- ☐ **4.** Using only tampons at night.

160. A client with a history of cystitis is admitted to the hospital with a diagnosis of pyelonephritis. Which of the following assessment findings specifically supports a diagnosis of pyelonephritis?
- ☐ **1.** Suprapubic pain.
- ☐ **2.** Dysuria.
- ☐ **3.** Urine retention.
- ☐ **4.** Costovertebral tenderness.

161. A woman is taking oral contraceptives. The nurse teaches the client that medications that may interfere with oral contraceptive efficacy include:
- ☐ **1.** Antihypertensives.
- ☐ **2.** Antibiotics.
- ☐ **3.** Diuretics.
- ☐ **4.** Antihistamines.

162. A 28-year-old female client is prescribed danazol (Danocrine) for endometriosis. Which of the following should the nurse include as an adverse effect when teaching the client about the drug?
- ☐ **1.** Headaches.
- ☐ **2.** Weight loss.
- ☐ **3.** Increased libido.
- ☐ **4.** Hair loss.

163. To which of the following unlicensed personnel should the nurse assign a male client of Mexican American descent who needs complete morning care?
- ☐ **1.** Mary, who has two complete morning care clients.
- ☐ **2.** Joe, who has one complete morning care client.
- ☐ **3.** Jill, who has four partial morning care clients.
- ☐ **4.** Jim, who has five partial morning care clients.

164. A client with chronic renal failure is experiencing central nervous system changes caused by uremic toxins. Which nursing intervention would be *most* appropriate for addressing the changes?
- ☐ **1.** Allow the client to grieve for body image changes.
- ☐ **2.** Restrict foods that are high in potassium.
- ☐ **3.** Restrict fluid intake to 1,000 ml/day.
- ☐ **4.** Assess the client's mental status regularly.

165. The nurse is preparing to give a subcutaneous injection to an elderly, emaciated client. Which needle length and angle should the nurse plan to use to administer the injection safely?
- ☐ **1.** A ⅜-inch needle at a 90-degree angle.
- ☐ **2.** A ⅝-inch needle at a 45-degree angle.
- ☐ **3.** A ½-inch needle at a 15-degree angle.
- ☐ **4.** A ⅝-inch needle at a 90-degree angle.

166. A young female client comes into the emergency department with complaints of flank pain, dysuria, urinary frequency, burning on urination, and malaise. The nurse obtains a urine specimen because the nurse anticipates that the client's symptoms are related to:
- ☐ **1.** Pelvic inflammatory disease.
- ☐ **2.** Renal calculi.
- ☐ **3.** Urinary tract infection.
- ☐ **4.** Renal failure.

167. A multigravid client at 38 weeks' gestation is admitted to the hospital's birthing center with dark, scant vaginal bleeding and abdominal pain. The nurse observes frequent low-amplitude uterine activity while the client's contraction pattern is externally monitored. Which of the following should the nurse suspect?
- ☐ **1.** Abruptio placentae.
- ☐ **2.** Placenta accreta.
- ☐ **3.** Placenta previa.
- ☐ **4.** Battledore placenta.

168. A female client is treated for trichomoniasis with metronidazole (Flagyl). The nurse instructs the client that:
- ☐ **1.** The medication should not alter the color of the urine.
- ☐ **2.** She should discontinue oral contraceptive use during this treatment.
- ☐ **3.** She should avoid alcohol during treatment and for 24 hours after completion of the drug.
- ☐ **4.** Her partner does not need treatment.

169. A client is in the advanced stages of osteoarthritis. Which of the following best describes the pain that occurs in the advanced stage of the disease?
- ☐ **1.** Pain occurs with minimal activity.
- ☐ **2.** Crepitation develops and intensifies pain.
- ☐ **3.** Joints are symmetrically affected by pain.
- ☐ **4.** Fatigue accompanies pain.

170. A family may request to have a client of Vietnamese descent transferred to die at home because it is traditionally believed that:
- ☐ **1.** It is disloyal to leave their loved one in the hospital.
- ☐ **2.** The hospital cannot be trusted.
- ☐ **3.** The family can provide more comfort at home.
- ☐ **4.** Reincarnation will not occur in the hospital.

171. A client has just been admitted with acute delirium of unknown etiology. The client's daughter states that she is worried about her mom because she has never been this sick before. Which of the following should be the most helpful statement to make to the daughter?

☐ 1. "Please don't worry. We will take good care of your mother."

☐ 2. "The doctor will order tests to find out what is causing her condition."

☐ 3. "We can help you learn how to take care of her after she is discharged."

☐ 4. "It helps if you avoid arguing when she talks about seeing people who aren't there."

172. A client with Alzheimer's dementia is going to live with his daughter who does not work outside of the home. The nurse evaluates that the daughter needs further education when she makes which of the following statements?

☐ 1. "I've put special locks on all the doors that Dad won't be able to unlock."

☐ 2. "Dad said that what he missed most while he was here was using his aftershave."

☐ 3. "Dad will be in a bedroom that has nothing for him to trip over getting to the bathroom."

☐ 4. "I've taken the knobs off of the stove so he won't be able to turn it on."

173. Allopurinol (Zyloprim) is prescribed for a client who has chronic gout. Which of the following comments indicates that the client understands how to take the allopurinol?

☐ 1. "I will take the medication whenever my joints hurt."

☐ 2. "I must take this drug on an empty stomach."

☐ 3. "I should drink plenty of fluids when taking allopurinol."

☐ 4. "I should not take aspirin when taking allopurinol."

174. A client complains of severe vulvar itching. The nurse recognizes that a client with candidiasis (*Candida albicans* infection) has a vaginal discharge that is:

☐ 1. Yellow-green in color.

☐ 2. Thick and white.

☐ 3. Fishy smelling.

☐ 4. Purulent.

175. The next-door neighbor of a nurse comes over to say that her toddler just got burned on the arm. The nurse should advise the mother to *first:*

☐ 1. Pack the arm in ice, then take the child to the closest emergency department.

☐ 2. Rub the burned area with an antibacterial ointment, then call the doctor.

☐ 3. Run cool water over the burned area, then wrap it in a clean cloth.

☐ 4. Call the child's health care provider immediately, then wrap the arm in a clean cloth.

176. The nursing assessment of a client with osteomyelitis of the left great toe reveals pain with partial weight-bearing, unsteady gait, and complaints of general weakness. Based on these data, the priority nursing diagnosis for the client is:

☐ 1. *Impaired physical mobility.*

☐ 2. *Impaired skin integrity.*

☐ 3. *Ineffective coping.*

☐ 4. *Risk for injury.*

177. A client receiving a blood transfusion begins to complain of chills and headache within the first 15 minutes of the transfusion. Based on these data, what should be the nurse's first response to the client's complaints?

☐ 1. Administer acetaminophen.

☐ 2. Take the client's blood pressure.

☐ 3. Discontinue the transfusion.

☐ 4. Check the infusion rate of the blood.

178. A 72-year-old client is referred for counseling. During the initial nursing assessment, the client denies the need for counseling. The nurse would agree with the client if she made which of the following comments?

☐ 1. "My doctor just put me on an antidepressant, and I'll be fine in a week or so."

☐ 2. "My daughter sent me here. She's mad because I don't have the energy to take care of my grandkids."

☐ 3. "Since I've gotten over the death of my husband, I've had more energy and been more active than before he died."

☐ 4. "My son got worried because I made this silly comment about wanting to be with my husband in heaven."

179. A client takes isosorbide dinitrate (Isordil) as an antianginal medication. Which of the following statements indicates that the client understands the adverse effects of the drug?

☐ 1. "I should take my pulse before taking the medication."

☐ 2. "I should take Isordil with food."

☐ 3. "I will need to change positions slowly so I won't get dizzy."

☐ 4. "It is important that I report any swelling in my ankles."

180. The nurse is working on discharge plans with a client who is diagnosed with intermittent explosive disorder, characterized by sudden angry outbursts. The nurse determines that the client is ready for discharge when he makes which of the following comments?
- [ ] 1. "I'm just not going to let myself get angry anymore."
- [ ] 2. "Drinking doesn't help, but I like being with my buddies at the bar."
- [ ] 3. "I'll be taking valproic acid (Depakote) and propranolol (Inderal) to help stay in control."
- [ ] 4. "It would help if my mom would stop getting on my case all the time."

181. The nurse walks into a client's room to administer the 9:00 a.m. medications and notices that the client is in an awkward position in bed. What is the nurse's first action?
- [ ] 1. Ask the client his name.
- [ ] 2. Check the client's name band.
- [ ] 3. Straighten the client's pillow behind his back.
- [ ] 4. Give the client his medications.

182. Which of the following is an expected outcome for a client 24 hours after an abdominal hysterectomy?
- [ ] 1. Bowel sounds will be heard on auscultation.
- [ ] 2. The perineal pad will have a minimal amount of serous drainage.
- [ ] 3. The client will express feelings of a positive body image.
- [ ] 4. The client will perform leg exercises hourly.

183. A client has been prescribed furosemide (Lasix) 80 mg twice daily. The cardiac monitor technician informs the nurse that the client has started having rare premature ventricular contractions followed by runs of bigeminy lasting 2 minutes. During the assessment, the nurse determines that the client is asymptomatic and has stable vital signs. Which of the following actions should the nurse perform next?
- [ ] 1. Call the physician.
- [ ] 2. Check the client's potassium level.
- [ ] 3. Summon the nurse-manager.
- [ ] 4. Administer potassium.

184. During a home visit 3 weeks after delivery of a term neonate, a primiparous client tells the nurse that she has had tremendous mood swings, uncontrollable crying, loss of energy, and no appetite. Based on an analysis of the client's assessment findings, which of the following should the nurse suspect?
- [ ] 1. Postpartum blues.
- [ ] 2. Postpartum depression.
- [ ] 3. Postpartum psychosis.
- [ ] 4. Normal postpartum adjustment.

185. After a child with leukemia dies, the mother asks the nurse, "What if we had brought her in when she first complained of an earache?" Which of the following would be the nurse's best response to the mother?
- [ ] 1. Explain that nothing could have helped the child.
- [ ] 2. Provide comfort by saying that the child is no longer suffering with an incurable illness.
- [ ] 3. Reassure the mother that all possible care was given.
- [ ] 4. Explain that infections are often the result of leukemia rather than the cause of it.

186. The nurse has received the following information from unlicensed assistive personnel about various clients. Which of the following clients should the nurse assess immediately?
- [ ] 1. A postoperative client who has a temperature of 100° F (37.8° C).
- [ ] 2. A client who had transurethral resection of the prostate (TURP) and complains of bladder spasms with 60 ml of urine output from his catheter.
- [ ] 3. A client with an ileal conduit who has a urinary appliance pouch that is one-third full of urine.
- [ ] 4. A client recovering from a bronchoscopy with a biopsy who expectorates a small amount of bloody sputum.

187. The physician orders 500 ml of dextrose 5% in water to be administered over 10 hours. Using a microdrip administration set, the nurse should adjust the I.V. flow rate to how many drops per minute?

_____ gtt/minute

188. A client who had been taking phenelzine (Nardil) is being switched to fluoxetine (Prozac) by the physician. Which of the following facts should the nurse emphasize with the client?
- [ ] 1. The client must wait 14 days before he can start taking fluoxetine (Prozac).
- [ ] 2. The client must have his blood levels drawn every week while taking fluoxetine (Prozac).
- [ ] 3. The client must notify his physician before taking any over-the-counter medication.
- [ ] 4. The client must report headache and nausea to the physician immediately.

189. The nurse should evaluate that a client is coughing effectively after surgery if the nurse observes which of the following activities?
- [ ] 1. The client breathes through her nose, holds her breath, and then exhales slowly before coughing.
- [ ] 2. The client takes short, panting breaths and coughs from the throat to expectorate sputum.
- [ ] 3. The client takes a deep abdominal breath and then "huff" coughs three or four times.
- [ ] 4. The client takes three deep breaths and then coughs forcefully.

190. A 14-year-old nulligravid client with no history of prenatal care is admitted to the birthing unit in active labor. On admission, the client's cervix is dilated to 9 cm, completely effaced, at 1 + station. The client is thrashing in the bed, screaming and crying, and tells the nurse, "Do something for the pain!" Which of the following should the nurse do first?

- ☐ **1.** Tell the client to calm down immediately.
- ☐ **2.** Tell the client to breathe deeply with each contraction.
- ☐ **3.** Get the client's attention by looking her in the eyes.
- ☐ **4.** Call the physician for an order for analgesia.

Correct Answers and Rationales

The letter in parentheses after each rationale identifies the client need addressed in the item, including management of care (M), safety and infection control (S), health promotion and maintenance (H), psychosocial adaptation (P), basic care and comfort (C), pharmacological and parenteral therapies (D), reduction of risk potential (R), and physiological adaptation (A).

1. 4. Heartburn is caused when stomach contents enter the distal end of the esophagus, producing a burning sensation. To avoid heartburn during pregnancy, the client should avoid spicy foods; eat smaller, more frequent meals; and avoid lying down after eating. Peristalsis usually decreases during the latter half of pregnancy. Displacement of the stomach by the uterus, not the diaphragm, may contribute to heartburn. Increased, not decreased, secretion of hydrochloric acid also contributes to heartburn during pregnancy. (C)

2. 2. Acknowledging the anger and its source encourages communication about the client's feelings. Although anger at God is common after a loss, the client is displacing the anger that she needs to deal with more directly. Telling the client that the miscarriage was an accident or that she is a strong person and will get through this ignores the client's feelings of anger and loss, thereby cutting off communication. (P)

3. 4. Asking the client to speak about his concerns encourages open discussion. Telling the client that he is making a mistake is judgmental of the client's wishes and eliminates opportunities for the client to explore the situation and discuss various treatment options. Saying that herbal treatments have not been approved by the FDA or that they have not been researched is irrelevant, places a value judgment on the client's wishes, and provides no opportunity for discussion. (M)

4. 3. The most important aspect of teaching a preschooler is to have the family members there for support. Preschoolers are able to understand information that is individualized to their level. Including a plastic model of the heart and a catheter as part of the preoperative preparation may be helpful. The other family members will understand the heart model and catheter better than the preschooler will. (R)

5. 4. Massaging an area that is reddened due to pressure is contraindicated because it further reduces blood flow to the area. In the past, massaging reddened areas was thought to improve blood flow to the area, and some nursing personnel may still believe that massaging the area is effective in preventing pressure ulcer formation. (M)

6. 3. Asking the mother to talk about her concerns acknowledges the mother's rights and encourages open discussion. The other responses negate the parent's concerns. (M)

7. 1, 3. The breast-feeding mother is encouraged to avoid potentially allergic foods, such as fish and peanuts, during the first several months. (H)

8. 3. The Meals on Wheels program delivers meals to clients once a day in their homes. In addition to the improved nutrition, it is commonly valued as a means to check on elderly persons who live alone. Hospice care involves daily needs for the terminally ill at home. VNA provides skilled nursing care to clients at home. AARP is a national organization for retired people, not a health care organization. (M)

9. 1. The cardiovascular status of the client is the first information documented, and will validate the effectiveness of the temporary pacemaker. The client's emotional state and the type of sedation are important but not a high priority. The nurse will need to document the pacemaker information (settings of the pacemaker); this will be considered part of the cardiovascular information. (A)

10. 3. Using a special feeding table or modified high chair is the best method for an infant who is used to sitting up for feedings. The child should not be flat because of the danger of aspiration. Raising the child's head will not work as well as using a feeding table because the child is not used to lying down to eat. Two people are not necessary. (H)

11. 4. Ventricular tachycardia is recognized by a wide QRS complex; the rhythm may be regular or irregular. The P waves, if observed, are not related to the QRS complex. Ventricular tachycardia is a major arrhythmia and must be treated immediately. (A)

12. **3.** Although coordinating documentation, resolving negative feelings, and calming down are goals of debriefing after a restraint, the ultimate outcome is to improve restraint procedures. (P)

13. **3.** ARDS frequently develops after a major insult to the body. The major diagnostic indicator is low arterial oxygen levels that are not responsive to the administration of high concentrations of oxygen. Early recognition of ARDS is important to increase the client's chances of recovery. The oxygen levels of clients with hospital-acquired pneumonia, hypovolemic shock, or asthma would be expected to improve with oxygen administration. (A)

14. **2.** By federal law, all clients entering a hospital or hospice program are offered the chance to make an advance directive, so that their wishes will be known and followed in an emergency. The directive is not a substitute for informed discussion with the physician. Worry about extraordinary means being taken can be discussed with the client later, but the client needs to be informed that the directive is a federal requirement to protect the client's autonomy. (M)

15. **4.** The role of the nurse in witnessing the signing of the consent is not to witness that the client is fully aware of the rehabilitation process. The nurse's role is to witness that the client is informed of the procedure, understands the information, and is signing of his or her own free will. (M)

16. **1.** Temporal arteritis, commonly seen in the elderly, can result in blindness if not treated quickly with steroids. The dose is individualized and depends on the elevation of the sedimentation rate. The client may need to take steroids for several weeks to months. Naproxen and aspirin may be used to treat headaches. Azathriopine is used to prevent rejection of transplanted organs. (D)

17. **4.** Doxycycline is contraindicated in pregnancy because it can stain the teeth of the developing fetus when given during the last half of pregnancy. The nurse should withhold the drug and notify the physician to change the order. All neonates are given prophylactic ophthalmic ointment for the prevention of ophthalmic neonatorum, conjunctivitis caused by gonorrhea. Naprosyn and aspirin may be used to treat headaches. Imuran is used to prevent rejection of transplanted organs. (D)

18. **3.** The contraction stress test simulates labor and determines the fetal response to the labor process and the mother's contractions. Therefore, determining that contractions have ceased after the test is important. Although spontaneous rupture of membranes is a possibility after a contraction stress test, it is not a typical occurrence. The test should not affect the viability of the fetus. Fetal viability is related to gestational age. A fetus of at least 23 weeks' gestation is considered viable, or capable of extrauterine life. A negative contraction stress test should not affect or alter fetal heart rate variability. (R)

19. **1.** A postoperative ileus is a functional obstruction of the bowel. Assessment of bowel sounds, the first stool, and the amount of gastric output provide information about the return of gastric function. Measurement of urine specific gravity provides information about fluid and electrolyte status. (R)

20. **2.** Salmeterol (Serevent) is a beta$_2$-agonist, a maintenance drug that the asthmatic client uses twice daily, every 12 hours. Albuterol (Proventil) is used as the "rescue inhaler" for bronchospasms. Serevent can be used to prevent exercise-induced bronchospasms, but it should be taken 30 to 60 minutes before exercise. If the client is taking Serevent twice daily, it should not be used in additional doses before exercise; twice daily is the maximum dosage. Indications for Serevent include only asthma and bronchospasm induced by chronic obstructive pulmonary disease. (D)

21. **1, 2, 4.** Nephrotic syndrome is characterized by massive proteinuria, hypoalbuminemia, edema, and hyperlipidemia and normal or lower than normal blood pressure. Elevated streptococcal antibody titers are associated with poststreptococcal glomerulonephritis, an immune complex disease. (A)

22. **4.** Because clozapine can cause tachycardia, the nurse should withhold the medication if the pulse rate is greater than 140 bpm and notify the physician. Giving the drug or telling the client to exercise could be detrimental to the client. (D)

23. **3.** The client has ventricular fibrillation, an arrhythmia that can lead to cardiac arrest. Given the client's history, the nurse should call the rapid response team to initiate interventions to avoid cardiac arrest. After calling the team, the nurse can administer oxygen. Taking time to inspect the incision delays the necessary intervention. This ECG strip does not show loose electrodes. (M)

24. **2.** The best approach by the mother is not to interfere. The children need to learn how to solve disagreements on their own. If the parent always intervenes, then the children do not learn how to do this. Siblings will disagree and argue as part of normal development. Punishment, including telling the children that they will not go out to lunch, is not warranted. (H)

25. **4.** Hyperventilation causes the excessive loss of carbon dioxide. This results in a decreased carbonic acid content of the blood. The kidneys will try to compensate by eliminating bicarbonate to maintain a normal ratio of carbonic acid to bicarbonate, but this takes several days. If compensatory efforts are insufficient, the client will develop respiratory alkalosis. Hyperventilation does not deplete oxygen levels. Arterial blood gas studies do not evaluate sodium or potassium levels. (A)

26. 2. Managing stressful life events can decrease the incidence of outbreaks of HSV-2. Occlusive ointments should not be applied. Antiviral therapies will not cure herpes, but they can manage symptoms and decrease the incidence of outbreaks. Clients with HSV-2 should use condoms to prevent HSV transmission. Cells can be shed at other times, not only when the vesicles are weeping. (A)

27. 2. Tinnitus, or a ringing in the ears, is a clinical manifestation of altered function of the auditory branch of the eighth cranial nerve, not the vestibular branch. Ototoxic adverse effects affecting the vestibular branch of the acoustic nerve include vertigo, nausea and vomiting with motion, and ataxia. (D)

28. 1. Tetanus toxoid is indicated, since there has been no booster in the last 5 years. With a human bite there is a risk of severe infection. Application of a steroid cream does not prevent infection. The closure of the wound should be delayed until it is determined that there is no infection, in approximately 24 to 48 hours. (D)

29. 3, 4, 5. Before discussing the use of Depo-Provera as a birth control option, the nurse should determine if the woman is or has been depressed because Depo-Provera can increase depression in a client with depression. The drug can be transmitted in breast milk, and the long-term effects on the baby are not known. Women who are pregnant should not take Depo-Provera. Depo-Provera does not treat or prevent sexually transmitted diseases, so this information is not essential when considering its use. Although the husband should be a part of birth control decisions, the final decision is made by the client. (D)

30. 3. The benefits of ACE inhibitors in the treatment of all stages of heart failure have been well documented. ACE inhibitors are useful in systolic and diastolic failure and are the first-line therapy. Examples of ACE inhibitors include captopril (Capoten), benazepril (Lotensin), and enalapril (Vasotec). SSRIs are used to treat depression. Steroids and NSAIDs are not used to treat heart failure. (D)

31. 3. With a parent who is visibly upset, it is best to try to determine the cause. Therefore, asking the mother about why she wants to take the child home can provide insight into the problem. The nurse cannot stop the mother from taking her child home. However, the physician should be notified about the mother's decision and efforts are needed to explain the ramifications of taking the child home. It is inappropriate for the nurse to say "I know how you feel" or "I can imagine how hard this is" unless the nurse has had the same experience. (P)

32. 2. Prolonged inactivity causes the body to excrete excessive calcium. This leads to breakdown of bone tissue; as a result, the bones become brittle and fracture easily, a condition known as osteoporosis. The excessive calcium excretion that occurs during bed rest also predisposes the client to formation of renal calculi. Prolonged bed rest does not increase sodium retention, insulin use, or red blood cell production. (A)

33. 1. Normal urine output for an infant is 1 to 2 ml/kg/hour. (A)

34. 2. Based on the data given, the most appropriate nursing diagnosis is *Activity intolerance* related to severe left leg pain. The other diagnoses are not supported by the data presented. There is no clinical indication that the leg will need to be amputated or that the client is experiencing a disturbance in body image. A temperature of 101° F (38.3° C) would be unlikely to produce a fluid volume deficit in this client. (A)

35. 3. After vasectomy, a sperm analysis will be performed every 4 to 6 weeks. A sperm-free analysis is necessary before the man can be considered sterile. Sperm gradually disappear from the ejaculate. Clients must be informed that conception is possible in the immediate postvasectomy period. (A)

36. 3. Gentamicin (Garamycin) is ototoxic; therefore, the client should have a vestibular and auditory check 3 to 4 weeks after discontinuing the drug. This is the most likely time for deafness to occur. It is not necessary to check the client's hemoglobin level, white blood cell count, or serum potassium level solely on the basis of having taken gentamicin. The blood urea nitrogen level and the creatinine level will be checked to assess renal function, if necessary. (D)

37. 1, 2, 4. Classic signs of meningitis in an infant include fever, poor feeding, vomiting, and irritability. Abdominal pain and diarrhea are not usual signs of meningitis; they are more commonly associated with gastroenteritis. (A)

38. 2. Deep-breathing exercises and use of incentive spirometry are more effective when pain is minimal. A client in severe pain tends to limit movement and to breathe shallowly to decrease the pain. Enough pain medication should be given to decrease pain without depressing respirations. Administration of oxygen or forcing fluids will not prevent atelectasis or pneumonia. Deep-breathing exercises and use of incentive spirometry should be done 10 times every hour while awake. The client's position should be changed every 1 to 2 hours to allow for full chest expansion. Ambulation, not just sitting in the chair, should be implemented as soon as physician approval is obtained. (R)

39. **2.** A child who has had rheumatic fever is likely to develop the illness again after a future streptococcal infection. Therefore, it is advised that the child receive antibiotic prophylaxis for at least 5 years and sometimes even longer after the acute attack to prevent recurrence. (A)

40. **4.** Crowning occurs when the fetal head is visible. Anterior-posterior slit occurs as the perineum flattens and is followed by an oval opening. As labor progresses, the perineum takes on a circular shape, followed by crowning. (A)

41. **1.** The first action is to increase the oxygen flow rate from 2 to 4 L/minute to help ensure adequate oxygenation for the client. Although it is important to notify the physician for additional orders and to obtain further assessment data, such as arterial blood gas measurements, it is a priority to support the client's cardiopulmonary system. It would be appropriate to reassure the client while these other interventions are occurring. (R)

42. **2.** Although a cool air vaporizer may be recommended to humidify the environment, using saline nose drops and then a bulb syringe before meals and at nap and bed times will allow the child to breathe more easily. Saline helps to loosen secretions and keep the mucous membranes moist. The bulb syringe then gently aids in removing the loosened secretions. Blowing into the child's mouth to clear the nose introduces more organisms to the child. A nonprescription vasoconstrictive nasal spray is not recommended for infants because if the spray is used for longer than 3 days a rebound effect with increased inflammation occurs. (R)

43. **3.** Hoarseness may indicate metastatic disease to the recurrent laryngeal nerve and is commonly noted with left upper lobe lung tumors. Diarrhea and constipation are not associated with lung cancer. Weight loss, not weight gain, can be a symptom of extensive disease. (A)

44. **1.** A client with metabolic alkalosis may exhibit irritability or nervousness. Hyperventilation is a clinical manifestation of respiratory alkalosis. Diarrhea is a possible clinical finding in metabolic acidosis. Edema is not specifically associated with an acid-base imbalance. (A)

45. **2.** An initial sign of hemorrhaging after a tonsillectomy is swallowing frequently as mucus and blood combine to increase secretions. Mouth breathing is expected after surgery because the child's mouth is very dry and the throat is sore. Because the child has been without fluids for some time, the child usually is thirsty and asks for a drink. Increased pulse rate is a later sign of hemorrhage. (R)

46.

1. Stop the transfusion.
3. Keep the vein open with normal saline solution.
4. Administer an antihistamine as directed.
2. Send the blood bag and blood slip to the blood bank.

The nurse should first stop the transfusion. The nurse should next keep the I.V. open at the original blood transfusion site with normal saline at a keep-vein-open rate. Then, the nurse should administer an antihistamine. Last, the nurse should return the blood bag and blood slip to the blood bank for testing. (D)

47. **33**

The flow rate is determined by the rate of infusion and the number of drops per milliliter of the fluid being administered: gtt/ml × ml/minute = I.V. flow rate (gtt/minute).

Therefore:

10 gtt/ml × 100 ml/30 minutes = 33 gtt/minute.

(D)

48. **4.** Delusions of grandeur provide the client with an exaggerated sense of self-esteem that is unrelated to the client's actual achievements. Other, less grandiose, religious delusions may provide comfort or meaning for the client. Delusions of persecution are frequently related to safety issues. Delusions may also be related to sexual issues. (P)

49. **3.** Loss of electrolytes from the gastrointestinal tract through vomiting, diarrhea, or nasogastric suction is a common cause of potassium loss, resulting in hypokalemia. Hypermagnesemia does not result from excessive loss of gastrointestinal fluids. Common causes of hypernatremia are water loss (as in diabetes insipidus or osmotic diuresis) and excessive sodium intake. Common causes of hypocalcemia include chronic renal failure, elevated phosphorus concentration, and primary hypoparathyroidism. (A)

50. **3.** It is a normal variation for women to have long-term, bilateral nipple inversion. A woman who has a unilateral nipple inversion that is a new change is at risk for a tumor; the weight of the tumor causes pulling on the nipple. A pronounced unilateral venous pattern, peau d'orange breast tissue, and breast tissue darker than the areolae are definite warning signals for breast cancer that must be reported to the physician immediately. (H)

51. **1.** It is important for children with sickle cell disease to drink lots of fluids to help prevent a crisis. Dehydration precipitates sickling and a crisis. Although taking the child's temperature may provide information about the child's status, it will do nothing to prevent a crisis, nor will weighing the child daily. Offering the child a high-protein diet will not prevent a crisis, nor is it recommended. (R)

52. **1.** The nurse notifies the pediatrician because a short, webbed neck is associated with genetic deviations or chromosomal disorders such as Turner's syndrome. Cleft palate is associated with embryonic developmental failures and an abnormal opening in the palate. Potter's syndrome (renal agenesis) is characterized by an atypical facial appearance consisting of a flat nose, recessed chin, epicanthal folds, low-set abnormal ears, limb abnormalities, and pulmonary hypoplasia. Neural tube defects are associated with spina bifida or myelomeningocele. (A)

53. **3.** Clinical manifestations of hypokalemia include an irregular pulse, fatigue, muscle weakness, flabby muscles, decreased reflexes, nausea, vomiting, and ileus. Muscle spasms are not seen in hypokalemia. Thirst is a symptom of hypernatremia. Confusion can be seen in hyponatremia and hypocalcemia. (A)

54. **2.** Pruritus, or skin itching, is not one of the assessment findings associated with a superinfection, which is a new infection caused by microorganisms different from the ones causing the initial infection. A black, hairy tongue; glossitis; and anal itching are manifestations of a superinfection. (A)

55. **2.** The client's self-report of pain is the most reliable indicator of the existence and intensity of the pain. Client response to pain is highly individualized and subjective. The nurse must respect the client's self-report. (A)

56. **2.** Excessive milk consumption can lead to the displacement of iron-rich foods in the diet. This can result in iron deficiency anemia. Drinking excess milk will not cause vitamin C, biotin, or folate deficiencies. (H)

57. **2.** Although all the symptoms listed can occur in cases of fat embolism syndrome, confusion is the earliest symptom noted. The confusion is caused by a low arterial oxygen level. (A)

58. **1.** An idea of reference is a person's view that other people recognize that she has an important characteristic or power. Thought insertion refers to a person's belief that others, or a specific other, can put thoughts into her mind. Visual hallucinations involve seeing objects or persons not based in reality. A neologism is a word or phrase that has meaning only to the person using it. (P)

59. **3.** The American Academy of Pediatrics and the American College of Obstetrics and Gynecology recommend hearing screening for all newborns. Currently more than 30 states mandate screening, which is done by otoacoustic emissions or auditory brainstem response. Newborns can hear as soon as the amniotic fluid drains from the ear canal. Even though hearing problems are not common in newborns, the mother's concerns should be addressed. Clapping to elicit a response is crude and unreliable. If done for minimal screening, the distance should be no more than 12 inches. (H)

60. **4.** The equianalgesic dose of oral meperidine hydrochloride is up to four times the I.M. dose. Meperidine hydrochloride (Demerol) can be given orally, but it is much more effective when given I.M. (D)

61. **1, 2, 3.** Children tend to be impulsive, which contributes to head injuries. Also, the larger size of the heads of infants and toddlers causes them to fall more easily than older children. Falls account for one-third of all head injuries. Motor vehicle accidents account for about 80% of all severe head injuries in children. Children age 5 to 15 are most likely to be involved in bicycle accidents as a result of only about 50% wearing helmets. Child abuse and tumors involve a much smaller number of children. (H)

62. **1.** In order to prevent disuse osteoporosis, it is important to implement weight-bearing activities as soon as medically allowed. Increasing the client's calcium intake will not prevent the development of osteoporosis without the inclusion of weight-bearing activity. Passive ROM exercises and isometric exercises do not provide the bone stress necessary to reduce the risk of osteoporosis. (R)

63. **3.** Toddlers have temper tantrums in their attempt to develop autonomy. Toddlers should be left alone as long as they are safe during a tantrum. Moving the child to a time-out chair or punishing the child reinforces the behavior and is to be avoided. Attempting to talk to the toddler also reinforces the behavior. Additionally, at this cognitive level, toddlers do not understand as well as older children do. (H)

64. **1.** When a nurse has been stuck by a used needle and has not completed the hepatitis B vaccination, he or she should receive both active and passive immunization. For postexposure prophylaxis, the hepatitis B virus vaccine and hepatitis B immune globulin (HBIG) are used. HBIG contains antibodies and confers temporary passive immunity. (S)

65. **2.** Daily skin inspection is essential in preventing pressure ulcers. Hot water is irritating to skin and should be avoided. Massaging bony prominences is contraindicated and may actually promote skin breakdown. Prolonged, uninterrupted chair sitting should be avoided; the client's position should be adjusted at least every hour. (R)

66. **3.** Skeletal pins should not be loose and able to move. Any pin loosening should be reported immediately. Slight serous drainage is normal and may crust around the insertion site or be present on the dressing. The pin insertion site should be cleaned with aseptic technique according to facility policy. Pin insertion sites are typically not painful; pain may be indicative of an infection and should be reported. (A)

67. **4.** Acknowledging the basic feeling that the client expressed and asking an open-ended question allows the client to explain her fears. Saying, "It's normal to be scared. We'll help you through it," does not focus on the client's feelings; rather, it gives reassurance. Asking if the client feels guilty for having smoked assumes guilt, which might be present, but additional information is needed to confirm. Telling the client not to be so hard on herself does not acknowledge the client's feelings at all. (P)

68. **3.** It is important that clients with rheumatoid arthritis maintain proper posture and body alignment to support joints and decrease pain and stiffness. Clients with hip pain will be most comfortable when sitting in a straight-back chair with an elevated seat. Elevated seats avoid excessive hip flexion and place less stress on the hip joints. (C)

69. **3.** Giving away personal items has consistently been shown to be an indicator of suicidal plans in the depressed and suicidal individual. The other behaviors indicate a return of interest in normal adolescent activities. (P)

70. **3.** When a neonate dies, the mother should be allowed to stay with the baby as long as she wants and say anything she wants. She is grieving and needs time with the neonate. A photograph should be taken in case the mother wants a photograph at a later time. Telling the mother that this is for the best is inappropriate because such a statement discounts the mother's feelings. Advising the mother to get pregnant again to get over the loss is not helpful because the mother needs time to grieve and be with the neonate. The nurse should remain near the mother and not delegate this responsibility to the hospital's chaplain. A chaplain or other religious member can be contacted if the mother desires. (P)

71. **3, 4, 5.** Spastic CP is the most common type, characterized by poor coordination and balance, gross motor skills impairment, and hypertonicity. CP is nonprogressive and is caused by a variety of prenatal, perinatal, and postnatal factors. Dyskinetic or athetoid CP is the next most common type and is characterized by abnormal involuntary movements and wormlike writhing movements. (A)

72. **4.** Serum albumin levels help determine whether protein intake is sufficient. Proteins are broken down into amino acids during digestion. Amino acids are absorbed in the small intestine, and albumin is built from amino acids. The red blood cell count, bilirubin levels, and reticulocyte count do not indicate protein intake. (A)

73. **2.** The client who is taking desmopressin (DDAVP) nasal spray should not use the same nares for administration each time. The client should alternate nares every dose. The client should observe for and report promptly signs and symptoms of nasal ulceration, congestion, or respiratory infection. (D)

74. **0.5**

$$500 \text{ mg/ml} = 250 \text{ mg}/X\,\text{ml}$$

$$X = 0.5 \text{ ml.}$$

(D)

75. **3.** Common clinical manifestations of hypokalemia include ventricular arrhythmias; weak and irregular pulse; soft and flabby muscles; and decreased deep tendon reflexes. Hypercalcemia causes confusion and decreased memory, bone pain, polyuria, and nausea, vomiting, and constipation. Hypernatremia causes signs of fluid volume deficit. Hypomagnesemia is manifested by tremors, confusion, hyperactive deep tendon reflexes, and seizures. (A)

76. **3.** As with other contraceptives that are adverse progestin-based, heavy menstrual bleeding may occur. Other adverse effects include rash, acne, alopecia, fluid retention, edema, and sudden loss of vision. Depression and weight gain have been reported. For clients taking this drug, the risk of endometrial or ovarian cancer is decreased. Amenorrhea has been reported in clients after receiving four injections 3 months apart for 1 year. Depression and loss of energy have been reported. (D)

77. **4.** Clients with burns are susceptible to the development of Curling's ulcer, a gastroduodenal ulcer that is caused by a generalized stress response. The stress response results in increased gastric acid secretion and a decreased production of mucus. Prevention is the best treatment, and clients are frequently treated prophylactically with antacids and H_2 histamine blockers such as famotidine (Pepcid). (R)

78. **2.** Fever is a cardinal manifestation of infection in people with AIDS. Because the major physiologic alteration in AIDS is generalized immune system dysfunction, typical indicators of the body's response to infection (e.g., erythema, warmth, tenderness) may be absent. (A)

79. 2. To care effectively for clients with depression, the nurse should teach the importance of demonstrating empathetic concern. Caregivers must accept clients as they are even though many will be angry and negative, acknowledge their emotional pain, and offer to help them work through their pain. For the client who is depressed, using a cheerful demeanor or a humorous, light-hearted approach may be overwhelming because the client will be unable to meet the caregiver's expectations, subsequently leading to decreased self-worth. A serious, business-like affect may threaten the client and inhibit the development of trust. (P)

80. 4. When a child is ready to take fluids by mouth postoperatively, clear liquids are given initially. If clear liquids are tolerated, the concentration and amount of oral feedings are gradually increased. This means advancing to half-strength and then to full-strength formula while increasing the amount given with each feeding. (C)

81. 2. The nurse should monitor the client taking paroxetine, a selective serotonin reuptake inhibitor, for sexual problems, such as decreased libido, impotence, and ejaculatory disturbances, because these adverse effects can occur frequently and lead to medication noncompliance. Sleep disturbances can occur with an SSRI such as paroxetine. However, this client is taking the drug every morning, which would not affect nighttime sleep. Hypertensive crisis is associated with the ingestion of foods rich in tyramine when a client is taking a monoamine oxidase inhibitor. Orthostatic hypotension is a potential adverse effect of tricyclic antidepressants. (D)

82. 1. This diet is based on research indicating that diets low in potassium are often associated with hypertension. Higher-potassium diets appear to prevent and correct hypertension. Magnesium deficiency causes artery walls and capillaries to constrict and therefore raises blood pressure. Magnesium intake within the normal range lowers blood pressure. Vitamin C helps to normalize blood pressure. Calcium lowers blood pressure in healthy people and in those with hypertension. (H)

83. 2. In the progressive stage of shock, the client can display listlessness or agitation, confusion, and slowed speech. Restlessness occurs in the compensatory stage. Incoherent speech and unconsciousness are clinical manifestations of the irreversible stage. (A)

84. 1, 4, 5. Common adverse effects of nafcillin include vomiting, diarrhea, sore mouth, fever, and gastritis. Pain with urination and headache are not associated with this drug. (D)

85. 1. When the crash cart arrives, ECG electrodes are applied to the client's chest. If the client is found to be in ventricular fibrillation, the immediate priority is to defibrillate the client. Pulse oximetry is not an immediate priority. The client's oxygenation is evaluated in a code situation using arterial blood gas analysis. The client's blood pressure is evaluated after the ECG rhythm has been established. A portable Doppler ultrasound unit may be needed to check for the presence of a pulse or to check the blood pressure in a code situation. (A)

86. 2. Heroin causes pinpoint pupils. Marijuana causes the eyes to appear red and bloodshot. Cocaine use causes pupils to dilate. Drooping of the eyelids is not typically associated with the use of any substance. (D)

87. 3. A typical sign of pediculosis capitis (head lice) is frequent scratching of the scalp because the condition causes severe itching. Scratch marks are usually easily visible. Because head lice are easily transmitted to others, the child's family members and peers also should be examined for infestation. Spotty baldness, wheals, and scaly lesions are often allergic in nature. (A)

88. 1. Passing flatus indicates the return of peristalsis, as does active bowel sounds. Hunger is not the best indicator of peristaltic return. Hypoactive bowel sounds indicate that there is some peristaltic activity but it is limited and not yet normal. Palpation is not an appropriate method of assessing bowel activity. (A)

89. 3. The pH of 7.24 indicates that the client is acidotic. The $Paco_2$ value of 49 mm Hg is elevated. The HCO_3^- value of 24 mEq/L is normal. The client is in uncompensated respiratory acidosis. Hypoventilation and a flushed appearance are additional clinical manifestations of respiratory acidosis. (A)

90. 2. It is essential for the nurse to evaluate the effects of pain medication after it has had time to act. Although other interventions may be appropriate, continual reassessment is most important to determine the effectiveness and need for additional intervention, if any. Repositioning could provide some comfort, but assessment of the client's pain level is essential. Reassuring the client is important, but it will be of no value unless the nurse evaluates the client's pain level. To readjust the pain dosage is appropriate only if titration is prescribed by the physician. (A)

91. 1. Barrier contraceptives must be used to protect against STDs. Birth control pills and douching are not effective for prevention of STDs. Prophylactic antibiotics are not used to prevent the acquisition of STDs. (S)

92. 2. A purplish blue discoloration of the vagina and cervix is termed Chadwick's sign; it is caused by increased vascularity of the vagina during pregnancy and is considered a probable sign of pregnancy. Goodell's sign, also considered a probable sign of pregnancy, refers to a softening of the cervix during pregnancy. Hegar's sign, also a probable sign of pregnancy, refers to a softening of the lower uterine segment. Melasma, the mask of pregnancy, refers to the pigmentation of the skin on the face during pregnancy. Melasma is considered a presumptive sign of pregnancy. (H)

93. **3.** Initially, the nurse would tell the client to seek out staff when feeling agitated or upset to prevent violent episodes. Doing so helps the client to redirect negative feelings in an appropriate manner (e.g., talking). Encouraging the client to stay in his room is inappropriate because it does not help the client to deal with his feelings. Secluding the client at the first sign of agitation is not indicated and may be perceived by the client as punishment. Instructing the client to ask for medication when agitated would not be the initial course of action. The nurse would interact with the client and direct the client to an activity to decrease his anxiety before intervening with any required medication. (P)

94. **3.** The nurse should use short words, sentences, and paragraphs and avoid medical jargon. Correct terminology should be used when appropriate (e.g., type 1 diabetes, not "sugar diabetes"). The format should be as simple as possible; charts are not necessary and may be confusing to some clients. Information should be prepared at a fifth-grade reading level. The information should be presented in large-sized type. (P)

95. **4, 5.** Rapid pulse, heat intolerance, diarrhea, exophthalmos, and accelerated linear growth are more characteristic of hyperthyroidism, which is caused by an autoimmune response to thyroid-stimulating hormone receptors. Weight gain, dry skin, and constipation are characteristic of hypothyroidism, which results from a deficiency in secretion of thyroid hormone. (A)

96. **4.** It is normal for the client to feel pressure on the palms of the hands when walking with crutches. The client should move her affected (right) leg forward first as she swings forward with the crutches. Leaning on the crutches can apply pressure to the axillae, leading to neurovascular impairment. If the client's arms are tingling after she uses her crutches, she is probably applying pressure on her axillae when walking. (R)

97. **2.** Because clients are discharged as soon as possible from the hospital, it is essential to evaluate the support for assistance and self-care at home. If the client has support at home, the distance from the hospital may be irrelevant. The client or support team will monitor vital signs as needed, but blood pressure monitoring is not specifically indicated. It is more important at this point for the client to understand how to manage his care at home, rather than knowing the causes of lung cancer. (M)

98. **3.** If the client begins breast-feeding early and often after delivery, the breasts begin to fill with milk within 48 to 96 hours, or 2 to 4 days. The breasts secrete colostrum for the first 24 to 48 hours, which is beneficial to the neonate because of the immunoglobulins contained in colostrum. (H)

99. **3.** The predominant clinical finding in elderly or debilitated clients indicating that they have developed pneumonia is confusion, which results from hypoxia. Fever and chills, productive cough, and pleuritic chest pain could be present, but confusion is the predominant development. (A)

100. **1.** It is important for the child and family to understand that chorea associated with rheumatic fever is not permanent. Therefore, the nurse should explain that the chorea will disappear over time. It is not necessary to assess the child's neurologic status because the chorea is self-limited and nonprogressive. Because the child has cardiac involvement, ambulation is contraindicated. Aspirin is used primarily as an anti-inflammatory drug and secondarily for pain relief. A slightly cool environment is unnecessary. Environmental temperature does not affect the child's polyarthritis and chorea. (A)

101. **1.** When the gestation is less than 13 weeks, an elective abortion is usually performed by the dilatation and curettage method. Menstrual extraction, or suction evacuation, is the easiest method, but it is used only when the client is between 5 and 7 weeks' gestation. Dilatation and vacuum extraction is used when clients are between 12 and 16 weeks' gestation. Saline induction, used for clients between 16 and 24 weeks' gestation, involves instillation of a hypertonic saline solution into the amniotic sac to initiate expulsion. Oxytocin infusion may also be used with saline induction. (H)

102. **1.** A pleural effusion is a collection of fluid between the pleural layers of the lung. The effusion decreases chest wall movement on the affected side. The nurse should expect the breath sounds to be decreased or diminished over the affected area. Because of the presence of fluid, percussion would elicit dullness, not hyperresonance. Fever may be present if empyema (purulent pleural fluid with bacterial infection) has developed, but not in the case of a nonpurulent pleural effusion. (A)

103. **1.** An expected client outcome relative to the nursing diagnosis of *Acute pain* related to cramping is that the client exhibits no manifestations of discomfort, such as crying or drawing the legs to the abdomen. Being very still may indicate either a pain state or a state of relaxation. (A)

104. **0.6**

$$40 \text{ mg}/\text{ml} = 25 \text{ mg}/X \text{ ml}$$

$$X = 0.6 \text{ ml}.$$

(D)

105. **4.** The client is exhibiting symptoms of herpes genitalis, which include painful blisters or vesicles that appear 2 to 20 days after transmission of the disease. The client was most likely exposed from her new partner. Vulvar pain, dyspareunia, dysuria, and flulike symptoms also may be present. HIV infection is commonly manifested by numerous signs and symptoms, such as persistent candidiasis, anogenital condyloma, and herpes simplex infections. *Chlamydia trachomatis* infection is asymptomatic, commonly going undetected by affected women. Signs and symptoms, when present, include a grayish white discharge and vulvar itching. Syphilis typically is manifested by a chancre occurring about 10 days after exposure. The chancre is usually deep but painless. (A)

106. **2.** It has been found that parents are more grieved when optimism is followed by defeat. The nurse should recognize this when planning various ways to help the parents of a dying child. It is not necessarily true that knowing about a poor prognosis for years helps prepare parents for a child's death, that trust in health personnel is destroyed when a death is untimely, or that it is more difficult for parents to accept the death of an older child than that of a younger child. (P)

107. **3.** The child is having a reaction to the blood transfusion. The priority is to stop the blood transfusion but maintain an open venous access for medication or high fluid volume delivery. Thus, switching the transfusion to normal saline solution would be done first. Since the child is having difficulty breathing, applying oxygen would be the next action. Additionally, vital signs are taken to determine the extent of circulatory involvement. Then the physician would be notified and, if necessary, the crash cart would be obtained. (D)

108. **1.** A client who has an allergy to penicillin may have a cross-sensitivity to cefazolin (Ancef), a first-generation cephalosporin, and the drug should be given with caution. The nurse should ask the client whether he has taken cefazolin before. The nurse should inform the pharmacy of the client's allergy after asking the client about prior use of cefazolin. The medication should not be administered until the nurse first inquires about the client's exposure to cefazolin and then consults the pharmacist or physician. Observing the client for urticaria is appropriate but is not an initial response. (S)

109. **3.** Clients with chronic renal failure are susceptible to uremia, an accumulation of nitrogenous waste products in the blood. Clinical manifestations include dry, itchy skin that can be severe in nature. Because of the irritation of the skin and the inclination to scratch, clients are prone to impaired skin integrity. The pruritus is not a result of poor hygiene. Chronic pain is not a likely result of the pruritus and is not a priority nursing diagnosis. The data do not support the nursing diagnosis of *Ineffective coping.* (A)

110. **1.** The nurse would teach the client taking lithium and his family about the importance of maintaining adequate sodium intake to prevent lithium toxicity. Because lithium is a salt, reduced sodium intake could result in lithium retention with subsequent toxicity. Increasing sodium in the diet is not recommended and may be harmful. Increased sodium levels result in lower lithium levels. Therefore, the drug may not reach therapeutic effectiveness. (D)

111. **3.** Mucositis is an inflammation of the oral mucosa caused by radiation therapy. It is important that the client with mucositis receive meticulous mouth care, including flossing, to prevent the development of an infection. Mouth care should be provided before and after each meal, at bedtime, and more frequently as needed. Extremes of temperature should be avoided in food and drink. Half-strength hydrogen peroxide is too harsh to use on irritated tissues. (R)

112. **3.** Acetaminophen ingestion can cause severe liver disease. The child should be evaluated in the emergency department. The child should not be offered any fluids, and the parents should not attempt to induce vomiting with syrup of ipecac. Assessing the child's respirations for 24 hours will delay needed emergency treatment. (A)

113. **1.** The best approach by the nurse is to determine why the parent thinks the child is hyperactive. Some children are very active but do not have the necessary defining characteristics of hyperactivity. Asking what the parent thinks needs to be done or how the child behaves normally would be an appropriate follow-up question once more information is gathered from the parent to determine whether the child indeed is hyperactive. Telling the parent to wait for the physician ignores the parent's concern and does not deal with the parent's issue. (A)

114. **2.** Dilatation at the anastomosis site is needed during the first years of childhood in about 50% of children who have had corrective surgery for TEF. Recurrent mild diarrhea with dehydration is not likely to develop with this surgery. Speech problems can occur if other abnormalities are present to produce them; the larynx and structures of speech are not affected by TEF. Dysphagia and strictures may decrease food intake, and poor weight gain may be noted, but gastric ulcers should not develop from surgery to repair TEF. (R)

115. **1.** Terminally ill clients most often describe feelings of isolation because they feel ignored. The terminally ill client may sense any discomfort that family and friends feel in the client's presence. Nursing interventions include spending time with the client, encouraging discussion about feelings, and answering questions openly and honestly. Reducing fear of pain or fear of more aggressive therapies is secondary to lessening the client's feelings of isolation. Reducing feelings of social inadequacy is not relevant to the terminally ill client. (P)

116. **2.** When the fetus is in a breech position, the fetal heart rate most often is located above the umbilicus because the fetal heart is near the top of the mother's uterus. The heart of a fetus in the cephalic position is typically located on either the left or the right side of the client's uterus. Also, because the fetal heart typically is located in the lower portion of the mother's uterus, the sounds would be heard below the umbilicus. With a face presentation, fetal heart sounds are typically located on either the left or the right side of the client's uterus; in addition, because the fetal heart typically is located in the lower portion of the mother's uterus, the sounds would be heard below the umbilicus. When the fetus is in a transverse position, the fetal heart sounds typically would be located below the umbilicus and in the midline. (H)

117. **4.** Clients who have been diagnosed with pernicious anemia are lacking adequate amounts of the intrinsic factor (IF) that is secreted by the gastric mucosa. IF is necessary for the absorption of cobalamin (vitamin B_{12}) in the distal ileum. Without the presence of IF, dietary intake of vitamin B_{12} is useless because it cannot be absorbed. Treatment of pernicious anemia includes I.M. injections of cobalamin, at first daily for 2 weeks, then weekly until the anemia is corrected. A maintenance schedule of monthly injections is then implemented. The injections will need to be continued for the rest of the client's life. (A)

118. **2.** The nurse should first assess the client because a hypoglycemic reaction is likely to occur. The nurse should provide a fast-acting simple carbohydrate. The nurse (charge nurse or otherwise) should notify the physician for orders to prevent or treat severe hypoglycemia. The nurse could consult the clinical pharmacist until able to contact the physician. The nurse should ask for assistance so that the client can be monitored by a nurse while someone prepares a longer-acting carbohydrate or protein. (R)

119. **4.** Safety is the priority in caring for this infant. Infants adapt easily, increasing mobility even with a splint in place. Therefore, the mother needs to ensure that the area in which the infant is mobile is safe. There is no need to contact the physician to alter the treatment plan. Confining the infant to one room may not allow the child to achieve normal development. The child needs different environments for maximum development. The infant needs to wear the splint as ordered by the physician to ensure optimal healing. (S)

120. **1.** Anxiety in a preoperative client may be caused by many different fears, such as fear of the effects of anesthesia, the effects of surgery on body image, separation from family and friends, job loss, disability, pain, or death. However, fear of the unknown is most likely to be the greatest fear because the client feels helpless. Therefore, an important part of preoperative nursing care is to assess the client for anxieties and explore possible causes. Emotional support can then be offered, so that the client is in the best possible psychological condition for surgery. (P)

121. **1.** An important nursing responsibility is preoperative teaching. The recommended guide for teaching is to tell the client as much as she wants to know and is able to understand. Delaying discussion of issues or concerns will most likely increase the client's anxiety. Telling the client to discuss questions with the physician avoids acknowledging the client's concerns. (P)

122. **3.** The client must have adequate disclosure of the risks associated with the surgery before signing the consent form. It is the physician's responsibility to explain the risks of any procedures and to obtain the client's informed consent. If the nurse suspects that the client has not been truly informed, it is the responsibility of the nurse to act as a client advocate and contact the surgeon to provide additional information to the client. It is not appropriate to have the client sign the consent form if the client has questions. The nurse should not minimize the procedure or dismiss the client's concerns. (M)

123. **4.** In right occipital anterior lie, the occiput faces the right anterior segment of the woman's pelvis. In left occipital transverse lie, the occiput faces the woman's left hip. In left occipital anterior lie, the occiput faces the left anterior segment of the woman's pelvis. In right occipital transverse lie, the occiput faces the woman's right hip. (A)

124. **2.** Urinary tract infections in infants are a bit hard to diagnose because signs and symptoms may be subtle, such as loss of appetite and fussiness. Dysuria and fever may also occur, but dysuria is harder to recognize in an infant. Increased urine output may occur, but it would be very difficult for the parent to actually determine this. Typically, urine is cloudy in appearance in an infant with a urinary tract infection. Feeding problems may occur, but jaundice would be a late sign. (A)

125. **3.** A positive Babinski's reflex in a neonate is a normal finding demonstrating the immaturity of the central nervous system in corticospinal pathways. A neonate's muscle coordination is immature, but the Babinski's reflex does not help determine this immaturity. A positive Babinski's reflex does not indicate a defect in the spinal cord or an injury to nerves that innervate the legs. There is no evidence to suggest partial paralysis. A positive Babinski's reflex in an adult indicates disease. (H)

126. **2.** The nurse should instruct the client who is taking dexamethasone (Decadron) and furosemide (Lasix) to observe for signs and symptoms of hypokalemia, such as malaise, muscle weakness, vomiting, and a paralytic ileus, because both dexamethasone and furosemide deplete serum potassium. This combination of drugs does not cause the client to become excitable or have diarrhea or thirst. (D)

127. **2.** After a bronchoscopy with a biopsy, the nurse should monitor the client for signs of pneumothorax as well as hemorrhage. The client should not gargle with oral lidocaine; this will not allow the gag reflex to return. The client should not have any mediastinal discomfort after a bronchoscopy; if pain does occur it should be reported promptly to the physician. It is not necessary to tell the client not to talk until the gag reflex returns. (R)

128. **42**

The number of drops the client should receive each minute is determined as follows:

500 ml/12 hours = between 41 and 42 ml
to be infused each hour

42 ml × 60 (drop factor) = 2,520 drops
to be infused each hour

2,520 drops/60 minutes = 42 drops
to be infused every minute.

(D)

129. **2.** Subcutaneous injections are administered at an angle of 45 to 90 degrees, depending on the size of the client. Subcutaneous needles are typically ⅜ to ⅝ inches in length. The skin should be pinched up at the injection site to elevate the subcutaneous tissue. Air is not drawn into the syringe for a subcutaneous injection. (D)

130. **3.** *Acute pain* is a priority nursing diagnosis for the client with pelvic inflammatory disease because the disease is associated with severe pain. *Imbalanced nutrition: Less than body requirements*, *Self-care deficit*, and *Impaired skin integrity* are not priority nursing diagnoses associated with pelvic inflammatory disease. (A)

131. **3.** Children with difficult temperaments do better in structured environments than in environments with daily changes. This helps to teach them what to expect. Easy children do well with flexible feeding times. Children with easy temperaments do not cry often, and parents need to remember to feed them. Children with high activity levels, another type of temperament, who are always on the go, need to be watched more closely and need extra safety precautions taken around the house. (H)

132. **4.** The position of the tube should be verified before the feeding is implemented. Warming the solution is not necessary or desirable because it can encourage bacterial growth. The client should be lying down with the head elevated or sitting upright during administration of the feeding. Gastric residual should be aspirated and then reinstilled to prevent electrolyte losses. (R)

133. **4.** The cramping is caused by the baby's sucking and subsequent stimulation for the release of oxytocin. This cramping is normal. With each subsequent pregnancy, the uterus becomes "stretched" and the release of oxytocin causes the uterus to contract, resulting in the feeling of cramping. Continued moderate to large amounts of lochia rubra is indicative of retained placental fragments. Cramping indicates that the uterus is contracting and most likely firm. A boggy uterus, continued moderate to heavy lochia, mild vasoconstriction, and restlessness and anxiety suggest delayed postpartum hemorrhage due to subinvolution of the placental site, retained placental tissue, or infection. Most clients receive a standard dose of oxytocin (Pitocin) after delivery. Oxytocin has a duration of action of 60 minutes. Therefore, the effects of the drug would have worn off by 24 hours postpartum. (H)

134. **4.** The current recommendations for children experiencing mild to moderate diarrhea are to continue the child's regular diet. With this diet plan, children seem to get well faster. Clear liquids, such as juices, colas, and gelatin, are high in carbohydrates but low in electrolytes, as are foods such as bananas, rice, applesauce, and toast. Foods low in fat also typically lack the electrolytes that the child needs. (A)

135. **2.** When performing tracheostomy care, it is important that the tracheostomy ties be securely tied to prevent dislodgment of the tube. It is not necessary to remove the inner cannula every 2 hours for cleaning. Routine cleaning is usually performed every 8 hours. The nurse should use precut tracheostomy dressings under the neck plate to protect the skin surrounding the stoma. Cutting and using a gauze dressing can cause loose gauze fibers to enter the airway. The inner cannula should be suctioned before cleaning, not afterward. (R)

136. **2.** The nurse should send the sealed container of I.V. 50% dextrose found in the catch-all bin to the pharmacy. A concentrated medication such as 50% dextrose could be lethal if inadvertently administered and should not be stored outside the pharmacy. An incident report is not necessary in this situation. The sharps container is not the appropriate method for disposal of this medication. (M)

137. **3.** The client who is wheelchair-bound with a spinal cord injury should be taught to make small weight shifts, lifting off the sacral area every 15 minutes. This decreases the risk of pressure ulcer formation. Bathing daily promotes skin cleanliness, but by itself will not prevent pressure ulcer formation. Eating a well-balanced diet that includes proteins and carbohydrates promotes good skin integrity. Moving from the bed to the wheelchair every 2 hours is not desirable because the client should not spend excessive amounts of time in bed. Pressure sores can develop in less than 2 hours. (R)

138. **1.** Anatomically, the squatting position enlarges the pelvic outlet and uses the force of gravity during pushing. The mother should curve her body into a C shape for the greatest effectiveness. (H)

139. **2.** Saying, "If you punch people out, you'll get into trouble," helps the client by pointing out the negative consequences of his behavior. Clients with antisocial personality disorder are aggressive, impulsive, and reckless; engage in illegal activities; and lack guilt or remorse. The nurse teaches the client that there are consequences to his irresponsible behavior and that the way to stay out of trouble is to change his behavior. Saying, "It's wrong to punch others," is not helpful since the client does not feel guilt or remorse. Saying, "I wouldn't do that again if I were you" or "Don't ever do that again," is authoritative and scolds the client without helping him. (P)

140. **3.** Self-mutilation is a way to express anger and rage, commonly seen in clients with borderline personality disorder. It typically is a cry for help, an expression of intense anger, helplessness, or guilt. When a client is experiencing numbness or feelings of unreality, self-mutilation induces physical pain which validates the person's being alive because of the ability to feel the physical pain. Self-mutilation is not a means of getting what the person wants. It is not used as a form of manipulation, although it is often misinterpreted as such. Self-mutilation is a serious behavior that is harmful to the self and cannot be ignored. (P)

141. **3.** Hepatitis C is transferred by percutaneous exposure, such as tattooing. Hepatitis A is acquired through contaminated water, exposure in underdeveloped countries, or shellfish in contaminated waters. (A)

142. **1.** Lorazepam (Ativan), a benzodiazepine, is commonly used to decrease the symptoms of central nervous system irritability in the client who is experiencing symptoms of alcohol withdrawal. Diazepam (Valium) and chlordiazepoxide (Librium), also benzodiazepines, may be used in some instances. Naltrexone (ReVia) is an opioid receptor antagonist that interferes with opioid functioning and reduces the craving for alcohol and opioids. It is used as an adjunct for treating alcohol or opioid dependence. Methadone (Dolophine) is an opioid similar to morphine. It is used to treat opioid dependence. Imipramine (Tofranil) is a tricyclic antidepressant used to treat major depression. It also may be used as a substitute for heroin and opioids in clients who want to terminate drug use. (D)

143. **2, 3.** Appropriate diet instructions for the client in the early stages of cirrhosis include ensuring an adequate intake of protein and eating small, frequent meals. There is no need to limit protein intake unless the patient has evidence of hepatic encephalopathy. Additionally, fluid intake is not restricted unless the client has significant ascites or edema (these typically occur later in the disease). Because of gastrointestinal dysfunction, small, frequent meals are frequently better tolerated than three regular meals. Clients with cirrhosis should be encouraged to increase their caloric intake instead of restricting it. Alcohol intake in any amount is discouraged. (A)

144. **3.** After surgery, the nurse's initial assessment is the surgical site dressing to determine whether there is any bleeding or drainage. Once this assessment is completed, then the nurse would assess the other areas such as the I.V. access site, pain, and nasogastric tube function. (A)

145. **1.** The nurse should use the radial artery to obtain blood gas samples because it is easier to maintain firm pressure there than on the femoral artery. Nursing interventions to protect the client who has received t-PA or alteplase recombinant (Activase) therapy include maintaining arterial pressure for 30 seconds because it takes longer for coagulation to occur with the thrombolytic agent on board. I.M. injections are contraindicated during thrombolytic therapy. The nurse should prevent physical manipulation of the client, which can cause bruising. (R)

146. **3.** Experimental and epidemiologic research indicates that approximately 50% of all patients with hypertension can lower their blood pressure through dietary sodium reduction. (H)

147. **4.** Serum amylase and lipase are increased in pancreatitis, as is urine amylase. Other abnormal laboratory values include decreased calcium level and increased glucose and lipid levels. (A)

148. 2. For the client with an alcohol or drug problem, group sessions are helpful in dealing with emotions and concerns about alcohol and drugs. Clients with substance abuse problems identify with each other's similar experiences and can best help each other deal with these feelings and emotions. Additionally, the members of the group are able to support and confront each other. Individual therapy is not as helpful as group sessions because group members offer peer support and confrontation when needed. Solitary activities and recreation lead to increased avoidance of the issues that must be faced and dealt with by the client. These are often areas that the client must learn to develop and manage while in recovery. (P)

149. 4. Foul-smelling urine is indicative of cystitis. Other symptoms include dysuria and urinary frequency and urgency. Flank pain, nausea, and vomiting indicate pyelonephritis. (A)

150. 4. By saying, "You couldn't have prevented the tornado; it just happened," the nurse helps the client to develop an objective perspective and promotes a better understanding of the event. The other statements tell the client how to feel, possibly causing resistance and thus delay therapeutic healing. Guilt and self-blame will not be decreased. (P)

151. 3. In many Asian cultures, the 30 days after the birth of the neonate is a time for the mother to heal from the delivery. The appropriate action by the nurse is to determine whether this is a cultural practice for this client and her family. If so, the client is behaving within her cultural practices. Teaching should be provided to both the mother and her mother-in-law. There is no indication that bonding is not taking place. Lack of bonding might be indicated if the client did not show any interest in the neonate. Documenting the client's maternal behavior in her chart is a routine task. However, the nurse should not assume that this behavior is unusual because it may be reflective of the client's cultural framework. A home visit is not warranted unless there is evidence of infant neglect or the family needs additional follow-up or teaching. (H)

152. 1. A creatinine clearance test is a 24-hour urine test that measures the degree of protein breakdown in the body. The collection is not maintained in a sterile container. There is no need to insert an indwelling urinary catheter as long as the client is able to control urination. It is not necessary to force fluids. (R)

153. 4. The statement, "Your eyes look dark," is the least sensitive statement because it points out an obvious difference for no real purpose. The nurse has a reason to ask the client about favorite foods and needs to know about past health problems. Also, it is appropriate for the nurse to ask the client how she wishes to be addressed. (P)

154. 2. Insight into the illness is demonstrated when the client recognizes the relationship between the chemical imbalance and his illness and symptoms. Stating that the olanzapine is the best medicine or that the client's mother is proud of him for staying on his medicines reflects awareness about the effect of medications and the need for compliance. Stating that he may be able to get a part-time job indicates an awareness of his increased capacity for work. (P)

155. 3. Carpal tunnel syndrome is a condition in which the median nerve becomes compressed in the wrist. The brachial nerve is not affected. Carpal tunnel syndrome may be the result of a systemic disease, such as rheumatoid arthritis or diabetes mellitus, or it may be an occupational hazard for people whose jobs require repetitive hand movements. It is not a condition resulting from disuse. The wrists do not develop flexion contractures with carpal tunnel syndrome. (A)

156. 1. Seventy-five percent of all food allergies are caused by milk, eggs, or peanuts. (A)

157. 3. Clients who have undergone TURP need to be instructed to maintain an adequate fluid intake despite urinary dribbling or incontinence. The client should be advised to drink at least eight glasses of water a day to dilute the urine and help prevent urinary tract infections. Maintaining a voiding schedule of every 2 hours can help decrease incidents of incontinence. Teaching the client Kegel exercises is also beneficial for strengthening sphincter tone. The nurse should not encourage the client to decrease fluids. It is not necessarily true that a decreased intake will cause renal calculi. Threatening the client with a catheter is not beneficial, and it is not the treatment of choice for a client who is experiencing incontinence from TURP. (R)

158. 1. *Risk for infection* would be a priority nursing diagnosis after surgery. With any type of incision, the immediate concern is preventing infection at the site. *Acute pain* is also a diagnosis of concern and would be next in order of priority. The infant would be partially restrained to prevent disturbance of the intravenous infusion and nasogastric tube. Bowel elimination should begin in a few days. (A)

159. 4. Risk factors for TSS include the use of tampons at night, when the tampon would be in place for 7 to 9 hours. TSS can occur in other situations, but it is commonly associated with women during menses, particularly women who use tampons. The longer the tampon is left in place, the greater the risk for TSS. Changing tampons every 3 hours or more frequently, avoiding use of deodorized tampons, and alternating tampons with sanitary pads are actions that decrease the risk of TSS. (R)

160. **4.** Costovertebral tenderness occurs on the side of the affected kidney in pyelonephritis. Dysuria, suprapubic pain, and urine retention may occur in pyelonephritis but do not specifically support a diagnosis of pyelonephritis. Dysuria, suprapubic pain, and urine retention are symptoms of cystitis, which can lead to pyelonephritis if not treated. (A)

161. **2.** Broad-spectrum antibiotics can cause decreased efficacy of oral contraceptives, placing the client at risk for an unplanned pregnancy. When a client is prescribed a course of antibiotics, a back-up method of contraception should be used. Antihypertensives, diuretics, and antihistamines do not interfere with oral contraceptive efficacy. (D)

162. **1.** Adverse effects of danazol (Danocrine) include headaches, dizziness, irritability, and decreased libido. Masculinization effects, such as deepened voice, facial hair, and weight gain, also may occur. (D)

163. **2.** The nurse should assign the male client of Mexican American descent who needs complete morning care to Joe. Modesty is a high priority for this client. The nurse must also consider case load, and Joe has the lightest assignment. (M)

164. **4.** Central nervous system changes include such symptoms as apathy, lethargy, and decreased concentration. Seizures and coma can also occur. The nurse should assess the client's level of consciousness at regular intervals and maintain client safety. Allowing the client to express feelings related to body image changes and restricting foods high in potassium and fluid intake are all appropriate activities, but they are not related to the central nervous system changes. (A)

165. **3.** Elderly individuals have less subcutaneous tissue. An elderly, emaciated client will require a short needle and a shallow angle to avoid hitting an underlying bone. The nurse should choose the shortest subcutaneous needle available, and use the least angle. (D)

166. **3.** This situation describes the classic symptoms of urinary tract infection. Urinalysis and culture and sensitivity studies would be helpful information for this diagnosis. Pelvic inflammatory disease is manifested by severe suprapubic pain and vaginal discharge. Renal calculi are accompanied by severe, colicky flank pain and hematuria. Renal failure is manifested by hypertension, pruritus, anorexia, nausea, and vomiting. (A)

167. **1.** Scant, dark vaginal bleeding; abdominal pain; and frequent low-amplitude uterine activity are associated with abruptio placentae. The client needs a cesarean delivery to prevent hypovolemic shock. Placenta accreta is an unusually deep attachment of the placenta to the myometrium and usually is not discovered until delivery.

Hysterectomy is usually the treatment. Placenta previa refers to an abnormal implantation of the placenta. Typically, painless, bright red vaginal bleeding is seen with this condition. Battledore placenta occurs when the cord is inserted marginally rather than centrally, and it is of no clinical significance. (A)

168. **3.** Metronidazole (Flagyl) can cause a disulfiram (Antabuse)-like reaction if it is taken with alcohol. Tachycardia, nausea, vomiting, and other serious interaction effects can occur. Flagyl will make the urine a darker color. Oral contraceptives should never be discontinued with trichomoniasis. The partner also requires treatment to prevent retransmission of infection. (D)

169. **1.** In the advanced stages of osteoarthritis, pain can occur with minimal activity or even when the client is at rest. Crepitation can be present at any stage of the disease and does not exacerbate pain. Joints are not symmetrically affected by the disease. Symmetric joint involvement and fatigue are characteristics of rheumatoid arthritis. (A)

170. **3.** The traditional belief of Vietnamese Americans is that the family can provide more comfort for their loved one at home. It is not seen as being disloyal if their loved one dies in the hospital. The request is not based on a feeling that the hospital cannot be trusted. Vietnamese Americans accept death as a part of life and do not think that reincarnation is prevented in the hospital. (P)

171. **2.** It is important for the daughter to know that there is an underlying cause for what her mother is experiencing and that it is treatable. Telling her not to worry is a useless cliché and does nothing to inform the daughter. Talking about care after discharge implies that the delirium is irreversible. Delirium is a reversible condition. Although not arguing with hallucinations is valid, this response ignores the daughter's concern. (P)

172. **2.** The client with Alzheimer's dementia should not have access to toiletries that could be swallowed (such as aftershave) unless closely supervised. Putting special locks on all the doors is appropriate to prevent wandering, thus maintaining the client's safety. Placing the client in a room that has nothing to trip over is appropriate to reduce the client's risk of falling. Taking the knobs off of the stove is appropriate to prevent possible burns. (P)

173. **3.** It is important that the client force fluids to 3,000 ml/day to avoid the development of renal calculi when taking allopurinol. Allopurinol must be taken consistently to be effective in the treatment of gout. The drug should be taken after meals to avoid gastrointestinal distress. Although the client can take aspirin when taking allopurinol, both drugs can cause gastrointestinal irritation and the practice is not recommended if the client is sensitive to the medications. (D)

174. 2. A white, cottage cheese–like discharge accompanied by severe itching is characteristic of candidal infection. Trichomonal infection has a yellow-green discharge. Bacterial vaginosis often has a positive, fishy odor. A purulent discharge should be investigated, cultured, and treated immediately. (A)

175. 3. The best advice for the nurse to give the child's mother is to run cool water over the burned area to stop the burning process. Then the area should be wrapped in a clean cloth. Once these initial actions are completed, the mother can call the child's physician. Packing the arm in ice may cause more damage to the burned area because cold can cause burns just as heat can. For most burns, it is not advised to apply ointment until the area has been evaluated. (R)

176. 4. The priority nursing diagnosis for this client is *Risk for injury*. The goal in this situation is to prevent falling. *Impaired physical mobility* contributes to the risk of injury and is an applicable diagnosis but does not address the client's safety needs, which are the priority. *Impaired skin integrity* and *Ineffective coping* are not applicable diagnoses at this time. (R)

177. 3. Chills and headache are signs of a febrile, non-hemolytic blood transfusion reaction and the nurse's first action should be to discontinue the transfusion as soon as possible and then notify the physician. Antipyretics and antihistamines may be ordered. The nurse would not administer acetaminophen without an order from the physician. The client's blood pressure should be taken after the transfusion is stopped. Checking the infusion rate of the blood is not a pertinent action; the infusion needs to be stopped regardless of the rate. (D)

178. 3. Resolving grief and having increased energy and activity convey good mental health, indicating that counseling is not necessary at this time. Taking an antidepressant or having less energy and involvement with grandchildren reflects possible depression and the need for counseling. Wanting to be with her dead husband suggests possible suicidal ideation that warrants serious further assessment and counseling. (P)

179. 3. Common adverse effects of isosorbide are light-headedness, dizziness, and orthostatic hypotension. Clients should be instructed to change positions slowly to prevent these adverse effects and to avoid fainting. Ankle swelling is not related to isosorbide administration. The client does not need to take his pulse before taking the medication. The client does not need to take the medication with food. (D)

180. 3. Valproic acid (Depakote) and propranolol (Inderal) are often prescribed to help manage explosive anger. Recognizing the need for medications indicates readiness for discharge. Not ever getting angry is difficult, impractical, and unrealistic without specific anger management strategies. Drinking does not address anger control and suggests a risk of continued drinking. Blaming others, such as the client's mother, does not address anger control and indicates a lack of responsibility for the client's own behavior. (D)

181. 3. The nurse should first help the client into a position of comfort even though the primary purpose for entering the room was to administer medication. After attending to the client's basic care needs, the nurse can proceed with the proper identification of the client, such as asking the client his name and checking his armband, so that the medication can be administered. (C)

182. 4. During the first 24 hours after an abdominal hysterectomy, the client is at risk for development of thrombophlebitis because of potential interference with pelvic and leg circulation. Leg exercises are essential to promote circulation and prevent a thrombus. Bowel sounds may not be heard immediately after surgery. It may take up to 48 hours for peristalsis to return. Perineal pads are used after a vaginal hysterectomy, not an abdominal hysterectomy. In the early phases of recovery, the client will be more likely to focus on expressing feelings of discomfort rather than a positive body image. (A)

183. 2. The client is asymptomatic but has had a change in heart rhythm. More information is needed before calling the physician. Because the client is taking furosemide (Lasix), a potassium-wasting diuretic, the next action would be to check the client's potassium level. The nurse would then call the physician with a more complete database. The physician will need to be notified after the nurse checks the latest potassium level. Calling the nurse-manager is not indicated at this time. Administering potassium requires a physician's order. (R)

184. 2. Depression is the most common affective disorder during the postpartum period, affecting 10% to 15% of all women. It is characterized by mood swings, uncontrollable crying, anorexia, and feelings of sadness. It is diagnosed when the transient "blues" persists beyond 2 weeks postpartum. Postpartum blues generally last only a few days and then resolve. Postpartum psychosis exists when the client loses touch with reality and requires hospitalization. Commonly, postpartum adjustment is resolved within a few days after delivery. (P)

185. **4.** Just as with a child, it is best to answer relatives honestly when they ask questions about their loved one's condition. The nurse answers the questions honestly when explaining that infections are often a result of leukemia rather than a cause of it. It is less satisfactory to tell the parents that everything possible has been done for their child, that the child is no longer suffering from the illness, or that nothing could have helped their child. (P)

186. **2.** After TURP, a client can be prone to bladder spasms. Because of the spasms and the decreased urine output, it is important for the nurse to evaluate the client to determine whether the bladder spasms have been caused by blood clots that are obstructing the flow of urine from the catheter. The client will be acutely uncomfortable until the situation is resolved. The febrile client will need to be assessed for the possible source of the fever, but this assessment can be delayed until the client with bladder spasms has received care. The client with the ileal conduit needs to have the pouch emptied of urine; this activity can be delegated to the assistant. A small amount of hemoptysis after a bronchoscopy with biopsy is to be expected and does not require immediate follow-up. (R)

187. **50**

Microdrip administration sets have a drop factor of 60 gtt/ml. Therefore,

60 gtt/ml × 500 ml/600 minutes = 50 gtt/minute.

(D)

188. **1.** The client must wait 14 days between stopping phenelzine and starting fluoxetine because of the risk of serotonin syndrome, a potentially lethal condition manifested by hyperreflexia, hyperthermia, myoclonus, and other signs and symptoms suggesting neuroleptic malignant syndrome. The client does not need to have blood levels drawn every week while taking fluoxetine. Weekly blood draws are especially needed when lithium or clozapine therapy is initiated. Notifying the physician before taking any over-the-counter medication is not usually necessary unless other conditions warrant it. Headache and nausea are common adverse effects of fluoxetine and do not require immediate physician notification. However, severe headaches or nausea should be reported. (D)

189. **3.** Taking a deep abdominal breath and then "huff" coughing is the most effective manner of coughing. This technique helps facilitate removal of secretions and conserves energy for the client. The client should breathe slowly but not hold her breath. Short, panting breaths and then coughing from the throat do not promote expectoration of sputum from the lungs. Coughing forcefully can cause alveoli to collapse; "huff" coughing prevents this. (R)

190. **3.** The first objective is for the nurse to get the client's attention. This can be done by looking the client in the eyes and speaking in a calm voice. Once the nurse has her attention, the nurse can instruct the client in breathing techniques. Modified pace breathing can be used during the contractions. The nurse may need to assist the client to breathe with each contraction. Telling the client to calm down or to breathe with each contraction is not helpful if the client isn't listening to the nurse. The nurse needs to get the client's attention first. Analgesia is not warranted at this phase of labor because the neonate may experience respiratory depression if delivery occurs within 1 to 2 hours. (P)

1. A nurse has been working with a battered woman who is being discharged and returning home with her husband. The nurse says, "All this work with her has been useless. She's just going back to him as usual." Which of the following statements by a nursing colleague would be *most* helpful to this nurse?

☐ **1.** "Her reasons for staying are complex. She can leave only when she is ready and can be safe."

☐ **2.** "I know it is frustrating to work with clients who don't follow our advice."

☐ **3.** "You did your best. You will see her again and have another chance."

☐ **4.** "These women almost never leave for good because of their emotional and financial dependency."

2. Ergonovine maleate (Ergotrate) 200 µg I.M. has been ordered. The ampule label reads 0.2 mg/ml. The nurse should administer how many milliliters?

_____ ml

3. The nurse in a community hospital has been notified that a 6-month-old infant is being admitted from the emergency department with dehydration secondary to viral gastroenteritis. Which of the following room assignments is the most appropriate for this infant?

☐ **1.** A semiprivate room with an 8-year-old child who has had an appendectomy.

☐ **2.** A semiprivate room with a 10-year-old child with a closed head injury.

☐ **3.** A private room.

☐ **4.** A semiprivate room with a 4-year-old child with leukemia.

4. For which of the following should the nurse be especially alert when caring for a term neonate, who weighed 10 lb at birth, 1 hour after a vaginal delivery?

☐ **1.** Hypoglycemia.

☐ **2.** Hypercalcemia.

☐ **3.** Hypermagnesemia.

☐ **4.** Hyperbilirubinemia.

5. A female client with infertility related to anovulatory cycles is prescribed menotropins (Pergonal). Which of the following, if stated by the client as a possible adverse effect of this medication, indicates successful teaching?

☐ **1.** Pulmonary edema.

☐ **2.** Ovarian enlargement.

☐ **3.** Visual disturbances.

☐ **4.** Breast tenderness.

6. A family has been notified that their son is brain dead, and the physician has discussed the possibility of donating organs. The nurse is aware that the referral sources responsible for organ recovery in the United States are the:

☐ **1.** Organ and Tissue Procurement Organizations.

☐ **2.** American Transplant Association.

☐ **3.** American Hospice Foundation.

☐ **4.** American Association of Critical-Care Nurses.

7. The nurse is involved in preoperative teaching with a client who will be undergoing a lung resection. The client is told that two chest tubes will be placed during surgery. The nurse explains that the purpose of the lower chest tube is to:

☐ **1.** Prevent clots.

☐ **2.** Remove air.

☐ **3.** Remove fluid.

☐ **4.** Facilitate "milking" of the tubes.

8. A nurse is assessing an 82-year-old for depression. Depression in an older adult differs from depression in a younger person in which way?

☐ **1.** Sadness of mood is usually present but it is masked by other symptoms.

☐ **2.** Impairment of cognition usually is not present.

☐ **3.** Psychosomatic tendencies do not tend to dominate.

☐ **4.** Antidepressant therapies are less effective.

9. A primary concern of the hospitalized adolescent would be:

☐ **1.** Respect for the need for privacy.

☐ **2.** Allowing parents to visit after hours.

☐ **3.** Wearing a hospital gown.

☐ **4.** The fear of loss of control when in pain.

10. A 20-year-old single parent brings her 3-year-old son into the emergency department because he "fell." The child has bruises on his face, arms, and legs; his mother says that she did not witness the fall. The nurse suspects child abuse. While examining the child, the mother says, "Sometimes I guess I'm pretty rough with him. I'm alone, and I just don't know how to manage him." The nurse should anticipate referring the mother to which of the following types of programs?

☐ **1.** A program for single parents.

☐ **2.** A parenting education program.

☐ **3.** A women's support group.

☐ **4.** A support group for abusive parents.

11. A nurse who fails to check a client's armband before administering his medications is:
- ☐ **1.** Res judicata.
- ☐ **2.** Negligent.
- ☐ **3.** Stare decisis.
- ☐ **4.** Vicariously liable.

12. Before administering morphine to a client, the nurse should assess the client's:
- ☐ **1.** Blood pressure.
- ☐ **2.** Respiration rate.
- ☐ **3.** Pulse.
- ☐ **4.** Temperature.

13. A client is to receive 1 unit of packed red blood cells over 2 hours. The I.V. administration infusion set delivers 10 gtt/ml. At what flow rate (in drops per minute) should the nurse run the infusion?

_____ gtt/minute

14. A mother states that she is very angry with the physician who diagnosed her child with leukemia. Which statement helps the nurse understand this mother's reaction?
- ☐ **1.** Anger is a natural result of a sense of loss and helplessness.
- ☐ **2.** Parents of sick children are usually unable to control their anger.
- ☐ **3.** Anger is rarely demonstrated by parents when coping with a sick child.
- ☐ **4.** The mother cannot overcome her anger in an acceptable manner.

15. Which of the following nursing strategies would be effective in managing a resident in a long-term care facility who has Alzheimer's disease and wanders?
- ☐ **1.** Encourage participation in activities such as board games.
- ☐ **2.** Discourage wandering by allowing the behavior at selected intervals.
- ☐ **3.** Involve the client in activities that promote walking.
- ☐ **4.** Promote safety by restricting the client in a geriatric chair.

16. A child who had a cast applied to his arm earlier this morning is complaining that his fingers are numb. Which of the following actions by the nurse would be most appropriate?
- ☐ **1.** Notify the physician who applied the cast.
- ☐ **2.** Cut the cast to loosen it.
- ☐ **3.** Assess the circulation to the fingers.
- ☐ **4.** Ensure that the arm is positioned correctly.

17. The major advantage of second-generation antihistamines such as loratadine (Claritin) and fexofenadine (Allegra) is:
- ☐ **1.** Decreased cost.
- ☐ **2.** Increased effectiveness.
- ☐ **3.** Delayed absorption.
- ☐ **4.** They are nonsedating.

18. The client with newly diagnosed low back pain (LBP) is very worried. The nurse emphasizes that the most common cause of LBP is:
- ☐ **1.** Osteoporosis.
- ☐ **2.** Herniated disk.
- ☐ **3.** Muscle strain.
- ☐ **4.** Spondylosis.

19. While helping clients brought to a crisis center during a severe flood, the nurse interviews a client whose pregnant wife is missing and whose home has been destroyed. The client keeps talking rapidly about his experience and says, "I can't see how I can ever rebuild my life." Which of the following responses by the nurse would be most appropriate?
- ☐ **1.** "If you start organizing your life now, I'm sure all will be fine."
- ☐ **2.** "This has been a terrible experience. Tell me more about how you feel."
- ☐ **3.** "Let me note a few of the things you said before you continue with your story."
- ☐ **4.** "Tonight, think some more of what happened, so that we can continue with this tomorrow."

20. A client with asthma has been prescribed beclomethasone (Beclovent) via metered-dose inhaler. The nurse instructs the client to rinse her mouth after using the beclomethasone inhaler to help prevent:
- ☐ **1.** Gingival hyperplasia.
- ☐ **2.** Oral candidiasis.
- ☐ **3.** Absorption of too large a dose.
- ☐ **4.** Dental caries.

21. The nurse finds a client lying on the floor next to the bed. After returning the client to bed, assessing for injury, and notifying the physician, the nurse fills out an incident report. Which of the following is the nurse's next action?
- ☐ **1.** Give the incident report to the nurse-manager.
- ☐ **2.** Place the incident report on the chart.
- ☐ **3.** Call the family to inform them.
- ☐ **4.** Omit mentioning the fall in the chart documentation.

22. The mother of 2-year-old who has been bitten by the family dog asks the nurse what to do about the bite. Which of the following would be the most appropriate recommendation to this mother?

☐ **1.** "You need to take the child to the local urgent care center immediately."

☐ **2.** "Wash the bite area with lots of running water, and then check the injury."

☐ **3.** "Determine when the child's latest tetanus vaccine was administered."

☐ **4.** "Make an appointment to see the child's physician now to start rabies shots."

23. A multigravid client at 36 weeks' gestation who has type 1 diabetes is scheduled for a biophysical profile in the morning. The nurse explains to the client that which of the following is one of the fetal parameters to be assessed?

☐ **1.** Biparietal diameter.

☐ **2.** Bilirubin levels.

☐ **3.** Contraction stress test.

☐ **4.** Breathing movements.

24. A schoolteacher calls the nurse and asks whether all the children at school need treatment after exposure to a 7-year-old child with bacterial meningitis. The nurse responds that chemoprophylaxis should be given to:

☐ **1.** All children at the school.

☐ **2.** All household contacts and close contacts.

☐ **3.** The entire community.

☐ **4.** Household contacts only.

25. The mother of an 18-month-old boy is concerned about the number of persons with heart disease in her family. She asks the nurse when she should start her infant on a diet to lower the risk of heart disease. The nurse tells her that the American Heart Association provides recommendations for children to prevent heart disease. For what age do they begin providing recommendations?

☐ **1.** At birth.

☐ **2.** At age 2.

☐ **3.** At age 5.

☐ **4.** At age 10.

26. A client is being treated for severe pediculosis. The nurse teaches the client to treat the problem in the eyebrows and eyelashes by:

☐ **1.** Applying petroleum jelly to lashes and brows three to four times a day.

☐ **2.** Applying a pediculicide with a cotton-tipped swab three to four times a day.

☐ **3.** Applying lindane ointment to the lashes and eyebrows three times a day.

☐ **4.** Applying bacitracin ointment to the lashes and brows three times a day.

27. The nurse is discussing safety and accident prevention with the mother of a 9-month-old. The nurse knows that the teaching has been effective when the mother states which of the following?

☐ **1.** "I make sure that I keep my cleaning supplies locked up."

☐ **2.** "Sometimes she plays in the bathroom when I'm cleaning in there."

☐ **3.** "Occasionally she gets under the chair and plays with the telephone cord."

☐ **4.** "I've found that those child-protective cabinet locks don't work very well."

28. The nurse knows that atypical signs and symptoms of appendicitis could occur in:

☐ **1.** Children older than age 5.

☐ **2.** Pregnant women in the first trimester.

☐ **3.** Adolescents.

☐ **4.** Clients who are taking steroids.

29. When assessing a child receiving tobramycin sulfate (Nebcin), which findings would indicate that the child is experiencing adverse effects? Select all that apply.

☐ **1.** Increased blood pressure.

☐ **2.** Weight gain.

☐ **3.** Rash.

☐ **4.** Fever.

☐ **5.** Ringing in the ears.

☐ **6.** Decreased heart rate.

30. The nurse instructs the client who is taking gentamicin to monitor factors related to renal function. The nurse determines that the client needs additional instruction when he makes which of the following statements?

☐ **1.** "I should call you if I notice that I'm not urinating as much."

☐ **2.** "I should call you if my urine looks dark or unusual."

☐ **3.** "I should call you if my legs swell or I notice my skin looks puffy around my eyes."

☐ **4.** "I should call you if I have a fever."

31. A 15-month-old child is admitted to the pediatric unit with the diagnosis of pneumonia and is placed in a mist tent. Which of the following toys would be appropriate for this child?

☐ **1.** A pull toy.

☐ **2.** Storybooks.

☐ **3.** Crayons and paper.

☐ **4.** Plastic blocks.

32. When teaching a group of parents about the potential for febrile seizures in children, which of the following facts should the nurse include?

☐ **1.** The exact cause is known.

☐ **2.** The seizures occur as the fever rises.

☐ **3.** Children older than age 3 are most at risk.

☐ **4.** These seizures commonly occur after immunization administration.

33. The nurse should instruct a woman taking folic acid supplements for folic acid-deficiency anemia that:

☐ **1.** It will take several months to notice an improvement.

☐ **2.** Folic acid should be taken on an empty stomach.

☐ **3.** Iron supplements are contraindicated with folic acid supplementation.

☐ **4.** Oral contraceptive use, pregnancy, and lactation increase daily requirements.

34. The nurse makes a home visit to a primiparous client and her neonate at 1 week after a vaginal delivery. Which of the following findings should be reported to the physician?

☐ **1.** A scant amount of maternal lochia serosa.

☐ **2.** The presence of a neonatal tonic neck reflex.

☐ **3.** A nonpalpable maternal fundus.

☐ **4.** Neonatal central cyanosis.

35. Which of the following is the most common systemic antibiotic used in the treatment of severe acne?

☐ **1.** Isotretinoin (Accutane).

☐ **2.** Cephalexin (Keflex).

☐ **3.** Azithromycin (Zithromax).

☐ **4.** Tetracycline (Achromycin).

36. Which of the following is not a risk factor for osteoporosis?

☐ **1.** Heavy use of alcohol.

☐ **2.** Excessive antacid use.

☐ **3.** A diet very high in fiber.

☐ **4.** Adequate vitamin K intake.

37. The nurse tells a rape victim that even if she was protected against pregnancy by a contraceptive and has no intention of taking any legal action against her assailant, she should still be checked by a physician. The nurse recommends this postrape physical examination primarily for early detection of which of the following?

☐ **1.** Sexually transmitted disease.

☐ **2.** Anxiety reaction.

☐ **3.** Periurethral tears.

☐ **4.** Menstrual difficulties.

38. A client in a private room fell on the floor and sustained a small laceration on her hand that required stitches. The intern asks for bupivacaine (Marcaine) with epinephrine and a suture kit in order to suture the laceration. The nurse should question which of the following?

☐ **1.** The intern's ability to suture.

☐ **2.** The client's room as an aseptic environment.

☐ **3.** Marcaine with epinephrine as the local anesthetic.

☐ **4.** The cosmetic effect from suturing.

39. Which of the following signs and symptoms experienced by a child with suspected appendicitis should the nurse correctly judge to be unrelated to the transient sympathetic effects caused by the acute abdominal pain?

☐ **1.** Tachycardia.

☐ **2.** Chills.

☐ **3.** Rapid breathing.

☐ **4.** Dilated pupils.

40. When assessing a dark-skinned client for cyanosis, the nurse should examine which of the following?

☐ **1.** The client's retinas.

☐ **2.** The client's nail beds.

☐ **3.** The client's oral mucous membranes.

☐ **4.** The inner aspects of the client's wrists.

41. Betamethasone (Celestone) syrup 0.9 mg has been ordered. It is available in a 0.6 mg/5 ml solution. How many milliliters should the nurse administer?

_____ ml

42. A client at 37 weeks' gestation is scheduled for a biophysical profile. Which of the following should the nurse instruct the client to do before the test?

☐ **1.** Drink 1 to 2 L of fluid.

☐ **2.** Take nothing by mouth after midnight before the test.

☐ **3.** Plan to remain in the clinic for 4 hours after the test.

☐ **4.** Eat a high-fiber meal after the test.

43. The nurse on the obstetric unit has been notified by staff in the emergency department that a primigravid client with a history of sickle cell disease is to be admitted at 32 weeks' gestation with a diagnosis of sickle cell crisis. The nurse anticipates that the physician will order an infusion of which of the following?

☐ **1.** Platelets.

☐ **2.** Granulocytes.

☐ **3.** Packed red blood cells (RBCs).

☐ **4.** Whole blood.

44. A working mother is concerned about the amount of snacking her teenage boy is doing. She is concerned that this behavior could lead to obesity. Which of the following is an appropriate percentage of the daily diet to be obtained from snacks?

☐ **1.** 10%.

☐ **2.** 25%.

☐ **3.** 40%.

☐ **4.** 50%.

45. The client complains of sore nares while a nasogastric (NG) tube is in place. Which of the following nursing measures would be most appropriate to help alleviate the client's discomfort?
- ☐ 1. Reposition the tube in the nares.
- ☐ 2. Irrigate the tube with a cool solution.
- ☐ 3. Apply a water-soluble lubricant to the nares.
- ☐ 4. Have the client change position more frequently.

46. The nurse is instructing a Hindu client to increase protein in the diet. Which of the following meal plans is appropriate for a Hindu client?
- ☐ 1. Lentil soup and fish sandwich.
- ☐ 2. Hamburger.
- ☐ 3. Steak.
- ☐ 4. Veal cutlet.

47. A child with partial- and full-thickness burns is admitted to the pediatric unit. Which of the following should be the priority at this time?
- ☐ 1. Preventing wound infection.
- ☐ 2. Evaluating vital signs frequently.
- ☐ 3. Maintaining fluid and electrolyte balance.
- ☐ 4. Managing the child's pain.

48. A normal, healthy infant is brought to the clinic for the first immunization against polio. The nurse should administer this vaccine by what route?
- ☐ 1. Oral route.
- ☐ 2. I.M. route.
- ☐ 3. Subcutaneous route.
- ☐ 4. Intradermal route.

49. A child has been prescribed diphenhydramine hydrochloride (Benadryl) to help control the itching from atopic dermatitis. Which adverse effects should the nurse include as most common when teaching the family about this drug? Select all that apply.
- ☐ 1. Weight loss.
- ☐ 2. Drowsiness.
- ☐ 3. Thickened bronchial secretions.
- ☐ 4. Upset stomach.
- ☐ 5. Bradycardia.

50. The nurse observes that a client who has received midazolam (Versed) for local anesthesia is having shallow respirations. Which of the following actions is inappropriate for the nurse to do?
- ☐ 1. Encourage the client to deep-breathe.
- ☐ 2. Have respiratory resuscitation equipment in the room.
- ☐ 3. Administer oxygen as ordered.
- ☐ 4. Administer naloxone (Narcan).

51. The nurse is planning to assist the physician with a thoracentesis for a client who has a pleural effusion. Which of the following positions would be appropriate for the client to assume?
- ☐ 1. Lying supine with the arms extended.
- ☐ 2. Lying prone with the head supported by the arms.
- ☐ 3. Sitting upright and leaning on an overbed table.
- ☐ 4. Side-lying with the knees drawn up to the abdomen.

52. The nurse is preparing a presentation on nutrition to a group of pregnant adolescents. Which of the following would be important for the nurse to include in the teaching plan?
- ☐ 1. Spinach is an excellent source of calcium in the diet.
- ☐ 2. Two to four servings of whole-grain products is recommended.
- ☐ 3. Three or more servings of dairy products meet the calcium requirement.
- ☐ 4. Vitamin A supplements may be necessary for clients who are vegetarian.

53. The nurse anticipates an expected outcome of a viral (coxsackie B) or trypanosomal (parasite) infection is:
- ☐ 1. Myocarditis.
- ☐ 2. Myocardial infarction.
- ☐ 3. Renal failure.
- ☐ 4. Liver failure.

54. Which of the following compensatory actions by the body would occur if a client were in respiratory acidosis?
- ☐ 1. Excretion of bicarbonate (HCO_3^-) by the kidneys.
- ☐ 2. Retention of HCO_3^- by the kidneys.
- ☐ 3. Increase in respiratory rate by the lungs.
- ☐ 4. Decrease in respiratory rate by the lungs.

55. A client has started taking amiodarone (Cordarone). The nurse should inform the client that periodic laboratory tests will be done to monitor the client's:
- ☐ 1. Hemoglobin.
- ☐ 2. Liver enzymes.
- ☐ 3. Creatine kinase (CK) concentration.
- ☐ 4. Renal function.

56. The father of a 9-month-old child diagnosed with a first ear infection asks whether he should do anything else to help the child. Which of the following would be the nurse's best response?
- ☐ 1. "Your child should also take an antihistamine."
- ☐ 2. "The antibiotic is the only medicine necessary."
- ☐ 3. "Cotton in the ears helps the discomfort."
- ☐ 4. "Over-the-counter eardrops often are helpful."

57. A child's plan of care lists increasing protein intake as a goal. Which of the following foods that the child likes should the nurse encourage the child to eat?
☐ **1.** A bacon, lettuce, and tomato sandwich.
☐ **2.** Fruit-flavored yogurt.
☐ **3.** Nacho chips and salsa.
☐ **4.** Crackers with butter and jelly.

58. The clinical findings of prominent neck veins, hypertension, and bounding pulse are specifically indicative of fluid excess in which body compartment?
☐ **1.** Interstitial compartment.
☐ **2.** Intravascular compartment.
☐ **3.** Intracellular compartment.
☐ **4.** Extracellular compartment.

59. Which of the following laboratory findings should the nurse anticipate will not be affected by ciprofloxacin (Cipro)?
☐ **1.** Theophylline level.
☐ **2.** Prothrombin time (PT).
☐ **3.** Partial thromboplastin time (PTT).
☐ **4.** Total iron-binding capacity.

60. A 10-year-old child is diagnosed with pediculosis. The mother is concerned about the spread of the lice to children who have been in contact with her child. Which of the following activities would cause the most concern?
☐ **1.** Sharing craft supplies.
☐ **2.** Having contact during a swimming class.
☐ **3.** Sharing batting helmets.
☐ **4.** Showering after football practice.

61. A 24-year-old nulligravid client with a history of irregular menstrual cycles visits the clinic because she suspects that she is "about 6 weeks pregnant." An ultrasound is scheduled for the client 2 weeks from today. When teaching the client about the procedure, which of the following should the nurse include as the most likely reason for this client to have the procedure?
☐ **1.** Assessment of gestational age.
☐ **2.** Determination of a multifetal pregnancy.
☐ **3.** Identification of the gender of the fetus.
☐ **4.** Assessment of maternal pelvic adequacy.

62. A client with a history of peptic ulcer disease is admitted to the hospital. Initial assessment reveals that his blood pressure is 96/60 mm Hg, his pulse rate is 120 bpm, and he has vomited coffee-ground material. Based on this assessment, what is the nurse's priority action?
☐ **1.** Administer an antiemetic.
☐ **2.** Prepare to insert a nasogastric (NG) tube.
☐ **3.** Collect data regarding recent client stressors.
☐ **4.** Place the client in a modified Trendelenburg position.

63. A male client has intermittent episodes of third-degree heart block and complains of shortness of breath and chest pain. The nurse anticipates that the client will undergo:
☐ **1.** Cardiac catheterization.
☐ **2.** Coronary artery bypass surgery.
☐ **3.** Insertion of a temporary pacemaker.
☐ **4.** Insertion of an aortic balloon pump.

64. As of 1999, all refined grain products, such as cereal, pasta, flour, rolls, buns, farina, grits, and rice, are fortified with which of the following?
☐ **1.** Vitamin C.
☐ **2.** Niacin.
☐ **3.** Vitamin B_{12}.
☐ **4.** Folic acid.

65. In the early postoperative period, the nurse notes a bright red, $3'' \times 5''$ area of drainage on the client's abdominal laparotomy dressing. What should be the nurse's first action in response to this observation?
☐ **1.** Ignore it because drainage is normal.
☐ **2.** Increase the I.V. flow rate.
☐ **3.** Take the client's vital signs.
☐ **4.** Change the dressing.

66. Knowing that the infant with pyloric stenosis is at risk because of decreased circulating fluid volume, the nurse should assess for which of the following disorders?
☐ **1.** Inappropriate antidiuretic hormone release.
☐ **2.** Acute renal failure.
☐ **3.** Paralytic ileus.
☐ **4.** Adrenal insufficiency.

67. A client has massive bleeding from esophageal varices. In what order should the nurse and care team provide care for this client?

1. Control hemorrhaging.

2. Replace fluids.

3. Relieve the client's anxiety.

4. Maintain a patent airway.

68. Which of the following areas would be most important for the nurse to include in the teaching plan for a client who is taking phenelzine (Nardil)?
- ☐ **1.** Eating a normal amount of salt in the diet.
- ☐ **2.** Drinking 10 to 12 glasses of water each day.
- ☐ **3.** Allowing 10 days to achieve therapeutic effects.
- ☐ **4.** Avoiding foods high in tyramine.

69. The nurse should closely monitor the client with an open fracture for which of the following complications?
- ☐ **1.** Avascular necrosis.
- ☐ **2.** Compartment syndrome.
- ☐ **3.** Osteomyelitis.
- ☐ **4.** Fat embolism syndrome.

70. Which of the following should be a priority nursing diagnosis for a client who has had a total laryngectomy?
- ☐ **1.** *Risk for impaired skin integrity.*
- ☐ **2.** *Excess fluid volume.*
- ☐ **3.** *Ineffective thermoregulation.*
- ☐ **4.** *Impaired verbal communication.*

71. When conducting a screening session for hypertension at a retirement center, the nurse encounters a client who has a long history of uncontrolled hypertension. The nurse should teach the client that chronic hypertension can damage which area of the eye?
- ☐ **1.** Iris.
- ☐ **2.** Cornea.
- ☐ **3.** Retina.
- ☐ **4.** Sclera.

72. While preparing to provide neonatal care instructions to a primiparous client who delivered a term neonate 24 hours ago, which of the following should the nurse be include in the client's teaching plan?
- ☐ **1.** Term neonates generally have few creases on the soles of their feet.
- ☐ **2.** Strawberry hemangiomas—deep, dark red discolorations—require laser therapy for removal.
- ☐ **3.** Milia are white papules from plugged sebaceous ducts that disappear by age 2 to 4 weeks.
- ☐ **4.** If erythema toxicum is present, it will be treated with antibiotic therapy.

73. Two days after the fracture of his femur, a client suddenly complains of chest pain and dyspnea. The nurse also notes some confusion and an elevated temperature. Based on these assessment findings, the nurse suspects which of the following complications?
- ☐ **1.** Osteomyelitis.
- ☐ **2.** Compartment syndrome.
- ☐ **3.** Venous thrombosis.
- ☐ **4.** Fat embolism syndrome.

74. Which findings should the nurse assess as late signs of a large overdose of sympathomimetic agents? Select all that apply.
- ☐ **1.** Hypotension.
- ☐ **2.** Bradycardia.
- ☐ **3.** Seizures.
- ☐ **4.** Profound pyrexia.
- ☐ **5.** Hypertension.

75. While assessing a neonate at 4 hours after birth, the nurse observes an indentation with a small tuft of hair at the base of the neonate's spine. The nurse should document this finding as which of the following?
- ☐ **1.** Spina bifida cystica.
- ☐ **2.** Spina bifida occulta.
- ☐ **3.** Meningocele.
- ☐ **4.** Myelomeningocele.

76. The primary purpose of instilling 5 ml of normal saline before suctioning a tracheostomy tube is to:
- ☐ **1.** Thin the secretions to be suctioned.
- ☐ **2.** Stimulate the client to cough.
- ☐ **3.** Help the catheter to slide down the tracheostomy tube.
- ☐ **4.** Provide humidification to the respiratory tract.

77. A client with emphysema is receiving continuous oxygen therapy. Depressed ventilation is likely to occur unless the nurse ensures that the oxygen is administered in which of the following ways?
- ☐ **1.** Cooled.
- ☐ **2.** Humidified.
- ☐ **3.** At a low flow rate.
- ☐ **4.** Through nasal cannula.

78. A client at 12 weeks' gestation tells the nurse that she is a vegetarian and eats "lots of rice." To help meet the client's need for protein during pregnancy, the nurse suggests that the client combine the rice with which of the following?
- ☐ **1.** Beans.
- ☐ **2.** Soy milk.
- ☐ **3.** Yogurt.
- ☐ **4.** Corn.

79. A client with rheumatoid arthritis tells the nurse that she feels "quite alone" in adjusting to changes in her lifestyle. Which of the following nursing actions is most appropriate in response to this statement?
- ☐ **1.** Refer the client and her husband for counseling to decrease her sense of isolation.
- ☐ **2.** Suggest that the client develop a hobby to occupy her time.
- ☐ **3.** Tell the client about her community's arthritis support group.
- ☐ **4.** Suggest that the client discuss her feelings with her minister.

80. Which of the following should the nurse expect to include in the plan of care to ensure adequate nutrition for a very active, talkative, and easily distractible client who is unable to sit through meals?
☐ **1.** Direct the client to his room to eat.
☐ **2.** Offer the client nutritious finger foods.
☐ **3.** Ask the client's family to bring his favorite foods from home.
☐ **4.** Ask the client about his food preferences.

81. A client is very dependent on the staff but is able to make simple decisions. The client asks, "Would you do my laundry? I don't know how the machine works." Which of the following responses would be best?
☐ **1.** "Sure, I have time; I can do it for you."
☐ **2.** "You'll have to wait; I don't have time now."
☐ **3.** "Can your family do it for you?"
☐ **4.** "Get your laundry; I'll show you how the machine works."

82. The nurse is caring for a client with chronic renal failure. Knowing that the client is a candidate for development of hypermagnesemia, for which of the following signs and symptoms should the nurse closely monitor the client?
☐ **1.** Flushed skin.
☐ **2.** Lethargy.
☐ **3.** Severe thirst.
☐ **4.** Tremors.

83. A newly diagnosed diabetic informs the nurse that she has not been eating to try and better control her blood sugar. The nurse tells her that this is not a solution to blood glucose control because blood glucose is regulated not only by insulin but by glucagon, which is stimulated to raise the blood glucose level when a person has not eaten. Glucagon causes a rise in the glucose level by stimulating:
☐ **1.** Glycogen breakdown and release from the muscles.
☐ **2.** The intestine to absorb glucose.
☐ **3.** The liver to release glucose into the blood.
☐ **4.** The brain to release glucose.

84. When giving a change of shift report, which of the following statements by the nurse is not considered appropriate?
☐ **1.** "Randi Smith is a 38-year-old female client of Dr. Born with cholecystitis and cholelithiasis."
☐ **2.** "Mrs. Jones' pain is best relieved in the left lateral Sims position."
☐ **3.** "Mr. Levi is just contrary today and nothing is going to please him."
☐ **4.** "Mr. Emmert was able to walk around the unit twice today with no complaint of dizziness."

85. The nurse is teaching unlicensed personnel about caring for a client who is withdrawing from alcohol and street drugs. Which of the following communication techniques should the nurse include in the teaching?
☐ **1.** Matter-of-fact manner and short sentences.
☐ **2.** Cheerful tone and humor.
☐ **3.** Abstract terms and a loud voice tone.
☐ **4.** Clear, lengthy explanations in a quiet voice.

86. When obtaining the diet history from a client with anemia, the nurse should include questions specifically about which of the following vitamins or minerals that are most likely missing in this client's diet? Select all that apply.
☐ **1.** Vitamin B_6.
☐ **2.** Vitamin K.
☐ **3.** Vitamin B_{12}.
☐ **4.** Iron.
☐ **5.** Vitamin C.

87. What is the primary goal of nursing care during the emergent phase after a burn injury?
☐ **1.** Replace lost fluids.
☐ **2.** Prevent infection.
☐ **3.** Control pain.
☐ **4.** Promote wound healing.

88. The nurse assesses for euphoria in a client with multiple sclerosis, looking for which of the following characteristic clinical manifestations?
☐ **1.** Inappropriate laughter.
☐ **2.** An exaggerated sense of well-being.
☐ **3.** Slurring of words when excited.
☐ **4.** Visual hallucinations.

89. The client with a burn injury is assessed using the "rule of nines" to determine which of the following?
☐ **1.** Amount of body surface area burned.
☐ **2.** Rehabilitation needs.
☐ **3.** Respiratory needs.
☐ **4.** Type of intravenous fluids required.

90. When assessing a 2-month-old infant, the nurse feels a "click" when abducting the infant's left hip. Which of the following should the nurse do next?
☐ **1.** Document the finding as normal for a 2-month-old.
☐ **2.** Check the lengths of the femurs to see if they are equal.
☐ **3.** Instruct the mother to keep the leg in an adducted position.
☐ **4.** Reschedule the child for a follow-up assessment in 3 weeks.

91. Which of the following laboratory tests should the nurse monitor when the client is receiving warfarin sodium (Coumadin) therapy?
- ☐ **1.** Partial thromboplastin time (PTT).
- ☐ **2.** Serum potassium.
- ☐ **3.** Arterial blood gas (ABG) values.
- ☐ **4.** Prothrombin time (PT).

92. A client who had transurethral resection of the prostate (TURP) 2 days earlier is complaining of lower abdominal pain. Which nursing intervention should the nurse perform first?
- ☐ **1.** Auscultate the abdomen for bowel sounds.
- ☐ **2.** Administer an oral analgesic.
- ☐ **3.** Have the client use a sitz bath for 15 minutes.
- ☐ **4.** Assess the patency of the urethral catheter.

93. The nurse should identify which of the following as a priority nursing diagnosis for the family of a neonate with cleft lip?
- ☐ **1.** *Impaired parenting.*
- ☐ **2.** *Grieving.*
- ☐ **3.** *Ineffective coping.*
- ☐ **4.** *Anxiety.*

94. The nurse is ready to administer a partial fill of imipenem-cilastatin (Primaxin) in the I.V. pump when a full partial fill bag of imipenem-cilastatin is found hanging at the client's bedside. Which of the following is not an appropriate response for the nurse when recognizing that the previous dose was not administered 8 hours ago to the client with pneumonia?
- ☐ **1.** Discard the full partial fill of imipenem-cilastatin found hanging at the client's bedside.
- ☐ **2.** Check the identifying information of the full partial fill of imipenem-cilastatin found hanging at the client's bedside.
- ☐ **3.** Follow up on the legal documentation of the client's previous administration of imipenem-cilastatin.
- ☐ **4.** Administer the new partial fill of imipenem-cilastatin.

95. A client with a moderate level of anxiety is pacing quickly in the hall. As the nurse approaches, he states, "Help me. I can't take it anymore." Which of the following would be the best response initially?
- ☐ **1.** "It would be best if you would lie down until you're calmer."
- ☐ **2.** "Let's go to a quieter area where we can talk if you want."
- ☐ **3.** "Try doing your relaxation exercises to calm down."
- ☐ **4.** "I'll get some medicine to help you relax."

96. The nurse should plan to teach a client who is taking warfarin sodium (Coumadin) to do which of the following?
- ☐ **1.** Consult the physician before undergoing dental work.
- ☐ **2.** Avoid the use of a toothbrush during oral hygiene.
- ☐ **3.** Use rectal suppositories to treat constipation.
- ☐ **4.** Eat green leafy vegetables.

97. A 30-year-old client is hospitalized with a fractured femur, which is being treated with skeletal traction. He states that he has not had a bowel movement for 2 days. Which of the following interventions is most appropriate at this time?
- ☐ **1.** Administer a tap water enema.
- ☐ **2.** Place the client on the bedpan every 2 to 3 hours.
- ☐ **3.** Increase the client's fluid intake to 3,000 ml/day.
- ☐ **4.** Perform range-of-motion movements to all extremities.

98. A client is receiving a tube feeding and has developed diarrhea, cramps, and abdominal distention. Which of the following interventions would be most appropriate? Select all that apply.
- ☐ **1.** Make sure to change the feeding apparatus every 24 hours.
- ☐ **2.** Use a higher volume of formula because the formula may be too hypotonic.
- ☐ **3.** Slow the administration rate.
- ☐ **4.** Use a diluted formula, gradually increasing the volume and concentration.
- ☐ **5.** Anticipate changing to a lactose-free formula.

99. A 62-year-old client with a 29-pack per year history is admitted with a diagnosis of lung cancer. She reports "no appetite" and exhibits symptoms of anorexia. The client is 5 feet, 8 inches tall and weighs 112 lb. The client is now scheduled for a left lung lobectomy. Which of the following would increase the client's risk of developing postoperative pulmonary complications?
- ☐ **1.** The client tends to keep her real feelings to herself.
- ☐ **2.** The client ambulates and can climb one flight of stairs without dyspnea.
- ☐ **3.** The client is age 62.
- ☐ **4.** The client is 5 feet, 8 inches tall and weighs 112 lb.

100. When developing the plan of care for a 12-year-old child who is to receive 48 hours of chemotherapy that is associated with nausea and vomiting, at which of the following times should the nurse anticipate administering an antiemetic?
☐ **1.** 30 minutes after the chemotherapy has started, then every 4 to 6 hours.
☐ **2.** 30 minutes before the chemotherapy starts, then every 4 to 6 hours.
☐ **3.** When the 12-year-old requests medication for nausea, then every 4 hours as needed.
☐ **4.** On starting the chemotherapy infusion, and then routinely every 8 hours.

101. The membranes of a multigravid client in active labor rupture spontaneously, revealing greenish colored amniotic fluid. The nurse interprets this finding as related to which of the following?
☐ **1.** Passage of meconium by the fetus.
☐ **2.** Maternal intrauterine infection.
☐ **3.** Rh incompatibility between mother and fetus.
☐ **4.** Maternal sexually transmitted disease.

102. A client's arterial blood gas values are as follows:

LABORATORY RESULTS	
Test	**Result**
pH	7.24
$Paco_2$	35 mm Hg
HCO_3^-	15 mEq/L

These findings indicate which of the following acid-base imbalances?
☐ **1.** Metabolic acidosis.
☐ **2.** Metabolic alkalosis.
☐ **3.** Respiratory acidosis.
☐ **4.** Respiratory alkalosis.

103. A client is suspected of having a slow gastrointestinal bleed. The nurse should evaluate the client for which sign or symptom?
☐ **1.** Increased pulse.
☐ **2.** Nausea.
☐ **3.** Tarry stools.
☐ **4.** Abdominal cramps.

104. Which of the following suggestions should the nurse give to an adolescent football player with Osgood-Schlatter disease of the left knee?
☐ **1.** Apply ice on the knee after playing.
☐ **2.** Use crutches until healing has occurred.
☐ **3.** Stop playing until healing has occurred.
☐ **4.** Make an appointment with a physical therapist.

105. The nurse instructs a client who is taking iron supplements that:
☐ **1.** Iron supplements should be taken on an empty stomach.
☐ **2.** A daily bulk laxative such as psyllium hydrophilic mucilloid (Metamucil) should be avoided.
☐ **3.** The stools will become darker.
☐ **4.** Liquid iron supplements will not discolor teeth.

106. Which of the following should the nurse teach a client with generalized anxiety disorder to help the client cope with anxiety?
☐ **1.** Cognitive and behavioral strategies.
☐ **2.** Issue avoidance and denial of problems.
☐ **3.** Rest and sleep.
☐ **4.** Withdrawal from role expectations and role relationships.

107. After a lobectomy, clients are instructed to perform deep-breathing exercises to:
☐ **1.** Decrease blood flow to the lungs for rest and increased surface alveoli ventilation.
☐ **2.** Elevate the diaphragm to enlarge the thorax so that the lung surface area available for gas exchange is increased.
☐ **3.** Control the rate of air flow to the remaining lobe to decrease the risk of hyperinflation.
☐ **4.** Expand the alveoli and increase lung surface available for ventilation.

108. Which of the following would demonstrate the correct technique for applying an elastic bandage to a leg?
☐ **1.** Increase tension with each successive turn of the bandage.
☐ **2.** Start at the distal end of the extremity and move toward the trunk.
☐ **3.** Secure the bandage with clips over the area of the inner thigh.
☐ **4.** Overlap each layer twice when wrapping.

109. A nulliparous client says that she and her husband plan to use a diaphragm with spermicide to prevent conception. Which of the following should the nurse include as the action of spermicides when teaching the client?
☐ **1.** Destruction of spermatozoa before they enter the cervix.
☐ **2.** Prevention of spermatozoa from entering the uterus.
☐ **3.** A change in vaginal pH from acidic to alkaline.
☐ **4.** Slowing of the movement of the migrating spermatozoa.

110. A client with acquired immunodeficiency syndrome (AIDS) is admitted because of paranoia and visual hallucinations probably related to progressive dementia. In addition to continuing all of the client's AIDS-related medications, which of the following medications should the nurse expect the physician to add?

☐ **1.** Methylphenidate (Ritalin).
☐ **2.** Lorazepam (Ativan).
☐ **3.** Nefazodone (Serzone).
☐ **4.** Sertraline (Zoloft).

111. Which of the following assessment findings should a nurse expect to find in a client with bacterial pneumonia?

☐ **1.** Increased fremitus.
☐ **2.** Bilateral expiratory wheezing.
☐ **3.** Resonance on percussion.
☐ **4.** Vesicular breath sounds.

112. A client is admitted with complaints of severe abdominal pains and the diagnosis of acute pancreatitis. The plan of care during the acute phase of pancreatitis will involve interventions targeting which of the following problems?

☐ **1.** Drug and alcohol abuse.
☐ **2.** Risk for injury.
☐ **3.** Severe pain.
☐ **4.** Ineffective airway clearance.

113. A diabetic client who takes insulin is being seen by the nurse for a low blood glucose level. Which of the following would be the best choices to begin to raise the blood glucose level? Select all that apply.

☐ **1.** One-half cup of orange juice.
☐ **2.** One cup of milk.
☐ **3.** One ounce of tuna.
☐ **4.** One tablespoon of peanut butter.
☐ **5.** One piece of bread.
☐ **6.** One-half cup of regular soda.

114. An infant with increased intracranial pressure (ICP) on a regular diet vomits while eating dinner. Which of the following should the nurse do next?

☐ **1.** Put the child on nothing-by-mouth (NPO) status for 4 hours.
☐ **2.** Call to report this event to the physician.
☐ **3.** Wait a few minutes, then refeed the child.
☐ **4.** Administer the prescribed antiemetic.

115. When preparing to draw up 8 units of a short-acting insulin and 20 units of a long-acting insulin in the same syringe, the nurse should:

☐ **1.** Inject air in the vial with the long-acting insulin first.
☐ **2.** Draw up the long-acting insulin first.
☐ **3.** Draw up either insulin first.
☐ **4.** Use a high-dose insulin syringe.

116. The mother of an infant with iron deficiency anemia asks the nurse what she could have done to prevent the anemia. The nurse should teach the mother that it is helpful to introduce solid foods into the infant's diet at age:

☐ **1.** 1 to 2 months.
☐ **2.** 5 to 6 months.
☐ **3.** 8 to 10 months.
☐ **4.** 10 to 12 months.

117. The nurse is caring for a client who is having an acute asthma attack. Which of the following symptoms should the nurse be most concerned about while caring for the client?

☐ **1.** Loud wheezing.
☐ **2.** Tenacious, thick sputum.
☐ **3.** Decreased breath sounds.
☐ **4.** Persistent cough.

118. A client who is in the end stage of cardiomyopathy asks the nurse about having a transplant. The nurse explains that the client could be a candidate for a:

☐ **1.** Heart transplant.
☐ **2.** Liver transplant.
☐ **3.** Lung transplant.
☐ **4.** Kidney transplant.

119. Which of the following skin care instructions would be appropriate for a client receiving radiation therapy?

☐ **1.** Avoid shaving with straight-edge razors.
☐ **2.** Clean the skin daily with antibacterial soap.
☐ **3.** Apply moisturizing lotion before and after each treatment.
☐ **4.** Keep the radiated area covered with a sterile gauze dressing.

120. A client has returned to the unit after a cardiac catheterization. Her left femoral dressing has a moderate amount of bloody drainage, and the client is complaining of severe pain in that area. What is the priority nursing intervention?

☐ **1.** Assess the airway.
☐ **2.** Administer oxygen.
☐ **3.** Apply pressure to the site.
☐ **4.** Assess the pulse in the left extremity.

121. The nurse tells the parent of a child who is taking valproic acid (Depakene) that the child will need to have routine blood analyses consisting of which of the following?

☐ **1.** Complete blood count (CBC)and alkaline phosphate level.

☐ **2.** Cholesterol and platelet levels.

☐ **3.** Electrolytes and CBC.

☐ **4.** Platelet and fibrinogen levels.

122. Bacterial conjunctivitis has affected several children at a local day care center. A nurse should advise which measure to minimize the risk of infection?

☐ **1.** Close the day care center for 1 week to control the outbreak.

☐ **2.** Restrict the infected children from returning for 48 hours after treatment.

☐ **3.** Perform thorough hand washing before and after touching any child in the day care center.

☐ **4.** Set up a conference with the parents of each child to explain the situation carefully.

123. The nurse is evaluating the client's potential for development of a pressure sore. Which of the following individual characteristics would be the best indicator of risk for the client's developing a pressure sore?

☐ **1.** The client's nutritional status.

☐ **2.** The client's circulatory status.

☐ **3.** The client's mobility status.

☐ **4.** The client's orientation status.

124. A patient with acute pancreatitis is put on nothing-by-mouth status, with the intent of not stimulating the pancreas. The client is prescribed an I.V. infusion of dextrose 5% in half-normal saline solution at 120 ml/hour. After 3 days of this regimen, the nurse should observe the client for which of the following metabolic conditions?

☐ **1.** Ketosis.

☐ **2.** Hyperglycemia.

☐ **3.** Metabolic syndrome.

☐ **4.** Lactic acidosis.

125. The nurse is assisting a client to ambulate as part of his cardiac rehabilitation program. He complains of midsternal burning. From an earlier assessment, the nurse knows that this is a typical complaint of the client and decides to:

☐ **1.** Stop and assess the client further.

☐ **2.** Measure the client's blood pressure and heart rate.

☐ **3.** Call for help and place the client in a wheelchair.

☐ **4.** Administer nitroglycerin.

126. The nurse is counseling a client about the prevention of coronary heart disease. Which of the following vitamins should the nurse recommend the client include in his diet to reduce homocysteine levels? Select all that apply.

☐ **1.** Vitamin K.

☐ **2.** Vitamin B_6.

☐ **3.** Folate.

☐ **4.** Vitamin B_{12}.

☐ **5.** Vitamin D.

127. The nurse evaluates a client's knowledge as deficient when the client makes which of the following statements about the drug dexamethasone (Decadron)?

☐ **1.** "I cannot stop the Decadron all at one time."

☐ **2.** "If I forget a dose, it's no big deal; I'll just take it when I remember it."

☐ **3.** "When I get a cold, I need to let my doctor know."

☐ **4.** "I need to watch for an allergic reaction when I first start taking Decadron."

128. A 3-month-old is admitted to the pediatric unit with moderate dehydration. Which of the following should the nurse expect to assess?

☐ **1.** Oliguria.

☐ **2.** Rapid, thready pulse.

☐ **3.** Decreased skin elasticity.

☐ **4.** Pale skin color.

129. The nurse is assessing a client who is suspected of being in the early symptomatic stages of human immunodeficiency virus (HIV) infection. Which of the following signs and symptoms of infection should the nurse detect during this stage?

☐ **1.** Whitish yellow patches in the mouth.

☐ **2.** Dyspnea.

☐ **3.** Bloody diarrhea.

☐ **4.** Raised, hyperpigmented lesions on the legs.

130. A primiparous client who is breast-feeding develops endometritis on the third postpartum day. Which of the following instructions should the nurse give to the mother?

☐ **1.** The neonate will need to be bottle-fed for the next few days.

☐ **2.** The condition typically is treated with I.V. antibiotic therapy.

☐ **3.** The client's uterus may become "boggy," requiring frequent massage and oxytocics.

☐ **4.** The client needs to remain in bed in a side-lying position as much as possible.

131. After instructing a primiparous client who is breast-feeding on how to prevent nipple soreness during feedings, the nurse determines that the client needs *further* instruction when she states which of the following?
☐ **1.** "I should position the baby the same way for each feeding."
☐ **2.** "I should make sure the baby grasps the entire areola and nipple."
☐ **3.** "I should air dry my breasts and nipples for 10 to 15 minutes after the feeding."
☐ **4.** "I shouldn't use a hand breast pump if my nipples get sore."

132. A client who has Ménière's disease is experiencing an acute attack of vertigo. Which of the following interventions should the nurse include in the plan of care?
☐ **1.** Darken the client's room and provide a quiet environment.
☐ **2.** Provide a low-sodium, bland diet.
☐ **3.** Administer an opioid to relieve headache.
☐ **4.** Encourage fluid intake to prevent dehydration.

133. During a home visit to a primiparous client 1 week postpartum who is bottle-feeding her neonate, the client tells the nurse that her mother has suggested that she feed the neonate cereal so he will sleep through the night. Which of the following would be the nurse's best response?
☐ **1.** "It is permissible to give the baby cereal if it is thinned with formula."
☐ **2.** "The time for starting cereal varies, so check with your pediatrician."
☐ **3.** "Formula is the food best digested by the baby until about 4 to 6 months of age."
☐ **4.** "If cereal is given too early in life, the undigested food can lead to a need for surgery."

134. When a client states that he is allergic to amoxicillin (Ampicillin) even though his medication administration record and armband do not indicate medication allergies, the nurse should perform which action?
☐ **1.** Administer the prescribed medication.
☐ **2.** Withhold the amoxicillin (Ampicillin).
☐ **3.** Administer another, similarly acting antibiotic.
☐ **4.** Call the family to verify the client's statement.

135. While assessing a term neonate on a home visit to a primiparous client 2 weeks after a vaginal delivery, the nurse observes that the neonate is slightly jaundiced and the stool is a pale, light color. The nurse notifies the physician because these findings should indicate which of the following?
☐ **1.** Biliary atresia.
☐ **2.** Rh isoimmunization.
☐ **3.** ABO incompatibility.
☐ **4.** Esophageal varices.

136. A 6-year-old child is admitted to the hospital for heart surgery to repair tetralogy of Fallot. The nurse should anticipate that when the child goes home the parents will most likely have a concern about:
☐ **1.** Allowing the child to lead a normal, active life.
☐ **2.** Persuading the child to get enough rest.
☐ **3.** Having the child develop postoperative complications.
☐ **4.** Having the child out of school for a month.

137. A client is recovering from abdominal surgery and has a nasogastric (NG) tube inserted. The nurse understands that the primary reason the tube is in place is to achieve which of the following functions in the gastrointestinal tract?
☐ **1.** Compression.
☐ **2.** Lavage.
☐ **3.** Decompression.
☐ **4.** Gavage.

138. The nurse teaches the mother of a toddler who has had cleft palate repair that her child is at risk for developing which of the following in the future?
☐ **1.** Hearing problems.
☐ **2.** Poor self-concept.
☐ **3.** A speech defect.
☐ **4.** Chronic sinus infections.

139. The nurse assesses a client who is receiving a tube feeding. Which of the following situations would require prompt intervention from the nurse?
☐ **1.** The client is sitting upright in bed while the feeding is infusing.
☐ **2.** The feeding that is infusing has been hanging for 8 hours.
☐ **3.** The client has a gastric residual of 25 ml.
☐ **4.** The feeding solution is at room temperature.

140. A client has been taking furosemide (Lasix) for 2 days. The nurse realizes that a possible adverse effect of this type of diuretic is:
☐ **1.** An elevated blood urea nitrogen (BUN) level.
☐ **2.** An elevated potassium level.
☐ **3.** A decreased potassium level.
☐ **4.** An elevated sodium level.

141. When suctioning the respiratory tract of a client, it is recommended that the suctioning period not exceed how many seconds?
☐ **1.** 5 seconds.
☐ **2.** 10 seconds.
☐ **3.** 15 seconds.
☐ **4.** 20 seconds.

142. An 80-year-old client with severe kidney damage is placed on life support and dialysis. Care decisions are being made by his wife, who is showing signs of early Alzheimer's disease. The client's daughter arrives from out of town with a copy of the client's living will, which states that the client did not want to be on life support. Which of the following is *most* appropriate for the nurse to do?
- ☐ **1.** Immediately inform the physician about the living will.
- ☐ **2.** Suggest to the daughter that she discuss her father's wishes with her mother.
- ☐ **3.** Prepare to remove the client from life support.
- ☐ **4.** Make a copy of the living will and give it to the client's wife.

143. Clients must meet certain criteria to be eligible for plasminogen activator (t-PA) or alteplase recombinant (Activase) therapy. Which of the following conditions makes the client ineligible to receive t-PA or alteplase recombinant therapy?
- ☐ **1.** Age greater than 65 years.
- ☐ **2.** No symptoms of stroke.
- ☐ **3.** Hypotension.
- ☐ **4.** Current active internal bleeding.

144. When caring for a client with myasthenia gravis who is receiving anticholinesterase drug therapy, the nurse must be able to distinguish cholinergic crisis from myasthenic crisis. Which of the following symptoms is not present in cholinergic crisis?
- ☐ **1.** Improved muscle strength after I.V. administration of edrophonium chloride (Tensilon).
- ☐ **2.** Increased weakness.
- ☐ **3.** Diaphoresis.
- ☐ **4.** Increased salivation.

145. The nurse identifies the type of presentation shown below as which of the following?
- ☐ **1.** Frank breech.
- ☐ **2.** Compound breech.
- ☐ **3.** Complete breech.
- ☐ **4.** Incomplete breech.

146. Which of the following client statements indicates that the client with hepatitis B understands his discharge teaching?
- ☐ **1.** "I will not drink alcohol for at least 1 year."
- ☐ **2.** "I must avoid sexual intercourse."
- ☐ **3.** "I should be able to resume normal activity in a week or two."
- ☐ **4.** "Because hepatitis B is a chronic disease, I know I will always be jaundiced."

147. Which of the following examples should the nurse use to describe bulimia to a group of parents at a local community center?
- ☐ **1.** An adolescent male who uses calorie-counting to maintain his weight in the desirable range for his height.
- ☐ **2.** A college-age male who uses regular exercise to be able to eat and drink what he wants without gaining weight.
- ☐ **3.** A middle-aged female who uses diet pills occasionally to help her lose 10 pounds.
- ☐ **4.** A college-age female who binges and then purges to prevent weight gain.

148. An early sign of Hodgkin's disease is:
- ☐ **1.** Difficulty breathing.
- ☐ **2.** Swollen cervical lymph nodes.
- ☐ **3.** Difficulty swallowing.
- ☐ **4.** Feeling of fullness over the liver.

149. A client who has been taking diazepam (Valium) for 3 months for skeletal muscle spasms and lower back pain states that he stopped taking the medication 2 days ago because it was no longer helping him, but now he feels terrible. The nurse should assess the client for which of the following? Select all that apply.
- ☐ **1.** Insomnia.
- ☐ **2.** Euphoria.
- ☐ **3.** Bradycardia.
- ☐ **4.** Diaphoresis.
- ☐ **5.** Tremor.
- ☐ **6.** Vomiting.

150. An I.V. infusion is to be administered through a scalp vein on an infant's head. What should the nurse tell the parents to prepare them for the procedure?
- ☐ **1.** It may be necessary to remove a small amount of hair from the infant's scalp.
- ☐ **2.** A sedative will be given to the infant to help keep the child quiet.
- ☐ **3.** Visiting the infant will be delayed until the infusion has been completed.
- ☐ **4.** Holding the infant will be contraindicated while the infusion is being administered.

151. Which of the following goals would be most expected for a client with acute pancreatitis?
- [ ] 1. The client reports minimal abdominal pain.
- [ ] 2. The client regains a normal pattern for bowel movements.
- [ ] 3. The client limits alcohol intake to two to three drinks per week.
- [ ] 4. The client maintains normal liver function.

152. A nurse is caring for a child with diabetes mellitus at camp. The child is irritable and complains of a headache. Which of the following should the nurse do first?
- [ ] 1. Administer 2 ounces of orange juice.
- [ ] 2. Notify the physician about the child's complaints.
- [ ] 3. Check the child's blood glucose level.
- [ ] 4. Send the child back to the planned activities.

153. A client tells the nurse that her bra fits more snugly at certain times of the month and she is concerned this may be a sign of breast cancer. The *best* response for the nurse is to explain that:
- [ ] 1. A change in breast size should be checked by her physician.
- [ ] 2. Benign cysts tend to cause the breast to vary in size.
- [ ] 3. It is normal for the breast to increase in size before menstruation begins.
- [ ] 4. A difference in the size of her breasts is related to normal growth and development.

154. Which of the following is an example of traditional Chinese medicine found in Asian-American culture?
- [ ] 1. Health is described as harmony between family members.
- [ ] 2. Illness is caused by an imbalance of the yin and yang.
- [ ] 3. Exercise to the point of overexertion can improve health.
- [ ] 4. Illness is caused by a change in eating habits.

155. A client is scheduled for an intravenous pyelogram (IVP). Which of the following questions would be most important for the nurse to ask the client in preparation for the procedure?
- [ ] 1. "Have you ever had an IVP before?"
- [ ] 2. "Do you have any allergies to shellfish?"
- [ ] 3. "When was your last bowel movement?"
- [ ] 4. "Have you ever experienced urinary incontinence?"

156. Which oral contraceptive is considered safe for use while breast-feeding because it will not affect the breast milk or breast-feeding?
- [ ] 1. Estrogen.
- [ ] 2. Estrogen and progestin.
- [ ] 3. Progestin.
- [ ] 4. Testosterone.

157. A multigravid client at 36 weeks' gestation who is visiting the clinic for a routine visit begins to sob and tells the nurse, "My boyfriend has been beating me up once in a while since I became pregnant—but I can't bring myself to leave him because I don't have a job and I don't know how I would take care of my other children." Which of the following actions should be the priority by the nurse at this time?
- [ ] 1. Contact a social worker for assistance and family counseling.
- [ ] 2. Help the client make concrete plans for the safety of herself and her children.
- [ ] 3. Tell the client that she shouldn't allow anyone to hit her or her children.
- [ ] 4. Provide the client with brochures on the statistics about violence against women.

158. Sulfadiazine has been ordered for a client who has a urinary tract infection. Which of the following nursing interventions is most appropriate for administering sulfonamides?
- [ ] 1. Encourage the client to take the medication with meals.
- [ ] 2. Instruct the client to drink at least 8 glasses of water a day.
- [ ] 3. Measure the client's urine output.
- [ ] 4. Instruct the client that the urine may turn reddish orange.

159. A client with chronic undifferentiated schizophrenia is having an acute exacerbation of symptoms. The client states, "Black cats and black hats. Where does the time go?" Which of the following would be most important for the nurse to say?
- [ ] 1. "Halloween is getting close, isn't it."
- [ ] 2. "Do you have a black cat?"
- [ ] 3. "What's the connection between cats, hats, and time?"
- [ ] 4. "Time certainly does go faster these days."

160. A client has been diagnosed with multi-infarct (or vascular) dementia (MID). Although there is no cure, there are ways to slow the progression of the disease. When preparing a teaching plan for the client and family, which of the following should the nurse indicate as the most critical factor for slowing MID?

☐ **1.** Administering anticoagulants such as warfarin (Coumadin).

☐ **2.** Administering benzodiazepines such as lorazepam (Ativan) to decrease choreiform movements.

☐ **3.** Managing related symptoms such as depression.

☐ **4.** Managing the symptoms by increasing dopamine availability.

161. While performing cardiopulmonary resuscitation (CPR) on a 5-year-old child, the nurse palpates for a pulse. Which of the following sites is best for checking the pulse during CPR in a 5-year-old child?

☐ **1.** Femoral artery.

☐ **2.** Carotid artery.

☐ **3.** Radial artery.

☐ **4.** Brachial artery.

162. A nurse is assessing a client with nephrotic syndrome. The nurse should assess the client for which condition?

☐ **1.** Hematuria.

☐ **2.** Massive proteinuria.

☐ **3.** Increased serum albumin level.

☐ **4.** Weight loss.

163. A child with tetralogy of Fallot and a history of severe hypoxic episodes is to be admitted to the pediatric unit. Which of the following would be most important for the nurse to have at the bedside?

☐ **1.** Morphine sulfate in a syringe ready to administer.

☐ **2.** Oxygen tubing and gauge plugged in.

☐ **3.** Blood pressure cuff and stethoscope.

☐ **4.** Suction tubing and equipment.

164. Which statement would most likely be made by a Mexican-American client with pain?

☐ **1.** "Enduring pain is a part of God's will."

☐ **2.** "This pain is killing me."

☐ **3.** "I've got to see a doctor right away."

☐ **4.** "I can't go on in pain like this any longer."

165. A client tells the nurse that he is voiding small amounts of urine every 30 to 60 minutes. Which of the following actions is the nurse's first priority?

☐ **1.** Palpate for a distended bladder.

☐ **2.** Catheterize the client for residual urine.

☐ **3.** Request a urine specimen for culture.

☐ **4.** Encourage an increased fluid intake.

166. Which of the following interventions would be most appropriate for a client with chronic renal failure?

☐ **1.** Apply corticosteroid creams to relieve itching.

☐ **2.** Achieve pain control with analgesics.

☐ **3.** Maintain a low-sodium diet.

☐ **4.** Measure abdominal girth daily.

167. An 18-month-old, previously well child is brought to the physician's office with severe respiratory distress. The father was baby-sitting and does not think the child choked. Which of the following should the nurse do first?

☐ **1.** Perform the abdominal thrust maneuver.

☐ **2.** Call an ambulance to take the toddler to the emergency department.

☐ **3.** Determine the child's oxygen saturation level.

☐ **4.** Carry the child next door for a chest radiograph.

168. The nurse is assessing a child's skeletal traction and notices that the weights are on the floor. Which of the following should the nurse do next?

☐ **1.** Raise the weights so that the child can move up in bed.

☐ **2.** Notify the physician immediately.

☐ **3.** Put the foot of the bed on blocks.

☐ **4.** Move the child up in bed.

169. Some parents ask about food requirements for school-age children. The nurse explains that, compared with the food requirements of preschoolers and adolescents, the food requirements of school-age children are not as great because these children have a lower:

☐ **1.** Growth rate.

☐ **2.** Metabolic rate.

☐ **3.** Level of activity.

☐ **4.** Hormonal secretion rate.

170. When assessing a 17-year-old client with depression for suicide risk, which of the following questions would be best?

☐ **1.** "What movies about death have you watched lately?"

☐ **2.** "Can you tell me what you think about suicide?"

☐ **3.** "Has anyone in your family ever committed suicide?"

☐ **4.** "Are you thinking about killing yourself?"

171. Which of the following is a major risk factor for having a low-birth-weight baby?

☐ **1.** Heredity.

☐ **2.** Age.

☐ **3.** Drug use during pregnancy.

☐ **4.** Poor nutrition.

172. Which of the following techniques is best for the nurse to use in evaluating the parents' ability to administer eardrops correctly?
- ☐ **1.** Observe the parents instilling the drops in the child's ear.
- ☐ **2.** Listen to the parents as they describe the procedure.
- ☐ **3.** Ask the parents to list the steps in the procedure.
- ☐ **4.** Ask the parents whether they have read the handout on the procedure.

173. Ibuprofen (Motrin) is prescribed for a client with osteoarthritis. Which of the following instructions about ibuprofen should the nurse include in the client's teaching plan?
- ☐ **1.** Report the development of tinnitus.
- ☐ **2.** Increase vitamin B_{12} intake.
- ☐ **3.** Take with food or antacids.
- ☐ **4.** Have the complete blood count (CBC) monitored monthly.

174. When a client has had surgery for a ruptured appendix, the nurse should document the wound as:
- ☐ **1.** Clean.
- ☐ **2.** Clean-contaminated.
- ☐ **3.** Contaminated.
- ☐ **4.** Infected.

175. A staff member states, "I don't know why Mary is so depressed. She lives in an exclusive part of town and has gorgeous clothes. Her husband seems to care about her very much. She really has it all." Which of the following should the nurse conclude from the staff member's statement?
- ☐ **1.** An accurate assessment of the client has been made.
- ☐ **2.** The staff member is jealous of the client.
- ☐ **3.** There is no reason for the client to be depressed.
- ☐ **4.** The staff member needs teaching about major depression.

176. The mother tells the nurse that she does not understand why her child had another asthma attack. He was not around any of the things that trigger his asthma. The nurse explains to the mother that asthma attacks may be triggered by various mechanisms, including certain food allergies, and states that which of the following foods would most likely be responsible for such an allergic reaction?
- ☐ **1.** Whitefish.
- ☐ **2.** Tossed salad.
- ☐ **3.** Hamburger patty.
- ☐ **4.** Fudge brownies.

177. When preparing to administer a tap water enema, in which position should the nurse place the client?
- ☐ **1.** Supine.
- ☐ **2.** Semi-Fowler's.
- ☐ **3.** Right lateral.
- ☐ **4.** Left Sims.

178. Which of the following is a risk factor for the development of pressure ulcers?
- ☐ **1.** Ambulating less than twice a day.
- ☐ **2.** An indwelling urinary catheter.
- ☐ **3.** Decreased serum albumin level.
- ☐ **4.** Elevated white blood cell count.

179. A 42-year-old woman was admitted to the hospital with a hemoglobin of 6.5 g/dl. She is experiencing signs and symptoms of cerebral tissue hypoxia. Which of the following nursing interventions would be most important?
- ☐ **1.** Plan frequent rest periods throughout the day.
- ☐ **2.** Assist the client in ambulating to the bathroom.
- ☐ **3.** Check the temperature of the water before the client showers.
- ☐ **4.** Refer the client to occupational therapy for energy conservation interventions.

180. A client has been diagnosed with multiple myeloma. Which of the following laboratory values should the nurse expect to find in a client with multiple myeloma?
- ☐ **1.** Polycythemia vera.
- ☐ **2.** Decreased serum protein.
- ☐ **3.** Decreased calcium level.
- ☐ **4.** Bence Jones protein.

181. The nurse is caring for a multigravid client in active labor who has contractions occurring 2 to 3 minutes apart and lasting 45 seconds. After the administration of an epidural anesthetic, the client's blood pressure drops from 124/80 to 84/60 mm Hg. What should the nurse have available to improve this situation?
- ☐ **1.** Atropine sulfate.
- ☐ **2.** Ephedrine.
- ☐ **3.** Methylergonovine.
- ☐ **4.** Oxytocin.

182. A major intervention for the prevention of lung cancer is to:
- ☐ **1.** Encourage the public to install high-efficiency particulate air (HEPA) filters in their homes.
- ☐ **2.** Encourage cigarette smokers to have yearly chest radiographs.
- ☐ **3.** Offer strategies for smoking cessation.
- ☐ **4.** Recommend that homes and apartments be checked for asbestos leakage.

183. A client diagnosed with tuberculosis (TB) is taking medication for the treatment of TB. The nurse should instruct the client that he will be safe from infecting others approximately how long after initiation of the chemotherapy regimen?
- ☐ **1.** Within 48 hours after initiation of bacteriocidal drugs.
- ☐ **2.** Two to 3 weeks after initiation of bacteriocidal drugs.
- ☐ **3.** Results vary with each client, so it is difficult to predict.
- ☐ **4.** After completion of 6 months of bacteriocidal drugs.

184. Which of the following client statements indicates that a client with major depression and suicidal ideation is improving?
- ☐ **1.** "I'll go to group when I have more energy."
- ☐ **2.** "I only think about killing myself at night."
- ☐ **3.** "My kids need me to be around."
- ☐ **4.** "I want everyone to leave me alone."

185. A client at 34 weeks' gestation visits the clinic complaining of flulike symptoms and a bull's eye–like rash. She reports that she went camping last weekend and may have gotten a tick bite. The client is diagnosed with Lyme disease. Which of the following medications should the nurse expect the physician to order?
- ☐ **1.** Tetracycline (Panmycin).
- ☐ **2.** Doxycycline (Vibramycin).
- ☐ **3.** Penicillin (Pen-Vee K).
- ☐ **4.** Gentamicin (Garamycin).

186. The physician orders an amnioinfusion for a multigravid client in active labor. When preparing the client's teaching plan, the nurse should include which of the following as a likely reason for using this procedure?
- ☐ **1.** Early decelerations.
- ☐ **2.** Meconium-stained fluid.
- ☐ **3.** Very short umbilical cord.
- ☐ **4.** Multifetal pregnancy.

187. A client is scheduled for a surgical procedure. When planning the client's care, the nurse should consider that which of the following conditions will increase the client's risk of complications after surgery?
- ☐ **1.** A history of diabetes.
- ☐ **2.** A history of sensitivity to aspirin.
- ☐ **3.** A history of osteoarthritis.
- ☐ **4.** A history of chronic low back pain.

188. A 36-year-old man is receiving three different chemotherapeutic agents for Hodgkin's disease. The nurse explains to the client that the three drugs are given over an extended period because:
- ☐ **1.** The three drugs can be given at lower doses.
- ☐ **2.** The second and third drugs increase the effectiveness of the first drug.
- ☐ **3.** The first two drugs are toxic to cancer cells, and the third drug promotes cell growth.
- ☐ **4.** The three drugs have a synergistic effect and act on the cancer cells with different mechanisms.

189. Which of the following should the nurse write on the parents' plan of care as an expected client outcome for the nursing diagnosis of *Grieving* related to their child's death? The parents will:
- ☐ **1.** Keep to themselves until 3 months after the baby's death.
- ☐ **2.** Be able to discuss their feelings with each other.
- ☐ **3.** Immerse themselves in work and outside activities.
- ☐ **4.** Act as if nothing has happened.

190. A nurse is assessing an older adult with pneumonia. Where should the nurse place the stethoscope to listen for breath sounds that will indicate the client is fully oxygenating the lung on the right side?

Correct Answers and Rationales

The letter in parentheses after each rationale identifies the client need addressed in the item, including management of care (M), safety and infection control (S), health promotion and maintenance (H), psychosocial adaptation (P), basic care and comfort (C), pharmacological and parenteral therapies (D), reduction of risk potential (R), and physiological adaptation (A).

1. 1. The colleague needs to provide the nurse with information about spouse abuse. Giving information about reasons for staying is useful for decreasing the nurse's frustration. Although expressing empathy is appropriate, it does not help the nurse understand the client's needs and behaviors. Telling the nurse that there will be another chance is not helpful and fails to educate the other nurse about the dynamics of abuse. Although dependence is a problem, women who are abused can overcome this and leave if they have support, not criticism. Saying that abused women almost never leave does not help the nurse understand the client's needs and behaviors. (P)

2. 1

First, convert micrograms to milligrams:

$$200 \text{ mcg} = 0.2 \text{ mg.}$$

Then:

$$0.2 \text{ mg}/X \text{ ml} = 0.2 \text{ mg}/1 \text{ ml}$$

$$X = 1 \text{ ml.}$$

(D)

3. 3. Viral gastroenteritis may be communicable, and all of the other children are already at risk for infection. The infant should be placed in a private room. (S)

4. 1. The neonate would be considered large for gestational age (LGA) because the neonate weighs more than 4,000 g (90th percentile). Therefore, the nurse needs to assess for the possibility of complications. Hypoglycemia is a problem for the LGA neonate because glycogen stores are quickly used to maintain the weight. Other common complications for an LGA neonate include hyperbilirubinemia from the bruising and polycythemia, cephalhematoma, caput succedaneum, molding, phrenic nerve paralysis, and a fractured clavicle. However, hyperbilirubinemia would not be evident 1 hour after birth. Hypercalcemia is not usually found in the LGA neonate. Hypocalcemia is common in infants of diabetic mothers. Hypermagnesemia may occur in neonates whose mothers received large doses of magnesium sulfate to treat severe preeclampsia. (A)

5. 2. Ovarian enlargement, hyperstimulation syndrome, febrile reaction, and multiple pregnancies are considered adverse effects of menotropins. If ovarian enlargement occurs, the drug should be discontinued to prevent damage to the ovary. Pulmonary edema is not associated with menotropin use. Visual disturbances and breast tenderness are associated with the use of clomiphene citrate (Clomid), another drug prescribed for infertility. (D)

6. 1. Organ and Tissue Procurement Organizations are responsible for organ recovery in the United States. These organizations have offices in major cities, and provide services on a local, state, and regional basis. The agency is the repository for information about tissues and organs and their distribution. The American Transplant Association coordinates recipients of transplants. The American Hospice Foundation is involved with hospice care. The American Association of Critical-Care Nurses is involved with professional critical care nurses. (M)

7. 3. Fluid accumulates in the base of the pleura postoperatively. The lower chest tube, called the posterior or lower tube, will drain serous and serosanguineous fluid that accumulates as a result of the surgical procedure. A larger-diameter tube is usually used for the lower tube to ensure drainage of clots. Air rises, and the anterior or upper tube is used to remove air from the pleural space. The practice of "milking" the tubes to prevent clots is becoming less common; the surgeon's orders must be followed regarding this procedure. (A)

8. 1. Elderly clients are a high-risk group for depression. The classic symptoms of depression frequently are masked, and depression presents differently in the aging population. Depression in late life is underdiagnosed because the symptoms are incorrectly attributed to aging or medical problems. Impairment of cognition in a previously well elderly client or psychosomatic complaints may be the presenting symptom of depression. Antidepressant therapy is usually effective. (P)

9. 4. Fears of the adolescent include body changes and loss of control. The young adolescent is typically concerned about the inability to control body changes and feelings and about embarrassment. The typical adolescent is more concerned about being separated from the peer group than from the family and schoolwork and is realistically worried about experiencing pain and loss of control. The adolescent may prefer to wear her own clothes, but this is not a primary concern. The nurse should respect the client's privacy, but this is not a primary concern for this client. (H)

10. **2.** The mother's statements reveal that she is having problems with parenting. Therefore, a referral to a parenting education program is the most appropriate measure at this time. (P)

11. **2.** The nurse acts in a reasonable and prudent manner to correctly identify a client by checking the client's armband and asking the client's name. Omitting to do so is an act of negligence. *Res judicata* and *stare decisis* are legal doctrines used to guide the courts in making decisions. Vicarious liability is a concept in which the employer is held liable for the nurse's act. It was established after precedent-setting cases in the 1960s. (H)

12. **2.** Morphine can cause respiratory depression, leading to respiratory arrest. The nurse should assess the client's respiratory rate before administration and throughout the course of analgesic treatment. Morphine does not affect blood pressure, pulse rate, or temperature. (D)

13. **21**

One unit of packed red blood cells contains 250 ml, and this is to infuse over 2 hours (120 minutes). First, determine the number of ml/minute by dividing 250 ml by 120 minutes:

$$250/120 = 2.1 \text{ ml/minute}.$$

Then multiply by the drop factor of 10 gtt/ml:

$$2.1 \times 10 = 21 \text{ gtt/minute}.$$

(D)

14. **1.** Anger is a natural result of feelings of loss and helplessness in normal, healthy people. It is a natural response to coping with a sick child. Nurses should recognize anger in clients and families. Parents are usually able to control their anger in a socially acceptable manner. Nurses can assist clients and families to overcome helplessness and anger in an acceptable manner. (P)

15. **3.** Supervised activities that promote walking are behavioral management strategies that help a client such as this. The client's cognitive and memory impairment would not be conducive to playing board games. Allowing the behavior at selected intervals would further encourage the client to wander. The client should not be restrained in a chair. (P)

16. **3.** With a new complaint of numbness in the fingers, the nurse needs to first assess the circulation to evaluate color, evidence of swelling, and presence of pulses to determine whether there is any circulatory compromise. Once the nurse had evaluated the child's circulatory status, the next action would be to verify the arm's position above the level of the heart. Notifying the physician would not be done until the child's neurovascular status and position are checked. Cutting the cast would be done only with a physician's order. (A)

17. **4.** The second-generation antihistamines do not cross the blood-brain barrier and therefore do not cause sedation or psychomotor dysfunction. They are much more expensive than first-generation antihistamines. The effectiveness is similar. The medications are rapidly absorbed in 1 to 2 hours after oral administration on an empty stomach. (D)

18. **3.** LBP is commonly associated with overuse or an injury to the soft-tissue structures. It is estimated that 50% to 70% of people will experience musculoskeletal back pain at some time. Although the other causes of pain must be excluded, the initial treatment of LBP is usually aimed at decreasing the inflammatory response to the tissue injury. (A)

19. **2.** At the time of a major crisis, the client suffering a great loss is best helped by being encouraged to talk about his experience and describe his feelings. Crisis interventions focus on reestablishing emotional equilibrium and preventing decompensation. Telling the client that everything will be fine is a cliché and inappropriate. Asking the client to stop talking so that the nurse can write notes places more emphasis on the nurse's needs than on the client's needs. Telling the client to think more about what happened for further discussion the next day is not helping him with the crisis. (P)

20. **2.** Beclomethasone is an inhaled steroid used for the maintenance treatment of asthma. The steroid can precipitate overgrowth of fungus, such as oral *Candida albicans*. Rinsing the mouth well after each use decreases the incidence of oral fungal infections. Beclomethasone does not cause gingival hyperplasia or caries. The dose is dependent on effective inhalation of the medication. (D)

21. **1.** The incident report should be given to the nurse-manager. The incident report should not be placed on the chart because it is considered a confidential communication and cannot be subpoenaed by a client or used as evidence in lawsuits. It is appropriate, ethical, and legally required that the fall be documented in the chart. Unless there is a change in the client's condition reflecting an injury from the fall, there is no need to notify the family. If the family does need to be notified, the nurse-manager or the physician should place the call. (M)

22. **2.** General wound care is appropriate initially. This includes washing the bite area with lots of water because infections occur frequently with animal bites, especially those on the arms or hands. Next, the mother should be advised to determine the extent of the injury and then to follow-up with the child's physician if needed. A trip to the local care center would be warranted if the bite injury was extensive or there was severe bleeding. Although knowledge of when the child last had a tetanus vaccination is important, the child's wound takes priority. For rabies injections, there needs to be a history of rabies or unusual behavior in the pet. (A)

23. 4. The biophysical profile uses a sonogram to assess five parameters, including fetal breathing movements, fetal movements, fetal tone, amniotic fluid volume, and fetal heart rate activity. A nonstress test is used to evaluate fetal heart rate activity. (H)

24. 2. Chemoprophylaxis should be given to household contacts and close contacts only. To prevent community outbreaks, chemoprophylaxis with rifampin 600 mg twice a day for 2 days or a single dose of Cipro 500 mg is indicated. (D)

25. 2. Infants and toddlers younger than age 2 should not be placed on a fat-restricted diet because cholesterol and other fatty acids are required for continued neural growth. After age 2 it is believed that no harm is done by encouraging a child to eat a variety of foods, maintain a desirable body weight, limit saturated fat and cholesterol, and increase fiber. (H)

26. 1. Petroleum jelly is thought to smother the lice. A pediculicide should not be applied to the face or close to the eyes. Bacitracin ointment will not kill the lice. (D)

27. 1. A major goal of safety and accident prevention focuses on having all cleaning supplies and medications locked up. Toddlers are great climbers and can very quickly get into what they should not. The child should not play in the bathroom even if the parent is present because the child will think that it is okay to play with these items when the parent is not present. Playing with cords could lead to possible strangulation. The child-protective cabinet locks should work unless they were installed incorrectly or are defective. (S)

28. 4. Steroid therapy can mask the signs of infection, making an atypical presentation. Age (adolescent or child) and pregnancy do not mask the signs of appendicitis. (D)

29. 3, 4, 5. Common adverse effects of tobramycin include nephrotoxicity, ototoxicity, fever, and rash. Hypertension, weight gain, and decreased heart rate are not associated with this drug. (D)

30. 4. Fever is generally not thought to be a sign of impaired renal function related to long-term use of gentamicin. The client should report signs of decreasing urinary function, such as decreased output, unusual appearance of the urine, or edema. (D)

31. 4. Plastic blocks are the most appropriate toy for a toddler in a mist tent. Because the blocks are plastic, they can be washed. For the pull toy to be used, the child would need to leave the mist tent, which is not advisable at this time. Although crayons may be appropriate for a mist tent, any paper, including storybooks, would become damp, crumble, and provide an environment for the growth of microorganisms. (H)

32. 2. Febrile seizures commonly occur as the fever rises. The exact cause of febrile convulsions is not known. Infants and young toddlers are the age-groups primarily affected. Febrile seizures typically do not follow immunization administration. (H)

33. 4. Oral contraceptive use, pregnancy, and lactation are situations that increase demand for folic acid. With supplementation, a response should cause the reticulocyte count to increase within 2 to 3 days after therapy has begun. It is not necessary to take folic acid on an empty stomach. A client may safely take both iron and folic acid supplementation. (D)

34. 4. Although acrocyanosis may be present for 24 to 48 hours after birth, central cyanosis of the trunk indicates decreased oxygenation from respiratory distress or another disease state (e.g., cardiac anomalies). This should be reported to the physician and evaluated further. Maternal lochia serosa in scant amount is a normal finding 1 week postpartum, as is a nonpalpable maternal fundus. Presence of a neonatal tonic neck reflex is a normal finding in a 1-week-old neonate. (A)

35. 4. Severe inflammatory acne is commonly treated with tetracycline or erythromycin. Isotretinoin is a retinoic acid derivative. Cephalexin and azithromycin are not used to treat acne. (A)

36. 4. People with hip fractures have been found to have low vitamin K intakes; vitamin K plays an important role in production of at least one bone protein. Heavy alcohol use is a risk factor because it causes fluid excretion resulting in heavy losses of calcium in urine. If the antacid contains aluminum or magnesium, a net loss of calcium can occur. High-fiber diets bind up some of the dietary calcium. (H)

37. 1. The postrape examination is important for detecting the possibility of sexually transmitted disease, which can be spread through rape. Additionally, if the victim or the rapist was not using a contraceptive, postcoital contraceptive methods should be discussed. The information provided does not indicate anxiety or physical injury, such as periurethral tears, and these are not the primary reason for the examination. Menstrual difficulties are not a common result of rape. (S)

38. 3. The nurse should question the use of a local anesthetic agent with epinephrine on the hands or feet because the epinephrine is a vasoconstrictor and can cause ischemia and gangrene of extremities. The nurse should suggest that the intern use bupivacaine (Marcaine) without epinephrine as the local anesthetic agent. An intern should be trained in suturing small superficial incisions, and the cosmetic effect should be acceptable. The client's room should be a sufficiently aseptic environment because there is no other client in the room. (M)

39. **2.** Chills are a normal response of the body's immune system to infection and are not a response of the sympathetic nervous system to pain. Tachycardia, increased respiratory rate, and dilated pupils are sympathetic effects. (A)

40. **3.** In dark-skinned clients, cyanosis can best be detected by examining the conjunctiva, lips, and oral mucous membranes. Examining the retinas, nail beds, or inner aspects of the wrists is not an appropriate assessment for determining cyanosis in any client. (H)

41. **7.5**

$$0.9 \text{ mg}/X \text{ ml} \times 0.6 \text{ mg}/5 \text{ ml}$$

$$X = 7.5 \text{ ml.}$$

(D)

42. **1.** A biophysical profile includes a nonstress test; evaluation of fetal breathing movements, gross body movements, and fetal tone; and amniotic fluid volume measurement. Because an ultrasound analysis is used during the test, the client should plan to drink 1 to 2 L of fluid before the test to ensure a full bladder, which provides better visualization of the fetus. The client does not need to be on nothing-by-mouth status before the test. The client does not need to remain in the clinic for 4 hours after the test. However, if the client were scheduled for a contraction stress test, she would be observed as an outpatient for 1 to 4 hours after the test to make certain that the contractions had stopped. The client does not need to eat a high-fiber meal after the test. A high-fiber meal typically is indicated after certain radiographic procedures, such as an upper gastrointestinal series. (R)

43. **3.** The physician will most likely order packed RBCs to alleviate the anemia of sickle cell disease. During pregnancy, sickle cell crises are more common and produce excruciating pain due to ischemia and infarction of various organs. Infections and pulmonary complications are also more common. Morphine or meperidine may be used to treat the client's pain. A transfusion of platelets may be ordered for clients exhibiting symptoms of HELLP syndrome (hemolysis, elevated liver enzymes, and low platelets). An infusion of granulocytes may be ordered for a pregnant client diagnosed with aplastic anemia who develops an infection. RBC and platelet transfusions also may be ordered to treat anemia or to control hemorrhage. Whole blood typically is used for a client who is hemorrhaging (e.g., postpartum hemorrhage). The whole blood not only treats the anemia but also replaces blood volume. (A)

44. **2.** About 25% of the teenager's diet can come from snacks. This is a way for teenagers to obtain protein, thiamine, riboflavin, vitamin B_6, magnesium, and zinc. Although not all snacks are low in fat or contain these nutrients, the nurse should encourage the mother to provide snacks with these nutrients. (H)

45. **3.** Applying a water-soluble lubricant to the nares helps alleviate sore nares when an NG tube is in place. Repositioning the tube does not eliminate the possibility of irritating the nares. Irrigating the tube with a cool solution or changing positions will not relieve the local irritation from the NG tube.(C)

46. **1.** Hindus do not eat beef. Sufficient protein can be obtained from lentils and fish. (C)

47. **3.** Although monitoring vital signs frequently is important, for the first few days the primary concern in burn care is fluid and electrolyte balance, with the goal being to replace fluid and electrolytes lost. With burns, fluid and electrolytes move from the interstitial spaces to the burn injury and are lost. These must be replaced. Once the child's fluid and electrolyte status has been addressed and fluid resuscitation has begun, preventing wound infection is a priority and efforts to control the child's pain can be initiated. (A)

48. **2.** Inactivated polio vaccine is given intramuscularly, usually with other vaccines. A killed virus is given to immunocompromised children. (D)

49. **2, 3, 4.** Diphenhydramine hydrochloride is an antihistamine that blocks the effects of histamine at receptor sites and has atropine-like effects, such as dry mouth, nausea, drowsiness, tachycardia, and thickened bronchial secretions. Weight loss and bradycardia are not adverse effects of this medication. (D)

50. **4.** The nurse does not administer naloxone because naloxone is the antidote for morphine, not midazolam. The benzodiazepine-receptor antagonist for midazolam is flumazenil (Romazicon). The nurse can promote oxygenation by encouraging deep breathing and administering oxygen. Resuscitation equipment should be accessible if needed. (D)

51. **3.** The client should be seated upright with the arms raised and crossed in front and supported by the overbed table. The client's head should rest on the arms. This position allows for outward expansion of the chest wall and promotes collection of the pleural fluid at the base of the thorax. (R)

52. **3.** Three or more servings of dairy products meet the calcium requirement. These can be obtained through milk, cheese, yogurt, and foods such as tofu. Spinach contains oxalates, which decrease the availability of calcium. Six to eleven servings of whole grains are recommended. Vitamin A supplements are not necessary in vegetarian diets because most vegetarian diets are rich in vitamin A. Vitamin A supplements can lead to anorexia, irritability, hair loss, and damage to the fetus. (C)

53. **1.** Intracellular microorganisms, such as viruses and parasites, invade the myocardium to survive. These microorganisms damage the vital organelles and cause cell death in the myocardium. The myocardium becomes weak, leading to heart failure; then T lymphocytes invade the myocardium in response to the viral infection. The T lymphocytes respond to the viral infection by secreting cytokines to kill the virus, but they also kill the virus-infected myocardium. Myocardial infarction, renal failure, and liver failure are not direct consequences of a viral or parasitic infection. (S)

54. **2.** The compensatory mechanism for respiratory acidosis is the renal system. In respiratory acidosis, the kidneys will conserve HCO_3^- in an attempt to correct the acidosis. Excretion of HCO_3^- would exacerbate the body's acidosis. The lungs cannot compensate for a problem that arises in the respiratory system. (A)

55. **2.** Amiodarone is metabolized in the liver and excreted in the bile and feces. Liver toxicity has been reported with the use of this drug, so the nurse will want to monitor the client's liver enzymes. Amiodarone does not affect hemoglobin, CK, or renal function. (D)

56. **2.** Antibiotics are the drug of choice in treating otitis media. Antihistamines, eardrops, and cotton in the ears are not helpful and are not recommended. (A)

57. **2.** Yogurt is high in protein because it is made from milk. The other choices are much higher in carbohydrates than protein except for bacon, which is higher in fat. (R)

58. **2.** The extracellular fluid compartment consists of two divisions, interstitial and intravascular. Prominent neck veins, hypertension, and bounding pulse indicate fluid excess in the intravascular (plasma) compartment. Fluid excess occurring in the interstitial compartment would lead to clinical findings related to tissue edema. Extra fluid in the intracellular compartment would lead to central nervous system changes such as confusion. (A)

59. **3.** Ciprofloxacin (Cipro) does not affect the PTT. It increases the theophylline level by 15% to 30% and may increase the PT. Iron decreases the absorption of ciprofloxacin. (D)

60. **3.** Pediculosis capitis, or head lice, can be spread by close contact or sharing of head gear or combs and brushes with other children. Sharing craft supplies, swimming, or showering usually does not provide close enough contact to permit transmission. (A)

61. **1.** In the first trimester, ultrasound scanning typically is ordered to determine the gestational age. This is especially important for a client with a history of irregular menstrual cycles to establish an accurate delivery date. There is no reason at this point in pregnancy to determine whether twins are present. This might be indicated if the fundal height were larger than the gestational age may indicate. Identifying the gender of the fetus is not a reason for an ultrasound examination unless there is a history of sex-linked genetic disorders. Pelvic adequacy can be determined by physical examination. If the client has a borderline pelvis, an ultrasound scan cannot confirm this. Pelvimetry can be done, but it is not performed as frequently as it once was. (H)

62. **2.** The nurse should prepare to insert an NG tube. The data collected provide evidence that the client is experiencing an upper gastrointestinal bleed secondary to a peptic ulcer. The client will be placed on nothing-by-mouth status and an NG tube will be inserted to provide gastric decompression and alleviate vomiting. Administering antiemetics is not a priority action for a client who is hypotensive and vomiting coffee-ground emesis. Assessment of client stressors is appropriate after emergency care has been provided and the client stabilized. A modified Trendelenburg position is inappropriate for clients who are vomiting. (R)

63. **3.** If the client is symptomatic, suggesting decreased cardiac output, he will need to be treated because maintaining circulation is the key goal. A temporary pacemaker can be inserted until the client is stable and the underlying etiology is determined. Cardiac catheterization with an electrophysiology study would follow insertion of the pacemaker. Bypass surgery is done when the arteries are occluded by plaque. An aortic balloon pump is used when pump failure is the problem. (A)

64. **4.** Refined grains are fortified with folic acid. Folic acid fortification is expected to prevent more than half of all neural tube defects. Vitamin C, which has multiple functions, is already added to many beverages and is widely available in many foods. Niacin maintains the normal functioning of the digestive tract and aids in energy metabolism. It is already added to enriched bread products and is widely available from many food sources. Vitamin B_{12} is involved in many metabolic processes. It is essential for the development of normal red blood cells. Many cereals, juices, soy, and bread products are fortified with vitamin B_{12}. (C)

65. **3.** The sudden onset of bright red drainage of this magnitude needs to be further assessed. Assessing vital signs is an important nursing action to determine whether there have been any changes in the client's status. Additional steps would include reinforcing the dressing and notifying the physician. Increasing the I.V. flow rate does not address the bleeding. Changing the dressing would be done only if the physician ordered it. (R)

66. **2.** Acute renal failure can occur secondary to a decrease in circulating fluid volume because of renal hypoperfusion. Paralytic ileus, adrenal insufficiency, and inappropriate antidiuretic hormone release can result in fluid volume alterations but do not occur secondary to a decrease in circulating fluid volume. (A)

67.

4. Maintain a patent airway.
1. Control hemorrhaging.
2. Replace fluids.
3. Relieve the client's anxiety.

The goal that has the highest priority when a client has a massive bleed from esophageal varices is to maintain a patent airway. The nurse should position the client to prevent aspiration and assess respirations and oxygen saturation. The nurse should then assist the health care provider in controlling the hemorrhage by using esophageal balloon tamponade. Octreotide (Sandostatin) may be administered to reduce portal pressure. The third priority is to restore circulating blood volume with blood and I.V. fluids. Esophageal bleeding is an anxiety-provoking event for the client and, although life-saving measures are the priority, the nurse and health care team should explain procedures to the client and provide reassurance as needed. (A)

68. **4.** A client who is taking phenelzine (Nardil), a monoamine oxidase inhibitor, needs to avoid foods that are rich in tyramine because this food-drug combination can cause hypertensive crisis. The client should be given a list of foods to avoid and should report headaches, palpitations, and a stiff neck to the physician immediately. The client does not need to restrict or add salt to the diet. Drinking 10 to 12 glasses of water each day is important to teach the client who is receiving lithium therapy. Antidepressant drugs take 2 to 4 weeks to achieve therapeutic effects. (D)

69. **3.** Clients with open fractures are particularly susceptible to infections. If not treated promptly, these infections can lead to the development of osteomyelitis. Localized symptoms of osteomyelitis include tenderness, swelling, and warmth at the site of infection, as well as unrelieved severe bone pain. Systemic symptoms include fever, chills, night sweats, and malaise. Avascular necrosis occurs when the blood supply to a bone is interrupted, most commonly in intracapsular hip fractures. Compartment syndrome is most commonly associated with fractures of the distal humerus and proximal tibia; it results from an increase in pressure on the nerves and blood supply within a closed tissue compartment. Fat embolism syndrome is associated most frequently with fractures of the long bones, ribs, and pelvis, which may or may not be open fractures. (R)

70. **4.** *Impaired verbal communication* is a priority nursing diagnosis after a total laryngectomy because the client will have a tracheostomy. The client frequently requires teaching on methods of communication after surgery. *Risk for impaired skin integrity, Excess fluid volume,* and *Ineffective thermoregulation* are not priority nursing diagnoses associated with a laryngectomy. (A)

71. **3.** The retina is especially susceptible to damage in a client with chronic hypertension. The arterioles supplying the retina are damaged. Such damage can lead to vision loss. The iris, cornea, and sclera are not affected by hypertension. (A)

72. **3.** Milia are white papules resulting from plugged sebaceous ducts that disappear by age 2 to 4 weeks. Parents should be instructed to avoid scratching them to prevent secondary infection. Term neonates generally have many creases on the soles of their feet. Preterm neonates may have only a few creases due to their immaturity. Strawberry hemangiomas are elevated areas formed by immature capillaries that will disappear over time. Port wine stains are deep, dark red discolorations that require laser therapy for removal. Erythema toxicum is a newborn rash or "flea bite" rash that requires no treatment and disappears over time. (H)

73. **4.** Clients with fractures of the long bones such as the femur are particularly susceptible to fat embolism syndrome (FES). Signs and symptoms include chest pain, dyspnea, tachycardia, and cyanosis. Changes in mental status are caused by hypoxemia and can be the first symptoms noted in FES. The client can also be restless and febrile and can develop petechiae. Osteomyelitis is infection of the bone; signs and symptoms of osteomyelitis do not include respiratory symptoms. Compartment syndrome causes signs of localized neurovascular impairment, not systemic symptoms. Venous thrombosis occurs in the lower extremities and is caused by venous stasis. (R)

74. **1, 3, 4.** As the homeostatic responses begin to decompensate, late clinical manifestations from a large overdose of sympathomimetic agents include loss of function of the hypothalamus such as temperature regulation, leading to profound pyrexia, and ectopic brain activity leading to seizures. Hypotension is a late sign that occurs as the vascular system collapses. Hypertension, an earlier sign, precedes hypotension. Tachycardia occurs as a reflex to hypotension, a late sign. (D)

75. **2.** A small tuft of hair and an indentation at the base of the neonate's spine is termed spina bifida occulta. This condition usually occurs between the L5 and S1 vertebrae with failure of the vertebrae to completely fuse. There are usually no sensory or motor deficits with this condition. Spina bifida cystica includes meningocele, myelomeningocele, and lipomeningocele. Meningocele is characterized by a saclike protrusion filled with spinal fluid and meninges. Usually, this condition is associated with sensory and motor deficits. Myelomeningocele is characterized by a saclike protrusion filled with spinal fluid, meninges, nerve roots, and spinal cord. With myelomeningocele, there are usually sensory and motor deficits. (H)

76. **1.** The primary purpose of instilling 5 ml of normal saline solution before suctioning a tracheostomy tube is to thin the secretions to be suctioned. The saline may stimulate a cough; however, this is not the reason for using saline. The tracheostomy tube is larger than the catheter and will easily pass into the tube. Humidification is provided by a nebulizer if needed. (R)

77. **3.** The client with emphysema has a chronically elevated carbon dioxide level. As a result, the normal stimulus for breathing in the medulla becomes ineffective. Instead, peripheral pressoreceptors in the aortic arch and carotid arteries, which are sensitive to oxygen blood levels, stimulate respirations. This is in response to low oxygen levels that have developed over time. If the client receives high concentrations of oxygen, the blood level of oxygen will rise excessively, the stimulus for respiration will decrease, and respiratory failure may result. Oxygen is not cooled. Humidification or administration of the oxygen through nasal cannula will not prevent depressed ventilation if the flow rate of the oxygen is too high. (A)

78. **1.** Protein intake is a concern in all vegetarian diets. Combining two incomplete proteins to make a complete protein (with all of the essential amino acids) can improve the client's protein intake. Rice with beans or tofu provides a complete protein. Soy milk would provide vitamin D and calcium, not protein. Yogurt provides vitamin D and calcium, not sufficient protein. Corn and rice do not make up a complete protein. However, corn and beans would be a complete protein. (C)

79. **3.** The client should be encouraged to join the community arthritis support group so that she can share her feelings with others who are facing similar experiences with this chronic illness and can identify with her concerns. A hobby will not help her resolve her feelings of being alone. Seeking counseling or discussing her feelings with a minister may be helpful, but these activities will not necessarily help the client to understand that there are many individuals who must adjust their lifestyles because of arthritis and that she is not alone. (H)

80. **2.** For the client who is unable to sit through meals to maintain adequate nutrition, the nurse should offer the client nutritious finger foods and fluids that he can consume while "on the run." Foods high in protein and carbohydrates, such as half of a peanut butter sandwich, will help to maintain nutritional needs. Adequate fluid intake is necessary, especially if the client has been started on lithium therapy. Directing the client to his room to eat is not helpful because the client will not stay in his room long enough to eat. Asking the client's family to bring his favorite foods or asking the client about his food preferences is not helpful in ensuring adequate nutrition for the hyperactive client who is unable to sit and eat. (P)

81. **4.** Telling the client to get her laundry and then showing her how to use the machine helps keep the client from becoming overly dependent on the nurse, establishes boundaries between the client and the nurse, and promotes positive self-worth. The statement, "Sure, I have time; I'll do it for you," is not therapeutic because it increases the client's dependency. Telling the client that she will have to wait because the nurse doesn't have time dismisses the client and insinuates that the nurse will do the laundry later, thus fostering dependency. Asking, "Can your family do it for you?" is not appropriate because the client is capable of doing her own laundry. This statement places responsibility on the family instead of the client. (P)

82. **2.** Early signs and symptoms of hypermagnesemia include drowsiness, lethargy, nausea, and vomiting. Flushed skin is a sign of hypernatremia. Severe thirst is associated with hyperglycemia. Tremors are associated with hypomagnesemia. (A)

83. **3.** When the blood glucose level drops, the pancreas secretes the hormone glucagon. The glucagon travels to the liver, where it stimulates the liver to release glucose. Muscles do not release glucose into the bloodstream. Glucagon does not stimulate intestinal absorption of glucose. Glucagon works only in the liver. (A)

84. **3.** Calling a client "contrary" is critical in nature and judgmental on the nurse's part. It is inappropriate for the nurse to make a comment like this at shift report or at any time. The other statements provide important and appropriate information (diagnosis, physician's name, pain relief strategies, and evaluation of ambulation). (M)

85. **1.** The nurse would teach personnel to communicate with these clients in a calm, matter-of-fact manner, using short sentences and a moderate tone of voice. This approach promotes orientation, reinforces cognitive-perceptual functions, and decreases anxiety. A cheerful tone and humor are inappropriate, possibly leading to misperceptions by the client with cognitive-perceptual impairment. Using abstract terms and a loud tone of voice increases anxiety and may lead to misunderstanding. Lengthy explanations delivered with a quiet voice will lead to frustration and increased anxiety. (P)

86. **1, 3, 4.** Vitamins B_6, B_{12}, and iron are important in the production of red blood cells. Therefore, the nurse should question the client specifically about food intake that contains these vitamins and minerals. Vitamins K and C have little role in the production of red blood cells. (H)

87. **1.** During the emergent phase of burn care, one of the most significant problems is hypovolemic shock. The development of hypovolemic shock can lead to impaired blood flow through the heart and kidneys, resulting in decreased cardiac output and renal ischemia. Efforts are directed toward replacing lost fluids and preventing hypovolemic shock. Preventing infection and controlling pain are important goals, but preventing circulatory collapse is a higher priority. It is too early in the stage of burn injury to promote wound healing. (A)

88. **2.** A client with multiple sclerosis may have a sense of optimism and euphoria, particularly during remissions. Euphoria is characterized by mood elevation with an exaggerated sense of well-being. Inappropriate laughter, slurring of words, and visual hallucinations are uncharacteristic of euphoria. (P)

89. **1.** The "rule of nines" is used to determine the percentage of the client's body surface area that was burned. Medical treatment, including fluid volume replacement therapy, is based on the percentage of body surface area burned. (A)

90. **2.** The "click" the nurse feels when abducting the femur is made by the head of the femur as it slips into the acetabulum. This is Ortolani's sign and indicates a dislocated hip. This is not a normal finding for a 2-month-old. The nurse needs to gather additional information by checking for unequal leg lengths and asymmetry of the gluteal and thigh folds. Once the nurse has obtained additional assessment information, the nurse would notify the physician. Usual medical treatment involves keeping the hip joint in an abducted position through triple diapering or a Pavlik harness. The goal of treatment is to keep the head of the femur centered in the acetabulum. Treatment needs to begin as soon as possible. Usually, the earlier treatment is started, the better the outcome. (H)

91. **4.** Warfarin sodium (Coumadin) interferes with clotting. The nurse should monitor the PT and evaluate for the therapeutic effects of Coumadin. A therapeutic PT is between 1.5 and 2.5 times the control value; the PT should be established by the health care provider. It may also be reported as an International Normalized Ratio, a standardized system that provides a common basis for communicating and interpreting PT results. The PTT is monitored in clients who are receiving heparin therapy. Serum potassium levels and ABG values are not affected by Coumadin. (D)

92. **4.** The lower abdominal pain is most likely caused by bladder spasms. A common cause of bladder spasms after TURP is blood clots obstructing the catheter; therefore, the nurse's first action should be to assess the patency of the catheter. Auscultating the abdomen for bowel sounds would be appropriate after patency of the catheter has been established. The nurse should assess for bladder spasms before administering an analgesic. A sitz bath would not relieve bladder spasms that are caused by an obstructed catheter. (A)

93. **2.** The parents of an infant with a congenital defect are frequently in a state of shock when the child is first born. The parents go through a period of grieving for the normal child they did not have. There are no data yet to support the other nursing diagnoses. (P)

94. **1.** The nurse should not automatically discard the partial fill of imipenem-cilastatin (Primaxin) found at the client's bedside until further investigation is done. The nurse should recognize the cost of medications such as imipenem-cilastatin and consult the pharmacist after identifying information on the partial fill that was found. The nurse should also ascertain whether the client received the last dose of imipenem-cilastatin. If the client did not receive the last dose, the nurse should notify the physician that the client did not receive the dose, receive orders, document, implement the orders, and complete an incident report. The nurse should administer the new partial fill of imipenem-cilastatin so that the client can receive the antibiotic on time. (S)

95. **2.** For a client with moderate anxiety, the nurse should initially lead the client to a less stimulating environment and help him discuss his feelings. Doing so helps the client to gain control over anxiety that could be overwhelming. Telling the client that it would be best to lie down until he is calmer is not appropriate because the client is too anxious to benefit from this intervention. Suggesting that the client try relaxation exercises could be helpful after the nurse takes the client to a less stimulating environment and allows the client to vent and discuss his feelings. Getting some medication to help the client relax is an intervention that the nurse would carry out later after trying to help the client decrease anxiety through ventilation and relaxation exercises. (P)

96. 1. Clients who are receiving anticoagulant therapy should consult the physician before undergoing any dental work. The dentist should also be aware that the client is taking anticoagulants. A soft toothbrush is desirable for oral hygiene if the client is receiving anticoagulant therapy; it helps prevent the gums from bleeding. Rectal suppositories are contraindicated during anticoagulant therapy because their insertion may cause bleeding. Stool softeners may be used instead to prevent straining, which also may promote bleeding. Green leafy vegetables should not be eaten in excess because of their vitamin K content, which may alter the effectiveness of the anticoagulant therapy. (D)

97. 3. Increasing the client's fluid intake to 3,000 ml/day, unless contraindicated, is the most appropriate action. Typically, clients who are immobilized by skeletal traction are given stool softeners. Treating constipation with diet, increased fluids, and stool softeners is preferred to the administration of an enema. Placing the client on the bedpan will not encourage a bowel movement. Range-of-motion movements maintain joint mobility but do not stimulate peristalsis. (R)

98. 1, 3, 4, 5. Although about 50% of diarrhea in clients receiving tube feedings is caused by sorbitol-containing medications, the nurse should assess for other possible causes. Diarrhea can occur as a result of bacterial contamination if fresh formula is not used or stored in a refrigerator, or if the feeding apparatus is not changed at least every 24 hours. Lactose intolerance, rapid formula administration, low serum albumin level, and hypertonic solutions may also cause diarrhea. Hypotonic solutions would not be a likely cause of diarrhea, abdominal distention, or cramping. (C)

99. 4. Risk factors for postoperative pulmonary complications include malnourishment, which is indicated by the client's height and weight. Although keeping feelings inside can be problematic, it would not be considered a postoperative risk for pulmonary complications. The absence of dyspnea on exertion is not indicative of postoperative complications. The client's age does not necessarily place her at increased risk. (H)

100. 2. Administering an antiemetic before beginning chemotherapy and then routinely around the clock helps prevent nausea and vomiting. Waiting until the client requests it may be too late because nausea is already present. (D)

101. 1. Greenish colored amniotic fluid is caused by the passage of meconium, usually secondary to a fetal insult during labor. Meconium passage also may be related to an intact gastrointestinal system of the neonate, especially those neonates who are full term or of postdate gestational age. Amnioinfusion may be used to treat the condition and dilute the fluid. Cloudy amniotic fluid is associated with an infection caused by bacteria or a sexually transmitted disease. Severe yellow-colored fluid is associated with Rh incompatibility or erythroblastosis fetalis. (H)

102. 1. The pH of 7.24 indicates that the client is acidotic. The carbon dioxide level is normal, but the HCO_3^- level is decreased. These findings indicate that the client is in metabolic acidosis. (A)

103. 3. Black, tarry stools indicate the presence of a slow upper gastrointestinal bleed. The longer the blood is in the system, the darker it becomes as the hemoglobin is broken down and iron is released. Vital sign changes, such as an increased pulse, are not evident with slow gastrointestinal bleeds. Nausea and abdominal cramps can occur but are not definitive signs of gastrointestinal bleeding. (A)

104. 1. Most adolescents with Osgood-Schlatter disease are able to continue to exercise and use ice afterward. Ibuprofen also may be ordered. Because Osgood-Schlatter disease is self-limited, crutches or physical therapy is usually unnecessary, and the adolescent usually does not need to stop playing sports. Only in severe cases would the adolescent have to stop playing sports. (A)

105. 3. Iron supplements will darken the stools. Iron supplements should not be taken on an empty stomach because they can cause gastric irritation. Iron is constipating, and a daily bulk-forming laxative should be started prophylactically. A straw should be used when taking liquid iron to avoid discoloring the teeth. (D)

106. 1. A client with generalized anxiety disorder needs to learn cognitive and behavioral strategies to cope with anxiety appropriately. In doing so, the client's anxiety decreases and becomes more manageable. The client may need assertiveness training, reframing, and relaxation exercises to adaptively deal with anxiety. (P)

107. 4. Deep breathing helps prevent microatelectasis and pneumonitis and also helps force air and fluid out of the pleural space into the chest tubes. It does not decrease blood flow to the lungs or control the rate of air flow. The diaphragm is the major muscle of respiration; deep breathing causes it to descend, thereby increasing the ventilating surface. (R)

108. 2. When applying an elastic bandage to a leg, start at the distal end and move toward the trunk in order to support venous return. Tension should be kept even and not increased with each turn to prevent circulatory impairment. Overlapping each layer twice when wrapping can also impair circulation. The clips securing the bandage should be placed on the outer aspect of the leg to avoid creating a pressure point on the other leg. (R)

109. **1.** Spermicidal agents work by destroying the spermatozoa before they enter the cervix. In addition, some spermicides alter the vaginal pH to a strong acidic environment, which is not conducive to survival of spermatozoa. Spermicides do not prevent the spermatozoa from entering the uterus, but the diaphragm or condom is a barrier. (D)

110. **4.** A low dosage of sertraline is helpful in controlling dementia-induced paranoia and hallucinations. Methylphenidate would be indicated for attention deficit hyperactivity disorder. Lorazepam would be ordered if the client were anxious and agitated. Nefazodone would be used if depression were prominent. (D)

111. **1.** Increased fremitus can be present in bacterial pneumonia, indicating the presence of pulmonary consolidation. Additional findings would include crackles, bronchial breath sounds, and dullness on percussion. Bilateral expiratory wheezing and resonance on percussion are not present in bacterial pneumonia. Vesicular breath sounds are normal and would not be an expected finding in bacterial pneumonia. (A)

112. **3.** Acute pancreatitis is very painful; management involves interventions for pain. Although alcohol abuse is often implicated in pancreatitis, drug and alcohol counseling will be an individual consideration. Risk for injury and ineffective airway clearance are not typically associated with acute pancreatitis. (C)

113. **1, 2, 5, 6.** To treat a low blood glucose level, the nurse should provide the client with approximately 15 g of carbohydrate and monitor the blood glucose level within 15 minutes. The orange juice, milk, bread, and soda would provide approximately 15 g of carbohydrate. Meat or fish, such as tuna, does not contain carbohydrate, although some of it can be converted to carbohydrate if sufficient carbohydrate from other sources is not provided. Processed peanut butter may contain small amounts of carbohydrate, but it is also high in fat and protein. To raise a blood glucose level in a timely manner, peanut butter is not a good option. (R)

114. **3.** Increased ICP can cause vomiting, particularly in children whose fontanels are closed. An infant with an open anterior fontanel may have less vomiting because the cranium can respond, expanding with increased ICP. The best course of action is to wait a few minutes and then refeed the child. Putting the child on NPO status may not be helpful because this is not a gastrointestinal problem. Because this is an expected event, notifying the physician is not necessary. Antiemetics frequently make a client sleepy, making neurologic checks difficult to interpret. (A)

115. **1.** The air is injected into the long-acting insulin first. Air is then injected into the short-acting insulin and the short-acting insulin is withdrawn. Then the long-acting insulin is withdrawn. It does matter which insulin is drawn up first because the nurse does not want to contaminate the short-acting insulin with the long-acting insulin. It is not necessary to use a high-dose insulin syringe to prepare 28 units of insulin. (D)

116. **2.** Solids should be introduced at about age 5 to 6 months. Full-term infants use up their prenatal iron stores within 4 to 6 months after birth. Cow's milk contains insufficient iron. (H)

117. **3.** Diminished breath sounds during an acute asthma attack are a serious sign of airway obstruction, fatigue, and impending respiratory failure. Wheezing, coughing, and the production of sputum indicate the presence of airflow through the lungs and are less ominous symptoms. (A)

118. **1.** Cardiomyopathies can be treated medically for a period of time. The only other treatment for the disease is a heart transplant. (A)

119. **1.** Clients should use an electric razor, instead of a straight-edge razor, on any skin areas that are receiving radiation. The skin should be cleaned daily with a mild soap, not harsh antibacterials. Lotion should be removed from the skin before any treatment and then reapplied after the treatment. The radiated skin area needs to be kept clean, dry, and open to air. (C)

120. **3.** A moderate amount of bloody drainage could indicate active bleeding. The priority action would be to apply pressure to the area and call for help. Assessing the airway or pulse or administering oxygen does not address the bleeding. (R)

121. **4.** Because valproic acid is associated with thrombocytopenia and hypofibrinogenemia, routine follow-up blood work would consist of monitoring platelet and fibrinogen levels for decreases. A CBC count and serum electrolyte level are not necessary. Aspartate transaminase, not alkaline phosphatase, is routinely monitored to evaluate for hepatic toxicity, a possible but rare effect of valproic acid. Valproic acid has no effect on cholesterol levels. (D)

122. **3.** Bacterial conjunctivitis is very contagious. Attention should be paid to thorough hand washing, a major means of stopping the transmission of the disease. Closing the day care center for 1 week is not necessary because thorough hand washing will stop the spread of the infection. Keeping the children out for 48 hours is not necessary. A child may return to day care after being treated for 24 hours. Although the parents of each child should be told about the outbreak, doing so will not help to curtail or prevent the spread of the infection. (S)

123. **3.** The client's mobility status is the best indicator of risk for development of a pressure sore. Nutritional and circulatory status are other factors that can contribute to pressure sore development, but immobility, even in the presence of adequate nutrition and circulation, is the leading cause of pressure sores. Disorientation can cause a client to neglect making needed position changes, but the underlying factor will be immobility. (R)

124. **1.** Ketosis is an adaptation to prolonged fasting or carbohydrate deprivation. The body takes partially broken-down fat fragments and combines them into ketone bodies, which the brain can then use for energy. Hypoglycemia is more likely to occur than hyperglycemia, although glucagon assists in preventing this. Metabolic syndrome refers to syndrome X, which includes an abnormal lipid profile and a tendency to gain weight in the abdomen. Lactic acidosis is a metabolic reaction that occurs when oxygen is reduced or not present. (A)

125. **1.** The nurse should stop and assess the client further. A chair should be available for the client to sit down. Obtaining the client's blood pressure and heart rate are important when exercising. These values can be used to predict when the oxygen demand becomes greater than the oxygen supply. Calling for help is not necessary for the complaint of midsternal burning. If the physician has ordered nitroglycerin, the nurse can administer it; however, stopping the activity may restore the oxygen balance. (A)

126. **2, 3, 4.** Vitamin B_6, folate, and vitamin B_{12} have been shown to reduce homocysteine levels. The effects of vitamins K and D have not been established with regard to homocysteine. (H)

127. **2.** The statement, "If I forget a dose, it's no big deal, I'll just take it when I remember it," indicates a knowledge deficit. The nurse should reinforce that the client should take dexamethasone as prescribed and at the same time each day. The drug has to be tapered off and cannot be stopped abruptly. The physician should be notified when the client is under additional stress (e.g., infection, surgery, illness). The client can have an allergic reaction to inactive ingredients contained in dexamethasone. (D)

128. **1.** A child with moderate dehydration, described as a loss of 50 to 90 ml/kg of body fluid, would have oliguria, gray skin color, increased pulse rate, and poor skin elasticity. A child with severe dehydration, described as a loss of more than 100 ml/kg of body fluid, would have a rapid and thready pulse, very poor skin elasticity, and mottled skin color. A child with mild dehydration, described as a loss of less than 50 ml/kg of body fluid, would have pale skin color, decreased skin elasticity, decreased urine output, and normal or increased pulse rate. (A)

129. **1.** Oropharyngeal candidiasis, or thrush, is the most common infection associated with the early symptomatic stages of HIV infection. Thrush is characterized by whitish yellow patches in the mouth. Various other opportunistic diseases can occur in clients with HIV infection, but they tend to occur later, after the diagnosis of acquired immunodeficiency syndrome has been made. Dyspnea can be indicative of pneumonia, which is caused by a variety of infective organisms. Bloody diarrhea is indicative of cytomegalovirus infection. Hyperpigmented lesions are indicators of Kaposi's sarcoma. (A)

130. **2.** Postpartum infection is a leading cause of maternal mortality in the United States. Typical treatment for the condition is I.V. antibiotic therapy with drugs such as clindamycin, gentamicin, or both. Cultures of the lochia will also be obtained. The neonate can continue to breastfeed as long as the mother desires. A switch to bottle-feeding is not necessary. The uterus tends to be firm, with increased cramping to rid the uterus of the infection. The client should be encouraged to remain in Fowler's position when in bed to allow for drainage of the lochia. (A)

131. **1.** The mother needs further instruction when she says, "I should position the baby the same way for each feeding." This can contribute to sore nipples. The position should vary for each feeding to prevent repeated pressure on the same area each time. Grasping the entire areola and nipple will help to decrease nipple soreness. Air drying the breasts and not using a hand pump will help to decrease nipple soreness. (H)

132. **1.** During an acute attack of vertigo, it is best for the client to lie down in a darkened, quiet room and to avoid sudden position changes. A low-sodium diet may be helpful in decreasing the number of attacks, but it is not recommended during the attack. Headaches are not a component of the vertigo attack. Because vertigo is frequently accompanied by nausea and vomiting, the client will not want to eat or drink. Fluids are usually administered parenterally to maintain hydration and administer medications. (A)

133. **3.** The American Academy of Pediatrics recommends that all neonates should receive only formula or breast milk for the first 4 to 6 months of life. Cereal will not help the neonate sleep through the night and may result in allergies and other digestive disorders. (H)

134. **2.** Once the client has stated that he is allergic to a substance, the nurse would be negligent to ignore the client's statement and administer the substance. The nurse should check the chart for allergies and call the physician for an alternative antibiotic prescription. (M)

135. **1.** Jaundice that persists past the third or fourth day of life and pale, light stools are associated with biliary atresia. Alkaline phosphatase levels will also be elevated. Surgical intervention is necessary to remove the blockage. Rh isoimmunization and ABO incompatibility are associated with neonatal anemia as the red blood cells are hemolyzed by the antibodies. Esophageal varices are associated with cirrhosis of the liver and large amounts of bleeding when the vessels rupture. The child with esophageal varices will exhibit manifestations of anemia such as pallor, and may experience hemorrhage and shock. (A)

136. **1.** Most parents find it especially difficult to allow a child who was unable to be normally active before corrective heart surgery to lead a normal and active life after surgery. These parents are less likely to be apprehensive about persuading the child of the need for rest, about postoperative complications, or having the child out of school for a month. (A)

137. **3.** After abdominal surgery, the reason for inserting a NG tube is to decompress the gastrointestinal tract until peristaltic action returns. Compression may be used to control bleeding esophageal varices. Lavage is used to remove substances from the stomach or control bleeding. Gavage is used to provide enteral feedings. (A)

138. **3.** The most common long-term problem experienced by children with cleft palate repair is speech problems. These children frequently need speech therapy for a period of time. Hearing problems may occur as a result of chronic ear infections and the placement of myringotomy tubes. A poor self-concept may develop in any child. However, if a child with a cleft palate receives adequate parenting and support, this should not occur. Chronic sinus infections are more commonly associated with asthma, not with this defect. (A)

139. **2.** Feeding solutions that have not been infused after hanging for 8 hours should be discarded because of the increased risk of bacterial growth. Sitting the client upright during the feeding helps prevent aspiration of the feeding. A gastric residual of 25 ml is considered acceptable. A gastric residual of 100 to 150 ml, or a residual greater than 100% of the previous hour's intake, indicates delayed emptying. The feeding solution should be at room or body temperature. (D)

140. **3.** Furosemide is a loop diuretic and inhibits the reabsorption of sodium and chloride from the proximal and distal renal tubules and the loop of Henle. Furosemide promotes sodium diuresis, resulting in a loss of potassium and serious electrolyte imbalances. Furosemide does not affect the BUN level. (D)

141. **3.** Suctioning the respiratory tract for prolonged periods depletes the client's oxygen supply and causes hypoxia. It is recommended that each suctioning period not exceed 15 seconds. (R)

142. **2.** The most appropriate action is to encourage the daughter to talk to her mother about the end-of-life issues first to reach a consensus or agreement. This is a family decision. Immediately informing the physician or preparing to remove the client from life support would be premature if the family is not in agreement. Although a copy of the living will should be on the client's chart, it is up to the daughter to show it to her mother. (P)

143. **4.** Contraindications for t-PA or alteplase recombinant therapy include current active internal bleeding, 3 hours or longer since the onset of symptoms of a stroke, and severe hypertension. Age greater than 65 years is not a contraindication for the therapy. (D)

144. **1.** Extreme muscle weakness is present in both cholinergic crisis and myasthenic crisis. In cholinergic crisis, I.V. edrophonium chloride (Tensilon), a cholinergic agent, does not improve muscle weakness; in myasthenic crisis, it does. Diaphoresis and increased salivation are not present in cholinergic crises. (A)

145. **3.** For a complete breech, the buttocks present, the feet and legs are flexed on the thighs, and the thighs are flexed on the abdomen. For a frank breech, the buttocks present with the hips flexed and the legs extended against the abdomen and chest. This is the most common type of breech presentation. For a compound breech, the buttocks present together with another part, such as a hand. This is a rare occurrence. For an incomplete breech, one or both feet or the knees extend below the buttocks. This can also be termed a single footling or double footling breech. (H)

146. **1.** It is important that the client understand that alcohol should be avoided for at least 1 year after an episode of hepatitis. Sexual intercourse does not need to be avoided, but the client should be instructed to use condoms until the hepatitis B surface antigen measurement is negative. The client will need to restrict activity until liver function test results are normal; this will not occur within 1 to 2 weeks. Jaundice will subside as the client recovers; it is not a permanent condition. (R)

147. **4.** The individual who is bulimic is most commonly female and age 15 to 24. She binges and purges to control her weight and to prevent weight gain. Sometimes excessive exercise is also used. Use of regular exercise and calorie counting and occasional use of diet medication to maintain normal weight are not considered dysfunctional in our society. (P)

148. 2. Swollen cervical lymph nodes are characteristic of early Hodgkin's disease. Difficulty breathing and swallowing are not early signs. The disease originates in the lymphatic system, not the liver. (A)

149. 1, 4, 5, 6. Diazepam (Valium) is a benzodiazepine that causes symptoms of withdrawal when stopped abruptly. The nurse should assess the client for tremors, agitation, irritability, insomnia, vomiting, sweating, tachycardia, headache, anxiety, and confusion. Euphoria or elevated mood is not a symptom of benzodiazepine withdrawal. (D)

150. 1. Parents are typically quick to notice changes in their infant's physical appearance. The removal of the infant's hair may be upsetting to them if they have not been told why it is being done. Hair may be removed on the scalp at the site of needle insertion for I.V. therapy to provide better visualization and a smooth surface on which to attach tape to secure the needle. Sedatives are not ordinarily prescribed before I.V. fluid administration. In most instances, it is acceptable for parents to visit their infant while the I.V. solution is infusing. Holding the infant is encouraged to provide comfort. (D)

151. 1. Abdominal pain can be a significant problem in acute pancreatitis. An expected outcome is to decrease or eliminate the pain the client is experiencing. Patterns of bowel elimination and liver function are not typically affected by pancreatitis. The client should avoid alcohol. (A)

152. 3. The most appropriate initial response by the nurse would be to test the child's blood glucose level. The child's symptoms are consistent with hypoglycemia but could also be used by the child to avoid participation in planned activities. Administering milk or fruit juice during a mild reaction may also be appropriate if testing cannot be done. Notifying the physician may be appropriate after the child's glucose level has been obtained and emergency treatment has been initiated if the child is experiencing hypoglycemia. Returning the child to previous activities is not appropriate until either testing or administering treatment has been done. (A)

153. 3. Normally, breasts are about the same size. They can vary in size before menstruation due to breast engorgement caused by hormonal changes. It is not necessary for a physician to check this slight change in breast size. The changes in breast size this client described are most likely caused by hormonal changes, not a benign cyst or normal growth and development. (H)

154. 2. Traditional Chinese medicine describes health as the balance of yin and yang. It describes health as harmony between the mind, body, and soul. (H)

155. 2. Before an IVP, the client should be assessed for allergies to iodine. Shellfish is a source of iodine, so people who are allergic to shellfish should not receive an IVP. Asking the client whether he or she has ever had an IVP before can help determine the degree of teaching needed before the procedure, but that is not the most important question. Neither the client's last bowel movement nor urinary incontinence has any relationship to an IVP. (R)

156. 3. Progestin alone has no effect on breast milk or breast-feeding once the milk supply is well established. Estrogen suppresses milk output. Testosterone is not given as an oral contraceptive. (D)

157. 2. In this situation, the client has indicated that she is not willing to leave the abusive boyfriend because of potential economic concerns and other children in the household. The nurse should explain the cycle of abuse (e.g., tension-building phase, battering incident, and honeymoon phase). The priority intervention is to assist the client to make concrete plans for the safety of herself and her children. The client should identify the safest, quickest routes out of the house and be able to identify where she will go once the cycle of violence escalates. Contacting a social worker at this time is not appropriate because the client is not ready to leave the abusive situation. The nurse can tell the client that these services are available, but it is up to the client to determine whether a referral is necessary. Telling the client that she shouldn't allow anyone to hit her or her children does not assist the client to make plans for her safety and the children's safety should the violence escalate. The client may have a flat affect or feel extreme humiliation from the abuse. The client may also be feeling that the abuse is her fault. When the client is ready to leave the abusive situation and receive continuous counseling, efforts can be taken to increase her self-esteem and prevent additional violence. The client should be made aware of the available services in the community for women who are involved in abusive relationships. The location and phone numbers for available shelters should be provided to the client. Giving her a brochure related to the statistics about violence against women is not helpful and, if found by the abuser, may lead to further violence. (P)

158. 2. The client who is taking sulfadiazine should be instructed to drink at least 8 glasses of water a day to prevent the development of crystalluria. Sulfadiazine should be taken on an empty stomach with a full glass of water. It does not require that the client's urine output be measured and does not affect the color of the urine. (D)

159. **3.** The client is demonstrating loose associations. Therefore, the nurse needs to clarify the meaning of and the connection between ideas. The nurse's statement about Halloween makes the assumption that the client is talking about Halloween from the mention of black cats and black hats. Asking if the client has a black cat is not helpful. The statement about time going faster ignores the client's statement entirely. (P)

160. **1.** MID results from multiple small blood clots in the brain. Therefore, the most critical factor is using anticoagulants to reduce the risk of more infarcts. Administering benzodiazepines such as lorazepam to decrease choreiform movements is associated with Huntington's disease. Although depression is common with MID, managing depression-related symptoms will not slow the progression of MID. Managing symptoms by increasing dopamine availability is appropriate for clients with Parkinson's disease. (D)

161. **2.** Checking the carotid artery pulse in a child during CPR provides information about perfusion of the brain. The brachial pulse is checked in an infant because the infant's short and typically fat neck makes it difficult to palpate the carotid pulse. The femoral and radial arteries might indicate perfusion to the peripheral body sites, but the critical need is for adequate circulation to the brain. (A)

162. **2.** Nephrotic syndrome is characterized by massive proteinuria caused by increased glomerular membrane permeability. Other symptoms include peripheral edema, hyperlipidemia, and hypoalbuminemia. Because of the edema, clients retain fluid and may gain weight. Hematuria is not a symptom related to nephrotic syndrome. (A)

163. **2.** Because the child has a history of severe hypoxic episodes, having oxygen readily available at the bedside is most important. Should the child experience another hypoxic episode, oxygen could be administered easily and quickly. Although morphine causes peripheral dilation, which causes the blood to remain in the periphery, decreasing system volume, oxygen administration is the priority. Typically a child with tetralogy of Fallot with episodes of hypoxia does not require suctioning. (A)

164. **1.** Although individuals differ, the most likely attitude of a Mexican-American client is to bear pain stoically, to endure pain as a part of God's will, and to delay seeking treatment. (C)

165. **1.** When a client voids frequent, small amounts, the nurse should suspect that the client is retaining urine. Palpating for a distended bladder is the first assessment that the nurse should perform to verify this suspicion. Obtaining an order to catheterize for residual urine may be appropriate as a follow-up activity. Obtaining a urine specimen for culture is not a first priority. The nurse would not encourage an increased fluid intake until further assessment of the situation is completed. (A)

166. **3.** It is appropriate for the client to be on a low-sodium diet to help decrease fluid retention. Dry skin and pruritus are common in renal failure. Lotions are used to relieve the dry skin, and antihistamines may be used to control itching; corticosteroids are not used. Pain is not a major problem in chronic renal failure, but analgesics that are excreted by the kidneys must be avoided. It is not necessary to measure abdominal girth daily because ascites is not a clinical problem in renal failure. (R)

167. **1.** The most frequent cause of respiratory distress in a toddler with no history of an illness is foreign body aspiration. The nurse should immediately begin abdominal thrusts. The nurse cannot wait for the ambulance or chest radiography report. Someone other than the nurse can check the oxygen saturation level. (S)

168. **4.** The traction weights should be hanging freely to maintain pull. The child needs to be moved up in bed with the weights left untouched to continue countertraction. Then the nurse can determine whether blocks are necessary to maintain the child in the correct position. Raising the weights is inappropriate because doing so interferes with countertraction. The physician does not need to be notified. The nurse can easily correct the problem by moving the child up in bed. (A)

169. **1.** Children ages 6 to 12 have a slower growth rate than do younger children and adolescents. As a result, their food requirements are comparatively less. (H)

170. **4.** Asking whether the client is thinking about killing herself is the most direct and therefore the best way to assess suicide risk. Knowing whether the client has recently watched movies on suicide and death, what the client thinks about suicide, or about previous suicides of family members will not tell the nurse whether the client herself is thinking about committing suicide right now. (P)

171. **4.** Proper nutrition before and during pregnancy helps to ensure that the uterus will be able to support the growth of a healthy placenta. If the placenta never develops properly, the fetus will fail to thrive and the infant may have a low birth weight. (H)

172. **1.** Return demonstrations are the best way to evaluate a person's ability to perform a skill. This technique enables the teacher to observe not only the learner's sequencing of steps of the procedure but also the learner's ability to perform the skill. (D)

173. **3.** Ibuprofen (Motrin) should be taken with food or antacids to avoid the development of gastrointestinal distress. Tinnitus is not an adverse effect of ibuprofen; it is a sign of salicylate toxicity. There is no need to increase vitamin B_{12} intake. The CBC is not typically monitored monthly, although clients should be told to report signs of unusual bleeding because ibuprofen can prolong bleeding time. (D)

174. **4.** When the client has a ruptured appendix, the nurse should document the surgical wound as an infected wound because bacterial organisms are present in the wound and there are signs of infection (e.g., inflammation, skin separation, purulent drainage). A clean wound is documented when no cavities have been entered and there is a low risk of infection. A clean-contaminated wound is recorded when a cavity, such as the gastrointestinal, genitourinary, or respiratory tract, has been entered under controlled conditions and there is greater risk of an infection than with a clean wound. A contaminated wound is when a traumatic, open, accidental wound has occurred or when a break in sterile technique occurred in a surgical wound and there is a high risk of infection. (S)

175. **4.** The nurse concludes that the staff member needs teaching about depression, specifically the biological basis of major depression, when the staff member states the client has no reason to be depressed because "she really has it all." Major depression, or endogenous depression, is caused by alterations of neurotransmitters, primarily serotonin and norepinephrine. Genetics and hereditary also predispose an individual to develop depression. Therefore, there may not be an external cause or a reason for depression to develop. Depression that occurs from an external cause is known as reactive depression and it could be caused by a loss or a life stress. (P)

176. **4.** In asthma, the airways react to certain external and internal stimuli, including allergens, infections, exercise, and emotions. Food allergens commonly associated with asthma include wheat, egg white, dairy products, citrus fruits, corn, and chocolate. (A)

177. **4.** When administering an enema, the nurse should position the client in a left Sims position. Placing the client in this position facilitates the flow of fluid into the rectum and colon. It also allows the client to flex the right leg forward, adequately exposing the rectal area. (D)

178. **3.** Risk factors for the development of pressure ulcers include poor nutrition, indicated by a decreased serum albumin level. According to the *Guidelines for Pressure Ulcers* published by the Agency for Healthcare Research and Quality, other risk factors include immobility, incontinence, and decreased sensation. A client who does not ambulate often can be repositioned frequently to prevent pressure ulcers. Having an indwelling urinary catheter does not normally increase the risk of developing a pressure ulcer unless pressure from the tubing impinges on urethral or other tissue. An elevated white blood cell count does not place a client at risk for pressure ulcers. (R)

179. **2.** Cerebral hypoxia is commonly associated with dizziness. The greatest risk of injury to a client with dizziness is a fall. Frequent rests and energy conservation measures should be included in the client's plan of care, but safety from falls is the greatest need. Checking the shower water temperature is not critical for this client, who will not be showering because of her fall risk. (R)

180. **4.** A characteristic finding in multiple myeloma is Bence Jones protein in the urine. Other laboratory findings include increased serum protein level, hypercalcemia, anemia, thrombocytopenia, and hyperuricemia. Polycythemia vera is not found in multiple myeloma. (A)

181. **2.** Ephedrine is the drug of choice when the client's blood pressure falls after administration of an epidural anesthetic. Atropine sulfate is used with general anesthesia to dry the secretions and prevent aspiration. It is the antidote for poisoning by several species of mushrooms. It is also used to treat cardiovascular collapse from cholinergic drugs. Methylergonovine is used for severe postpartum hemorrhage. It does exert an antihypotensive effect. Oxytocin, a vasoconstrictor, is used to stimulate uterine contractions. It is not as effective as ephedrine in raising the client's blood pressure, and the client does not need additional uterine stimulation. (D)

182. **3.** Epidermoid cancer involving the larger bronchi is almost entirely associated with heavy cigarette smoking. The American Cancer Society reports that smoking is implicated in more than 80% of lung cancers in men and women. The prevalence of lung cancer is related to the duration and intensity of the smoking. The best intervention for nurses is to encourage smoking cessation. HEPA filters can reduce allergens, but they do not prevent lung cancer. Chest radiographs aid in detection of lung cancer but do not prevent it. Exposure to asbestos has been implicated as a risk factor, but cigarette smoking is the major risk factor. (H)

183. **2.** The client needs to take the prescribed medications for approximately 2 to 3 weeks before discontinuing precautions against infecting others. Effectiveness of the drug therapy is determined by negative sputum smears obtained on three consecutive days. Although results can vary among clients, the majority respond to therapy within 2 to 3 weeks. (D)

184. **3.** The statement, "My kids need me," indicates an improvement in the client's condition because the client is stating a reason for wanting to live rather than exhibiting hopelessness and worthlessness. Stating that he will go to group when he has more energy conveys the presence of fatigue and withdrawal, key features of depression. Saying that he only thinks about killing himself at night indicates the presence of suicidal ideation and recurrent thoughts of death, and thus continued depression. Stating, "I want everyone to leave me alone," indicates the presence of withdrawal, depressed mood, and a lack of focus on present activities. (P)

185. **3.** Penicillin is the drug of choice to treat Lyme disease in pregnant women. Tetracycline and doxycycline are contraindicated during pregnancy because they have been associated with fetal defects. Gentamicin is not used for Lyme disease but is useful for treating gram-negative bacterial infections. It may be teratogenic to the fetus and is not used during pregnancy. (D)

186. **2.** Amnioinfusion is the addition of sterile fluid into the uterus to supplement or dilute amniotic fluid that is meconium-stained. Amnioinfusion may be used when there is evidence of variable decelerations caused by cord compression, not early decelerations. Amnioinfusion is not used for short umbilical cords; there is no treatment for an abnormally short umbilical cord. Electronic fetal monitoring, not amnioinfusion, is used for multifetal pregnancies. (R)

187. **1.** As chronic condition that affects many body systems, diabetes is a risk factor for surgical complications. The client's blood glucose level and insulin requirements need to be closely monitored before and after surgery. Being sensitive to aspirin does not pose a risk for the client in surgery. Osteoarthritis is not a systemic condition and does not place the client at risk during surgery. Chronic low back pain is not a systemic condition that places the client at risk during surgery; however, it can be exacerbated by positioning on the operating room table. (A)

188. **4.** Multiple drug regimens are used because the drugs have a synergistic effect. The drugs have different cell-cycle lysis effects, different mechanisms of action, and different toxic adverse effects. They are usually given in combination to enhance therapy. Dosage is not affected by giving the drugs in combination. The second and third drugs do not increase the effectiveness of the first. It is not true that the first two drugs are toxic to cancer cells while the third drug promotes cell growth. (D)

189. **2.** The parents need to discuss their feelings with each other to begin the healing process. Avoiding discussing their feelings causes each one to become isolated and to grieve without support. Keeping to themselves does not allow an opportunity for social support and would promote isolation. Working long hours is detrimental to the grieving process; there is no time to come to terms with what has occurred. Acting as if nothing has happened is avoiding the issue. (P)

190. The nurse should auscultate the right lower lobe and listen as the client inhales and exhales. The nurse should be able to hear vesicular breath sounds. (A)

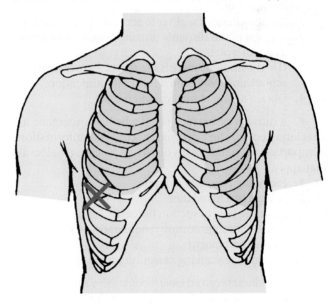

1. A client returns to the recovery room following left supratentorial surgery for treatment of a brain tumor. The nurse should place the client in which position to facilitate venous drainage?

- ☐ **1.** Lying flat without a pillow with his head turned to the right.
- ☐ **2.** Lying flat with his head elevated on three pillows.
- ☐ **3.** Head of the bed elevated to 30 degrees with his head in a neutral position.
- ☐ **4.** Side-lying on his left side.

2. A 57-year-old Hispanic woman with breast cancer who does not speak English is admitted for a lumpectomy. Her daughter, who speaks English, accompanies her. In order to obtain admission information from the client, what should the nurse do?

- ☐ **1.** Ask the client's daughter to serve as an interpreter.
- ☐ **2.** Ask one of the Hispanic nursing assistants to serve as an interpreter.
- ☐ **3.** Use the limited Spanish she remembers from high school along with nonverbal communication.
- ☐ **4.** Obtain a trained medical interpreter.

3. A nurse is caring for a client who has undergone a total laryngectomy for laryngeal cancer. What information is important to include in his discharge teaching? Select all that apply.

- ☐ **1.** Providing humidity at home.
- ☐ **2.** Following a bland diet.
- ☐ **3.** Learning how to suction himself.
- ☐ **4.** Having communication rehabilitation with a speech pathologist
- ☐ **5.** Attending a smoking cessation program.

4. The client received electroconvulsive therapy (ECT) an hour ago and tells the nurse that he has a headache. Which response by the nurse is best?

- ☐ **1.** "A headache is common after ECT."
- ☐ **2.** "I will get some acetaminophen (Tylenol) for you."
- ☐ **3.** "A nap will help you feel better."
- ☐ **4.** "Eat your breakfast and then let me know how you feel."

5. When assessing speech development, which of the following children should the nurse refer for further examination?

- ☐ **1.** A 4-month-old who laughs out loud.
- ☐ **2.** A 10-month-old who says "dada" and "mama."
- ☐ **3.** A 1-year-old who says 3 to 5 words.
- ☐ **4.** An 18-month-old who only says "no."

6. During a clinic visit for a postpartum examination, the mother of a 2-week-old infant tearfully tells the nurse she feels very tired and thinks she is not a good mother to her baby. Which statement by the nurse would be best?

- ☐ **1.** "The hormonal changes your body is experiencing are causing you to feel this way."
- ☐ **2.** "Most new mothers feel the same way that you do. I hear that a lot from others."
- ☐ **3.** "You need to have your husband and family help you so that you can get some rest."
- ☐ **4.** "I'm concerned about what you are experiencing. Tell me more about what you are thinking and feeling."

7. A client is to receive 2 g of metronidazole (Flagyl) orally in a single dose. The medication is available in 500-mg tablets. How many tablets should the nurse administer?

_____ tablets

8. A college student is asking the nurse about his grandfather, who just received a diagnosis of Huntington's disease. The student wants to know if he will have the disease, too. What should the nurse tell the student? Select all that apply.

- ☐ **1.** "Huntington's disease affects men more than women."
- ☐ **2.** "Huntington's disease is an autosomal dominant disease."
- ☐ **3.** "Huntington's disease does not skip a generation."
- ☐ **4.** "Huntington's disease is a treatable disease."
- ☐ **5.** "There is a 75% chance you will have the disease."

9. A client is admitted with numbness and tingling of the feet and toes after having an upper respiratory infection and flu for the past 5 days. Within 1 hour of admission, the client states that his legs are numb all the way up to his hips. The nurse should do which of the following next? Select all that apply.

- ☐ **1.** Call his family to come in to visit with him.
- ☐ **2.** Notify his health care provider of the change.
- ☐ **3.** Place respiratory resuscitation equipment in the client's room.
- ☐ **4.** Check for advancing levels of paresthesia.
- ☐ **5.** Perform ankle pumps to increase circulation and relieve numbness.

10. The nurse is caring for a client with an injury to the thalamus. The nurse should plan to:
- ☐ **1.** Give higher doses of pain medication.
- ☐ **2.** Keep patches on the client's eyes to prevent corneal abrasion.
- ☐ **3.** Monitor the temperature of the bathwater.
- ☐ **4.** Avoid turning the client.

11. A client who voluntarily admitted herself to the in-patient mental health unit adamantly demands to be discharged immediately. What is the most appropriate response by the nurse?
- ☐ **1.** "We hate to see you go, but that is your right. I'll get the forms for you so you can go."
- ☐ **2.** "I'm sorry, but your lawyer or family must request such forms when you are hospitalized."
- ☐ **3.** "I will get the forms, but your psychiatrist will need to see you before you leave."
- ☐ **4.** "Are you sure we can't convince you to stay here a few days longer? Your insurance is still valid and there are several issues we need to address."

12. A client in an outpatient clinic tells the nurse that he is going to harm his brother-in-law, who called the police on him for threatening to hurt his ex-wife. The nurse should document the situation after notifying all of the following persons except whom?
- ☐ **1.** Clinic administrator.
- ☐ **2.** Ex-wife.
- ☐ **3.** Police.
- ☐ **4.** Intended victim.

13. The nurse is assigned a client who has sustained a spinal cord injury. When assessing the client the nurse will expect the client to experience:
- ☐ **1.** Complete anesthesia below the level of the injury.
- ☐ **2.** Tingling in the fingers.
- ☐ **3.** Pain below the site of the injury.
- ☐ **4.** Loss of position and vibratory sense.

14. A client who is paraplegic cannot feel her lower extremities and has been positioned on her side. The nurse should anticipate that which of the following areas would be a pressure point in this position?
- ☐ **1.** Sacrum.
- ☐ **2.** Occiput.
- ☐ **3.** Ankles.
- ☐ **4.** Heel.

15. Which of the following is appropriate in promoting the development of a preschooler? Select all that apply.
- ☐ **1.** Providing anticipatory guidance for parents.
- ☐ **2.** Helping the parents understand their child's behavior.
- ☐ **3.** Identifying deviations from normal growth and development patterns.
- ☐ **4.** Determining the child's future development.
- ☐ **5.** Sending the child to a day care center.

16. A neonate is to receive an I.V. infusion of normal saline solution at 3 ml/hour. The nurse is setting the alarms on an I.V. infusion pump. How should the nurse set the alarms?
- ☐ **1.** At 5% above and 5% below the keep-vein-open rate.
- ☐ **2.** Within a 15% range of the keep-vein-open rate
- ☐ **3.** To sound when the infusion is infiltrating.
- ☐ **4.** At the exact drip rate as prescribed.

17. A nurse is interpreting a client's telemetry strip. If the QRS measures six small blocks, how many seconds is the QRS interval?

_____ seconds

18. A client is admitted to the inpatient unit and is exhibiting pressured speech, a labile affect, euphoria, and hyperactivity. The client states, "I am the Savior of the city." The family states that the client has hardly slept or eaten for days. Which of the following client needs is a priority in the nurse's plan of care?
- ☐ **1.** Physical.
- ☐ **2.** Social.
- ☐ **3.** Spiritual.
- ☐ **4.** Cultural.

19. A neonate is receiving an I.V. infusion of dextrose 10% in water administered by an infusion pump. The nurse should verify the alarm settings on the infusion pump at which times? Select all that apply.
- ☐ **1.** When the infusion is started.
- ☐ **2.** At the beginning of each shift.
- ☐ **3.** When the neonate returns from X-ray.
- ☐ **4.** When the neonate moves in the crib.
- ☐ **5.** After the parents have visited.

20. The nurse is planning care for a neonate to prevent neonatal heat loss immediately after delivery. Which situation would conserve heat and help the infant maintain a stable temperature?
- ☐ **1.** The neonate is nestled against the crib wall.
- ☐ **2.** The neonate has a hat and blanket on.
- ☐ **3.** Bathe the neonate with warm water.
- ☐ **4.** The neonate is lying in an open crib with a diaper on.

21. The pain associated with migraine headaches is believed to be caused by:
- ☐ **1.** Dilation of the cranial arteries.
- ☐ **2.** A temporary decrease in intracranial pressure (ICP).
- ☐ **3.** Irritation and inflammation of the openings of the sinuses.
- ☐ **4.** Sustained contraction of muscles around the scalp and face.

22. The nurse observes that the client's right eye does not close completely. Based on this finding, which of the following nursing interventions would be *most* appropriate?

☐ **1.** Making sure the client wears her eyeglasses at all times.

☐ **2.** Placing an eye patch over her right eye.

☐ **3.** Instilling artificial tears once every shift.

☐ **4.** Cleaning the eye with a clean washcloth every shift.

23. The nurse is administering an injection to an infant. Indicate the appropriate site for administering medication to an infant via injection.

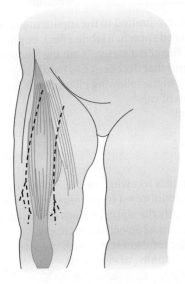

24. A 14-year-old with rheumatic fever who is on bed rest is receiving an I.V. infusion of dextrose 5% in water administered by an infusion pump. The nurse should verify the alarm settings on the infusion pump at which of the following times? Select all that apply.

☐ **1.** When the infusion is started.

☐ **2.** At the beginning of each shift.

☐ **3.** When the child returns from X-ray.

☐ **4.** When the child moves in the bed.

☐ **5.** When the child is sleeping.

25. A potential concern when caring for an older adult who has diminished hearing and vision would be the client's:

☐ **1.** Feelings of disorientation.

☐ **2.** Cognitive impairment.

☐ **3.** Sensory overload.

☐ **4.** Social isolation.

26. Which of the following children should be referred for further assessment regarding language development?

☐ **1.** A 2-year-old who has a vocabulary of 300 words and can combine two or three words in a phrase.

☐ **2.** A 3-year-old who has a vocabulary of 900 words and can make a complete sentence of three or four words.

☐ **3.** A 2-year-old who has a vocabulary of 100 words and can point to objects.

☐ **4.** A 1-year-old who has a vocabulary of 8 words and can say "mommy" and "daddy" with specific reference to the correct person.

27. A nurse is taking a medication history on a client with multiple sclerosis before administering an initial dose of baclofen (Lioresal). What should the nurse check before administering the drug? Select all that apply.

☐ **1.** Presence of muscle weakness.

☐ **2.** History of muscle spasms.

☐ **3.** Serum creatinine level.

☐ **4.** Serum potassium level.

☐ **5.** Blood glucose.

28. A client has been taking carbamazepine (Tegretol) for 2 years. The nurse should assess the client for which of the following? Select all that apply.

☐ **1.** Bruising.

☐ **2.** Sore throat.

☐ **3.** Urine retention.

☐ **4.** Light-colored stool.

☐ **5.** Hydration status.

29. A 12-year-old client says, "Give me my pajamas. I'm not putting your silly gown on." An appropriate response by the nurse should be:

☐ **1.** "I know they're funny but everyone here wears them."

☐ **2.** "You don't mean that, now. A big guy like you knows how hospitals are."

☐ **3.** "You're upset because you feel awkward and embarrassed in these gowns."

☐ **4.** "You're upset because you think we're unreasonable."

30. A nursing assistant is taking care of a child in the arm restraint shown below. To provide care for this child, what should the assistant do?
- ☐ **1.** Unpin the restraint and perform range-of-motion exercises.
- ☐ **2.** Unwrap the restraint and bathe the arm using warm water.
- ☐ **3.** Leave the restraint in its current position.
- ☐ **4.** Remove one tape at a time while bathing the child's arm.

31. The nurse is administering prednisone to a child with nephrosis. To assure that the nurse has identified the child correctly, the nurse should do which of the following. Select all that apply.
- ☐ **1.** Ask another nurse to confirm that this is the correct dose and correct client for whom the prednisone has been prescribed.
- ☐ **2.** Check the child's identification band against the medical record number.
- ☐ **3.** Verify the date of birth from the medical record with the date of birth on the client's identification band.
- ☐ **4.** Compare the room number on the bed with the number on the client's identification band.
- ☐ **5.** Ask the client to state his first name.

32. The nurse is administering propranolol (Inderal) to a client for control of migraine headaches. The client's pulse rate is 56 bpm. What should the nurse do next?
- ☐ **1.** Contact the physician immediately.
- ☐ **2.** Assess blood pressure.
- ☐ **3.** Administer oxygen.
- ☐ **4.** Ask for a relative to contact.

33. When a child is able to grasp the idea that a ball continues to exist even though his parent placed the ball under a hat, the child is in which of the following stages in the development of logical thinking, according to Piaget?
- ☐ **1.** Sensorimotor.
- ☐ **2.** Preoperational.
- ☐ **3.** Concrete operations.
- ☐ **4.** Formal operations.

34. A nurse discusses with parents the procedures that will be performed on their neonate immediately after delivery. The nurse determines that the instructions have been understood when the client states that what will be done to the neonate first?
- ☐ **1.** The neonate will be suctioned.
- ☐ **2.** The neonate will be dried and stimulated to cry.
- ☐ **3.** The neonate will be given oxygen.
- ☐ **4.** The neonate's umbilical cord will be cut.

35. An infusion of lidocaine hydrochloride (Xylocaine) is running at 30 ml/hour. The dilution is 1,000 mg/250 ml. What dosage is the client receiving per minute?

_____ mg/minute

36. A nurse is instructing a client about the use of nitroglycerin patches. The nurse should instruct the client to:
- ☐ **1.** Remove the patch every night.
- ☐ **2.** Use the patch only when chest pain occurs.
- ☐ **3.** Change the site of the patch every day.
- ☐ **4.** Apply the patch only on alternate days.

37. The nursing staff has safely and successfully secluded and restrained a client with acute mania who threatened the nurse and threw a chair against the wall in the community room. Which statement by the nurse is most helpful to the client at this time?
- ☐ **1.** "Threatening others and throwing furniture is not allowed."
- ☐ **2.** "You have been restrained until you can manage your behavior."
- ☐ **3.** "Since you have been here before, you know what the rules are."
- ☐ **4.** "We are only doing this for your own good, so calm down."

38. A client is taking 600 mg of valproic acid (Depakene) twice daily. Which adverse effect is least associated with valproic acid?
- ☐ **1.** Tremors.
- ☐ **2.** Hair loss.
- ☐ **3.** Gastrointestinal upset.
- ☐ **4.** Anorexia.

39. A client has a cerclage placed at 16 weeks' gestation. She has had no contractions and her cervix is dilated 2 centimeters. The nurse is preparing the client for discharge. Which statement by the client should indicate to the nurse that the client needs further instruction?

☐ **1.** "I will need more frequent prenatal visits."
☐ **2.** "I should call if I am leaking fluid or have bleeding or contractions."
☐ **3.** "I can have sex again in about 2 weeks."
☐ **4.** "I can have nothing in my vagina until I am at term."

40. Calculate the I.V. infusion rate in milliliters per hour for a 70-kg client requiring 50 mcg/minute of nitroglycerin (Tridil), using a nitroglycerin dilution of 50 mg in 250 ml of dextrose 5% in water.

_____ ml/hour

41. Which of the following conditions is a potential consequence of a prolonged QT interval?

☐ **1.** Serious electrolyte imbalance.
☐ **2.** Predisposition to torsades de pointes.
☐ **3.** Predisposition to atrial fibrillation.
☐ **4.** Development of orthostatic hypotension.

42. A client is taking nonsteroidal anti-inflammatory drugs (NSAIDs) to manage pain from rheumatoid arthritis. What instruction should the nurse give the client about NSAIDs?

☐ **1.** Take the prescribed medication with food and fluids.
☐ **2.** Gradually decrease the medication dosage.
☐ **3.** Rinse the mouth with water after taking NSAIDs.
☐ **4.** Avoid driving and using machinery while taking NSAIDs.

43. The nurse is assessing a neonate at 5 minutes after birth. The nurse records the Apgar score based on the findings in the chart below.

FLOW SHEETS

APGAR AT 5 MINUTES AFTER BIRTH

Heart rate	100 bpm
Respirations	Irregular
Color	Pink
Muscle tone	Moving all four extremities
Reflexes	Cough

The nurse compares these findings to the Apgar score obtained at birth, as determined by the findings in the chart below.

FLOW SHEETS

APGAR AT BIRTH

Heart rate	120 bpm
Respirations	Slow
Color	Blue extremities
Muscle tone	Flexion of extremities
Reflexes	Grimace

What should the nurse do next?

☐ **1.** Notify the neonatologist on call.
☐ **2.** Continue to assess the neonate.
☐ **3.** Apply an oxygen mask.
☐ **4.** Rub the neonate's extremities.

44. Communicating with parents and children about health care has become increasingly significant because:

☐ **1.** Consumers of health care cannot keep up with rapid advances in science.
☐ **2.** The influence of the media and specialization have increased the complexity of managing health.
☐ **3.** Nurse educators have recognized the value of communication.
☐ **4.** Clients are more demanding that their rights be respected.

45. The most appropriate toys to give to a 5-month-old infant are:
- ☐ **1.** Plastic toy cars.
- ☐ **2.** Wooden puzzles.
- ☐ **3.** Stuffed animals.
- ☐ **4.** Soft, washable toys.

46. The nurse is beginning the shift and is assessing the oxygen exchange on a neonate. The nurse reviews the chart for pulse oximetry reading for the last 8 hours.

FLOW SHEETS

PULSE OXIMETRY

Time	7 am	9 am	11 am	1 pm	3 pm
Reading	95%	90%	90%	85%	80%

The pulse oximetry reading at 3:30 p.m. is 75%. What should the nurse do first?
- ☐ **1.** Administer oxygen via mask.
- ☐ **2.** Swaddle the neonate in heated blankets.
- ☐ **3.** Reassess the oximetry reading in 30 minutes.
- ☐ **4.** Draw blood gases for oxygen and carbon dioxide levels.

47. The nurse reviews the client's laboratory report to determine the client's blood level of valproic acid (Depakene), which is 35 mcg/ml. Based on this report, what should the nurse do first?
- ☐ **1.** Withhold the next dose of valproic acid.
- ☐ **2.** Notify the physician.
- ☐ **3.** Give the next dose as ordered.
- ☐ **4.** Take the client's vital signs.

48. After 2 days on a psychiatric unit, a client is still isolating himself in his room, except for meals. The client says he is uncomfortable around crowds of people. Which nursing intervention is the most appropriate initially?
- ☐ **1.** Play a game of checkers with the client in his room.
- ☐ **2.** Ask the client to attend a group session with the nurse.
- ☐ **3.** Invite the client to go for a walk with the nurse and one other client.
- ☐ **4.** Talk with the client in a corner of the crafts room.

49. A nurse is caring for a woman who delivered a term neonate at 6 a.m. At 4 p.m., the woman has a distended bladder and is reporting pain of 5 on a scale of 1 to 10. The nurse reviews the client's output record.

INTAKE AND OUTPUT

OUTPUT RECORD

Time	8 am	10 am	11 am	4 pm
	30 ml	50 ml	30 ml	60 ml

What should the nurse do first?
- ☐ **1.** Apply a warm, moist towel over the bladder.
- ☐ **2.** Ask the woman to sit on the toilet while the nurse runs water from the faucet.
- ☐ **3.** Administer Tylenol with codeine.
- ☐ **4.** Use an in-and-out catheter to empty the bladder.

50. A client who tested positive for group B streptococcus has an order for 2 g of ampicillin I.V. in 100 ml of normal saline solution to be administered over 20 minutes. The nurse should set the infusion to run at how many drops per minute using tubing that delivers 10 gtt/minute?

_____ gtt/minute

51. The father of a 3-week-old infant who has developed sepsis says that he feels guilty because he did not realize his infant was sick. Which of the following responses by the nurse would be *most* appropriate?
- ☐ **1.** "You should have realized something was wrong; he is your son."
- ☐ **2.** "Did you read the booklet on newborns that was sent home with you from the hospital?"
- ☐ **3.** "What you are feeling is normal; next time, you will know what to look for."
- ☐ **4.** "Babies can get sick quickly, and parents do not always realize it."

52. A mother brings a 15-month-old child to the well-baby clinic. She states the child has been taking approximately 18 to 20 oz of whole milk per day from a bottle with meals and at bedtime. The nurse should suggest that she begin weaning the child from the bottle to avoid risking:
- ☐ **1.** Malnutrition.
- ☐ **2.** Anemia.
- ☐ **3.** Dental caries.
- ☐ **4.** Malocclusion.

53. The physician orders 20 units of oxytocin (Pitocin) I.V. in 1,000 ml of normal saline solution to run at 600 ml/hour. How many drops per minute should the nurse set for the infusion rate for tubing that delivers 10 gtt/minute?

_____ gtt/minute

54. Diuretic therapy with torsemide (Demadex) is started for a client with heart failure. When calling the client 2 days after the drug therapy is started, the nurse evaluates the torsemide as effective when the client says she has experienced which of the following outcomes?
- ☐ **1.** She has an improved appetite and is eating better.
- ☐ **2.** She weighs 6 pounds less than she did 2 days ago.
- ☐ **3.** She is less thirsty than she was before the drug therapy.
- ☐ **4.** She has clearer urine since starting torsemide.

55. Which of the following techniques is correct for the nurse to use when inserting a rectal suppository for an adult client?
- ☐ **1.** Insert the suppository while the client bears down.
- ☐ **2.** Place the client in a supine position.
- ☐ **3.** Position the suppository along the rectal wall.
- ☐ **4.** Insert the suppository 2 inches into the rectum.

56. A client receiving digoxin (Lanoxin) for heart failure undergoes cardiac catheterization to evaluate his condition further. The procedure reveals a cardiac output of 2.2 L/minute. How should the nurse evaluate this cardiac output?
- ☐ **1.** High, because of the effects of digoxin.
- ☐ **2.** Within normal limits, because of the effects of digoxin.
- ☐ **3.** Within normal limits, but not adequate to support strenuous activity.
- ☐ **4.** Low, requiring further medical intervention.

57. A young woman is brought from the emergency department (ED) to the psychiatric unit. ED staff report that she is not answering questions and has been sitting in the same position in the wheelchair for 45 minutes. When her arm was extended to draw blood, she did not move her arm back to a natural position. The client's brother says he found her this way yesterday and couldn't get her to move on her own. Which nursing interventions have a high priority in this case? Select all that apply.
- ☐ **1.** Ask her to describe her stressors.
- ☐ **2.** Monitor her body positions to prevent injury.
- ☐ **3.** Offer her nutritional shakes every 3 hours.
- ☐ **4.** Encourage her to talk about her feelings.
- ☐ **5.** Assist her to the bathroom every 2 hours.
- ☐ **6.** Protect her from intrusions by other clients.

58. A client who had a total hip placement at 9 a.m. is receiving an autologous blood transfusion that was started at 11 a.m. At the change of shift (3 p.m.), the day nurse reports that there is 50 ml of the unit of blood remaining to be infused. Which of the following is a priority action for the evening nurse?
- ☐ **1.** Keep the blood transfusing at the same rate.
- ☐ **2.** Increase the rate so it will infuse by 4 p.m.
- ☐ **3.** Discontinue the blood transfusion at the beginning of the shift.
- ☐ **4.** Maintain the current rate and discontinue the blood transfusion at 5 p.m.

59. A client is admitted with fatigue, shortness of breath, pale skin, and dried, cracked lips, tongue, and mouth. Her hemoglobin is 9 g/dl and red blood cell count is 3.5 million cells/mm³. Which of the following foods should the nurse teach this client to include in her diet?
- ☐ **1.** Beef, beets, and cabbage.
- ☐ **2.** Lamb, applesauce, and mint jelly.
- ☐ **3.** Chicken, dumplings, and biscuits.
- ☐ **4.** Fish, wine, and apples.

60. A nurse is preparing to administer 13 mg of gentamicin sulfate (Garamycin) every 36 hours to a neonate who is 5 hours old and weighs 7 lb (3.2 kg). The pharmacy sends 20 mg/2 ml of gentamicin. How many milliliters should the nurse administer?

_____ ml

61. When assessing a neonate 1 hour after birth, the nurse observes that the neonate exhibits slight cyanosis when quiet but becomes pink when crying. The nurse is unable to pass a catheter through the left nostril. The nurse notifies the pediatrician because the neonate most likely is exhibiting signs and symptoms of which of the following?
- ☐ **1.** Esophageal reflux disorder.
- ☐ **2.** Unilateral choanal atresia.
- ☐ **3.** Respiratory distress syndrome.
- ☐ **4.** Tracheoesophageal fistula.

62. When teaching parents of toddlers about poisonous substances, the nurse should emphasize which of the following safety points? Select all that apply.
- ☐ **1.** Toddlers should be adequately supervised at all times.
- ☐ **2.** All poisonous substances should be kept out of the reach of children and stored in a locked cabinet if necessary.
- ☐ **3.** The difference between pediatric and adult dosages of medicines is significant and adult dosages given to children can have serious, harmful effects.
- ☐ **4.** Syrup of ipecac should be administered following all ingestions of poisonous substances.
- ☐ **5.** Following any poisoning, the parents should call the Poison Control Center for instructions for appropriate treatment.

63. A client on a psychiatric care unit approaches the nurse and complains of muscle spasms in his neck, stiffness in other muscles, and that his eyes are rolling upward. The client had two p.r.n. doses of haloperidol (Haldol) in the last 6 hours. What should the nurse administer?
- ☐ **1.** Lorazepam (Ativan) I.M.
- ☐ **2.** Amantadine (Symmetrel) P.O.
- ☐ **3.** Diphenhydramine (Benadryl) P.O.
- ☐ **4.** Benztropine (Cogentin) I.M.

64. After delivery of a male neonate at 38 weeks' gestation, the nurse dries the neonate and places him under the radiant warmer. The nurse performs this action based on the understanding that one neonatal response to cold stress involves which of the following?
- ☐ **1.** Metabolism of brown adipose tissue.
- ☐ **2.** Decreased utilization of glycogen stores.
- ☐ **3.** Decreased utilization of calorie stores.
- ☐ **4.** Increased shivering to keep warm.

65. When developing the teaching plan for a primiparous client who is bottle-feeding her term neonate for the first feeding, which of the following instructions should the nurse expect to include?
- ☐ **1.** Fill the entire nipple of the bottle with formula.
- ☐ **2.** All term babies have well-developed sucking skills.
- ☐ **3.** Bubble the baby after 2 oz of formula have been taken.
- ☐ **4.** Propping of the bottle results in too much air being taken in by the baby.

66. A client complains of back pain 10 minutes after a unit of packed red blood cells (RBCs) was started. The client's pulse, blood pressure, and respirations are stable, and similar to vital signs obtained before infusing the RBCs. What should the nurse do? Select all that apply.
- ☐ **1.** Turn off the infusion of the packed RBCs.
- ☐ **2.** Flush the Y-tubing with normal saline to clear the line.
- ☐ **3.** Insert an indwelling urinary catheter.
- ☐ **4.** Prepare for cardiopulmonary resuscitation.
- ☐ **5.** Obtain a urine specimen to send to the laboratory.

67. A primiparous client at 4 hours after a vaginal delivery and manual removal of the placenta voids for the first time. The nurse palpates the fundus, noting it to be 1 cm above the umbilicus, slightly firm, and deviated to the left side, and notes a moderate amount of lochia rubra. The nurse notifies the physician based on the interpretation that the assessment indicates which of the following?
- ☐ **1.** Perineal lacerations.
- ☐ **2.** Retained placental fragments.
- ☐ **3.** Cervical lacerations.
- ☐ **4.** Urine retention.

68. While performing a gestational age assessment for a newly delivered male neonate who was delivered vaginally at 37 weeks' gestation, which of the following should the nurse expect to find?
- ☐ **1.** An anterior transverse crease on the soles.
- ☐ **2.** Extensive rugae on the scrotum.
- ☐ **3.** Some cartilage in the ear lobes.
- ☐ **4.** Coarse and silky scalp hair.

69. Two family members are visiting their father who is experiencing acute delirium. They are upset that their father is so disoriented. "He knows who we are, but that's about it. We don't know what to say to him." What should the nurse tell the family? Select all that apply.
- ☐ **1.** "Answer his questions simply, honestly, slowly, and clearly."
- ☐ **2.** "Correct him when he is hearing and seeing things that are not there."
- ☐ **3.** "Occasionally remind him of the time, day, and place when he doesn't remember."
- ☐ **4.** "Include him in your conversation, instead of talking about him while he is present."
- ☐ **5.** "Raise your voice a bit so you are sure he hears you."

70. A 26-year-old male client is being admitted for treatment of delirium due to acute alcohol intoxication. The client is restless, does not want to stay seated, and has a staggering gait. What should the nurse do?
- ☐ **1.** Place the client in a chair with a waist restraint.
- ☐ **2.** Provide one-to-one supervision of the client until detoxification treatment can begin.
- ☐ **3.** Ask the client to sit in a chair next to the nurses' station.
- ☐ **4.** Decrease stimuli by putting the client in bed with his room door closed.

71. The nurse is monitoring a client receiving a blood transfusion when the client develops a cough with shortness of breath. The client also complains of a headache and a racing heart. What should the nurse do first?
- ☐ **1.** Slow the infusion rate.
- ☐ **2.** Replace the blood with saline.
- ☐ **3.** Administer an antihistamine.
- ☐ **4.** Place the client flat with the feet elevated.

72. A nurse is obtaining an ankle-brachial index for a client with arteriosclerosis. Identify the correct order for obtaining the ankle-brachial index.

1.	Place a Doppler probe at a 45-degree angle to the correct pulse (dorsalis pedis or posterior tibial).

2.	Place the client in the supine position.

3.	Record the highest systolic blood pressure readings in both arms.

4.	Record the ankle systolic blood pressure reading when the Doppler sound returns.

73. A nurse is analyzing a client's intake and output. The client has a temperature of 102° F (38.9° C) and is receiving I.V. fluid therapy because of his nothing-by-mouth status due to acute pancreatitis. Before planning nursing actions, the nurse should first consider which of the following details?
☐ **1.** The client's body mass index.
☐ **2.** Insensible fluid loss through the lungs and skin.
☐ **3.** When the client last ate.
☐ **4.** The number of bags of I.V. fluid for the client.

74. Two toddlers are arguing over a toy in the playroom. The nurse should say to the children:
☐ **1.** "If you can't play together, I'll have to put you back in your rooms."
☐ **2.** "Give the toy to me. Now neither of you will have it."
☐ **3.** "Let me see if I can get both of you a similar toy."
☐ **4.** "Let one of you play with it for awhile, then give it to the other."

75. A 4-year-old child continues to come to the nurses' station after being told children are not allowed there. What need is the child's behavior exhibiting?
☐ **1.** Attention-seeking behavior.
☐ **2.** Aggressive behavior.
☐ **3.** Resistive behavior.
☐ **4.** Exaggerated stress behavior.

76. A 5-month-old infant is brought to the emergency department with vomiting and diarrhea, which the mother states started 3 days ago. Which of the following are signs of dehydration in a child who has had vomiting and diarrhea for 3 days? Select all that apply.
☐ **1.** Decreased or absent tearing.
☐ **2.** Dry mucous membranes.
☐ **3.** Sunken fontanel.
☐ **4.** Clear, pale yellow urine.
☐ **5.** Bounding pulse.

77. A neonate of a primiparous client delivered at 36 weeks' gestation in a small, rural hospital is to be transferred by ambulance to a level III nursery. To prepare the parents for the transfer, which of the following should the nurse include in the plan of care?
☐ **1.** Instruct the parents that the neonate is in critical condition.
☐ **2.** Obtain the mother's consent for the neonate's transfer.
☐ **3.** Allow the parents to touch the neonate before transfer.
☐ **4.** Ask the father if he desires to ride in the ambulance during the transfer.

78. A multiparous client delivers a neonate at 24 weeks' gestation. After 12 hours, the neonate's condition deteriorates, and death appears likely within the next few minutes. The parents are Roman Catholic, and they request that the neonate be baptized. Which of the following actions would be most appropriate?
☐ **1.** Contact the hospital chaplain to perform the baptism.
☐ **2.** Alert the hospital's director that a neonatal death is imminent.
☐ **3.** Find a health care provider who is Roman Catholic to perform the baptism.
☐ **4.** Baptize the neonate, regardless of the nurse's own religious beliefs.

79. A client has bursitis in the subacromial bursa. A nurse determines that the client understands teaching when he makes which of the following statements?
☐ **1.** "I will apply moist heat to my shoulder for 20 minutes three times each day."
☐ **2.** "I will lift 30-pound weights at least three times each day."
☐ **3.** "I will apply dry ice to my shoulder for 20 minutes three times each day."
☐ **4.** "I will perform 360-degree circles with my arms extended at least three times daily."

80. A client has just undergone a lumbar puncture. Which finding should the nurse immediately report to the physician?
- ☐ **1.** The client's oral intake was 1,200 ml in the past 8 hours.
- ☐ **2.** The client required analgesia for headache.
- ☐ **3.** A moderate amount of serous fluid was noted on the lumbar dressing.
- ☐ **4.** The client is concerned about the test results.

81. A hospice nurse is caring for a client with breast cancer and brain metastasis. The nurse is reviewing the lab report below. According to the information in the chart, what should the nurse do next?

LABORATORY RESULTS

Test	Result
Potassium	4.0 mEq/L
Sodium	142 mEq/L
Chloride	100 mEq/L
Calcium	12.4 mg/dl

- ☐ **1.** Document these results on the medical record.
- ☐ **2.** Report the elevated potassium level immediately.
- ☐ **3.** Report the elevated calcium level immediately.
- ☐ **4.** Refrain from reporting the results because the client is in hospice care.

82. The nurse on the postpartum unit has delegated the care of a multiparous client and her term neonate at 4 hours postpartum to the licensed practical nurse (LPN). Which of the following findings should the LPN report to the nurse immediately?
- ☐ **1.** Neonatal regurgitation of 1 tablespoon after a feeding.
- ☐ **2.** Maternal pulse rate of 100 bpm at rest.
- ☐ **3.** Neonatal heart rate of 140 bpm while at rest.
- ☐ **4.** Increased maternal lochia rubra with initial ambulation.

83. The squatting position is commonly assumed by a child with a cardiac defect because it:
- ☐ **1.** Increases venous return.
- ☐ **2.** Decreases venous return.
- ☐ **3.** Relieves abdominal pressure.
- ☐ **4.** Increases muscle tone.

84. An I.V. infusion of 1,000 ml is to run over 20 hours. How many drops per minute would there be using a macrodrip with 10 gtt/ml?

_____ gtt/minute

85. The physician orders 100 ml of dextrose 5% in water to be administered to a child in 1 hour. The solution is to be infused by microdrip. The nurse should adjust the rate to deliver how many drops per minute?

_____ gtt/minute

86. A client was brought to the emergency department following a motor vehicle accident. The physician determines that there is phrenic nerve involvement. The nurse should anticipate which of the following conditions and plan accordingly?
- ☐ **1.** Alteration in level of consciousness.
- ☐ **2.** Altered cardiac functioning.
- ☐ **3.** Ineffective breathing pattern.
- ☐ **4.** Alteration in urinary elimination.

87. A client with a peritonsillar abscess has been hospitalized. Upon assessment, the nurse determines the following: a temperature of 103° F (39.4° C), body chills, and leukocytosis. The client begins to complain of difficulty breathing. In what order should the nurse perform the following actions?

1. Call the physician.
2. Open the airway.
3. Start an I.V. access site.
4. Explain the situation to the family.

88. The nurse is teaching a client who has deep vein thrombosis from limited mobility that caused a pulmonary embolus, which has resolved. Which of the following instructions should nurse give to this client?
- ☐ **1.** "Report such signs as leg swelling, discomfort, redness, or warmth."
- ☐ **2.** "Sit with your legs lower than the rest of your body."
- ☐ **3.** "Walk at least every other day."
- ☐ **4.** "Limit your fluids to 1 liter each day."

89. A multiparous client and her neonate, who has been cared for in the intensive care nursery for the past 3 days because of being small for gestational age, are to be discharged. Before their release, the mother tells the nurse, "I've been living in my car for the past 2 weeks." Which of the following should the nurse do next?

☐ **1.** Notify the director of the birthing unit.
☐ **2.** Contact the hospital's social worker.
☐ **3.** Contact the client's physician.
☐ **4.** Notify the client's family members.

90. A nurse is assessing a client who is having her 14th laser surgery for removal of a birthmark from her left cheek. The nurse should ask this client about which food allergy associated with a surgery risk given the circumstance of multiple surgeries?

☐ **1.** Canned peas.
☐ **2.** Frozen carrots.
☐ **3.** Tomatoes.
☐ **4.** Organ meats.

91. The nurse is assessing a teenage girl. According to the figure below, the nurse should note that the girl has:

☐ **1.** Kyphosis.
☐ **2.** Arthritis.
☐ **3.** Developmental dysplasia of the hip.
☐ **4.** Scoliosis.

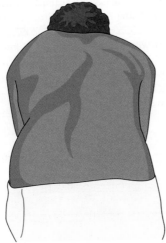

92. A client in surgery has an endotracheal tube (ET) in place. The nurse should call a time-out if which of the following requirements is not in place? Select all that apply.

☐ **1.** An identification band.
☐ **2.** Postoperative pain medication.
☐ **3.** An I.V. line.
☐ **4.** Oxygen administration.
☐ **5.** An anesthesiologist.

93. A multiparous client at 16 weeks' gestation is diagnosed as having a fetus with probable anencephaly. The client is a devout Baptist and has decided to continue the pregnancy and donate the neonatal organs after the death of the neonate. Which of the following actions by the nurse would be most appropriate?

☐ **1.** Explore his or her own feelings about the issues of anencephaly and organ donation.
☐ **2.** Contact the client's minister to discuss the client's options related to the pregnancy.
☐ **3.** Advise the client that the prolonged neonatal death will be very painful for her.
☐ **4.** Ask the client if she has discussed this with her family.

94. A 3-month-old infant is being discharged on digoxin (Lanoxin). The nurse should instruct the parents to report which of the following? Select all that apply.

☐ **1.** Signs of constipation or painful straining.
☐ **2.** Decrease in the amount of infant formula taken or a refusal to take it.
☐ **3.** Pulse rate greater than 140 bpm or less than 100 bpm.
☐ **4.** Signs that the infant is not following moving objects.
☐ **5.** Sudden vomiting or sudden drowsiness.

95. The nurse receives a report of a serum potassium level on an infant of 6.0 mEq/L. The nurse should:

☐ **1.** Notify the physician of the abnormal level.
☐ **2.** Call the laboratory to see how the specimen was obtained.
☐ **3.** Connect the infant to a cardiac monitor.
☐ **4.** Check the infant's last 24-hour output.

96. A client with suicidal thoughts is admitted to an adult inpatient behavioral health unit. What should the nurse do first?

☐ **1.** Initiate suicide precautions with face-to-face observation of the client at all times.
☐ **2.** Place the client on suicide watch and have a family member remain with the client.
☐ **3.** Question the client further about his suicidal thoughts and plans.
☐ **4.** Confine the client to his room and post a staff member at the door to observe his actions.

97. A nurse is planning care for a regressed, chronically ill client diagnosed with schizophrenia. What is the most appropriate milieu?
- [ ] 1. Confrontation and peer pressure to break down the client's denial.
- [ ] 2. Reminder that all clients must participate fully in unit self-governance.
- [ ] 3. Required attendance at group activities with equal participation from all clients.
- [ ] 4. Nurturance and supportive interaction focusing on individual needs.

98. Assessment of a primigravid client in active labor reveals cervical dilation at 9 cm with complete effacement and the fetus at +1 station. Which of the following should the nurse do when the physician orders meperidine (Demerol) 50 mg I.M. for the client?
- [ ] 1. Administer the medication in the left ventrogluteal muscle.
- [ ] 2. Be certain that naloxone (Narcan) is at the client's bedside.
- [ ] 3. Ask the physician to validate the dosage of the drug.
- [ ] 4. Refuse to administer the medication to the client.

99. A client has been hospitalized with a diagnosis of myasthenia gravis. A friend is visiting the client during lunch. The nurse enters the room after the client recovered from choking on lunch. What should the nurse do next?
- [ ] 1. Instruct the client to sit at a 30-degree angle in bed when eating.
- [ ] 2. Tell the client to swallow when her chin is tipped down on her chest.
- [ ] 3. Remind the client to rest after eating.
- [ ] 4. Encourage the client to eat alone.

100. A nurse is assessing a client with a brain injury. What is a client's cerebral perfusion pressure (CPP) when the blood pressure (BP) is 90/50 mm Hg and the intracranial pressure (ICP) is 21?

_____ mm Hg

101. A client with a T2-to-T3 spinal cord injury suddenly complains of a throbbing headache and blurred vision. The nurse assesses that he is flushed and sweating on his upper trunk and face, and the hairs on his arms are raised. What should the nurse do first?
- [ ] 1. Raise the head of the bed.
- [ ] 2. Assess for hypotension.
- [ ] 3. Check the client for a distended bladder.
- [ ] 4. Logroll the client to see if he is lying on a foreign object.

102. A 17-year-old unmarried primigravida client at 10 weeks' gestation tells the nurse that her family doesn't have much money and her dad just got laid off from his job. Which of the following would be the nurse's most appropriate action?
- [ ] 1. Instruct the client in methods for low-cost, highly nutritious meal preparation.
- [ ] 2. Determine whether the client qualifies for state assistance programs.
- [ ] 3. Refer the client to a social worker for enrollment in the Women, Infants, and Children (WIC) program.
- [ ] 4. Ask the client if she has a job and the amount of income earned.

103. A client has impairments in immediate recall and short-term memory. A nurse is planning for the client's daily activities. Which action by the nurse would be most effective?
- [ ] 1. Write out the client's schedule in large print, and show the client where the schedule is placed.
- [ ] 2. Describe each activity and the time of the events at the beginning of the day.
- [ ] 3. Lead the client to each activity if he does not attend on time.
- [ ] 4. Tell the client about each activity 10 minutes before it begins.

104. A 17-year-old male client is being admitted to the adolescent psychiatric unit. He was brought in by the police after beating up two male peers. The client says, "They said I was gay because I had sex with an older neighbor when I was 8 years old. I am not gay!" Which of the following nursing interventions would be appropriate? Select all that apply.
- [ ] 1. Monitor the client's level of anger and potential aggression.
- [ ] 2. Help the client express anger safely.
- [ ] 3. Assist the client in processing his feelings about the sexual abuse.
- [ ] 4. Ask the client if he would like to attend a support group.
- [ ] 5. Discuss the client's attitude about going to jail after discharge.

105. The nurse has been assigned to care for several postpartum clients and their neonates on a birthing unit. Which of the following clients should the nurse assess first?
- [ ] 1. A multiparous client at 48 hours postpartum who is being discharged.
- [ ] 2. A primiparous client at 2 hours postpartum who delivered a term neonate vaginally.
- [ ] 3. A multiparous client at 24 hours postpartum whose infant is in the special care nursery.
- [ ] 4. A primiparous client at 48 hours after cesarean delivery of a term neonate.

106. A client is admitted to the hospital with malaise, headache, and cough followed by fever, chills, dyspnea, chest discomfort, myalgia, anorexia, vomiting, and diarrhea. The physician makes the diagnosis of legionellosis (legionnaires' disease). The client asks, "How did I get this?" Which response by the nurse is the most accurate?

☐ **1.** "The bacteria thrive in warm water environments and are inhaled from contaminated water droplets."

☐ **2.** "You inhaled the bacteria from secondary smoke."

☐ **3.** "As ceiling fans circulate, bacteria are dispersed into the air."

☐ **4.** "You may have swallowed contaminated water."

107. A client is scheduled to undergo an upper GI series. Which of the following instructions should the nurse give the client in preparation for the test? Select all that apply.

☐ **1.** "You will need to take a stool softener before the test to promote evacuation of the barium."

☐ **2.** "Do not eat or drink for 8 hours before the test."

☐ **3.** "You can expect white stools for about 48 hours after the test."

☐ **4.** "You will experience mild stomach pain during the test."

☐ **5.** "It is okay for you to smoke before the test."

108. A client with metastatic cancer of the liver is concerned about his progress. Which of the following nursing interventions is most appropriate?

☐ **1.** Provide information for the client to consider a liver transplantation.

☐ **2.** Assure the client that the prescribed medications will shrink all tumor sites.

☐ **3.** Explain the effects of chemotherapy.

☐ **4.** Place emphasis on providing symptomatic and comfort measures.

109. The nurse must run 250 ml of lactated Ringer's solution and 150 ml of normal saline solution over the next 6 hours. Using a microdrip set (60 gtt/ml), how many drops per minute will be administered?

☐ **1.** 33 gtt/minute.

☐ **2.** 49 gtt/minute.

☐ **3.** 67 gtt/minute.

☐ **4.** 83 gtt/minute.

110. The nurse is to administer meperidine hydrochloride (Demerol) 9 mg I.M. to a client. If the drug is available in a concentration of 25 mg/ml, how much should the client receive?

_____ ml

111. The nurse is preparing to give an I.M. injection. Which of the following sites has the least amount of blood vessels and major nerves located in the area?

☐ **1.** Deltoid.

☐ **2.** Dorsogluteal.

☐ **3.** Vastus lateralis.

☐ **4.** Triceps.

112. The nurse is planning to teach the client how to properly use a metered-dose inhaler to treat asthma. Which of the following instructions should the nurse include in the teaching plan?

☐ **1.** Rinse the mouth after each use of a steroid inhaler.

☐ **2.** Inhale quickly when administering the medication.

☐ **3.** Inhale the medication and then exhale through the nose.

☐ **4.** Cough and deep-breathe before inhaling the medication.

113. A client is receiving a transfusion of packed red blood cells. Which of the following actions should the nurse implement to safely administer the blood?

☐ **1.** Keep the blood refrigerated on the nursing unit until ready to administer.

☐ **2.** Stay with the client during the first 15 minutes to detect signs or symptoms of a reaction.

☐ **3.** Do not infuse blood that has been hanging for more than 6 hours.

☐ **4.** Administer the blood quickly to prevent wasting it if the client develops a fever.

114. A client is receiving a blood transfusion when he begins to complain of difficulty breathing. The nurse notes an elevated blood pressure and a cough. Based on these signs, the nurse suspects which of the following complications?

☐ **1.** Anaphylactic reaction.

☐ **2.** Circulatory overload.

☐ **3.** Sepsis.

☐ **4.** Acute hemolytic reaction.

115. A client has had sucralfate (Carafate) ordered as treatment for peptic ulcer disease. Which of the following statements indicates that the client understands how to take the medication?

☐ **1.** "I should take the Carafate every evening at bedtime."

☐ **2.** "It is important that I take this drug on an empty stomach."

☐ **3.** "I should avoid milk products while taking this drug."

☐ **4.** "I should have my hemoglobin checked monthly while taking Carafate."

116. During the admission interview, an adult client reveals that, as a child, she was sexually abused by her uncle and a male cousin. She reports that when she has flashbacks of this abuse she cuts her arms, legs, and abdomen. In addition to having the client sign a no-harm contract, which nursing intervention is most important?
- ☐ 1. Assist the client with finding safe ways to express her anger.
- ☐ 2. Talk with the client about confronting her uncle and cousin directly.
- ☐ 3. Defer talking about the abuse to prevent further self-mutilation.
- ☐ 4. Discuss the possibility of the client suing her relatives for their abuse.

117. An adult client has bacterial conjunctivitis. What should the nurse teach him to do? Select all that apply.
- ☐ 1. Use warm saline soaks four times per day to remove crusting.
- ☐ 2. Apply topical antibiotic without touching the tip of the tube to his eye.
- ☐ 3. Wash his hands after touching his eyes.
- ☐ 4. Avoid touching his eyes.
- ☐ 5. Observe isolation procedures and confine himself to his bedroom until the redness in the eye disappears.

118. Which of the following actions by the nurse will most likely ensure that the correct client receives a medication? Select all that apply.
- ☐ 1. Have the client state his or her name.
- ☐ 2. Check the name on the arm band with the name on the medication.
- ☐ 3. Learn to recognize the client.
- ☐ 4. Check the client's room number.
- ☐ 5. Compare the date of birth on the client's chart to the date of birth on the client's armband.

119. The nurse is preparing to administer digoxin (Lanoxin) 0.125 mg. Scored 0.25-mg tablets are available. How many tablets should the nurse administer?

_____ tablets

120. A nurse is counseling a mother with young children after the mother left her abusive husband 6 months ago. The mother says, "My 6-year-old, Kevin, is starting to act just like his father. I just don't know how to handle this." Which response by the nurse is most appropriate?
- ☐ 1. "You'll have to limit Kevin's contact with his father."
- ☐ 2. "Counseling for Kevin would be helpful."
- ☐ 3. "Most boys outgrow these behaviors."
- ☐ 4. "Setting limits on his behavior is all you need to do now."

121. A 13-year-old male was kidnapped and held for ransom by two criminals. His parents asked to have him admitted to the adolescent psychiatric unit. He is sleep-deprived, filthy, alternating between sobbing and making threats to kill his captors, suspicious, and easily startled. He signs a no harm contract and then asks to go to sleep. What is the best initial plan for this client?
- ☐ 1. Encourage him to talk with the Federal Bureau of Investigation (FBI) about the crime details.
- ☐ 2. Develop trust and allow him to talk about his memories and feelings.
- ☐ 3. Help him and his parents prepare for the future trial.
- ☐ 4. Discourage him from making threats toward his captors.

122. A 16-year-old primiparous client has decided to place her baby for adoption. The adoptive parents are on their way to the hospital when the mother says, "I want to see the baby one last time." Which of the following should the nurse do?
- ☐ 1. Tell the client that it would be best if she didn't see the baby.
- ☐ 2. Allow the client to see the baby through the nursery window.
- ☐ 3. Contact the physician for advice related to the client's visitation.
- ☐ 4. Allow the client to see and hold the baby for as long as she desires.

123. The nurse received an order to administer atropine 0.1 mg. The drug is available in 0.4 mg/ml. How much should the client receive?
- ☐ 1. 0.125 ml.
- ☐ 2. 0.25 ml.
- ☐ 3. 0.4 ml.
- ☐ 4. 0.5 ml.

124. A 10-year-old child is admitted with a brain tumor. Which assessment made by the nurse is most critical to report to the child's physician?
- ☐ 1. Vomiting after lunch.
- ☐ 2. Difficulty in recalling the day of the week.
- ☐ 3. Blood pressure of 102/62 mm Hg.
- ☐ 4. 100 ml of concentrated urine voided at one voiding.

125. The nurse is teaching a 17-year-old girl who has a severe gonorrheal infection. The nurse realizes that the girl understands the implications of her disease when she tells the nurse:
- ☐ 1. "Once I'm treated, I'll have immunity."
- ☐ 2. "My partner doesn't need treatment."
- ☐ 3. "I won't have any more problems once I learn to protect myself."
- ☐ 4. "I could have trouble getting pregnant."

126. The nurse-manager on the medical unit is teaching the staff about the medication reconciliation policy. The nurse teaches the staff that reconciliation is needed to ensure that clients are on the correct medications in which situations? Select all that apply.
- ☐ **1.** Admission to the hospital.
- ☐ **2.** Transfer to the nursing home.
- ☐ **3.** Transfer of a client from surgery to the surgical unit.
- ☐ **4.** Admission to a home health agency from the hospital.
- ☐ **5.** Move from a double room to a single room on the same unit.

127. A client is admitted with dehydration and oliguria. The physician orders 1,000 ml of 5% dextrose solution I.V. to be infused within an 8-hour period. The I.V. set delivers 15 gtt/ml. The nurse should regulate the flow rate so it delivers how many drops of fluid per minute?

_____ gtt/minute

128. A client was treated for a streptococcal throat infection 2 weeks ago. The client now has been diagnosed with acute poststreptococcal glomerulonephritis. The client asks the nurse how he could have prevented this condition. What should the nurse tell the client?
- ☐ **1.** "See your physician for an early diagnosis and treatment of a sore throat."
- ☐ **2.** "As long as you do not have a fever, it is sufficient to gargle daily with an antibacterial mouthwash."
- ☐ **3.** "You may continue to utilize the previously prescribed antibiotics until they are gone."
- ☐ **4.** "Unscented bar soap may be used in showers."

129. Assessment of a primigravid client in active labor reveals a cervix dilated to 5 cm and completely effaced, with the fetus at –1 station. The client has indicated that she wants a "natural childbirth" with no analgesia or anesthesia. The client's husband has been present since their arrival at the birthing unit. The physician enters the room and tells the client that it is time for an epidural anesthetic. Which of the following would be the nurse's best action at this time?
- ☐ **1.** Ask the client if she desires an epidural anesthetic.
- ☐ **2.** Tell the physician that the client desires a "natural childbirth."
- ☐ **3.** Tell the client that her labor will be more comfortable with an anesthetic.
- ☐ **4.** Ask the client to discuss this with her husband and then make a decision.

130. A client is ready to be discharged from same-day surgery following an inguinal hernia repair. Which criteria must the client meet before the nurse can discharge the client?
- ☐ **1.** The client has transportation home via a taxicab.
- ☐ **2.** The client has pain no greater than 5 on a scale of 1 to 10.
- ☐ **3.** The client can walk to the bathroom by himself.
- ☐ **4.** The client states he will urinate later when he has more fluids.

131. The client is to receive an I.V. infusion at 100 ml/hour. The infusion set delivers 15 gtt/ml. What is the flow rate (in gtt/minute) of the infusion?

_____ gtt/minute

132. Procaine penicillin G 600,000 units I.M. has been ordered. The nurse has available a 1-ml prefilled syringe labeled 600,000 units/ml. How many milliliters should the nurse administer?

_____ ml

133. The nurse is administering eyedrops to a client with glaucoma. Which of the following is a correct technique for instilling the eyedrops? The eyedrops are placed:
- ☐ **1.** In the lower conjunctival sac.
- ☐ **2.** Near the opening of the lacrimal ducts.
- ☐ **3.** On the cornea.
- ☐ **4.** On the scleral surface.

134. A client has an anaphylactic reaction to penicillin that results in respiratory distress. Which of the following medications should the nurse anticipate administering first?
- ☐ **1.** Dopamine (Intropin).
- ☐ **2.** Diphenhydramine (Benadryl).
- ☐ **3.** Cimetidine (Tagamet).
- ☐ **4.** Epinephrine.

135. A client is using an over-the-counter nasal spray containing pseudoephedrine to treat allergic rhinitis. Which instruction about this medication would be most appropriate for the nurse to provide for the client?
- ☐ **1.** Prolonged use of nasal spray can lead to nasal infections.
- ☐ **2.** Pseudoephedrine is an addictive drug and must be used cautiously.
- ☐ **3.** Overuse of pseudoephedrine can lead to increased nasal congestion.
- ☐ **4.** A common side effect of pseudoephedrine nasal spray is thrush.

136. A 6-year-old child is admitted for an appendectomy. What is the most appropriate way for the nurse to prepare the child for surgery?

☐ **1.** Explain how to use a patient-controlled analgesia (PCA) pump for pain control.

☐ **2.** Permit the child to play with the blood pressure cuff, electrocardiogram (ECG) pads, and a face mask.

☐ **3.** Show the child a video about the surgery.

☐ **4.** Show the child a visual analog scale (VAS) based on a scale from 0 to 10.

137. The nurse is working on a hospital's birthing unit when a primigravid client in active labor is ordered to receive meperidine (Demerol) 75 mg I.M. As the nurse enters the medication room, the nurse observes a female coworker slipping a vial of morphine into the side pocket of her uniform. Which of the following actions would be most appropriate?

☐ **1.** Contact the hospital's security chief.

☐ **2.** Notify the supervisor of the unit.

☐ **3.** Tell the coworker of the incident.

☐ **4.** Notify the federal drug agents about the incident.

138. Which of the following medications should the nurse expect to administer to a client who is experiencing an oculogyric crisis?

☐ **1.** Chlorpromazine (Thorazine) 50 mg.

☐ **2.** Procyclidine (Kemadrin) 5 mg.

☐ **3.** Thioridazine (Mellaril) 100 mg.

☐ **4.** Benztropine (Cogentin) 1 mg.

139. Which of the following should the nurse include when teaching the family and a client who was prescribed benztropine (Cogentin), 1 mg P.O. twice daily, about the drug therapy?

☐ **1.** The drug can be used with over-the-counter cough and cold preparations.

☐ **2.** The client should not discontinue taking the drug abruptly.

☐ **3.** Antacids can be used freely when taking this drug.

☐ **4.** Alcohol consumption with benztropine therapy need not be restricted.

140. Which of the following should the nurse include in a teaching plan that addresses the adverse effects of antipsychotic medication?

☐ **1.** Information about all potential adverse effects.

☐ **2.** Research data about rare adverse effects.

☐ **3.** Adverse effects that can be seen or felt.

☐ **4.** Percentages associated with each adverse effect.

141. A client has nephrotic syndrome. To aid in the resolution of the client's edema, the physician orders 25% albumin. In addition to an absence of edema, the nurse should evaluate the client for which expected outcome?

☐ **1.** Crackles in the lung bases.

☐ **2.** Blood pressure elevation.

☐ **3.** Cerebral edema.

☐ **4.** Cool skin temperature in lower extremities.

142. A client has been diagnosed with acute prostatitis. The physician orders 1 g of nafcillin sodium (Unipen) every 4 hours. The pharmacy has 250-mg capsules available. How many capsules should the nurse administer every 4 hours?

_____ capsules

143. A client has polycystic kidney disease. The client asks the nurse, "How did I get these fluid-filled bubbles on my kidneys? I have not had any X-ray type tests." How should the nurse respond to help the client understand risk factors for this disease process?

☐ **1.** "Second-hand smoke puts you at greater risk for developing cysts."

☐ **2.** "Exposure to dyes used to color fruits and vegetables increases the risk of polycystic kidney disease."

☐ **3.** "There is a higher incidence of polycystic kidney disease among blood relatives."

☐ **4.** "Drinking alcohol daily allows the kidneys to develop cysts."

144. A nurse is administering I.V. fluids to a dehydrated client. When administering an I.V. solution of 3% sodium chloride, what should the nurse do? Select all that apply.

☐ **1.** Measure the intake and output.

☐ **2.** Inspect the jugular veins for distention.

☐ **3.** Evaluate the client for neurologic changes.

☐ **4.** Force fluids, especially water.

☐ **5.** Insert an indwelling urinary catheter.

145. The nurse is working on a birthing unit that has several unlicensed assistive personnel (UAP). The nurse expects the UAP assigned to several clients in labor to notify the nurse if the UAP notes which of the following about one of the clients?

☐ **1.** An episode of nausea after administration of an epidural anesthetic.

☐ **2.** Contractions 3 minutes apart and lasting 40 seconds.

☐ **3.** Evidence of spontaneous rupture of the membranes.

☐ **4.** Sleeping after administration of I.V. nalbuphine (Nubain).

146. A 9-year-old child is scheduled for an electromyelogram. To prepare the child for this procedure, what should the nurse do?
- ☐ **1.** Wait until just before the test to tell the child what will be done.
- ☐ **2.** Ask the child to draw a picture of the body structures involved.
- ☐ **3.** Show the child the equipment that will be used in the test.
- ☐ **4.** Verbally explain what will be done during the test.

147. A 10-year-old client with rheumatic fever is on bed rest. Which of the following would be an appropriate diversional activity for the nurse to encourage?
- ☐ **1.** Watching television with his roommate.
- ☐ **2.** Coloring picture books with his brother.
- ☐ **3.** Keeping up with his school work.
- ☐ **4.** Building a bird house.

148. Clients who are receiving total parenteral nutrition (TPN) are at risk for development of which of the following complications?
- ☐ **1.** Hypostatic pneumonia.
- ☐ **2.** Pulmonary hypertension.
- ☐ **3.** Orthostatic hypotension.
- ☐ **4.** Fluid imbalances.

149. The nurse is to administer a bolus starting dose of heparin to a child who is taking penicillin. What should the nurse do? Select all that apply.
- ☐ **1.** Check that the dose is appropriate for the child's weight.
- ☐ **2.** Note that the onset of the medication will be immediate.
- ☐ **3.** Follow the administration of the bolus of heparin with an I.V. infusion of heparin 10 units/kg/hour.
- ☐ **4.** Monitor partial thromboplastin time (PTT).
- ☐ **5.** Discontinue the penicillin until the PTT is at a therapeutic level.

150. The client is receiving propantheline bromide (Pro-Banthine) to treat cholecystitis. The nurse should evaluate the client's response to the medication by observing for which of the following adverse effects?
- ☐ **1.** Urine retention.
- ☐ **2.** Diarrhea.
- ☐ **3.** Hypertension.
- ☐ **4.** Diaphoresis.

151. The nurse is preparing to start an I.V. infusion. Before inserting the needle into a vein, the nurse should apply a tourniquet to the client's arm to accomplish which of the following?
- ☐ **1.** Distend the veins.
- ☐ **2.** Stabilize the veins.
- ☐ **3.** Immobilize the arm.
- ☐ **4.** Occlude arterial circulation.

152. Prochlorperazine (Compazine) is prescribed postoperatively. The nurse should evaluate the drug's therapeutic effect when the client expresses relief from which of the following?
- ☐ **1.** Nausea.
- ☐ **2.** Dizziness.
- ☐ **3.** Abdominal spasms.
- ☐ **4.** Abdominal distention.

153. A 17-year-old client has been admitted to the hospital for a biopsy to confirm the diagnosis of bone cancer. The nurse should assess the client for which conditions? Select all that apply.
- ☐ **1.** Cough.
- ☐ **2.** Dyspnea.
- ☐ **3.** Pain.
- ☐ **4.** Swelling.
- ☐ **5.** Fever.
- ☐ **6.** Anorexia.
- ☐ **7.** Decreased range of motion.

154. A nurse on the labor-and-delivery unit transfers a primiparous client and her term neonate to the mother-baby unit 2 hours after the client delivered the neonate by vaginal delivery. Which of the following information is a priority for the nurse to report to the nurse receiving the client on the mother-baby unit?
- ☐ **1.** Firm fundus when gentle massage is used.
- ☐ **2.** Evidence of bonding well with the neonate.
- ☐ **3.** Labor that lasted 12 hours with a 1-hour second stage.
- ☐ **4.** Temperature of 99° F (37.4° C) and pulse rate of 80 bpm.

155. A client who underwent cardiac surgery 2 days ago is recovering well. His wife, who is assisting with his care, says, "He is doing too much. I told him to let me help, but he won't let me." The nurse says to the wife, "It sounds like you need to feel you can be more helpful to him." What nurse action would be most effective in complementing her words?
- ☐ **1.** Directing her eyes at the client.
- ☐ **2.** Directing her position and eyes at the wife and client.
- ☐ **3.** Avoiding direct eye contact with the client and wife.
- ☐ **4.** Shifting her eyes back and forth between the client and wife.

156. A nurse is having difficulty establishing a relationship with an aggressive client. What strategy will most likely improve the relationship?
- ☐ **1.** The nurse and the client agree to work to improve their involvement in the therapeutic relationship.
- ☐ **2.** The nurse establishes goals for having only positive interactions with the client.
- ☐ **3.** The nurse agrees to be submissive so the client can dominate the relationship.
- ☐ **4.** The nurse seeks assistance from colleagues to become more aware of the quality of the interactions and more sensitive to the dynamics of communication.

157. A nurse is about to conduct a sexual history for a 16-year-old female who is accompanied by her mother. What is an appropriate question for the nurse to ask this client or her mother?
- ☐ **1.** "What do you think about having your mother leave the room now?"
- ☐ **2.** "Mother, do you think your daughter is sexually active?"
- ☐ **3.** "Mother, I am going to ask you to wait a few minutes in the waiting room now so I can complete the health history with your daughter."
- ☐ **4.** "The two of you seem like you share everything. I am going to ask questions about sexual history now."

158. A nurse is admitting an older female client to the gynecology surgical unit. When the nurse asks the client what medication she is taking at home, the client responds that she is taking a little red pill in the morning and a white capsule at night for her blood pressure. What action by the nurse is focused on safe, effective care of this client?
- ☐ **1.** Consult the pharmacist regarding identification of the medications.
- ☐ **2.** Show pictures to the client from the *Physician's Desk Reference* to identify the medications.
- ☐ **3.** Consult the previous medical record from 2 years ago and notify the physician regarding medications that must be ordered.
- ☐ **4.** Ask a family member to bring the medications from home in the original vials for proper identification and administration times.

159. A client who had undergone an abdominal hysterectomy is in the recovery room. The surgeon has ordered a 250-ml bolus of normal saline over 1 hour to replace blood loss. The I.V. solution infusing in the client was 1,000 ml normal saline with 40 mEq of potassium chloride at 100 ml/hour. What actions should the nurse implement? Select all that apply.
- ☐ **1.** Increase the I.V. infusion rate to 250 ml/hour for 1 hour.
- ☐ **2.** Add 250 ml of normal saline to the current infusion bag and continue at 100 ml/hour.
- ☐ **3.** Connect a 250-ml bag of normal saline to the Y-connection and calculate to infuse over 1 hour.
- ☐ **4.** Contact the physician regarding continuation of the primary I.V. infusion during the bolus infusion.
- ☐ **5.** Administer the normal saline bolus via an I.V. infusion pump.

160. The nurse is working in a newborn nursery and caring for several neonates. Precautions that should be taken to prevent an infant abduction include which of the following?
- ☐ **1.** Notifying the hospital's security staff about anyone who appears unusual.
- ☐ **2.** Taking several neonates to their mothers at the same time.
- ☐ **3.** Placing the infant near the doorway of the mother's room.
- ☐ **4.** Contacting the hospital's security staff if an exit alarm is triggered.

161. Clozapine (Clozaril) therapy has been initiated for a client with schizophrenia who has been unresponsive to other antipsychotics. The client states, "Why do I have to have a blood test every week?" Which of the following responses by the nurse would be *most* appropriate?
- ☐ **1.** "Weekly blood tests are necessary to determine safe dosage and to monitor the effect of the medication on the blood."
- ☐ **2.** "Weekly blood tests are done so that you can receive another week's supply of the medication."
- ☐ **3.** "Your physician will want to know how well you are progressing with the medication therapy."
- ☐ **4.** "Everyone taking clozapine (Clozaril) has to go through the same procedure because it is required by the drug company."

162. The nurse administers an intradermal injection to a client. Proper technique has been used if the injection site demonstrates which of the following?
- ☐ **1.** Minimal leaking.
- ☐ **2.** No swelling.
- ☐ **3.** Tissue pallor.
- ☐ **4.** Evidence of a bleb.

163. The client is prescribed ketorolac (Toradol) 15 mg I.M. for pain. The nurse has a 1-ml preloaded syringe of Toradol labeled 30 mg/ml. How many milliliters of the medication should the nurse administer?

_____ ml

164. The sudden onset of which of the following signs or symptoms indicates a potentially serious complication for the client receiving an I.V. infusion?
☐ **1.** Noisy respirations.
☐ **2.** Pupillary constriction.
☐ **3.** Halitosis.
☐ **4.** Moist skin.

165. The nurse is planning to initiate a blood transfusion. Which of the following solutions should the nurse select to prime the tubing when preparing to administer the blood?
☐ **1.** Lactated Ringer's solution.
☐ **2.** Normal saline.
☐ **3.** 5% dextrose in half-normal saline.
☐ **4.** 5% dextrose in water.

166. When preparing to insert an I.V. catheter to administer fluids to a client who is going to surgery, the nurse selects the median cubital vein. Identify the location of the median cubital vein on the illustration below.

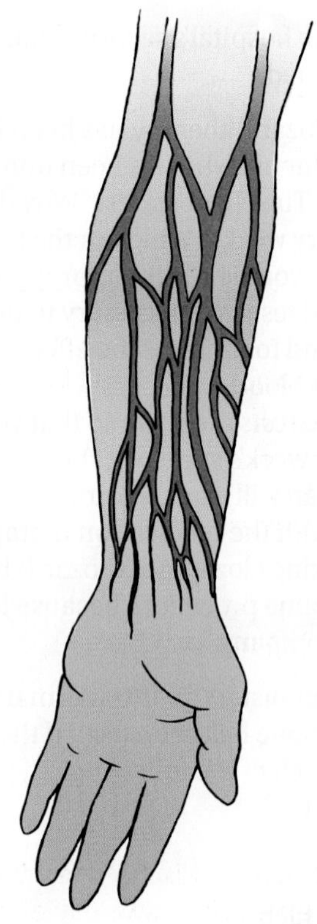

167. The mother of a 28-year-old client who is taking clozapine (Clozaril) states, "Something is wrong. My son is drooling like a baby." Which of the following responses by the nurse would be *most* helpful?
☐ **1.** "I wonder if he's having an adverse reaction to the medicine."
☐ **2.** "Excess saliva is common with this drug; here's a paper cup for him to spit into."
☐ **3.** "Don't worry about it; this is only a minor inconvenience compared to its benefits."
☐ **4.** "I've seen this happen to other clients who are taking Clozaril."

168. A client taking clozapine (Clozaril) states, "I think I'm getting the flu. I have a fever and feel weak." Which of the following should the nurse do *next*?
☐ **1.** Tell the client to wait another day to see if other symptoms of the flu appear.
☐ **2.** Advise the client to take over-the-counter medication for the flu.
☐ **3.** Discuss the importance of maintaining an adequate fluid intake.
☐ **4.** Report the client's symptoms to the physician after taking the client's temperature.

169. Which of the following medications should the nurse anticipate administering in the event of a heparin overdose?
☐ **1.** Warfarin sodium (Coumadin).
☐ **2.** Protamine sulfate.
☐ **3.** Acetylsalicylic acid (ASA).
☐ **4.** Atropine sulfate.

170. Chloral hydrate 1,000 mg has been ordered. It is available in a syrup containing 0.5 g/5 ml. How many milliliters should the nurse give?

_____ ml

171. The client is supposed to receive 500 ml of 5% dextrose in half-normal saline with 20 mEq of potassium chloride over the next 6 hours. The infusion set administers 10 gtt/ml. To what flow rate should the nurse adjust the I.V. flow? Round to the nearest whole number.

_____ gtt/minute

172. What is the primary purpose of administering aminophylline to a client with emphysema?
☐ **1.** To relieve spasms of the diaphragm.
☐ **2.** To relax smooth muscles in the bronchioles.
☐ **3.** To promote efficient pulmonary circulation.
☐ **4.** To stimulate the medullary respiratory center.

173. The nurse is conducting health assessments for school-age children. A characteristic behavior of a 7-year-old girl is that she:
☐ **1.** Likes to play only with other girls.
☐ **2.** Prefers to play with her sister.
☐ **3.** Prefers to play team games.
☐ **4.** Likes to play alone.

174. A nurse is planning care for a 7-year-old who is hospitalized for a hernia repair. Which of the following fears is the most common fear for this type of client?
☐ **1.** Separation from parents.
☐ **2.** Trying something new.
☐ **3.** Injury and pain.
☐ **4.** Opposite-sex relationships.

175. Before inserting a nasogastric (NG) tube in an adult client, the nurse estimates the length of tubing to insert. Identify the point on the illustration below where the nurse would end the measurement.

176. A woman who delivered a healthy baby 6 hours ago tells the nurse that she is having cramps in her legs. Upon further assessment, the nurse identifies leg pain on dorsiflexion. The nurse should:
☐ **1.** Tell the woman to massage the area.
☐ **2.** Apply warm compresses to the area.
☐ **3.** Instruct the woman on how to do ankle pumps.
☐ **4.** Notify the physician.

177. The nurse interprets the rhythm strip below from a client's bedside monitor as which of the following?
☐ **1.** Normal sinus rhythm.
☐ **2.** Sinus tachycardia.
☐ **3.** Ventricular tachycardia.
☐ **4.** Ventricular fibrillation.

178. A young adult is hospitalized with a seizure disorder. The client, who is in a bed with padded side rails, has a tonic-clonic seizure. In what order should the nurse take the following actions?

| **1.** Loosen clothing around the client's neck. |
| **2.** Turn the client on his or her side. |
| **3.** Clear the area around the client. |
| **4.** Suction the airway. |

| |
| |
| |
| |

179. The nurse interprets the rhythm strip below from a client's bedside monitor as which of the following?
☐ **1.** Normal sinus rhythm.
☐ **2.** Sinus tachycardia.
☐ **3.** Atrial fibrillation.
☐ **4.** Ventricular tachycardia.

180. An older woman has a history of a left radical mastectomy and now presents with a swollen left arm. The nurse understands that it is appropriate to:
☐ **1.** Take the blood pressure only in the unaffected arm.
☐ **2.** Start an I.V. line in the affected arm.
☐ **3.** Encourage a dependent position of the affected arm.
☐ **4.** Allow blood draws in the affected arm.

181. A 36-month-old child weighing 44 pounds is to receive ceftriaxone (Rocephin) 2 g I.V. every 12 hours. The recommended dose of Rocephin is 50 to 75 mg/kg/day in divided doses. The nurse should:
- [ ] **1.** Administer the medication as ordered.
- [ ] **2.** Administer half the ordered dose.
- [ ] **3.** Call the laboratory to check the therapeutic serum level of Rocephin.
- [ ] **4.** Withhold administering the Rocephin and notify the child's physician.

182. The nurse has provided an in-service presentation to ancillary staff about standard precautions on the birthing unit. The nurse determines that one of the staff members needs further instructions when the nurse observes which of the following?
- [ ] **1.** Use of protective goggles during a cesarean delivery.
- [ ] **2.** Placement of bloody sheets in a container designated for contaminated linens.
- [ ] **3.** Wearing of sterile gloves to bathe a newly delivered neonate at 1 hour of age.
- [ ] **4.** Disposal of used scalpel blades in a puncture-resistant container.

183. The client is prescribed olanzapine and fluoxetine (Symbyax) for bipolar disorder, depressive phase. Which adverse effects of Symbyax should the nurse include in the teaching plan? Select all that apply.
- [ ] **1.** Orthostatic hypotension.
- [ ] **2.** Drowsiness.
- [ ] **3.** Weight loss.
- [ ] **4.** Sore throat.
- [ ] **5.** Tremor.
- [ ] **6.** Weakness.

184. The physician orders Ringer's lactate solution to replace the fluid losses of a client. While the solution is infusing, the nurse should assess for which of the following symptoms that might indicate that fluid overload is developing?
- [ ] **1.** Increased abdominal girth.
- [ ] **2.** Rapid, thready pulse.
- [ ] **3.** Moist crackles on auscultation.
- [ ] **4.** Increased urine output.

185. The nurse is administering albumin solution to a client. During administration of this solution, the nurse should evaluate the client closely for which of the following complications?
- [ ] **1.** Excessive diuresis.
- [ ] **2.** Fluid overload.
- [ ] **3.** Abnormal weight loss.
- [ ] **4.** Dehydration.

186. As part of the management of constipation, the client is instructed to take 30 ml of mineral oil orally. Mineral oil facilitates bowel evacuation by:
- [ ] **1.** Lubricating and softening the stool.
- [ ] **2.** Increasing the volume of intestinal contents.
- [ ] **3.** Irritating nerve endings in the intestinal mucosa.
- [ ] **4.** Decreasing water retention of stool.

187. A 20-year-old client visiting the clinic requests the use of oral contraceptives. When reviewing the client's history, which of the following should alert the nurse to a possible contraindication to using these agents?
- [ ] **1.** Thrombophlebitis.
- [ ] **2.** Urinary tract infections.
- [ ] **3.** Ulcerative colitis.
- [ ] **4.** Menorrhagia.

188. A 30-year-old multiparous client has been prescribed oral contraceptives as a method of birth control. The nurse instructs the client that decreased effectiveness may occur if the client is prescribed which of the following?
- [ ] **1.** Indomethacin (Indocin).
- [ ] **2.** Amitriptyline (Elavil).
- [ ] **3.** Ampicillin.
- [ ] **4.** Omeprazole (Prilosec).

189. A client with a urinary tract infection has been prescribed phenazopyridine (Pyridium) to relieve the dysuria. The nurse tells the client to expect which of the following effects as a result of taking this drug?
- [ ] **1.** A slight fever.
- [ ] **2.** Thrush.
- [ ] **3.** Urinary frequency.
- [ ] **4.** Reddish orange urine.

190. The client has been prescribed aripiprazole (Abilify). Which client statements indicate an understanding of this medication? Select all that apply.
- [ ] **1.** "I can take the drug with or without food."
- [ ] **2.** "Abilify stabilizes dopamine."
- [ ] **3.** "I need to take it twice a day."
- [ ] **4.** "Abilify can give me a headache."
- [ ] **5.** "I might feel sleepy after taking the drug,"

Correct Answers and Rationales

The letter in parentheses after each rationale identifies the client need addressed in the item, including management of care (M), safety and infection control (S), health promotion and maintenance (H), psychosocial adaptation (P), basic care and comfort (C), pharmacological and parenteral therapies (D), reduction of risk potential (R), and physiological adaptation (A).

1. 3. The head of the bed should be elevated 30 degrees to promote venous drainage and decrease intracranial pressure. The client's head should be in a midline, or neutral, position. Clients with supratentorial surgery should be positioned on the nonoperative side to prevent displacement of the cranial contents by gravity. (R)

2. 4. A trained medical interpreter is required to ensure safety, accuracy of history data, and client confidentiality. The medical interpreter knows the client's rights and is familiar with the client's culture. Using the family member as interpreter violates the patient's confidentiality. Using the nursing assistant or limited Spanish and nonverbal communication do not ensure accuracy of interpretation and back-translation into English. (M)

3. 1, 3, 4, 5. Home care for a client with a total laryngectomy should include a high-humidity environment, laryngectomy tube care and suctioning, speech rehabilitation, and smoking cessation. The client is not restricted to a bland diet. (M)

4. 2. Administering acetaminophen to the client with a post ECT headache is the best action. Stating a headache is common after ECT and that napping will help the client feel better may be true, but it does not offer the client pain relief. Telling the client to eat breakfast and then to let the nurse know how the client feels conveys a lack of understanding to the client and dismisses the client's concern. (P)

5. 4. An 18-month-old child should be able to say 10 or more words. Lack of speech development may indicate a lack of social stimulation, a hearing deficiency, or developmental delay. Referring the child for an evaluation may increase the child's chance of reaching his potential. A 4-month-old child with a healthy central nervous system and normal mental development should be able to laugh out loud if his environment has been caring and his needs are met safely and consistently. Children at age 10 months should be able to say the words "dada" and "mama" in response to the appropriate person. A 1-year-old child should have the ability to speak 3 to 5 words plus "mama" and "dada." (H)

6. 4. The nurse should convey empathy and invite the client to share more about her thoughts and feelings so that the nurse can assess the mother for possible postpartum depression, which usually occurs between 2 weeks and 3 months after the baby's birth but also can occur later. Postpartum depression is a mood disorder with symptoms of tearfulness, mood swings, despondency, feelings of inadequacy, inability to cope with the baby, and guilt about performance as a mother. Postpartum depression commonly goes undetected because of poor recognition and lack of knowledge. Hormonal changes during and after childbirth may account for some of the symptoms; however, the nurse should not assume that that is the case. Stating the client's husband and family should help her is an assumption that they are not and dismisses the client's concerns. Saying most new mothers feel the same way minimizes the client's concerns and decreases the likelihood of further disclosure by the client. (P)

7. 4

$$1,000 \text{ mg} = 1 \text{ g}$$

$$2 \text{ g} = 2,000 \text{ mg}$$

$$2,000 \text{ mg} \div 500 \text{ mg} = 4$$

(D)

8. 2, 3. Huntington's disease, or *Huntington's chorea*, is an autosomal dominant genetic neurologic disease that affects descendants of an affected person at a 50% rate. Huntington's disease does not skip generations and affects men and women equally. Huntington's disease is genetically transmitted on chromosome 4, and death usually results from respiratory complications related to aspiration. (A)

9. 2, 3, 4. A client who has been admitted for numbness and tingling in his lower extremities that advances upward, especially after having a viral infection, has clinical manifestations characteristic of Guillain-Barré syndrome. The health care provider must be notified of the change immediately because this disease is progressively paralytic and should be treated before paralysis of the respiratory muscles occurs. The nurse must assess the client continuously to determine how fast the paralysis is advancing. The family does not need to be called in to visit until the client is stabilized and emergency equipment is placed at the bedside. Performing ankle pumps will not relieve the numbness or change the course of the disease. (M)

10. 3. The spinal cord connects the brain to the periphery. The thalamus is located in the midbrain and integrates all sensory impulses except olfaction. The afferent impulses are received and then transmitted from the thalamus. Destruction or interruption of the neurosensory pathway results in loss of communication between the two systems. Monitoring the temperature of the bathwater is important because the client cannot feel whether the water is too hot or too cold. Damage to the thalamus does not result in loss of the corneal reflex. Loss of position and vibratory sense usually occurs with degeneration of the posterior column of the spinal cord; therefore, turning every 2 hours is critical to prevent skin breakdown related to increased capillary pressure. The nurse can give only the prescribed dosage of pain medication. (A)

11. 3. The client needs to know her request is being met but also should be informed that discharge will not be immediate and that the client's psychiatrist will be notified to discuss the matter with the client. While it is true that a client admitted voluntarily has the right to leave, the client cannot leave immediately. It is inaccurate that a lawyer or family member must request forms for release against medical advice. Although it is acceptable for the nurse to try to convince the client to stay, the mention of insurance implies the client is hospitalized because of having insurance, rather than the psychiatric issues being treated. (M)

12. 2. Compliance with the Tarasoff rule involves wide notification and careful documentation of the notification. The nurse should notify the potential victim. The police must be notified, making it less possible for the client to follow through on his threat. The nurse must also notify key administrators in the health care facility so they are aware of the issue and the potential hazards related to the client's threat. The client is not a threat to the ex-wife at this time so she does not need to be notified. (M)

13. 1. The spinal cord connects the brain to the periphery. Destruction or interruption of the neurosensory pathway results in loss of communication between the two systems. Transection of the spinal cord renders the individual in a complete state of anesthesia below the level of injury. Tingling in the fingers may be related to spinal cord disease or to improper positioning of the extremity. Loss of position and vibratory sense usually occurs when the individual has degeneration of the posterior column of the spinal cord. (A)

14. 3. Common pressure points in the side-lying position include the ears, shoulders, ribs, greater trochanter, medial and lateral condyles, and ankles. The sacrum, occiput, and heel are pressure points in the supine position. (A)

15. 1, 2, 3. Goals for promoting healthy development in preschoolers include anticipatory guidance, helping parents understand their child's behavior, identifying deviations from the norm, and assessing parent-child interaction. No one can assess or determine the child's future development and trying to do so can limit the potential the child may achieve. Although learning to interact with others is important, sending the child to a day care center is not essential to promote healthy development. The nurse can encourage the parents to provide opportunities for the child to play with others. (P)

16. 1. Alarms on infusion pumps should be set at 5% above and 5% below the prescribed infusion rate. A wider range is not safe. The alarms must be set to indicate a change in the drip rate, not infiltration. Setting the alarms for the exact drip rate will cause the alarms to trigger when the client moves, and this exact range is not needed to alert the nurse to an unsafe rate. (S)

17. 0.24

Each small box on the telemetry strip represents 0.04 second. So, six blocks multiplied by 0.04 second equals 0.24 second. (R)

18. 1. The client's physical needs are a priority in the nurse's plan of care. The lack of fluid and caloric intake can lead to dehydration and cardiac collapse. The lack of sleep and rest can lead to exhaustion and death. Social, spiritual, and cultural needs are important client needs but not as important as the physical needs during an acute manic episode. (P)

19. 1, 2, 3. The alarm settings on infusion pumps should be verified at the time the infusion is started, at the beginning of each shift, and when the client is moved. The neonate can move in bed, but if the alarm is triggered, the nurse should verify the settings. Unless the neonate has moved or been taken out of the crib, it is not necessary to check alarm settings after the parents visit. (S)

20. 2. Thermoregulation of the neonate is a critical intervention for the nurse caring for neonates. A hat on the neonate conserves heat as the majority of heat is lost through the top of the head. Wrapping will also conserve heat and prevent heat loss. With the neonate lying against a crib wall, heat transfers away from the infant to the cooler surface (conduction). If the neonate is wet, the warmer water on the surface of the neonate evaporates to the cooler air (evaporation). If the neonate is lying in an open crib with a diaper on, the body naturally loses heat to the surrounding cooler air as it radiates from the warm body to the cooler room (radiation). (M)

21. 1. A vascular disturbance involving branches of the carotid artery is believed to cause migraine attacks. Vasoconstriction of blood vessels apparently occurs first. The extracranial and intracranial arteries then dilate, causing the headache. A family history of migraine headaches is present in more than half of all people who experience migraines. Migraine headache pain is not caused by increased ICP, inflammation in the sinuses, or facial muscle contraction. (A)

22. **2.** When the blink reflex is absent or the eyes do not close completely, the cornea may become dry and irritated. Placing a patch over the eye is the most appropriate intervention to prevent eye injury. Making sure the client wears her eyeglasses at all times will not help protect the eye from injury. A once-per-shift intervention will not adequately relieve the potential for injury from a dry and irritating ocular environment. A normal saline solution should be used to moisten the eye, not tap water. (H)

23. The rectus femoris is a safe site for injections for infants. The site is free from most nerves and blood vessels. The nurse should use a needle that is 1 inch or smaller, and inject the needle at a 45-degree angle. (S)

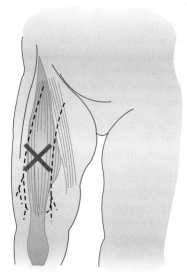

24. **1, 2, 3.** The alarm settings on infusion pumps should be verified at the time the infusion is started, at the beginning of each shift, and when the client is moved. The child can move in bed or sleep, but if the alarm is triggered, the nurse should verify the settings. (S)

25. **4.** Social isolation is a concern for an older adult who has diminished hearing and vision. Feeling disoriented may be related to cognitive problems rather than diminished hearing and vision. Diminished hearing and vision is related to the aging process and does not result in impairment of the older adult's thought processes. The client with impaired hearing and vision is unlikely to experience sensory overload. (P)

26. **3.** According to the Denver Developmental Screening Examination, a child age 2 years should have a vocabulary of 300 words, be able to combine two or three words, and ask for what he wants by name. By age 3, the child should have a vocabulary of 900 words and can use a com-

plete sentence of three or four words. A 1-year-old has a vocabulary of at least 8 words and can reference people and objects. (H)

27. **1, 2, 3, 5.** The nurse should ask the client with multiple sclerosis about areas of muscle weakness because baclofen may increase the weakness. The nurse should ask the client about a history of muscle spasms. Baclofen is effective against involuntary spasms resistant to passive movement for clients with multiple sclerosis and paralysis. Baclofen is not effective against the spasticity of cerebral origin, such as with cerebral palsy and Parkinson's disease. The nurse should ask the client about his liver and renal function because baclofen is metabolized and excreted by these organs. The nurse should check the laboratory values reflecting the function of the kidneys and liver, which include serum creatinine and blood urea nitrogen levels. The nurse should also check blood glucose levels because baclofen can increase blood glucose. Clients with diabetes taking antidiabetic medication may need to adjust the dosage. Potassium is not affected by the drug, so the nurse does not need to check the serum potassium level. (D)

28. **1, 2, 4.** The nurse should assess the client for signs of bone marrow depression, manifested by bruising or unusual bleeding, and signs of infection such as a sore throat. The nurse should also assess the client for signs of hepatic dysfunction, such as light-colored stool or dark-colored urine. Although the nurse may want to check the client's urinary function and hydration status, urine output and hydration are not specific monitoring needs related to long-term use of carbamazepine (Tegretol). (D)

29. **3.** The nurse uses active listening, in which the client's feelings are reflected back to him. Telling the client that everyone wears them does not consider the client's feelings. Telling the client that what he said is not what he meant discounts the validity of his statement. Interpreting the reason for the client being upset as the rule being unreasonable does not take into account how it affects the client personally. (P)

30. **3.** The restraint should remain in position. Removing the restraint or untaping the restraint will risk dislodging the I.V. (S)

31. **2, 3.** The nurse should use at least two sources of identification before administering medication to any client. The identification can include the medical record number and the client's date of birth. It is not necessary to check the client and dose for this drug with another nurse. It is also not safe to use the room number or bed number as a source of identification as clients' locations in the hospital are frequently changed. The nurse should not assume that the child will give a correct first name. (S)

32. **2.** One of the actions of propranolol (Inderal), a drug used in the treatment of migraine headaches, is to decrease the heart rate. The nurse should assess the client's blood pressure to evaluate overall circulatory response to the medication. Until the blood pressure value is assessed, there is no immediate need to contact the physician. The nurse should complete the blood pressure assessment before administering the drug. There is no immediate need to administer oxygen or contact a relative because a slowed pulse rate is an expected action of propranolol. (D)

33. **1.** During the tertiary circular reaction stage of the sensorimotor stage (12 to 18 months of age), the infant comes to understand causality and object performance, recognizing that objects placed out of sight continue to exist. During the preoperational stage (ages 2 to 6), the child's perception is based on how he views an event. The concrete operational stage (ages 6 to 12) is the beginning of concrete, logical thinking. During the formal operations stage (ages 13 to 18), the child is able to perform abstract reasoning. (H)

34. **2.** The neonate will be simultaneously dried and stimulated to cry immediately upon delivery. If the neonate does not cry as a result of these measures, the ABCs (airway, breathing, and circulation) of cardiopulmonary resuscitation will be followed. Positioning the neonate and suctioning or clearing the airway ensure that the airway is clear so that the first breath the neonate takes is air, rather than fluid or particulate matter. Breathing will be stimulated once the airway is clear and then heart rate will be validated either apically or through the cord. The cord may be cut in order to hand the neonate to the mother for nursing. In many instances, the infant is placed on the mother's abdomen before the cord is cut. (H)

35. **2**

First, calculate the concentration of mg/ml:

$$\frac{\overset{4}{\cancel{1,000}}\text{ mg}}{\underset{1}{\cancel{250}}\text{ ml}} = 4\text{ mg/ml}.$$

Next, multiply the number of milligrams per milliliter by the pump setting in milliliters per hour:

$$\frac{4\text{ mg}}{1\text{ }\cancel{ml}} \times \frac{30\text{ }\cancel{ml}}{1\text{ hour}} = 120\text{ mg/hour}.$$

Next, divide the milligrams per hour by 60 to obtain milligrams per minute:

$$120\text{ mg/hour} \div 60\text{ minutes} = 2\text{ mg/minute}.$$

(D)

36. **1.** The client may become tolerant of the antianginal effects of nitrates. Removing nitrates for 8 hours each day is usually effective in preventing tolerance. Nitrate patches should not be used on an as-needed basis. Sites should be rotated daily to prevent skin irritation, but this is not related to tolerance. Removing the patch for only 8 hours is sufficient to prevent tolerance and skipping days could impact the drug's effectiveness. (D)

37. **2.** The nurse should tell the client in a simple, matter-of-fact manner the purpose of the restraints to help the client understand why restraints are necessary. Long explanations and interactions with the acutely manic and agitated client are not appropriate or therapeutic at this time because the client with a high level of anxiety has difficulty focusing and processing. Saying "threatening others and throwing furniture is not allowed" could lead the client to believe he is being punished. Reminding the client that he's "been here before and knows what the rules are" and "we are only doing this for your own good, so calm down" are condescending and verbalizing the expectation that he can control his illness. (P)

38. **4.** Anorexia or loss of appetite is not associated with valproic acid. Adverse effects include tremors, transient hair loss, gastrointestinal upset, and weight gain. (D)

39. **3.** Intercourse commonly stimulates uterine contractions. The prostaglandins found in semen can also initiate contractions. After placement of a cerclage for advanced dilation and contractions, the client is considered at high risk for preterm delivery and should be seen by her health care provider more frequently. The client should call the health care provider immediately if she sees signs of complications, such as leaking fluid (rupture of membranes), vaginal bleeding, and contractions (particularly with a cerclage in place). Anything in the vagina may initiate contractions and the labor process. (R)

40. **15**

First, calculate the concentration of the drug in 1 ml:

$$\frac{\overset{0.2}{\cancel{50}}\text{ mg}}{\underset{1}{\cancel{250}}\text{ ml}} = 0.2\text{ mg/ml or }200\text{ mcg/ml}.$$

Next, calculate ml/hour:

$$\frac{50\text{ mcg}}{1\text{ }\cancel{minute}} \times \frac{60\text{ }\cancel{minutes}}{1\text{ hour}} = \frac{3,000\text{ mcg}}{\text{hour}}$$

$$3,000\text{ mcg/hour} \div 200\text{ mcg/ml} =$$

$$\frac{\overset{15}{\cancel{3,000}\text{ mcg}}}{1\text{ hour}} \times \frac{1\text{ ml}}{\underset{1}{\cancel{200}\text{ mcg}}} = 15\text{ ml/hour}.$$

(D)

41. **2.** A prolonged QT interval is significant because it can lead to the development of polymorphic ventricular tachycardia, also known as *torsades de pointes*. A prolonged QT interval may result from electrolyte imbalance but it does not lead to the development of an electrolyte imbalance, atrial fibrillation, or orthostatic hypotension. (A)

42. **1.** Gastric upset is an adverse effect of NSAIDs. Taking these drugs with food and fluids minimizes this effect. The dosage of NSAIDs does not need to be tapered. Because NSAIDs do not cause drowsiness or stomatitis, the patient does not need to restrict driving or rinse the mouth. (D)

43. **2.** The neonate's Apgar score has been improving since birth. (The birth score is 6; the current score is 9.) The nurse should continue to assess the neonate. There is no indication that oxygen is needed since the color is improving, and stimulating the baby is not necessary as the he is now flexing his extremities. (M)

44. **2.** Today's health care network includes many specialized areas, such as respiratory therapy, medicine, laboratory, social services, and technical monitoring, to name a few. Due to expanded media coverage of health care issues, parents are more aware of health care issues but cannot understand all the ramifications of possible health care decisions. Because of this expanded media coverage, health care consumers are more aware of advances in the science of health care. Nurses have always recognized the value of communication and that all nurses are teachers. Clients are more aware of their rights through media exposure and information disseminated by health care facilities. However, respect for the client's rights should be the nurse's concern as well and communicating with parents and children should not be impacted by a client's knowledge or demand for those rights. (H)

45. **4.** Soft, washable toys are appropriate for infants, who tend to place everything in their mouths. These toys are not harmful. Plastic toys cannot be manipulated by a child of this age and the child would put the car in his mouth, which may not be safe due to small parts that may be swallowed or aspirated. Games and puzzles are too advanced for a 5-month-old and he could put the pieces in his mouth and swallow them. Some stuffed animals have eyes that can be swallowed or aspirated. (R)

46. **1.** The oxygen levels for this neonate have dropped during the last 8 hours; the nurse should administer oxygen, as the neonate is not obtaining adequate oxygenation on room air. The recommended pulse oximetry reading in a term neonate is 95% to 100%. Keeping the neonate warm may improve the oxygen saturation if that is the cause of the poor gas exchange, but overheating with warm blan-

kets may increase oxygen demand. Waiting to reassess the neonate could cause the neonate to have inadequate oxygen levels unnecessarily. While blood gases may be drawn, the first action is to administer the oxygen. (M)

47. **3.** The nurse should give the next dose as ordered because the blood level is 35 mcg/ml, which is lower than the normal range of 50 to 100 mcg/ml. Withholding the next dose, notifying the physician, and taking the client's vital signs are not indicated in this situation. (D)

48. **3.** Going for a walk with the nurse and another client is a more gradual introduction to being with others. The goal is to gradually encourage interaction with others; playing games in the client's room promotes continued isolation. Going to a group session and participating in crafts is exposing the client to large groups too rapidly. (P)

49. **4.** The client is not emptying her bladder after repeated attempts. The nurse should now use an in-and-out catheter to empty the bladder. While the other comfort measures may be helpful, this client has not completely emptied her bladder since delivery and will be at risk for a urinary tract infection. (M)

50. **50**

Convert milliliters per minute to drops per minute:

$$100 \text{ ml}/20 \text{ minutes} \times 10 \text{ (drop factor)} = X \text{ gtt/minute}$$

$$5 \times 10 = 50 \text{ gtt/minute.}$$

(D)

51. **4.** The signs and symptoms of sepsis in a neonate, such as changes in appearance and behavior, are almost imperceptible. Often, the parents' only complaint is that the neonate does not look "right." Fever and localized response, which are clues to infections in older children, are often absent in the neonate. Telling the father that he should have realized something was wrong is condescending and serves only to further the father's guilt feelings. Asking the father whether he read the booklet from the hospital implies that the father is at fault. One experience would not necessarily ensure that the father would be able to detect sepsis another time. (P)

52. **3.** Nursing bottle caries occur when a child is routinely given a bottle of milk or juice at nap and bedtime. When teeth become coated in sugar before sleep, the lack of activity in the child's mouth for several hours during sleep allows the sugar to convert to acid, leading to decay. A child drinking 18 to 20 oz of whole milk in a day should not be malnourished, although she may lack essential vitamins and iron. Anemia may occur if she is only drinking milk because it contains no iron; however, the mother indicates she is eating meals. Regardless, children of this age should be taking no more than 16 oz of milk per day, and most children at this age should be drinking from a cup. The mother should be instructed to wean the child to a cup one feeding at a time until the child is completely weaned to a cup for all feedings. The last bottle-feeding to be replaced is usually the night bottle. Malocclusion of the teeth does not occur at 15 months. If the child were to continue to suck on a bottle until age 4 years or later, then malocclusion may occur. (P)

53. 100

Convert milliliters per minute to drops per minute:

$$600 \text{ ml}/60 \text{ minutes} \times 10 \text{ (drop factor)} = X \text{ gtt/minute}$$

$$10 \times 10 = 100 \text{ gtt/minute.}$$

(D)

54. 2. The primary reason to give a diuretic to a client with heart failure is to promote sodium and water excretion through the kidneys. As a result, the excessive body water that tends to accumulate in a client with heart failure is eliminated, which causes the client to lose weight. Monitoring the client's weight daily helps evaluate the effectiveness of diuretic therapy. The client should be advised to weigh herself daily. An increased appetite or decreased thirst does not establish the effectiveness of the diuretic therapy, nor does having clearer urine after starting torsemide. (D)

55. 3. The client should be placed in a side-lying position and encouraged to take a deep breath during the insertion of the suppository. Placing the suppository along the rectal wall promotes absorption of the medication and helps avoid placing it into a stool mass. The nurse should insert the suppository 3 to 4 inches into the rectum of an adult client. (R)

56. 4. Normal cardiac output is 4 to 8 L/minute. The value does vary with body size, but 2.2 L/minute is very low and can be life-threatening. For the client with a cardiac output of 2.2 L/minute, the nurse should anticipate that the physician would adjust the medication regimen. The client may experience symptoms of dyspnea and fatigue, requiring nursing intervention. (R)

57. 2, 3, 5, 6. Safety and physiological needs are crucial initially for a client who is unable to meet her own needs. Identifying her stressors and feelings will be important later when she is responding to questions and her environment. (P)

58. 4. In most agencies, it is a policy to discard the autologous blood after 4 hours of transfusing, due to an increased risk of infection. Increasing the infusion rate could cause fluid overload. Monitoring blood transfusions is a serious nursing responsibility, and because it is the change of shift, there is increased risk of error. (S)

59. 1. The client is demonstrating signs of anemia. Beef, beets, and cabbage are good sources of iron. Chicken, dumplings, biscuits, fish, applesauce, jelly, and wine are not major iron sources. (H)

60. 1.3

$$13 \text{ mg}/X \text{ ml} = 20 \text{ mg}/2 \text{ ml}$$

$$20 \text{ mg} \times X = 13 \text{ mg} \times 2 \text{ ml}$$

$$\frac{13 \text{ mg}}{X} = \frac{20 \text{ mg}}{2 \text{ ml}}$$

$$X = \frac{13 \text{ mg} \times 2 \text{ ml}}{20 \text{ mg}}$$

$$X = 26 \text{ ml} \div 20$$

$$X = 1.3 \text{ ml.}$$

(D)

61. 2. Infants are obligatory nose breathers except when crying. The observation that the infant has slight cyanosis when quiet but becomes pink when crying and the inability to pass a catheter through the left nostril suggest that the neonate is exhibiting symptoms of unilateral choanal atresia. With this condition, one of the nasal passages is blocked by an abnormality of the septum. Surgical intervention is necessary to open the nostril. Typically, a neonate with esophageal reflux disorder exhibits episodes of apnea and vomiting after eating. Respiratory distress syndrome commonly occurs in preterm neonates who lack surfactant to maintain lung expansion. Common findings include sternal retractions, tachypnea, grunting respirations, nasal flaring, cyanosis, pallor, hypotonia, and bradycardia. A neonate with tracheoesophageal fistula commonly exhibits cyanosis during feedings and vomiting. (R)

62. 1, 2, 3, 5. Safety measures for poisonous substances include close supervision of children, safely storing toxic substances, teaching proper dosages and differences between adult and child doses, and the proper way to contact the Poison Control Center for instructions. Poison Control should be notified as soon as the poisoning has occurred and airway and circulation have been assessed. Poison Control will direct any further treatment. Syrup of ipecac is rarely used today in the treatment of ingested substances due to the potential for aspiration. It is contraindicated in cases of arsenic poisoning, seizures, and the ingestion of petroleum or corrosive substances. (S)

63. **4.** Dystonic adverse effects of haloperidol, especially oculogyric crises, are painful and frightening. I.M. benztropine is the fastest and most effective drug for managing dystonia. Lorazepam is an antianxiety medication and is not effective for treatment of dystonia. Although amantadine and diphenhydramine can be used for extrapyramidal symptoms, oral medications do not work as quickly, and amantadine may worsen psychotic symptoms. (P)

64. **1.** Neonates burn brown adipose tissue (fat) as a response to cold stress. In addition, there is increased utilization of glycogen and calorie stores. Hypoglycemia may result from becoming stressed by a cold environment. Neonates do not have the ability to shiver. (H)

65. **1.** Formula should fill the entire nipple of the bottle while the baby is sucking. This decreases the amount of air taken in by the baby; taking in too much air can lead to regurgitation. Not all babies at term are born with well-developed sucking skills. Some neonates are sleepy and do not suck well. For the first feeding, the baby should be bubbled after taking one-fourth to one-half ounce of formula and then again when the infant has finished the feeding. Bottle propping can lead to aspiration, decreased infant bonding, and aspiration of formula. However, it is not associated with the intake of too much air. (H)

66. **1, 4, 5.** When a client complains of back pain with administration of blood, the nurse should suspect a hemolytic reaction, and the blood transfusion should be stopped immediately. The nurse should prepare for a reaction from mild to severe, including the need for cardiopulmonary resuscitation, because even a small amount of mismatched blood can lead to a major reaction. The nurse should obtain a urine specimen to send to the laboratory to check for hemoglobin because RBC hemolysis filters through the kidneys from the reaction. The nurse should stop the I.V. line with the Y-tubing for the blood and not flush the line with saline so that the client does not receive any more blood. The tubing should be changed so that a tube without blood can be used for infusions. The nurse should anchor an indwelling urinary catheter to monitor hourly urine output. (D)

67. **2.** At 4 hours postpartum, the fundus should be midline and at the level of the umbilicus. Whenever the placenta is manually removed after delivery, there is a possibility that all of the placenta has not been removed. Sometimes small pieces of the placenta are retained, a common cause of late postpartum hemorrhage. The client is exhibiting signs and symptoms associated with retained placental fragments. The client will continue to bleed until the fragments are expelled. Perineal and cervical lacerations are characterized by bright red bleeding and a firmly contracted fundus at the level that is expected. Urine retention is characterized by a full bladder, which can be ob-served by a bulge or fullness just above the symphysis pubis. Also, the client's fundus would be deviated to one side and boggy to the touch. (R)

68. **3.** A neonate born at 37 weeks' gestation will have some cartilage in the ear lobes, fine and fuzzy hair, scant to moderate rugae in the scrotum, and a breast nodule diameter of 4 mm. Neonates born before 36 weeks' gestation will have only an anterior transverse crease on the soles of the feet. Extensive rugae on the scrotum are a typical finding in neonates born at 39 weeks' gestation or later. Coarse and silky scalp hair typically is found in neonates that are born at 39 weeks or later. (H)

69. **1, 3, 4.** Clear communication is crucial for a client with delirium. The family must include the client in all conversations and keep him oriented to time and place. It is inappropriate to argue with a client's hallucinations because they are real to the client. Speaking more loudly will not help this client hear more distinctly and may increase his confusion. (M)

70. **2.** One-to-one supervision provides safety until appropriate detoxification can be given. Restraints are the last intervention after less restrictive alternatives have been tried. It is unlikely that the client can cooperate with staying in a chair. Putting the client in bed in his room puts him at risk for falling and a closed door prevents close observation. (S)

71. **1.** The nurse should recognize that the client's clinical manifestations indicate fluid overload, and decrease the infusion rate so the client's circulation can handle the extra fluid. Antihistamines are used for allergic reactions. The nurse should place the client in an upright position with his feet down so that blood or fluid volume can drain to his lower extremities and relieve some of the extra fluid load on his heart. The nurse does not need to replace the blood with another type of fluid because the client's response is not a blood transfusion reaction. (D)

72.

2.	Place the client in the supine position.

3.	Record the highest systolic blood pressure readings in both arms.

1.	Place a Doppler probe at a 45-degree angle to the correct pulse (dorsalis pedis or posterior tibial).

4.	Record the ankle systolic blood pressure reading when the Doppler sound returns.

The nurse should first place the client in a supine position. Next the nurse should assess blood pressures in both arms and record the highest systolic blood pressure as the brachial pressure. To obtain the brachial pressure, the nurse should place the blood pressure cuff around the affected leg just above the malleolus and then place a Doppler probe at a 45-degree angle to the dorsalis pedis or posterior tibial pulse. The nurse should then inflate the blood pressure cuff until the Doppler sound stops and then deflate it until the Doppler sound returns. The point when sound returns is recorded as the ankle systolic pressure. The ankle-brachial index is the ankle (dorsalis pedis or posterior tibial) pressure divided by the highest arm pressure. A pressure above .90 is normal; anything lower indicates obstruction. (A)

73. **2.** Insensible fluid loss is invisible vaporization from the lungs and skin, and assists in regulating body temperature. The amount of water loss is increased by accelerated body metabolism, which occurs with increased body temperature. The client's body mass index does not directly influence calculating fluid therapy. When the client's last meal was consumed and the availability of I.V. fluids have no influence on the analysis of intake and output. (M)

74. **3.** A toddler has not developed the concept of sharing, so two similar toys must be provided to prevent disagreements. Playing together in harmony is not the developmental level of a toddler. They play side by side, but not together. Threatening to put the children in their rooms does not solve the problem, nor does taking away the toy. (H)

75. **1.** The child wants attention from the nurse, even if the behavior is met by a negative response. Aggression, resistance against authority, and exaggerated stress are behaviors that can be associated with a 4-year-old. However, coming to the nurses' station after being told not to do so is not an example of these behaviors. (P)

76. **1, 2, 3.** Clinical manifestations of dehydration include decreased tearing; dry mucous membranes; sunken fontanelles; weight loss; behavioral changes; scanty, concentrated urine; and a thready, fast pulse. Clear, pale yellow urine would indicate adequate hydration. A bounding pulse would indicate fluid volume excess. (A)

77. **3.** When a neonate is being transferred to a neonatal care center (level III nursery), the parents should be allowed to see and touch the neonate, if possible, before transfer. The parents should be given the location and telephone number of the unit to which the neonate is being transferred. This helps to keep the parents informed. The parents are already aware of the neonate's condition and should recognize that it is critical if the neonate is being transferred to a neonatal care center. The parents have signed consent for treatment on admission, and in most states another consent is not necessary. Asking whether the father would like to ride in the ambulance with the neonate during the transfer is inappropriate. Most ambu-

lances or transferring vehicles (e.g., helicopters, airplanes) do not allow family members to accompany the ill client. Space in the motor vehicle, helicopter, or plane is limited. In addition, most transferring vehicles do not have insurance to cover family members should an accident occur during transfer. (M)

78. **4.** Tenets of the Roman Catholic Church hold that it is acceptable for anyone, regardless of religious belief, to baptize a neonate. For Roman Catholic families, baptism ensures entry into heaven. Local practice may vary, and in some situations the parents may prefer to have a Roman Catholic person perform the rites; however, this person may not be available until after the death. The parents may wish to have a priest contacted for grief support. Notification of the hospital's director is not necessary. (M)

79. **1.** Moist heat is a nonpharmacologic pain management strategy that may alleviate pain and reduce the dose of analgesic, if required. Heat dilates blood vessels, and decreases inflammation. Lifting and circular exercises will aggravate the already-inflamed joint. Cold constricts blood vessels, and dry ice is not used on the body. (C)

80. **3.** For a lumbar puncture (LP), a needle is inserted into the subarachnoid space to obtain a specimen of spinal fluid for diagnostic testing. Fluid on the lumbar dressing indicates cerebrospinal fluid (CSF) leakage, and must be reported to the physician immediately. The client should be encouraged to drink fluids after an LP to facilitate production of CSF. It is normal to have a mild headache due to the removal of CSF samples for laboratory analysis. Although the concerns of the client should be discussed with the physician at some point, the CSF leakage is a priority and should be reported immediately. (R)

81. **3.** The normal calcium level is 9.0 to 10.5 mg/dl. Hypercalcemia is commonly seen with malignant disease and metastases. The other laboratory values are normal. Hypercalcemia can be treated with fluids, furosemide (Lasix), or administration of calcitonin. Failure to treat hypercalcemia can cause muscle weakness, changes in level of consciousness, nausea, vomiting, abdominal pain, and dehydration. Although the client is on hospice care, she will still need palliative treatment. Comfort and risk reduction are components of hospice care. (R)

82. **2.** The LPN should report a maternal pulse rate of 100 bpm at rest because it could potentially indicate shock or hemorrhage. Typically, the pulse rate of a postpartum client slows after delivery and continues to be slow for about 1 week because of an increase in central circulation that results in increased stroke volume to provide adequate maternal circulation. The normal pulse rate is 60 to 70 bpm. Neonatal regurgitation of 1 tablespoon after a feeding, a neonatal heart rate of 140 bpm at rest, and increased maternal lochia rubra when the mother initially ambulates are normal findings. (M)

83. **2.** A child with a cardiac defect finds that squatting decreases venous return and workload to the heart and increases comfort and blood flow to the lungs. Squatting traps blood in the lower extremities so less blood is returned to the right atrium. Squatting would not relieve abdominal pressure; it may even increase it slightly. Squatting has no effect on muscle tone. When done by a child with a cardiac defect, it is not meant as an exercise but is a compensatory process used to reduce dyspnea. (A)

84. 8.33

$$20 \text{ hours} = 20 \times 60 \text{ minutes} = 1{,}200 \text{ minutes}$$

$$\frac{1{,}000 \text{ ml}}{1{,}200 \text{ minutes}} \times \frac{10 \text{ gtt}}{\text{ml}} = \frac{X \text{ gtt}}{\text{minutes}}$$

$$\frac{10{,}000 \text{ gtt}}{1{,}200 \text{ minutes}} = \frac{X \text{ gtt}}{\text{minutes}}$$

$$\frac{8.33 \text{ gtt}}{\text{minute}} = X$$

(P)

85. 60

A microdrip set infuses 60 microdrops/ml. There are 60 minutes in 1 hour. Use the formula:

(total volume to be to be delivered $\times$ drop factor) ÷ total time in minutes = drops per minute.

(D)

86. **3.** The diaphragm is the major muscle of respiration; it is made up of two hemidiaphragms, each innervated by the right and left phrenic nerves. Injury to the phrenic nerve results in hemidiaphragm paralysis on the side of the injury and an ineffective breathing pattern. Consciousness, cardiac function, and urinary elimination are not affected by the phrenic nerve. (M)

87.

2. Open the airway.
3. Start an I.V. access site.
1. Call the physician.
4. Explain the situation to the family.

An open airway is essential to survival. The nurse should first ensure an open airway. Next, the nurse should start an I.V. and then notify the physician. Finally, the nurse should inform the family of the situation and, if appropriate, allow them to remain with the client. (M)

88. **1.** Prevention of another pulmonary embolus is important; the nurse should teach the client to observe for signs of clot formation to prevent a potentially fatal episode and maintain cardiopulmonary integrity and adequate ventilation and perfusion. Elevation of the lower extremities, not lowering them, promotes venous return to the heart. Ambulation must be done several times each day. Limiting fluid intake increases blood viscosity, promoting clot formation. (H)

89. **2.** When a client is being released from the hospital with her neonate and the nurse learns that the client is homeless, the nurse should contact the hospital's or unit's social worker. Social workers have access to resources to assist the client to find temporary shelter in emergencies. The director of the birthing unit does not need to be notified. The director's responsibilities are primarily administrative. The client's physician can be notified once the social worker has offered assistance to the client. The physician may cancel the release of the neonate until temporary housing is located. Notifying the client's family is inappropriate. The client may not have any immediate family members, or there may be some stress between the client and family. (M)

90. **2, 3.** A client who has had numerous surgical or medical procedures is more prone to latex exposure and thus latex sensitivity or allergy. People who are allergic to latex may also have an allergy to fresh fruits and vegetables such as tomatoes. If a client denies a latex allergy, the nurse should ask about food allergies to fresh fruits and vegetables as well as for latex allergies and shellfish for iodine allergies. The client with one allergy commonly has more than one allergy, so the nurse must specifically ask the client about food allergies related to other allergies. (R)

91. **4.** The teenage girl has scoliosis, the lateral deviation of the spine. Kyphosis is noted by a forward curvature of the shoulders. Arthritis is diagnosed by radiographs. Hip dysplasia is noted in older children by pain, but is usually diagnosed before the child walks by noting excessive gluteal folds and limited hip abduction. (H)

92. **1, 3, 4, 5.** The nurse is responsible for the patient's safety in the operating room. The nurse should call a time-out if the client is not properly identified with an identification band. In addition, an I.V. line and oxygen should always be established when an ET tube is placed. This practice applies whenever a client's airway is compromised enough for intubation to occur, not only in the operating room environment. An anesthesiologist should be present during surgery to manage the airway. Postoperative pain medication is administered in the recovery room. (S)

93. **1.** Anencephaly is a neural tube defect that is not compatible with life, although some infants with anencephaly live for several days before death occurs. When the client has decided to continue the pregnancy and donate the neonatal organs after the death of the neonate, the nurse should remain nonjudgmental. The nurse should explore his or her feelings about the issue of anencephaly and organ donation. The nurse should not make judgments about the client's position, nor should the nurse try to persuade the client to terminate the pregnancy. Contacting the client's minister to explore the client's options is not appropriate. As a devout Baptist, the client probably has already discussed the matter with her minister. Telling the client that the neonatal death will be prolonged and painful to her is not helpful. Death may occur very soon after birth. Contacting the client's family members is not appropriate. The client may wish to maintain confidentiality and privacy related to the birth. (M)

94. **2, 3, 4, 5.** Anorexia is commonly the first indication of digoxin toxicity. Arrhythmias are also common with digoxin toxicity. Although bradycardia is the most common sign of toxicity, other tachycardic arrhythmias can occur. A normal pulse rate for a 3-month-old child at rest is about 120 bpm. Blurred vision can be associated with digoxin toxicity and may be detected in an infant if he stops following moving objects. Sudden vomiting or drowsiness can be associated with digoxin toxicity. Constipation is not associated with digoxin toxicity and is not an adverse effect of digoxin. (D)

95. **2.** If the specimen was from a fingerstick and not a venous sample, the potassium level can be falsely elevated. Because the finger is squeezed to obtain the sample, cells may have been broken from the pressure of squeezing. When the cells break, they release potassium, which will falsely elevate the potassium level in the result. Calling the physician without first checking the source of the sample would not give the physician accurate and complete information. A cardiac monitor would not be necessary if the potassium level is falsely elevated. The last 24-hour output would only indicate that the infant is voiding in an adequate amount. This may or may not have an influence on the infant's potassium level. (R)

96. **3.** The level of lethality of a client's suicidal thoughts depends on the presence or absence of a plan. If the client has a plan, the nurse must know what it is and whether or not the client has access to the means to complete suicide. The initiation of suicide precautions is necessary whenever a client threatens suicide, but first it is important to discover more information about what the client is thinking and planning. Unless the client has at his disposal the means to harm himself or is constantly trying to harm himself with objects on the unit, placing him on a suicide watch or confining him to his room are overreactions to the client's disclosure of suicidal ideation. (S)

97. **4.** Due to the client's psychosis and difficulties coping, a positive, supportive environment is essential to limit further regression and help the client engage in her own treatment. Confrontation and peer pressure are the type of milieu more suited to a chemically dependent client. While involvement in self-governance can be therapeutic, forcing a psychotic client to participate in self-governance before she is ready could actually hinder treatment and recovery. Although group activities are commonly required in treatment programs, a client who is very disturbed or confused is not forced to attend. Also, the client must participate when and how she feels comfortable, rather than mandating a specific amount of participation. Equal participation by clients does not ensure a therapeutic milieu or speed the client's recovery. (P)

98. **4.** The nurse should refuse to administer the medication to the client because of the risk of respiratory depression in the neonate. Meperidine, given I.M., peaks in 30 to 60 minutes and lasts 2 to 4 hours. Based on the assessment findings, the client most likely will be delivering within that time frame, increasing the risk of respiratory depression in the neonate, a serious consequence. Therefore, the nurse should not administer the drug. Naloxone (Narcan) should be readily available whenever opioids that can result in respiratory depression are used. Asking the physician to validate the dosage is not necessary. For clients in early labor, meperidine can be given I.M. in dosages ranging from 50 to 100 mg. (M)

99. **2.** Bending the chin down toward the chest decreases the risk of food entering the trachea and causing aspiration into the lungs. The client should sit up at a 90-degree angle when eating. Although eating and talking increase the risk of aspiration as well as muscle fatigue, the nurse should encourage the client to have visitors but avoid talking while chewing and swallowing. The client should rest before eating because muscle fatigue can contribute to choking. (R)

100. **42.3**

To obtain CPP, use this formula:

$$CPP = \text{mean arterial pressure (MAP)} - ICP.$$

To obtain the MAP, use this formula:

$$MAP = [\text{systolic BP} + (2 \times \text{diastolic BP})] \div 3$$

$$MAP = [90 + (2 \times 50)] \div 3 = 63.3$$

$$CPP = 63.3 - 21 = 42.3 \text{ mm Hg.}$$

(A)

101. **1.** The client with a spinal cord injury above T6 who suddenly experiences clinical manifestations of autonomic stimulation, such as flushing, sweating, and pilocarpia, is demonstrating life-threatening autonomic dysreflexia. The cluster of manifestation results from noxious stimuli, such as a full bladder, or lying on a foreign object, such as a plastic cap or crinkled paper, which the client cannot feel. As soon as the noxious stimulus is removed, the manifestations begin to subside. When the client demonstrates clinical manifestations of autonomic dysreflexia, the nurse should first elevate the head of the bed immediately to decrease the intracerebral pressure caused by the hypertension that developed from autonomic stimulation. The nurse can next check for a distended bladder or foreign object. The client's blood pressure will be elevated; the nurse should assess vital signs frequently. (M)

102. **3.** The nurse should refer the client to a social worker for assistance in enrolling in the WIC program. This program provides assistance for foods such as milk, cereal, and infant formula. Instructing the client in low-cost, highly nutritious meal preparation will not meet the client's need for additional funds for food. Determining whether the client qualifies for state assistance is part of the role of the social worker, not the nurse. Asking the client if she has a job and the amount of income earned is not within the role of the nurse. The social worker can determine whether the family income guidelines are met for state and federal assistance. (M)

103. **4.** Telling the client about one activity at a time with 10 minutes' notice gives the client time to prepare for that activity. Writing out the schedule does not ensure that the client will remember to look at it. It is overwhelming to explain an entire day's schedule all at once to a client diagnosed with dementia. Leading a client to an activity after the fact doesn't allow the client to prepare. (P)

104. **1, 2, 3, 4.** Safety of others is a priority and the nurse must monitor the client's anger and potential for aggression. The nurse should also find safe ways for the client to express his anger and any other feelings about the abuse. A referral to a support group is appropriate because anger management groups are one way to assist the client in learning to manage anger. Nothing about jail is mentioned in the question. Discussion of jail does not help the client address his issues with anger and the abuse causing the anger. (M)

105. **2.** The primiparous client at 2 hours postpartum who delivered a term neonate vaginally should be assessed first because this client is at risk for postpartum hemorrhage. Early postpartum hemorrhage typically occurs during the first 24 hours postpartum. Once the nurse has assessed the client's fundus, lochia, and vital signs, a determination about the stability of the client can be made. After this assessment, the nurse can provide care to the other clients, who are of lesser priority than the newly delivered primiparous client. (M)

106. **1.** Legionellosis is a pneumonia caused by the bacterium *Legionella pneumophilia* that thrives in water that is 95° to 115° F (35° to 46° C). When a building's hot water plumbing has water at this temperature, the bacteria thrive; then they may be transmitted via inhalation from air conditioning, showers, spas, and whirlpools. The bacteria are not transmitted via smoke or ceiling fan blades or by swallowing contaminated water. (H)

107. **2, 3.** The client should be instructed not to eat or drink for 8 to 12 hours before the test. Stools will be white for up to 72 hours following the procedure as the barium is eliminated from the body. Laxatives and fluids will be encouraged after the procedure to help prevent barium impaction, but the client will not be given stool softeners or laxatives before the procedure. The client should not experience pain during the procedure. The nurse should also instruct the client to stop smoking at midnight the night before the test. (R)

108. **4.** There is no cure for metastatic cancer of the liver; palliative nursing care is required. Liver transplants are not recommended for the client with widespread malignant disease. Prescribed medications will not make metastatic lesions shrink. There is nothing to indicate that the client is receiving chemotherapy; therefore, explaining its effects would not be helpful. (A)

109. **3.**

$$250 \text{ ml} + 150 \text{ ml} = 400 \text{ ml}/6 \text{ hours}$$

$$\frac{400 \text{ ml}}{6 \text{ hours}} = \frac{66.67 \text{ ml}}{1 \text{ hour}} = 67 \text{ gtt/minute.}$$

With a microdrip set, the milliliters per hour is the same as the drops per minute. (D)

110. **0.36**

$$\frac{25 \text{ mg}}{1 \text{ ml}} = \frac{9 \text{ mg}}{X \text{ ml}}$$

$$25 \text{ mg} \times X \text{ ml} = 9 \text{ mg} \times 1 \text{ ml}$$

$$X \text{ ml} = \frac{9 \text{ mg} \times 1 \text{ ml}}{25 \text{ mg}}$$

$$X \text{ ml} = 9 \div 25 = 0.36$$

$$X = 0.36 \text{ ml.}$$

(D)

111. **3.** The vastus lateralis site is the preferred I.M. site for all ages because it does not have any major nerves or blood vessels located near it. The deltoid and dorsogluteal muscles have major nerves and blood vessels located nearby. The triceps is not an acceptable muscle for I.M. injections because it is not well developed in most clients. (D)

112. **1.** Clients should be instructed to rinse their mouths after using a steroid inhaler to avoid developing thrush. Clients should also be instructed to inhale slowly through the mouth and then hold the breath as they count to 10 slowly. It is not necessary for the client to cough and deep-breathe before using the inhaler. (D)

113. **2.** The nurse should stay with the client during the first 15 minutes of a blood transfusion because this is when reactions are most likely to occur. Blood products should never be refrigerated on the nursing unit. Blood that has not been infused after 4 hours should not be infused. The blood should be infused over the specific time ordered by the physician. If a fever develops, the transfusion should be stopped immediately and the blood reaction policy of the facility should be followed. (D)

114. **2.** The symptoms of difficulty breathing, elevated blood pressure, and cough are indicative of circulatory overload. Circulatory overload occurs when blood is infused more rapidly than the circulatory system can accommodate. Anaphylactic reactions are manifested by urticaria, wheezing, and shock. Sepsis begins with a rapid onset of chills and fever. Acute hemolytic reaction is typically manifested by chills, fever, low back pain, and flushing. (D)

115. **2.** Sucralfate (Carafate) should be taken on an empty stomach 1 hour before or 2 hours after meals, and at bedtime. It is usually taken four times a day. There is no need to avoid milk products while taking the drug. Sucralfate does not affect hemoglobin levels. (D)

116. **1.** Anger is a common feeling that may lead to self-mutilation. Anger must be expressed in safe ways to diminish self-mutilation. Confronting the abusers directly is rarely successful and must be done with much preparation. Talking about the abuse typically decreases, not increases, self-mutilation. Civil suits are possible, but should only be undertaken after significant recovery from the abuse. (P)

117. **1, 2, 3, 4.** The client with conjunctivitis can use warm soaks to remove crusting. The nurse should teach the client to dispose of the soaks by wrapping them in a separate bag to avoid spreading bacteria. Topical antibiotics are used to treat the infection. The client should avoid contaminating the tip of the medication dispenser. Bacterial conjunctivitis requires containing the spread of the infection. The client should wash his hands after touching his eyes, but he does not need to be isolated. (R)

118. **2, 5.** Two sources of identification must be confirmed before administering medication to a client. A source of information can be the client's record number, name, or date of birth, as noted on the client's armband. A client may be confused or hard of hearing and may give a wrong name or answer to a wrong name, thus having the client state his name or respond to his name is not safe practice. Client recognition is not sufficient identification for administering medication. Clients change rooms frequently, so a room number is not a source of identification for administering medication. (D)

119. **0.5**

$$0.125 \text{ mg}/X \text{ tablets} = 0.25 \text{ mg}/1 \text{ tablet}$$

$$X = 0.5 \text{ tablets.}$$

(D)

120. **2.** Children who witness domestic violence commonly grow up to be victims or abusers. Counseling helps interrupt the pattern of violence in families. Limiting contact between the father and child does not address the child's behavior, and outgrowing violent behaviors is not likely without other interventions. Setting limits on violent behaviors alone does not address the child's feelings and needs. (P)

121. **2.** After such a crime, talking about his memories and feelings is an early part of the emotional recovery process. Encouraging him to talk to the FBI and helping him prepare for the trial may be appropriate later as he reorganizes his life for a trial. It is important for him to express his anger, even fantasies of revenge, rather than repress it. (P)

122. **4.** The nurse should allow the client to see and hold the baby for as long as she desires. Such activities provide memories for the mother and assist in the grieving process. There is a possibility that the client may change her mind about the adoption. In most states, there is a defined period (6 months to 1 year or longer) before an adoption becomes final. If the client changes her mind about the adoption, the nurse should accept the client's decision and notify the physician and social worker. Telling the client that it would be best if she didn't see the baby is imposing the nurse's value system on the client. Allowing the client to see the baby through the nursery window is inappropriate because the client should be allowed to touch and hold the baby. Contacting the physician for advice related to the client's visitation is not necessary. (M)

123. **2.**

$$\frac{0.4 \text{ mg}}{1 \text{ ml}} = \frac{0.1 \text{ mg}}{X}$$

$$0.4 \text{ mg} \times X = 0.1 \text{ mg} \times 1 \text{ ml}$$

$$X = \frac{0.1 \text{ mg} \times 1 \text{ ml}}{0.4 \text{ mg}}$$

$$X = 0.25 \text{ ml.}$$

(D)

124. **2.** A decrease or change in the level of consciousness is an early indication of increased intracranial pressure (ICP) and should be reported to the child's physician as soon as possible to try and control the pressure so it doesn't increase further. Vomiting can be a sign of increased ICP that occurs with a brain tumor, but it usually occurs unrelated to food and in the morning upon arising. Blood pressure increases with a brain tumor due to pressure on the brain stem. Concentrated urine is a sign of dehydration and is not related to the signs of a brain tumor. (A)

125. **4.** With a severe gonorrheal infection, scarring of the fallopian tubes may occur, and becoming pregnant may be difficult or impossible. If the girl's partner is not treated, she can be reinfected. There is no immunity against gonorrhea and, if exposed again, the girl can again become infected. Although a condom may provide some protection against contracting gonorrhea, it is not an adequate protection against the condition and will not help clear up an existing infection. It is only with proper antibiotic administration that the condition can be eradicated. (S)

126. **1, 2, 3, 4.** The goal of "medication reconciliation" is to ensure that clients are on the right medication after any transfer, admission, or going in and out of a health care facility. It is not necessary to reconcile the medications if the client moves to a different room on the same floor. It is estimated that more than half of medication errors occur during these transitions, and medication reconciliation can reduce errors by 70% or more. The Joint Commission requirements mandate medication reconciliation programs. (D)

127. **31**

Use this formula to obtain the correct answer:

$$\frac{\text{Total volume} \times \text{drop factor}}{\text{Total time in minutes}}$$

$$\frac{1,000 \times 15}{8 \times 60 \text{ minutes}} = \frac{\overset{31.25}{\cancel{15,000}} \text{ drops}}{\underset{1}{\cancel{480}} \text{ minutes}} = 31 \text{ gtt/minute.}$$

(D)

128. **1.** Acute poststreptococcal glomerulonephritis usually follows a streptococcal throat or skin infection by 1 to 2 weeks. Streptococcus-type infections require medical intervention with antibiotics. Antibacterial mouthwashes do not kill streptococci. Previously prescribed antibiotics may not be effective against streptococci, and may also be expired. Bar soap fragrance has no impact on its ability to kill bacteria that reside on skin. (H)

129. **1.** To be a true client advocate, the nurse should ask the client if she desires an epidural anesthetic even though the client has indicated a desire for "natural childbirth." The client has a right to change her mind and also a right to refuse treatment. The client, not the nurse, should be the one to tell the physician that she does not want an epidural anesthetic; the nurse should support the client's decision. Although telling the client that her labor will be more comfortable with an anesthetic provides the client with information, a statement such as this can be viewed as an attempt to change the client's mind. The client may wish to discuss this situation with her husband, but she does not have to do so. (M)

130. **2, 3.** In order to meet the criteria for discharge from same-day surgery, the postoperative client must be able to take fluids by mouth, walk without hypotension, void, and be escorted by a responsible adult who will drive him home. Transportation home via a taxicab is not a sufficient escort to assist a client home after surgery. The client may be discharged with severe pain. The nurse should make sure the client has a prescription for pain medication. Because a client has been on nothing-by-mouth status and thinks he is dry is not a sufficient reason for being unable to urinate postoperatively. The inability to void in the first 8 hours after surgery is one of the potential complications for all surgical patients and is related to the stress response. (S)

131. **25**

The I.V. flow rate is determined by the rate of infusion and the number of drops per milliliter of the fluid being administered: gtt/ml × ml/minute = gtt/minute (the I.V. flow rate).

$$15 \text{ gtt/ml} \times 100 \text{ ml/60 minutes} = 25 \text{ gtt/minute.}$$

(D)

132. **1**

$$600,000 \text{ units/1 ml} = 600,000 \text{ units/}X \text{ ml}$$

$$X = 1 \text{ ml.}$$

(D)

133. **1.** Eyedrops are correctly instilled by placing them in the lower conjunctival sac. Eyedrops should not be placed near the lacrimal ducts, to decrease the chance of the medication's being systemically absorbed. Placing the drops on the cornea or sclera is uncomfortable for the client and may cause the medication to run out of the eye socket instead of being absorbed. (D)

134. **4.** To treat anaphylactic reactions, epinephrine is administered to counteract the effects of histamine. Epinephrine is a rapid-acting sympathomimetic drug that has a bronchodilator effect. Dopamine may be used if hypotension develops. Diphenhydramine may also be given, but not as the initial drug of choice. Cimetidine is not administered to treat an anaphylactic reaction resulting in shortness of breath. (D)

135. **3.** Overuse of nasal spray containing pseudoephedrine can lead to rhinitis medicamentosa, which is a rebound effect causing increased swelling and congestion. Use of pseudoephedrine nasal spray does not cause infections or thrush. Pseudoephedrine is not addictive. (D)

136. **2.** The best way to teach a child about surgery is through play. The nurse can let the child handle the items that will be used for monitoring, such as the blood pressure cuff and the ECG pads. The child will become more familiar with the face masks he sees the surgical team wearing in the operating room after playing with one and wearing it before surgery. A child of this age-group does not understand detailed explanations of how to use equipment, such as a PCA, a VAS, or even a video. The pain scale that should be used for children is the FACES scale. (C)

137. **2.** When a nurse observes the theft of an opioid, it is the responsibility of the nurse to report the incident to the supervisor of the unit. The supervisor of the unit can confront the coworker and notify the hospital's chief of security about the incident. In some situations, the drug-abusing coworker may be offered drug counseling. In situations in which the drugs are being sold, the police should be notified. The nurse should not confront the coworker because this may put the nurse in danger. It is not the responsibility of the nurse to notify federal drug agents about the incident. (M)

138. **4.** An oculogyric crisis is a severe dystonic reaction typically caused by the older generation of antipsychotics. The nurse would administer 1 to 2 mg of benztropine intramuscularly to provide a prompt onset of action and offer the client reassurance. Cogentin is generally used to treat drug-induced extrapyramidal side effects. Chlorpromazine and thioridazine are traditional antipsychotic agents that would intensify the client's oculogyric crisis. Although procyclidine is effective for treating the rigidity and sialorrhea associated with antipsychotics, it is available only in oral form and would not be used in a crisis, when a parenteral form is needed for quicker onset of action. (D)

139. **2.** The nurse should teach the client and family the importance of not discontinuing benztropine abruptly. Rather, the drug should be tapered slowly over a 1-week period. Benztropine should not be used with over-the-counter cough and cold preparations because of the risk of an additive anticholinergic effect. Antacids delay the absorption of benztropine, and alcohol in combination with benztropine causes an increase in central nervous system depression; concomitant use should be avoided. (D)

140. **3.** The nurse needs to focus on adverse effects that can be seen or felt, using a simple, brief, written description of the benefits of the medication and a list of common adverse effects and how to cope with them. The written format helps the client and family feel more in control by participating in treatment. They also can use the written information as a helpful resource for review. Information about all potential adverse effects, including percentages associated with each, will cause undue anxiety in the client and possibly overwhelm the client and family, negatively affecting compliance. The nurse should use discretion in selecting the content of educational sessions. (H)

141. **2.** Albumin is a colloid that remains in the intravascular space, pulling fluid out of the intracellular and interstitial space. The client with nephrotic syndrome loses excessive amounts of protein, mainly albumin, in the urine. Because fluid is drawn into the intravascular space, blood pressure will increase. Crackles in the lung bases and cerebral edema are signs of circulatory overload or fluid volume excess. When edema is present in lower extremities, the skin feels cool to the touch unless an infection is present. (A)

142. **4**

$$1 \text{ g} = 1,000 \text{ mg}$$
$$250 \text{ mg} : 1 \text{ capsule} = 1,000 \text{ mg} : X \text{ capsules}$$
$$250 \times X = 1,000 \times 1$$
$$X = 1,000 \div 250$$
$$X = 4 \text{ capsules.}$$

(D)

143. **3.** Although inherited, it is not clearly understood why cysts form in polycystic kidney disease. Environmental exposures promote development of bladder cancer. Although drinking alcohol requires the kidneys to excrete the alcohol, it is not thought to cause the kidneys to develop cysts. (A)

144. **1, 2, 3.** A 3% sodium chloride solution is hypertonic; it will pull fluid into the intravascular compartment and may increase renal perfusion, so intake and output should be monitored. As fluid is pulled into the vasculature, the client may demonstrate signs of fluid overload such as jugular vein distention. Hypernatremia and hyperchloremia will produce neurologic signs and symptoms. Fluids should not be forced in a client with fluid overload. There is no need for an indwelling urinary catheter. (R)

145. **3.** The nurse expects the UAP assigned to several clients in labor to notify the nurse if the UAP observes that one of the clients has evidence of spontaneous rupture of the membranes. When the membranes rupture spontaneously, there is danger of a prolapsed cord, a medical emergency requiring a cesarean delivery. Nausea may occur after administration of an epidural anesthetic, but this is not a priority or emergency. Having contractions that are 3 minutes apart and last for 40 seconds is normal during active labor. Because nalbuphine (Nubain) is an analgesic, it is normal for a client to fall asleep after I.V. administration of this drug. (M)

146. **2.** Before teaching a school-age child about a medical or nursing procedure, it is best to become familiar with the child's knowledge level. The nurse can then begin by explaining about the body structure involved in the procedure. Children of this age should be told about the unknown procedures far enough in advance for them to prepare for what is going to happen to them. Showing the child the equipment and explaining what is going to be done during the test should be done after the child is allowed to express what he knows about what is going to happen to him. (P)

147. **3.** The client should be encouraged to keep up with his school work. The developmental task of the school-age child is industry versus inferiority. Keeping up with his peers is very important to this age-group. Watching television does provide rest, but it does not lead to a feeling of accomplishment. Coloring pictures is not an appropriate pastime for this age-group. Making crafts may be too strenuous of an activity for a client on bed rest. (H)

148. **4.** Clients receiving TPN are at risk for a number of complications, including fluid imbalances such as fluid overload and hyperosmolar diuresis. Other common complications include hyperglycemia, sepsis, pneumothorax, and air embolism. Hypostatic pneumonia, pulmonary hypertension, and orthostatic hypotension are not complications of TPN. (D)

149. **1, 2, 4.** Heparin dosage in children is based on the child's weight. A bolus of heparin is administered by the I.V. route and the onset of action is immediate. The PTT is an indicator of the effectiveness of heparin. Following the heparin with a continuous infusion of heparin would cause life-threatening anticoagulation in this child. Penicillin and cephalosporins potentiate the effects of heparin, so the heparin must be carefully titrated to obtain maximum effect without causing an overdose. However, the antibiotic should not be discontinued. (D)

150. **1.** Propantheline bromide (Pro-Banthine) is an anticholinergic drug. Common adverse effects include urine retention and constipation; flushed, dry skin; and dry mouth, nose, and throat. Orthostatic hypotension may also occur. Diarrhea and diaphoresis are adverse effects of cholinergic drugs. (D)

151. **1.** Applying a tourniquet obstructs venous blood flow and, as a result, distends the veins. A tourniquet does not stabilize veins or immobilize the arm, nor is it applied to occlude arterial circulation. (D)

152. **1.** Prochlorperazine is administered postoperatively to control nausea and vomiting. Prochlorperazine is also used in psychotherapy because of its effects on mood and behavior. It is not used to treat dizziness, abdominal spasms, or abdominal distention. (D)

153. **1, 2, 3, 4.** Cough and dyspnea can be present at the time of diagnosis of bone cancer, indicating that the cancer has metastasized to the lungs. About one-quarter of all adolescents with bone cancer have lung metastasis at the time of diagnosis. Pain and swelling result from the inflammation caused by the bone tumor and the increased vascularity of the tumor. At the time of diagnosis, fever, anorexia, and decreased range of motion have not occurred. The tumor involves the bone, so there is pain when pressure is exerted on the involved bone, but range of motion is not affected. Fever and anorexia can occur if extensive metastasis has occurred. (H)

154. **1.** The priority assessment is that the client has a firm fundus when gentle massage is used. This indicates that the client's fundus may be soft or "boggy" when it is not massaged. The receiving nurse should assess the client's fundus soon after admission and continue to monitor the client's fundus, lochia, and pulse rate. Postpartum hemorrhage is associated with uterine atony. Maternal-infant bonding is a process that usually starts on day 2 and ends at week 1. A 12-hour labor is normal. The temperature and pulse are within normal limits. (M)

155. **2.** Assuming cultural appropriateness of eye contact with the client and his wife, this body language would make the nurse's nonverbal message congruent with the nurse's verbal message and demonstrate empathy. Directing her eyes only toward the client, rather than including the wife, ignores the wife. Avoiding eye contact with the client and wife or shifting her gaze between the client and wife conveys a lack of assurance about the nurse's focus and comments. (P)

156. **4.** Colleagues can be a source of suggestions and validation of communication strategies. The nurse has identified difficulty with the relationship and should seek assistance before discussing improved involvement with the client because improved involvement may not be the most appropriate approach. Positive and negative interactions occur in relationships. The frequency of both types of interactions determines the quality of an interpersonal relationship. In a therapeutic relationship, both parties contribute to the relationship; neither one should dominate or be submissive. (P)

157. **3.** Confidentiality and privacy are critical developmental needs for the adolescent. These needs are important to enable the nurse to establish a relationship of trust with the adolescent. A sexual history should be conducted with a teen without parents. Therefore, the nurse should not ask the mother to provide information or put the daughter in a position of having to make a decision about her mother remaining in the room. Inform the adolescent that this information is confidential, and will not be shared with the parent. Inform the adolescent that issues of abuse or life-threatening issues are required by law to be disclosed to the authorities, and all other information is private. (M)

158. **4.** It is critical for medication safety to know the name, dosage, and times of administration of the medication taken at home. The family should bring the medication bottles to the hospital. The nurse should document the medication on the medical record from the bottles to ensure accuracy before the medication is ordered and administered. The pharmacist is a helpful resource, but the safest way to identify the medication is in its original container. It is not safe to assume the client could correctly identify the medications from a drug book. The medication regimen may have changed since the record 2 years ago. (D)

159. **3, 4, 5.** The additional fluids should run through a separate line using a Y connector. The nurse must contact the surgeon to clarify if the client should receive the additional 100 ml/hour of I.V. fluids containing potassium chloride during the bolus infusion. Rapid infusion of potassium chloride can cause hyperkalemia with adverse cardiac outcomes such as arrhythmias. Bolus infusions of I.V. fluids should be run via an infusion pump to avoid excess fluid administration. Increasing the current I.V. infusion rate or adding additional fluids to the existing infusion is not safe because the current infusion contains potassium. (D)

160. **1.** The nurse should notify the hospital's security staff about anyone who appears unusual. Typically the abductor is an older woman who wishes to have a baby. The nurse should take only one baby at a time to a mother to prevent the neonate being taken to the wrong mother. Infants should never be left in the hallway. When in the mother's room, the infant should be placed away from the doorway to prevent or minimize the risk of abduction of the neonate. If an exit alarm is triggered, it is possible that an abductor is running away with an infant. Staff members should investigate the alarm immediately and stop the potential abductor. Hospital security can be alerted if someone is seen exiting the unit carrying a large bag or an infant. (M)

161. **1.** The client needs specific information about the effects of the drug, specifically its effect on the blood. The statement about weekly blood tests to determine safe dosage and monitoring for effects on the blood gives the client specific information to ensure follow-up with the required protocol for clozapine (Clozaril) therapy. Lack of accurate knowledge can lead to noncompliance with necessary follow-up procedures and noncompliance with medication. The supply of medication is not dependent on blood testing. Telling the client that his physician wants to know the progress does not provide specific information for this client. The blood tests are not required by the drug company. (D)

162. **4.** A properly administered intradermal injection shows evidence of a bleb at the injection site. There should be no leaking of medication from the bleb; it needs to be absorbed into the tissue. Lack of swelling at the injection site means that the injection was given too deeply. The presence of tissue pallor does not indicate that the injection was given correctly. (D)

163. **0.5**

$$30 \text{ mg}/1 \text{ ml} = 15 \text{ mg}/X \text{ ml}$$

$$X = 0.5 \text{ ml.}$$

(D)

164. **1.** A serious complication of I.V. therapy is fluid overload. Noisy respirations can develop as a result of pulmonary congestion. Additional symptoms of fluid overload include dyspnea, crackles, hypertension, bounding pulse, and distended neck veins. (D)

165. **2.** Only isotonic (normal) saline should be used when administering a blood transfusion. The use of dextrose or lactated Ringer's will cause the hemolysis of red blood cells. (D)

166. **3.** The median cubital vein is located in the approximate center of the antecubital space. (D)

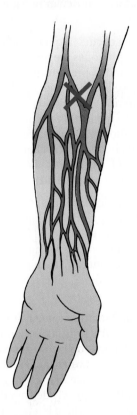

167. **2.** Telling the mother that excess saliva is a common adverse effect of the drug is most helpful because it gives her information about the problem, thereby helping to decrease her anxiety about what is occurring with her son. By offering the paper cup, the nurse also demonstrates concern for the client, thereby leading to increased trust. Saying "I wonder if he's having an adverse reaction to the medicine" shows the nurse's lack of knowledge about the drug, decreases confidence in the nurse, and indicates poor judgment. Saying, "Don't worry about it, it's only a minor inconvenience compared to its benefits," or telling the mother that the nurse has seen this happening to other clients is insensitive and does not assuage the mother's anxiety. (D)

168. **4.** The nurse should take the client's temperature and report the symptoms to the physician. Flulike symptoms of weakness, malaise, fever, sore throat, and lethargy may indicate leukopenia. An elevated temperature could also indicate an infection. Either condition requires medical intervention by the physician. Telling the client to wait another day or to take over-the-counter flu medication is inappropriate because the client is at risk for leukopenia secondary to clozapine therapy and serious consequences could occur. Although it would be important to encourage the client to consume adequate fluids, the priority is to report the symptoms and check the temperature. (D)

169. **2.** Protamine sulfate is a heparin antagonist. It is administered intravenously very slowly (over at least 10 minutes). Warfarin sodium and ASA have anticoagulant properties and would be contraindicated. Atropine sulfate is an anticholinergic drug and would not be effective in treating a heparin overdose. (D)

170. **10**

First, convert grams to milligrams:

$$0.5\text{ g} = 500\text{ mg.}$$

Then:

$$1{,}000\text{ mg}/X\text{ ml} = 500\text{ mg}/5\text{ ml}$$

$$X = 10\text{ ml.}$$

(D)

171. **14**

The I.V. flow rate is determined by the rate of infusion and the number of drops per milliliter of the fluid being administered: gtt/ml × ml/minute = gtt/minute (the I.V. flow rate).

$$10\text{ gtt/ml} \times 500\text{ ml}/360\text{ minutes} = 13.8\text{ gtt/minute.}$$

(D)

172. **2.** Aminophylline, a bronchodilator that relaxes smooth muscles in the bronchioles, is used in the treatment of emphysema to improve ventilation by dilating the bronchioles. Aminophylline does not have an effect on the diaphragm or the medullary respiratory center and does not promote pulmonary circulation. (D)

173. **1.** Seven-year-olds like to play with friends of the same sex. In early school-age years, children enjoy the company of same-sex friends. Relatives become second-choice friends to those from school. Team games can be competitive, and the ego of a 7-year-old may be too fragile to endure losing the game without losing self-confidence. Infants enjoy solitary play. The school-age child enjoys cooperative play with friends of the same sex and age. (H)

174. **2.** Trying something new is usually frightening for a 7-year-old. Separation anxiety is the most common fear between the ages of 5 months and 5 years of age. Injury and pain are a common fear of the preschool child. Fear of the opposite sex is common during adolescence. (H)

175. When measuring for NG tube insertion, the nurse would end the measurement at the xiphoid process. (S)

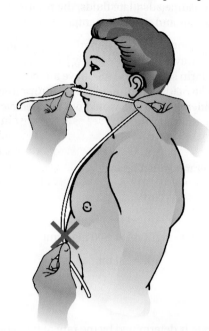

176. **4.** The client is experiencing signs of thrombophlebitis. The nurse should notify the physician because emboli formation is a potential risk. Massaging the area may cause the thrombus to dislocate and become an embolus. Warm compresses will increase circulation to the area and may precipitate embolus formation. Ankle pump exercises are helpful in preventing thrombophlebitis but will not prevent further risk of embolus formation at this time. (R)

177. **3.** This rhythm is ventricular tachycardia, which is characterized by an absent P wave and a heart rate of 140 to 220 bpm. Ventricular tachycardia requires immediate intervention, usually with lidocaine (Xylocaine). (A)

178.

3. Clear the area around the client.

1. Loosen clothing around the client's neck.

2. Turn the client on the side.

4. Suction the airway.

The goal of care for a client who is having a seizure is to prevent respiratory arrest and aspiration. The nurse should first clear the area around the client. Next, she should loosen clothing around the client's neck and turn the client on the side. As needed, the nurse can then suction the airway and administer oxygen. (R)

179. **3.** This rhythm is atrial fibrillation. It is characterized by an irregular QRS interval, no definite P waves before the QRS waves, and a ventricular rate greater than 100 bpm. (R)

180. **1.** Lymphedema occurs frequently after radical mastectomy when lymph nodes are removed. Aplasia, or the absence of lymph nodes, prevents proper lymph drainage. The tissue swelling is caused by obstructed lymph flow in the extremity. The blood pressure is taken in the unaffected arm to avoid further accumulation of lymphedema. An I.V. line should not be started in the affected arm. The nurse would encourage the client to elevate the extremity above the level of the heart. Blood draws in the affected arm should not be allowed. (A)

181. **4.** The child's physician should be notified because the maximum daily recommended dosage for ceftriaxone (Rocephin) for this child's weight would be 3.3 g/day and giving this dose would administer 4 g/day. The nurse cannot administer a different dose than that ordered by the physician. There is no therapeutic serum level of Rocephin. (D)

182. **3.** One of the staff members needs further instructions when the nurse observes the staff member wearing sterile gloves to bathe a newly delivered neonate at 1 hour of age. Clean gloves should be worn, not sterile gloves. Sterile gloves are more expensive than clean gloves and are not necessary when bathing a newly delivered neonate. Goggles should be worn when there is a possibility of blood and body fluid spatter. Bloody sheets should be placed in labeled containers for contaminated linens. Scalpel blades are disposed of in specified containers. (S)

183. **1, 2, 4, 5, 6.** Symbyax is a combination of olanzapine (Zyprexa) 6 mg and fluoxetine (Prozac) 25 mg and is used for the treatment of bipolar disorder, depressive phase. Adverse effects include orthostatic hypotension, drowsiness, weight gain, increased appetite, weakness, swelling, tremor, sore throat, and difficulty concentrating. The drug works to decrease depressive symptoms while guarding against the client moving into mania. (D)

184. **3.** Fluid overload or a positive fluid balance can result in increased blood pressure, pulse, and respirations. With fluid volume overload, there can be moist crackles, which may be heard on auscultation. The pulse rate is bounding because of the extra fluid. Increased abdominal girth is usually the result of ascites, which does not develop as a result of intravascular fluid excess from administration of too much I.V. fluid. An increased urine output is not an indicator of fluid volume excess. It would be expected that the administration of I.V. fluids in a client with a negative fluid balance would eventually increase the urine output. (D)

185. **2.** The client is at risk for development of fluid overload. Albumin is a hyperosmolar solution and acts to move fluid from the extravascular space into the intravascular space. The solution should be given slowly enough to prevent rapid plasma volume expansion. The client should be monitored closely for signs of fluid overload, such as shortness of breath and moist crackles on auscultation. Administration of albumin would not cause excessive diuresis, abnormal weight loss, or dehydration. (A)

186. **1.** Mineral oil is used to soften impacted stool in the management of constipation. It coats the surface of stool and intestine with a lubricant film to allow passage of stool through the intestine. Mineral oil also improves water retention of stool, thereby softening stool and facilitating bowel evacuation. Mineral oil does not work by irritating nerve endings in the intestinal mucosa. Saline cathartics, such as magnesium sulfate and citrate, increase the volume of intestinal content, thus stimulating evacuation. (R)

187. **1.** Oral contraceptives are contraindicated for clients with a history of thrombophlebitis because a serious adverse effect of oral contraceptives is thrombus formation. Other contraindications include stroke and liver disease. Oral contraceptives are used cautiously in clients with migraines, hypertension, or diabetes. Close follow-up of these clients is essential. (D)

188. **3.** Oral contraceptives may interact with other medications and the effectiveness may be decreased if the client is prescribed ampicillin, tetracycline, or anticonvulsants such as phenytoin (Dilantin). Indomethacin (Indocin), an anti-inflammatory agent; amitriptyline (Elavil), an antidepressant agent; and omeprazole (Prilosec), a drug used to suppress gastric acid secretion, do not decrease the effectiveness of oral contraceptives. (D)

189. **4.** Phenazopyridine (Pyridium) is used as a urinary tract analgesic and can cause the urine to turn reddish orange. A fever is not expected with phenazopyridine administration. If a fever develops, the client should report it because it could be an indication of drug toxicity. Thrush occurs with antibiotic therapy. Phenazopyridine should relieve urinary frequency, not cause it. (D)

190. **1, 2, 4, 5.** Aripiprazole (Abilify) is a dopamine system stabilizer. It functions as an antagonist in hyperdopaminergic areas of the brain and as an agonist in hypodopaminergic areas. Once-daily dosing is required and the drug can be taken with or without food. Adverse effects include headache, anxiety, insomnia, nausea, vomiting, somnolence, light-headedness, akathisia, and constipation. (D)

Appendices

Alabama
Alabama Board of Nursing
770 Washington Ave.
RSA Plaza, Suite 250
Montgomery, AL 36130-3900
Phone: 334-242-4060
Fax: 334-242-4360
Web site: www.abn.state.al.us

Alaska
Alaska Board of Nursing
550 W. 7th Ave., Suite 1500
Anchorage, AK 99501-3567
Phone: 907-269-8161
Fax: 907-269-8196
Web site: www.dced.state.ak.us/occ/pnur.htm

Arizona
Arizona State Board of Nursing
4747 N. 7th St., Suite 200
Phoenix, AZ 85014
Phone: 602-889-5150
Fax: 602-889-5155
Web site: www.azbn.gov

Arkansas
Arkansas State Board of Nursing
University Tower Building
1123 S. University, Suite 800
Little Rock, AR 72204-1619
Phone: 501-686-2700
Fax: 501-686-2714
Web site: www.arsbn.org

California
California Board of Registered Nursing
1625 N. Market Blvd., Suite N-217
Sacramento, CA 95834-1924
Phone: 916-322-3350
Fax: 916-574-8637
Web site: www.rn.ca.gov

Colorado
Colorado Board of Nursing
1560 Broadway, Suite 1370
Denver, CO 80202
Phone: 303-894-2430
Fax: 303-894-2821
Web site: www.dora.state.co.us/nursing

Connecticut
Connecticut Board of Examiners for Nursing
Department of Public Health
410 Capitol Ave., MS# 13PHO
P.O. Box 340308
Hartford, CT 06134-0328
Phone: 860-509-7624
Fax: 860-509-7553
Web site: www.state.ct.us/dph

Delaware
Delaware Board of Nursing
861 Silver Lake Blvd.
Cannon Building, Suite 203
Dover, DE 19904
Phone: 302-739-4522
Fax: 302-739-2711
*Web site: www.professionallicensing.state.
de.us/boards/nursing/index.shtml*

District of Columbia
District of Columbia Board of Nursing
Department of Health
Health Professional Licensing Administration
District of Columbia Board of Nursing
717 14th St., NW, Suite 600
Washington, DC 20005
Phone: 877-672-2174
Fax: 202-727-8471
Web site: www.hpla.doh.dc.gov

Florida
Florida Board of Nursing
Capital Circle Officer Center
4052 Bald Cypress Way BIN C02
Tallahassee, FL 32399-3252
Phone: 850-245-4125
Fax: 850-245-4172
Web site: www.doh.state.fl.us/mqa

Georgia
Georgia Board of Nursing
237 Coliseum Dr.
Macon, GA 31217-3858
Phone: 478-207-2440
Fax: 478-207-1354
Web site: www.sos.state.ga.us/plb/rn

Hawaii

Hawaii Board of Nursing
King Kalakaua Bldg., 3rd floor
335 Merchant St.
Honolulu, HI 96813
Phone: 808-586-3000
Fax: 808-586-2689
Web site: www.hawaii.gov/dcca/areas/pvl/boards/nursing

Idaho

Idaho Board of Nursing
280 N. 8th St., Suite 210
P.O. Box 83720
Boise, ID 83720-0061
Phone: 208-334-3110
Fax: 208-334-3262
Web site: www2.state.id.us/lbn

Illinois

Illinois Department of Professional Regulation
James R. Thompson Center
100 W. Randolph, Suite 9-300
Chicago, IL 60601
Phone: 312-814-2715
Fax: 312-814-3145
Web site: www.dpr.state.il.us

Indiana

Indiana State Board of Nursing
Professional Licensing Agency
402 W. Washington St., Room W072
Indianapolis, IN 46204
Phone: 317-234-2043
Fax: 317-233-4236
Web site: www.in.gov/pla

Iowa

Iowa Board of Nursing
RiverPoint Business Park
400 S.W. 8th St., Suite B
Des Moines, IA 50309-4685
Phone: 515-281-3255
Fax: 515-281-4825
Web site: www.state.ia.us/government/nursing

Kansas

Kansas State Board of Nursing
Landon State Office Bldg.
900 S.W. Jackson, Suite 1051
Topeka, KS 66612-1230
Phone: 785-296-4929
Fax: 785-296-3929
Web site: www.ksbn.org

Kentucky

Kentucky Board of Nursing
312 Whittington Parkway, Suite 300
Louisville, KY 40222-5172
Phone: 502-429-3300
Fax: 502-429-3311
Web site: www.kbn.ky.gov

Louisiana

Louisiana State Board of Nursing
5207 Essen Lane, Suite 6
Baton Rouge, LA 70809
Phone: 225-763-3570
Fax: 225-763-3580
Web site: www.lsbn.state.la.us

Maine

Maine State Board of Nursing
#158 State House Station
Augusta, ME 04333
Phone: 207-287-1133
Fax: 207-287-1149
Web site: www.maine.gov/boardofnursing

Maryland

Maryland Board of Nursing
4140 Patterson Ave.
Baltimore, MD 21215-2254
Phone: 410-585-1900
Fax: 410-358-3530
Web site: www.mbon.org

Massachusetts

Massachusetts Board of Registration in Nursing
Commonwealth of Massachusetts
239 Causeway St., 2nd floor
Boston, MA 02114
Phone: 617-973-0800
Fax: 617-973-0984
Web site: www.mass.gov/dpl/boards/rn

Michigan

Michigan/DCH/Bureau of Health Services
Ottawa Towers North
611 W. Ottawa, 1st floor
Lansing, MI 48933
Phone: 517-335-0918
Fax: 517-373-2179
Web site: www.michigan.gov/healthlicense

Minnesota

Minnesota Board of Nursing
2829 University Ave. SE, Suite 200
Minneapolis, MN 55414
Phone: 612-617-2770
Fax: 612-617-2190
Web site: www.nursingboard.state.mn.us

Mississippi
Mississippi Board of Nursing
1935 Lakeland Dr., Suite B
Jackson, MS 39216-5014
Phone: 601-987-4188
Fax: 601-364-2352
Web site: www.msbn.state.ms.us

Missouri
Missouri State Board of Nursing
3605 Missouri Blvd.
P.O. Box 656
Jefferson City, MO 65102-0656
Phone: 573-751-0681
Fax: 573-751-0075
Web site: www.pr.mo.gov/nursing.asp

Montana
Montana State Board of Nursing
301 South Park
P.O. Box 200513
Helena, MT 59620-0513
Phone: 406-841-2345
Fax: 406-841-2305
Web site: www.nurse.mt.gov

Nebraska
Nebraska Dept. of Health and Human Services
Regulations and Licensure
Nursing and Nursing Support
301 Centennial Mall South
Lincoln, NE 68509-4986
Phone: 402-471-4376
Fax: 402-471-1066
Web site: www.hhs.state.ne.us/crl/nursing/
nursingindex.htm

Nevada
Nevada State Board of Nursing
5011 Meadowood Mall Way, Suite 300
Reno, NV 89502
Phone: 775-688-2620
Fax: 775-688-2628
Web site: www.nursingboard.state.nv.us

New Hampshire
New Hampshire Board of Nursing
21 S. Fruit St., Suite 16
Concord, NH 03301-2341
Phone: 603-271-2323
Fax: 603-271-6605
Web site: www.state.nh.us/nursing

New Jersey
New Jersey Board of Nursing
P.O. Box 45010
124 Halsey St., 6th floor
Newark, NJ 07101
Phone: 973-504-6430
Fax: 973-648-3481
Web site: www.state.nj.us/lps/ca/medical/nursing.htm

New Mexico
New Mexico Board of Nursing
6301 Indian School NE, Suite 710
Albuquerque, NM 87110
Phone: 505-841-8340
Fax: 505-841-8347
Web site: www.bon.state.nm.us/index.html

New York
New York State Board of Nursing Education Bldg.
89 Washington Ave., 2nd floor, West Wing
Albany, NY 12234
Phone: 518-474-3817, ext. 280
Fax: 518-474-3706
Web site: www.nysed.gov/prof/nurse.htm

North Carolina
North Carolina Board of Nursing
3724 National Dr., Suite 201
Raleigh, NC 27602
Phone: 919-782-3211
Fax: 919-781-9461
Web site: www.ncbon.com

North Dakota
North Dakota Board of Nursing
919 S. 7th St., Suite 504
Bismarck, ND 58504-5881
Phone: 701-328-9777
Fax: 701-328-9785
Web site: www.ndbon.org

Ohio
Ohio Board of Nursing
17 S. High St., Suite 400
Columbus, OH 43215-3413
Phone: 614-466-3947
Fax: 614-466-0388
Web site: www.nursing.ohio.gov

Oklahoma
Oklahoma Board of Nursing
2915 N. Classen Blvd., Suite 524
Oklahoma City, OK 73106
Phone: 405-962-1800
Fax: 405-962-1821
Web site: www.youroklahoma.com/nursing

Oregon
Oregon State Board of Nursing
800 N.E. Oregon St., Suite 465, Box 25
Portland, OR 97232-2162
Phone: 971-673-0685
Fax: 971-673-0684
Web site: www.osbn.state.or.us

Pennsylvania
Pennsylvania State Board of Nursing
P.O. 2649
Harrisburg, PA 17105-2649
Phone: 717-783-7142
Fax: 717-783-0822
Web site: www.dos.state.pa.us/bpoa/cwp

Rhode Island
Rhode Island Board of Nurse Registration
        and Nursing Education
105 Cannon Building
3 Capitol Hill
Providence, RI 02908
Phone: 401-222-5700
Fax: 401-222-3352
Web site: www.healthri.org/hsr/professions/nurses.htm

South Carolina
South Carolina State Board of Nursing
P.O. Box 2367
Columbia, SC 29211
Phone: 803-896-4550
Fax: 803-896-4525
Web site: www.llr.state.sc.us/pol/nursing

South Dakota
South Dakota Board of Nursing
4305 S. Louise Ave., Suite 201
Sioux Falls, SD 57106-3115
Phone: 605-362-2760
Fax: 605-362-2768
Web site: www.state.sd.us/doh/nursing

Tennessee
Tennessee State Board of Nursing
227 French Landing, Suite 300
Nashville, TN 37243
Phone: 615-532-3202
Fax: 615-741-7899
Web site: www.tennessee.gov/health

Texas
Texas Board of Nurse Examiners
333 Guadalupe, Suite 3-460
Austin, TX 78701
Phone: 512-305-7400
Fax: 512-305-7401
Web site: www.bne.state.tx.us

Utah
Utah State Board of Nursing
Heber M. Wells Bldg., 4th floor
160 E. 300 South
Salt Lake City, UT 84111
Phone: 801-530-6628
Fax: 801-530-6511
Web site: www.doplutah.gov/licensing/nurse.html

Vermont
Vermont State Board of Nursing
81 River Rd., Heritage Bldg.
Montpelier, VT 05609-1106
Phone: 802-828-2396
Fax: 802-828-2484
Web site: www.vtprofessionals.org/opr1/nurses

Virginia
Virginia Board of Nursing
6603 W. Broad St., 5th floor
Richmond, VA 23230-1712
Phone: 804-662-9909
Fax: 804-662-9512
Web site: www.dhp.virginia.gov/nursing/

Washington
Washington State Nursing Care Quality
        Assurance Commission
Department of Health, HPQA #6
310 Israel Rd. SE
Tumwater, WA 98501-7864
Phone: 360-236-4700
Fax: 360-236-4738
Web site: fortress.wa.gov/doh/hpqa1/
        hps6/nursing/default.htm

West Virginia
West Virginia Board of Examiners
        for Registered Professional Nurses
101 Dee Dr.
Charleston, WV 25311-1620
Phone: 304-558-3596
Fax: 304-558-3666
Web site: www.wvrnboard.com

Wisconsin
Wisconsin Department of Regulation and Licensing
1400 E. Washington Ave., Rm. 173
Madison, WI 53708
Phone: 608-266-0145
Fax: 608-261-7083
Web site: www.drl.state.wi.us

Wyoming
Wyoming State Board of Nursing
1810 Pioneer Ave.
Cheyenne, WY 82002
Phone: 307-777-7601
Fax: 307-777-3519
Web site: nursing.state.wy.us

Bibliography

1. The Nursing Care of the Childbearing Family

Klossner, N.J., & Hatfield, N. (2005). *Introduction to maternity and pediatric nursing.* Philadelphia: Lippincott Williams & Wilkins.

Pillitteri, A. (2006). *Maternal & child health nursing: Care of the childbearing and childrearing family* (5th ed.). Philadelphia: Lippincott Williams & Wilkins.

Simpson, K.R., & Creehan, P.A. (2007). *Association of women's health, obstetric, and neonatal nurses (AWHONN) perinatal nursing* (3rd ed.). Philadelphia: Lippincott Williams & Wilkins.

Witt, C. (2007). *Advances in neontal care.* Philadelphia: Lippincott Williams & Wilkins.

2. The Nursing Care of Children

Hatfield, N. (2006). *Broadribb's introductory pediatric nursing.* Philadelphia: Lippincott Williams & Wilkins.

Pillitteri, A. (2006). *Maternal & child health nursing: Care of the childbearing and childrearing family* (5th ed.). Philadelphia: Lippincott Williams & Wilkins.

Wong, D.L., et al. (2006). *Maternal child nursing care.* St. Louis: Mosby.

3. The Nursing Care of Adults with Medical and Surgical Health Problems

Altman, G. (2004). *Delmar's fundamental and advanced nursing skills* (2nd ed.). Albany, NY: Delmar.

Ellis, J., & Hartley, C. (2005). *Managing and coordinating nursing care.* Philadelphia: Lippincott Williams & Wilkins.

Karch, A. (2006). *Lippincott's nursing drug guide.* Philadelphia: Lippincott Williams & Wilkins.

Nursing 2008 drug handbook. Ambler, PA: Lippincott Williams & Wilkins.

Purnell, L., & Paulanka, B. (Eds.). (2003). *Transcultural healthcare: A culturally competent approach.* Philadelphia: F.A. Davis.

Smeltzer, B., et al. (2006). *Brunner and Suddarth's textbook of medical-surgical nursing* (11th ed.). Philadelphia: Lippincott Williams & Wilkins.

Taylor, C. et al. (2006). *Fundamentals of nursing.* Philadelphia: Lippincott Williams & Wilkins.

Weber, J.R., & Kelley, J. (2007). *Nurses handbook of health assessment.* Philadelphia: Lippincott Williams & Wilkins

Yarbro, C.H., Frogge, M., & Goodman, M. (2004). *Cancer symptom managemnt* (3rd ed.). Sudbury, MA: Jones and Bartlett.

4. The Nursing Care of Clients with Psychiatric Disorders and Mental Health Problems

Andrews, M., & Boyle, J. (2007). *Transcultural concepts in nursing care* (4th ed.).Philadelphia: Lippincott Williams & Wilkins.

Boyd, M.A. (2007). *Psychiatric nursing contemporary practice* (3rd ed.). Philadelphia: Lippincott Williams & Wilkins.

Karch, A. (2006). *Lippincott's nursing drug guide.* Philadelphia: Lippincott Williams & Wilkins.

Shives, L.R. (2007) *Basic concepts of psychiatric mental health nursing.* Philadelphia: Lippincott Williams & Wilkins.

Videbeck, S. (2007). *Psychiatric mental health nursing.* Philadelphia: Lippincott Williams & Wilkins.

About the CD-ROM

This *Lippincott's Q&A Review for NCLEX-RN®* CD-ROM is just another reason why the book in your hands is so highly regarded by students and faculty. With more than 1,300 additional NCLEX-style questions (traditional multiple-choice *and* alternate formats), this easy-to-use program provides even more practice that is sure to lead you to exam excellence!

Minimum system requirements

- Windows XP-Home
- Pentium 4
- 512 MB RAM
- 10 MB of free hard-disk space
- SVGA monitor with high color (16-bit)
- CD-ROM drive
- mouse.

Installation

Place the *Lippincott's Q&A Review for NCLEX-RN®* CD-ROM into your CD-ROM drive. After a few moments, the install process will automatically begin. *Note:* If the install process doesn't automatically begin, click the Start button on your computer and select "Run." At the command line, type *D:\setup.exe*, where the letter D represents your CD-ROM drive. If your drive is designated by a different letter, use the letter of your drive instead. Then click OK. Follow the installation instructions.

Technical support

For technical support, call toll-free 1-800-638-3030, Monday through Friday, 8:30 a.m. to 5 p.m. Eastern Time. You may also write to Lippincott Williams & Wilkins Technical Support, 351 W. Camden Street, Baltimore, MD 21201-2436, or e-mail support at *wkhealth-support@wolterskluwer.com*.